SAUNDERS

Comprehensive
Review for
NCLEX-PN

SAUNDERS
Comprehensive
Review for
NCLEX-PN

Linda Anne Silvestri, MSN, RN

Assistant Professor of Nursing
Clinical Coordinator, Nursing Program
Salve Regina University
Newport, Rhode Island

President
Professional Nursing Seminars, Inc.
Charlestown, Rhode Island

W.B. Saunders Company
An Imprint of Elsevier Science
Philadelphia London New York St. Louis Sydney Toronto

W.B. SAUNDERS COMPANY
An Imprint of Elsevier Science

The Curtis Center
Independence Square West
Philadelphia, Pennsylvania 19106

Library of Congress Cataloging-in-Publication Data

Saunders comprehensive review for NCLEX-PN / Linda Anne Silvestri.

p.   cm.

ISBN 0–7216–7794–0

1. Practical nursing examinations, questions, etc.   I. Title.   II. Title:
Comprehensive review for NCLEX-PN.   [DNLM: 1. Nursing, Practical
Examination Questions.   WY 18.2 S587s 2000]

RT62.S53 2000   610.73′06′93076—dc21

DNLM/DLC   99–23882

SAUNDERS COMPREHENSIVE REVIEW FOR NCLEX-PN   ISBN 0–7216–7794–0

Printed in the United States of America.

Last digit is the print number: 9   8   7   6   5   4

To my parents,
To my mother, Frances Mary, and in loving memory of my father, Arnold Lawrence,
who taught me to always love, care, and be the best that I could be.

To my grandmother,
Beatrice Elizabeth Profiglio, my memories of her caring and love will remain in my heart
forever.

About the Author

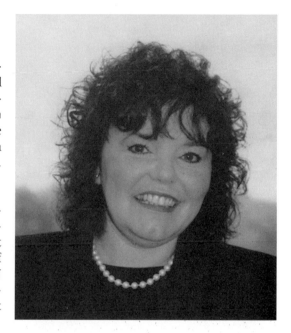

Linda Anne Silvestri received her diploma in nursing at Cooley Dickinson Hospital School of Nursing in Northampton, Massachusetts. She worked at Baystate Medical Center in the trauma center and in the pediatric and acute care units. She later received her BSN from American International College in Springfield, Massachusetts.

A native of Springfield, Massachusetts, Linda began her teaching career as an instructor of medical-surgical nursing and leadership-management nursing at Baystate Medical Center School of Nursing in 1981. In 1985, she earned her MSN from Anna Maria College, Paxton, Massachusetts, with a dual major in Nursing Management and Patient Education.

Linda moved to Rhode Island in 1989 and began teaching advanced medical-surgical nursing and psychiatric nursing to RN and LPN students at the Community College of Rhode Island. While teaching at the Community College of Rhode Island, a group of students approached Linda, asking her to help them prepare for the NCLEX. Based on her past experience as an NCLEX item writer, she developed a comprehensive review course and hired faculty from the University of Rhode Island, Community College of Rhode Island, and Rhode Island College to teach specific clinical areas for the courses.

In 1991, Linda established Professional Nursing Seminars, Inc., dedicated to conducting NCLEX-RN review courses and assisting nursing graduates to achieve their goals of becoming Registered Nurses. The next year, her company began conducting NCLEX-PN review courses. During 1994, she was courted by Salve Regina University in Newport, Rhode Island, to conduct review courses for their program. Later that same year, Salve Regina University invited her to work as an Assistant Professor and Clinical Coordinator of the Nursing Program, where she teaches in the areas of acute care, community and family health, and NCLEX review. She is currently matriculated at the University of Rhode Island in the PhD in Nursing Program.

Today, Linda Silvestri's company conducts NCLEX review courses throughout New England. She is the successful author of numerous NCLEX-RN and NCLEX-PN review products, including *Saunders Comprehensive Review for NCLEX-RN, Saunders Q&A Review for NCLEX-RN, Saunders Computerized AssessTest for NCLEX-RN, Saunders Instructor's Resource Package for NCLEX-RN, Saunders Comprehensive Review for NCLEX-PN, Saunders Q&A Review for NCLEX-PN,* and *Saunders Instructor's Resource Package for NCLEX-PN.*

Contributors

Alicia M. Adams, MN, RN, CEN
Director, Practical Nursing and Allied Health, Uintah Basin Applied Technology Center, Roosevelt, Utah

Carol Boswell, EdD, RN
Chairperson, Odessa College Nursing Program, Odessa, Texas

Sharen Brady, MSN, RN
Early Intervention Specialist and Associate Professor of Nursing in PN/ADN Program, Weber State University, Ogden, Utah

Brenda E. Caranicas, MS, RN
Director, Practical Nursing Program, Fort Berthold Community College, New Town, North Dakota

Jean DeCoffe, MSN, RN
Assistant Professor of Nursing, Salve Regina University, Newport, Rhode Island

Mary Ann Hogan, MSN, RN
Clinical Faculty, University of Massachusetts, Amherst, Massachusetts

Lisa Ivers, BSN, RN
Instructor, Indiana University, Butler County Program of Practical Nurse Education, Hamilton, Ohio

Lula Johnson, MSN, RN
Director, JTPA School of Practical Nursing, Detroit, Michigan

Mary T. Kowalski, MSN, BA, RN
Director of Vocational Nursing and Health Career Programs, Cerro Coso Community College, Ridgecrest, California

Beverly McNeese, RN
Department Head, Practical Nursing Program, Louisiana Technical College, Baton Rouge Campus, Baton Rouge, Louisiana

Jan H. Mearkle, MSN, RN, CSNP
Instructor, S.W. Mississippi Community College, Summit, Mississippi

Jo Ann Barnes Mullaney, PhD, RN, CS
Professor of Nursing, Salve Regina University, Newport, Rhode Island

Joann E. Potts Peuterbaugh, MSN, RN
LPN Coordinator, F. W. Olin Vocational School of Practical Nursing, Alton, Illinois

Ann Leiphart Unholz, MS, RN
Director, Henrico County, St. Mary's Hospital School of Practical Nursing, Highland Springs, Virginia

Laurent W. Valliere, BS
Vice President, Professional Nursing Seminars, Inc., Charlestown, Rhode Island; Area Manager, Training Services, Henkels & McCoy, Inc., Blue Bell, Pennsylvania

Paula A. Viau, PhD, RN
Assistant Professor of Nursing, College of Nursing, University of Rhode Island, Kingston, Rhode Island

Margaret Wafstet, MN, RN
Director, Practical Nursing Program, University of Montana/College of Technology-Missoula, Missoula, Montana

Mona Louise White, MSN, RN
Clinical Nurse Specialist, Delta College, University Center, Michigan

Mary E. Wright
Student, Department of Nursing, Rhode Island College, Providence, Rhode Island

Reviewers

Carolyn Bailey, MSN, RN
Assistant Professor, Coppin State
College, Baltimore, Maryland

Heidi Hartenstein Benoit, MS, RN
School of Health Sciences, Practical
Nursing Program, Lafayette General
Medical Center, Lafayette, Louisiana

Sue Boedeker, MSN, RN, FNP
Gateway Technical College, Kenosha,
Wisconsin

Bonita E. Broyles, EdD, RN
Piedmont Community College,
Roxboro, North Carolina

Jane Bruker, MSN, RNCS
Chair, Health Careers, University of
New Mexico–Gallup, Gallup, New
Mexico

Mary L. Centa, BA, RN, CNOR
Assistant Professor and Program
Coordinator, Surgical Technology and
Perioperative Nursing, Community
College of Denver, Denver, Colorado

Melissa L. Charlie, MS, RN
Adjunct Faculty, University of New
Mexico–Gallup, Gallup, New Mexico

Karen E. B. Evans, MSN, RN
Assistant Professor, Coppin State
College, Baltimore, Maryland

Margaret M. Gingrich, MSN, RN
Associate Professor, Harrisburg Area
Community College, Harrisburg,
Pennsylvania

Brenda P. Johnson, MSN
Doctoral Candidate, Southeast
Missouri State University, Cape
Girardeau, Missouri

Cheryl Karvonen, MSN, RN
Northern Michigan University,
Marquette, Michigan

Nancy Jo Kastor, BSN, RN
Portage Lakes Career Center, Green,
Ohio

Mary Beth Kiefner, MS, RN
Illinois Central College, East Peoria,
Illinois

Marquita Lindsey, BSN, RNC
Caddo-Kiowa Vo-Tech Center, Ft.
Cobb, Oklahoma

Mary Jo Melby, BS, RN
Department of Nursing, Great Plains
Area Vo-Tech School, Lawton,
Oklahoma

Kim Rengstorf, MS, RN
Edmond, Oklahoma

Leslie Robbins, MSN, RNCS
Assistant Professor and Coordinator,
Nursing Program, Doña Ana Branch
Community College, Las Cruces, New
Mexico

Susan T. Sanders, MSN, RN, CNAA
Motlow State Community College,
Tullahoma, Tennessee

B. J. O'Connor Schevers, MS, RN
Fox Valley Technical College,
Appleton, Wisconsin

Mary Sletten, BSN, RN
Doña Ana Branch Community
College, Las Cruces, New Mexico

Marian I. Stewart, MSN, RN
Motlow State Community College,
Tullahoma, Tennessee

Student Reviewers

Karen Downs
Salve Regina University, Newport, Rhode Island

Sharon Gittens
Salve Regina University, Newport, Rhode Island

Elizabeth Houghton
Salve Regina University, Newport, Rhode Island

Carolyn Kerns
Salve Regina University, Newport, Rhode Island

Lisa Rego
Salve Regina University, Newport, Rhode Island

Nicole Valliere
Saint Anselm College, Manchester, New Hampshire

Sarah Wilson
Salve Regina University, Newport, Rhode Island

Mary Wright
Rhode Island College, Providence, Rhode Island

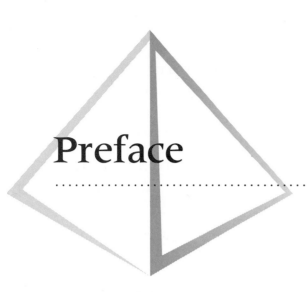

Preface

"To know that even one life has breathed easier because you have lived, this is to have succeeded."

RALPH WALDO EMERSON

Welcome to *Saunders Pyramid to Success*!

The *Saunders Comprehensive Review for NCLEX-PN* is one of a series of products designed to assist you in achieving your goal of becoming a licensed practical/vocational nurse. The *Saunders Comprehensive Review for NCLEX-PN* will provide you with a comprehensive review of all of the nursing content areas specifically related to the new 1999 CAT NCLEX-PN test plan implemented in April 1999 by the National Council of State Boards of Nursing.

ORGANIZATION

The *Saunders Comprehensive Review for NCLEX-PN* contains 20 units and 65 chapters. The chapters are designed to identify specific components of nursing content. Each chapter contains practice questions reflective of the content of the chapter and of the 1999 CAT NCLEX-PN test plan.

In the new test plan implemented in April 1999, the National Council of State Boards of Nursing has identified a test plan framework based on *Client Needs*. These Client Needs categories include Safe, Effective Care Environment; Health Promotion and Maintenance; Psychosocial Integrity; and Physiological Integrity. All of the chapters in this book address all components of the test plan framework. However, Units I through IV include content that specifically addresses the Client Needs category of Safe, Effective Care Environment; Units V through VII and Unit XX provide a focus on Health Promotion and Maintenance; Units VIII through XVIII emphasize Physiological Integrity; and Unit XIX focuses on Psychosocial Integrity.

UNIT I: NCLEX-PN PREPARATION

Chapter 1 addresses all of the information related to the 1999 CAT NCLEX-PN test plan and the testing procedures related to the examination. This chapter answers questions that you may have regarding the testing procedures.

Chapter 2 discusses the issue of NCLEX-PN preparation from a nonacademic view and provides an emphasis on a holistic approach for your individual test preparation. This chapter identifies the components of a structured study plan and pattern, anxiety reduction techniques, and personal focus issues.

Nursing students want to hear what other students have to say about their experiences with NCLEX-PN to learn what it is "really like" to take the examination. Chapter 3 is written by a nursing student who recently took the NCLEX-PN examination. The chapter addresses the issue of what the examination is all about and includes the student's "story of success."

Test-taking strategies are an important component of success in taking such an important examination. Chapter 4, *Test-Taking Strategies*, includes all of those important strategies that will teach you how to read a question, how not to read into a question, and how to use the process of elimination and various other strategies to select the correct response from the options presented.

UNIT II: ISSUES IN NURSING

Unit II addresses relevant nursing issues reflective of the components of the CAT NCLEX-PN test plan. Chapter 5, *Cultural Diversity*, identifies the specific common cultures and the related factors that promote maintenance of cultural identity when caring for culturally diverse clients. Chapter 6, *Ethical and Legal Issues*, provides a review of the ethical and legal considerations important to the practice of nursing and relevant to the components of the test plan. Chapter 7, *Leadership Issues and Priorities of Care*, identifies issues pertinent to the practice of nursing.

UNIT III: NURSING SCIENCES

The chapters in this unit specifically address content that students have identified as areas requiring review. Chapter 8, *Fluids and Electrolytes*, and Chapter 9, *Acid-Base Balance*, highlight the key components of the physiology, then move towards the necessary data collection and nursing interventions required to identify alterations that can occur in a client. Chapter 10, *Laboratory Values*, identifies the common laboratory studies, the normal values, and significant information related to the specific laboratory test. Chapter 11, *Nutritional Components of Care,* addresses the various food groups and important nutritional components of specific diet therapy. This chapter will assist you with your review of the selection of the correct food or the foods to avoid with certain physiological conditions, as these types of questions are certainly addressed in the CAT NCLEX-PN test plan. Chapter 12, *Intravenous Therapy and Blood Administration,* focuses on the nurse's role in monitoring these therapies and complications.

UNIT IV: FUNDAMENTAL SKILLS

Chapter 13, *Hygiene and Safety,* addresses nursing care specific to client safety and the measures that promote environmental safety. Chapter 14, *Medication and Intravenous Administration,* includes the important components related to conversion tables, calculation of medication dosages, and intravenous (IV) solutions and flow rates. Chapter 15, *Basic Life Support,* has been included to assist you in reviewing the steps in cardiopulmonary resuscitation and the Heimlich maneuver and to refresh your memory on the priorities to be addressed in emergency situations. Chapter 16, *Perioperative Nursing Care,* addresses the key components related to caring for the client requiring surgery. Chapter 17, *Positioning Clients,* identifies safe client positions specific to various surgical and diagnostic procedures. Chapter 18, *Care of a Client with a Tube,* addresses the various types of tubes, such as chest tubes, gastrointestinal tubes, or renal tubes, that have always been very confusing to students, particularly in terms of their purpose and the nursing care involved.

UNITS V, VI, AND VII: GROWTH AND DEVELOPMENT ACROSS THE LIFE SPAN AND MATERNITY AND PEDIATRIC NURSING

Units V, VI, and VII address many of the components of the Health Promotion and Maintenance category of Client Needs. Unit V, *Growth and Development Across the Life Span,* addresses the common theories of growth and development utilized in nursing. Unit VI, *Maternity Nursing,* includes chapters that address care of the pregnant client, care of the newborn, and maternity and newborn medications. Unit VII, *Pediatric Nursing,* focuses on the components of pediatric care and on the specifics related to administering medication to the child.

UNITS VIII THROUGH XVIII: ADULT HEALTH

Units VIII through XVIII address the components of Adult Health and are divided based on specific body system, including the integumentary, endocrine, gastrointestinal, respiratory, cardiovascular, renal, eye and ear, neurological, musculoskeletal, and immune, and oncology nursing. These chapters incorporate all of the Client Needs components of the CAT NCLEX-PN test plan with a particular emphasis on Physiological Integrity. Each unit includes a pharmacology chapter that provides a comprehensive review of the medications specific to the body system.

UNIT XIX: MENTAL HEALTH NURSING

This unit primarily addresses the Psychosocial Integrity of the Client Needs component of the test plan. Specific mental health disorders are addressed. A chapter that provides a comprehensive review of the psychiatric medications is included.

UNIT XX: THE GERONTOLOGICAL CLIENT

Unit XX focuses on the variations related to caring for the gerontological client.

SPECIAL FEATURES OF THE BOOK

PYRAMID TERMS

Each content area begins with *Pyramid Terms,* the definitions of important related terms significant to the content contained in the chapter. Additionally, these *Pyramid Terms* are in bold type throughout the content section.

PYRAMID TO SUCCESS

The *Pyramid to Success,* a unit or chapter introduction, provides you with an overview of the chapter, guidance, and direction regarding the focus of review in the particular content area, and its relative importance to the CAT 1999 NCLEX-PN test plan. Specific nursing content areas, as specified in the test plan, are identified.

Nursing Process. The steps of the Nursing Process provide a systematic and organized method of providing care to clients. Although the 1999 CAT NCLEX-PN test plan addresses Nursing Process as an integrated concept or process in the test plan, each chapter or unit introduction provides a general nursing care plan specific to the content area. This has been incorporated to provide you with the highlights of care related to Nursing Process that you need to keep in mind as you are moving through the content area of the chapter.

Client Needs. Client Needs are identified at the beginning of each unit or chapter. This section identifies the significant content of the unit or chapter that is representative of the CAT NCLEX-PN test plan. These points are the specific components or content areas to which you should pay particular attention.

PYRAMID POINTS

Pyramid Points ◆ are the bullets that are placed at specific content areas throughout the chapters. The *Pyramid Points* provide you with immediate recognition of content that is important in preparation for CAT NCLEX-PN. These bullets identify areas of content most likely to be addressed in the examination.

PRACTICE QUESTIONS

While preparing for NCLEX-PN, it is crucial for students to practice questions. This book contains 1600 practice questions. The accompanying software includes all the questions from the book, plus an additional 1400 questions, for a total of 3000 test questions. Each of the 65 chapters is followed by practice questions in NCLEX format. The answer section for the practice questions include the correct answer and the rationale for the correct and incorrect answers. The structure of the answer section is unique and provides the following information for every question:

Rationale. The rationale provides you with the significant information regarding both correct and incorrect options.

Test-Taking Strategy. The test-taking strategy provides you with the logical path in selecting the correct option and assists you in selecting an answer to a question should you need to guess. Specific suggestions for review are identified in the test-taking strategy.

Question Categories. Each question is identified based on the categories used by the CAT NCLEX-PN test plan. Additional content categories are provided with each question to assist you in identifying areas in need of review. The categories identified with each question include Level of Cognitive Ability, Phase of Nursing Process, Client Needs, and the specific nursing Content Area. All categories are identified by their full names, so that you do not need to memorize codes or abbreviations.

Reference Source. The reference source and page number are provided so you can easily find the information that you need to review in your nursing textbooks.

PHARMACOLOGY AND MEDICATION CALCULATIONS REVIEW

Students consistently ask for assistance with pharmacology. The 1999 CAT NCLEX-PN is incorporating pharmacology into the examination to a greater extent than in the past. Therefore, these chapters have been included for your review and practice. This book includes 13 pharmacology chapters, a medication and intravenous administration chapter, and a pediatric medication calculation chapter. Each of these chapters is followed by a practice test using the same question format as described above. This book contains over 400 pharmacology questions.

BOXES, TABLES, AND FIGURES

Several boxes, tables, and figures have been included to provide you with the visualization of significant content areas represented in the CAT NCLEX-PN test plan.

NCLEX-PN REVIEW SOFTWARE

Packaged in the back of this book you will find a CD-ROM containing NCLEX-PN review software. This software contains 3000 questions, 1600 from the book and 1400 additional questions. This Windows- and Macintosh-compatible program offers three testing modes for review:

Quiz—10 randomly chosen questions on a specific content area. Results are provided after you answer all 10 questions.

Study—10 randomly chosen questions on a specific content area. The answer, comprehensive rationale, and test-taking strategy appear after your answer. Results are provided after you answer all 10 questions.

Examination—100 randomly selected questions from the pool of 3000 questions. Results are provided and review is offered after you answer all 100 questions.

The software allows you to customize your review and determine your areas of strength and weakness. It also provides you with a wealth of practice test questions while at the same time simulating the NCLEX-PN experience on computer.

HOW TO USE THIS BOOK

Saunders Comprehensive Review for NCLEX-PN is especially designed to help you with your successful journey to the peak of the *Saunders Pyramid to Success*, becoming a licensed practical/vocational nurse.

As you begin your journey through this book you will be introduced to all of the important points regarding the CAT NCLEX-PN examination, the process of testing, and the unique and special tips regarding how to prepare yourself for this important examination.

You should begin your process through the *Saunders Pyramid to Success* by reading all of Unit I and becoming familiar with the important points regarding the CAT NCLEX-PN examination, the process of testing, and the unique and special tips regarding how to prepare yourself for this examination. Read the chapter from the nursing graduate who recently passed NCLEX-PN and pay attention to what this graduate has to say about the examination. Read the chapter on test-taking strategies and practice these strategies as you proceed through your journey with this book. Continue on your journey by reading each of the chapter content areas. Review the Pyramid Terms, the Nursing Process and specific components of the nursing process that are general to the content area, and identify the Client Needs specific to the test plan in that area. Read each of the content areas, focusing on the Pyramid Points that identify those areas most likely to be tested on CAT NCLEX-PN.

As you read each chapter, identify your strengths and those areas in need of further review. Highlight those areas and test your strength and ability by taking all of the practice tests provided at the end of each chapter. Be sure to read all of the rationales and the test-taking strategies. The rationale offers significant information regarding both the correct and incorrect options. The test-taking strategy provides you with the logical path to selecting the correct option. The strategy also identifies the content area that you need to review if you had difficulty with the question. Use the reference source provided so that you can easily find the information that you need to review.

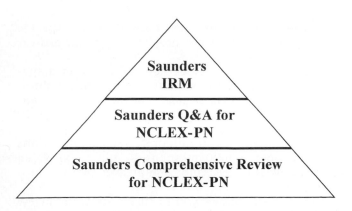

After using this book to review specific content areas, continue on your journey through *Saunders Pyramid to Success* with the companion book, *Saunders Q&A Review for NCLEX-PN*. This companion book and its accompanying software offer you 3000 practice questions on specific areas outlined by the CAT NCLEX-PN test plan. With practice questions uniquely focused on steps of the Nursing Process and categories of Client Needs, you can assess your level of competence on these types of questions. The final component of the *Saunders Pyramid to Success* is the *Saunders Instructor's Resource Package for NCLEX-PN*. Be sure to ask your nursing program director and nursing faculty about the CD-ROM and its usefulness as a review course or a self-paced review in your school's computer laboratory.

Good Luck with your journey through the *Saunders Pyramid to Success*. I wish you continued success throughout your new career as a licensed practical/vocational nurse.

Linda Anne Silvestri, MSN, RN

To All Future Licensed Practical/Vocational Nurses:

Congratulations to you!

You should be very proud and pleased with yourself on your most recent accomplishment of completing your nursing program to become a licensed practical/vocational nurse. I know that you have worked very hard to become successful and you have proved to yourself that you indeed can achieve your goals.

In my opinion, you are about to enter the most wonderful and rewarding profession that exists. Your willingness, desire, and ability to assist those who need nursing care will bring great satisfaction to your life.

In the profession of nursing, your learning will be a lifelong process. This aspect of the profession makes it stimulating and dynamic. Your learning process will continue to expand and grow as the profession continues to evolve. Your next very important endeavor will be the learning process involved to achieve success in your examination to become a licensed practical/vocational nurse.

I am excited and pleased to be able to provide you with the *Saunders Pyramid to Success* products that will prepare you for your next important professional goal of becoming a licensed practical/vocational nurse. I want to thank all of my former nursing students that I have assisted in preparing for NCLEX-PN for their willingness to offer ideas regarding their needs in preparing for NCLEX-PN. Student ideas have certainly added a special, unique aspect to all of the products available in the *Saunders Pyramid to Success.*

Saunders Pyramid to Success products provide you with everything that you need to prepare for the NCLEX-PN. These products have been designed to include material that is required for all nursing students who are preparing to take the NCLEX-PN, regardless of the educational background, specific strengths, areas in need of improvement, or clinical experience during the nursing program.

So, let's get started and begin our journey through the *Saunders Pyramid to Success.* Welcome to the wonderful profession of nursing!

Sincerely,

Linda Anne Silvestri MSN, RN

Linda Anne Silvestri, MSN, RN

Acknowledgments

Sincere appreciation and warmest thanks is extended to many individuals who in their own way have contributed to the publication of this book.

First, I want to thank all of my nursing students at the Community College of Rhode Island in Warwick, Rhode Island who approached me in 1991 and persuaded me to assist in preparing them to take the NCLEX examination. Their enthusiasm and inspiration led to the commencement of my professional endeavors in conducting NCLEX review courses for nursing students. I also thank the numerous nursing students who have attended my review courses for their willingness to share their needs and ideas. Their input has certainly added a special uniqueness to this publication. I wish to acknowledge all of the nursing faculty who have taught in my NCLEX review courses. Their commitment, dedication, and expertise has certainly assisted the nursing students in achieving success with the NCLEX examination. Additionally, I want to acknowledge Laurent W. Valliere for his contribution to this publication, for teaching in my NCLEX review courses, and for his commitment and dedication in assisting my nursing students to prepare for this examination from a nonacademic point of view.

I want to acknowledge all of the staff at the W.B. Saunders Company for their tremendous assistance throughout the preparation and production of this publication. A special thank you to all of them.

I would also like to acknowledge Patricia Mieg, Senior Educational Representative, who encouraged me to submit my ideas and initial work to the W.B. Saunders Company and for initiating my meeting with Maura Connor.

I sincerely acknowledge and thank Maura Connor, former Senior Acquisitions Editor, for the opportunity to provide this unique and exciting comprehensive review book to all nursing students. Her commitment to facilitating nursing students in achieving success complemented my professional expectations for this publication. I thank Maura for her expert professional guidance, extraordinary support, and for her patience as I prepared the manuscript. Her caring and warm personality, along with her energy, enthusiasm, and

professional direction have certainly led me to success.

I would also like to thank Victoria Legnini, Assistant Developmental Editor, for her assistance throughout this project. Her expert organizational skills maintained order for all of the work that I submitted for manuscript production. I also thank all of the special people in the production department and Agnes Byrne, Project Supervisor, whose consistent editing assisted in finalizing this publication. I also had the fortunate opportunity to work with Janet Blanner from the Marketing Department, whose support and special creativity assisted with this publication. Additionally, I wish to acknowledge David Saracco, Manager, Electronic Productions, and David Murphy, Production Manager/Electronic Products, of W.B. Saunders, and Jeffrey Babin from Corporate Technology Ventures for their work in producing the CD-ROM.

I want to acknowledge my parents who opened my door of opportunity in education. I thank my mother, Frances Mary, for all of her love, support, and assistance as I continuously worked to achieve my professional goals. I thank my father, Arnold Lawrence, who always provided insightful words of encouragement, and my memories of his love and support will always remain in my heart. I also thank my sister, Dianne Elodia, my brother, Lawrence Peter, and my niece, Gina Marie, who were supportive, giving, and helpful during my research and the preparation of this publication.

A very special thank you to Sarah Miller, for her support and dedication to my work and for her assistance each and every moment as I prepared my work for publication. I want to acknowledge all of the contributors who provided many of the practice questions contained in this publication, and to the many faculty and student reviewers for their thoughts and ideas. I sincerely thank Mary Ann Hogan, MSN, RN, who has always encouraged and supported me through my professional endeavors. Her numerous contributions to this publication are a reflection of her dedication to the profession of nursing and to nursing students.

A special thank you to Dr. Jo Ann Mullaney from

Salve Regina University in Newport, Rhode Island, for her numerous and expert contributions and to Mary Wright, LPN, for providing a chapter regarding her experiences with NCLEX-PN. I want to thank Salve Regina University for the opportunity to educate nursing students in the baccalaureate nursing program and for its support during my research and writing. I would like to especially acknowledge Dr. Louise Murdock and Dr. Ellen McCarty, Co-Chairpersons of the Department of Nursing at Salve Regina University, for their continuous support and encouragement.

I wish to acknowledge the University of Rhode Island, College of Nursing, for providing me with the opportunity for professional growth in my nursing education, particularly Dr. Donna Schwartz Barcott and Dr. Suzie Kim, my academic advisors in the doctoral program at the university.

I wish to acknowledge the Community College of Rhode Island for providing me with the opportunity to educate nursing students in the Associate Degree of Nursing program. A special thank you to Patricia Miller, MSN, RN, and Michelina McClellan, MS, RN, from Baystate Medical Center, School of Nursing in Springfield, Massachusetts who were my very first mentors in nursing education.

Lastly, a very special thank you to all my nursing students, past, present, and future. Your love and dedication to the profession of nursing and your commitment to provide health care will bring never ending rewards!

Linda Anne Silvestri, MSN, RN

Contents

xxvi   Contents

UNIT I

NCLEX-PN Preparation

CHAPTER 1

NCLEX-PN Preparation

THE PYRAMID TO SUCCESS

Welcome to the Pyramid to Success!

Saunders Comprehensive Review for NCLEX-PN is specially designed to help you begin your successful journey to the peak of the Pyramid, becoming a Licensed Practical Nurse! As you begin your journey, you will be introduced to all of the important points regarding the NCLEX-PN examination, the process of testing, and the unique and special tips regarding how to prepare yourself for this very important exam. You will read what a nursing graduate, who recently passed NCLEX-PN, has to say about the exam. All of those important Test-Taking Strategies are detailed. These details will guide you in selecting the correct option or assist you in selecting an answer to a question you must guess at.

Each of the content areas in this book begins with the Pyramid to Success. The Pyramid to Success addresses specific points related to NCLEX-PN including the Pyramid Terms, the Nursing Process, and Client Needs. Pyramid Terms are key words that are defined and are bolded throughout each chapter to attract you toward those significant NCLEX points. The Nursing Process is outlined as a guide and includes the significant areas to address in a particular content area. The Client Needs area lists the related content that is a component of the NCLEX-PN.

Throughout each chapter, you will find the Pyramid Points that identify those areas most likely to be tested on NCLEX-PN. Read each content chapter and identify your strengths and areas in need of further review. Test your strengths and abilities by taking all of the practice tests provided to you in this book. Be sure to read all of the rationales and the test-taking strategies. The rationales provide you with significant information regarding both the correct and incorrect options. The test taking strategies provide you with the logical path to selecting the correct option. The test-taking strategies also identify the content area to review, if required. The reference source and page number are provided so that you can easily locate the information that you need to review. Each question is coded based on the Level of Cognitive Ability, the

Phase of Nursing Process, the Client Needs category, and the Nursing Content Area.

Following the completion of your comprehensive review in this book, continue your journey though the Pyramid to Success with the companion book, *Saunders Q & A Review for NCLEX-PN*, which provides you with 3000 practice questions based on the NCLEX-PN test plan.

Let's begin our journey through the Pyramid to Success.

THE EXAMINATION PROCESS

An important step in the Pyramid to Success is to become as familiar as possible with the examination process. A significant amount of anxiety can occur in candidates facing the challenge of this examination. Knowing what the examination is all about and knowing what you will encounter during the process of testing will assist in alleviating fear and anxiety. The information contained in this chapter addresses the procedures related to the development of the NCLEX-PN Test Plan, the components of the test plan and the answers to the questions most commonly asked by nursing students and graduates preparing to take the NCLEX-PN. The information related to the development of the NCLEX-PN Test Plan, the components of the test plan, and the testing procedures were adapted from the *National Council Detailed Test Plan for the NCLEX-PN Examination*, National Council of State Boards of Nursing, Chicago, 1998; and *The NCLEX Process*, National Council of State Boards of Nursing, Chicago, 1995.

DEVELOPMENT OF THE TEST PLAN

In the test development process, the National Council of State Boards of Nursing considers the legal scope of nursing practice as governed by state laws and regulations, including the Nurse Practice Act. The National Council uses these laws to define the areas on NCLEX-PN that will assess the competence of candidates for nurse licensure.

The National Council of State Boards of Nursing

also conducts a Job Analysis study, which guides the selection of content and behaviors to be tested on NCLEX-PN. Because nursing practice continues to change, this study is conducted every 3 years. The results of this study, most recently conducted in 1997, provided the framework for the new test plan implemented in April 1999.

JOB ANALYSIS STUDY

The participants of this study are selected by a stratified random sampling process and include newly licensed practical nurses. In this study, the participants are provided a list of identified nursing activities that are then analyzed by the National Council in relation to their frequency of performance in the clinical setting, their impact on maintaining client safety, and the settings where the activities were performed. This analysis guides the development of a framework for the NCLEX-PN that delineates specific Client Needs, and Integrated Concepts and Processes for entry level practice.

THE TEST PLAN

The content on NCLEX-PN reflects the knowledge, skills, and abilities essential for the practical/vocational nurse to meet the needs of clients requiring the promotion, maintenance, and restoration of health. The questions are written to address the Levels of Cognitive Ability, Client Needs, and Integrated Concepts and Processes as identified in the Test Plan.

LEVELS OF COGNITIVE ABILITY

The NCLEX-PN examination includes questions at the cognitive levels of knowledge, comprehension, application, and analysis (Box 1–1).

CLIENT NEEDS

In the new Test Plan implemented in April 1999, the National Council of State Boards of Nursing has identified a Test Plan framework based on Client Needs. This framework was selected based on the analysis of the findings in the Job Analysis study, and because Client Needs provides a universal structure for defining nursing actions and competencies for a variety of clients across a variety of settings, and is congruent with state laws and statutes. The National Council of State Boards of Nursing identifies four major categories of Client Needs. These categories are further divided into subcategories, and the percentage of test questions in each subcategory is identified (Box 1–2).

Safe, Effective Care Environment

The Safe, Effective Care Environment category includes two subcategories, Coordinated Care, and Safety and Infection Control. Coordinated Care (6%–12%) addresses content related to facilitating effective client care through collaboration with other health care team members. Safety and Infection Control (7%–13%) addresses content that tests the knowledge, skills, and ability required to protect clients and

---

BOX 1–1. Level of Cognitive Ability

The nurse is collecting data from a perinatal client with a history of left-sided heart failure. The nurse notes that the client is experiencing unusual episodes of a cough on minimal exertion. The nurse recognizes this finding as significant and associated with the first indicator of which of the following important cardiac problems?

1 Orthopnea
2 Decreased blood volume
3 Right-sided heart failure
4 Pulmonary edema

ANSWER: 4
RATIONALE: This question requires the test taker to analyze the data provided in order to recognize the client's problem. The test taker needs to know the complications of left-sided heart failure and the signs and symptoms of pulmonary edema. The analysis of the data provided in the question will direct the test taker to the correct option.
LEVEL OF COGNITIVE ABILITY: Analysis
REFERENCE
Gorrie, T., McKinney, E., & Murray, S. (1998). *Foundations of maternal-newborn nursing* (2nd ed.). Philadelphia: W. B. Saunders, p. 725.

---

health care personnel from environmental hazards (Box 1–3).

Health Promotion and Maintenance

The Health Promotion and Maintenance category includes two subcategories, Growth and Development Through the Life Span, and the Prevention and Early Detection of Disease. Growth and Development

---

BOX 1–2. Client Needs and the Percentage of Test Questions

SAFE, EFFECTIVE CARE ENVIRONMENT	
Coordinated Care	6%–12%
Safety and Infection Control	7%–13%
HEALTH PROMOTION AND MAINTENANCE	
Growth and Development Through the Life Span	4%–10%
Prevention and Early Detection of Disease	4%–10%
PSYCHOSOCIAL INTEGRITY	
Coping and Adaptation	6%–12%
Psychosocial Adaptation	4%–10%
PHYSIOLOGICAL INTEGRITY	
Basic Care and Comfort	10%–16%
Pharmacological Therapies	5%–11%
Reduction of Risk Potential	11%–17%
Physiological Adaptation	13%–19%

BOX 1–3. Safe, Effective Care Environment

COORDINATED CARE

The nurse observes that a client becomes agitated and incoherent and suspects that the client is experiencing a reaction to medication. In planning a safe environment for this client, the most appropriate intervention is to:
1 Request that the physician order restraints and sedation.
2 Ask the family to stay with the client.
3 Ask a nursing assistant to stay with the client.
4 Collaborate with the registered nurse to plan safe care.

ANSWER: 4
RATIONALE: This question addresses the subcategory, Coordinated Care, in the Client Needs category, Safe, Effective Care Environment. The nurse has the responsibility to facilitate safe and effective client care through collaboration with other health care team members.
CLIENT NEEDS: Safe, Effective Care Environment
REFERENCE
Hill, S., & Howlett, H. (1997). *Success in practical nursing: Personal and vocational issues* (3rd ed.). Philadelphia: W. B. Saunders, p. 322.

SAFETY AND INFECTION CONTROL

The nurse is assigned to care for a client receiving an intravenous (IV) infusion. While caring for the client, the nurse implements which of the following nursing actions to decrease the risk for infection?
1 Take the vital signs at 4-hour intervals
2 Change the IV dressing every shift
3 Administer acetaminophen (Tylenol) every 4 hours
4 Use aseptic technique when handling the intravenous solution and tubing

ANSWER: 4
RATIONALE: This question addresses the subcategory, Safety and Infection Control, in the Client Needs category, Safe, Effective Care Environment. It addresses content related to surgical asepsis and protecting the client from infection.
CLIENT NEEDS: Safe, Effective Care Environment
REFERENCE
deWit, S. (1998). *Essentials of medical-surgical nursing* (4th ed.). Philadelphia: W. B. Saunders, p. 125.

BOX 1–4. Health Promotion and Maintenance

GROWTH AND DEVELOPMENT THROUGH THE LIFE SPAN

The nurse is assisting in planning a health maintenance program for a group of older adults. Which of the following activities best promotes health and maintenance among this group?
1 Gardening every day for an hour
2 Cycling three times a week for 20 minutes
3 Sculpting once a week for 40 minutes
4 Walking three to five times a week for 30 minutes

ANSWER: 4
RATIONALE: This question addresses the subcategory, Growth and Development Through the Life Span, in the Client Needs category, Health Promotion and Maintenance. The content addresses the aging process. Exercise and activity are essential for health promotion and maintenance in the older adult and to achieve an optimal level of functioning. One of the best exercises for an older adult is walking, progressing to 30-minute sessions three to five times each week.
CLIENT NEEDS: Health Promotion and Maintenance
REFERENCE
deWit, S. (1998). *Essentials of medical-surgical nursing* (4th ed.). Philadelphia: W. B. Saunders, p. 284.

PREVENTION AND EARLY DETECTION OF DISEASE

The nurse is reinforcing teaching points provided to a client by the registered nurse regarding measures that can be taken to prevent thrombophlebitis. Which of the following statements indicates that the client understands these measures?
1 "I need to sit with my legs elevated for most of the day."
2 "I need to avoid sitting in one position for prolonged periods."
3 "I'm glad I don't need to wear those ugly stockings anymore."
4 "I have decreased my fluid consumption to one glass of water a day."

ANSWER: 2
RATIONALE: This question addresses the subcategory, Prevention and Early Detection of Disease, in the Client Needs category, Health Promotion and Maintenance. The content addresses measures that will prevent thrombophlebitis. Avoidance of sitting or standing for a prolonged period is one of the measures for the prevention of venous stasis and thrombophlebitis.
CLIENT NEEDS: Health Promotion and Maintenance
REFERENCE
Luckmann, J. (1997). *Saunders manual of nursing care.* Philadelphia: W. B. Saunders, p. 1019.

Through the Life Span (4%–10%) addresses content that tests the knowledge, skills, and ability required to assist the client and significant others in the normal expected stages of growth and development from conception through advanced old age. Prevention and Early Detection of Disease (4%–10%) addresses content that tests the knowledge, skills, and ability required to provide client care related to prevention and early detection of health problems (Box 1–4).

Psychosocial Integrity

The Psychosocial Integrity category includes two subcategories, Coping and Adaptation and Psychosocial Adaptation. Coping and Adaptation (6%–12%) addresses content that tests the knowledge, skills, and ability required to promote the client's ability to cope, adapt, and/or problem solve situations related to illnesses or stressful events. Psychosocial Adaptation (4%–10%) addresses content that tests the knowledge, skills, and ability required to participate in providing care for clients with acute or chronic mental illnesses (Box 1–5).

BOX 1–5. Psychosocial Integrity

COPING AND ADAPTATION

The nurse is assigned to care for a client with ovarian cancer. While giving morning care, the client says, "If I can just live long enough to attend my daughter's graduation, I'll be ready to die." Which phase of coping is this client experiencing?
1 Isolation
2 Bargaining
3 Depression
4 Acceptance

ANSWER: 2
RATIONALE: This question addresses the subcategory, Coping and Adaptation in the Client Needs category, Psychosocial Integrity. The content addresses coping mechanisms. Bargaining is the phase of coping in which the dying person tries to negotiate, as in this case, making deals with their god or fate.
CLIENT NEEDS: Psychosocial Integrity
REFERENCE
deWit, S. (1998). *Essentials of medical-surgical nursing* (4th ed.). Philadelphia: W. B. Saunders, p. 301.

PSYCHOSOCIAL ADAPTATION

The nurse is collecting data regarding the lethality risk of a suicidal client. The best question for the nurse to ask the client is which of the following?
1 "Do you ever think about ending it all?"
2 "Have you ever thought of killing yourself?"
3 "Do you wish your life were over?"
4 "Do you have a death wish?"

ANSWER: 2
RATIONALE: This question addresses the subcategory, Psychosocial Adaptation in the Client Needs category, Psychosocial Integrity. The question addresses Mental Illness Concepts and Crisis Intervention. A lethality assessment requires direct communication between the client and the nurse concerning the client's intent. It is important to provide a question that is directly related to lethality.
CLIENT NEEDS: Psychosocial Integrity
REFERENCE
deWit, S. (1998). *Essentials of medical-surgical nursing* (4th ed.). Philadelphia: W. B. Saunders, p. 1003.

Physiological Integrity

The Physiological Integrity category includes four subcategories, Basic Care and Comfort, Pharmacological Therapies, Reduction of Risk Potential, and Physiological Adaptation. Basic Care and Comfort (10%–16%) addresses content that tests the knowledge, skills, and ability required to provide comfort and assistance in the performance of activities of daily living. Pharmacological Therapies (5%–11%) addresses content that tests the knowledge, skills, and ability required to provide care related to the administration of medications and monitoring clients receiving parenteral therapies. Reduction of Risk Potential (11%–17%) addresses content that tests the knowledge, skills, and ability required to reduce the client's potential for developing complications or health problems related to existing conditions, treatments, or procedures. Physiological Adaptation (13%–19%) addresses content that tests the knowledge, skills, and ability required to participate in providing care to clients with acute, chronic, or life-threatening physical health conditions (Box 1–6).

INTEGRATED CONCEPTS AND PROCESSES OF THE TEST PLAN

The National Council of State Boards of Nursing has identified seven concepts and processes that are fundamental to the practice of nursing. These concepts, principles, and processes are a component of the Test Plan and are integrated throughout the categories of Client Needs (Box 1–7).

CAT NCLEX-PN

The term NCLEX-PN stands for National Council Licensure Examination for Practical Nurses. CAT NCLEX-PN is a computer-administered, multiple-choice examination that the nursing graduate must take and pass in order to practice in the role as a practical/vocational nurse. This examination measures the competency needed to practice safely and effectively as a newly licensed entry level practical/vocational nurse.

COMPUTER ADAPTIVE TESTING (CAT)

The acronym CAT stands for Computer Adaptive Testing. CAT provides a uniqueness to the examination that the candidate will take, as the examination adapts to each test taker's skill level. The CAT is an examination that is assembled interactively as the candidate answers the questions. All of the test questions are stored in a large test bank and are categorized based on the test plan structure and the level of difficulty of the question. With the CAT method of testing, an examination is created and tailored to test the candidate's knowledge and abilities while fulfilling test plan requirements. Candidates will not waste time answering questions that are far above or below their competency level.

When you answer a question on CAT NCLEX-PN,

BOX 1–6. Physiological Integrity

BASIC CARE AND COMFORT

The nurse notes that the client has slight weakness in the right leg. Based on this observation, the nurse recognizes that the client would benefit most from the use of a:

1 Walker.
2 Wooden crutch.
3 Lofstrand crutch.
4 Straight-leg cane.

ANSWER: 4
RATIONALE: This question addresses the subcategory, Basic Care and Comfort in the Client Needs category, Physiological Integrity. It addresses content related to mobility and assistive devices. A straight-leg cane is useful for the client with slight weakness in one leg.
CLIENT NEEDS: Physiological Integrity
REFERENCE
Monahan, F., & Neighbors, M. (1998). *Medical-surgical nursing: Foundations for clinical practice* (2nd ed.). Philadelphia: W. B. Saunders, p. 880.

PHARMACOLOGICAL THERAPIES

The nurse is caring for a client with a diagnosis of chronic angina pectoris who is receiving sotalol (Betapace) 80 mg PO daily. Which of the following indicates to the nurse that the client is experiencing a side effect related to the medication?

1 Difficulty swallowing
2 Diaphoresis
3 Dry mouth
4 Bradycardia

ANSWER: 4
RATIONALE: This question addresses the subcategory, Pharmacological Therapies in the Client Needs category, Physiological Integrity. It addresses side effects of a medication. Sotalol (Betapace) is a beta-adrenergic blocking agent. Side effects include bradycardia, palpitations, difficulty breathing, irregular heartbeat, signs of congestive heart failure, and cold hands and feet. Gastrointestinal disturbances, anxiety and nervousness, and unusual tiredness and weakness can also occur.
CLIENT NEEDS: Physiological Integrity
REFERENCE
Hodgson, B., & Kizior, R. (1999) *Saunders nursing drug handbook 1999*. Philadelphia: W. B. Saunders, p. 939.

REDUCTION OF RISK POTENTIAL

The nurse is assigned to assist in caring for a client who has undergone cystoscopy. The nurse recognizes that which of the following are abnormal signs if noted during the first few hours after the procedure?

1 Pink-tinged urine
2 Bloody urine with clots
3 Clear yellow urine
4 Urine with a bluish or green tinge

ANSWER: 2
RATIONALE: This question addresses the subcategory, Reduction of Risk Potential in the Client Needs category, Physiological Integrity. It relates to potential complications and alterations in body systems. Bloody urine with clots is always an abnormal finding, and should be reported immediately.
CLIENT NEEDS: Physiological Integrity
REFERENCE
Monahan, F., & Neighbors, M. (1998). *Medical-surgical nursing: Foundations for clinical practice* (2nd ed.). Philadelphia: W. B. Saunders, p. 1352.

PHYSIOLOGICAL ADAPTATION

The nurse is assigned to care for a client with a diagnosis of pheochromocytoma. The nurse is told in report that the client's magnesium level is 7 mEq/L. Based on this laboratory result, the nurse recognizes which of the following signs as significant?

1 Drowsiness
2 Hypertension
3 Hyperpnea
4 Hyperactive reflexes

ANSWER: 1
RATIONALE: This question addresses the subcategory, Physiological Adaptation in the Client Needs category, Physiological Integrity. It addresses an alteration in body systems. Neurologic manifestations begin to occur at magnesium levels of 6 to 7 mEq/L and are noted as symptoms of neurologic depression, such as drowsiness, sedation, lethargy, respiratory depression, muscle weakness, and areflexia.
CLIENT NEEDS: Physiological Integrity
REFERENCE
deWit, S. (1998). *Essentials of medical-surgical nursing* (4th ed.). Philadelphia: W. B. Saunders, p. 110.

---

the computer will calculate a competency skill estimate based on the answer that you selected. If you selected a correct answer to a question, the computer scans the test bank and selects a more difficult question. If you selected an incorrect answer, the computer scans the test bank and selects an easier question. This process continues until the test plan requirements are met and a reliable pass or fail decision is made.

THE PROCESS OF REGISTRATION

The initial step in the registration process is that you apply to the State Board of Nursing in the state in which you intend to obtain licensure. (The addresses and telephone numbers of Boards of Nursing in all states and territories of the United States are provided at the end of this chapter.) You need to obtain information from the Board of Nursing regard-

BOX 1–7. Integrated Concepts and Processes of the Test Plan

Caring	Nursing Process
Communication	Teaching/Learning
Cultural Awareness	Self-Care
Documentation	

ing the specific registration process, as the process may vary from state to state. It is very important that you follow the registration instructions and complete the registration forms precisely and accurately. Registration forms not properly completed or not accompanied by the proper fees in the required method of payment, will be returned to you and will delay testing. The initial fee for the application process may vary from state to state. Each Board of Nursing will set its initial license fee according to its own needs. The registration forms will identify the registration and testing service fees. When the Board of Nursing receives the completed registration form, based on the criteria established by the Board, your eligibility is determined, and the Board authorizes your admission to the examination.

Once your eligibility to test has been determined by the Board of Nursing in the jurisdiction in which licensure is requested, the valid NCLEX registration is processed and an Authorization to Test form will be sent to you. You cannot make an appointment until the Board of Nursing declares eligibility and you receive an Authorization to Test form. The Authorization to Test form will provide you with an identification number and an authorization number, and these numbers will be needed to make an appointment with the testing center.

SPECIAL TESTING CIRCUMSTANCES

A candidate that is requesting special accommodations should contact the Board of Nursing prior to submitting a registration form. The Board of Nursing will provide the candidate with the procedures for the request. Testing accommodations for candidates with disabilities must be authorized by the Board of Nursing. Following Board of Nursing approval, the National Council of State Boards reviews the requested accommodations to ensure that the proposed modification does not affect the psychometric properties of NCLEX or cause a security risk.

MAKING AN APPOINTMENT TO TEST

The CAT NCLEX-PN examination is administered year-round. You will be provided with a list of testing centers and the telephone numbers. Note the expiration date on the Authorization to Test form. You must schedule and make an appointment prior to this expiration date. You may take the test at any approved testing center and do not have to test in the same jurisdiction in which you are seeking licensure.

An eligible candidate taking NCLEX for the first time will be offered an appointment date within 30 days of the telephone call to the testing center. Repeat candidates will be offered an appointment date within 45 days of the telephone call to the testing center. A confirmation notice will not be sent to you; therefore, it is important to note the date and time of the appointment. When the test center is called, it is also important to verify the address and the directions to the testing center.

CANCELING OR RESCHEDULING AN APPOINTMENT

If for any reason you need to cancel your appointment to test, remember that 3 business days' (Monday through Saturday) notice is required. The original appointment must be canceled before a new appointment can be scheduled.

LATE ARRIVALS TO THE TEST CENTER

It is important that you arrive at the testing center 30 minutes before the test is scheduled. Candidates arriving late for the scheduled testing appointment may be required to forfeit the NCLEX appointment. If it is necessary for the appointment to be forfeited, candidates will need to reregister for the examination and pay an additional fee. The Board of Nursing will be notified that the candidate will not test.

A few days prior to your scheduled date of testing, take the time to drive to the testing center to determine its exact location, the length of time required to arrive to that destination, and any potential obstacles that might delay you, such as road construction, traffic, or parking sites.

THE TESTING CENTER

The testing center is designed to ensure complete security of the testing process. Strict candidate identification requirements have been established. To be admitted to the testing center, it is imperative that you bring the Authorization to Test form, along with two forms of identification. Both forms of identification must be signed by you, and one must contain your photograph. The name on the photograph identification must bear the same name as stated on the Authorization to Test form. Examples of acceptable forms of identification will be included in the information received with the Authorization to Test form. You will be required to sign in and out on the test center log form. Each candidate will be thumbprinted and photographed at the testing center, and the photograph will accompany the NCLEX results to confirm the candidate's identity. Personal belongings are not allowed in the testing room. Secure storage will be provided for the candidate; however, storage space is small so you must plan accordingly. In addition, the testing center will not assume responsibility for your personal belongings. The testing waiting areas are generally small; therefore, friends or family members who accompany you are not permitted to wait in the testing center while you are taking the NCLEX-PN.

Once you have completed the admission process and a brief orientation, the proctor will escort you to the assigned computer. You will be seated at an individual table with an appropriate work space that includes computer equipment, appropriate lighting, scratch paper, and a pencil. Unauthorized scratch paper may not be brought into or removed from the testing room. Eating, drinking, and smoking are not allowed in the testing room. A video camera is located in the testing room for full sound and motion videotaping of all test sessions.

Keep your two forms of identification with you at all times. You cannot leave the testing room without the permission of the proctor. If you leave the testing room for any reason, you will be required to show two forms of identification in order to be readmitted. You must follow the directions given by the test center staff and must remain in your seat during the test, except when authorized to leave. If you feel that you have a problem with the computer, need more scratch paper, or need the proctor for any reason, you must raise your hand to notify the proctor.

THE COMPUTER

You do not need any computer experience to take a CAT NCLEX-PN examination. Only two computer keys are needed to take the CAT examination, the space bar and the enter key. The space bar key will allow you to scroll the options and the enter key will allow you to highlight and select an answer. The enter key must be struck twice in order to record the answer choice and to proceed to the next question. A key board tutorial is provided and administered to all test takers prior to the start of the examination. In addition, a proctor is present to assist in explaining the use of the computer to ensure your full understanding of how to proceed.

CAT NCLEX-PN TEST QUESTIONS

The examination is composed of individual or a "stand alone" test questions. This means that there is not a case situation followed by several related questions. With the stand alone test question, you can expect that the question will appear on the left-hand side of the screen with the four responses on the right-hand side of the screen, or the question appears across the top of the screen with the four responses below (Box 1–8).

You must answer the test question presented on the computer screen or the test will not move on. This means that you will not be able to skip questions, go back and review questions, or go back and change answers. Students preparing for CAT NCLEX-PN become anxious and frustrated because questions cannot be skipped and returned to at a later time during the examination process. Remember, in a CAT examination, once an answer is recorded, all subsequent questions administered depend to an extent, on the response selected for that question. Skipping and returning to earlier questions is not compatible with the logical methodology of a computerized adaptive test. Additionally, it is important to recall the number of times you may have changed a correct answer to an incorrect one on a pencil-and-paper nursing examination during your nursing education. The inability to skip questions or go back to change previous answers will not disadvantage you. Actually, you will not fall into that trap of changing a correct answer to an incorrect one with CAT. There is no penalty for guessing on CAT NCLEX-PN. Remember, the answer to the question will be right there in front of you. If you need to guess, utilize your nursing knowledge to its fullest extent, and all of the test-taking strategies provided to you in Chapter 4 of this book.

TESTING TIME

The maximum testing time will be 5 hours including the short keyboard tutorial and any rest breaks. There is no minimum amount of examination time. A mandatory 10-minute break will be taken after 2 testing hours and an optional 10-minute break can be taken after an additional 1.5 hours of testing. The computer screen will notify you of the time for these

---

BOX 1–8. Appearance of an Individual Test Item on the Computer Screen	
The most appropriate method for feeding the infant with cleft lip or palate is	1 With the infant's head in an upright position. 2 With the infant in a lying position. 3 With the infant in a side-lying position. 4 With the infant prone.
The client is admitted with a diagnosis of myasthenia gravis and is receiving pyridostigmine (Mestinon). The nurse recognizes that the client is experiencing an adverse effect of this medication if which of the following is noted? 1 Muscle cramps 2 Mouth ulcers 3 Depression 4 Unexplained weight gain	

breaks. You must leave the testing room during breaks. You may leave the room for additional un-scheduled breaks, but no additional testing time will be allowed.

THE LENGTH OF THE EXAMINATION

The minimum number of questions that you need to answer in order to meet adequate testing in all areas of the test plan is 75. Sixty of these questions will be real (scored) questions and 15 of these questions will be try-out (unscored) questions. The maximum number of questions you may need to answer will be 265. Again, of these 265 questions, 15 of these questions will be try-out (unscored) questions. The try-out questions are not identified as such. In other words, you do not know which questions are the unscored questions.

COMPLETING THE EXAMINATION

Once the test is completed, you will complete a brief computer-delivered questionnaire about your testing experience. After this questionnaire is completed, the test proctor will collect all scratch paper, sign you out, and permit you to leave.

PROCESSING RESULTS

Upon completion of the examination, results are transmitted electronically to the data center at the testing service. Your results are transmitted to the Board of Nursing in the state in which you applied for licensure. A paper copy of the results is mailed to the Board of Nursing within 48 hours after the examination is completed. The Board of Nursing will mail the results to you. You should not telephone the testing center, the National Council, or your State Board of Nursing for results. The results will not be given to you over the telephone.

INTERSTATE ENDORSEMENT

Since the CAT NCLEX-PN is a national examination, you can apply to take and sit for the examination in any state. Once licensure is received, the practical/vocational nurse can apply for Interstate Endorsement. The procedures and requirements for Interstate Endorsement may vary from state to state, and these procedures can be obtained from the State Board of Nursing in the state in which endorsement is sought.

STATE BOARDS OF NURSING

Alabama Board of Nursing
P.O. Box 303900
Montgomery, AL 36130-3900
(344) 242-4060

Alaska Board of Nursing
3601 C. Street, Suite 722
Anchorage, AK 99503
(907) 561-2878

American Samoa Board of Nursing
Health Services Regulatory Board
LBJ Tropical Medical Center
Pago Pago, American Samoa 96799
(684) 633-1222, Ext. 206

Arizona State Board of Nursing
1651 E. Morton, Suite 150
Phoenix, AZ 85020
(602) 255-5092

Arkansas State Board of Nursing
1123 South University, Suite 800
Little Rock, AR 72204
(501) 686-2700

California Board of Vocational Nursing & Psych.
  Tech Examiners
2535 Capital Oaks Drive, Suite 205
Sacramento, CA 95833
(916) 263-7840

Colorado State Board of Nursing
1560 Broadway, Suite 670
Denver, CO 80202-2410
(303) 894-2430

Connecticut Department of Public Health
Board of Examiners for Nursing
410 Capital Avenue
MS# 12 Nur.
P.O. Box 340308
Hartford, CT 06134-0308
(860) 509-7624

Delaware Board of Nursing
Cannon Bldg., P.O. Box 1401, Suite 203
Dover, DE 19903
(302) 739-4522, Ext. 217

District of Columbia Board of Nursing
614 H Street NW
Washington, DC 20013
(202) 727-7856

Florida State Board of Nursing
111 E. Coastline Drive East
Jacksonville, FL 32202
(904) 798-4215

Georgia Board of Examiners of
  Lic. Practical Nurse
166 Pryor Street, NW, Suite 300
Atlanta, GA 30303
(404) 656-3921

Guam Board of Nurse Examiners
P.O. Box 2816
Agana, Guam 96910
(671) 734-7295

Hawaii Board of Nursing
Box 3469
Honolulu, HI 99503
(808) 586-2695

Idaho State Board of Nursing
P.O. Box 83720
Boise, ID 83720-0061
(208) 334-3110

Illinois Department of Professional Regulations
320 W. Washington Street
Springfield, IL 62786
(217) 785-9465

Indiana State Board of Nursing
402 W. Washington Street
Indianapolis, IN 46204
(317) 233-4405

Iowa Board of Nursing
1223 E. Court Avenue
Des Moines, IA 50319
(515) 281-3255

Kansas State Board of Nursing
900 SW Jackson Street, Suite 551S
Topeka, KS 66612-1256
(913) 296-3782

Kentucky Board of Nursing
312 Whittington Parkway, Suite 300
Louisville, KY 40222-5172
(502) 329-7000, Ext. 235

Louisiana State Board of Practical Nurse Examiners
1440 Canal Street, Suite 1722
New Orleans, LA 70112
(504) 838-5791

Maine State Board of Nursing
35 Anthony Avenue
State House Station 158
Augusta, ME 04333-0158
(207) 624-5275

Maryland Board of Nursing
4140 Patterson Avenue
Baltimore, MD 21215-2254
(410) 764-5124

Massachusetts Board of Registration in Nursing
100 Cambridge Street, Room 150
Boston, MA 02202
(617) 727-3060

Michigan Board of Nursing
P.O. Box 30018
611 West Ottawa
Lansing, MI 48909
(517) 373-4674

Minnesota Board of Nursing
2700 University Avenue West 108
St. Paul, MN 55114
(612) 643-2565

Mississippi Health Occupation Education
Division of Vocational Education
Department of Education
P.O. Box 771
3825 Ridgewood Road
Jackson, MS 39205
(601) 359-3461

Missouri State Board of Nursing
3605 Missouri Blvd.
Jefferson City, MO 65102
(573) 751-1416

Montana State Board of Nursing
Arcade Building
111 Jackson
Helena, MT 59620-0513
(406) 444-2071

Nebraska Bureau of Examining Board
P.O. Box 95007
Lincoln, NE 68509
(402) 471-4917

Nevada State Board of Nursing
4335 S. Industrial Road #420
Las Vegas, NV 89103
(702) 739-1575

New Hampshire State Board of Nursing
Division of Public Health
6 Hazen Drive
Concord, NH 03301
(603) 271-2323

New Jersey Board of Nursing
P.O. Box 45010
Newark, NJ 07101
(201) 504-6493

New Mexico Board of Nursing
4206 Louisiana NE, Suite A
Albuquerque, NM 87109
(505) 841-8340

New York State Board of Nursing
The Cultural Center, Room 3023
Albany, NY 12230
(518) 486-2967

North Carolina Board of Nursing
P.O. Box 2129
Raleigh, NC 27602
(919) 782-3211

North Dakota Board of Nursing
919 S. 7th Street, Suite 504
Bismarck, ND 58504-5881
(701) 328-9777

Ohio Board of Nursing
77 S. High Street, 17th Floor
Columbus, OH 43266-0316
(614) 466-9800

Oklahoma Board of Nursing
2915 N. Classen Blvd., Suite 524
Oklahoma City, OK 73106
(405) 525-2076

Oregon State Board of Nursing
800 NE Oregon Street, #25
Portland, OR 97232
(503) 731-4745

Pennsylvania State Board of Nurses
P.O. Box 2649
Harrisburg, PA 17105
(717) 783-7142

Puerto Rico Board of Nursing Licensure Office
General Council on Education
P.O. Box 195429
San Juan, PR 00919-5429
(809) 764-0101

Rhode Island Board of Nursing Education and
  Nurse Registration
3 Capital Hill
Providence, RI 02908-5097
(401) 277-2827

State Board of Nursing for South Carolina
220 Executive Center Drive, Suite 220
Columbia, SC 29210
(803) 731-1648

South Dakota Board of Nursing
3307 South Lincoln
Sioux Falls, SD 57105
(605) 367-5940

Tennessee Board of Nursing
283 Plus Park Boulevard
Nashville, TN 37217
(615) 367-6232

Texas Board of Vocational Nurse Examiners
9101 Burnett Road, Suite 105
Austin, TX 78758
(512) 305-8100

Utah State Board of Nursing
160 E. 300 South, Box 45805
Salt Lake City, UT 84145
(801) 530-6789

Vermont Board of Nursing
Licensing and Registration Division
109 State Street
Montpelier, VT 05602
(802) 828-2396

Virgin Islands Board of Nurse Licensure
P.O. Box 4247
Charolotte Amalie, VI 00803
(809) 776-7397

Virginia State Board of Nursing
6606 W. Broad Street, 4th Floor
Richmond, VA 23230-1717
(804) 662-9951

Washington State Nursing Care
Quality Assurance Commission
1300 Quince, P.O. Box 47864
Olympia, WA 98504-7864
(360) 664-4208

West Virginia State Board of Examiners for Licensed
  Practical Nurses
101 Dee Drive
Charleston, WV 25311-1688
(304) 558-3572

Wisconsin Department of Regulation & Licensing
P.O. Box 8935
Madison, WI 53708-8935
(608) 267-2357

State of Wyoming Board of Nursing
2301 Central Avenue, Barrett Bldg.
Cheyenne, WY 82002
(307) 777-7601

BIBLIOGRAPHY

Bonilla, E., & Trotman, S. (1996). *State approved schools of nursing LPN/LVN* (38th ed.). New York: Center for Research in Nursing Education and Community Health, National League for Nursing.

deWit, S. (1998). *Essentials of medical-surgical nursing* (4th ed.). Philadelphia: W. B. Saunders.

Gorrie, T., McKinney, E., & Murray, S. (1998). *Foundations of maternal-newborn nursing* (2nd ed.). Philadelphia: W. B. Saunders.

Hill, S., & Howlett, H. (1997). *Success in practical nursing: Personal and vocational Issues* (3rd ed.). Philadelphia: W. B. Saunders.

Hodgson, B., & Kizior, R. (1999). *Saunders nursing drug handbook 1999*. Philadelphia: W. B. Saunders.

Luckmann, J. (1997). *Saunders manual of nursing care*. Philadelphia: W. B. Saunders.

Monahan, F., & Neighbors, M. (1998). *Medical-surgical nursing: Foundations for clinical practice* (2nd ed.). Philadelphia: W. B. Saunders.

National Council of State Boards of Nursing. (1995). *The NCLEX process*. Chicago: Author.

National Council of State Boards of Nursing. (1998). *National Council Detailed Test Plan for the NCLEX-PN Examination*.

CHAPTER 2

Pathways To Success

Laurent W. Valliere, B.S.

FOUNDATION TO SUCCESS

The foundation to success begins with a positive attitude about your ability to succeed, and with developing your own short- and long-term goals. Without these components, your Pathway to Success leads to nowhere, and you will expend energy and valuable time and will experience exhaustion without any accomplishment. Therefore, your first step is to take the time to develop and maintain that positive attitude, and to establish your list of short- and long-term goals.

THE LIST OF GOALS

At this time, you may or may not have a scheduled date for taking the NCLEX-PN. Regardless, it is time to create "The List." The List is your set of goals. Begin by developing the goals you wish to accomplish today, tomorrow, and into the future. Where do you start? To begin, find a comfortable position, close your eyes, inhale, hold your breath to a count of four, exhale slowly, and relax. Repeat this breathing exercise several times until you begin to feel relaxed, free from anxiety, and in control of your pathway to success. Allow yourself the opportunity to list all that is flowing from your uninhibited thought process. Develop three columns on a piece of paper, identifying a column for your goals for today, tomorrow, and the future. Start writing your goals. When the list is complete, it is time to bank the List away for 2 or 3 days, then retrieve and review it and begin the process of planning for preparing for the licensing examination.

A POSITIVE ATTITUDE

Confidence and the belief that you have the ability to achieve success will bring your goals to fruition. Reflect on the pathway that you maintained during your nursing education. Your confidence and belief in yourself, along with your academic achievements, have brought you to the status of a graduate from a nursing program. Now you are facing one more important challenge. Can you meet this challenge successfully? Yes, you can! There is no reason to think otherwise if you have taken all the necessary steps to ensure that pathway to success.

Obtain a large blank card, write your name on the card and the letters LPN or LVN after your name. Post the card where you will see it every morning. Each morning, place your feet on the floor, stand tall, take a deep breath, and believe. Take both hands and brush any negatives that you may be feeling off of you. Look at your card and tell yourself, "Yes, I can. I believe!"

THE PLAN FOR STUDY

The first task is to decide what study pattern works best for you. Review what has worked most successfully for you in the past. The following questions must be addressed in order to establish the correct Plan for Study. Ask yourself:

Do I work better alone or in a group study environment?

If I work best in a group, does the group consist of one, two, or more study partners?

Who are these study partners?

How long should my study sessions last?

Does the time of day that I study make a difference for me?

Do I retain more if I study in the morning?

How does my work schedule affect my study pattern?

How do I balance my family obligations with my need to study?

Do I have a comfortable study area at home or do I need to find an environment that is conducive to my study needs?

The Plan for Study must include how you will manage your study needs with the demands of your family and friends. Think about how you will balance your everyday commitments with your plan for study. Your family and friends are key players in your life and are going to become a part of your Pyramid to Success. After you have established your study needs, communicate these needs, and the importance of your study plan in achieving your goal of becoming a Licensed Practical/Vocational Nurse, with your family and friends.

A difficult part of the Plan for Study may be how you will deal with those family and friends who choose not to participate in your Pyramid to Success. What if someone chooses not to be part of the Pyramid? Then you are faced with a decision, and you must weigh all the factors carefully. Keep your goals in mind and remember that your need for positive momentum is critical. Your decision may not be an easy one but must be one that will help ensure that your goal of becoming a Licensed Practical/Vocational Nurse is achieved. Remember, your positive momentum and goal achievement must to be shared by all who support you.

The Plan for Study must include a schedule. Establish a realistic schedule that includes your daily, weekly, and future goals, and adhere to it. This consistency will provide advantages to you and to those supporting you. A daily schedule allows you to plan your topic areas for study more carefully. Adherence to the plan helps you develop a rhythm that can only enhance your retention and positive momentum. Those who are supporting you will share this rhythm and will be able to schedule their activities and life better because you are consistent with your study plan. Remember, you are moving forward and you are in control!

POSITIVE PAMPERING

Positive momentum can be maintained only if you are properly balanced. This means that you must continue to care for yourself. Proper exercise, diet, and positive mental stimulation are critical to achieving your goal of becoming a Licensed Practical/Vocational Nurse.

Just as you have developed a plan for study, you should develop a plan that includes fun and some form of physical activity—aerobics, running, weight lifting, bowling, tennis, or whatever makes you feel good about yourself. Time spent away from the difficult study schedule and devoted to some form of fun and physical exercise pays its rewards one hundred-fold. You will feel alive and more energetic with a plan that includes these activities.

Establish good eating habits. Stay away from fatty foods because they will slow you down. Eat three balanced and lighter meals each day, including healthy snacks throughout the day. Include complex carbohydrates in your daily diet for energy and be careful not to include too much caffeine.

Feel good about yourself because you are in control. Take the time to pamper yourself with activities that make you feel even better about who you are. Make dinner reservations at your favorite restaurant with someone who is special and is supporting your goal to become a Licensed Practical/Vocational Nurse. Take walks in a place that provides a special tranquillity and enables you to reflect on the positive momentum you have maintained. Whatever it is, wherever it takes you, allow yourself the time to do some Positive Pampering.

FINAL PREPARATION

You have established the foundation of your Pyramid to Success. You are moving forward and you are in control. When you receive your date and time for the NCLEX-PN you may immediately think, "I am not ready!"

Stop! Reflect on all that you have achieved. Think about your goals and the organization of the positive life momentum that you have surrounded yourself with. Think about all of those individuals who support your effort to be a Licensed Practical/Vocational Nurse. Believe that the challenge that awaits you is one that you have successfully prepared for and will lead you to your goal, becoming a Licensed Practical/Vocational Nurse! Take a deep breath and organize the remaining days so that they support your educational and personal needs. Support your positive momentum. Look at your card that bears your name with the letters LPN or LVN after it, and tell yourself, "Yes, I can. I believe!"

Through all that you have accomplished to this point, it is imperative that you do not fall into the trap of expecting too much of yourself. The idea of perfection must not drive you to a point that causes your positive momentum to hesitate. You must believe in who you are, as you are, and stay focused on your goals. Allow yourself the opportunity to continue to carry out your plan in a manner that is most conducive to who you are, not someone else. When the day and time of the examination is scheduled, write it down and underneath write the word "Yes," and post it next to your name plus LPN/LVN. Make sure you know how to get to the testing center. A test run is a must. Time the drive and allow for road construction or whatever may occur that slows down the traffic. On the test run, once you arrive at the test facility, you may want to walk into the facility to become familiar with the lobby and the surroundings. This may help to alleviate some of the peripheral nervousness associated with entering an unknown facility. Remember, you must do whatever it takes to keep yourself in control. If familiarizing yourself with the facility will help you to maintain a positive momentum, by all means, be sure to do so! Who is in control? You are!

Now that a scheduled date and time for the examination is set, check your study plan and make the necessary adjustments. Adjust your review so that it flows to your needs and that your study plan ends 1 to 2 days before the examination. Remember that the mind is like a muscle—if it is overworked, it has no strength or stamina. Your strategy is to rest the body and the mind on the day before the examination. Stay in control and allow yourself the opportunity to be absolutely fresh and attentive on the day of the examination. This will help you control the nervousness that is natural, achieve the clear thought process required, and maintain the confidence that you have done all that is necessary to prepare and conquer this challenge.

Plan the day before the examination just as you have planned your study schedule. This day is to be one of pleasure. Treat yourself to what you enjoy the most. Relax! You have prepared yourself well for the challenge of tomorrow. Get a good night's sleep and wake up the day of the examination knowing you are absolutely ready to succeed. Look at your name with the letters LPN/LVN after it and the word, "Yes!" Wake up believing in yourself and that all that you have accomplished is about to propel you to the level of Licensed Practical/Vocational Nurse. Allow yourself plenty of time, eat a nutritious breakfast, and groom yourself for success. You are ready to meet the challenges of the day and overcome any obstacle that may face you. Today will soon be history and tomorrow will bring you the envelope that reads your name with the words, Licensed Practical/Vocational Nurse, after it.

Be proud and confident of your achievements. You have worked hard to achieve your goal of becoming a Licensed Practical/Vocational Nurse. If you believe in yourself, no one person or obstacle can move you off the pathway that leads to success, to the peak of the Pyramid!

Congratulations and I wish you the very best in your career as a Licensed Practical/Vocational Nurse!

CHAPTER 3

The NCLEX-PN Examination: From a Student's Perspective

Mary E. Wright, LPN

When I graduated from nursing school, I was 32 years old. My three best friends graduated at the same time from the same nursing program, and all of us were the older students of the class. There were many commitments that we had to contend with during our education. We had many hats to wear, so to speak, and several roles and responsibilities: We were mothers, wives, friends, nursing students, and support systems to each other and everyone around us. Our path through the learning process in nursing school was not an easy one. There were many obstacles and many commitments to meet, but the perseverance and desire to become a nurse made all of the obstacles challenges—challenges that we all knew would lead to many rewards.

When we graduated from nursing school, we knew that we had one more major challenge to meet and that was to pass the NCLEX examination. My three friends and I lived quite a distance from the test site so we decided that we would pack up our bags, register at a luxurious hotel, and take the test together. We arrived at the hotel on the day before our scheduled and dreaded examination with our nerves in a state of high anxiety. Were we ready to meet this last challenge? Yes, we were.

Suggestions about preparing for this examination were fortunately shared by the nursing graduates who took it the previous year, and by my nursing instructors. Whenever I became anxious, nervous, or felt as though I was losing confidence in my abilities to succeed, I thought about all of their suggestions, which helped get me back on track.

I want to share with you some of the tips I received from others regarding the preparation for this important examination as well as add my own hints.

To begin, it is important to listen to what others have to say about preparing for this examination because their input will be very helpful. But remember that this test is all about you and you must meet your own needs in preparing yourself.

You need to remember that balance in life can bring success. A study plan is important but it needs to be structured and realistic to meet your needs and all of the commitments that you have in your life. An immediate instinct is to study every minute that you can right up to the time of the examination. My suggestion is that you spend 2 hours each day for intensive review. If you feel as though you can spend more than 2 hours, then do so; but I found that after the 2 hours, I became distracted and fatigued. How do you proceed with your study? Practice questions—do as many as you possibly can. Read the rationales for the correct and incorrect answers and learn how to answer the question if you are unfamiliar with the content area. Make a list of the content that you will need to read, and refresh your memory on these areas from your nursing textbooks. But again, practice with as many questions as you can. Do you study right up to the time of the examination? No. You need to relax and enjoy yourself the day before the examination. Remember, no cramming at the last minute. Be confident that you have what it takes to pass this test to become a licensed practical or vocational nurse. I needed to remember that I would not be taking this important examination if I didn't have what it takes.

In addition to your 2 hours' study time, make sure that you spend time having some fun. Each day, spend time doing what you like to do, whatever that may be. It is also very important that you save time for exercise and to prepare healthy meals for yourself. You need to be prepared physically and mentally.

On the night before the examination, don't study, have fun, and get a good night sleep. Again, remember that you are prepared. My nursing instructors told me that if I had difficulty sleeping, to try deep- and slow-breathing exercises because they would relax my body. That is what I did, and it helped. In fact, whenever I became distracted and nervous during the examination, I began to deep breathe and became relaxed so that I could proceed.

On the night before the examination, my friends and I went out for dinner and a relaxing evening; but as soon as we ordered our meals, they began asking questions about medications, medication calculations, and various other topics related to nursing. I could feel my stomach beginning to knot, and I finally told my friends that there would be no nursing conversations at this dinner table. I reminded them that we knew what we needed to know and that these last hours were not going to make a difference.

On the morning of the examination, we had a wake-up call in addition to four alarm clocks going off at the crack of dawn. You want to get up early enough to have time to prepare yourself physically and mentally. Eat a light, healthy breakfast and take something to eat for breaktime during the examination. It may be difficult to eat because your stomach may feel as though it is a big knot. But remember to feed your brain because your brain is what you will really need.

When you arrive at the testing center, you will need to complete all of the pretesting rituals. This will make you nervous because all you want to do is get on with it and get this test over with. Take those deep breaths and don't become frustrated because you will begin to block your thought process. You haven't started the test yet. Be patient.

As you have probably been told, all of the questions are multiple choice. You will, just as I did, receive questions about nursing content that you do not know or have never heard of. When this happens, don't get nervous. Take a deep breath and remember this happens to everyone. Also, remember that the answer is right there in front of you, so read the question again, and make an educated quess just as you had to with all of your practice questions.

When the examination was completed, I felt relieved, yet I kept experiencing ambivalent feelings. One minute I felt as though I did great, and then I would begin to feel nervous and anxious as though I had failed. You are likely to experience these same feelings. Remember, it is over with, you did the best that you could, now go on with your life.

The final component is the waiting game, waiting for the results. This is as difficult as any other part of the process. Keep yourself busy. Anxiously, I checked my mailbox every day awaiting the news. Finally, it came. It was a white, thin envelope. I could see my name through a clear opening in the envelope, but I could not see the letters LPN, so I feared opening it. But I remembered that I was told—a thin envelope is a good sign. So I carefully and anxiously opened it and saw my name with LPN following it. I ran back into my house yelling "Yes!" all the way. I immediately called everyone that I knew to spread the great news. And then, I called my three friends. They passed too. Now, we could begin our careers that we have dreamed for.

As a final thought, always remember that belief and a positive attitude will help guide you to your goal of becoming a Licensed Practical Nurse.

Congratulations to you and I wish you continued success in your new career as a Licensed Practical Nurse.

CHAPTER 4

Test-Taking Strategies

. . . .

I. The Pyramid to Success (Box 4–1)

II. The Components of the Question

A. Strategy 1
1. Identify the components of the question
2. Identify the "Case situation" from the "Stem" of the question
3. Read all of the options carefully and thoroughly
B. The case situation
1. The case situation gives you the information about a clinical health problem and the information you need to consider in answering the question
2. It is extremely important to read all of the information and every word in the case situation
C. The stem
1. The stem usually comes after the case situation and asks you something about it
2. The stem asks you to solve a problem and select an answer
3. Read the stem very carefully and specifically identify exactly what the question is asking
D. The options
1. The options are all of the answers and you must select one
2. Read all of the options very carefully and then reread the stem of the question before selecting the answer

---

BOX 4–1. The Pyramid to Success

Read the questions and options thoroughly and carefully!
   Ask yourself, "What is the question really asking me?"
   Be alert to key words and true and false stems!
   Eliminate the incorrect options!
   Use all of your nursing knowledge, your clinical experiences, and your test-taking skills to answer the question!

---

3. Use the process of elimination and eliminate the incorrect options
4. Once you have eliminated the incorrect options, reread the stem again to identify specifically what the question is asking before selecting your answer from the remaining options

III. The Critical Elements of the Question

A. Strategy 2
1. Identify the critical elements of the case situation and the stem of the question
2. The critical elements are the key words or phrases in the case situation and the stem of the question
B. Key words or phrases
1. The key words or phrases focus your attention on critical ideas in the case, stem, and in the options
2. Some of the key words or phrases that you should look for and focus your attention on include
   a. Early or late
   b. Immediately
   c. Most likely or least likely
   d. Initial
   e. First
   f. Best
   g. Most appropriate
   h. On the day of
   i. After several days
3. The key words will make a difference in your selection of an answer (Box 4–2)

IV. The Client of the Question

A. Strategy 3
1. Identify the client of the question
2. The client is the person who is the focus of the question
B. The client
1. It is important to remember that the client of the question may not necessarily be the person with the health problem

> **BOX 4–2. Key Words in the Question**
>
> Which of the following is an EARLY sign of shock?
>
> Which of the following is a LATE SIGN of shock?
>
> ON THE DAY OF surgery, immediately following a transurethral resection of the prostate (TURP), the nurse observes that the client's urine is bright red. Which of the following nursing actions is appropriate?
>
> AFTER SEVERAL DAYS, following a TURP, the nurse observes that the client's urine is bright red. Which of the following nursing actions is appropriate?
>
> Noting the key words or phrases in each of these situations will assist in directing you to select the correct option.
>
> The EARLY signs of shock are quite different from the LATE signs of shock!
>
> Bright red urine might be expected ON THE DAY OF surgery immediately following a TURP, but would not be expected AFTER SEVERAL DAYS!

2. In the test question, the client may be a relative, friend, spouse, significant other, or even another nurse
3. Identify the client of the question and select an answer that relates to and most directly addresses that client

V. The Issue of the Question

A. Strategy 4
   1. Identify the issue of the question
   2. The issue of the question is the specific subject content that the question is asking about
B. The issue
   1. Identifying the issue of the question will assist in eliminating the incorrect options and direct you to selecting the correct answer
   2. The issue of the question can include
      a. A medication
      b. A side effect or toxic effect of a medication
      c. A procedure
      d. A complication
      e. A specific nursing action

VI. The Type of Stem in the Question

A. Strategy 5
   1. Identify the type of stem in the question
   2. The stem can be either a true response stem or a false response stem
B. True response stem
   1. True response stems use key words that ask you to select an answer that is true regarding the situation and the question
   2. True response stems may use the following key words or phrases
      a. Most
      b. Best
      c. Best judgment

      d. Initial
      e. First
      f. Chief
      g. Immediate
C. False response stem
   1. False response stems use key words that ask you to select an answer that is *not* true regarding the situation and question
   2. False response stems may use the following key words or phrases
      a. Except
      b. Not
      c. Least likely
      d. Need for further education
      e. Lowest priority
      f. Incorrect
      g. Unsafe

VII. Eliminating the Incorrect Options

A. Strategy 6
   1. Using the process of elimination, eliminate the incorrect options before selecting an answer
   2. Be alert to the key words or phrases and to the true and the false response stems
B. Distracters
   1. Distracters are options that are made to look like correct answers but, in fact, are not
   2. They are intended to distract you from answering questions correctly
   3. There are three distracters and one correct answer
   4. Use the process of elimination and eliminate the incorrect options
   5. Be alert to the key words and to the true and the false response stems
   6. Once you have eliminated the incorrect options, reread the stem again and identify specifically what the question is asking before selecting your answer

VIII. Questions That Require Prioritizing

A. Strategy 7
   1. Identify the key words in the question that indicate the need for you to prioritize
   2. Key words include the following
      a. Initial
      b. Essential
      c. Vital
      d. Immediate
      e. Highest
      f. Best
      g. Most
B. Strategy 8
   1. Use Maslow's Hierarchy of Needs Theory to prioritize
   2. Physiological needs come *first*, so select an answer that addresses physiological needs
   3. When a physiological need is not addressed in the question, safety needs receive priority, and

in this situation select an answer that
addresses safety

C. Strategy 9
 1. Use the ABCs when selecting an answer
 2. Remember the order of priority of AIRWAY,
    BREATHING AND CIRCULATION

D. Strategy 10
 1. Use the Nursing Process to prioritize
 2. Remember that data collection is the first step
    in the Nursing Process
 3. When you are asked to select your first and
    initial nursing action, use and follow the steps
    of the Nursing Process to select your answer
 4. If an answer contains the concept of data
    collection related to the client, select that
    answer

IX. The Nursing Process (Box 4–3)

A. Data Collection
 1. Data collection questions will address the
    process of gathering subjective and objective
    data relative to the client, communicating
    information gained in data collection, and
    contributing to the formulation of nursing
    diagnoses
 2. Remember that data collection is the first step
    in the nursing process
 3. When you are asked a question regarding
    your initial or first nursing action, select the
    option that addresses the process of data
    collection
 4. If a data collection action is not one of the
    options, follow the steps of the nursing
    process as your guide to select your initial or
    first action
 5. When answering questions that focus on data
    collection, look for key words in the options
    that reflect the collection of data relative to
    the client
 6. Key words or phrases that reflect data
    collection
    a. Gather
    b. Collect
    c. Recognize
    d. Observe

    e. Check
    f. Monitor
    g. Obtain information
    h. Find out
    i. Determine

B. Planning
 1. Planning questions will require providing
    input into plan development, assisting in the
    formulation of the goals of care, and assisting
    in the development of a plan of care
 2. Remember that this is a nursing examination
    and the answer to the question involves
    something that is included in the nursing care
    plan, rather than the medical plan

C. Implementation
 1. This examination is about NURSING, so focus
    on the nursing action rather than on the
    medical action, unless the question is asking
    you what prescribed action is anticipated
 2. Implementation questions address the process
    of assisting with organizing and managing
    care, providing care to achieve established
    goals, and communicating and documenting
    nursing interventions thoroughly and
    accurately
 3. On NCLEX-PN, the only client that you need
    to be concerned about is the client in the
    question you are answering
 4. When you are answering a question,
    remember that this client is your only
    assigned client
 5. Answer the question as if the situation were
    textbook and ideal and the nurse had all the
    time and resources needed and readily
    available at the client's bedside

D. Evaluation
 1. Evaluation questions focus on comparing the
    actual outcomes of care with the expected
    outcomes, and communicating and
    documenting findings
 2. These questions focus on assisting in
    determining the client's response to care, and
    identifying factors that may interfere with
    implementation of the plan of care
 3. In an evaluation question, be alert to false
    response stems because they are frequently
    used in evaluation-type questions
 4. The question may ask for the client's
    statement that indicates INACCURATE
    information regarding the issue in the
    question

X. Client Needs

A. Safe, Effective Care Environment
 1. These questions address the provision that the
    nurse collaborates with other health care team
    members to facilitate effective client care, and
    that the nurse protects clients and health care
    personnel from environmental hazards
 2. Be alert to safety needs addressed in a
    question

BOX 4–3. Steps of the Nursing Process	
Data Collection ↓	Use the nursing process to answer questions
Planning ↓	Follow the steps of the nursing process to select an answer
Implementation ↓	The first step of the nursing process is data collection
Evaluation	When the question asks you what the nurse's first or most appropriate action is, select the answer that relates to data collection relative to the client

3. Remember the importance of handwashing, side rails, and call bells

B. Health Promotion and Maintenance
   1. These questions address the provision that the nurse assists the client and significant others in the normal expected stages of growth and development from conception through advanced old age
   2. It includes providing client care related to prevention and early detection of health problems
   3. Be alert to those true and false response stems with questions that address health promotion and maintenance

C. Psychosocial Integrity
   1. These questions address the provision that the nurse promotes the client's ability to cope, adapt, and problem solve situations related to illnesses or stressful events, and that the nurse participates in providing care for clients with acute and chronic mental illness
   2. Communication questions
      a. Identify the use of therapeutic communication tools
      b. When answering communication questions, use of communication tools indicates a CORRECT answer
      c. When answering communication questions, use of communication blocks indicates an INCORRECT answer (Table 4–1)

D. Physiological Integrity
   1. These questions address the provision that the nurse provides comfort and assistance in the performance of activities of daily living, provides care related to the administration of medications, and monitors clients receiving parenteral therapies
   2. These questions also address the nurse's ability to reduce the client's potential for developing complications or health problems related to treatments, procedures, or existing conditions, and the nurse's role in participating in providing care to clients with acute, chronic, or life-threatening physical health conditions
   3. Be careful not to read into the question

Table 4–1. **Communication Tools and Blocks**

Tools	*Blocks*
Being silent	Giving advice
Offering to assist client	Showing approval/disapproval
Showing empathy	Using cliché and false reassurance
Focusing	Requesting an explanation, "Why?"
Restatement	Devaluing the client's feelings
Validation/clarification	Being defensive
Giving information	Focusing on inappropriate issues
Dealing with the here and now	Placing the client's issues on "hold"

Always focus on the client's feelings *first*!
If an option reflects the client's feelings, select that option!

BOX 4–4. Pyramid Points

- If the question asks for an immediate action or response, all answers may be correct; therefore, base your selection on priorities
- Reword a difficult question, but if you do so, be careful not to change the intent of the question
- Look for the most common or typical response
- Relate the situation to something that you are familiar with and try to visualize the client as you go through the case situation and the question
- Look for answers that focus on the client as a worthy human being or that are directed toward feelings
- With medication calculations, talk yourself through each step and be sure the answer makes sense
- If there are words in the stem that are unfamiliar, try to figure out the meaning in terms of the context of the sentence or break down the word using your medical terminology skills
- If one option includes qualifiers such as *generally, usually, may,* and *tends to,* and other options do not, select that option
- Absolute terminology such as *always, never, all, every, none,* and *must,* tends to make a statement false
- Unusual or highly technical language typically indicates that the option is not correct
- Remember that lengthy questions are not always the most difficult
- Answer all questions as if the situation were ideal and the nurse had all the time and resources needed
- Remember, the only client you need to be concerned about is the one in the question you are answering
- Pace yourself and concentrate and focus on one item at a time
- Do not become frustrated
- Be patient with yourself

SMILE!
BELIEF!
CONFIDENCE!
CONTROL!
SUCCESS!

---

4. Remember that physiological needs are a priority and are addressed first
5. Remember to use the ABCs when selecting an answer addressing physiological integrity
6. Remember the order of priority of AIRWAY, BREATHING, AND CIRCULATION

XI. Pyramid Points

A. Unfamiliar content
   1. Answer questions using your nursing knowledge, clinical experience, and test-taking skills
   2. If the content of the question is unfamiliar and you are unable to answer questions using your nursing knowledge, look for a Global

Response, Similar Distracters, or Similar Words in the question and in the options
B. The global option
1. When more than one option appears to be correct, look for a global option
2. A global option is one that is a general statement and may include the ideas of other options within it
C. Similar distracters
1. If you don't know the answer, try looking for similar distracters
2. Remember that there is only ONE answer
3. If two options say the same thing or include the same idea, then NEITHER OF THESE OPTIONS can be the answer
4. The answer has to be the option that is different

D. Similar words
1. If you do not know the answer, look for a similar word or phrase used in the stem or the case situation and in one of the options
2. If you find a word, feeling, or behavior that is used in the stem or the case situation and is repeated in one of the options, that option MAY be the correct answer (Box 4–4)

BIBLIOGRAPHY

deWit, S. (1998). *Essentials of medical-surgical nursing* (4th ed.). Philadelphia: W. B. Saunders.

Hill, S., & Howlett, H. (1997). *Success in practical nursing: Personal and vocational issues* (3rd ed.). Philadelphia: W. B. Saunders.

National Council of State Boards of Nursing. (1998) *National Council detailed test plan for the NCLEX-PN examination.* Chicago: Author.

Varcarolis, E. (1998). *Foundations of psychiatric mental health nursing* (3rd ed.). Philadelphia: W. B. Saunders.

UNIT II

Issues in Nursing

CHAPTER 5

Cultural Diversity

. . . .

PYRAMID TERMS

Acculturation—Process of learning norms, beliefs, and behavioral expectations of a group.

Belief—Something accepted as true and accepted by an ethnocultural group.

Cultural Assimilation—Occurs when individuals from a minority group are absorbed by the dominant culture and take on the characteristics of the dominant culture.

Cultural Competence—Having the knowledge, understanding, and skills regarding a diverse culture that allows one to provide acceptable care.

Cultural Diversity—The differences among people that result from ethnic, racial, and cultural variables.

Cultural Imposition—The tendency to impose one's own beliefs, values, and patterns of behavior on individuals from another culture.

Culture—Refers to the structures of knowledge, beliefs, behaviors, ideas, attitudes, values, habits, customs, languages, symbols, rituals, ceremonies, and practices that are unique to a particular group of people.

Dominant Culture—The group whose values prevail within society.

Ethnic—A group of people who has had different experiences from those of the dominant culture by status, background, residence, religion, education, or other factors that functionally unify the group.

Ethnicity—A cultural group's perception of themselves, or the group identity. This self-perception influences how the group members are perceived by others.

Ethnocentrism—An assumption of cultural superiority, and an inability to accept another culture's ways.

Minority Group—An ethnic, racial, or religious group that constitutes less than a numerical majority of the population.

Oppression—Is based on cultural biases and stems from values, beliefs, traditions, and cultural expectations. Occurs when the rules, modes, and ideals of one group are imposed on another group.

Race—Refers to a grouping of people based on biological similarities. Members of a racial group have similar physical characteristics, such as blood group, facial features, and color of skin, hair, and eyes.

Racism—Discrimination directed toward individuals who are misperceived to be inferior due to biological differences. A form of oppression.

Stereotyping—An expectation that all people within the same racial, ethnic, or cultural group act alike and share the same beliefs and attitudes.

Subculture—A group of people with characteristic patterns of behavior that distinguish the group from the larger culture or society.

Values—Principles and standards that have meaning and worth to an individual, family, group, or community.

◆ PYRAMID TO SUCCESS

Often, nurses are caring for clients who come from different ethnic, cultural, and religious backgrounds from their own. Awareness of and sensitivity to the unique health and illness beliefs and practices are essential in the delivery of safe and effective care. Acknowledgment and acceptance of cultural differences with a nonjudgmental attitude are essential in providing culturally sensitive care. The belief underlying the NCLEX-PN test plan is that people are unique individuals and define their own systems of daily living, which reflects their values, motives, and life-styles. Cultural awareness is a concept and process that is fundamental to the practice of nursing, and is integrated throughout the categories of Client Needs, the framework for NCLEX-PN.

NURSING PROCESS

DATA COLLECTION

Ethnic heritage
Native language
Religious practices
Food preferences
Health care beliefs

Family role and function
Family patterns of health care
Social networks and supports
Educational experiences

PLANNING
Assist in developing the plan of care based on the unique characteristics of the individual. Include the client, family, and community in the plan of care as appropriate. Discuss the plan of care with the client and family. Respect client and family needs based on their cultural practices and preferences.

IMPLEMENTATION
Use data collection findings to adjust interventions in order to meet the unique needs of the client. Incorporate interventions that are compatible with the client's cultural heritage, educational level, and language. Provide care using a nonjudgmental approach.

EVALUATION
Assist in determining the compatibility of plan with client and family in meeting needs based on cultural practices and preferences.

◆ CLIENT NEEDS

SAFE, EFFECTIVE CARE ENVIRONMENT

Cultural awareness
Caring
Communication
Advocacy
Client rights
Confidentiality
Ethical practice and legal responsibilities
Consultation and referrals

HEALTH PROMOTION AND MAINTENANCE

Cultural awareness
Caring
Communication
Family planning and family interaction patterns
Health and wellness
Lifestyle choices

PSYCHOSOCIAL INTEGRITY

Cultural awareness
Caring
Communication
Coping mechanisms
Religious and spiritual influences on health
Support systems

PHYSIOLOGICAL INTEGRITY

Cultural awareness
Caring
Communication
Nutritional preferences (Box 5–1)
Comfort practices
Practices or restrictions related to procedures and treatments

I. African-Americans

A. Communication
   1. Languages include English or black English
   2. Head nodding does not necessarily mean agreement

BOX 5–1. Dietary Practices and Preferences

AFRICAN-AMERICANS
Fried foods
Pork, greens, rice
Some pregnant African-Americans engage in pica

ASIAN-AMERICANS
Soy sauce
Raw fish
Rice

EUROPEAN AMERICANS
Carbohydrates (potatoes)
Red meat

HISPANIC-AMERICANS
Beans
Fried foods
Spicy foods
Chili
Carbonated beverages

NATIVE AMERICANS
Blue cornmeal
Fish
Game
Fruits and berries

3. Direct eye contact is often viewed as being rude
4. Nonverbal communication is very important
5. It is considered to be intrusive to ask personal questions of someone on initial contact or meeting

B. Space
1. Close personal space is important
2. Touching another's hair is sometimes viewed as offensive

C. Social Roles
1. Large extended family networks are important
2. Women serve as both breadwinners and caretakers
3. Religion is usually Protestant (Baptist) (Box 5–2)
4. Strong church affiliation with community is important
5. Social organizations are strong within communities

D. Health and illness
1. Harmony with nature
2. No separation of body, mind, and spirit
3. Illness is a disharmonious state that may be caused by demons or spirits
4. Illness can be prevented by nutritious meals, rest, and cleanliness

E. Health risks
1. Lactose intolerance
2. Keloid formation
3. Sickle cell anemia
4. Hypertension
5. Cancer (especially stomach and esophageal)
6. Coronary heart disease

F. Implementation
1. Avoid **stereotyping**
2. Do not label black English as an unacceptable form of language
3. Clarify meaning of client's verbal and nonverbal behavior
4. Be flexible and avoid rigidity in scheduling care
5. Encourage involvement with family
6. A folk healer or herbalist may be consulted before the individual seeks medical treatment

---

BOX 5–2. Religions and Dietary Practices

SEVENTH-DAY ADVENTIST (CHURCH OF GOD)

Alcohol, coffee, and tea are prohibited
Some groups prohibit meat

BAPTIST

Alcohol is prohibited
Consumption of coffee and tea is discouraged

BUDDHISM

Alcohol and drug use are discouraged
Some sects are vegetarian

ROMAN CATHOLICISM

Fasting on Ash Wednesday and Good Friday
Optional fasting during Lent season
During Lent, meat is discouraged on Friday
Children and the ill are exempt from fasting

CHURCH OF JESUS CHRIST OF LATTER-DAY SAINTS (MORMON)

Alcohol, coffee, and tea are prohibited
Limited consumption of meat
First Sunday of the month is time for fasting

HINDUISM

Beef and veal are prohibited
Many individuals are vegetarians
Limited consumption of meat
Fasting occurs on specific days of the week according to which god the person worships
Children are not allowed to participate in fasting
Fasting rituals vary from complete abstinence to consumption of only one meal per day

ISLAM

Pork is prohibited
Any meat product not ritually slaughtered is prohibited

Alcohol or drugs avoided
During Ramadan (Ninth month of Mohammedan year), fasting occurs during daytime

JEHOVAH'S WITNESS

Prohibition of any foods to which blood has been added
Can consume animal flesh that has been drained

JUDAISM

Dietary kosher laws must be adhered to by Orthodox believers
Meats allowed include animals that are vegetable eaters, cloven-hoofed animals, and animals that are ritually slaughtered
Fish that have scales and fins are allowed
Any combination of meat and milk is prohibited
During Yom Kippur, 24-hour fasting
Pregnant women and those who are seriously ill are exempt from fasting
During Passover week, only unleavened bread is eaten

PENTECOSTAL (ASSEMBLY OF GOD)

Alcohol is prohibited
Avoid consumption of anything to which blood has been added
Some individuals avoid pork

RUSSIAN ORTHODOX

Abstention from meat and dairy products on Wednesday, Friday, and during Lent
During Lent, all animal products, including dairy products, are forbidden
Fasting during Advent
Exceptions from fasting include illness and pregnancy

II. Asian-Americans

A. Communication
1. Languages include Chinese, Japanese, Korean, Vietnamese, English
2. Silence is valued
3. Eye contact is considered rude
4. Criticism or disagreement is not expressed verbally
5. The word "no" is interpreted as disrespect for others

B. Space
1. Social distance is important
2. Usually do not touch others during conversation
3. Touch is unacceptable with members of opposite sex
4. The head is considered to be sacred; therefore, touching someone on the head is disrespectful

C. Social roles
1. Immediate and extended family loyalty and honor are valued
2. Family unit is very structured and hierarchical
3. Men have the power and authority, and the women are expected to be obedient
4. Education is viewed as important
5. Religions include Taoism (Buddhism), Islam, Christianity (see Box 5–2)

D. Health and illness
1. Health is a state of physical and spiritual harmony with nature and a balance between positive and negative energy forces (yin and yang)
2. A healthy body is viewed as a gift from ancestors
3. Illness is viewed as an imbalance between yin and yang
4. Illness is attributed to prolonged sitting or lying, or to overexertion

E. Health risks
1. Lactose intolerance
2. Hypertension
3. Cancer (stomach and liver)

F. Implementation
1. Avoid physical closeness and excessive touch and touch the client's head only when necessary, informing the client before doing so
2. Limit eye contact
3. Avoid gesturing with hands
4. Clarify responses to questions
5. Be flexible and avoid rigidity in scheduling care
6. Encourage involvement with family
7. A traditional healer may be consulted before the individual seeks medical treatment

III. European Americans

A. Communication
1. Languages include national languages, English
2. Silence can be used to show respect or disrespect for another, depending on the situation

3. Eye contact is viewed as indicating trustworthiness

B. Space
1. Aloof and tend to avoid close physical contact
2. Handshakes are used for formal greetings

C. Social roles
1. The nuclear family is the basic unit; the extended family is important
2. The man is the dominant figure
3. Religion includes Judeo-Christian (see Box 5–2)
4. Community social organizations are important

D. Health and illness
1. Health is usually viewed as an absence of disease or illness
2. Have a tendency to be stoical when expressing physical concerns

E. Health risks
1. Heart disease
2. Thalassemia
3. Breast cancer
4. Diabetes

F. Implementation
1. Monitor client's body language
2. Respect client's personal space
3. Home remedies may be the first method of treatment used

IV. Hispanic-Americans

A. Communication
1. Languages include Spanish or Portuguese, with various dialects
2. Tend to be verbally expressive, yet confidentiality is important
3. Eye behavior is significant; for example, the "evil eye" can be given to a child if a person looks at and admires a child without touching the child
4. Avoiding eye contact indicates respect and attentiveness
5. Direct confrontation is disrespectful and the expression of negative feelings is impolite
6. Dramatic body language, such as gestures or facial expressions, is used to express emotion or pain

B. Space
1. Comfortable with proximity to others
2. Very tactile and uses embraces and handshakes
3. Value the physical presence of others
4. Politeness and modesty are essential

C. Social roles
1. The nuclear family is the basic unit; the extended family is highly regarded
2. Needs of the family take precedence over individual family members' needs
3. Man is the decision maker and breadwinner, and the woman is the caretaker and homemaker
4. Religion includes Catholicism (see Box 5–2)

D. Health and illness
1. Health may be a reward from God or be a result of good luck
2. Health results from a state of balance between "hot and cold" forces and "wet and dry" forces
3. Illness occurs as a result of God's punishment for sins

E. Health risks
1. Lactose intolerance
2. Diabetes
3. Parasites

F. Implementation
1. Communicate with male head of family
2. Protect privacy
3. Offer to call priest or other clergy because of the significance of religious practices related to illnesses
4. Always touch a child during care
5. Be flexible and avoid rigidity in scheduling care

V. Native Americans

A. Communication
1. Languages include English, Navajo, and other tribal languages
2. Silence indicates respect for the speaker
3. Speak in a low tone of voice and expect others to be attentive
4. Eye contact is avoided because it is a sign of disrespect
5. Body language is important

B. Space
1. Personal space is very important
2. Will lightly touch another person's hand during greetings
3. Massage is used for the newborn to promote bonding between infant and mother
4. Touching a dead body may be prohibited

C. Social roles
1. Very family orientated
2. Basic family unit is the extended family and often includes people from several households
3. In some tribes, grandparents are viewed as family leaders
4. Elders are honored
5. Children are taught to respect traditions
6. The father does all the work outside the home, and the mother assumes responsibility for domestic duties
7. Sacred myths and legends provide spiritual guidance
8. Religion and healing practices are integrated
9. Community social organizations are important

D. Health and illness
1. Health is a state of harmony between the person, the family, and the environment
2. Illness is caused by supernatural forces and disequilibrium between a person and the environment

E. Health risks
1. Tuberculosis
2. Diabetes

3. Heart disease
4. Arthritis
5. American Eskimos are susceptible to glaucoma

F. Implementation
1. Clarify communication
2. Understand that the client may be attentive even when eye contact is absent
3. Be attentive to own use of body language
4. Obtain input from extended family members
5. Encourage client to personalize space in which health care is delivered, for example, to bring personal items or objects to the hospital
6. In the home, monitor for the availability of running water, and modify infection control and hygiene practices as necessary

PRACTICE QUESTIONS

1. The nurse is assisting in collecting data on an African-American client admitted to the ambulatory care unit who is scheduled for a hernia repair. Which of the following information about the client is of least priority during the data collection?
   1 Cardiovascular
   2 Neurological
   3 Respiratory
   4 Psychosocial

2. The nursing instructor is providing a session on cultural beliefs related to health and illness. Following the session, the instructor asks the nursing student to describe the beliefs of an African-American in regard to illness. Which of the following is the most appropriate response made by the student?
   1 "Illness is due to an imbalance between yin and yang."
   2 "Illness is a punishment for sins."
   3 "Illness is a disharmonious state that may be caused by demons and spirits."
   4 "Illness is due to lack of exercise."

3. The nurse is planning to reinforce instructions to the African-American client about nutrition. When developing the plan, the nurse is aware that a common dietary practice of African-Americans is to
   1 Eat fried foods
   2 Eat rice as the basis for all meals
   3 Eat red meat
   4 Eat raw fish

4. The nurse is assigned to care for an Asian-American client. The nurse plans care knowing that which of the following most appropriately describes the Asian-American's view of illness?
   1 Illness is caused by supernatural forces
   2 Illness is a punishment for sins
   3 Illness is a disharmonious state that may be caused by demons and spirits
   4 Illness is due to an imbalance between yin and yang

5. The nurse assists in developing a plan of care for an Asian-American client. Which of the following is not a component of the plan of care for this client?
   1 Avoid physical closeness
   2 Limit eye contact
   3 Avoid hand gestures
   4 Light touch to the head for comfort

6. The nurse consults with a nutritionist regarding the dietary preferences of an Asian-American client. Which of the following foods does the nurse most appropriately plan to include in the diet plan?
   1 Red meat
   2 Rice
   3 Fried foods
   4 Fruits

7. The nurse assists in developing a plan of care for a European American client and considers the practices and preferences of the culture. Which of the following cultural practices or preferences are not considered when planning care?
   1 Community social organizations are important
   2 Health is often viewed as an absence of disease or illness
   3 Appears stoic when expressing physical concerns

4 The woman is the dominant figure

8. A Hispanic-American mother brings her child to the clinic for an examination. Which of the following is most important when gathering data about the child?
   1 Avoiding eye contact
   2 Touching the child during the examination
   3 Avoiding speaking to the child
   4 Using body language only

9. The nurse assists in developing a plan of care for the Native American client considering the practices and preferences of the culture. Which of the following practices and preferences is not normally a characteristic of this ethnic group?
   1 Religion and healing practices
   2 Touching the body of a dead family member
   3 Avoiding eye contact
   4 Use of healing practices

10. The nurse caring for an Orthodox Jewish client plans a diet that adheres to the practices of Judaism. The nurse plans the diet knowing that which of the following is not a practice of Judaism?
   1 Eating fish with scales and fins is allowed
   2 Meat is allowed if ritually slaughtered
   3 Only unleavened bread is eaten during Passover week
   4 Meat and milk can be eaten together

ANSWERS

1. **4**

RATIONALE: The psychosocial data is the least priority during the initial admission data collection. In the African-American culture, it is considered to be intrusive to ask personal questions on the initial contact or meeting. Additionally, cardiovascular, neurological, and respiratory data include physiological assessments that would be the priority.
TEST-TAKING STRATEGY: Note the key words "least priority." Use Maslow's Hierarchy of Needs theory to answer the question. Options 1, 2, and 3 address physiological needs. Review the characteristics of the African-American culture if you had difficulty with this question.
LEVEL OF COGNITIVE ABILITY: Comprehension
PHASE OF NURSING PROCESS: Data Collection
CLIENT NEEDS: Physiological Integrity
CONTENT AREA: Fundamental Skills
REFERENCE
deWit, S. (1998). *Essentials of medical-surgical nursing* (4th ed.). Philadelphia: W. B. Saunders. pp. 39–40.

2. **3**

RATIONALE: In the African-American culture, illness is viewed as a disharmonious state that may be caused by demons and spirits. The goal of treatment, from the traditional African perspective, is to remove the harmful spirit from the body of the ill person. Asian-Americans believe that illness is due to an imbalance between yin and yang and due to prolonged sitting or lying, or to overexertion.
TEST-TAKING STRATEGY: Knowledge regarding the beliefs related to health and illness of the various cultures assists in answering the question. From this point, use the process of elimination to determine the correct option. If you had difficulty with the question, take time now to review these various beliefs.
LEVEL OF COGNITIVE ABILITY: Comprehension
PHASE OF NURSING PROCESS: Evaluation
CLIENT NEEDS: Psychosocial Integrity
CONTENT AREA: Fundamental Skills
REFERENCE
Potter, P., & Perry, A. (1997). *Fundamentals of nursing: Concepts, process, and practice* (4th ed.). St. Louis: Mosby–Year Book. p. 362.

3. **1**

RATIONALE: African-American food preferences include pork, greens, rice, and fried foods. Asian-Americans eat raw fish, rice, and soy sauce. Hispanic-Americans prefer beans, fried foods, spicy foods, chili, and carbonated beverages. European Americans prefer carbohydrates and red meat.
TEST-TAKING STRATEGY: Knowledge regarding the food practices and preferences related to the various cultures is required to answer the question. Knowledge that African-Americans are at risk for hypertension and coronary artery disease may assist in directing you to option 1. If you had difficulty with this question, take time now to review the food preferences associated with the African-American culture.

LEVEL OF COGNITIVE ABILITY: Comprehension
PHASE OF NURSING PROCESS: Planning
CLIENT NEEDS: Physiological Integrity
CONTENT AREA: Fundamental Skills
REFERENCE
Leahy, J., & Kizilay, P. (1998). *Foundations of nursing practice: A nursing process approach.* Philadelphia: W. B. Saunders. p. 1105.

4. 4

RATIONALE: Asian-Americans believe that illness is due to an imbalance between yin and yang, and due to prolonged sitting or lying, or to overexertion. In the African-American culture, illness is viewed as a disharmonious state that may be caused by demons and spirits. Native Americans believe that illness is caused by supernatural forces.
TEST-TAKING STRATEGY: Knowledge regarding the beliefs related to health and illness of the various cultures assists in answering the question. From this point, use the process of elimination in determining the correct option. If you had difficulty with the question, take time now to review these various beliefs.
LEVEL OF COGNITIVE ABILITY: Comprehension
PHASE OF NURSING PROCESS: Planning
CLIENT NEEDS: Psychosocial Integrity
CONTENT AREA: Fundamental Skills
REFERENCE
Luckmann, J. (1997). *Saunders manual of nursing care.* Philadelphia: W. B. Saunders. p. 41.

5. 4

RATIONALE: Avoiding physical closeness, limiting eye contact, avoiding hand gestures, and clarifying responses to questions are all a component of the plan of care for an Asian-American client. In the Asian-American culture, the head is considered to be sacred; therefore, touching someone on the head is disrespectful. Touch the client's head only when necessary, and inform the client before doing so.
TEST-TAKING STRATEGY: Note the key word "not" in the stem of the question. Note that options 1, 2, and 3 are similar in that they all address a lack of physical contact. Option 4 is the different option. If you had difficulty with this question, take time now to review the beliefs associated with this culture.
LEVEL OF COGNITIVE ABILITY: Comprehension
PHASE OF NURSING PROCESS: Planning
CLIENT NEEDS: Psychosocial Integrity
CONTENT AREA: Fundamental Skills
REFERENCE
Luckmann, J. (1997). *Saunders manual of nursing care.* Philadelphia: W. B. Saunders. p. 474.

6. 2

RATIONALE: Asian-Americans' food preferences include raw fish, rice, and soy sauce. African-American food preferences include pork, greens, rice, and fried foods. Hispanic-Americans prefer beans, fried foods, spicy foods, chili, and carbonated beverages. European Americans prefer carbohydrates and red meat.
TEST-TAKING STRATEGY: Knowledge regarding the food practices and preferences related to the various cultures is required to answer the question. Correlate rice with Asian-Americans. This may assist when answering other questions similar to this one. If you had difficulty with this question, take time now to review the food preferences associated with the Asian-American culture.

LEVEL OF COGNITIVE ABILITY: Comprehension
PHASE OF NURSING PROCESS: Planning
CLIENT NEEDS: Physiological Integrity
CONTENT AREA: Fundamental Skills
REFERENCE
Leahy, J., & Kizilay, P. (1998). *Foundations of nursing practice: A nursing process approach.* Philadelphia: W. B. Saunders. p. 1106.

7. 4

RATIONALE: In the European American culture, the man is the dominant figure. Community social organizations are important in this culture. European Americans tend to be aloof and avoid physical contact and appear stoic when expressing physical concerns.
TEST-TAKING STRATEGY: Use knowledge regarding the practices and beliefs associated with the European American culture to answer the question. If you had difficulty with this question, take time now to review the practices and beliefs of the European American culture.
LEVEL OF COGNITIVE ABILITY: Comprehension
PHASE OF NURSING PROCESS: Planning
CLIENT NEEDS: Psychosocial Integrity
CONTENT AREA: Fundamental Skills
REFERENCE
Potter, P., & Perry, A. (1997). *Fundamentals of nursing: Concepts, process, and practice* (4th ed.). St. Louis: Mosby–Year Book. pp. 364, 366.

8. 2

RATIONALE: In the Hispanic-American culture, eye behavior is significant. The "bad (evil) eye" can be given to a child if a person looks at and admires a child without touching the child. Therefore, touching the child during the examination is very important. Although avoiding eye contact indicates respect and attentiveness, this is not the most important intervention. Avoiding speaking to the child, and using body language only, are not therapeutic interventions.
TEST-TAKING STRATEGY: Use the process of elimination. Eliminate options 3 and 4 first, as they are basically similar. For the remaining two options, select the intervention that is most therapeutic, that being touch. If you had difficulty with this question, take time now to review the characteristics associated with Hispanic-Americans.
LEVEL OF COGNITIVE ABILITY: Application
PHASE OF NURSING PROCESS: Implementation
CLIENT NEEDS: Psychosocial Integrity
CONTENT AREA: Fundamental Skills
REFERENCE
Potter, P., & Perry, A. (1997). *Fundamentals of nursing: Concepts, process, and practice* (4th ed.). St. Louis: Mosby–Year Book. p. 364.

9. 2

RATIONALE: In the Native American culture, touching a dead body is normally prohibited. The use of religion and healing practices is integrated into health care and illness practices. Eye contact is avoided because it is a sign of disrespect.
TEST-TAKING STRATEGY: Use the process of elimination based on knowledge of the beliefs of this cultural group. Eliminate options 1 and 4 first because they are similar. Remembering that eye contact is a sign of disrespect will direct you to option 2. If you had difficulty with this question, take time now to review the traditional beliefs of the Native American culture.

LEVEL OF COGNITIVE ABILITY: Comprehension
PHASE OF NURSING PROCESS: Planning
CLIENT NEEDS: Psychosocial Integrity
CONTENT AREA: Fundamental Skills
REFERENCE
Leahy, J., & Kizilay, P. (1998). *Foundations of nursing practice: A nursing process approach.* Philadelphia: W. B. Saunders. p. 1109.

10. **4**

RATIONALE: Dietary kosher laws must be adhered to by Orthodox believers. Meats allowed include animals that are vegetable eaters, cloven-hoofed animals, and animals that are ritually slaughtered. Fish that have scales and fins are allowed; however, any combination of meat and milk is prohibited. During Passover week, only unleavened bread is eaten.
TEST-TAKING STRATEGY: Note the key word "not" in the stem of the question. Knowledge regarding the dietary practices in Judaism is required to answer the question. If you had difficulty with the question, take time now to review the dietary practices of this cultural group.
LEVEL OF COGNITIVE ABILITY: Comprehension
PHASE OF NURSING PROCESS: Planning
CLIENT NEEDS: Psychosocial Integrity
CONTENT AREA: Fundamental Skills
REFERENCE
Potter, P., & Perry, A. (1997). *Fundamentals of nursing: Concepts, process, and practice* (4th ed.). St. Louis: Mosby–Year Book. p. 359.

BIBLIOGRAPHY

deWit, S. (1998). *Essentials of medical-surgical nursing* (4th ed.). Philadelphia: W. B. Saunders.
Hill, S., & Howlett, H. (1997). *Success in practical nursing: Personal and vocational issues* (3rd ed.). Philadelphia: W. B. Saunders.
National Council of State Boards of Nursing. (1998) *National Council detailed test plan for the NCLEX-PN examination.* Chicago: Author.
Luckmann, J. (1997). *Saunders manual of nursing care.* Philadelphia: W. B. Saunders.
Leahy, J., & Kizilay, P. (1998). *Foundations of nursing practice: A nursing process approach.* Philadelphia: W. B. Saunders.
Potter, P., & Perry, A. (1997). *Fundamentals of nursing: Concepts, process, and practice* (4th ed.). St. Louis: Mosby–Year Book.

CHAPTER 6

Ethical and Legal Issues

. . . .

PYRAMID TERMS

Advance directive—Written document, recognized by state law, that provides directions concerning the provision of care when a person is unable to make his or her own treatment choices.

Advocacy—Acting on the behalf of clients, protecting the clients' right to make their own decisions.

Consent—Voluntary act by which a person agrees to allow someone else to do something.

Ethics—Deals with the rules of conduct and what the nurse should do in a particular situation.

Informed consent—The client understands the reason for the proposed intervention, with its benefits and risks, and agrees to the treatment by signing a consent form.

Law—In nursing, the rules and regulations that control the practice of nursing.

Malpractice—Failure to meet the standards of acceptable care, which results in harm to another person.

Negligence—Failure to provide care that a reasonable person would ordinarily use in a similar circumstance.

Nurse Practice Act—Legal guideline in nursing.

Patient's Bill of Rights—Includes the rights and responsibilities of clients receiving care.

Values—Beliefs and attitudes that may influence behavior and the process of decision making.

◆ PYRAMID TO SUCCESS

Across all settings in the practice of nursing, nurses are frequently confronted with ethical and legal issues related to client care. It is the responsibility of the nurse to be aware of the ethical principles, laws, and guidelines related to providing safe and quality care to clients. In the Pyramid to Success, focus on ethical practices; the Nurse Practice Act; client rights, particularly confidentiality; and informed consent, advocacy, documentation, advance directives, death and dying, and organ donation.

NURSING PROCESS

DATA COLLECTION

Client values
Cultural and religious beliefs
Client rights
Standards of Care
Ethical and legal responsibilities

PLANNING

Assist in developing the plan of care based on the ethical and legal considerations related to the client. Include the client and family in the plan of care as appropriate. Discuss the plan of care with the client and family.

IMPLEMENTATION

Identify own value system. Function within the guidelines of the Nurse Practice Act, Standards of Care, Code of Ethics, and agency policies and procedures and legal system. Identify cultural and religious preferences of the client. Develop a caring and nonjudgmental relationship with the client. Provide care functioning as a client advocate and protect client rights. Respect client and family needs based on their value system.

EVALUATION

Determine compatibility of plan with client and family in meeting needs based on their value system and legal responsibilities. Client rights are upheld.

◆ **CLIENT NEEDS**

SAFE, EFFECTIVE CARE ENVIRONMENT

Advance directives
Advocacy
Client rights
Confidentiality
Ethical practice
Incident reports
Informed consent
Legal responsibilities
Organ donation

HEALTH PROMOTION AND MAINTENANCE

Developmental stages and transitions
Family interaction patterns
Lifestyle choices

PSYCHOSOCIAL INTEGRITY

Abuse/neglect
Chemical dependency
Grief and loss
Support systems

PHYSIOLOGICAL INTEGRITY

Basic care and comfort
Alterations in body systems
Potential complications of tests and procedures

I. Ethics and Values

A. **Ethics:** The branch of philosophy that deals with the distinction between right and wrong on the basis of a body of knowledge, not just on the basis of opinions
B. Morality: Behavior in accordance with customs or tradition, usually reflecting personal or religious beliefs
C. Ethical principles: Codes that direct or govern a nurse's actions (Box 6–1)
D. **Values:** Beliefs and attitudes that may influence behavior and the process of decision making
E. **Values** clarification: Process of analyzing one's own **values** to better understand what is truly important
F. Ethical codes
 1. Provide broad principles for determining and evaluating client care
 2. Are not legally binding, but in most states, the board of nursing has authority to reprimand nurses for unprofessional conduct that results from violation of the ethical code
 3. Specific ethical codes
  a. National Federation of Licensed Practical Nurses (NFLPN) Code for Licensed Practical/Vocational Nurses
  b. NFLPN Nursing Practice Standards
  c. NFLPN Specialized Nursing Practice Standards
  d. National Association of Practical Nurse Education and Service (NAPNES) code of ethics

BOX 6–1. Ethical Principles	
Autonomy	Respect for an individual's right to maintain control over health care decisions
Nonmaleficence	The obligation to do or cause no harm to another
Beneficence	The obligation of doing good with nursing actions and preventing and removing harm. Paternalism is an undesirable outcome of beneficence, in which the health care provider decides what is best for the client and attempts to encourage the client to act against his or her own choices
Justice	Providing fair and equitable treatment to clients
Veracity	The obligation to tell the truth
Fidelity	The duty to do what one has promised

  e. NAPNES Standards of Practice for Practical/Vocational Nurses
G. Ethical dilemma
 1. Occurs when there is a conflict between two or more ethical principles
 2. There is no correct decision
 3. The nurse must make a choice between two alternatives that are equally unsatisfactory
 4. Ethical reasoning is the process of thinking through what one ought to do in an orderly and systematic manner to provide justification of actions based on principles
 5. The licensed practical/vocational nurse must confirm his or her final ethical decision with the registered nurse before acting
H. **Advocate**
 1. A person who speaks up for or acts on the behalf of the client, protects the client's right to make his or her own decisions, and upholds the principle of fidelity
 2. Represents the client's viewpoint to others
 3. Avoids letting personal **values** influence **advocacy** for the client
 4. Supports a client's decision even when it conflicts with own preferences or choices
I. **Ethics** committee
 1. Multidisciplinary approach to facilitate dialogue regarding ethical dilemmas
 2. Develop and establish policies and procedures for the prevention and resolution of dilemmas

II. Regulation of Nursing Practice

A. Nurse Practice Act
 1. On a state level, defines the duties and functions that the nurse can perform

2. Defines what nursing is, what it is not, and under what circumstances nursing can be practiced for compensation

3. Additional issues covered by the Nurse Practice Act include licensure requirements for protection of the public, grounds for disciplinary action, rights of the nurse licensee if a disciplinary action is taken, and related topics

4. All nurses are responsible for knowing the provisions of the act of the state or province in which they work

5. No physician, registered professional nurse, or agency can give the licensed practical/vocational nurse the right to do more than can be performed legally

B. Standards of care
   1. Guidelines by which the nurse should practice
   2. Guidelines for determining whether nurses performed duties in an appropriate manner
   3. Based on what an ordinary prudent nurse with similar education and experience would do in similar circumstances
   4. If nurses do not perform duties within accepted standards of care, they place themselves in jeopardy of legal action
   5. If a nurse is named as defendant in a **malpractice** lawsuit and it is shown that neither the accepted standards of care outlined by the state or province nursing practice act nor the policies of the employing institution were followed, the nurse's legal liability is clear

C. Employee guidelines
   1. Respondent superior: Employer will be held liable for any negligent acts of an employee if the alleged negligent act occurred during the employment relationship and was within the scope of the employee's responsibilities
   2. Contracts
      a. Nurses are responsible for carrying out the terms of contractual agreement with the employee agency and the client
      b. The nurse employee relationship is governed by established employee handbooks and client care policies and procedures that create obligations, rights, and duties between those parties
   3. Institutional policies
      a. Written policies and procedures of the employing institution that detail how nurses are to perform their duties
      b. Policies and procedures are usually quite specific and are located in manuals in most health care facilities
      c. Although policies are not **laws,** courts generally rule against nurses who violate policies
      d. If the nurse practices nursing in accordance with the client care policies and procedures established by the employer, functions within the job responsibility, and provides

care consistent with the care in a nonnegligent manner, the potential for liability is minimized
      e. The employer may sue the nurse to recover fees and other monies involved while defending the employee in a lawsuit

D. Hospital staffing
   1. Nurses should not walk out when staffing is inadequate because charges of abandonment can be made
   2. Nurses in short staffing situations are obligated to notify the nursing supervisor

E. Floating
   1. An acceptable legal practice used by hospitals to solve their understaffing problems
   2. Legally, a nurse cannot refuse to float unless a union contract guarantees that nurses can only work in a specified area or the nurse can prove lack of knowledge for the performance of assigned tasks
   3. Nurses in a floating situation must not assume responsibility beyond their level of experience or qualification
   4. Nurses who float should inform the supervisor of any lack of experience in caring for the type of clients on the new nursing unit
   5. The nurse should request and be given orientation to the new unit

F. Disciplinary action
   1. Boards of nursing may deny, revoke, or suspend any license to practice as a practical/vocational nurse in accordance with their statutory authority
   2. Causes for disciplinary action
      a. Unprofessional conduct
      b. Conduct that could adversely affect the health and welfare of the public
      c. Breach in client confidentiality
      d. Failure to use sufficient knowledge, skills, or nursing judgment
      e. Physically or verbally abusing a client
      f. Assuming duties without sufficient preparation
      g. Knowingly delegating nursing care to unlicensed personnel that places the client at risk for injury
      h. Failure to accurately maintain a record for each client
      i. Falsifying a client's record
      j. Leaving a nursing assignment without properly notifying appropriate personnel

III. Legal Liability

A. **Laws**
   1. Nurses are governed by civil and criminal **law** in roles as providers of services, employees of institutions, and private citizens
   2. A nurse has a personal and legal obligation to provide a standard of client care expected of a reasonably competent nurse
   3. Nurses are held responsible (liable) for harm

resulting from their negligent acts, or omissions to act

B. Types of **laws** (Box 6–2)

C. **Negligence** and **Malpractice**
1. Unintentional torts
2. Conduct that falls below the standard of care
3. Can include act of commission (was not done correctly) as well as act of omission (was not done)
4. If a nurse gives care that does not meet appropriate standards, he or she may be held liable for **negligence**
5. **Malpractice** is **negligence** on the part of a nurse
6. **Malpractice** is determined if the nurse owed a duty to the client and did not carry out the duty, and the client was injured because the nurse failed to perform the duty
7. Proof of liability
    a. Duty: The nurse's responsibility to provide care in an acceptable way
    b. Breach of duty: The nurse did not adhere to the nursing standard of practice
    c. Causation: The breach of the duty was the legal cause of injury to the client
    d. Injury: The client experienced injury or damages or both and can be compensated by **law**

D. Professional liability insurance
1. Nurses need their own liability insurance for protection against **malpractice** lawsuits
2. Having one's own insurance provides the nurse protection as an individual and in a lawsuit allows the nurse to have an attorney present who has only the nurse's interests in mind

BOX 6–2. Types of Laws	
Contract law	Concerned with enforcement of agreements among private individuals
Civil law	Concerned with relationships among people and the protection of a person's rights
	Violation may cause harm to an individual or property, but no grave threat to society exists
Criminal law	Concerned with relationships between individuals and governments and with acts that threaten society and its order
	A crime is an offense against society that violates a law and is defined as a misdemeanor (less serious nature) or felony (serious nature)
Tort law	Civil wrong, other than a breach in contract, in which the law allows an injured person to seek damage from a person who caused the injury

E. Good Samaritan **Laws**
1. Passed by a state legislature
2. These **laws** limit liability and offer legal immunity for people helping at the scene of an accident, providing they give reasonable care
3. Immunity from suit applies only when all of the conditions of the state **law** are met, such as the caregiver receives no compensation for the care provided and the care given is not intentionally negligent

F. Controlled substances
1. The nurse must adhere to facility policies and procedures concerning administration of controlled substances, which is governed by federal and state **laws**
2. Controlled substances must be kept securely locked, and only authorized personnel should have access to them

IV. Legal Risk Areas

A. Assault and battery
1. Intentional torts
2. Assault is an unjustified attempt or threat to touch someone else
3. Battery constitutes touching another's body without the other's **consent**

B. Invasion of privacy: Includes violating confidentiality, intruding on private client or family matters, and sharing client information with unauthorized persons

C. False Imprisonment
1. Occurs when a client is not allowed to leave a health care facility when there is no legal justification to detain the client
2. Occurs when restraining devices are used without an appropriate clinical need
3. A client can sign an Against Medical Advice form when the client is competent to make decisions, refuses care, and is requesting to leave the health care facility
4. Document circumstances in the medical record to avoid allegation by the client that cannot be defended

D. Defamation: Occurs when information is communicated to a third party that causes damage to someone's reputation, either written (libel) or verbally (slander)

E. Fraud: Results from a deliberate deception intended to produce unlawful gains

V. Client Rights

A. **Patient's Bill of Rights**
1. Increases health care providers' awareness of the need to treat clients in an ethical and legal manner and encourages protection of rights
2. Key elements of a client's rights with which nurses should be familiar include **informed consent** and confidentiality

B. Confidentiality
   1. A special relationship exists between two people in which information discussed will not be shared with a third party who is not directly involved in the client's care
   2. Nurses are bound to protect client confidentiality by most nurse practice acts, by ethical principles and standards, and by institutional and agency policies and procedures
   3. Treatment records cannot be released to any third party without the client's written **consent** and only after agency policies and procedures are followed
   4. Information release may be mandatory when ordered by a court, or when state statutes require reporting child abuse, communicable diseases, or other associated incidents

C. **Informed consent**
   1. **Consent** is the client's approval to have his or her body touched by a specific individual
   2. Legally, the client must be mentally competent to give **consent** for procedures
   3. Prior to granting **consent,** the client must be fully informed regarding treatment, tests, surgery, and so on, and must understand both the intended outcome and the potentially harmful results
   4. **Consent** must be obtained by the physician, surgeon, or other medical practitioner performing the treatment or procedure
   5. In most states, when a nurse is involved in the **informed consent** process, the nurse is only witnessing the signature of the client on the **informed consent**
   6. If a client is determined by a court to be unable to make decisions and is declared incompetent or under a legal disability, a personal guardian is appointed by the court to make decisions
   7. An **informed consent** can be waived for urgent medical and surgical intervention as long as institutional policy so indicates
   8. Parental or guardian **consent** should be obtained before treatment is initiated on a minor except in an emergency, in situations where the **consent** of the minor is sufficient such as treatment of a sexually transmitted disease, or if a court order or other legal authorization has been obtained
   9. Minors who are married or emancipated from parents and those seeking treatment for sexually transmitted diseases can sign a **consent** form
   10. A client has the right to refuse information and waive the **informed consent** and undergo treatment, but this decision must be documented in the medical record

VI. Legal Safeguards

A. Risk management

   1. A method of identifying risks followed by a plan to reduce client injuries
   2. Programs are based on a systematic reporting system of incidence or unusual occurrences

B. Incident reports
   1. A tool used as a means of identifying and improving client care
   2. Required by federal **law**
   3. Written as soon as possible after the occurrence by the person who witnessed the incident
   4. The report should be legible, factual, and objective
   5. No reference should be made to the report form in a client's record, although the incident itself is recorded in the client's chart

C. Physician's orders
   1. The nurse is obligated to carry out a physician's orders except when the nurse believes the order is inappropriate
   2. A nurse carrying out an inaccurate order may be legally responsible for any harm suffered by the client
   3. A nurse must clarify an unclear or inappropriate order with the physician
   4. If no resolution occurs regarding the order in question, the nursing supervisor needs to be contacted
   5. Verbal physician's orders should not be accepted except in an emergency
   6. Check the agency's policy regarding accepting a physician's orders
   7. See Box 6–3 concerning telephone orders

D. Documentation
   1. Legally required by accrediting agencies, state licensing **laws,** and state nurse and medical practice acts
   2. Follow agency guidelines and procedures (Box 6–4)

E. Client/family teaching
   1. Client and family teaching is the responsibility of the registered nurse (RN), and the practical nurse reinforces teaching once the instruction and education has been started by the RN
   2. The practical nurse initiates client teaching in the area of basic health care
   3. Provide complete instructions in a language the client can understand

---

BOX 6–3. Telephone Orders

Date and time the entry
Repeat the order to the physician and record the order given
Sign the order beginning with t.o. (telephone order), write the physician's name, and sign the order
If another nurse witnessed the order, that signature follows
The physician needs to countersign the order within a time frame according to agency policy

BOX 6–4. Documentation Guidelines

NARRATIVE

Use a black pen with permanent ink
Date and time entries
Provide objective, factual, accurate, and specific documentation
Document entries in chronological order
Document care, medications, treatments, and procedures as soon as possible after completed
Document client responses to interventions
Document consent for or refusal of treatments
Document calls made to other health care providers
Do not document for others or change documentation for other individuals
Do not sign off charts for nursing students
Sign and title each entry made
Use quotes as appropriate for subjective data
Use correct spelling, grammar, and punctuation
Avoid unacceptable abbreviations
Avoid judgmental or evaluative statements, such as "uncooperative client"
Do not leave blank spaces on documentation forms
Follow agency policies when an error is made (draw one line through the error, initial, and date)
Follow agency guidelines regarding late entries

COMPUTERIZED

Use only the user ID code, name, or password
Never lend access ID to another
Maintain privacy and confidentiality of documented information printed from the computer

4. Document client and family teaching, what was taught, evaluation of understanding, and who was present during the teaching
5. Inform the client of what would happen if information shared during teaching is not followed

VII. Legal Documents for Decision Making

A. Wills
   1. Some agencies have specific policies that prohibit the nurse from signing as witness to this legal document for a client
   2. If a nurse witnesses a legal document, the nurse must document the event and factual circumstances surrounding the signing in the medical record
   3. Documentation should include who was present, any significant comments by the client, and the nurse's observations of the client's conduct during the process
B. Advance directives
   1. Written document recognized by state **law** that provides directions concerning the provision of care when a person is unable to make his or her own treatment choices
   2. It must be made part of the medical record
   3. A physician must be notified of its presence so

orders can be written consistent with the client's wishes
C. Living will: Document prepared by a competent adult that provides direction regarding medical care in the event of a person's incapacitation or otherwise becoming unable to make decisions personally
D. Durable power of attorney
   1. Also called health care proxy
   2. An authorization that enables any competent individual to name someone to exercise decision-making authority under specific circumstances on the individual's behalf

VIII. Death and Dying

A. Right of informed refusal: A competent adult has the right to refuse treatment, even life-sustaining treatment
B. Do not resuscitate (DNR) orders
   1. Written order must be present and must be reviewed on a regular basis
   2. Specific agency guidelines must be followed regarding when and under what circumstances an oral DNR order is acceptable
   3. The client or legal representative must provide **informed consent** for the DNR status
   4. Both DNR and CPR (cardiopulmonary resuscitation) orders must be clearly defined so that other treatment not refused by the client will be continued
   5. There is no such thing as a partial or slow code
C. Organ transplant: The option to accept an organ transplant can be refused
D. Organ donation
   1. Any person 18 or older may become an organ donor by written **consent**
   2. Informed choice to donate an organ can take place with the use of a written document signed by the client prior to death, a will, donor card, or **advance directive**
   3. A family member or legal guardian may authorize donation of the decedent's organs in the absence of appropriate documentation
   4. All 50 states have adopted the Uniform Anatomical Gift Act for cadaveric organ donation
E. Autopsy
   1. Medical examination of the body after death for the purpose of determining the cause of death
   2. Required by state **law** in certain circumstances such as a sudden death or a death that occurs under suspicious circumstances
   3. If no oral or written instructions were given by the decedent, state **law** determines who has the authority to **consent** for any autopsy requested on a voluntary basis
   4. Documentation regarding **consent** must be

present before the body can be released for autopsy
F. Assisted suicide
 1. Legal support exists for a client to refuse life-sustaining procedures and for health care providers to honor the client's voluntary and informed decision by withdrawing or withholding treatment
 2. Taking an active role in assisting a client to die is a criminal offense in many states

IX. Reporting Responsibilities

A. Requirements: Nurses are required to report certain communicable diseases or criminal activities such as abuse, gunshot or stab wounds, assaults, homicides, and suicides to the appropriate authorities
B. The impaired nurse
 1. If a nurse suspects that a coworker is abusing chemicals, the nurse must report the individual to nursing administration in a confidential manner with the goal of treatment being the priority issue
 2. Nursing administration then notifies the board of nursing regarding the nurse's behavior
C. Occupational Safety and Health Administration (OSHA)
 1. Requires that an employer provide a safe workplace for employees according to regulations
 2. Employees can confidentially report working conditions that violate regulations
 3. An employee who does not report unsafe working conditions can be retaliated against by the employer
D. Sexual harassment
 1. Prohibited by state and federal **laws**
 2. Includes unwelcome conduct of a sexual nature
 3. Follow agency policies and procedures to handle reporting a concern or complaint

PRACTICE QUESTIONS

1. The nurse enters a client's room and finds the client lying on the floor. The nurse checks the client and then calls the nursing supervisor and the physician to inform them of the occurrence. The nursing supervisor instructs the nurse to complete an incident report. The nurse completes the incident report, understanding that it allows the analysis of adverse client events through
 1 A method of promoting quality care and risk management.
 2 Determining the effectiveness of interventions in relation to outcomes.
 3 The appropriate method of reporting to local, state, and federal agencies.
 4 Providing clients with necessary stabilizing treatments.

2. The nurse observes that the client received pain medication 1 hour ago from another nurse, but that the client still has severe pain. The nurse has previously observed this same occurrence. Based on the Nurse Practice Act, the observing nurse plans to do which of the following?
 1 Talk with the nurse who gave the medication
 2 Report the information to a nursing supervisor
 3 Call the Impaired Nurse Organization
 4 Report the information to the police

3. A client has died and a family member is asked about the funeral arrangements. The family member refuses to discuss the issue. The nurse's most appropriate action is to
 1 Provide information needed for decision making.
 2 Identify a risk of harm to self and refer to a mental health professional.
 3 Show acceptance of liability of feelings.
 4 Remain with family member without discussing funeral arrangements.

4. A client arrives in the emergency room and is staggering, confused, and verbally abusive. The client complains of a headache from drinking alcohol and is asking for medication. The nurse explains to the client that the physician will need to perform an assessment prior to the administration of medication. When the client becomes verbally abusive, the nurse obtains leather restraints and threatens to place the client in the restraints. With which of the following can the client legally charge the nurse as a result of the nursing action?
 1 Assault
 2 Battery
 3 Negligence
 4 Invasion of privacy

5. A nurse lawyer provides an education session to the nursing staff regarding client rights. A nurse asks the lawyer to describe an example that might relate to invasion of client privacy. A nursing action that indicates a violation of this right is
 1 Taking photographs of the client without consent.
 2 Telling the client that he or she cannot leave the hospital.
 3 Threatening to place a client in restraints.
 4 Performing a surgical procedure without consent.

6. The nurse calls the physician of a client scheduled for a cardiac catherization because the client has numerous questions regarding the procedure and has requested to speak to the physician. The physician is very upset and arrives at the unit to visit the client after prompting by the nurse. The nurse is outside the client's room and hears the physician tell the client in a derogatory manner that the nurse "doesn't know anything." The nurse plans to address the physician's remark

because the physician has violated which legal tort?

1 Libel
2 Slander
3 Assault
4 Negligence

7. The nurse employed in a long-term care facility calls the physician regarding a new medication order because the dosage prescribed is higher than the recommended dosage. The nurse is unable to locate the physician and the medication is due to be administered. Which of the following actions does the nurse take?

1 Hold the medication until the physician can be contacted
2 Administer the dose prescribed
3 Administer the recommended dose until the physician can be located
4 Contact the nursing supervisor

8. The nurse enters a client's room and finds the client sitting on the floor. The nurse checks the client thoroughly and then assists the client back to bed. The nurse completes an incident report and notifies the nursing supervisor and the physician of the incident. Which of the following is the next appropriate nursing action regarding the incident?

1 Make a copy of the incident report for the physician
2 Place the incident report in the client's chart
3 Document a complete entry in the client's record concerning the incident
4 Document in the client's record that an incident report has been completed

9. A nursing graduate who recently passed NCLEX-PN is employed as a licensed practical nurse (LPN) in a local hospital. During orientation, the nurse educator asks the LPN about his or her understanding of the need to obtain professional liability insurance. The most appropriate response by the LPN is

1 "The hospital's liability insurance will cover my actions."
2 "It is very expensive and not necessary."
3 "Nurses are encouraged to have their own malpractice insurance."
4 "The majority of suits are filed against physicians and the hospital."

10. A nurse witnesses an automobile accident and provides care to an open wound at the scene of the accident to a young child. The family is extremely grateful and insists that the nurse accept monetary compensation for the care provided to the child. Because of the family insistence, the nurse accepts the compensation to avoid offending the family. The child develops an infection and sepsis, and is hospitalized. The family files suit against the nurse who provided care

to the child at the scene of the accident. The nurse understands that which of the following is accurate regarding immunity from this suit?

1 The Good Samaritan Law will protect the nurse
2 The Good Samaritan Law will protect the nurse if the care given at the scene was not negligent
3 The Good Samaritan Law will not provide immunity from suit if the nurse accepted compensation for the care provided
4 The Good Samaritan Law protects laypersons and not professional health care providers

11. A client is brought to the emergency room after a serious accident, unconscious and bleeding profusely. Surgery is required immediately in order to save the client's life. In regard to informed consent for the surgical procedure, which of the following is the best action?

1 Try calling the client's spouse to obtain telephone consent prior to the surgical procedure
2 Transport the client to the operating room immediately as required by the physician without obtaining an informed consent
3 Ask the friend that accompanied the client to the emergency room to sign the consent form
4 Call the nursing supervisor to initiate a court order for the surgical procedure

12. The LPN arrives at work and is told to report (float) to the pediatric unit for the day because the unit is understaffed and needs additional nurses to care for the children. The LPN has never worked in the pediatric unit. Which of the following is the most appropriate nursing action?

1 Refuse to float to the pediatric unit
2 Call the hospital lawyer
3 Call the nursing supervisor
4 Report to the pediatric unit and identify tasks that can be safely performed

13. The nurse enters a client's room and notes that the client's lawyer is present and that the client is preparing a living will. The living will requires that the client's signature is witnessed and the client asks the nurse to witness the signature. Which of the following is the most appropriate nursing action?

1 Sign the living will as a witness to signature only
2 Sign the will, clearly identifying credentials and employment agency
3 Decline from signing the will
4 Call the hospital lawyer prior to signing the will

14. An elderly women is brought to the emergency room. When caring for the client, the nurse notes old and new ecchymotic areas on both arms and buttocks. The nurse asks the client how the bruises were sustained. The client, although re-

luctant, tells the nurse in confidence that the daughter frequently hits her if she gets in the way. Which of the following is the most appropriate nursing response?
1 "I promise I will not tell anyone but let's see what we can do about this."
2 "I have a legal obligation to report this type of abuse."
3 "Let's talk about ways that will prevent your daughter from hitting you."
4 "This should not be happening, and if it happens again you must call the emergency room."

15. A client tells the nurse of his or her decision to refuse external cardiac massage. Which of the following is the most appropriate nursing action?
1 Notify the physician of the client's request
2 Document the client's request in the client's record
3 Conduct a client conference to share the client's request
4 Discuss the client's request with the family

16. A client is brought to the emergency room by the ambulance team following collapse at home. Cardiopulmonary resuscitation is attempted but is unsuccessful. The wife of the client tells the nurse that the client is an organ donor and that the eyes are to be donated. Which of the following is the most appropriate nursing action?
1 Elevate the head of the bed of the deceased and place dry sterile dressings over the eyes
2 Call the National Donor Association to confirm that the client is a donor
3 Close the deceased client's eyes and place wet saline gauze pads and an ice pack on the eyes
4 Ask the wife to obtain the legal documents regarding organ donation from the lawyer

17. A client asks the nurse how to become an organ donor. Which of the following is not a component of the nurse's response?
1 A donor must be 18 years or older
2 The donation is done by written consent
3 The family is responsible for making that decision at the time of death

4 The client has the right to donate own organs for transplantation

18. The nurse recognizes that which of the following interventions is unlikely to facilitate effective communication between the dying client and the client's family?
1 The nurse encourages the client and family to openly identify and discuss feelings
2 The nurse makes decisions for the client and family in order to relieve them of unnecessary demands
3 The nurse assists the client and family in carrying out spiritually meaningful practices
4 The nurse maintains a calm attitude and one of acceptance when the family or client expresses anger

19. The client had a colon resection. A Levin tube was in place when a regular diet was brought to the client's room. The client did not want to eat solid food and asked that the physician be called. The nurse persisted in the belief that the solid food was the correct diet. The client ate two meals and subsequently had additional surgery due to complications. The nurse understands that the determination of negligence in this situation is based on
1 A duty existed, and it was breached.
2 Not calling the physician.
3 The dietary department sending the wrong food.
4 The nurse's beliefs.

20. A 39-year-old man learned today that his 36-year-old wife has an incurable cancer, and is expected to live not more than a few weeks. The nurse identifies which of these responses by the husband as indicative of effective individual coping?
1 He states that he will not allow his wife to come home to die
2 He immediately arranges for their three teenaged children to live with relatives in another state
3 He expresses his anger at God and the physicians for allowing this to happen
4 He refuses to visit his wife in the hospital or to discuss her illness

ANSWERS

1. **1**

RATIONALE: Proper documentation of unusual occurrences, incidents, and accidents, and the nursing actions taken as a result of the occurrence, are internal to the institution or agency and allows the nurse and administration to review the quality of care and determine any potential risks present. Option 2, 3, and 4 are incorrect.

TEST-TAKING STRATEGY: Use the process of elimination to eliminate options 2 and 4 because incident reports are not routinely filled out for interventions or treatment measures. Eliminate option 3 because incident reports are not used to report occurrences to other agencies. Medical records are used for this purpose. If you had difficulty with this question, take time now to review the purpose of incident reports.
LEVEL OF COGNITIVE ABILITY: Comprehension
PHASE OF NURSING PROCESS: Implementation

CLIENT NEEDS: Safe, Effective Care Environment
CONTENT AREA: Fundamental Skills
REFERENCE
Hill, S., & Howlett, H. (1997). *Success in practical nursing: Personal and vocational issues* (3rd ed.). Philadelphia: W. B. Saunders. pp. 308–309.

2. **2**

RATIONALE: Nurse Practice Acts require reporting the suspicion of impaired nurses. The board of nursing has jurisdiction over the practice of nursing and may develop plans for treatment and supervision. This suspicion needs to be reported to the nursing supervisor, who will then report to the board of nursing. Option 1 may cause a conflict. Options 3 and 4 are inappropriate.
TEST-TAKING STRATEGY: Use the principles of prioritizing when answering this question. By reporting the information, the nurse alerts the institution to the potential problem and sets the stage for further investigation and appropriate action.
LEVEL OF COGNITIVE ABILITY: Application
PHASE OF NURSING PROCESS: Planning
CLIENT NEEDS: Safe, Effective Care Environment
CONTENT AREA: Fundamental Skills
REFERENCE
Hill, S., & Howlett, H. (1997). *Success in practical nursing: Personal and vocational issues* (3rd ed.). Philadelphia: W. B. Saunders. pp. 158–159.

3. **4**

RATIONALE: The family member is exhibiting the first stage of grief—denial. Option 1 may be an appropriate intervention for the bargaining stage. Option 2 may be an appropriate intervention for the depression stage. Option 3 is an appropriate intervention for the acceptance or reorganization and restitution stage.
TEST-TAKING STRATEGY: Note the key words "most appropriate." Use the therapeutic communication techniques to direct you to option 4. Remember to address client and family feelings first. Review the grieving process and therapeutic communication techniques now if you had difficulty with this question.
LEVEL OF COGNITIVE ABILITY: Application
PHASE OF NURSING PROCESS: Implementation
CLIENT NEEDS: Psychosocial Integrity
CONTENT AREA: Fundamental Skills
REFERENCE
Leahy, J., & Kizilay, P. (1998). *Foundations of nursing practice: A nursing process approach*. Philadelphia: W. B. Saunders. p. 226.

4. **1**

RATIONALE: An assault occurs when a person puts another person in fear of a harmful or offensive contact. For this intentional tort to be actionable, the victim must be aware of the threat of harmful or offensive contact. Battery is the actual contact with one's body. Negligence involves actions below the standards of care. Invasion of privacy occurs when the individual's private affairs are unreasonably intruded.
TEST-TAKING STRATEGY: Note the key word "threatens" in the question. This should easily direct you to option 1. If you had difficulty with this question, take time now to review the descriptions associated with the terms in each option.
LEVEL OF COGNITIVE ABILITY: Comprehension

PHASE OF NURSING PROCESS: Evaluation
CLIENT NEEDS: Safe, Effective Care Environment
CONTENT AREA: Fundamental Skills
REFERENCE
Leahy, J., & Kizilay, P. (1998). *Foundations of nursing practice: A nursing process approach*. Philadelphia: W. B. Saunders. p. 66.

5. **1**

RATIONALE: Invasion of privacy takes place when an individual's private affairs are unreasonably intruded upon. Not allowing a client to leave the hospital constitutes false imprisonment. Threatening to place a client in restraints constitutes assault. Performing a surgical procedure without consent is an example of battery.
TEST-TAKING STRATEGY: The key words are "invasion of client privacy." These words should easily direct you to option 1. If you had difficulty with this question, take time now to review those situations that include invasion of privacy.
LEVEL OF COGNITIVE ABILITY: Application
PHASE OF NURSING PROCESS: Implementation
CLIENT NEEDS: Safe, Effective Care Environment
CONTENT AREA: Fundamental Skills
REFERENCE
Leahy, J., & Kizilay, P. (1998). *Foundations of nursing practice: A nursing process approach*. Philadelphia: W. B. Saunders. p. 67.

6. **2**

RATIONALE: Defamation takes place when something untrue is said (slander) or written (libel) about a person resulting in injury to that person's good name and reputation. An assault occurs when a person puts another person in fear of a harmful or an offensive contact. Negligence involves professionals' actions that fall below the standard of care for a specific professional group.
TEST-TAKING STRATEGY: You should easily eliminate options 3 and 4 first. Recalling that slander constitutes verbal defamation will easily direct you to option 2. If you had difficulty with this question, review the torts identified in each option.
LEVEL OF COGNITIVE ABILITY: Application
PHASE OF NURSING PROCESS: Planning
CLIENT NEEDS: Safe, Effective Care Environment
CONTENT AREA: Fundamental Skills
REFERENCE
Leahy, J., & Kizilay, P. (1998). *Foundations of nursing practice: A nursing process approach*. Philadelphia: W. B. Saunders. p. 68.

7. **4**

RATIONALE: If the physician writes an order that requires clarification, it is the nurse's responsibility to contact the physician for clarification. If there is no resolution regarding the order, because the physician cannot be located, or because the order remains as it was written after talking with the physician, the nurse should then contact the nurse manager or supervisor for further clarification as to what the next step should be. Under no circumstances should the nurse proceed to carry out the order until clarification is obtained.
TEST-TAKING STRATEGY: Eliminate options 2 and 3 first because they are similar and unsafe actions. Holding the medication can result in client injury. The nurse needs to take action. Option 4 clearly identifies the required action in this situation. Review nursing responsibilities related to physician's orders now if you had difficulty with this question.

LEVEL OF COGNITIVE ABILITY: Application
PHASE OF NURSING PROCESS: Implementation
CLIENT NEEDS: Safe, Effective Care Environment
CONTENT AREA: Fundamental Skills
REFERENCE
Leahy, J., & Kizilay, P. (1998). *Foundations of nursing practice: A nursing process approach.* Philadelphia: W. B. Saunders. p. 70.

8. 3

RATIONALE: The incident report is confidential and privileged information and should not be copied, placed in the chart, or have any reference made to it in the client's record. The incident report is not a substitute for a complete entry in the client's record concerning the incident.
TEST-TAKING STRATEGY: Eliminate options 2 and 4 first because they are similar. Recalling that incident reports should not be copied will direct you to option 3. Review nursing responsibilities related to incident reports now if you had difficulty with this question.
LEVEL OF COGNITIVE ABILITY: Comprehension
PHASE OF NURSING PROCESS: Implementation
CLIENT NEEDS: Safe, Effective Care Environment
CONTENT AREA: Fundamental Skills
REFERENCE
Leahy, J., & Kizilay, P. (1998). *Foundations of nursing practice: A nursing process approach.* Philadelphia: W. B. Saunders. p. 72.

9. 3

RATIONALE: Nurses need their own liability insurance for protection against malpractice law suits. Nurses erroneously assume that they are protected by an agency's professional liability policies. Usually when a nurse is sued, the employer is also sued for the nurse's actions or inactions. Even though this is the norm, nurses are encouraged to have their own malpractice insurance.
TEST-TAKING STRATEGY: Note that the issue of the question relates to "professional liability insurance." This issue should easily direct you to option 3. Review liability related to malpractice insurance now if you had difficulty with this question.
LEVEL OF COGNITIVE ABILITY: Comprehension
PHASE OF NURSING PROCESS: Implementation
CLIENT NEEDS: Safe, Effective Care Environment
CONTENT AREA: Fundamental Skills
REFERENCE
Leahy, J., & Kizilay, P. (1998). *Foundations of nursing practice: A nursing process approach.* Philadelphia: W. B. Saunders. pp. 83–84.

10. 3

RATIONALE: A Good Samaritan Law is passed by a state legislature to encourage nurses and other health care providers to provide care to a person when an accident, emergency, or injury occurs, without fear of being sued for the care provided. Called immunity from suit, this protection usually applies only if all of the conditions of the law are met, such as the health care provider receives no compensation for the care provided, and the care given is not willfully and wantonly negligent.
TEST-TAKING STRATEGY: If you read the question carefully, you will note the key phrase "accept monetary compensation." This will easily direct you to option 3. Additionally, options 1, 2, and 4 are similar. Review the Good Samaritan Law now if you had difficulty with this question!
LEVEL OF COGNITIVE ABILITY: Comprehension
PHASE OF NURSING PROCESS: Evaluation

CLIENT NEEDS: Safe, Effective Care Environment
CONTENT AREA: Fundamental Skills
REFERENCE
Leahy, J., & Kizilay, P. (1998). *Foundations of nursing practice: A nursing process approach.* Philadelphia: W. B. Saunders. p. 73.

11. 2

RATIONALE: Generally there are only two instances in which the informed consent of an adult client is not needed. One instance is when an emergency is present and delaying treatment for the purpose of obtaining informed consent would result in injury or death to the client. The second instance is when the client waives the right to give informed consent. Options 1, 3, and 4 are inappropriate.
TEST-TAKING STRATEGY: Option 3 can be easily eliminated first. Note the key phrase "surgery is required immediately." Options 1 and 4 would delay treatment and should be eliminated. Review the issues surrounding informed consent now if you had difficulty with this question.
LEVEL OF COGNITIVE ABILITY: Application
PHASE OF NURSING PROCESS: Implementation
CLIENT NEEDS: Safe, Effective Care Environment
CONTENT AREA: Fundamental Skills
REFERENCE
Leahy, J., & Kizilay, P. (1998). *Foundations of nursing practice: A nursing process approach.* Philadelphia: W. B. Saunders. pp. 74–75.

12. 4

RATIONALE: Floating is an acceptable legal practice used by hospitals to solve their understaffing problems. Legally, a nurse cannot refuse to float unless a union contract guarantees that nurses can work only in a specified area, or the nurse can prove the lack of knowledge for the performance of assigned tasks. When encountered with this situation, nurses should set priorities and identify potential areas of harm to the client.
TEST-TAKING STRATEGY: Note the key words "most appropriate." Options 1 and 2 can be eliminated first because they are inappropriate. For the remaining options, it is premature to call the nursing supervisor. Option 4 is most appropriate. Review nursing responsibilities related to "floating" now if you had difficulty with this question.
LEVEL OF COGNITIVE ABILITY: Application
PHASE OF NURSING PROCESS: Implementation
CLIENT NEEDS: Safe, Effective Care Environment
CONTENT AREA: Fundamental Skills
REFERENCE
Hill, S., & Howlett, H. (1997). *Success in practical nursing: Personal and vocational issues* (3rd ed.). Philadelphia: W. B. Saunders. p. 311.

13. 3

RATIONALE: Living wills are required to be in writing and signed by the client. The client's signature either must be witnessed by specified individuals or notarized. Many states prohibit any employee, including a nurse of a facility where the declaring is receiving care, from being a witness.
TEST-TAKING STRATEGY: Note the key words "most appropriate." Options 1 and 2 are similar and should be eliminated first. From the remaining options, option 3 is most appropriate. Review legal implications associated with wills now if you had difficulty with this question.
LEVEL OF COGNITIVE ABILITY: Application
PHASE OF NURSING PROCESS: Implementation
CLIENT NEEDS: Safe, Effective Care Environment
CONTENT AREA: Fundamental Skills

REFERENCE
Hill, S., & Howlett, H. (1997). *Success in practical nursing: Personal and vocational issues* (3rd ed.). Philadelphia: W. B. Saunders. p. 310.

14. 2

RATIONALE: Confidential issues are not to be discussed with nonmedical personnel or the person's family or friends without the person's permission. Clients should be assured that information is kept confidential, unless it places the nurse under a legal obligation. The nurse must report situations related to child or elderly abuse, gunshot wounds, and certain infectious diseases.

TEST-TAKING STRATEGY: Option 4 can be eliminated first because this action does not protect the client from injury. Options 1 and 3 are similar and should be eliminated. Review the nursing responsibilities related to reporting obligations now if you had difficulty with this question!

LEVEL OF COGNITIVE ABILITY: Application
PHASE OF NURSING PROCESS: Implementation
CLIENT NEEDS: Psychosocial Integrity
CONTENT AREA: Fundamental Skills
REFERENCE
Luckmann, J. (1997). *Saunders manual of nursing care.* Philadelphia: W. B. Saunders. p. 84.

15. 1

RATIONALE: External cardiac massage is one type of treatment that a client can refuse. The most appropriate nursing action is to notify the physician because a written do not resuscitate (DNR) order from the physician must be present. The DNR order must be reviewed or renewed on a regular basis per agency policy.

TEST-TAKING STRATEGY: The key words "most appropriate" may indicate that more than one option may be correct. Prioritize the options. Although options 2, 3, and 4 may be appropriate, remember that first a written physician's order is necessary. Review DNR procedures now if you had difficulty with this question.

LEVEL OF COGNITIVE ABILITY: Application
PHASE OF NURSING PROCESS: Implementation
CLIENT NEEDS: Safe, Effective Care Environment
CONTENT AREA: Fundamental Skills
REFERENCE
Leahy, J., & Kizilay, P. (1998). *Foundations of nursing practice: A nursing process approach.* Philadelphia: W. B. Saunders. p. 76.

16. 3

RATIONALE: When a corneal donor dies, the eyes are closed and gauze pads wet with saline are placed over them with a small ice pack. Within 2 to 4 hours the eyes are enucleated. The cornea is usually transplanted within 24 to 48 hours. The head of the bed should also be elevated.

TEST-TAKING STRATEGY: Note that the key issue relates to donation of the eyes. This should assist in directing you to eliminating options 2 and 4. For the remaining options, knowledge regarding care to the eyes of the deceased who is a donor is required. This knowledge should direct you to option 3. Review this procedure now if you had difficulty with the question!

LEVEL OF COGNITIVE ABILITY: Application
PHASE OF NURSING PROCESS: Implementation
CLIENT NEEDS: Safe, Effective Care Environment
CONTENT AREA: Fundamental Skills
REFERENCE:
Monahan, F., & Neighbors, M. (1998). *Medical-surgical nursing: Foundations for clinical practice* (2nd ed.). Philadelphia: W. B. Saunders. p. 1954.

17. 3

RATIONALE: Clients have the right to donate their own organs for transplantation. Any person 18 or older may become an organ donor by written consent. In the absence of appropriate documentation, a family member or legal guardian may authorize donation of the decedent's organs.

TEST-TAKING STRATEGY: Note the key word "not" in the stem of the question. Using the process of elimination and the issues related to client rights will easily direct you to option 3. If you had difficulty with this question, take time now to review the procedure for organ donation.

LEVEL OF COGNITIVE ABILITY: Application
PHASE OF NURSING PROCESS: Implementation
CLIENT NEEDS: Safe, Effective Care Environment
CONTENT AREA: Fundamental Skills
REFERENCE:
Leahy, J., & Kizilay, P. (1998). *Foundations of nursing practice: A nursing process approach.* Philadelphia: W. B. Saunders. p. 76.

18. 2

RATIONALE: Maintaining effective and open communication among family members affected by death and grief is of the greatest importance. The nurse looks for ways to maintain and enhance communication as well as preserving the family's sense of self-direction and control. Option 1 describes encouraging discussion of feelings, and is likely to enhance communication. Option 3 is also an effective intervention, as spiritual practices give meaning to life and have an impact on how people react to crisis. Option 4 is also an effective technique, as the client and family need to know that someone will be there, supportive, and nonjudgmental. Option 2 describes the nurse removing autonomy and decision making from the client and family, who are already experiencing feelings of loss of control in that they cannot change the process of dying. This is an ineffective intervention that can further impair communication.

TEST-TAKING STRATEGY: Read the stem carefully, and note the key words "unlikely" and "facilitate." This question is asking you to identify the negative response, so it is important to read each possible answer carefully before deciding which to choose. Understanding that people in crisis usually feel helpless and unable to control their circumstances, you can then identify option 2 as a response that further removes control.

LEVEL OF COGNITIVE ABILITY: Comprehension
PHASE OF NURSING PROCESS: Implementation
CLIENT NEEDS: Psychosocial Integrity
CONTENT AREA: Fundamental Skills
REFERENCE:
Hill, S., & Howlett, H. (1997). *Success in practical nursing: Personal and vocational issues* (3rd ed.). Philadelphia: W. B. Saunders. p. 185.

19. 1

RATIONALE: For negligence to be proven, there must be a duty, a breach of duty, the breach of duty must cause the injury, and damages or injury must be experienced. Options 2, 3, and 4 do not fall under the criteria for negligence. Option 1 is the only response that fits the criteria of negligence.

TEST-TAKING STRATEGY: Options 2, 3, and 4 do not directly support the issue of negligence because it would be difficult to determine that these elements caused injury. The focus relates to what the nurse is responsible for. Option 1 is a broad, general response to the question. Review the legal elements of nursing practice and criteria for negligence now if you had difficulty with this question!

LEVEL OF COGNITIVE ABILITY: Comprehension
PHASE OF NURSING PROCESS: Evaluation
CLIENT NEEDS: Safe, Effective Care Environment
CONTENT AREA: Fundamental Skills
REFERENCE:

Hill, S., & Howlett, H. (1997). *Success in practical nursing: Personal and vocational issues* (3rd ed.). Philadelphia: W. B. Saunders. p. 305.

20. **3**

RATIONALE: The expression of anger is known to be a normal response to impending loss, and the anger may be directed toward the self, the dying person, God or other spiritual being, or toward the caregivers. Options 1 and 2 indicate possibly rash and unilateral decisions made by the husband, without taking into consideration anyone else's feelings. There is strong evidence of denial in option 4, as he refuses to see or discuss his wife. The only "normal" or expected response by the husband is option 3.

TEST-TAKING STRATEGY: Note the key words, "effective individual coping." Knowledge of the stages of grief associated with loss is essential in answering this question. Each of the four possible options seems negative unless carefully considered within the framework of responses to grief and loss. Look for the option that uses the same terminology as the stages of death and dying. Anger stands out as the only concept that matches the expected stages of coping with grief and loss.

LEVEL OF COGNITIVE ABILITY: Comprehension
PHASE OF THE NURSING PROCESS: Evaluation
CLIENT NEEDS: Psychosocial Integrity
CONTENT AREA: Fundamental Skills
REFERENCE:

deWit, S. (1998). *Essentials of medical-surgical nursing* (4th ed.). Philadelphia: W. B. Saunders. pp. 300–301.

BIBLIOGRAPHY

Brent, N. (1997). *Nurses and the law.* Philadelphia: W. B. Saunders.
deWit, S. (1998). *Essentials of medical-surgical nursing* (4th ed.). Philadelphia: W. B. Saunders.
Hill, S., & Howlett, H. (1997). *Success in practical nursing: Personal and vocational issues* (3rd ed.). Philadelphia: W. B. Saunders.

Leahy, J., & Kizilay, P. (1998). *Foundations of nursing practice: A nursing process approach.* Philadelphia: W. B. Saunders.
Luckmann, J. (1997). *Saunders manual of nursing care.* Philadelphia: W. B. Saunders.
Monahan, F., & Neighbors, M. (1998). *Medical-surgical nursing: Foundations for clinical practice* (2nd ed.). Philadelphia: W. B. Saunders.
National Council of State Boards of Nursing. (1998) *National Council Detailed Test Plan for the NCLEX-PN Examination.* Chicago: Author.

CHAPTER 7

Leadership Issues and Priorities of Care

PYRAMID TERMS

Accountability—A moral concept that involves acceptance by the nurse of the consequences of a decision or action

Case Management—Represents an interdisciplinary health care delivery system designed to promote appropriate use of hospital personnel and material resources to maximize hospital revenues while providing for optimal outcome of care

Critical Paths—Provide effective clinical management systems for monitoring care and for reducing or controlling the length of hospital stay

Delegation—Process of transferring a selected nursing task in a situation to an individual who is competent to perform that specific task

Leadership—The interpersonal process that involves motivating and guiding others to achieve goals

Management—The accomplishment of tasks either by oneself or by directing others

Prioritizing—Deciding which needs or problems require immediate action and which ones could be delayed because they are not urgent

Responsibility—The duty to act

Variances—Actual deviations or detours from the critical paths

THE PYRAMID TO SUCCESS

The nurse is both a leader and a manager. As described in the NCLEX-PN Test Plan, the nurse needs to collaborate with other health care team members to facilitate effective care. Pyramid points focus on the concepts of management and supervision, leadership responsibilities, resource management, making client care assignments, establishing priorities of care among a group of clients, and the principles of time management.

NURSING PROCESS

DATA COLLECTION

Health care setting
Multidisciplinary health care team
Support systems
Resources

PLANNING

Develop management and supervisory plan based on organizational goals. Plan client care based on client priorities.

IMPLEMENTATION

Identify organizational mission and goals. Manage the health care environment congruent with organizational mission and goals. Function within the guidelines of the Nurse Practice Act, Standards of Care, Code of Ethics, agency policies and procedures, and legal system. Plan client care assignments appropriately, considering client care needs and available staff members. Establish priorities of care for clients. Incorporate principles of time management when providing care.

EVALUATION

Care to the client is congruent with organizational mission and goals. Continuous quality improvement in client care occurs.

◆ CLIENT NEEDS

SAFE, EFFECTIVE CARE ENVIRONMENT

Concepts of management and supervision
Continuous quality improvement
Assignments
Consultation and referrals
Resource management

HEALTH PROMOTION AND MAINTENANCE

Family systems
Disease prevention
Health and wellness
Health screening
Health promotion programs

PSYCHOSOCIAL INTEGRITY

Religious, spiritual, and cultural influences on health
Support systems
Therapeutic environment

PHYSIOLOGICAL INTEGRITY

Prioritizing client care
Basic care and comfort

I. Health Care Delivery Systems

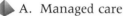

A. Managed care
1. Designed to control the cost of health services and promote a continuum of care through the development and use of integrated services
2. Emphasizes the promotion of health, client education and responsible self-care, early identification of disease, and the use of health care resources
B. Health maintenance organizations (HMOs)
1. Offers comprehensive coverage for hospital and physician services in exchange for a fixed, prepaid fee
2. Both an insurance company and a health care delivery system
C. Preferred provider organizations
1. Represent an arrangement between employers and insurance companies that provide member services from a selected group of providers
2. The choice of physicians is comprehensive and members can elect to see any participating physician
D. Exclusive provider organization: parallels preferred provider organization except that beneficiaries are limited to those providers who are participating physicians for any required health care service
E. **Case management:** represents an interdisciplinary health care delivery system designed to promote appropriate use of hospital personnel and material resources to maximize hospital revenues while providing for optimal outcome of care
F. **Critical paths**
1. Developed based on appropriate standards of care
2. Provide effective clinical **management**

systems for monitoring care and for reducing or controlling the length of hospital stay
3. The goal of **critical paths** is to anticipate and recognize negative **variance** early so that appropriate action can be taken and better client outcomes can be achieved
4. **Variances**
a. Actual deviations or detours from the **critical paths**
b. Positive **variance** occurs when the client achieves maximum benefit and is discharged earlier than anticipated on his or her **critical path**
c. Negative **variance** occurs when untoward events prevent a timely discharge and the length of stay is longer than planned for a client on a specific **critical path**
d. Accurate monitoring of **critical paths** with **variance** analysis can estimate the financial impact of client care
G. Levels of prevention
1. Primary prevention: relates to health promotion activities and specific protection from disease or illness
2. Secondary prevention: focuses on the early diagnosis and prompt treatment of disease
3. Tertiary prevention: represented by rehabilitative services
H. Health care settings
1. Hospital care
2. Home care
3. Hospice care
4. Long-term care
5. Surgical and ambulatory centers
6. Public health departments

II. Formal Organizations

A. Mission statement: communicates in broad terms the reason for existence, the geographical area the organization serves, and attitudes and beliefs within which the organization functions
B. Goals and objectives: measurable activities specific to the development of designated services and programs of an organization
C. Organizational chart: depicts and communicates how activities are arranged, how authority relationships are defined, and how communication channels are established
D. Procedures and protocols
1. Guides in defining appropriate courses of action
2. Procedure defines a task
3. Protocol signifies the definition of a clinical process
E. Centralization: when decisions are made by a limited number of individuals at the top of the organization or by managers of a department or unit and thereafter, communicated to the employees
F. Decentralization: authority is distributed throughout the organization to allow for

increased **responsibility** and **delegation** in decision making

III. Nursing Delivery Systems

A. Functional nursing: involves a task approach to client care, with major tasks being delegated by the charge nurse to individual members of the team

B. Team nursing: the team is generally led by a charge nurse and each staff member works fully within the realm of his or her educational and clinical expertise

C. Primary nursing: focuses on the client outcomes as opposed to nursing tasks and is concerned with keeping the nurse at the bedside and actively involved in individualized client care

IV. Nursing Responsibilities

A. Accountability
1. The process that mandates that individuals are answerable for their actions and have an obligation (or duty) to act
2. Assuming only the responsibilities that are within one's scope of practice
3. Not assuming **responsibility** for activities in which competency has not been achieved
4. Involves admitting mistakes rather than blaming others, and evaluating the outcomes of one's own actions
5. Includes a **responsibility** to the client to be competent, to render nursing services in accordance with standards of nursing practice, and to adhere to the professional ethic code

B. **Leadership**
1. The interpersonal process that involves motivating and guiding others to achieve goals
2. A method of modeling accountable behavior to others

C. **Management:** the accomplishment of tasks either by oneself or by directing others

D. Supervision: the process of being in charge of or directing others and activities

E. **Leadership** styles
1. Autocratic: leader maintains strong control, makes the decisions, and solves all problems
2. Democratic: also called participative **leadership,** based on the belief that every group member should have input into development of goals and problem solving
3. Laissez-faire: leader assumes a passive, nondirective, and inactive approach and all decision making is left to the group, with the leader giving little if any guidance, support, or feedback
4. Situational: utilizing a combination of styles based on current circumstances and events

F. **Leadership** qualities (Box 7–1)

BOX 7–1. Leadership Qualities

Communication
Credibility
Critical thinking
Initiating action
Risk taking

V. Assignments and Delegation

A. Process of transferring a selected nursing task in a situation to an individual who is competent to perform that specific task

B. Licensed practical nurses may be responsible, depending on the state Nurse Practice Act, to assign and delegate tasks to certified nursing assistants (CNA) and unlicensed assistive personnel (UAP)

C. Even though a task may be delegated to someone, the nurse who delegates maintains **accountability** for the overall nursing care of the client

D. Only the task, not the ultimate **accountability,** may be delegated to another

E. Guidelines for client care assignments
1. Determine which tasks can be delegated and to whom
2. Match the task to the health care worker based on the Nurse Practice Act and appropriate position descriptions
3. Communicate a feeling of confidence to the health care worker and provide feedback promptly after the task is performed
4. Maintain continuity of care as much as possible when assigning client care

VI. Empowerment

A. An interpersonal process of enabling others to do for themselves

B. Nurses can empower clients through advocacy

VII. Priorities of Care

A. Prioritizing—deciding which needs or problems require immediate action and which ones could be delayed because they are not urgent

B. Guidelines
1. The nurse and client mutually rank the client's needs in order of importance based on the client's desires, needs, and safety
2. Priorities are classified as high, intermediate, or low
   a. Client needs that are life-threatening or if untreated could result in harm to the client are high priorities
   b. Nonemergency and non–life-threatening client needs are intermediate priorities
   c. Client needs that are not directly related to the client's illness or prognosis are low priorities

3. When providing care, the nurse needs to decide which needs or problems require immediate action and which ones could be delayed because they are not urgent
4. Client problems that involve actual or life-threatening concerns are considered prior to potential health-threatening concerns
5. The nurse must consider time constraints and available resources when prioritizing care
6. Problems identified as important by the client must be given high priority
7. Priority setting may be guided by theories, models, and principles, such as Maslow's hierarchy of needs
8. Maslow's hierarchy of needs identifies levels of physiological needs, safety, love and belonging, self-esteem, and self-actualization; basic needs are met before moving to other needs in the hierarchy
9. Use the ABCs—airway, breathing, and circulation; client needs related to maintaining a patent airway is always the priority

VIII. Time Management

A. Description
   1. A technique designed to assist in completing tasks within a definite period
   2. Involves efficiency in completing tasks as quickly as possible, and effectiveness in deciding on the most important task to do and doing it correctly
B. Guidelines
   1. Keep a daily hour-by-hour log to assist in providing structure to the tasks that must be accomplished
   2. Organize the workday and prioritize client needs and daily tasks
   3. Focus on beginning the daily tasks while keeping goals in mind; looking at the final goal for the day will help to break down tasks into manageable parts
   4. Anticipate the needs and goals of the day and provide time for unexpected and unplanned tasks that may arise
   5. Use hospital resources wisely, anticipating resource needs and gathering these supplies prior to beginning the task
   6. Begin client rounds at the beginning of the shift, collecting data on each assigned client
   7. Organize paperwork and continuously document task completion and necessary client data throughout the day
   8. At the end of the day, evaluate the effectiveness of time management

PRACTICE QUESTIONS

1. The nurse is asked by another nurse about the definition of case management. Which of the following is not a component of the response?
   1 Represents a primary health prevention focus managed by a single case manager
   2 Manages client care by managing the client care environment
   3 Designed to promote appropriate use of hospital personnel and material resources
   4 Maximizes hospital revenues while providing for optimal outcome of client care

2. The nurse is assisting in reviewing the critical paths of the clients on the nursing unit. In performing a variance analysis, which of the following indicates the need for further action?
   1 A client's family attending a diabetic teaching session
   2 Canceling physical therapy sessions on the weekend
   3 Normal vital signs and absence of wound infection in a postoperative client
   4 A client demonstrating accurate medication administration following teaching

3. A licensed practical nurse (LPN) is attending an agency orientation regarding the nursing model of practice implemented in the facility. The nurse is told that the nursing model is a team nursing approach. The nurse understands that which of the following is a characteristic of this type of nursing model of practice?
   1 A task approach method is used to provide care to clients
   2 A single registered nurse (RN) is responsible for providing nursing care to a group of clients
   3 Managed care concepts and tools are used in providing client care
   4 Nursing personnel are led by an RN leader in providing care to a group of clients

4. A nurse is assigned to assist with working with food services in a rural, poor school setting. A goal for the school dietary program is to avoid nutritional deficiencies and enhance children's nutritional status through healthy dietary practices. In planning interventions by levels of prevention, which of the following is a primary prevention intervention that the nurse could suggest?
   1 Case finding in the school to identify dietary practices
   2 School screening programs for early detection of children with poor eating habits
   3 Providing educational programs, literature, and posters to promote awareness of healthy eating
   4 Conducting a community-wide dietary screening activity to detect community dietary trends

5. A nurse is assisting with working with disaster relief following a tornado. The nurse's goal with the overall community is to prevent as much injury and death as possible from the uncontrollable event. Finding safe housing for survivors, providing support to families, organizing counsel-

ing, and securing physical care when needed are all examples of which type of prevention?
1 The primary level of prevention
2 The secondary level of prevention
3 The tertiary level of prevention
4 Aggregate care prevention

6. The nurse is planning the client assignments. Which of the following is the least appropriate assignment for the unlicensed nursing assistant?
1 Assist a 12-year-old boy with Down syndrome, who is profoundly developmentally disabled, to eat lunch
2 Obtain frequent oral temperatures on a client
3 Accompany a 51-year-old man, being discharged to home following a bowel resection 8 days ago, to his transportation
4 Collect a urine specimen from a 70-year-old woman admitted 3 days ago

7. The nurse is assigned to care for four clients. In planning client rounds, which client does the nurse collect data on first?
1 A client receiving oxygen via nasal cannula who had difficulty breathing during the previous shift
2 A postoperative client preparing for discharge
3 A client scheduled for a chest x-ray
4 A client requiring daily dressing changes

8. The nurse employed in a long-term care facility is planning the client assignments for the shift. Which of the following clients does the nurse

most appropriately assign to the certified nursing assistant (CNA)?
1 A client requiring BID dressing changes
2 A client requiring frequent ambulation
3 A client on a bowel management program requiring rectal suppositories and a daily enema
4 A diabetic client requiring daily insulin and reinforcement of dietary measures

9. The nurse has received the client assignment for the day and is organizing the required tasks. Which of the following is not a component of the plan for time management?
1 Prioritizing client needs and daily tasks
2 Providing time for unexpected tasks
3 Gathering supplies prior to beginning a task
4 Documenting task completion at the end of the day

10. The nurse is giving a bed bath to an assigned client. A nursing assistant enters the client's room and tells the nurse that another assigned client is in pain and needs pain medication. The most appropriate action is which of the following?
1 Finish the bed bath and then administer the pain medication to the other client
2 Cover the client, raise the side rails, tell the client that you will return shortly, and administer the pain medication to the other client
3 Ask the nursing assistant to tell the client in pain that medication will be administered as soon as the bed bath is complete
4 Ask the nursing assistant to find out when the last pain medication was given to the client

ANSWERS

1. **1**

RATIONALE: Case management represents an interdisciplinary health care delivery system to promote appropriate use of hospital personnel and material resources to maximize hospital revenues while providing for optimal outcome of care. Options 2, 3, and 4 identify the components of managed care.
TEST-TAKING STRATEGY: Note the key word "not." Knowledge regarding the characteristics of case management is necessary to answer this question. Use the process of elimination. Also, note the key word "single" in the correct option to this question. Review the characteristics of case management now if you had difficulty with this question.
LEVEL OF COGNITIVE ABILITY: Comprehension
PHASE OF NURSING PROCESS: Planning
CLIENT NEEDS: Safe, Effective Care Environment
CONTENT AREA: Fundamental Skills
REFERENCE
Rocchiccioli, J., & Tilbury, M. (1998). *Clinical leadership in nursing.* Philadelphia: W. B. Saunders. pp. 38–39

2. **2**

RATIONALE: Variances are actual deviations or detours from the critical paths. Variances can be either positive or negative, avoidable or unavoidable, and can be caused by a variety of things. Positive variance occurs when the client achieves maximum benefit and is discharged earlier than anticipated. Negative variance occurs when untoward events prevent a timely discharge. Variance analysis occurs continually in order to anticipate and recognize negative variance early so that appropriate action can be taken.
TEST-TAKING STRATEGY: Use the process of elimination to identify the negative variance. Options 1, 3, and 4 identify positive outcomes. Option 2 identifies a negative outcome. Review the purpose of variance analysis now if you had difficulty with this question.
LEVEL OF COGNITIVE ABILITY: Comprehension
PHASE OF NURSING PROCESS: Evaluation
CLIENT NEEDS: Safe, Effective Care Environment
CONTENT AREA: Fundamental Skills
REFERENCE
Rocchiccioli, J., & Tilbury, M. (1998). *Clinical leadership in nursing.* Philadelphia: W. B. Saunders. p. 42.

3. **4**

RATIONALE: In team nursing, nursing personnel are led by an RN leader in providing care to a group of clients. Option 1 identifies functional nursing. Option 2 identifies primary nursing. Option 3 identifies a component of case management.
TEST-TAKING STRATEGY: Note that the issue of the question relates to team nursing. Keep this issue in mind and use the process of elimination. Option 4 is the only option that identifies the concept of a team approach. Review the various types of nursing delivery systems now if you had difficulty with this question.
LEVEL OF COGNITIVE ABILITY: Comprehension
PHASE OF NURSING PROCESS: Implementation
CLIENT NEEDS: Safe, Effective Care Environment
CONTENT AREA: Fundamental Skills
REFERENCE
Rocchiccioli, J., & Tilbury, M. (1998). *Clinical leadership in nursing.* Philadelphia: W. B. Saunders. p. 30.

4. **3**

RATIONALE: Primary prevention interventions are those measures that keep illness, injury, or potential problems from occurring. Option 1 is a tertiary prevention measure; options 2 and 4 are secondary prevention measures that seek to detect existing health problems or trends.
TEST-TAKING STRATEGY: Note the issue of the question "primary prevention intervention." Knowledge that primary prevention interventions are those measures that keep illness from occurring will direct you to option 3. If you had difficulty with this question, take time now to review the levels of prevention.
LEVEL OF COGNITIVE ABILITY: Comprehension
PHASE OF NURSING PROCESS: Planning
CLIENT NEEDS: Health Promotion and Maintenance
CONTENT AREA: Fundamental Skills
REFERENCE
Leahy, J., & Kizilay, P. (1998). *Foundations of nursing practice: A nursing process approach.* Philadelphia: W. B. Saunders. pp. 83–84.

5. **3**

RATIONALE: Tertiary prevention involves the reduction of the amount and degree of disability, injury, and damage following a crisis. Primary prevention means keeping the crisis from ever occurring and secondary prevention focuses on reducing the intensity and duration of the crisis during the crisis itself. There is no known aggregate care prevention level.
TEST-TAKING STRATEGY: Identify the scenario in the question. Focus on this scenario and use knowledge regarding the various levels of prevention to answer the question. If you had difficulty with this question, take time now to review the levels of prevention.
LEVEL OF COGNITIVE ABILITY: Application
PHASE OF NURSING PROCESS: Implementation
CLIENT NEEDS: Safe, Effective Care Environment
CONTENT AREA: Fundamental Skills
REFERENCE
Leahy, J., & Kizilay, P. (1998). *Foundations of nursing practice: A nursing process approach.* Philadelphia: W. B. Saunders. pp. 83–84.

6. **1**

RATIONALE: The nurse must determine the most appropriate assignment based on the skills of the staff member and the needs of the client. In this case, the least appropriate assignment for an unlicensed nursing assistant is assisting with feeding a profoundly developmentally disabled child. The child is likely to have difficulty eating and, therefore, has a higher potential for complications such as choking and aspiration. The remaining three options include nothing to indicate that these tasks carry any unforeseen risk.
TEST-TAKING STRATEGY: Note the key words "least appropriate." Use the process of elimination. Consider the ABCs and recall the principles of delegation and supervision of the work of others in answering the question. Work that is delegated to others must be done consistent with the individual's level of expertise and licensure or lack of licensure. Review the principles of assignments and delegation now if you had difficulty with this question.
LEVEL OF COGNITIVE ABILITY: Application
PHASE OF NURSING PROCESS: Planning
CLIENT NEEDS: Safe, Effective Care Environment
CONTENT AREA: Fundamental Skills
REFERENCE
Rocchiccioli, J., & Tilbury, M. (1998). *Clinical leadership in nursing.* Philadelphia: W. B. Saunders. p. 140.

7. **1**

RATIONALE: Airway is always a high priority and the nurse attends to the client who has been experiencing an airway problem first. The clients described in options 2, 3, and 4 are an intermediate priority.
TEST-TAKING STRATEGY: Use Maslow's hierarchy of needs and the ABCs to answer the question. Remember that airway is always the first priority.
LEVEL OF COGNITIVE ABILITY: Application
PHASE OF NURSING PROCESS: Planning
CLIENT NEEDS: Safe, Effective Care Environment
CONTENT AREA: Fundamental Skills
REFERENCE
Leahy, J., & Kizilay, P. (1998). *Foundations of nursing practice: A nursing process approach.* Philadelphia: W. B. Saunders. p. 168.

8. **2**

RATIONALE: Assignment of tasks needs to be implemented based on the job description of the CNA, the level of clinical competence, and state law. Options 1, 3, and 4 involve care that requires the skill of the licensed practical nurse.
TEST-TAKING STRATEGY: Use the process of elimination and knowledge regarding tasks that can be safely delegated to the CNA. Eliminate options 1, 3, and 4 because these clients require care that needs to be provided by the licensed practical nurse.
LEVEL OF COGNITIVE ABILITY: Application
PHASE OF NURSING PROCESS: Planning
CLIENT NEEDS: Safe, Effective Care Environment
CONTENT AREA: Fundamental Skills
REFERENCE
Hill, S., & Howlett, H. (1997). *Success in practical nursing: Personal and vocational issues* (3rd ed.). Philadelphia: W. B. Saunders. p. 283.

9. **4**

RATIONALE: The nurse should document task completion continuously throughout the day. Options 1, 2, and 3 identify accurate components of time management.
TEST-TAKING STRATEGY: Use the process of elimination and knowledge regarding the guidelines for time management to answer the question. If you had difficulty with

this question, take time now to review time management principles and the principles related to documentation.
LEVEL OF COGNITIVE ABILITY: Application
PHASE OF NURSING PROCESS: Planning
CLIENT NEEDS: Safe, Effective Care Environment
CONTENT AREA: Fundamental Skills
REFERENCE
de Wit, S. (1998). *Essentials of medical-surgical nursing* (4th ed.). Philadelphia: W. B. Saunders. p. 1055.

10. 2

RATIONALE: The nurse is responsible for the care provided to the assigned clients. The most appropriate action is to provide safety to the client who is receiving the bed bath and prepare to administer the pain medication. Options 1 and 3 delay the administration of medication to the client in pain. Option 4 is not a responsibility of the nursing assistant.
TEST-TAKING STRATEGY: Use the process of elimination and principles related to priorities of care. Options 1 and 3 delay the administration of pain medication, and option 4 is not a responsibility of the nursing assistant. The most appropriate action is to plan to administer the medication.
LEVEL OF COGNITIVE ABILITY: Application
PHASE OF NURSING PROCESS: Planning
CLIENT NEEDS: Safe, Effective Care Environment
CONTENT AREA: Fundamental Skills
REFERENCE
Leahy, J., & Kizilay, P. (1998). *Foundations of nursing practice: A nursing process approach.* Philadelphia: W. B. Saunders. p. 168.

BIBLIOGRAPHY

deWit, S. (1998). *Essentials of medical-surgical nursing* (4th ed.). Philadelphia: W. B. Saunders.
Hill, S., & Howlett, H. (1997). *Success in practical nursing: Personal and vocational issues* (3rd ed.). Philadelphia: W. B. Saunders.
Leahy, J., & Kizilay, P. (1998). *Foundations of nursing practice: A nursing process approach.* Philadelphia: W. B. Saunders.

National Council of State Boards of Nursing (1998). *National Council detailed test plan for the NCLEX-PN examination.* Chicago: Author.
O'Toole, M. (1997). *Miller-Keane encyclopedia & dictionary of medicine, nursing, & allied health* (6th ed.). Philadelphia: W. B. Saunders.
Rocchiccioli, J., & Tilbury, M. (1998). *Clinical leadership in nursing.* Philadelphia: W. B. Saunders.

UNIT III

Nursing Sciences

CHAPTER 8

Fluids and Electrolytes

. . . .

PYRAMID TERMS

Fluid volume deficit—Dehydration in which water and electrolytes are lost in the same proportion. The goal of treatment is to restore fluid volume, replace electrolytes as needed, and eliminate the cause of the fluid volume deficit.

Fluid volume excess—An actual excess of total body fluid or a relative fluid excess in one or more fluid compartments. Also called overhydration or fluid overload. The goal of treatment is to restore fluid balance, correct electrolyte imbalances if present, and eliminate or control the underlying cause of the overload.

Homeostasis—The tendency of biological systems to maintain relatively constant conditions in the internal environment while continuously interacting with and adjusting to changes originating within or outside the system.

Hypercalcemia—A high serum calcium level that exceeds 11 mg/dL or 5.5 mEq/L.

Hypocalcemia—A low serum calcium level, below 4.5 mEq/L or below 9 mg/dL.

Hyperkalemia—A high serum potassium level, greater than 5.1 mEq/L.

Hypokalemia—A low serum potassium level, below 3.5 mEq/L, or potassium deficit. Potassium deficit is the most common electrolyte imbalance and is potentially life threatening.

Hypermagnesemia—An increased serum magnesium level above 2.3 mEq/L or 2.6 mg/dL.

Hypomagnesemia—A decreased serum magnesium level of less than 1.5 mEq/L or 1.8 mg/dL.

Hypernatremia—A condition in which the serum sodium concentration is greater than 145 mEq/L.

Hyponatremia—A sodium deficit in which there is too little sodium in the serum, less than 135 mEq/L.

Hyperphosphatemia—A serum phosphate level greater than 4.5 mg/dL or 1.8 mEq/L.

Hypophosphatemia—A serum phosphate level below 3.0 mg/dL or below 1.8 mEq/dL.

Third space losses—A fluid shift from the intravascular space into another part of the body where the fluid is not functional.

PYRAMID TO SUCCESS

Pyramid points focus primarily on data collection related to a fluid and electrolyte imbalance, implementation, and evaluating the expected outcomes. Fluid and electrolytes constitute a content area that is complex and sometimes difficult to understand. It is important to understand cell functions and properties and the concepts related to body fluids as outlined in this chapter. Review this content. Pyramid points focus on the common fluid and electrolyte disturbances. Focus on the pyramid points related to the causes, data collection, and related treatments.

NURSING PROCESS

DATA COLLECTION

Vital signs
Clients at risk
Signs and symptoms
Laboratory results
Health maintenance patterns

PLANNING
Client tolerates measures initiated to maintain normal fluid and electrolyte balance. Client remains free of complications associated with the fluid and electrolyte imbalance. Client describes appropriate health care measures to prevent fluid and electrolyte imbalances.

IMPLEMENTATION
Identify clients at risk for an imbalance. Monitor vital signs. Monitor cardiovascular, respiratory, and neurological status. Monitor for signs and symptoms indicative of a fluid or electrolyte imbalance. Monitor laboratory results. Initiate measures as prescribed to treat the imbalance. Monitor for complications associated with the imbalance or interventions. Monitor for and document the outcomes of interventions. Reinforce client instructions regarding appropriate measures to prevent alterations in fluid and electrolyte balance.

EVALUATION
Fluid and electrolyte values are within normal limits. Client demonstrates compliance with prescribed treatment plan.

◆ CLIENT NEEDS

SAFE, EFFECTIVE CARE ENVIRONMENT

Accident prevention
Asepsis
Standard (Universal) precautions
Handling hazardous and infectious materials

HEALTH PROMOTION AND MAINTENANCE

Health screening and potential risk for a fluid and electrolyte imbalance
Instructions related to medication and diet management
Instructions related to the signs and symptoms of an imbalance
Measures to prevent an imbalance

PSYCHOSOCIAL INTEGRITY

Reassure the client experiencing symptoms related to a fluid and electrolyte imbalance
Provide support and continuously inform the client of the purpose for prescribed interventions

PHYSIOLOGICAL INTEGRITY

Identify clients at risk for a fluid or electrolyte imbalance
Monitor laboratory values
Monitor for complications related to the imbalance
Assist in managing emergencies
Identify the expected and unexpected responses to treatment and document accordingly.

I. Cell Properties (Box 8–1)

II. Concepts of Fluid and Electrolyte Balance

A. Electrolytes
   1. Description: When a substance is dissolved in solution and some of its molecules split or dissociate into electrically charged atoms or ions
   2. Measurement
      a. To measure volume of fluids, the metric system is used and measures liters (L) or milliliters (mL)
      b. The unit of measure that expresses the combining activity of an electrolyte is the milliequivalent (mEq)
B. Body fluid compartments (Box 8–2)
   1. Fluid in each of the body compartments contains electrolytes
   2. Each compartment has a particular composition of electrolytes, which differs from that of other compartments
   3. To function normally, body cells must have fluids and electrolytes
   4. The electrolytes must be in the right compartments in the right amounts
   5. A specific kind and amount of certain

BOX 8–1. Cell Properties

Atom—The smallest part of an element that still has the properties of the element.
   Composed of particles known as the proton (positive charge), neutron (neutral), and electron (negative charge).
   Protons and neutrons are in the nucleus of the atom; therefore, the nucleus is positively charged.
   Electrons carry a negative charge and revolve around the nucleus. As long as the number of electrons is the same as the number of protons, there is no net charge on the atom, that is, it is neither positive nor negative. Atoms may gain, lose, or share electrons and then no longer are neutral.
   Molecule—When two or more atoms combine to form a substance.
   Ion—When an atom carries an electrical charge because it has either gained or lost electrons. Some ions carry a negative electrical charge, and some carry a positive charge.
   Cation—When an ion carries a positive charge and it has given away or lost electrons. The result is fewer electrons than protons and a positive charge.
   Anion—An ion that has gained electrons and therefore carries a negative charge. When an ion has gained or taken on electrons, it assumes a negative charge and the result is a negatively charged ion.

BOX 8–2. Body Fluid Compartments

Intracellular compartment—Refers to all fluid inside the cells. Most of the body fluids are inside the cells.
   Extracellular compartment—Refers to all fluid outside the cells.
   Intravascular compartment—Fluid that is within blood vessels.
   Interstitial fluids—Fluid between the cells and blood vessels

electrolytes must be available for normal cell function

6. Whenever an electrolyte moves out of a cell, another electrolyte moves in to take its place
7. The number of cations and anions must be the same for homeostasis to exist
8. Compartments are separated by semipermeable membranes

C. Body fluid
   1. Description
      a. Provides transportation of nutrients to the cells and carries waste products from the cells
      b. Total body fluid amounts to about 60% of body weight
      c. A loss of 10% of body fluid in the adult is serious
      d. A loss of 20% of the body fluid in the adult is fatal
   2. Constituents of body fluids
      a. Body fluids consist of water and dissolved substances
      b. The largest single fluid constituent of the body is water

D. Body fluid transport
   1. Diffusion
      a. The movement of particles in all directions through a solution
      b. Occurs within fluid compartments and from one compartment to another if the barrier between the compartments is permeable to the diffusing substances
      c. Diffusion of a solute (substance that is dissolved) will spread the molecules from an area of high concentration to an area of lower concentration
      d. A permeable membrane will allow substances to pass through it without restriction
      e. A selectively permeable membrane will allow some solutes to pass through without restriction but will prevent other solutes from passing freely
   2. Osmosis
      a. Osmotic pressure is the force that draws the water from a less concentrated solution through a selectively permeable membrane into a more concentrated solution
      b. If a membrane is permeable to water but not to all the solutes present, it is a selective or semipermeable membrane
      c. When the solvent (solution in which the solute is dissolved) or water moves across this membrane, it is called osmosis
   3. Filtration
      a. Filtration is the movement of solutes and solvents by hydrostatic pressure
      b. Hydrostatic pressure is the force exerted by the weight of a solution
      c. The movement is from an area of greater pressure to an area of lesser pressure

4. Osmolality
   a. Refers to the number of osmotically active particles per kilogram of water
   b. In the body, osmotic pressure is measured in milliosmols
   c. The normal osmolality of plasma is 280 to 294 mOsm/kg
5. Hydrostatic pressure
   a. The force of the fluid pressing outward against some surface
   b. When there is a difference in the hydrostatic pressure on two sides of a membrane, water and diffusible solutes move out of the solution that has the higher hydrostatic pressure by the process of filtration
   c. At the arterial end of the capillary, the hydrostatic pressure is greater than the osmotic pressure; therefore, fluids and diffusible solutes move out of the capillary
   d. At the venous end, the osmotic pressure or pull is greater than the hydrostatic pressure, and fluids and some solutes move into the capillary
   e. The excess fluid and solutes remaining in the interstitial spaces are returned to the intravascular compartment by the lymph channels

E. Movement of body fluid
   1. Description
      a. Cell membranes separate the interstitial fluid from the intravascular fluid
      b. These barriers are selectively permeable, that is, the cell membrane and the capillary wall will allow water and some solutes free passage through them
      c. Several forces affect the movement of water and solutes through the walls of cells and capillaries
      d. The greater the number of particles in the concentrated solution, the more pull there will be to move the water through the membrane
      e. Fluids and electrolytes must be kept in balance for health; when they remain out of balance, death can occur
      f. If the body loses more electrolytes than fluids, as can happen in diarrhea, then the extracellular fluid will contain fewer electrolytes or solutes than the intracellular fluid
   2. Isotonic solutions (Table 8–1)
      a. When the solutions on both sides of a selectively permeable membrane have established equilibrium or are equal in concentration, they are then isotonic
      b. An isotonic solution is isotonic to human cells and thus there will be very little osmosis
   3. Hypotonic solutions (see Table 8–1)
      a. When a solution contains a lower concentration of salt than other solutions, it is hypotonic

Table 8–1. **Tonicity of IV Fluids**

Solution	Tonicity
0.45% saline (½ NS)	Hypotonic
0.9% saline (NS)	Isotonic
5% dextrose in water (5% D/W)	Isotonic
5% dextrose in 0.225% saline (5% D/¼ NS)	Isotonic
Lactated Ringer's solution (RL)	Isotonic
5% dextrose in lactated Ringer's solution	Hypertonic
5% dextrose in 0.45% saline (5% D/½ NS)	Hypertonic
5% dextrose in 0.9% saline (5% D/NS)	Hypertonic
10% dextrose in water (10% D/W)	Hypertonic

b. A hypotonic solution has less salt or more water than an isotonic solution
4. Hypertonic solutions: A solution that has a higher concentration of solutes than another solution (see Table 8–1)
5. Osmotic pressure
   a. The force that draws the solvent from a solution with more solvent activity through a selectively permeable membrane to a solution with less solvent activity
   b. When the solutions on each side of a selectively permeable membrane are equal in concentration, they are isotonic
   c. A hypotonic solution has less solute than an isotonic solution, whereas a hypertonic solution contains more solute
6. Active transport
   a. If an ion is to move through a membrane from an area of low concentration to an area of high concentration, an active transport system is necessary
   b. An active transport system moves molecules or ions uphill against concentration and osmotic pressure
   c. The energy for active transport is supplied by metabolic processes in the cell
   d. Substances that are actively transported through the cell membrane include ions of sodium, potassium, calcium, iron, hydrogen, some of the sugars, and the amino acids
F. Body fluid excretion (Box 8–3)
   1. Description
      a. Fluids leave the body by several routes including the skin, lungs, gastrointestinal (GI) tract, and kidneys
      b. The kidneys excrete the largest quantity of fluid

BOX 8–3. Daily Body Fluid Excretion

Skin by diffusion = 350 mL
Skin by perspiration = 100 mL
Lungs = 350 mL
Feces = 200 mL
Kidneys = 1400 mL

---

c. As long as all organs are functioning normally, the body is able to maintain balance in its fluid content
2. Skin
   a. Water is lost through the skin by diffusion in the amounts of 300 to 400 mL/day
   b. Water is also lost through the skin by perspiration
   c. The amount of water lost by perspiration will vary depending on the temperature of the environment and of the body
   d. Average amount of water lost by perspiration is 100 mL/day
3. Lungs
   a. Water is lost from the lungs through expired air that is saturated with water vapor
   b. The amount of water lost from the lungs will vary with the rate and the depth of respiration
   c. The average amount of water lost from the lungs is 300 to 400 mL/day
   d. Water lost from the lungs and the skin by diffusion is called insensible loss because the individual is unaware of losing that water
4. GI tract
   a. Large quantities of water are secreted into the GI tract, but almost all of this fluid is reabsorbed
   b. The average amount of water lost in the feces is 200 mL/day, equal to the amount of water gained through the oxidation of foods
   c. Severe diarrhea will result in the loss of large quantities of fluids and electrolytes
5. Kidneys
   a. Play a major role in regulating fluid and electrolyte balance
   b. Normal kidneys can adjust the amount of water and electrolytes leaving the body
   c. The usual quantity of urine output is approximately 1400 mL/day; however, this will vary greatly depending on fluid intake, amount of perspiration, and other factors
G. Body fluid replacement
   1. Description: Water enters the body through three sources: oral liquids, water in foods, and water formed by oxidation of foods
   2. Amounts
      a. The average total amount of water taken into the body by all three sources is 2400 mL/day
      b. About 10 mL of water is released by the metabolism of each 100 calories of fat, carbohydrates, or proteins
   3. Electrolytes
      a. Electrolytes are present in both foods and liquids
      b. With a normal diet, an excess of essential electrolytes is taken in and the unused electrolytes are excreted

H. Maintaining fluid and electrolyte balance
   1. Description
      a. **Homeostasis** is a term that indicates the relative stability of the internal environment
      b. Concentration and composition of body fluids must be nearly constant
      c. In the client, when one of the substances, either fluids or electrolytes, is deficient, it must be replaced either normally by the intake of food and water or by therapy such as IVs, and/or medications
      d. When the client has an excess of fluid or electrolytes, therapy is directed toward assisting the body to eliminate the excess
   2. Kidneys: Play a major role in controlling all types of balance in fluid and electrolytes
   3. Adrenal glands: Through the secretion of aldosterone, the adrenal glands also aid in controlling extracellular fluid volume by regulating the amount of sodium reabsorbed by the kidneys
   4. Antidiuretic hormone (ADH): ADH from the pituitary gland regulates the osmotic pressure of extracellular fluid by regulating the amount of water reabsorbed by the kidney

III. Fluid Volume Deficit

A. Description
   1. Dehydration in which water and electrolytes are lost in the same proportion
   2. The goal of treatment is to restore fluid volume, replace electrolytes as needed, and eliminate the cause

B. Causes
   1. Vomiting and/or diarrhea
   2. Continuous GI irrigation
   3. GI suctioning
   4. Ileostomy or colostomy drainage
   5. Draining wounds, burns, or fistulas
   6. Increased urine output from the use of diuretics
C. Data collection
   1. Thirst
   2. Poor skin turgor and dry mucous membranes
   3. Increased heart rate, thready pulse, postural hypotension
   4. Rapid weight loss
   5. Flat neck or hand veins
   6. Dizziness or weakness
   7. Decrease in urine volume and dark, concentrated urine
   8. Increased specific gravity of the urine
   9. Confusion
   10. Increased hematocrit
D. Implementation
   1. Monitor vital signs
   2. Check mucous membranes and skin turgor
   3. Monitor weight daily
   4. Monitor I&O (intake and output)

5. Test urine for specific gravity
6. Monitor hematocrit and electrolyte values
7. Replace fluids by PO, NG, or IV (lactated Ringer's solution, 0.9% normal saline) as prescribed

IV. Fluid Volume Excess

A. Description
   1. An actual excess of total body fluid or a relative fluid excess in one or more fluid compartments
   2. Also called overhydration or fluid overload
   3. The goal of treatment is to restore fluid balance, correct electrolyte imbalances if present, and eliminate or control the underlying cause of the overload
B. Causes
   1. Excessive administration of oral or IV fluids
   2. Excessive irrigation of body cavities such as tap-water enemas
   3. Decreased kidney function
   4. Conditions such as congestive heart failure (CHF), syndrome of inappropriate antidiuretic hormone (SIADH), cirrhosis, and Cushing's syndrome
C. Data collection
   1. Cough and dyspnea
   2. Lung crackles
   3. Increased respirations and heart rate
   4. Increased blood pressure and bounding pulse
   5. Pitting edema
   6. Weight gain
   7. Neck and hand vein distention
   8. Decreased hematocrit
   9. Confusion
D. Implementation
   1. Monitor vital signs
   2. Position client in semi-Fowler's position
   3. Check for edema
   4. Monitor I&O
   5. Monitor weight
   6. Administer diuretics as prescribed
   7. Monitor hematocrit and electrolyte values
   8. Restrict fluids as prescribed
   9. Provide a low-sodium diet as prescribed

V. Hypokalemia (Table 8–2)

A. Description (Box 8–4)
   1. A low serum potassium level below 3.5 mEq/L
   2. Potassium deficit is the most common electrolyte imbalance and is potentially life-threatening
B. Implementation
   1. Monitor vital signs
   2. Monitor neuromuscular activity
   3. Monitor I&O
   4. Check renal function before administering potassium

Table 8–2. Potassium Imbalances

Hypokalemia	*Hyperkalemia*
Causes	*Causes*
Use of nonpotassium-sparing diuretics	Renal failure
Diarrhea	Intestinal obstruction
Vomiting	Cell damage
Inadequate intake of potassium	Excessive oral or parenteral administration of potassium
Excessive gastric suction	Metabolic acidosis
Excessive fistula drainage	Addison's disease
Cushing's syndrome	Excessive use of potassium-based salt substitutes
Chronic use of corticosteroids	Transfusion of stored blood with red blood cell (RBC) release of potassium
Renal disease	
Total parenteral nutrition	
Uncontrolled diabetes	*Signs and Symptoms*
Alkalosis	Muscle weakness
Signs and Symptoms	Paresthesias
Leg and abdominal cramps	Hypotension
Lethargy and weakness	Diarrhea
Shallow respirations and thready pulse	Hyperactive bowel sounds
Confusion	Wide, flat P waves, widened QRS complex, prolonged PR interval, depressed ST segment, and narrow, peaked T waves
Decreased or absent reflexes	
Hypoactive bowel sounds and ileus	
Postural hypotension	
Peaked P waves, flat T waves, depressed ST segment, and U waves	

5. Administer potassium supplements as prescribed (orally or monitor by IV)
6. Oral potassium chloride has an unpleasant taste and should be taken with juice or other desired liquid
7. Oral potassium preparations can cause GI irritation and should not be taken on an empty stomach
8. If the client complains of abdominal pain, distention, nausea, vomiting, diarrhea, or GI bleeding, the oral potassium may need to be discontinued
9. When potassium is added to an IV solution, shake the bag and invert it to ensure that the potassium is evenly distributed

BOX 8–4. Potassium (K)

NORMAL VALUE

3.5 mEq/L to 5.1 mEq/L

POTASSIUM-CONTAINING FOODS

Apricots	Peaches
Avocados	Pork
Bananas	Potatoes
Beef	Prunes
Cantaloupes	Raisins
Carrots	Spinach
Chocolate	Tomatoes
Figs	Veal

10. An IV bolus injection of potassium is never administered, it is always diluted
11. A client receiving more than 10 mEq/hour should be placed on a cardiac monitor, and the infusion should be controlled by an infusion device
12. Monitor for cardiac changes during the administration of potassium
13. Monitor electrolyte values
14. Monitor IV site; if phlebitis or infiltration occurs, the IV should be stopped immediately and restarted at another site
15. Instruct the client not to use salt substitutes containing potassium unless prescribed by a physician

VI. Hyperkalemia (see Table 8–2)

A. Description: A high serum potassium level greater than 5.1 mEq/L (see Box 8–4)
B. Implementation
 1. Monitor vital signs
 2. Monitor for cardiac changes
 3. Decrease potassium intake
 4. Administer potassium excreting diuretics as prescribed
 5. Monitor I&O
 6. Monitor laboratory values
 7. Emergency treatment includes rapid IV administration of dextrose with regular insulin to move excess potassium into the cells
 8. Administer sodium polystyrene sulfonate (Kayexalate) orally or by enema as prescribed, which absorbs the potassium into the GI tract
 9. Monitor for calcium and magnesium loss when using sodium polystyrene sulfonate
 10. Monitor renal function
 11. Prepare for peritoneal or hemodialysis as prescribed
 12. When blood transfusions are prescribed for a client with a potassium imbalance, the client should receive fresh blood if possible because transfusions of stored blood may elevate the potassium level as the breakdown of older blood cells releases potassium
 13. Instruct the client to avoid foods high in potassium
 14. Instruct the client to avoid the use of salt substitutes or other potassium-containing substances

VII. Hyponatremia (Table 8–3)

A. Description: A sodium deficit in which there is too little sodium in the serum, less than 135 mEq/L (Box 8–5)
B. Implementation
 1. Monitor vital signs
 2. Monitor I&O
 3. Monitor weight

Table 8–3. Sodium Imbalances

Hyponatremia	Hypernatremia
Causes	*Causes*
Inadequate sodium intake (NPO, low-sodium diet)	Decreased water intake or excessive loss of water
Gastrointestinal suction	Fever
Excessive intake of water	Excessive perspiration
Irrigation of GI tubes with plain water	Dehydration
Potent diuretics	Hyperventilation
Increased perspiration	Watery diarrhea
Draining skin lesions	Enteral nutrition and TPN deplete the cells of water
Burns	Diabetes insipidus
Nausea and vomiting	Cushing's syndrome
Diabetic ketoacidosis (DKA)	Impaired renal function
SIADH	Use of corticosteroids
Retention of fluid such as with kidney or heart failure	Excessive administration of sodium bicarbonate
Signs and Symptoms	*Signs and Symptoms*
Rapid, thready pulse	Dry mucous membranes
Postural blood pressure changes	Loss of skin turgor
Weakness	Thirst
Abdominal cramping	Flushed skin
Poor skin turgor	Elevated temperature
Muscle twitching and seizures	Oliguria
Mental confusion	Muscle twitching
Apprehension	Fatigue
	Confusion
	Seizures

4. Assess skin turgor and mucous membranes
5. Restrict water intake and avoid tap-water enemas
6. Use normal saline rather than sterile water for irrigation
7. Administer sodium replacement as prescribed and monitor electrolyte values
8. Encourage foods high in sodium
9. If the client is taking lithium, monitor lithium level, as hyponatremia can cause diminished lithium excretion, resulting in toxicity

VIII. Hypernatremia (see Table 8–3)

A. Description: A condition in which the serum

sodium concentration is greater than 145 mEq/L (see Box 8–5)

B. Implementation
   1. Monitor vital signs
   2. Monitor I&O
   3. Monitor electrolyte values
   4. Increase water intake orally
   5. Encourage the client to drink 8 to 10 glasses of water daily
   6. Provide water between meals or tube feedings

IX. Hypocalcemia (Table 8–4)

A. Description: A calcium level below 4.5 mEq/L or below 9 mg/dL (Box 8–6)

B. Implementation
   1. Monitor vital signs
   2. Monitor for the presence of Chvostek's and Trousseau's signs
   3. Provide a quiet environment and avoid overstimulation
   4. Initiate seizure precautions
   5. Administer calcium orally or monitor IV as prescribed

Table 8–4. Calcium Imbalances

Hypocalcemia	Hypercalcemia
Causes	*Causes*
Inadequate dietary intake of calcium	Excessive intake of calcium supplements, milk, and antacids
Increased absorption of calcium from intestinal tract	Products containing calcium
Inadequate vitamin D consumption	Excessive intake of vitamin D
Diarrhea	Increased bone reabsorption or destruction from conditions such as bone tumors, fractures, osteoporosis, immobility
Long-term immobilization and bone demineralization	
Excessive GI losses from diarrhea or wound draining	Decreased excretion of calcium
End-stage renal disease	Renal failure
Calcium-excreting medications such as diuretics, caffeine, anticonvulsants, heparin, laxatives, nicotine	Use of thiazide diuretics
	Hyperparathyroidism
	Use of lithium
	Use of glucocorticoids
Decreased secretion of parathyroid hormone	Adrenal insufficiency
Acute pancreatitis	
Crohn's disease	*Signs and Symptoms*
Excessive administration of blood	Increased heart rate and blood pressure
Signs and Symptoms	Bounding pulse
Tachycardia	Shortened QT interval and widened T wave
Hypotension	Muscle weakness
Paresthesias	Diminished deep tendon reflexes
Twitching	
Cramps	Nausea and vomiting
Tetany	Constipation
Positive Chvostek's or Trousseau's sign	Abdominal distention
Diarrhea	Confusion, lethargy, coma
Hyperactive bowel sounds	
Prolongation of QT interval	

BOX 8–5. Sodium (Na)

NORMAL VALUE

135 to 145 mEq/L

SODIUM-CONTAINING FOODS

Bacon	Crackers
Bouillon cubes	Frankfurters
Bread stuffing mixes	Green olives
Canned crab	Lunch meat
Catsup	Pickles
Cheese	Pretzels
Common table salt	Processed oat cereals
Corn flakes	Processed salad dressings
Corned beef	Soy sauce

BOX 8–6. Calcium (Ca)

NORMAL VALUE
4.5 mEq/L to 5.5 mEq/L or 9 to 11 mg/dL

SOURCES

Almonds	Molasses
Antacids containing calcium salts	Mustard greens
	Oysters
Creamed soups	Rhubarb
Dairy products	Sardines
Kale	Spinach
Macaroni	Turnip greens
Milk	

---

6. Administer vitamin D as prescribed to aid in the absorption of calcium from the intestinal tract
7. Administer calcium supplements 1 to 2 hours after meals to maximize intestinal absorption
8. Keep 10% calcium gluconate available for acute calcium deficit
9. Monitor calcium levels closely after thyroid surgery
10. Instruct the client taking calcium excreting medications to have serum calcium levels checked periodically
11. Teach proper use of antacids or laxatives
12. Instruct the client to consume foods high in calcium

X. Hypercalcemia (see Table 8–4)

A. Description: A serum calcium level that exceeds 11 mg/dL or 5.5 mEq/L (see Box 8–6)
B. Implementation
   1. Monitor vital signs
   2. Monitor for dysrhythmias
   3. Restrict calcium intake
   4. Increase mobility
   5. Assist with passive range of motion exercises when ambulation is not possible
   6. Move clients carefully
   7. Monitor for the development of pathological fractures
   8. Strain urine to check for urinary stones
   9. Monitor for severe flank or abdominal pain
   10. Monitor level of consciousness
   11. Monitor for confusion and neurological changes
   12. Avoid large doses of vitamin D supplements
   13. Avoid the use of thiazide diuretics
   14. Prepare for administration of phosphate as prescribed
   15. Prepare for administration of calcitonin (Calcimar) as prescribed to increase incorporation of calcium into the bones

XI. Hypomagnesemia (Table 8–5)

A. Description: A decreased serum magnesium level of less than 1.5 mEq/L or 1.8 mg/dL (Box 8–7)

Table 8–5. Magnesium Imbalances

Hypomagnesemia	*Hypermagnesemia*
Causes	*Causes*
Malnutrition	Overuse of antacids or laxatives containing magnesium
Diarrhea	
Celiac disease	
Crohn's disease	Renal insufficiency and renal failure
Alcoholism	
Prolonged gastric suctioning	Treatment of toxemia of pregnancy with magnesium
Ileostomy or colostomy, intestinal fistulas	
Acute pancreatitis	
Diabetic ketoacidosis	*Signs and Symptoms*
Eclampsia	Hypotension
Chemotherapy	Bradycardia
Sepsis	Weak pulse
Signs and Symptoms	Sweating and flushing
Twitching	Respiratory depression
Paresthesias	Loss of deep tendon reflexes
Hyperactive reflexes	
Irritability	Peaked T waves, prolonged PR and QT intervals, widened QRS complexes
Confusion	
Positive Chvostek's or Trousseau's sign	
Shallow respirations	
Tetany	
Seizures	
Tachycardia	
Broadening of T waves, shortening of ST segment, prolonged QT interval, and widened QRS	
In severe deficiency, inverted T waves and prominent U waves	

B. Implementation
   1. Monitor vital signs
   2. Monitor for dysrhythmias
   3. Monitor for neuromuscular changes
   4. Monitor I&O
   5. Initiate seizure precautions
   6. Administer magnesium supplements and monitor laboratory values
   7. Monitor serum magnesium levels every 12 to 24 hours when the client is receiving magnesium by IV
   8. Monitor for reduced deep tendon reflexes

BOX 8–7. Magnesium (mg)

NORMAL VALUE
1.5 to 2.3 mEq/L or 1.8 to 2.6 mg/dL

SOURCES

Chocolate	Fish
Dairy products	Green leafy vegetables
Dried fruits	Legumes
Drinking water that has not been processed through a water softener	Meat
	Nuts
	Unprocessed cereal grains

suggesting **hypermagnesemia** during administration of magnesium
   9. Instruct the client to eat food high in magnesium

◆ **XII. Hypermagnesemia** (see Table 8–5)

A. Description: A magnesium level that exceeds 2.3 mEq/L or 2.6 mg/dL (see Box 8–7)
B. Implementation
   1. Monitor vital signs
   2. Monitor for respiratory depression
   3. Monitor for hypotension, bradycardia, and dysrhythmias
   4. Monitor neurological and muscular activity
   5. Monitor level of consciousness
   6. Remove the source of the excess magnesium
   7. Monitor laboratory values
   8. Increase renal excretion by forcing fluids or administering loop diuretics as prescribed
   9. Prepare for the administration of 10% calcium gluconate if serum levels are over 7 mEq/L
   10. Instruct clients regarding avoiding the use of laxatives and antacids containing magnesium

XIII. Hypophosphatemia (Table 8–6)

A. Description: A serum phosphate level below 3.0 mg/dL or below 1.8 mEq/L (Box 8–8)
B. Implementation
   1. Monitor vital signs
   2. Monitor respiratory status
   3. Move the client carefully
   4. Administer phosphate as prescribed

Table 8–6. Phosphorus Imbalances

Hypophosphatemia	Hyperphosphatemia
Causes	*Causes*
Decreased nutritional intake and malnutrition	Excessive dietary intake of phosphorus
Use of magnesium-based or aluminum hydroxide–based antacids	Overuse of phosphate-containing laxatives or enemas
Renal failure	Vitamin D intoxication
Hyperparathyroidism	Hypoparathyroidism
Malignancy	Renal insufficiency
Hypercalcemia	Chemotherapy
Alcohol withdrawal	
Diabetic ketoacidosis	*Signs and Symptoms*
Respiratory alkalosis	Neuromuscular irritability
	Muscle weakness
Signs and Symptoms	Hyperactive reflexes
Confusion	Tetany
Seizures	Positive Chvostek's or Trousseau's sign
Weakness	
Decreased deep tendon reflexes	
Shallow respirations	
Increased bleeding tendency	
Immunosuppression	
Bone pain	

BOX 8–8. Phosphorus (P)

NORMAL VALUE
3.0 to 4.5 mg/dL or 1.8 to 2.6 mEq/L

SOURCES

Almonds	Liver
Barley	Milk
Beef	Oatmeal
Bran	Peanuts
Cheese	Pork
Chocolate	Poultry
Cocoa	Pumpkin
Dried beans and peas	Sardines
Eggs	Soft drinks
Fish	Squash
Legumes	Walnuts
Lentils	Wheat and rye

   5. Check the renal system before administering phosphate
   6. Monitor calcium, phosphorus, sodium, and chloride levels
   7. Administer vitamin D
   8. Monitor for decreased neuromuscular activity
   9. Monitor for calcium excess and kidney stones
   10. Monitor for hematologic changes
   11. Decrease the intake of calcium-rich foods and increase the intake of meats and whole grains that contain phosphorus
   12. Instruct the client regarding the use of antacids

XIV. Hyperphosphatemia (see Table 8–6)

A. Description: A serum phosphate level greater than 4.5 mg/dL or 2.6 mEq/L (see Box 8–8)
B. Implementation
   1. Increase fecal excretion of phosphorus by binding phosphorus from food in the GI tract (aluminum hydroxide gel)
   2. Monitor laboratory values
   3. Prepare for dialysis if prescribed
   4. Monitor for signs of **hypocalcemia**
   5. Administer calcium as prescribed if **hypocalcemia** exists
   6. Monitor neuromuscular irritability
   7. Monitor for hyperreflexia, tetany, and seizures
   8. Monitor for Chvostek's and Trousseau's sign
   9. Instruct clients to avoid phosphate-containing medications, including laxatives and enemas
   10. Instruct clients to decrease their intake of foods high in phosphorus
   11. Instruct clients how to take phosphate-binding medications, emphasizing that these should be taken with meals or immediately after meals

PRACTICE QUESTIONS

1. Normal saline 0.9% 1000 mL IV solution is prescribed for the client. The IV is to run at 100 mL/hour. The nurse prepares the solution understanding that which of the following is not a characteristic of this type of solution?
   1 It's isotonic with the plasma and other body fluids
   2 It's hypotonic with the plasma and other body fluids
   3 It does not affect the plasma osmolarity
   4 It's the same solution as sodium chloride 0.9%

2. The RN tells the LPN that the physician has prescribed a hypotonic IV solution for the client. Which of the following IV solutions does the LPN plan to administer to the client?
   1 0.45% saline (½ NS)
   2 5% dextrose in water (5% D/W)
   3 10% dextrose in water (10% D/W)
   4 5% dextrose in 0.9% saline (5% D/NS)

3. Lactated Ringer's solution (RL) IV is prescribed for the postoperative client. A nursing student is caring for the client. The nursing instructor asks the student about the tonicity of the prescribed IV solution. The student tells the instructor that the solution is
   1 Isotonic
   2 Normotonic
   3 Hypotonic
   4 Hypertonic

4. The nurse is reading the physician's progress notes in the client's record and reads that the physician has documented "insensible fluid loss of approximately 800 mL daily." The nurse understands that this type of fluid loss can occur through
   1 The GI tract
   2 Urinary output
   3 Wound drainage
   4 The skin

5. The nurse is reviewing the health records of assigned clients. The nurse plans care knowing that which of the following clients is least likely at risk for the development of third spacing?
   1 The client with cirrhosis
   2 The client with diabetes mellitus
   3 The client with sepsis
   4 The client with renal failure

6. The nurse is reviewing the health records of assigned clients. The nurse plans care knowing that which of the following clients is at risk for fluid volume deficit?
   1 A client with a colostomy
   2 A client with cirrhosis
   3 A client with congestive heart failure (CHF)
   4 A client with decreased kidney function

7. The nurse is caring for a client who has been taking diuretics on a long-term basis. A fluid volume deficit is suspected. Which of the following findings is noted in the client with this condition?
   1 Rales
   2 Increased blood pressure
   3 Decreased hematocrit
   4 Increased specific gravity of the urine

8. The nurse is caring for a client with a fluid volume excess. Which of the following clients is at risk for fluid volume excess?
   1 The client with renal failure
   2 The client with an ileostomy
   3 The client on diuretics
   4 The client on GI suctioning

9. The nurse is caring for a client with cirrhosis. The nurse notes that the client is dyspneic and crackles are heard on auscultation of the lungs. The nurse suspects fluid volume excess. What additional signs should the nurse expect to note in this client if a fluid volume excess is present?
   1 Flat hand and neck veins
   2 A weak and thready pulse
   3 An increase in blood pressure
   4 An increased urine output

10. The nurse is caring for a client who has been taking diuretics on a long-term basis. The nurse reviews the medication record knowing that which of the following medications, if prescribed for this client, would place the client at risk for hypokalemia?
    1 Spironolactone (Aldactone)
    2 Bumetanide (Bumex)
    3 Triamterene (Dyrenium)
    4 Amiloride HCl (Midamor)

11. The nurse is reviewing the health records of assigned clients. The nurse plans care knowing that which of the following clients is at risk for a potassium deficit?
    1 The client on nasogastric (NG) suction
    2 The client with renal disease
    3 The client with Addison's disease
    4 The client in metabolic acidosis

12. The nurse is told that the client's potassium level is 3.2 mEq/L. Which of the following does the nurse note on the cardiac monitor as a result of the laboratory value?
    1 Elevated T waves
    2 Absent P waves
    3 Elevated ST segment
    4 U waves

13. The nurse is instructing a client how to decrease the intake of magnesium in the diet. The nurse plans to tell the client that which of the following

food items contains the least amount of magnesium?
1 Processed drinking water
2 Nuts
3 Spinach
4 Broccoli

14. The nurse instructs a client at risk for hypokalemia about the foods high in potassium that should be included in the daily diet. The nurse tells the client that which of the following foods provides the least likely source of potassium?
1 Spinach
2 Carrots
3 Apricots
4 Apples

15. The nurse reviews the electrolyte values and notes a potassium level of 5.5 mEq/L. The nurse understands that which of the following clients is at risk for the development of a potassium value at this level?
1 The client who sustained a traumatic burn
2 The client with Cushing's syndrome
3 The client with colitis
4 The client who has been overusing laxatives

16. The nurse reviews the electrolyte results and notes that the potassium level is 5.4 mEq/L. Which of the following does the nurse note on the cardiac monitor as a result of the laboratory value?
1 Narrow peaked T waves
2 Prominent U wave
3 ST elevation
4 Peaked P wave

17. The nurse prepares to administer sodium polystyrene sulfonate (Kayexalate) to the client. Prior to administering the medication, the nurse reviews the action of the medication and understands that it
1 Releases bicarbonate in exchange for primarily sodium ions
2 Releases sodium ions in exchange for primarily bicarbonate ions
3 Releases sodium ions in exchange for primarily potassium ions
4 Releases potassium ions in exchange for primarily sodium ions

18. The nurse reviews the electrolyte values and notes a sodium level of 130 mEq/L. The nurse understands that which of the following clients is at risk for the development of a sodium value at this level?
1 The client with syndrome of inappropriate antidiuretic hormone (SIADH)
2 The client with an inadequate daily water intake
3 The client with watery diarrhea
4 The client with renal disease

19. The nurse is caring for a client with leukemia. When caring for the client, the nurse notes that the client has poor skin turgor and has flat neck and hand veins. The nurse suspects hyponatremia. What additional signs does the nurse expect to note in this client if hyponatremia is present?
1 Dry, sticky mucous membranes
2 Postural blood pressure changes
3 Intense thirst
4 Slow, bounding pulse

20. The nurse is caring for a client with an NG tube. NG tube irrigations are prescribed to be performed once every shift. The serum electrolyte results indicate a potassium level of 4.5 mEq/L and a sodium level of 132 mEq/L. Based on these laboratory findings, which of the following solutions is the most appropriate to use for the NG irrigation?
1 Tap water
2 Distilled water
3 Sterile water
4 Normal saline

21. The clinic nurse reviews the serum sodium level and notes that the client's level is 150 mEq/L. The physician prescribes dietary instructions for the client based on the sodium level. Which of the following foods will the nurse instruct the client to avoid?
1 Spinach
2 Squash
3 Processed oat cereals
4 Molasses

22. The nurse reviews the serum calcium level and notes that the client's level is 4 mEq/L. The nurse understands that which of the following conditions most likely caused this serum calcium level?
1 Prolonged bed rest
2 Excessive administration of vitamin D
3 Renal disease
4 Multiple myeloma

23. The nurse is caring for a client with a suspected diagnosis of hypocalcemia. Which of the following signs is not an indication of this diagnosis?
1 Hypotonicity of the muscles
2 Tingling sensations
3 Hyperactive reflexes
4 Positive Trousseau's sign

24. The nurse is instructing a client how to decrease the intake of calcium in the diet. The nurse plans to tell the client that which of the following food items contains the least amount of calcium?
1 Butter
2 Milk
3 Spinach
4 Turnip greens

25. The nurse is caring for a client with hyperparathyroidism. The serum calcium level is 6.2 mEq/L. Which of the following medications does the nurse plan to administer as prescribed to the client?
    1 Calcium gluconate
    2 Calcium chloride
    3 Calcitonin (Calcimar)
    4 Large doses of vitamin D

26. The nurse is instructing a client how to decrease the intake of potassium in the diet. The nurse plans to tell the client that which of the following foods contains the least amount of potassium?
    1 Potatoes
    2 Apricots
    3 Avocados
    4 Lettuce

27. The nurse is caring for a client with renal failure. The laboratory results reveal a magnesium level of 6 mEq/L. Which of the following signs does the nurse most likely expect to note in the client based on this magnesium level?
    1 Tetany
    2 Muscular excitability
    3 Tremors
    4 Loss of deep tendon reflexes

28. The nurse reviews the serum phosphorus level and notes that the client's level is 1 mEq/dL. The nurse understands that which of the following conditions most likely caused this serum phosphorus level?
    1 Alcoholism
    2 Hypoparathyroidism
    3 Renal failure
    4 Acromegaly

29. The nurse is instructing a client how to decrease the intake of phosphorus in the diet. The nurse plans to tell the client that which of the following foods contains the least amount of phosphorus?
    1 Oranges
    2 Eggs
    3 Beans
    4 Almonds

30. The nurse is caring for a client with renal failure. The serum phosphate level is reported as 7 mg/dL. Which of the following medications does the nurse plan to administer as prescribed to the client?
    1 Calcium gluconate
    2 Calcium chloride
    3 Aluminum hydroxide gel (Amphojel)
    4 Calcitonin (Calcimar)

ANSWERS

1. **2**

RATIONALE: Sodium chloride 0.9% is the same solution as normal saline 0.9%. This solution is isotonic, and isotonic solutions are frequently used for intravenous infusion because they do not affect the plasma osmolarity. A fluid that does not affect the cell size is described as being isotonic with the cells.
TEST-TAKING STRATEGY: Use the process of elimination and knowledge regarding the concepts related to body fluids. If you know that normal saline is the same as sodium chloride, you can eliminate option 4. Note the word "normal" saline. This should provide you with the key that options 1 and 3 are incorrect for this question as stated. Remember "normal" is isotonic and does not affect plasma osmolarity.
LEVEL OF COGNITIVE ABILITY: Comprehension
PHASE OF NURSING PROCESS: Planning
CLIENT NEEDS: Physiological Integrity
CONTENT AREA: Fundamental Skills
REFERENCE
deWit, S. (1998). *Essentials of medical-surgical nursing* (4th ed.). Philadelphia: W. B. Saunders. p. 125.

2. **1**

RATIONALE: 5% dextrose in water (5% D/W) is an isotonic solution; 10% dextrose in water (10% D/W) and 5% dextrose in 0.9% saline (5% D/NS) are hypertonic solutions; 0.45% saline (½ NS) is hypotonic and is probably the only hypotonic solution used in clinical situations. Distilled water is another example of a hypotonic solution. Hypotonic solutions contain a lower concentration of salt or more water than an isotonic solution.
TEST-TAKING STRATEGY: Note the similarities in options 2, 3, and 4. All of these solutions contain dextrose. Option 1 is different than the others. If you had difficulty with this question, take time now to review the tonicity of the various IV solutions.
LEVEL OF COGNITIVE ABILITY: Analysis
PHASE OF NURSING PROCESS: Planning
CLIENT NEEDS: Physiological Integrity
CONTENT AREA: Fundamental Skills
REFERENCE
deWit, S. (1998). *Essentials of medical-surgical nursing* (4th ed.). Philadelphia: W. B. Saunders. p. 125.

3. **1**

RATIONALE: RL is an isotonic solution. Other isotonic solutions include 5% dextrose in water (5% D/W), 0.9% saline (NS), and 5% dextrose in 0.225% saline (5% D/¼ NS); 0.45% saline (½ NS) is hypotonic; 10% dextrose in water (10% D/W) and 5% dextrose in 0.9% saline (5% D/NS) and 5% dextrose in 0.45% saline (5% D/½ NS) are hypertonic solutions.
TEST-TAKING STRATEGY: Knowledge regarding the tonicity of the various IV solutions is required to answer the question. If you had difficulty with this question, take time now to review its content.
LEVEL OF COGNITIVE ABILITY: Comprehension
PHASE OF NURSING PROCESS: Planning
CLIENT NEEDS: Physiological Integrity
CONTENT AREA: Fundamental Skills

REFERENCE
deWit, S. (1998). *Essentials of medical-surgical nursing* (4th ed.). Philadelphia: W. B. Saunders. p. 125.

4. **4**

RATIONALE: Sensible losses are those that the person is aware of, such as through wound drainage, GI tract losses, and urination. Insensible losses may occur without the person's awareness. Insensible losses occur daily through the skin and the lungs.
TEST-TAKING STRATEGY: Using the process of elimination, note the similarity between options 1, 2, and 3 and that the issue of the question is fluid loss. In options 1, 2, and 3 these types of losses can be measured for accurate output. Fluid loss through the skin cannot be accurately measured, only approximated. If you had difficulty with this question, take time now to review the difference between sensible and insensible fluid loss.
LEVEL OF COGNITIVE ABILITY: Comprehension
PHASE OF NURSING PROCESS: Evaluation
CLIENT NEEDS: Physiological Integrity
CONTENT AREA: Fundamental Skills
REFERENCE
Lee, C., Barrett, C., & Ignatavicius, D. (1996). *Fluids and electrolytes: A practical approach* (4th ed.). Philadelphia: F. A. Davis. pp. 8–9.

5. **2**

RATIONALE: Fluid that shifts into the interstitial spaces and remains there is referred to as third space fluid. Common sites for third spacing include the abdomen, pleural cavity, peritoneal cavity, and the pericardial sac. Third space fluid is physiologically useless because it does not circulate to provide nutrients for the cells. Risk factors include clients with liver or kidney disease, major trauma, burns, sepsis, wound healing or major surgery, malignancy, GI malabsorption, malnutrition, and alcoholic or elderly clients.
TEST-TAKING STRATEGY: Use the process of elimination, and note the key words "least likely." Eliminate options 1 and 4 first, as it is likely that fluid balance disturbances will occur with these conditions. From the remaining two options, sepsis is the option that is most acute and therefore is most similar to options 1 and 4, the incorrect options. Take time now to review the risk factors associated with third spacing if you had difficulty with this question.
LEVEL OF COGNITIVE ABILITY: Comprehension
PHASE OF NURSING PROCESS: Planning
CLIENT NEEDS: Physiological Integrity
CONTENT AREA: Fundamental Skills
REFERENCE
deWit, S. (1998). *Essentials of medical-surgical nursing* (4th ed.). Philadelphia: W. B. Saunders. p. 104.

6. **1**

RATIONALE: Causes of a fluid volume deficit include vomiting, diarrhea, conditions that cause increased respirations or increased urinary output, insufficient IV fluid replacement, draining fistulas, or the client with an ileostomy or colostomy. A client with cirrhosis, CHF, or decreased kidney function is at risk for fluid volume excess.
TEST-TAKING STRATEGY: Read the question carefully, noting that it asks for the client at risk for a deficit. Read each option and think about the fluid imbalance that can occur in each. Use the process of elimination. The clients presented in options 2, 3, and 4 retain fluid. The only condition that can cause a deficit is that condition noted in option 1. If you had difficulty with this question, take time now to review the causes of fluid volume deficit.
LEVEL OF COGNITIVE ABILITY: Comprehension
PHASE OF NURSING PROCESS: Planning
CLIENT NEEDS: Physiological Integrity
CONTENT AREA: Fundamental Skills
REFERENCE
deWit, S. (1998). *Essentials of medical-surgical nursing* (4th ed.). Philadelphia: W. B. Saunders. p. 649.

7. **4**

RATIONALE: Findings in a client with a fluid volume deficit include increased respiration and heart rate, decreased central venous pressure (CVP), weight loss, poor skin turgor, dry mucous membranes, decreased urine volume, increased specific gravity of the urine, dark-colored and odorous urine, an increased hematocrit, and altered level of consciousness. The signs in options 1, 2, and 3 are seen in a client with fluid volume excess.
TEST-TAKING STRATEGY: Knowledge regarding the findings in fluid volume deficit is required to answer the question. Eliminate options 1 and 2 first. Rales are noted in fluid volume excess as is an increased BP. Remember that the specific gravity of the urine is increased in a client with a fluid volume deficit. If you had difficulty with this question, take time now to review the findings noted in fluid volume deficit.
LEVEL OF COGNITIVE ABILITY: Comprehension
PHASE OF NURSING PROCESS: Data Collection
CLIENT NEEDS: Physiological Integrity
CONTENT AREA: Fundamental Skills
REFERENCE
Lee, C., Barrett, C. & Ignatavicius, D. (1996). *Fluids and electrolytes: A practical approach* (4th ed.). Philadelphia: F. A. Davis. p. 23.

8. **1**

RATIONALE: The causes of fluid volume excess include decreased kidney function, CHF, cirrhosis, the use of hypotonic fluids to replace isotonic fluid losses, excessive irrigation of body fluids, and the excessive ingestion of table salt. The client with an ileostomy, the client on diuretics, and the client on GI suctioning are at risk for fluid volume deficit.
TEST-TAKING STRATEGY: Read the question carefully, noting that it asks for the client at risk for an excess. Read each option and think about the fluid imbalance that can occur in each. Use the process of elimination. The clients presented in options 2, 3, and 4 lose fluid. The only condition that can cause excess is the condition noted in option 1. If you had difficulty with this question, take time now to review the causes of fluid volume excess.
LEVEL OF COGNITIVE ABILITY: Comprehension
PHASE OF NURSING PROCESS: Data Collection
CLIENT NEEDS: Physiological Integrity
CONTENT AREA: Fundamental Skills
REFERENCE
deWit, S. (1998). *Essentials of medical-surgical nursing* (4th ed.). Philadelphia: W. B. Saunders. p. 726.

9. **3**

RATIONALE: Findings associated with fluid volume excess include cough, dyspnea, crackles, tachypnea, tachycardia, an elevated BP and a bounding pulse, an elevated central venous pressure, weight gain, edema, neck and

hand vein distention, altered level of consciousness, and a decreased hematocrit.
TEST-TAKING STRATEGY: Knowledge regarding the findings in fluid volume excess is required to answer the question. Note the similarities in options 1, 2, and 4. Each of these signs relates to a decrease in fluid volume. Option 3 reflects an increase. If you had difficulty with this question, take time now to review the assessment signs noted in fluid volume excess.
LEVEL OF COGNITIVE ABILITY: Comprehension
PHASE OF NURSING PROCESS: Data Collection
CLIENT NEEDS: Physiological Integrity
CONTENT AREA: Fundamental Skills
REFERENCE
deWit, S. (1998). *Essentials of medical-surgical nursing* (4th ed.). Philadelphia: W. B. Saunders. p. 726.

10. **2**

RATIONALE: Bumetanide (Bumex) is a loop diuretic. The client on this medication is at risk for hypokalemia. Spironolactone, triamterene, and amiloride HCl are potassium-sparing diuretics. Other potassium-sparing diuretics include amiloride HCl and hydrochlorothiazide (Moduretic), spironolactone and hydrochlorothiazide (Aldactazide), and triamterene and hydrochlorothiazide (Dyazide, Maxzide).
TEST-TAKING STRATEGY: Knowledge regarding the diuretics that are in the classification of potassium sparing is required to answer this question. It is important to know which medications are in this classification. Take time now to learn these medications if you had difficulty with this question.
LEVEL OF COGNITIVE ABILITY: Analysis
PHASE OF NURSING PROCESS: Data Collection
CLIENT NEEDS: Physiological Integrity
CONTENT AREA: Pharmacology
REFERENCE
Hodgson, B., & Kizior, R. (1999). *Saunders nursing drug handbook 1999.* Philadelphia: W. B. Saunders. pp. 41, 126, 494, 942, 1021.

11. **1**

RATIONALE: Potassium-rich GI fluids are lost through GI suction, placing the client at risk for hypokalemia. The client with renal disease, Addison's disease, and the client in metabolic acidosis are at risk for hyperkalemia.
TEST-TAKING STRATEGY: Read the question carefully, noting that it asks for the client at risk for hypokalemia. Read each option and think about the electrolyte loss that can occur in each. Option 1 clearly identifies a loss of body fluid. If you had difficulty with this question, take time now to review the causes of hypokalemia.
LEVEL OF COGNITIVE ABILITY: Comprehension
PHASE OF NURSING PROCESS: Planning
CLIENT NEEDS: Physiological Integrity
CONTENT AREA: Fundamental Skills
REFERENCE
deWit, S. (1998). *Essentials of medical-surgical nursing* (4th ed.). Philadelphia: W. B. Saunders. p. 108.

12. **4**

RATIONALE: A serum potassium level below 3.5 mEq/L is indicative of hypokalemia. Potassium deficit is the most common electrolyte imbalance and is potentially life threatening. Cardiac changes include peaked P waves, flat T waves, depressed ST segment, and prominent U waves.
TEST-TAKING STRATEGY: Knowledge of the normal po-

tassium level is required to answer this question. From the information in the question, you need to determine that this condition is a hypokalemic one. From this point, it is necessary to know the cardiac changes that are expected when hypokalemia exists. If you had difficulty with this question, take time now to review the cardiac changes that occur in hypokalemia.
LEVEL OF COGNITIVE ABILITY: Analysis
PHASE OF NURSING PROCESS: Data Collection
CLIENT NEEDS: Physiological Integrity
CONTENT AREA: Fundamental Skills
REFERENCE
deWit, S. (1998). *Essentials of medical-surgical nursing* (4th ed.). Philadelphia: W. B. Saunders. p. 108.

13. **1**

RATIONALE: Drinking water that has not been processed through a water softener is high in magnesium. Nuts, spinach, and broccoli are magnesium-containing foods and should be avoided by the client on a magnesium-restricted diet.
TEST-TAKING STRATEGY: Note the key word "least." Knowledge regarding the foods high in magnesium is required to answer the question. Eliminate options 3 and 4 first because they are similar. Recalling that unprocessed water is high in magnesium will easily direct you to option 1. If you had difficulty with the question, it is important to review the foods that are high in magnesium.
LEVEL OF COGNITIVE ABILITY: Application
PHASE OF NURSING PROCESS: Planning
CLIENT NEEDS: Health Promotion and Maintenance
CONTENT AREA: Fundamental Skills
REFERENCE
Peckenpaugh, N., & Poleman, C. (1999). *Nutrition essentials and diet therapy* (8th ed.). Philadelphia: W. B. Saunders. pp. 90, 104.

14. **4**

RATIONALE: An apple provides approximately 3 mEq of potassium per serving. Spinach and carrots (½ cup cooked) and 4 apricots provide approximately 7 mEq of potassium per serving.
TEST-TAKING STRATEGY: Knowledge regarding the potassium content of foods is required to answer this question. Take the time now to learn the foods that are high and low in potassium if you had difficulty with this question.
LEVEL OF COGNITIVE ABILITY: Application
PHASE OF NURSING PROCESS: Implementation
CLIENT NEEDS: Health Promotion and Maintenance
CONTENT AREA: Fundamental Skills
REFERENCE
Peckenpaugh, N., & Poleman, C. (1999). *Nutrition essentials and diet therapy* (8th ed.). Philadelphia: W. B. Saunders. p. 148.

15. **1**

RATIONALE: A serum potassium level greater than 5.1 mEq/L is indicative of hyperkalemia. Clients who experience cellular shifting of potassium as in the early stages of massive cell destruction, such as in trauma, burns, sepsis, or with metabolic or respiratory acidosis (with the exception of diabetic acidosis), are at risk for hyperkalemia. The client with Cushing's or colitis, and the client who has been overusing laxatives is at risk for hypokalemia.
TEST-TAKING STRATEGY: Eliminate options 3 and 4 first as they are similar, both being reflective of a GI loss. Remembering that cell destruction causes potassium shifts

may assist in directing you to the correct option. Remember that Cushing's presents a risk for hypokalemia and Addison's presents a risk for hyperkalemia. If you had difficulty with this question, take time now to review the risk factors associated with hyperkalemia.
LEVEL OF COGNITIVE ABILITY: Analysis
PHASE OF NURSING PROCESS: Data Collection
CLIENT NEEDS: Physiological Integrity
CONTENT AREA: Fundamental Skills
REFERENCE
deWit, S. (1998). *Essentials of medical-surgical nursing* (4th ed.). Philadelphia: W. B. Saunders. p. 110.

16. 1

RATIONALE: A serum potassium level above 5.4 mEq/L is indicative of hyperkalemia. Cardiac changes include a wide, flat P wave, prolonged PR interval, widened QRS complex, narrow, peaked T waves, and a depressed ST segment.
TEST-TAKING STRATEGY: Knowledge of the normal potassium level is required to answer this question. From the information in the question, you need to determine that this condition is a hyperkalemic one. From this point, it is necessary to know the cardiac changes that are expected when hyperkalemia exists. If you had difficulty with this question, take time now to review the cardiac changes that occur in hyperkalemia.
LEVEL OF COGNITIVE ABILITY: Analysis
PHASE OF NURSING PROCESS: Data Collection
CLIENT NEEDS: Physiological Integrity
CONTENT AREA: Fundamental Skills
REFERENCE
deWit, S. (1998). *Essentials of medical-surgical nursing* (4th ed.). Philadelphia: W. B. Saunders. p. 110.

17. 3

RATIONALE: Sodium polystyrene sulfonate is a cation exchange resin used in the treatment of hyperkalemia. The resin either passes through the intestine or is retained in the colon. It releases sodium ions in exchange for primarily potassium ions. The therapeutic effect occurs 2 to 12 hours after oral administration and longer after rectal administration.
TEST-TAKING STRATEGY: Knowledge regarding this medication is required to answer the question. Looking at the name of the medication (Kayexalate) closely may provide you with assistance regarding the action of the medication. If you had difficulty with this medication, take time now to review the action of this very important medication.
LEVEL OF COGNITIVE ABILITY: Comprehension
PHASE OF NURSING PROCESS: Planning
CLIENT NEEDS: Physiological Integrity
CONTENT AREA: Pharmacology
REFERENCE
Hodgson, B., & Kizior, R. (1999). *Saunders nursing drug handbook 1999.* Philadelphia: W. B. Saunders. p. 935.

18. 1

RATIONALE: Hyponatremia is evidenced by a serum sodium level of less than 135 mEq/L. Hyponatremia can result secondary to SIADH. The client with an inadequate daily water intake, watery diarrhea, or with renal disease is at risk for hypernatremia.

TEST-TAKING STRATEGY: Knowledge regarding the normal sodium levels and the causes of hyponatremia is required to answer the question. Take time now to review the normal laboratory value and the causes of hyponatremia if you had difficulty with this question.
LEVEL OF COGNITIVE ABILITY: Analysis
PHASE OF NURSING PROCESS: Data Collection
CLIENT NEEDS: Physiological Integrity
CONTENT AREA: Fundamental Skills
REFERENCE
deWit, S. (1998). *Essentials of medical-surgical nursing* (4th ed.). Philadelphia: W. B. Saunders. p. 107.

19. 2

RATIONALE: Postural blood pressure changes occur in the client with hyponatremia. Dry sticky mucous membranes and intense thirst are seen in clients with hypernatremia. A slow, bounding pulse is not indicative of hyponatremia. In hyponatremia, a rapid, thready pulse is noted.
TEST-TAKING STRATEGY: Knowledge regarding the signs of hyponatremia is helpful in answering the question. Note the information provided in the question. If the client has poor skin turgor, then the client is unlikely to have dry sticky mucous membranes. Eliminate option 3 next as it is similar to option 1. A client with dry, sticky mucous membranes is likely to have intense thirst. From this point, you need to rely on your knowledge to assist in selecting the correct option. If you have difficulty with this, take time now to review the assessment signs associated with hyponatremia.
LEVEL OF COGNITIVE ABILITY: Comprehension
PHASE OF NURSING PROCESS: Data Collection
CLIENT NEEDS: Physiological Integrity
CONTENT AREA: Fundamental Skills
REFERENCE
deWit, S. (1998). *Essentials of medical-surgical nursing* (4th ed.). Philadelphia: W. B. Saunders. p. 107.

20. 4

RATIONALE: A potassium level of 4.5 mEq/L is within normal range. A sodium level of 132 mEq/L is low, indicating hyponatremia. In clients with hyponatremia, normal (isotonic) saline should be used rather than sterile water for GI or urinary tract irrigations.
TEST-TAKING STRATEGY: Use the process of elimination. Note that sterile water, distilled water, and tap water are similar. The only option that is different is option 4. If you had difficulty with this question, take time now to review the care to the client experiencing hyponatremia.
LEVEL OF COGNITIVE ABILITY: Comprehension
PHASE OF NURSING PROCESS: Implementation
CLIENT NEEDS: Physiological Integrity
CONTENT AREA: Fundamental Skills
REFERENCE
Lee, C., Barrett, C., & Ignatavicius, D. (1996). *Fluids and electrolytes: A practical approach* (4th ed.). Philadelphia: F. A. Davis. p. 80.

21. 3

RATIONALE: The normal serum sodium level is 135 to 145 mEq/L. A serum sodium level of 150 mEq/L is indicative of hypernatremia. Based on this finding, the nurse instructs the client to avoid foods high in sodium. Spinach and molasses are good food sources of calcium. Squash is high in phosphorus.

TEST-TAKING STRATEGY: Note the key word "avoid." Knowledge regarding the normal serum sodium level is required to answer this question. After determining that the client has hypernatremia, determining the food to avoid is the issue. Elimination options 1 and 2 first because these are basically very healthy foods. From the remaining two options, note the word "processed" in option 3. Processed foods tend to be higher in sodium content. This is the food to avoid. Take time now to review foods high in sodium content if you had difficulty with this question.
LEVEL OF COGNITIVE ABILITY: Analysis
PHASE OF NURSING PROCESS: Planning
CLIENT NEEDS: Health Promotion and Maintenance
CONTENT AREA: Fundamental Skills
REFERENCE
Peckenpaugh, N., & Poleman, C. (1999). *Nutrition essentials and diet therapy* (8th ed.). Philadelphia: W. B. Saunders. pp. 146–147.

22. **1**

RATIONALE: The normal serum calcium level is 4.5 mEq/L to 5.5 mEq/L or 9 to 11 mg/dL. A client with a serum calcium level of 4.0 mEq/L is experiencing hypocalcemia. The excessive administration of vitamin D, renal disease, and multiple myeloma are causative factors associated with hypercalcemia. Although immobilization can initially cause hypercalcemia, the long-term effect of prolonged bed rest is hypocalcemia.
TEST-TAKING STRATEGY: Knowledge regarding the normal serum calcium level will assist in determining that the client is experiencing hypocalcemia. This should help to eliminate option 2. Knowledge regarding the causative factors associated with hypocalcemia is necessary to select the correct answer from the remaining options. If you had difficulty with this question, take time now to review the causative factors associated with hypocalcemia.
LEVEL OF COGNITIVE ABILITY: Comprehension
PHASE OF NURSING PROCESS: Data Collection
CLIENT NEEDS: Physiological Integrity
CONTENT AREA: Fundamental Skills
REFERENCE
deWit, S. (1998). *Essentials of medical-surgical nursing* (4th ed.). Philadelphia: W. B. Saunders. pp. 108–109.

23. **1**

RATIONALE: Hypotonicity of the muscles is seen in hypercalcemia. Signs of hypocalcemia include tingling sensations, hyperactive reflexes, and a positive Chvostek's or Trousseau's sign. Additional signs of hypocalcemia include increased neuromuscular excitability, muscle cramps, tetany, seizures, insomnia, irritability, memory impairment, and anxiety.
TEST-TAKING STRATEGY: Note the key word "not." Use the process of elimination, noting that options 2, 3, and 4 are similar in that they all reflect a hyperactivity of the neuromuscular system. The option that is different is option 1. Take time now to review the assessment signs noted in hypocalcemia if you had difficulty with this question.
LEVEL OF COGNITIVE ABILITY: Comprehension
PHASE OF NURSING PROCESS: Data Collection
CLIENT NEEDS: Physiological Integrity
CONTENT AREA: Fundamental Skills
REFERENCE
deWit, S. (1998). *Essentials of medical-surgical nursing* (4th ed.). Philadelphia: W. B. Saunders. pp. 108–109.

24. **1**

RATIONALE: Butter comes from milk fat and does not contain significant amounts of calcium. Milk, spinach, and turnip greens are calcium-containing foods and should be avoided by the client on a calcium-restricted diet.
TEST-TAKING STRATEGY: Note the key word "least." Knowledge regarding the foods high in calcium is required to answer the question. Option 2 can be easily eliminated. Eliminate options 3 and 4 next because they are similar. If you had difficulty with the question, it is important to review the foods that are high in calcium.
LEVEL OF COGNITIVE ABILITY: Application
PHASE OF NURSING PROCESS: Planning
CLIENT NEEDS: Health Promotion and Maintenance
CONTENT AREA: Fundamental Skills
REFERENCE
Peckenpaugh, N., & Poleman, C. (1999). *Nutrition essentials and diet therapy* (8th ed.). Philadelphia: W. B. Saunders. pp. 90, 104.

25. **3**

RATIONALE: The normal serum calcium level is 4.5 mEq/L to 5.5 mEq/L or 9 to 11 mg/dL. This client is experiencing hypercalcemia. Calcium gluconate and calcium chloride are medications used in the treatment of tetany that occurs from acute hypocalcemia. In hypercalcemia, large doses of vitamin D need to be avoided. Calcitonin, a thyroid hormone, decreases the plasma calcium level by increasing the incorporation of calcium into the bones, thus keeping it out of the serum.
TEST-TAKING STRATEGY: Knowledge regarding the normal serum calcium level will assist in determining that the client is experiencing hypercalcemia. With this knowledge, you can easily eliminate options 1 and 2 because you would not administer medication that adds calcium to the body. Remembering that excessive vitamin D is a causative factor of hypercalcemia will assist in eliminating option 4, leaving option 3 as the correct choice. If you had difficulty with this question, take time now to review the treatment for hypercalcemia.
LEVEL OF COGNITIVE ABILITY: Comprehension
PHASE OF NURSING PROCESS: Planning
CLIENT NEEDS: Physiological Integrity
CONTENT AREA: Pharmacology
REFERENCE
deWit, S. (1998). *Essentials of medical-surgical nursing* (4th ed.). Philadelphia: W. B. Saunders. p. 108.

26. **4**

RATIONALE: Lettuce contains less than 100 mg of potassium. Potatoes, apricots, and avocados are potassium-containing foods and should be avoided by the client on a potassium-restricted diet.
TEST-TAKING STRATEGY: Note the key word "least." Knowledge regarding the foods high in potassium is required to answer the question. The question asks for the food that contains the least amount of potassium. If you had difficulty with the question, it is important to review the foods that are high in potassium.
LEVEL OF COGNITIVE ABILITY: Application
PHASE OF NURSING PROCESS: Planning
CLIENT NEEDS: Health Promotion and Maintenance
CONTENT AREA: Fundamental Skills

REFERENCE
Peckenpaugh, N., & Poleman, C. (1999). *Nutrition essentials and diet therapy* (8th ed.). Philadelphia: W. B. Saunders. p. 238.

27. **4**

RATIONALE: The normal magnesium level is 1.5 to 2.3 mEq/L or 1.8 to 2.6 mg/dL. A client with a magnesium level of 6.0 mEq/L is experiencing hypermagnesemia. Signs include neurologic depression, drowsiness and lethargy, loss of deep tendon reflexes, respiratory paralysis, and loss of consciousness. Tetany, muscular excitability, and tremors are seen in a client with hypomagnesemia.
TEST-TAKING STRATEGY: Knowledge regarding the normal magnesium level and the associated signs related to an imbalance is helpful in answering the question. Use the process of elimination, noting that options 1, 2, and 3 are similar in that they reflect neurological excitability. If you had difficulty with this question, take time now to review the assessment signs found in magnesium imbalances.
LEVEL OF COGNITIVE ABILITY: Analysis
PHASE OF NURSING PROCESS: Data Collection
CLIENT NEEDS: Physiological Integrity
CONTENT AREA: Fundamental Skills
REFERENCE
deWit, S. (1998). *Essentials of medical-surgical nursing* (4th ed.). Philadelphia: W. B. Saunders. p. 110.

28. **1**

RATIONALE: The normal serum phosphorus level is 3.0 to 4.5 mg/dL or 1.8 to 2.6 mEq/L. The client in this question is experiencing hypophosphatemia. Causative factors relate to low or decreased nutritional intake, poor absorption from the bowel, or malabsorption syndrome. A poor nutritional state is associated with alcoholism. Hypoparathyroidism, renal failure, and acromegaly are causative factors of hyperphosphatemia.
TEST-TAKING STRATEGY: Knowledge regarding the normal phosphorus level is required to determine the condition that this client is experiencing. From this point, it is necessary to know the causes of hypophosphatemia. If you had difficulty with this question, take time now to review the causative factors associated with hypophosphatemia.
LEVEL OF COGNITIVE ABILITY: Analysis
PHASE OF NURSING PROCESS: Data Collection
CLIENT NEEDS: Physiological Integrity
CONTENT AREA: Fundamental Skills
REFERENCE
deWit, S. (1998). *Essentials of medical-surgical nursing* (4th ed.). Philadelphia: W. B. Saunders. p. 111.

29. **1**

RATIONALE: An orange contains 18 mg of phosphorus. One egg contains 86 mg, beans (½ cup) 137 mg, and almonds (¼ cup) 184 mg of phosphorus.
TEST-TAKING STRATEGY: Note the key word "least." Knowledge regarding the foods high in phosphorus is required to answer the question. The question asks for the food that contains the least amount of phosphorus. If you had difficulty with this question, it is important to review the foods that are high in phosphorus.
LEVEL OF COGNITIVE ABILITY: Application
PHASE OF NURSING PROCESS: Planning
CLIENT NEEDS: Health Promotion and Maintenance
CONTENT AREA: Fundamental Skills
REFERENCE
Peckenpaugh, N., & Poleman, C. (1999). *Nutrition essentials and diet therapy* (8th ed.). Philadelphia: W. B. Saunders. p. 147.

30. **3**

RATIONALE: The normal serum phosphate level is 3.0 to 4.5 mg/dL or 1.8 to 2.6 mEq/L. The client in this question is experiencing hyperphosphatemia. Certain medications can be given to increase fecal excretion of phosphorus by binding phosphorus from the food in the GI tract. Aluminum hydroxide gel is one such medication. Calcium gluconate and calcium chloride are medications used in the treatment of tetany that occurs from acute hypocalcemia. Calcitonin, a thyroid hormone, decreases the plasma calcium level by increasing the incorporation of calcium into the bones, thus keeping it out of the serum.
TEST-TAKING STRATEGY: Use the process of elimination in answering the question. Note the similarity in options 1, 2, and 4. All relate to calcium in some way. Option 3 is the one that is different. If you had difficulty with this question, take time now to review the treatments associated with phosphorus imbalances.
LEVEL OF COGNITIVE ABILITY: Comprehension
PHASE OF NURSING PROCESS: Planning
CLIENT NEEDS: Physiological Integrity
CONTENT AREA: Pharmacology
REFERENCE
Lee, C., Barrett, C., & Ignatavicius, D. (1996). *Fluids and electrolytes: A practical approach* (4th ed.). Philadelphia: F. A. Davis. p. 120.

BIBLIOGRAPHY

deWit, S. (1998). *Essentials of medical-surgical nursing* (4th ed.). Philadelphia: W. B. Saunders.
Hodgson, B., & Kizior, R. (1999). *Saunders nursing drug handbook 1999.* Philadelphia: W. B. Saunders.
Leahy, J., & Kizilay, P. (1998). *Foundations of nursing practice: A nursing process approach.* Philadelphia: W. B. Saunders.

Luckmann, J. (1997). *Saunders manual of nursing care.* Philadelphia: W. B. Saunders.
Lee, C., Barrett, C., & Ignatavicius, D. (1996). *Fluids and electrolytes: A practical approach* (4th ed.). Philadelphia: F. A. Davis.
National Council of State Boards of Nursing. (1998). *National Council Detailed Test Plan for the NCLEX-PN Examination.* Chicago: Author.
Peckenpaugh, N., & Poleman, C. (1999). *Nutrition essentials and diet therapy* (8th ed.). Philadelphia: W. B. Saunders.

CHAPTER 9

Acid-Base Balance

. . . .

PYRAMID TERMS

Allen's Test—Testing for collateral circulation to the hand before performing an arterial puncture in the radial artery.

Metabolic Acidosis—The total concentration of buffer base is lower than normal, with a relative increase in the H^+ concentration. It occurs as a result of losing buffer bases or retaining too many acids without sufficient bases. It occurs in conditions such as renal failure, diabetic ketoacidosis, and production of lactic acid, and from the ingestion of toxins, such as aspirin.

Metabolic Alkalosis—A deficit or loss of H^+ or acids or an excess of base (bicarbonate). It results from the accumulation of base or from a loss of acid without a comparable loss of base in the body fluids. It is caused by conditions resulting in hypovolemia, from the loss of gastric fluid, or excessive bicarbonate intake.

Respiratory Acidosis—The total concentration of buffer base is lower than normal with a relative increasing hydrogen ion (H^+) concentration, thus a greater number of H^+ are circulating in the blood than can be absorbed by the buffer system. Caused by primary defects in the function of the lungs or by changes in normal respiratory patterns due to secondary problems. Any condition that causes an obstruction of the airway or depresses respiratory status can cause respiratory acidosis.

Respiratory Alkalosis—A deficit of carbonic acid (H_2CO_3) or a decrease in H^+ concentration. It results from the accumulation of base or from a loss of acid without a comparable loss of base in the body fluids. It is caused by conditions that cause overstimulation of the respiratory status.

◆ PYRAMID TO SUCCESS

Acid-base imbalance is a content area that is sometimes viewed as complex to understand. It is important to understand the description of each imbalance and then review the causes of each disorder, correlating the pathophysiology to each cause. From this point, note the signs and symptoms related to each disorder and the treatment associated with the clinical manifestations.

NURSING PROCESS

DATA COLLECTION

Preexisting conditions
Vital signs
Respiratory status
Restlessness
Mental status changes
Nausea, vomiting, or diarrhea
Fruity-smelling breath due to improper fat metabolism
Diaphoresis
Cyanosis

Headache
Light-headedness
Visual disturbances
Paresthesias
Tetany
Convulsions
Cardiac changes
Abnormal electrolyte or blood gas values

PLANNING

Client will maintain a patent airway. Client requests breathing assistance when needed. Client maintains an adequate fluid balance. Client remains free from injury. Client is oriented to person, time, and place. Client demonstrates anxiety-reducing techniques.

IMPLEMENTATION

Monitor vital signs. Monitor for signs of respiratory distress. Administer oxygen as prescribed. Assist with breathing techniques and breathing aids as prescribed. Educate and encourage appropriate breathing patterns. Use caution when caring for ventilator clients so that the client is not forced to take breaths too deeply or rapidly. Monitor level of consciousness (LOC). Provide emotional support and reassurance to the client. Monitor laboratory values. Maintain I&O. Initiate safety precautions.

EVALUATION

Vital signs are within normal limits. Breathing patterns are effective. Client performs breathing techniques appropriately. Client remains oriented. Laboratory values are within normal range. Client remains free of injury. Anxiety is reduced.

◆ CLIENT NEEDS

SAFE, EFFECTIVE CARE ENVIRONMENT

Invasive procedures, such as arterial blood gas specimens or treatments, related to the various acid-base imbalances

Asepsis, standard (universal) precautions

Providing safety to the client when implementing various treatments for the acid-base disorders

HEALTH PROMOTION AND MAINTENANCE

Identify those clients at risk for an acid-base disturbance

Reinforce instructions to the client and family about the prevention, early detection, and treatment measures for health disorders

PSYCHOSOCIAL INTEGRITY

Provide emotional support to the client and to the family

Support systems

PHYSIOLOGICAL INTEGRITY

Identify clients at risk for an acid-base disturbance

Reduce the likelihood that an alteration will occur

Monitor for changes in status and complications

Administer and monitor medications, IV fluids, and other prescribed therapies

Document the expected and unexpected responses to the therapy

Assist with obtaining arterial blood gases

Provide wound care when blood is obtained for a blood gas determination

Assist with determining the results from an arterial blood gas study

I. Hydrogen Ions, Acids, and Bases

A. Hydrogen ions (H$^+$)
   1. Vital to life
   2. Expressed as pH
   3. pH of body fluid is normally alkaline (between 7.35 and 7.45)
B. Acids
   1. Produced as end products of metabolism
   2. Contain hydrogen ions
   3. Hydrogen ion donors, which means that acids give up H$^+$ to neutralize or decrease the strength of an acid or to form a weaker base
   4. The number of hydrogen ions in body fluid determines its acidity, alkalinity, or if it is neutral

C. Bases
   1. Contain no H$^+$
   2. Hydrogen ion acceptors
   3. Accept H$^+$ from acids to neutralize or decrease the strength of a base or to form a weaker acid

II. Regulatory Systems for H$^+$ Concentration in the Blood

A. Buffers
   1. The fastest-acting regulatory system
   2. Provide immediate protection against changes in H$^+$ concentration in the extracellular fluid
   3. Serve as a transport mechanism that carries excess H$^+$ to the lungs
   4. Once the primary buffer systems react, they are consumed, and this leaves the body less able to withstand further stress until they are replaced
B. Primary buffer systems in extracellular fluid
   1. Hemoglobin (Hgb) system
      a. In the red blood cells (RBCs)
      b. Maintains acid-base balance by a process called chloride shift
      c. Chloride shifts in and out of the cells in response to the level of oxygen (O$_2$) in the blood
   2. Plasma protein system
      a. Functions in conjunction with the liver to vary the amount of H$^+$ in the chemical structure of protein
      b. Plasma proteins have the ability to attract or release H$^+$
   3. Carbonic acid/bicarbonate system
      a. Maintains a pH of 7.4 with a ratio of 20 parts bicarbonate to 1 part carbonic acid (20:1)
      b. This ratio (20:1) determines H$^+$ concentration of body fluid
      c. Carbonic acid concentration is controlled by the excretion of CO$_2$ by the lungs; the rate and depth of respiration changes are the response to changes in CO$_2$
      d. Bicarbonate concentration is controlled by the kidneys, which selectively retain or secrete bicarbonates in response to the body needs
   4. Phosphate buffer system
      a. Present in the cells and body fluids

b. Especially active in the kidneys
c. Acts like bicarbonate and clears spare H^+

C. Lungs
1. Body's second defense that interacts with the buffer system to maintain acid-base balance
2. In acidosis, the pH goes down and the respiratory rate and depth go up in an attempt to blow off acids; the carbonic acid created by the neutralizing action of bicarbonate can be carried to the lungs, where it is reduced to CO_2 and water and exhaled, thus H^+ are inactivated and excreted
3. In alkalosis, the pH goes up and the respiratory rate and depth go down; the CO_2 is retained, and the carbonic acid builds to neutralize and decrease the strength of excess bicarbonate
4. The action of the lungs is reversible in controlling an excess or deficit
5. The lungs can hold H^+ until the deficit is corrected or can inactivate H^+, changing them to water molecules to be exhaled as CO_2, thus correcting the excess
6. The lungs are capable of inactivating only H^+ carried by carbonic acid (H_2CO_3); excess H^+ created by other problems must be excreted by the kidneys

D. Kidneys
1. The ultimate correction of acid-base disturbances is dependent on the kidneys, even though the renal excretion of acids and alkali occurs more slowly
2. Compensation requires a few hours to several days; however, it is more thorough and selective than that of other regulators
3. In acidosis, the pH goes down, and excess H^+ are secreted into the tubules and combine with buffers for excretion in the urine
4. In alkalosis, the pH goes up, and bicarbonate ions move into the tubules, combine with sodium, and are excreted in the urine
5. Selective regulation of bicarbonate in the kidneys
   a. The kidneys restore bicarbonate by the release of H^+ and holding bicarbonate ions
   b. Extra H^+ are excreted in the urine in the form of phosphoric acid
   c. The alteration of certain amino acids in the renal tubules results in a diffusion of ammonia into the kidneys, and the ammonia combines with extra H^+ and is excreted in the urine

E. Potassium
1. Plays an exchange role in maintaining acid-base balance
2. The body changes the potassium (K) level by drawing H^+ into the cell or by pushing them out of the cell
3. In acidosis, the body protects itself from the acid state by moving H^+ into the cell; therefore, K moves out to make room for H^+; the K level goes up

4. In alkalosis, the cells release H^+ into the blood in an attempt to increase the acidity of the blood and combat alkalinity; the K moves into the cells and the K level goes down

III. Respiratory Acidosis

A. Description: The total concentration of buffer base is lower than normal, with a relative increasing H^+ concentration; thus, a greater number of H^+ are circulating in the blood than can be absorbed by the buffer system

B. Causes
1. Due to primary defects in the function of the lungs or by changes in normal respiratory patterns from secondary problems
2. Remember that any condition that causes an obstruction of the airway or depresses respiratory status can cause **respiratory acidosis**
3. Hypoventilation
4. Chronic obstructive pulmonary disease (COPD)
5. Pulmonary edema
6. Pneumonia
7. Atelectasis
8. Asthma
9. Bronchitis or bronchiectasis
10. Infection
11. Medications such as sedatives, narcotics, or anesthetics
12. Brain trauma

C. Data collection
1. In an attempt to compensate, the respiratory rate and depth increase
2. pH less than 7.35 and pCO_2 greater than 45 mmHg
3. Mental status changes such as confusion
4. Drowsiness
5. Restlessness
6. Weakness
7. Dizziness
8. Dyspnea
9. Hyperkalemia

D. Implementation
1. Maintain patent airway
2. Monitor for signs of respiratory distress
3. Administer oxygen as prescribed
4. Place the client in semi-Fowler's position unless contraindicated
5. Encourage and assist the client to turn, cough, and deep breathe
6. Prepare to administer chest physiotherapy and postural drainage as prescribed
7. Encourage hydration to thin secretions unless excess fluid intake is contraindicated
8. Suction the client as necessary
9. Monitor electrolyte values
10. Avoid the use of tranquilizers, narcotics, and hypnotics because they further depress respirations

11. Administer antibiotics for infection as prescribed

IV. Respiratory Alkalosis

A. Description: A deficit of H_2CO_3 and a decrease in H^+ concentration; results from the accumulation of base or from a loss of acid without a comparable loss of base in the body fluids

B. Causes
1. Due to conditions that cause overstimulation of the respiratory status
2. Hyperventilation
3. Hypoxemia
4. Fever
5. Early stages of salicylate poisoning
6. Reactions to certain medications
7. Pain
8. Anxiety
9. Hysteria

C. Data collection
1. Initially the hyperventilation and respiratory stimulation will cause abnormal rapid and deep respirations (tachypnea); in an attempt to compensate, respiratory rate and depth then go down
2. pH is greater than 7.45 and pCO_2 is less than 35 mmHg
3. Mental status changes
4. Pallor around the mouth
5. Tingling of the fingers
6. Dizziness
7. Spasms of the muscles of the hands
8. Hypokalemia

D. Implementation
1. Maintain a patent airway
2. Provide emotional support and reassurance to the client
3. Encourage appropriate breathing patterns
4. Provide cautious care with ventilator clients so that the client is not forced to take breaths too deeply or rapidly
5. Monitor electrolyte values
6. Administer sedatives as prescribed

V. Metabolic Acidosis

A. Description: The total concentration of buffer base is lower than normal, with a relative increase in the H^+ concentration; occurs as a result of losing too many bases and holding too many acids without sufficient bases

B. Causes
1. Excessive burning of fats such as occurs in the diabetic client or in the client who is on a low-carbohydrate, high-protein diet to lose weight
2. Abnormal carbohydrate metabolism in which, in the absence of oxygen, lactic acid accumulates in the blood
3. Failure of the kidneys to reabsorb bicarbonate
4. Severe diarrhea: Intestinal and pancreatic

secretions are normally alkaline; therefore, excessive loss of base leads to acidosis
5. Malnutrition

C. Data collection
1. In an attempt to blow off the extra CO_2 and compensate for the acidosis, hyperpnea with Kussmaul's respirations occurs
2. pH less than 7.35 and a HCO_3 less than 22 mEq/L
3. Headache
4. Weakness
5. Malaise
6. Fruity-smelling breath
7. Hyperkalemia
8. Stupor, unconsciousness, coma, and death, if acidosis is not resolved

D. Implementation
1. Based on the cause of the acidosis
2. Maintain a patent airway
3. Prepare for the administration of IV bicarbonate or lactate
4. Monitor electrolyte values
5. Initiate safety precautions
6. Frequent mouth care using an alkaline mouthwash such as baking soda
7. Monitor the K level very closely; when acidosis is being treated, K will move back into the cell and the blood level will drop

E. Implementation in diabetes/diabetic ketoacidosis: Insulin is given to hasten the movement of serum glucose into the cell, thereby decreasing the concurrent ketosis

F. Implementation in renal failure: Dialysis may be used to remove protein and waste products, thereby lessening the acidotic state

VI. Metabolic Alkalosis

A. Description: A deficit of H_2CO_3 and a decrease in hydrogen ion concentration; results from the accumulation of base or from a loss of acid without a comparable loss of base in the body fluids

B. Causes
1. Hypokalemia
2. Vomiting
3. Gastric suction
4. Intestinal fistulas
5. Diuretics
6. Steroid therapy

C. Data collection
1. In an attempt to compensate, respiratory rate and depth go down to conserve carbon dioxide (CO_2)
2. Slow, shallow respirations
3. Decreased chest movements
4. Cyanosis
5. Irritability
6. Disorientation
7. Lethargy
8. Convulsions
9. Hypokalemia
10. Hypocalcemia

BOX 9–1. Normal Blood Gas Values

pH 7.35–7.45
PCO_2 35–45 mmHg
HCO_3 22–27 mEq/L
PO_2 80–100 mmHg

D. Implementation
1. Maintain a patent airway
2. Monitor vital signs
3. Monitor I&O
4. Monitor electrolyte values
5. Institute safety precautions
6. Prepare to replace K and calcium as prescribed
7. Prepare to administer medications as prescribed to promote the kidneys' excretion of bicarbonate
8. Prepare to administer acidifying solutions as prescribed

VII. Arterial Blood Gases (Box 9–1)

A. Description: Reflect the ability of the lungs to exchange oxygen and carbon dioxide, the effectiveness of the kidneys in balancing retention and elimination of bicarbonate, and the effectiveness of the heart as a pump
B. Obtaining an arterial blood gas specimen
1. Obtain vital signs
2. Perform **Allen's test** to determine the presence of collateral circulation (Box 9–2)
3. Identify factors that may affect the accuracy of the results, such as changes in the O_2 settings on respiratory-assistive devices, suctioning within the last 20 minutes, and client activities
4. Assist with the specimen draw by preparing a heparinized syringe
5. Provide emotional support to the client
6. Apply pressure immediately to the puncture site for 5 minutes, and for 10 minutes if the client is taking anticoagulants
7. Appropriately label the specimen and transport on ice to the laboratory
8. Record the client's temperature and the type of supplemental oxygen that the client is receiving on the laboratory form
C. Respiratory Imbalances (Box 9–3)

BOX 9–2. Performing Allen's Test

Ask client to make a tight fist
Apply direct pressure over the client's ulnar and radial arteries
While pressure is applied, ask the client to open the hand
Remove pressure from the ulnar artery and assess the color of the extremity distal to the pressure point

BOX 9–3. Analyzing Arterial Blood Gas Results

If you can remember the following pyramid points and steps, you will be able to analyze any blood gas report.

PYRAMID POINTS

In acidosis, the pH is down.
In alkalosis, the pH is up.
The respiratory function indicator is the PCO_2.
The metabolic function indicator is the HCO_3.

PYRAMID STEPS

Look at the blood gas report.

Pyramid Step 1

Look at the pH. Is it up or down? If it is up, it reflects alkalosis. If it is down, it reflects acidosis.

Pyramid Step 2

Look at the PCO_2. Is it up or down? If it reflects an opposite response as the pH, then you know that the condition is a respiratory imbalance. If it does not reflect an opposite response as the pH, then move on to Pyramid Step 3.

Pyramid Step 3

Look at the HCO_3. Does the HCO_3 reflect a corresponding response with the pH? If it does, then the condition is a metabolic imbalance.

1. Remember, the respiratory function indicator is the PCO_2
2. In a respiratory imbalance, you will find an opposite response between the pH and the PCO_2; in other words, the pH will be up with a PCO_2 down, or the pH will be down with an elevated PCO_2
3. Remember the pH is down in an acidotic condition and is elevated in an alkalotic condition
4. Look at the pH and the PCO_2 to determine if the condition is a respiratory problem
5. **Respiratory acidosis**
   a. The pH is down
   b. The PCO_2 is up
6. **Respiratory alkalosis**
   a. The pH is up
   b. The PCO_2 is down
D. Metabolic imbalances (see Box 9–3)
1. Remember, the metabolic function indicator is the bicarbonate (HCO_3)
2. In a metabolic imbalance, you will find a corresponding response between the pH and the HCO_3
3. In other words, the pH will be up and the HCO_3 will be up, or the pH will be down and the HCO_3 will be down
4. Remember, the pH is down in an acidotic condition and is elevated in an alkalotic condition
5. Look at the pH and the HCO_3 to determine if the condition is a metabolic problem

6. **Metabolic acidosis**
   a. The pH is down
   b. The HCO_3 is down
7. **Metabolic alkalosis**
   a. The pH is up
   b. The HCO_3 is up
E. Analyzing arterial blood gas results (see Box 9–3)

PRACTICE QUESTIONS

1. The nurse is caring for a client with a diagnosis of chronic obstructive pulmonary disease (COPD). The nurse monitors the client for which acid-base imbalance that most likely occurs in this condition?
   1 Respiratory acidosis
   2 Respiratory alkalosis
   3 Metabolic acidosis
   4 Metabolic alkalosis

2. The LPN is assigned to care for a client with Guillain-Barré syndrome. The RN reviews the results of the arterial blood gases with the LPN and tells the LPN that the client is experiencing respiratory acidosis. The LPN expects to note which of the following?
   1 pH 7.40, PCO_2 52 mmHg
   2 pH 7.35, PCO_2 40 mmHg
   3 pH 7.25, PCO_2 50 mmHg
   4 pH 7.50, PCO_2 30 mmHg

3. The nurse is caring for a client with respiratory insufficiency. Blood gas results indicate a pH of 7.50 and a PCO_2 of 30 mmHg, and the nurse is told that the client is experiencing respiratory alkalosis. Which of the following additional laboratory values does the nurse expect to note?
   1 Sodium level, 145 mEq/L
   2 Potassium level, 3.2 mEq/L
   3 Magnesium level, 2.0 mEq/L
   4 Phosphorus level, 2.3 mEq/L

4. The nurse is caring for a client with pneumonia. The nurse is told that the blood gas results indicate a pH of 7.50 and a PCO_2 of 30 mmHg. The nurse identifies that these results indicate
   1 Metabolic acidosis
   2 Metabolic alkalosis
   3 Respiratory alkalosis
   4 Respiratory acidosis

5. The client is scheduled for blood to be drawn from the radial artery for an arterial blood gas (ABG) determination. The nurse assists in performing Allen's test prior to drawing the blood gas to determine the adequacy of the
   1 Brachial circulation
   2 Ulnar circulation
   3 Femoral circulation
   4 Carotid circulation

6. The nurse is caring for a client with a nasogastric tube (NG) that is attached to low suction. The nurse monitors the client closely for which of the following acid-base disorders that is most likely to occur in this client?
   1 Respiratory acidosis
   2 Respiratory alkalosis
   3 Metabolic acidosis
   4 Metabolic alkalosis

7. The nurse is caring for a client with an ileostomy. The nurse monitors the client closely, understanding that this client is at risk for developing which of the following acid-base disorders?
   1 Respiratory acidosis
   2 Respiratory alkalosis
   3 Metabolic acidosis
   4 Metabolic alkalosis

8. The nurse is caring for a client with diabetic ketoacidosis and documents that the client is experiencing Kussmaul's respirations. Based on this documentation, which of the following did the nurse most likely observe?
   1 Respirations that are abnormally deep, regular, and increased in rate
   2 Respirations that are regular but abnormally slow
   3 Respirations that are labored and increased in depth and rate
   4 Respirations that cease for several seconds

9. The nurse is collecting data from a client with a suspected diagnosis of gastric ulcer. The client tells the nurse that oral antacids are taken frequently throughout the day. The nurse continues to collect data from the client, understanding that the client is at risk for which of the following acid-base disturbances?
   1 Respiratory alkalosis
   2 Respiratory acidosis
   3 Metabolic acidosis
   4 Metabolic alkalosis

10. The nurse is caring for a client with renal failure. The nurse is told that the blood gas results indicate a pH of 7.30 and a PCO_2 of 32 mmHg and that the client is experiencing metabolic acidosis. The nurse reviews the laboratory results and expects to note which of the following?
    1 Sodium level, 145 mEq/L
    2 Magnesium level, 2.0 mEq/L
    3 Potassium level, 5.2 mEq/L
    4 Phosphorus level, 2.3 mEq/L

ANSWERS

1. 1

RATIONALE: Respiratory acidosis is most often due to hypoventilation. Chronic respiratory acidosis is most commonly caused by COPD. Acute respiratory acidosis also occurs in these clients when superimposed respiratory infection or concurrent respiratory disease increases the work of breathing. Options 2, 3, and 4 are not likely to occur unless other conditions complicate the COPD.

TEST-TAKING STRATEGY: Knowledge regarding the causes of respiratory acidosis is necessary to answer this question. Remembering that hypoventilation results in respiratory acidosis will direct you toward the correct option. Review the causes of respiratory acidosis now if you had difficulty with this question.

LEVEL OF COGNITIVE ABILITY: Comprehension
PHASE OF NURSING PROCESS: Data Collection
CLIENT NEEDS: Physiological Integrity
CONTENT AREA: Fundamental Skills
REFERENCE

deWit, S. (1998). *Essentials of medical-surgical nursing* (4th ed.). Philadelphia: W. B. Saunders. pp. 120–121.

2. 3

RATIONALE: The normal pH is 7.35 to 7.45. The normal PCO_2 is 35 to 45 mmHg. In respiratory acidosis the pH is down and the PCO_2 is up.

TEST-TAKING STRATEGY: Remember that in a respiratory imbalance you will find an opposite response between the pH and the PCO_2. Also remember that the pH is down in an acidotic condition. Options 1 and 4 reflect an elevated pH, which indicates an alkalotic condition. Option 2 reflects a normal blood gas result. Option 3 is the only option that reflects an acidotic condition.

LEVEL OF COGNITIVE ABILITY: Analysis
PHASE OF NURSING PROCESS: Data Collection
CLIENT NEEDS: Physiological Integrity
CONTENT AREA: Adult Health/Neurological
REFERENCE

deWit, S. (1998). *Essentials of medical-surgical nursing* (4th ed.). Philadelphia: W. B. Saunders. p. 122.

3. 2

RATIONALE: Clinical manifestations of respiratory alkalosis include tachypnea, mental status changes, dizziness, pallor around the mouth, spasms of the muscles of the hands, and hypokalemia.

TEST-TAKING STRATEGY: Knowledge regarding the clinical manifestations of respiratory alkalosis, along with normal laboratory values, will assist you in answering the question. By the process of elimination, you can then determine that the only abnormal laboratory value is the K level, option 2. Review the clinical manifestations of respiratory alkalosis now if you had difficulty with this question.

LEVEL OF COGNITIVE ABILITY: Analysis
PHASE OF NURSING PROCESS: Data Collection
CLIENT NEEDS: Physiological Integrity
CONTENT AREA: Adult Health/Respiratory
REFERENCE

deWit, S. (1998). *Essentials of medical-surgical nursing* (4th ed.). Philadelphia: W. B. Saunders. p. 123.

4. 3

RATIONALE: The normal pH is 7.35 to 7.45. In respiratory conditions, an opposite effect will be seen between the pH and the PCO_2. In an alkalotic condition, the pH is up. Clients with pneumonia are also at risk for respiratory alkalosis as a result of hypoxemia.

TEST-TAKING STRATEGY: Remember that in a respiratory imbalance you will find an opposite response between the pH and the PCO_2. Therefore, options 1 and 2 can be eliminated. Also remember that the pH is up in an alkalotic condition. Review the steps related to reading blood gas values if you had difficulty with this question.

LEVEL OF COGNITIVE ABILITY: Analysis
PHASE OF NURSING PROCESS: Data Collection
CLIENT NEEDS: Physiological Integrity
CONTENT AREA: Adult Health/Respiratory
REFERENCE

deWit, S. (1998). *Essentials of medical-surgical nursing* (4th ed.). Philadelphia: W. B. Saunders. pp. 121–122.

5. 2

RATIONALE: Before radial puncture for obtaining an arterial specimen for ABGs, an Allen's test should be performed to determine adequate ulnar circulation. Failure to assess collateral circulation could result in severe ischemic injury to the hand, if damage to the radial artery occurs with arterial puncture.

TEST-TAKING STRATEGY: Knowledge regarding the purpose and procedure for the Allen's test is required to answer this question. Review the purpose and procedure of the Allen's test now, if you had difficulty with this question.

LEVEL OF COGNITIVE ABILITY: Analysis
PHASE OF NURSING PROCESS: Data Collection
CLIENT NEEDS: Physiological Integrity
CONTENT AREA: Adult Health/Cardiovascular
REFERENCE

Black, J., & Matassarin-Jacobs, E. (1997). *Medical-surgical nursing: Clinical management for continuity of care* (5th ed.). Philadelphia: W. B. Saunders. p. 339.

6. 4

RATIONALE: Loss of gastric fluid via nasogastric suction or vomiting causes metabolic alkalosis due to the loss of hydrochloric acid (HCl). This results in an alkalotic condition.

TEST-TAKING STRATEGY: If you can remember that HCl is lost when the client is on nasogastric suction, this will direct you to the option identifying an alkalotic condition. Since the question addresses a situation other than a respiratory one, the acid-base disorder is a metabolic condition. If you had difficulty with this question, review the causes of metabolic alkalosis now.

LEVEL OF COGNITIVE ABILITY: Analysis
PHASE OF NURSING PROCESS: Data Collection
CLIENT NEEDS: Physiological Integrity
CONTENT AREA: Adult Health/Gastrointestinal
REFERENCE

deWit, S. (1998). *Essentials of medical-surgical nursing* (4th ed.). Philadelphia: W. B. Saunders. pp. 120–121.

7. **3**

RATIONALE: Intestinal secretions high in HCO_3 may be lost through enteric drainage tubes, an ileostomy, or with diarrhea. The decreased HCO_3 level creates the actual base deficit of metabolic acidosis.
TEST-TAKING STRATEGY: Remembering that intestinal fluids are primarily alkaline will assist you in selecting the correct option. When excess HCO_3 is lost, acidosis will result. Note that the client described in the question has a gastrointestinal disorder. This will direct you toward a metabolic disorder. If you had difficulty with this question, review the causes of metabolic acidosis now.
LEVEL OF COGNITIVE ABILITY: Analysis
PHASE OF NURSING PROCESS: Data Collection
CLIENT NEEDS: Physiological Integrity
CONTENT AREA: Adult Health/Gastrointestinal
REFERENCE
deWit, S. (1998). *Essentials of medical-surgical nursing* (4th ed.). Philadelphia: W. B. Saunders. pp. 120–121.

8. **1**

RATIONALE: Kussmaul's respirations are abnormally deep, regular, and increased in rate. In bradypnea, respirations are regular but abnormally slow. In hyperpnea, respirations are labored and increased in depth and rate. Apnea is described as respirations that cease for several seconds.
TEST-TAKING STRATEGY: Knowledge regarding the descriptions for alterations in breathing pattern is required to answer the question. Kussmaul's respirations occur in diabetic ketoacidosis. Review the characteristics of these types of respirations now if you had difficulty with this question.
LEVEL OF COGNITIVE ABILITY: Comprehension
PHASE OF NURSING PROCESS: Data Collection
CLIENT NEEDS: Physiological Integrity
CONTENT AREA: Fundamental Skills
REFERENCE
Potter, P., & Perry, A. (1997). *Fundamentals of nursing: Concepts, process, and practice* (4th ed.). St. Louis: Mosby–Year Book. p. 624.

9. **4**

RATIONALE: Increases in base components occur as a result of oral or parenteral ingestion of bicarbonates, carbonates, acetates, citrates, and lactates. Excessive use of oral antacids containing sodium or calcium HCO_3 can cause a metabolic alkalosis.
TEST-TAKING STRATEGY: Remembering that antacids contain HCO_3 and that an excess oral intake will increase HCO_3 will assist in directing you to the correct option. Review the causes of metabolic alkalosis now if you had difficulty with the question.
LEVEL OF COGNITIVE ABILITY: Analysis
PHASE OF NURSING PROCESS: Data Collection
CLIENT NEEDS: Physiological Integrity
CONTENT AREA: Adult Health/Gastrointestinal
REFERENCE
deWit, S. (1998). *Essentials of medical-surgical nursing* (4th ed.). Philadelphia: W. B. Saunders. p. 121.

10. **3**

RATIONALE: Clinical manifestations of metabolic acidosis include weakness, malaise, and headache. Hyperkalemia will occur. The pH will be less than 7.35 and the HCO_3 lower than 22 mEq/L.
TEST-TAKING STRATEGY: Knowledge regarding the clinical manifestations of metabolic acidosis along with normal laboratory values will assist you in answering the question. By the process of elimination, you can then determine that the only abnormal laboratory value is the potassium level. Review the manifestations of metabolic acidosis now if you had difficulty with this question.
LEVEL OF COGNITIVE ABILITY: Analysis
PHASE OF NURSING PROCESS: Data Collection
CLIENT NEEDS: Physiological Integrity
CONTENT AREA: Adult Health/Renal
REFERENCE
deWit, S. (1998). *Essentials of medical-surgical nursing* (4th ed.). Philadelphia: W. B. Saunders. p. 123.

BIBLIOGRAPHY

Black, J., & Matassarin-Jacobs, E. (1997). *Medical-surgical nursing: Clinical management for continuity of care* (5th ed.). Philadelphia: W. B. Saunders.

deWit, S. (1998). *Essentials of medical-surgical nursing* (4th ed.). Philadelphia: W. B. Saunders.

Hodgson, B., & Kizior, R. (1999). *Saunders nursing drug handbook 1999.* Philadelphia: W. B. Saunders.

Lee, C., Barrett, C., & Ignatavicius, D. (1996). *Fluid and electrolytes: A practical approach* (4th ed.). Philadelphia: F. A. Davis.

Luckmann, J. (1997). *Saunders manual of nursing care.* Philadelphia: W. B. Saunders.

National Council of State Boards of Nursing (1998). *National Council Detailed Test Plan for the NCLEX-PN Examination.* Chicago: Author.

Potter, P., & Perry, A. (1997). *Fundamentals of nursing: Concepts, process, and practice* (4th ed.). St. Louis: Mosby–Year Book.

CHAPTER 10

Laboratory Values

. . . .

PYRAMID TERMS

Capillary Puncture—Preferred for a peripheral blood smear.

Plasma—The fluid substance; what remains after the cells have been removed from a sample of whole blood.

Serum—Blood plasma from which clotting agents have been removed.

Venipuncture—Allows for obtaining larger quantities of blood for testing; the antecubital veins are the veins of choice because of ease of access.

◆ PYRAMID TO SUCCESS

This chapter identifies the normal adult values of the most common laboratory tests. If you are familiar with the normal values, you will be able to determine if an abnormality exists. It is unlikely that a question on NCLEX-PN will simply ask you what a normal value may be. The questions on NCLEX-PN related to laboratory values will require you to identify whether the laboratory value is normal or abnormal, and then you will be required to think about the effects of the laboratory value in terms of the client.

Pyramid points focus on awareness of the normal values of the most common laboratory tests, therapeutic levels in the serum of commonly prescribed medications, and interventions based on the findings. When a question is presented on NCLEX-PN regarding a specific laboratory value, note the disorder presented in the question and the associated body organ that is affected as a result of the disorder. This process will assist you in determining the correct answer. For example, if the question is asking you about the immune status of a client receiving chemotherapy, assessment of laboratory values will focus on the white blood cell count and the neutrophils because

this client may be at risk for infection. In the client receiving chemotherapy who has a low white blood cell count, the plan of care focuses on the immune system and protecting the client from infection. Implementation focuses on preventive interventions related to infection, such as protective isolation measures. Evaluation may focus on maintenance of a normal temperature in the client.

Box 10–1 lists abbreviations found in laboratory values.

> **BOX 10–1. Pyramid Abbreviations**
>
> g/dL—gram per deciliter
> μg/dL—microgram per deciliter
> mg/dL—milligram per deciliter
> mEq/dL—milliequivalent per liter
> U/L—unit per liter
> mm/hr—millimeter per hour
> IU/L—international unit per liter
> μg/mL—microgram per milliliter
> ng/mL—nanogram per milliliter
> μu/mL—microunit per milliliter
> mL/kg—milliliter per kilogram

NURSING PROCESS

DATA COLLECTION

Specific client preparation required for test
Specific postprocedure measures
Significant laboratory value specific to the client's condition

Significant value as compared with a normal finding
Signs and symptoms in the client based on an abnormal laboratory value

PLANNING
Client identifies purpose of test. Client describes laboratory test preparation. Client describes postprocedure measures. Client identifies the need for follow-up testing.

IMPLEMENTATION
Explain purpose of test to client. Obtain informed consent if required. Inform client of specific test preparation. Use standard (universal) or other precautions as necessary. Maintain asepsis. Inform client of post-test procedures and need for follow-up. Note if the laboratory value is abnormal. Monitor for signs and symptoms that will occur as a result of the abnormality. Report significant results if noted. Initiate prescribed interventions, Document the effectiveness of interventions and follow-up laboratory studies.

EVALUATION
Client prepares for the laboratory study. Client performs postprocedure measures. Client complies with prescribed interventions. Client obtains follow-up testing as required.

◆ CLIENT NEEDS

SAFE, EFFECTIVE CARE ENVIRONMENT

Informed consent for specific procedures
Handling infectious materials
Asepsis
Standard (universal) and other precautions

HEALTH PROMOTION AND MAINTENANCE

Client preparation for laboratory test
Post-test procedures
Importance of follow-up laboratory studies
Community resources available for the follow-up

PSYCHOSOCIAL INTEGRITY

Communicate purpose of test to client
Provide psychosocial comfort during testing
Identify support systems
Describe specific interventions required based on the results

PHYSIOLOGICAL INTEGRITY

Comfort interventions
Normal values of the most common laboratory tests
Significant laboratory values
Therapeutic serum medication levels of commonly prescribed medications
Monitoring for clinical manifestations associated with the abnormal laboratory value
Monitoring for potential complications related to the test
Signs and symptoms that need to be reported

◆ I. Electrolytes (Table 10–1)

A. **Serum** sodium (Na)
  1. Description
     a. A major cation of extracellular fluid
     b. Maintains osmotic pressures and acid-base balance and transmits nerve impulses
     c. Absorbed from the small intestine and excreted in urine in amounts dependent on dietary intake

Table 10–1. **Normal Adult Electrolyte Values**

Sodium	136–145 mEq/l
Potassium	3.5–5.1 mEq/L
Chloride	98–107 mEq/L
Bicarbonate (venous)	22–29 mEq/L

     d. Minimum daily requirement is 15 mEq
  2. Nursing considerations
     a. Should not be drawn during hemodialysis
     b. Drawing blood samples proximal to intravenous (IV) infusion of sodium chloride will falsely elevate results

B. **Serum** potassium (K)
  1. Description
     a. A major intracellular cation
     b. Regulates cellular water balance, electrical conduction in muscle cells, and acid-base balance
     c. The body obtains K through dietary ingestion, and the kidneys either preserve or excrete K depending upon cellular need
     d. K levels are used to evaluate cardiac dysrhythmias, renal dysfunction, mental confusion, gastrointestinal (GI) distress, and the need for IV replacement therapy
  2. Nursing considerations
     a. Should not be drawn during hemodialysis
     b. Should not be drawn from a site where an IV infusion exists
     c. If the client is receiving K, note on the laboratory form
     d. Potassium level will decrease in clients taking potassium-wasting diuretics
     e. In kidney failure or during shock, K excess will occur
     f. Potassium shifts occur in acid-base imbalances

C. **Serum** chloride
  1. Description
     a. A hydrochloric acid salt that is the most abundant body anion in the extracellular fluid
     b. Functions in counterbalancing cations such as sodium, and acts as a buffer during oxygen (O_2) and carbon dioxide (CO_2) exchange in red blood cells
     c. Aids in digestion, maintaining osmotic pressure, and water balance
  2. Nursing considerations
     a. Should not be drawn during hemodialysis
     b. Should not be drawn from an extremity that has normal saline infusing into it
     c. Any condition accompanied by prolonged vomiting, diarrhea, or both will alter levels

II. Coagulation Studies (Table 10–2)

A. Activated partial thromboplastin time (aPTT)
  1. Description
    a. Evaluates how well the coagulation sequence is functioning by measuring the amount of time it takes for **plasma** to clot after partial thromboplastin is added to it
    b. Screens for deficiencies and inhibitors of all clotting factors except VII and XIII
    c. Most commonly used to monitor heparin therapy and screen for coagulation disorders
  2. Value: 20 to 36 seconds depending on the type of activator used
  3. Nursing considerations
    a. If client is on intermittent heparin therapy, the sample should be drawn 1 hour prior to next scheduled dose
    b. Should not be drawn during hemodialysis
    c. Should not be drawn from an extremity where heparin is infusing
    d. Transport the specimen to the laboratory immediately
    e. If value is prolonged, initiate bleeding precautions

B. Prothrombin time (PT) and International Normalized Ratio (INR)
  1. Description
    a. Prothrombin is a vitamin K–dependent glycoprotein produced by the liver that is necessary for firm fibrin clot formation
    b. Each laboratory establishes a normal value or control based on the method used to perform the test (PT)
    c. The PT measures the amount of time it takes for clot formation and is used to monitor the response to warfarin (Coumadin) therapy or to screen for dysfunctions resulting from liver disease, vitamin K deficiency, or disseminated intravascular coagulation (DIC)
    d. A PT value within 2 seconds (plus or minus) of the control is considered normal
    e. The INR standardized the PT ratio
  2. Values
    a. Normal PT is 9.6 to 11.8 seconds (adult male) and 9.5 to 11.3 seconds (adult female)
    b. INR of 2.0 to 3.0 for standard warfarin therapy
    c. INR of 3.0 to 4.5 for high-dose warfarin therapy

3. Nursing considerations
    a. Blood for baseline PT should be drawn before starting anticoagulation therapy
    b. Should not be drawn during hemodialysis
    c. Note time of collection on laboratory form
    d. Provide direct pressure to the site for 3 to 5 minutes if a coagulation defect is present
    e. Concurrent therapy with heparin can lengthen PT
    f. Diets high in green, leafy vegetables can increase the absorption of vitamin K, which shortens the PT
    g. A PT greater than 30 seconds places the client at risk for hemorrhage
    h. Oral anticoagulation therapy usually maintains the PT at 1.5 to 2 times the laboratory control value

C. Clotting time
  1. Description: measures the time required for the interaction of all factors involved in the clotting process
  2. Nursing considerations
    a. The client should not receive heparin therapy for 3 hours prior to specimen collection
    b. The test result is prolonged by any anticoagulant therapy, test tube agitation, or higher temperature changes

D. Platelet count
  1. Description
    a. Platelets function in hemostatic plug formation, clot retraction, and coagulation factor activation
    b. Platelets are produced by the bone marrow to function in hemostasis
  2. Nursing considerations
    a. Should not be drawn during hemodialysis
    b. Monitor site for bleeding in clients with known bleeding problems
    c. High altitudes, chronic cold weather, and exercise increase platelet counts
    d. Bleeding precautions should be instituted in clients with a low platelet count

III. Serum Gastrointestinal Studies (Table 10–3)

A. Albumin
  1. Description
    a. A major plasma protein of blood
    b. Maintains oncotic pressure and transports bilirubin, fatty acids, medications, hormones, and other substances that are insoluble in water
  2. Nursing considerations
    a. Draw from an extremity that does not have an IV infusing into it
    b. Instruct the client to consume a low-fat diet on the day of the test

B. Alkaline phosphatase
  1. Description
    a. An enzyme normally found in bone, liver, intestine, and placenta

Table 10–2. Coagulation Studies

aPTT	20–36 seconds
PT	9.6–11.8 seconds (male); 9.5–11.3 seconds (female)
INR	2–3 (standard warfarin therapy)
	3.0–4.5 (high-dose warfarin therapy)
Clotting time	8–15 minutes
Platelet count	150,000 to 400,000 cells/μL

Table 10–3. Gastrointestinal Studies

Albumin	3.4–5 g/dL
Alkaline phosphatase	4.5–13 King-Armstrong units/dL
Ammonia	15–45 μg/dL
Amylase	50–180 Somogyi U/dL in the adult
	20–160 Somogyi U/dL in the older adult
Bilirubin, direct	0–0.3 mg/dL
Bilirubin, indirect	0.1–1.0 mg/dL
Bilirubin, total	Less than 1.5 mg/dL
Total cholesterol	120–200 mg/dL
Lipase	31–186 U/L
Lipids, total	400–800 mg/dL
Triglycerides	Normal range: 10–190 mg/dL
	Borderline high: 200–400 mg/dL
	High: 400–1000 mg/dL
	Very high: >1000 mg/dL
Protein	6.0–8.0 g/dL
Uric acid	Male: 4.5–8 ng/dL
	Female: 2.5–6.2 ng/dL

  b. The level rises during periods of bone growth, liver disease, and bile duct obstruction

 2. Nursing considerations

  a. The client may be requested to fast 10 to 12 hours prior to the test

  b. Hepatotoxic medications administered within 12 hours prior to specimen collection invalidate the test

  c. Should not be drawn during hemodialysis

  d. Transport the specimen to the laboratory immediately

C. Ammonia

 1. Description

  a. A waste product from nitrogen breakdown that occurs during protein metabolism

  b. Metabolized by the liver and excreted by the kidneys as urea

  c. Elevated levels due to hepatic dysfunction may lead to encephalopathy

  d. Not a reliable indicator of hepatic coma

 2. Nursing considerations

  a. Instruct the client to fast, except for water, and refrain from smoking for 8 to 10 hours

  b. Should not be drawn during hemodialysis

  c. Place specimen in an ice-water bath

  d. Transport to the laboratory immediately

D. Amylase

 1. Description

  a. An enzyme produced by the pancreas and salivary glands that aids in the digestion of complex carbohydrates

  b. Excreted by the kidneys

  c. In acute pancreatitis, amylase starts rising at least 2 hours after the onset, peaks at about 24 hours, and returns to normal in 2 to 3 days after the onset

  d. Normal **serum** amylase may occur in pancreatitis, especially chronic pancreatitis

 2. Nursing considerations

  a. List medications that the client has taken 24 hours prior to the test on the laboratory form

  b. Results are invalidated if the specimen is obtained less than 72 hours after cholecystography with radiopaque dyes

E. Bilirubin

 1. Description

  a. Produced by the liver, spleen, and bone marrow and is also a by-product of hemoglobin breakdown

  b. Total bilirubin levels can be broken down into direct bilirubin, which is primarily excreted via the intestinal tract, and indirect bilirubin, which circulates primarily in the bloodstream

  c. Total bilirubin levels rise with any type of jaundice, whereas direct and indirect levels rise depending on the cause of the jaundice

 2. Nursing considerations

  a. Should not be drawn during hemodialysis

  b. Instruct the client to eat a diet low in yellow foods such as carrots, yams, yellow beans, and pumpkin, 3 to 4 days before sampling

  c. Instruct the client to fast for 4 hours before sampling

  d. Note that results will be elevated with the use of alcohol, morphine, theophylline, ascorbic acid, and aspirin

  e. Note that results are invalidated if the client received a radioactive scan within 24 hours prior to the test

F. Cholesterol, total

 1. Description: cholesterol is present in all body tissues and is a major component of low-density lipoproteins (LDL), brain and nerve cells, cell membranes, and some gallstones

 2. Nursing considerations

  a. Instruct the client to fast from foods and fluid, except for water, for 12 to 14 hours and from alcohol for 24 hours prior to the test

  b. Instruct the client that the evening meal prior to the test should be free of high-cholesterol foods; failure to follow dietary restrictions will interfere with test results

  c. Cholesterol levels tend to decrease temporarily with major illness or surgery

  d. Oral contraceptives will increase the level of cholesterol in the **serum**

G. Lipase

 1. Description

  a. A pancreatic enzyme that changes fats and triglycerides into fatty acids and glycerol

  b. In acute pancreatitis, **serum** lipase begins to increase in 2 to 6 hours, peaks at 12 to 30 hours, remains elevated, but slowly decreases in 2 to 4 days

 2. Nursing considerations

  a. Endoscopic retrograde cholangiopancreatography (ERCP) may increase lipase activity

b. Traumatic **venipuncture** can inhibit lipase activity

H. Lipids, total
1. Description
   a. Blood lipids consist of cholesterol, triglycerides, and phospholipids
   b. A lipid profile helps determine the risk factors in coronary artery disease
2. Nursing considerations
   a. Instruct the client to fast from food and fluids for 12 hours prior to the test
   b. Oral contraceptives may increase the levels of lipids in the **serum**

I. Triglycerides
1. Description
   a. Triglycerides comprise a major part of very-low-density lipoproteins (VLDL) and a small part of low-density lipoproteins (LDL)
   b. Synthesized in the liver from fatty acids, protein, and glucose, and are obtained from the diet
2. Nursing considerations
   a. Instruct the client to fast for 12 hours prior to the test
   b. Instruct the client to avoid alcohol and refined carbohydrates for 3 days prior to the test

J. Protein
1. Description
   a. Reflects the total amount of albumin and globulins in the **serum**
   b. Regulates osmotic pressure and is composed of coagulation factors for hemostasis, enzymes, hormones, tissue growth and repair, and pH buffers
2. Nursing considerations
   a. Should not be drawn during hemodialysis
   b. Should not be drawn in an extremity with an IV infusion
   c. Instruct the client to avoid a high-fat diet for 8 hours prior to the test

K. Uric acid
1. Description
   a. Formed as the purines adenine and guanine, and is continuously metabolized during the formation and degradation of DNA and RNA, and from the metabolism of dietary purines
   b. Elevated amounts deposited in joints and soft tissue can cause gout
   c. Conditions of fast cell turnover, as well as slowed renal excretion of uric acid, may cause uricemia
   d. Elevated amounts of urinary uric acid precipitate into urate stones in the kidneys
2. Nursing considerations
   a. Instruct the client to fast for 8 hours prior to the test
   b. Aminophylline, caffeine, and vitamin C may cause falsely elevated results

IV. **Glucose Studies** (Table 10–4)

A. Fasting blood glucose (FBS)
1. Description
   a. Glucose is a monosaccharide found in fruits and is formed from the digestion of carbohydrates and the conversion of glycogen by the liver
   b. Glucose is the body's main source of cellular energy and is essential for brain and erythrocyte function
   c. FBS levels are used to help diagnose diabetes mellitus and hypoglycemia
2. Nursing considerations
   a. Instruct the client to fast for 8 to 12 hours prior to the test
   b. Instruct the diabetic client to withhold morning insulin or oral hypoglycemic medication until after the blood is drawn

B. Glucose tolerance test (GTT)
1. Description
   a. Aids in the diagnosis of diabetes mellitus
   b. If the glucose levels peak at higher than normal at 1 and 2 hours after injection or ingestion of glucose, and are slower than normal to return to fasting levels, then diabetes mellitus is confirmed
2. Nursing considerations
   a. Instruct the client to eat a high-carbohydrate (200–300 g) diet for 3 days before the test
   b. Instruct the client to avoid alcohol, coffee, and smoking for 36 hours before testing
   c. Instruct the client to fast for 10 to 16 hours prior to the test
   d. Instruct the client to avoid strenuous exercise for 8 hours before and after the test
   e. Instruct a diabetic client to withhold morning insulin or oral hypoglycemic medication
   f. Instruct the client that the test will take 3 to 5 hours and requires intravenous or oral

Table 10–4. Glucose Studies

Glucose, fasting	70–105 mg/dL
Glucose monitoring (capillary blood)	60–110 mg/dL
Glucose Tolerance Test, Oral	
Baseline fasting	70–105 mg/dL
30-minute fasting	110–170 mg/dL
60-minute fasting	120–170 mg/dL
90-minute fasting	100–140 mg/dL
120-minute fasting	70–120 mg/dL
Glucose, 2-hour postprandial	<140 mg/dL
Glycosylated Hemoglobin	
Expressed as percentage of total hemoglobin	
Nondiabetic: 5.5–8.5%	
Diabetic with good control: 7.5–11.4%	
Diabetic with moderate control: 11.5–15%	
Diabetic with poor control: >15%	

administration of glucose and multiple blood samples
C. Glycosylated hemoglobin
1. Description
   a. Glycosylated hemoglobin is blood glucose bound to hemoglobin
   b. HbA_{1c} is a reflection of how well blood glucose levels have been controlled for up to the prior 4 months
   c. Hyperglycemia in diabetics is usually a cause of an increase in HbA_{1c}
2. Nursing consideration: fasting is not required

V. Renal Function Studies (Table 10–5)

A. **Serum** creatinine
1. Description
   a. A very specific indicator of renal function, revealing the balance between creatinine formation and excretion
   b. Increased levels indicate a slowing of the glomerular filtration rate
2. Nursing considerations
   a. Should not be drawn during hemodialysis
   b. Instruct the client to avoid excessive exercise for 8 hours and avoid excessive red meat intake for 24 hours before the test
   c. Ascorbic acid, barbiturates, and diuretics may cause a rise in levels
B. Blood urea nitrogen (BUN)
1. Description
   a. Urea nitrogen is the nitrogen portion of urea, a substance formed in the liver through an enzymatic protein breakdown process
   b. Urea is normally freely filtered through the renal glomeruli with a small amount reabsorbed in the tubules and the remaining excreted in the urine
   c. Elevated values may result from prerenal, renal, or postrenal causes
2. Nursing considerations
   a. Should not be drawn during hemodialysis
   b. Both creatinine levels and urea nitrogen levels should be analyzed when evaluating renal function
   c. Nephrotoxic medications can cause a rise in levels

VI. Serum Enzymes (Table 10–6)

A. Creatine phosphokinase (CPK)
1. Description
   a. An enzyme found in muscle and brain

Table 10–5. Renal Function Studies

Serum creatinine	0.6–1.3 mg/dL
BUN	5–20 mg/dL

Table 10–6. Serum Enzymes

Creatine Phosphokinase	
MM: 5–70 U/L	
MB: 0–7 U/L	
BB: 0.3 U/L	
Lactate Dehydrogenase	70–200 IU/L
Lactate Dehydrogenase Isoenzymes	
LDH_1	14–26%
LDH_2	29–39%
LDH_3	20–26%
LDH_4	8–16%
LDH_5	6–16%

tissue and reflects tissue catabolism due to cell trauma
   b. The test is performed to detect myocardial or skeletal muscle damage or central nervous system damage
   c. Isoenzymes include CK-BB (brain), CK-MB (heart), and CK-MM (muscles)
   d. CK-BB is found mainly in brain tissue, CK-MB is found mainly in cardiac muscle, and CK-MM is found mainly is skeletal muscle
2. Nursing considerations
   a. If the test is to evaluate skeletal muscle, instruct the client to avoid strenuous physical activity for 24 hours prior to the test
   b. Instruct the client to avoid ingestion of alcohol for 24 hours prior to the test
   c. Invasive procedures and IM injections may falsely elevate CK levels
   d. Failure to obtain samples at the scheduled times, missing peak levels, may interfere with accurate determination of test results
B. Lactate dehydrogenase (LD or LDH)
1. Description
   a. The isoenzymes that are particularly affected with acute myocardial infarction are LDH_1 and LDH_2
   b. This enzyme begins to elevate approximately 24 hours after myocardial infarction and peaks in 48 to 72 hours; thereafter, it returns to normal, usually within 7 to 14 days
   c. The presence of an LD flip (when LD_1 is greater than LD_2) is helpful in diagnosing an MI
2. Nursing considerations
   a. LDH isoenzymes should be interpreted in view of the clinical findings
   b. Testing should be repeated on 3 consecutive days
   c. Recent surgery or pregnancy can cause elevated LDH levels

VII. Erythrocyte Studies (Table 10–7)

A. Erythrocyte sedimentation rate (ESR)
1. Description

Table 10–7. Erythrocyte Studies

ESR	0–30 mm/hr
Hemoglobin	
Male	14–16.5 g/dL
Female	12–15 g/dL
Hematocrit	
Male	42–52%
Female	35–47%
Iron	
Male	65–175 µg/dL
Female	50–170 µg/dL
Red blood cell count	
Male	4.5–6.2 million/µL
Female	4–5.5 million/µL

   a. The rate at which erythrocytes settle out of
      anticoagulated blood in 1 hour
   b. Not diagnostic of any particular disease but
      indicates that a disease process is ongoing
   2. Nursing consideration: fasting is not necessary,
      but a fatty meal may cause **plasma**
      alterations
B. Hemoglobin and hematocrit
   1. Description
      a. Hemoglobin is the main component of
         erythrocytes and serves as the vehicle for
         the transportation of oxygen (O_2) and
         carbon dioxide (CO_2)
      b. Hemoglobin determinations are important
         in determining anemia
      c. Hematocrit determines red blood cell mass
         and is an important measurement in the
         determination of anemia or polycythemia
   2. Nursing consideration: fasting is not required
C. Serum iron
   1. Description
      a. Mostly found in hemoglobin
      b. Acts as a carrier of O_2 from the lungs to
         the tissues and indirectly aids in return of
         CO_2 to the lungs
      c. Aids in diagnosing anemias and hemolytic
         disorders
   2. Nursing considerations
      a. Should not be drawn during hemodialysis
      b. The level will be increased if the client has
         ingested iron prior to the test
D. Red blood cell (RBC) count
   1. Description
      a. RBCs function in hemoglobin transport,
         which results in delivery of O_2 to the body
         tissues
      b. RBCs are formed by red bone marrow,
         have a life span of 120 days, and are
         removed from the blood by the liver,
         spleen, and bone marrow
      c. Aids in diagnosing anemias and blood
         dyscrasias
      d. Evaluate the body's ability to produce red
         blood cells in sufficient numbers
   2. Nursing consideration: should not be drawn
      during hemodialysis

VIII. Elements (Table 10–8)

A. Calcium
   1. Description
      a. A cation that is absorbed into the
         bloodstream from dietary sources and
         functions in bone formation, nerve impulse
         transmission, and contraction of
         myocardial and skeletal muscles
      b. Aids in blood clotting by converting
         prothrombin to thrombin
   2. Nursing considerations
      a. Should not be drawn during hemodialysis
      b. Instruct the client to eat a diet with normal
         calcium levels (800 mg/day) for 3 days
         before test
      c. Instruct the client that fasting may be
         required for 8 hours prior to the test
B. Magnesium
   1. Description
      a. Used as an index to determine metabolic
         activity and renal function
      b. Magnesium is needed in the blood clotting
         mechanism, regulates neuromuscular
         activity, acts as a cofactor that modifies the
         activity of many enzymes, and has an
         effect on the metabolism of calcium
   2. Nursing considerations
      a. Should not be drawn during hemodialysis
      b. Prolonged use of magnesium products will
         cause falsely increased levels, especially if
         renal damage is present
      c. Prolonged IV or total parenteral nutrition
         (TPN) therapy, blood transfusions, or
         prolonged nasogastric suctioning may
         cause falsely decreased results
C. Phosphorus
   1. Description
      a. Phosphorus is important in bone
         formation, energy storage and release,
         urinary acid-base buffering and
         carbohydrate metabolism
      b. High concentrations of phosphorus are
         stored in bone and skeletal muscle
      c. Phosphorus is absorbed from food and
         excreted by the kidneys
   2. Nursing considerations
      a. Do not draw during hemodialysis
      b. Instruct the client to fast prior to the test

IX. Thyroid Studies (Table 10–9)

   1. Description
      a. Performed if a thyroid disorder is suspected
      b. Helpful to differentiate primary thyroid

Table 10–8. Elements

Calcium	8.6–10.2 mg/dL or 4.5–5.5 mEq/L
Magnesium	1.8–2.6 mg/dL or 1.5–2.3 mEq/L
Phosphorus	2.5–4.5 mg/dL or 1.8–2.6 mEq/dL

Table 10–9. Thyroid Studies

Thyroid stimulating hormone (thyrotropin; TSH)	0.2–5.4 µU/mL
Thyroxine (T₄)	5.0–12.0 µg/dL
Thyroxine, free (FT₄)	0.8–2.4 ng/dL
Triiodothyronine (T₃)	80–230 ng/dL

disease from secondary causes and from abnormalities in thyroxine-binding globulin levels

2. Nursing consideration: test results are invalid if client had undergone a radionuclide scan within 7 days prior to the test

X. White Blood Cells (WBC) (Table 10–10)

1. Description
   a. White blood cells function in the body's immune defense system
   b. The WBC count assesses each leukocyte distribution
2. Nursing considerations
   a. A "shift to the left" means there is an increased number of immature neutrophils in the peripheral blood
   b. A low total WBC count with a left shift indicates a recovery from bone marrow depression or an infection of such intensity that the demand for neutrophils in the tissue is greater than the capacity of the bone marrow to release them in the circulation
   c. A high total WBC count with a left shift indicates an increased release of neutrophils by the bone marrow in response to an overwhelming infection or inflammation
   d. A "shift to the right" means cells have more than the usual number of nuclear segments; found in liver disease, Down syndrome, or megaloblastic and pernicious anemia

XI. Hepatitis Tests

1. Description
   a. Tests include radioimmune assay (RIA) and enzyme-linked immunosorbent assay (ELISA)
   b. Serologic tests for specific hepatitis virus markers assist in defining the specific type of hepatitis

Table 10–10. White Blood Cells

Value: 4500–11,000/µL	
Differential:	
Neutrophils	56% or 1800–7800/µL
Bands	3% or 0–700/µL
Eosinophils	2.7% or 0–450/µL
Basophils	0.3% or 0–200/µL
Lymphocytes	34% or 1000–4800/µL
Monocytes	4% or 0–800/µL

2. Values
   a. The presence of IgM antibody to hepatitis A virus (IgM anti-HAV) and the total antibody to hepatitis A virus (total anti-HAV) identify the disease
   b. Detection of core antigen (HB$_c$Ag), envelope antigen (HB$_e$Ag), and surface antigen (HB$_s$Ag), or their corresponding antibodies, constitutes hepatitis B assessment
   c. Hepatitis C is confirmed by the presence of antibodies to hepatitis C (anti-HCV)
   d. Serologic hepatitis delta virus (HDV) determination is made by detection of the hepatitis D antigen (HDAg) early in the course of the infection and by detection of anti-HDV antibody in the later disease stages
   e. Hepatitis E virus (HEV) is serologically distinct
3. Nursing consideration: if using RIA technique, the injection of radionuclides within 1 week prior to the test may falsely elevate results

XII. Acquired Immunodeficiency Syndrome (AIDS) Testing

1. Description
   a. Detects human immunodeficiency virus (HIV) that causes AIDS
   b. Tests used to determine the presence of antibodies to HIV include ELISA, Western blot (WB), and indirect fluorescent antibody (IFA)
   c. A single reactive ELISA test by itself cannot be used to diagnose AIDS and should be repeated in duplicate with the same blood sample; if repeatedly reactive, follow-up tests using WB or IFA should be done
   d. A positive WB or IFA is considered confirmatory for HIV
   e. A positive ELISA that fails to be confirmed by WB or IFA should not be considered negative and repeat testing should take place in 3 to 6 months
2. Nursing considerations
   a. Maintain issues of confidentiality surrounding HIV testing
   b. Follow prescribed state regulations and protocols related to reporting positive test results

XIII. Urine Tests

A. See Table 10–11

Table 10–11. Normal Adult Values: Urine Tests

Chloride	110–250 mEq/24 hours
Magnesium	7.3–12.2 mg/dL/24 hours
Potassium	25–125 mEq/24 hours
Protein	40–150 mg/24 hours
Sodium	40–220 mEq/24 hours
Uric acid	250–750 mg/24 hours
pH	4.5–7.8
Specific gravity	1.016 and 1.022

Table 10–12. Therapeutic Serum Medication Levels

Medication	Therapeutic Range
Acetaminophen (Tylenol)	10–20 μg/mL
Carbamazepine (Tegretol)	5–12 μg/mL
Digoxin (Lanoxin)	0.5–2.0 ng/mL
Gentamicin (Garamycin)	5–10 μg/mL
Magnesium sulfate	4–7 mg/dL
Phenytoin (Dilantin)	10–20 μg/mL
Salicylate	100–250 μg/mL
Theophylline (Aminophylline, Theo-Dur)	10–20 μg/mL
Valproic acid (Depakene)	50–100 μg/mL

XIV. Therapeutic Serum Medication Levels

A. See Table 10–12

PRACTICE QUESTIONS

1. The nurse is assigned to a 40-year-old client admitted with chronic pancreatitis. The nurse reviews the client's record and expects to note a serum amylase level that is most similar to which of the following values?
   1 50 Somogyi U/dL
   2 100 Somogyi U/dL
   3 300 Somogyi U/dL
   4 500 Somogyi U/dL

2. The adult client with hepatic encephalopathy has a serum ammonia level of 95 μg/dL and receives treatment with lactulose syrup. The nurse evaluates that the client had the best and most realistic response if the level changed to which of the following after medication administration?
   1 80 μg/dL
   2 40 μg/dL
   3 10 μg/dL
   4 5 μg/dL

3. The nurse is reviewing the laboratory results of an adult client with Addison's disease. The nurse identifies that the magnesium level is normal if which of the following is noted?
   1 2 mEq/L
   2 3 mEq/L
   3 4 mEq/L
   4 5 mEq/L

4. The adult client has undergone lumbar puncture to obtain cerebrospinal fluid (CSF) for analysis. The nurse checks for which of the following negative values if the CSF is normal?
   1 Protein
   2 Glucose
   3 White blood cells
   4 Red blood cells

5. The client is suspected of having a myocardial infarction. The nurse expects elevations in which of the following isoenzyme values reported with the creatinine phosphokinase (CPK) level?

   1 MM
   2 MB
   3 BB
   4 MK

6. The adult male client has had laboratory work done as part of a routine physical examination. The nurse reviews the client's record and identifies that the client may have a mild degree of renal insufficiency if which of the following serum creatinine levels is found?
   1 0.6 mg/dL
   2 1.1 mg/dL
   3 1.9 mg/dL
   4 3.5 mg/dL

7. The client with a seizure disorder is taking phenytoin (Dilantin). A serum phenytoin level is drawn and the nurse evaluates that the medication therapy is effective if the laboratory result is
   1 3 μg/mL
   2 8 μg/mL
   3 16 μg/mL
   4 24 μg/mL

8. The client who takes theophylline for chronic obstructive pulmonary disease (COPD) is seen in the urgent care center for respiratory distress. Just prior to initiating therapy, a baseline theophylline (aminophylline) level is drawn. The nurse determines that the client may not be compliant with medication therapy if the result is
   1 6 μg/mL
   2 11 μg/mL
   3 15 μg/mL
   4 18 μg/mL

9. The nurse is told that the laboratory result for a serum digoxin level is 2.4 ng/mL. The nurse plans to do which of the following?
   1 Record the normal value on the client's flowsheet
   2 Administer the next dose of the medication as scheduled
   3 Check the client's last pulse rate
   4 Hold the medication

10. The client is receiving a continuous IV infusion of heparin in the treatment of deep vein thrombosis. The nurse is told that the client's activated partial thromboplastin time (aPTT) level is 65 seconds and that the client's baseline before the initiation of therapy was 30 seconds. The nurse identifies these results as
    1 Low
    2 Elevated
    3 Within the therapeutic range
    4 Abnormal

11. The client with atrial fibrillation who is receiving maintenance therapy of warfarin sodium (Coumadin) has a prothrombin time (PT) of 30 sec-

onds. The nurse anticipates that which of the following will be prescribed?
1 Holding the next dose of warfarin
2 Administering the next dose of warfarin
3 Increasing the next dose of warfarin
4 Adding a dose of heparin

12. The adult client who has had preadmission testing before surgery has had blood drawn for determination of serum electrolytes. The nurse identifies which of the following as an abnormal value?
1 Sodium of 148 mEq/L
2 Potassium of 3.8 mEq/L
3 Chloride of 101 mEq/L
4 Bicarbonate of 26 mEq/L

13. The adult client with a critically high potassium level has received sodium polystyrene sulfonate (Kayexalate). The nurse evaluates that the medication was most effective if the client's repeat serum potassium level is
1 6.2 mEq/L
2 5.8 mEq/L
3 5.4 mEq/L
4 4.9 mEq/L

14. The client with a history of cardiac disease is due for a morning dose of furosemide (Lasix). The nurse reviews the client's record and reports which of the following serum potassium levels before administering the dose of furosemide?
1 3.8 mEq/L
2 3.2 mEq/L
3 4.8 mEq/L
4 4.2 mEq/L

15. The diabetic client has had a fasting blood glucose drawn. The nurse identifies which of the following results as a critical value?
1 150 mg/dL
2 225 mg/dL
3 290 mg/dL
4 340 mg/dL

16. The adult client with a history of GI bleeding has a platelet count of 300,000 cells/μL. Which of the following actions by the nurse is most appropriate upon reading this report?
1 Report the abnormally low count
2 Report the abnormally high count
3 Place the client on bleeding precautions
4 Place the normal report in the client's medical record

17. The adult client with hepatic cirrhosis has been taking a diet with optimal amounts of protein, since neither excess nor deficiency of protein has been helpful. The nurse evaluates the client's status as most satisfactory if the total protein level is which of the following values in the normal range?

1 0.4 g/dL
2 3.7 g/dL
3 6.4 g/dL
4 9.8 g/dL

18. The client was seen in the urgent care center for complaints of chest pain 3 days ago. Since that time, the client has not been feeling well and fatigues easily. The nurse reviews the results of the laboratory tests and suspects myocardial infarction at the time of chest pain if which of the following isoenzymes for LDH came back positive?
1 LDH_1
2 LDH_3
3 LDH_4
4 LDH_5

19. The adult client was diagnosed with acute pancreatitis 9 days ago. The nurse interprets that the client is recovering from this episode if the serum lipase level drops to which of the following values, which is just beneath the upper limit of normal?
1 20 IU/L
2 80 IU/L
3 175 IU/L
4 350 IU/L

20. The client who suffered a crush injury to the leg has a highly positive urine myoglobin level. The nurse plans to monitor this particular client carefully for signs of
1 Cerebrovascular accident
2 Acute tubular necrosis
3 Respiratory failure
4 Myocardial infarction

21. The nurse has an order to test the stool of a client with Hemoccult slides. The nurse reviews the client's record, knowing that which of the following medications can cause false negative results?
1 Ascorbic acid
2 Colchicine
3 Iodine
4 Acetylsalicylic acid

22. The adult female client has a hemoglobin level of 10.8 g/dL. The nurse interprets that this result is most likely due to which of the following factors in the client's history?
1 Chronic obstructive pulmonary disease (COPD)
2 Heart failure
3 Dehydration
4 Iron deficiency anemia

23. The adult male client admitted with dehydration has received fluid volume replacement. The nurse evaluates that the client has had adequate fluid resuscitation if the client's repeat hematocrit

level has decreased to which of the following values in the normal range?
1 56%
2 48%
3 39%
4 34%

24. The diabetic client has a glycosylated hemoglobin A1c level of 8%. Based on this test result, the nurse plans to reinforce teaching measures with the client about the need to
1 Avoid infection
2 Take in adequate fluids
3 Prevent hyperglycemia
4 Prevent hypoglycemia

25. The client has been diagnosed as having syndrome of inappropriate antidiuretic hormone secretion (SIADH) following cranial surgery. The nurse interprets that this complication is not resolving if which of the following urine specific gravity measurements is obtained?
1 1.002
2 1.016
3 1.020
4 1.030

26. The nurse is caring for the client with a diagnosis of cancer who is immunosuppressed. The nurse knows that neutropenic precautions will be implemented if the client's white blood cell (WBC) count is
1 2,000/μL
2 5,800/μL
3 8,400/μL
4 11,500/μL

27. The nurse volunteering at the health screening clinic teaches a 22-year-old client that diet and exercise should be used as tools to keep the total cholesterol level under
1 150 mg/dL
2 200 mg/dL
3 250 mg/dL
4 300 mg/dL

28. A 78-year-old client has been admitted for urinary tract infection and dehydration. The nurse evaluates that the client has received adequate volume replacement if the blood urea nitrogen (BUN) level drops to
1 35 mg/dL
2 29 mg/dL
3 15 mg/dL
4 7 mg/dL

29. The client is at risk for developing disseminated intravascular coagulopathy (DIC). The nurse would become most concerned with which of the following fibrinogen levels?
1 390 mg/dL
2 290 mg/dL
3 190 mg/dL
4 90 mg/dL

30. The nurse is reviewing the laboratory results of a female adult client suspected of having iron deficiency anemia. The nurse reviews the results, knowing that the normal hemoglobin level for this client is
1 10 g/dL
2 14 g/dL
3 17 g/dL
4 19 g/dL

ANSWERS

1. **3**

RATIONALE: The normal serum amylase level is 50 to 180 Somogyi U/dL in the adult, and 20 to 160 Somogyi U/dL in the older adult. With chronic cases of pancreatitis, the rise in serum amylase levels usually does not exceed three times the normal value. In acute pancreatitis, the value may exceed five times the normal value.
TEST-TAKING STRATEGY: Familiarity with the normal serum amylase level is needed to answer this question. Note the key word "chronic." It is also necessary to understand the effects of pancreatitis on this laboratory value. Review these effects now if you had difficulty with this question.
LEVEL OF COGNITIVE ABILITY: Comprehension
PHASE OF NURSING PROCESS: Data Collection
CLIENT NEEDS: Physiological Integrity
CONTENT AREA: Adult Health/Gastrointestinal
REFERENCE
Chernecky, C., & Berger, B. (1997). *Laboratory tests and diagnostic procedures* (2nd ed.). Philadelphia: W. B. Saunders. pp. 186–187.

2. **2**

RATIONALE: The normal serum ammonia level is 15 to 45 μg/dL. In the client with hepatic encephalopathy, the serum level is not likely to drop below normal. The most optimal yet realistic change would be to 40 μg/dL, which falls into the high normal range. A level of 80 μg/dL represents insufficient effect of the medication.
TEST-TAKING STRATEGY: Familiarity with the normal serum ammonia level is needed to answer this question. It is also necessary to understand the association between hepatic encephalopathy and this laboratory value. Review this test and the desirable effects of this medication now if you had difficulty with this question.
LEVEL OF COGNITIVE ABILITY: Analysis
PHASE OF NURSING PROCESS: Evaluation
CLIENT NEEDS: Physiological Integrity
CONTENT AREA: Adult Health/Gastrointestinal
REFERENCE
Chernecky, C., & Berger, B. (1997). *Laboratory tests and diagnostic procedures* (2nd ed.). Philadelphia: W. B. Saunders. p. 179.

3. **1**

RATIONALE: The normal magnesium level in an adult client is 1.5 to 2.3 mEq/L or 1.8 to 2.6 mg/dL. Options 2, 3, and 4 indicate elevated values.
TEST-TAKING STRATEGY: Knowledge regarding the normal magnesium level in an adult client is required to answer this question. If you are unfamiliar with this level, take time now to review.
LEVEL OF COGNITIVE ABILITY: Comprehension
PHASE OF NURSING PROCESS: Data Collection
CLIENT NEEDS: Physiological Integrity
CONTENT AREA: Adult Health/Endocrine
REFERENCE
Chernecky, C., & Berger, B. (1997). *Laboratory tests and diagnostic procedures* (2nd ed.). Philadelphia: W. B. Saunders. p. 703.

4. **4**

RATIONALE: The adult with normal cerebrospinal fluid has no red blood cells in the CSF. The client may have small levels of white blood cells (0–3 per mm³). Protein (15–45 mg/dL) and glucose (40–80 mg/dL) are normally present in CSF.
TEST-TAKING STRATEGY: To answer this question accurately, it is necessary to understand which of the aforementioned components above are present and absent in the cerebrospinal fluid. If needed, take a few moments to review the basics of this procedure and the normal results.
LEVEL OF COGNITIVE ABILITY: Comprehension
PHASE OF NURSING PROCESS: Data Collection
CLIENT NEEDS: Physiological Integrity
CONTENT AREA: Adult Health/Neurological
REFERENCE
Chernecky, C., & Berger, B. (1997). *Laboratory tests and diagnostic procedures* (2nd ed.). Philadelphia: W. B. Saunders. pp. 346–347.

5. **2**

RATIONALE: CPK is a cellular enzyme that can be fractionated into three isoenzymes. The MM band reflects CPK from skeletal muscle. The MB band reflects CPK from cardiac muscle. This is the level that elevates with myocardial infarction. The BB band reflects CPK from the brain. There is no MK band.
TEST-TAKING STRATEGY: To answer this question correctly, it is necessary to have specific knowledge of the isoenzymes that are produced with elevations in this enzyme. If needed, take a few moments now to review this important laboratory value for detecting myocardial infarction.
LEVEL OF COGNITIVE ABILITY: Comprehension
PHASE OF NURSING PROCESS: Data Collection
CLIENT NEEDS: Physiological Integrity
CONTENT AREA: Adult Health/Cardiovascular
REFERENCE
Chernecky, C., & Berger, B. (1997). *Laboratory tests and diagnostic procedures* (2nd ed.). Philadelphia: W. B. Saunders. pp. 324–326.

6. **3**

RATIONALE: The normal serum creatinine level for a man is 0.6 to 1.3 mg/dL. The normal value for women is 0.5 to 1.0 mg/dL. The client with a mild degree of renal insufficiency would have a slightly elevated level, which would be the value of 1.9 mg/dL. Creatinine levels of 3.5 mg/dL may be associated with acute or chronic renal failure.

TEST-TAKING STRATEGY: Note the key word "mild." This tells you that the correct option will be an abnormal value, but perhaps not the most abnormal of all the options. Use your knowledge of this common laboratory test to choose correctly. Review the normal value of this laboratory test now if you had difficulty with this question.
LEVEL OF COGNITIVE ABILITY: Comprehension
PHASE OF NURSING PROCESS: Data Collection
CLIENT NEEDS: Physiological Integrity
CONTENT AREA: Adult Health/Renal
REFERENCE
Chernecky, C., & Berger, B. (1997). *Laboratory tests and diagnostic procedures* (2nd ed.). Philadelphia: W. B. Saunders. pp. 415–416.

7. **3**

RATIONALE: The therapeutic range for serum phenytoin (Dilantin) level is 10 to 20 μg/mL. If the level is below the therapeutic range, the client may continue to experience seizure activity. If the level is too high, the client could experience phenytoin toxicity.
TEST-TAKING STRATEGY: To answer this question accurately, specific knowledge is needed about the normal range of results for this laboratory test. If needed, take a few moments to review and learn this material at this time.
LEVEL OF COGNITIVE ABILITY: Comprehension
PHASE OF NURSING PROCESS: Evaluation
CLIENT NEEDS: Physiological Integrity
CONTENT AREA: Adult Health/Neurological
REFERENCE
Chernecky, C., & Berger, B. (1997). *Laboratory tests and diagnostic procedures* (2nd ed.). Philadelphia: W. B. Saunders. pp. 805–806.

8. **1**

RATIONALE: The therapeutic range for serum theophylline level is 10 to 20 μg/mL. If the level is below the therapeutic range, the client may experience frequent exacerbations of the disorder. If the level is within the therapeutic range, the client is most likely compliant with medication therapy.
TEST-TAKING STRATEGY: Note the key words "may not be compliant." Familiarity with the therapeutic level of theophylline is needed to select the correct option. Review this therapeutic range now if you had difficulty with this question.
LEVEL OF COGNITIVE ABILITY: Comprehension
PHASE OF NURSING PROCESS: Evaluation
CLIENT NEEDS: Physiological Integrity
CONTENT AREA: Adult Health/Respiratory
REFERENCE
Hodgson, B., & Kizior, R. (1999). *Saunders nursing drug handbook 1999*. Philadelphia: W. B. Saunders. pp. 44–47.

9. **4**

RATIONALE: The normal therapeutic range for digoxin is 0.5 to 2.0 ng/mL. A value of 2.4 exceeds the therapeutic range, and it could be toxic to the client. The most important action is to hold further doses of digoxin. Option 1 is incorrect because the value is not normal. The next dose should not be administered automatically. Checking the client's pulse is not incorrect but may have limited value. Depending on the time that has elapsed since the last pulse check, it may be more useful to do a current assessment of the client's status.

TEST-TAKING STRATEGY: To choose correctly, it is necessary to be familiar with the therapeutic range for this medication. If this question was difficult, take a few moments to review the information on this important and commonly used medication, and measurement of its therapeutic serum level.
LEVEL OF COGNITIVE ABILITY: Application
PHASE OF NURSING PROCESS: Planning
CLIENT NEEDS: Physiological Integrity
CONTENT AREA: Adult Health/Cardiovascular
REFERENCE
Hodgson, B., & Kizior, R. (1999). *Saunders nursing drug handbook 1999*. Philadelphia: W. B. Saunders. pp. 324–326.

10. 3

RATIONALE: The normal aPTT varies between 20 and 36 seconds, depending on the type of activator used in testing. The therapeutic dose of heparin for treatment of deep vein thrombosis is to keep the aPTT between 1.5 and 2.5 times normal. Thus, the client's aPTT is within the therapeutic range, and the dose should remain unchanged.
TEST-TAKING STRATEGY: Knowledge of the normal aPTT level is required to answer this question. Eliminate options 1, 2, and 4 because they are similar. If this question was difficult, review this important and frequently encountered content area now.
LEVEL OF COGNITIVE ABILITY: Analysis
PHASE OF NURSING PROCESS: Evaluation
CLIENT NEEDS: Physiological Integrity
CONTENT AREA: Adult Health/Cardiovascular
REFERENCE
Chernecky, C., & Berger, B. (1997). *Laboratory tests and diagnostic procedures* (2nd ed.). Philadelphia: W. B. Saunders. p. 780.

11. 1

RATIONALE: The normal PT is 9.6 to 11.8 seconds (adult male) and 9.5 to 11.3 seconds (adult female). A therapeutic PT level is 1.3 to 1.5 times greater than the client's control level. Since the value stated is extremely high (and perhaps near the critical range), the nurse should anticipate that the client would not receive further doses at this time. If the level were too high, then the antidote (vitamin K) may be prescribed.
TEST-TAKING STRATEGY: To answer this question accurately, it is necessary to be familiar with both the normal PT level and the therapeutic level needed following institution of warfarin therapy. If this question was difficult, review this important and frequently encountered content area now.
LEVEL OF COGNITIVE ABILITY: Analysis
PHASE OF NURSING PROCESS: Planning
CLIENT NEEDS: Physiological Integrity
CONTENT AREA: Adult Health/Cardiovascular
REFERENCE
Chernecky, C., & Berger, B. (1997). *Laboratory tests and diagnostic procedures* (2nd ed.). Philadelphia: W. B. Saunders. p. 847.

12. 1

RATIONALE: The normal serum electrolyte ranges for adults is as follows: sodium, 136 to 145 mEq/L; potassium, 3.5 to 5.1 mEq/L; chloride 98 to 107 mEq/L; bicarbonate (venous) 22 to 29 mEq/L. The only abnormal value identified above is the serum sodium.
TEST-TAKING STRATEGY: Familiarity with normal serum electrolyte values is needed to answer this question. If

this question was difficult, take the time to memorize these common laboratory values.
LEVEL OF COGNITIVE ABILITY: Comprehension
PHASE OF NURSING PROCESS: Data Collection
CLIENT NEEDS: Physiological Integrity
CONTENT AREA: Fundamental Skills
REFERENCE
Chernecky, C., & Berger, B. (1997). *Laboratory tests and diagnostic procedures* (2nd ed.). Philadelphia: W. B. Saunders. p. 470.

13. 4

RATIONALE: The normal serum potassium level in the adult is 3.5 to 5.3 mEq/L. Option 4 is the only option reflecting a value that has dropped down into the normal range.
TEST-TAKING STRATEGY: Note the key words "critically high." You would expect that this medication is administered to lower the potassium level. Familiarity with normal serum potassium levels is needed to answer this question. If this question was difficult, take the time to memorize this common laboratory value.
LEVEL OF COGNITIVE ABILITY: Analysis
PHASE OF NURSING PROCESS: Evaluation
CLIENT NEEDS: Physiological Integrity
CONTENT AREA: Pharmacology
REFERENCE
Chernecky, C., & Berger, B. (1997). *Laboratory tests and diagnostic procedures* (2nd ed.). Philadelphia: W. B. Saunders. p. 470.

14. 2

RATIONALE: The normal adult serum potassium level in the adult is 3.5 to 5.3 mEq/L. Option 2 is the only value that falls below the therapeutic range. Administering furosemide to a client with a low potassium level and a cardiac history could precipitate ventricular dysrhythmias in the client.
TEST-TAKING STRATEGY: Familiarity with the normal serum potassium level is needed to answer this question. This will assist you in identifying the value that is not within normal range. If this question was difficult, take the time to memorize this common laboratory value now.
LEVEL OF COGNITIVE ABILITY: Application
PHASE OF NURSING PROCESS: Implementation
CLIENT NEEDS: Physiological Integrity
CONTENT AREA: Pharmacology
REFERENCE
Chernecky, C., & Berger, B. (1997). *Laboratory tests and diagnostic procedures* (2nd ed.). Philadelphia: W. B. Saunders. p. 470.

15. 4

RATIONALE: The normal fasting blood glucose is 70 to 105 mg/dL in the adult client. A critical level is considered to be one that exceeds 300 mg/dL. This makes option 4 the correct choice.
TEST-TAKING STRATEGY: Note the key words "critical value." This will assist in directing you to option 4. Familiarity with the normal fasting serum glucose level is needed to answer this question. If this question was difficult, take the time to memorize this common laboratory value now.
LEVEL OF COGNITIVE ABILITY: Comprehension
PHASE OF NURSING PROCESS: Data Collection
CLIENT NEEDS: Physiological Integrity
CONTENT AREA: Adult Health/Endocrine
REFERENCE
Chernecky, C., & Berger, B. (1997). *Laboratory tests and diagnostic procedures* (2nd ed.). Philadelphia: W. B. Saunders. p. 565.

16. 4

RATIONALE: A normal platelet count ranges from 150,000 to 400,000 cells/μL. The nurse should place the report containing the normal laboratory value in the client's medical record.
TEST-TAKING STRATEGY: Remember that options that are similar are not likely to be correct. With this in mind, eliminate options 1 and 3 first. To discriminate between the final two options, it is necessary to be familiar with the normal range for this laboratory test. Since this is a common hematological study, the normal range is worth memorizing.
LEVEL OF COGNITIVE ABILITY: Application
PHASE OF NURSING PROCESS: Implementation
CLIENT NEEDS: Physiological Integrity
CONTENT AREA: Adult Health/Gastrointestinal
REFERENCE
Chernecky, C., & Berger, B. (1997). *Laboratory tests and diagnostic procedures* (2nd ed.). Philadelphia: W. B. Saunders. p. 815.

17. 3

RATIONALE: The normal range for total serum protein level in the adult client is 6.0 to 8.0 g/dL, making option 3 the correct choice. Options 1 and 2 indicate low levels. Option 4 indicates an elevated level.
TEST-TAKING STRATEGY: Familiarity with the normal total protein level is needed to answer this question. If needed, take a few moments to review this important laboratory range now!
LEVEL OF COGNITIVE ABILITY: Analysis
PHASE OF NURSING PROCESS: Evaluation
CLIENT NEEDS: Physiological Integrity
CONTENT AREA: Adult Health/Gastrointestinal
REFERENCE
Chernecky, C. & Berger, B. (1997). *Laboratory tests and diagnostic procedures* (2nd ed.). Philadelphia: W. B. Saunders. p. 843.

18. 1

RATIONALE: The isoenzymes that are particularly affected with acute myocardial infarction are LDH_1 and LDH_2. LDH begins to elevate approximately 24 hours after myocardial infarction and peaks in 48 to 72 hours. Thereafter, it returns to normal, usually within 7 to 14 days.
TEST-TAKING STRATEGY: Familiarity with the cardiac isoenzymes for LDH is needed to answer this question. If needed, take a few moments to review this important laboratory data now.
LEVEL OF COGNITIVE ABILITY: Comprehension
PHASE OF NURSING PROCESS: Data Collection
CLIENT NEEDS: Physiological Integrity
CONTENT AREA: Adult Health/Cardiovascular
REFERENCE
Luckmann, J. (1997). *Saunders manual of nursing care*. Philadelphia: W. B. Saunders. p. 1047.

19. 3

RATIONALE: The normal serum lipase level is 31 to 186 IU/L. The client who is recovering from acute pancreatitis usually has elevated lipase levels for approximately 10 days after onset of symptoms. This makes lipase a valuable test in monitoring the client's pancreatic function. Option 3 is the only option that contains a value just under the peak of normal.
TEST-TAKING STRATEGY: Familiarity with the serum lipase level is needed to answer this question. If needed,

take a few moments to review the range for this laboratory study now.
LEVEL OF COGNITIVE ABILITY: Comprehension
PHASE OF NURSING PROCESS: Evaluation
CLIENT NEEDS: Physiological Integrity
CONTENT AREA: Adult Health/Gastrointestinal
REFERENCE
Chernecky, C., & Berger, B. (1997). *Laboratory tests and diagnostic procedures* (2nd ed.). Philadelphia: W. B. Saunders. p. 674.

20. 2

RATIONALE: The normal urine myoglobin level is negative. After extensive muscle destruction or damage, myoglobin is released into the bloodstream, where it is cleared from the body by the kidneys. When there is a large amount of myoglobin being cleared from the body, there is risk of the renal tubules being clogged with myoglobin, causing acute tubular necrosis. This is one form of acute renal failure.
TEST-TAKING STRATEGY: Familiarity with this laboratory study is needed to answer this question. It is also necessary to understand the nature and consequences of crush injury. Note the relationship between the test identified in the question and the diagnosis in the correct option.
LEVEL OF COGNITIVE ABILITY: Comprehension
PHASE OF NURSING PROCESS: Planning
CLIENT NEEDS: Physiological Integrity
CONTENT AREA: Adult Health/Renal
REFERENCE
Chernecky, C., & Berger, B. (1997). *Laboratory tests and diagnostic procedures* (2nd ed.). Philadelphia: W. B. Saunders. p. 745.

21. 1

RATIONALE: Ascorbic acid can interfere with the result of occult blood testing, causing false negative findings. Colchicine and iodine can cause false positive results. Acetylsalicylic acid would either have no effect on results or could cause a positive result, since aspirin is irritating to the stomach lining.
TEST-TAKING STRATEGY: Specific knowledge of interfering factors with occult blood testing is needed to answer this question accurately. If this question was difficult, a brief review of this test may be useful.
LEVEL OF COGNITIVE ABILITY: Comprehension
PHASE OF NURSING PROCESS: Data Collection
CLIENT NEEDS: Physiological Integrity
CONTENT AREA: Adult Health/Gastrointestinal
REFERENCE
Jaffee, M., & McVan, B. (1997). *Davis's laboratory and diagnostic test handbook*. Philadelphia: F. A. Davis. p. 819.

22. 4

RATIONALE: The normal hemoglobin level for an adult female client is 12 to 15 g/dL. Iron deficiency anemia can result in lower hemoglobin levels. Heart failure and COPD may increase the hemoglobin level due to the need by the body for more oxygen-carrying capacity. Dehydration may increase the hemoglobin level by hemoconcentration.
TEST-TAKING STRATEGY: Evaluate each of the options in terms of whether each is likely to raise or lower the hemoglobin level. Review the normal hemoglobin level and the causes of a low level now if you had difficulty with this question.
LEVEL OF COGNITIVE ABILITY: Comprehension
PHASE OF NURSING PROCESS: Data Collection
CLIENT NEEDS: Physiological Integrity
CONTENT AREA: Fundamental Skills

REFERENCE
Chernecky, C., & Berger, B. (1997). *Laboratory tests and diagnostic procedures* (2nd ed.). Philadelphia: W. B. Saunders. p. 593.

23. 2

RATIONALE: The normal hematocrit level for an adult male is 42% to 52%. The client who is dehydrated has an elevated level owing to hemoconcentration. The client's level may be expected to drift back down to within the normal range once fluid volume has been adequately restored. Thus, option 2 is the only correct choice. Option 1 is too high, whereas options 3 and 4 are low.

TEST-TAKING STRATEGY: Familiarity with this laboratory study is needed to answer this question. Since this is a very common laboratory study, it would be useful to have this one committed to memory.

LEVEL OF COGNITIVE ABILITY: Comprehension

PHASE OF NURSING PROCESS: Evaluation

CLIENT NEEDS: Physiological Integrity

CONTENT AREA: Fundamental Skills

REFERENCE
Chernecky, C., & Berger, B. (1997). *Laboratory tests and diagnostic procedures* (2nd ed.). Philadelphia: W. B. Saunders. p. 591.

24. 3

RATIONALE: The normal level for glycosylated hemoglobin A1c is 3.5% to 6.0%. This test measures the amount of glucose that has become permanently bound to the RBCs from circulating glucose. Elevations in blood glucose will cause elevations in the amount of glycosylation. Thus, the test is useful in detecting clients who have periods of hyperglycemia that are undetected in other ways. Elevations indicate continued need for teaching related to prevention of hyperglycemic episodes.

TEST-TAKING STRATEGY: Familiarity with this test and its significance is needed to answer this question accurately. Take a few moments to review this increasingly common test now if you have the need.

LEVEL OF COGNITIVE ABILITY: Application

PHASE OF NURSING PROCESS: Planning

CLIENT NEEDS: Health Promotion and Maintenance

CONTENT AREA: Adult Health/Endocrine

REFERENCE
Chernecky, C., & Berger, B. (1997). *Laboratory tests and diagnostic procedures* (2nd ed.). Philadelphia: W. B. Saunders. p. 576.

25. 4

RATIONALE: The normal range for urine specific gravity is between 1.016 and 1.022. Elevations may occur with SIADH, because the kidneys are stimulated to reabsorb water, thus causing unusual concentration of the urine. Option 1 represents a low value, which may be seen with diabetes insipidus. Options 2 and 3 reflect normal values.

TEST-TAKING STRATEGY: Familiarity with this test and its significance is needed to answer this question accurately. Take a few moments to review this common urine measurement now if you have the need.

LEVEL OF COGNITIVE ABILITY: Analysis

PHASE OF NURSING PROCESS: Evaluation

CLIENT NEEDS: Physiological Integrity

CONTENT AREA: Adult Health/Neurological

REFERENCE
Chernecky, C., & Berger, B. (1997). *Laboratory tests and diagnostic procedures* (2nd ed.). Philadelphia: W. B. Saunders. p. 921.

26. 1

RATIONALE: The normal WBC count ranges from 4500 to 11,000/μL. The client who is immunosuppressed has a decrease in the number of circulating WBCs. The nurse implements neutropenic precautions when the client's values fall sufficiently under the low normal level.

TEST-TAKING STRATEGY: Familiarity with this test and its significance is needed to answer this question accurately. Take a few moments to review this common hematological test now if you have the need.

LEVEL OF COGNITIVE ABILITY: Comprehension

PHASE OF NURSING PROCESS: Planning

CLIENT NEEDS: Safe, Effective Care Environment

CONTENT AREA: Adult Health/Oncology

REFERENCE
Chernecky, C., & Berger, B. (1997). *Laboratory tests and diagnostic procedures* (2nd ed.). Philadelphia: W. B. Saunders. p. 451.

27. 2

RATIONALE: The client should be counseled to keep the total cholesterol level under 200 mg/dL. This will aid in prevention of atherosclerosis, which can lead to a number of cardiovascular disorders later in life.

TEST-TAKING STRATEGY: To answer this question accurately, it is necessary to be familiar with this specific laboratory value. Because of the importance of the health problems resulting from atherosclerosis, it is a helpful value to memorize.

LEVEL OF COGNITIVE ABILITY: Application

PHASE OF NURSING PROCESS: Implementation

CLIENT NEEDS: Health Promotion and Maintenance

CONTENT AREA: Adult Health/Cardiovascular

REFERENCE
Chernecky, C., & Berger, B. (1997). *Laboratory tests and diagnostic procedures* (2nd ed.). Philadelphia: W. B. Saunders. p. 364.

28. 3

RATIONALE: The normal BUN for the older adult is 5 to 20 mg/dL. Thus option 3 is correct. Values such as those in options 1 and 2 reflect continued dehydration. Option 4 reflects a lower than normal value, which may occur with fluid overload, among other conditions.

TEST-TAKING STRATEGY: To answer this question accurately, it is necessary to be familiar with this specific laboratory value. Because it is such a common laboratory study, this one is quite useful to memorize.

LEVEL OF COGNITIVE ABILITY: Analysis

PHASE OF NURSING PROCESS: Evaluation

CLIENT NEEDS: Physiological Integrity

CONTENT AREA: Adult Health/Renal

REFERENCE
Chernecky, C., & Berger, B. (1997). *Laboratory tests and diagnostic procedures* (2nd ed.). Philadelphia: W. B. Saunders. p. 1003.

29. 4

RATIONALE: The normal fibrinogen level is 180 to 340 mg/dL for men and 190 to 420 mg/dL for women. A critical value is one that is less than 100 mg/dL. With DIC, the fibrinogen level drops because fibrinogen is used up in the clotting process. For these reasons, the nurse is most concerned with the level of 90 mg/dL.

TEST-TAKING STRATEGY: Note the key words "most concerned." Knowing that DIC causes the value to fall, you

would select the value that is the lowest. Review this normal value and manifestations that occur in DIC now if you had difficulty with this question.
LEVEL OF COGNITIVE ABILITY: Analysis
PHASE OF NURSING PROCESS: Data Collection
CLIENT NEEDS: Physiological Integrity
CONTENT AREA: Adult Health/Cardiovascular
REFERENCE
Jaffee, M., & McVan, B. (1997). *Davis's laboratory and diagnostic test handbook* Philadelphia: F. A. Davis. p. 1369.

30. **2**
RATIONALE: The normal hemoglobin level for an adult

female is 12 to 15 g/dL. Option 1 indicates a low value and indicates an anemia. Options 3 and 4 are elevated values.
TEST-TAKING STRATEGY: Knowledge regarding the normal hemoglobin level is required to answer this question. If you are unfamiliar with this laboratory value, take time now to review.
LEVEL OF COGNITIVE ABILITY: Comprehension
PHASE OF NURSING PROCESS: Data Collection
CLIENT NEEDS: Physiological Integrity
CONTENT AREA: Fundamental Skills
REFERENCE
Chernecky, C., & Berger, B. (1997). *Laboratory tests and diagnostic procedures* (2nd ed.). Philadelphia: W. B. Saunders. p. 593.

BIBLIOGRAPHY

Chernecky, C., & Berger, B. (1997). *Laboratory tests and diagnostic procedures* (2nd ed.). Philadelphia: W. B. Saunders.
deWit, S. (1998). *Essentials of medical-surgical nursing* (4th ed.). Philadelphia: W. B. Saunders.
Hodgson, B., & Kizior, R. (1999). *Saunders nursing drug handbook 1999.* Philadelphia: W. B. Saunders.
Jaffee, M., & McVan, B. (1997). *Davis's laboratory and diagnostic test handbook* Philadelphia: F. A. Davis.

Leahy, J., & Kizilay, P. (1998). *Foundations of nursing practice: A nursing process approach.* Philadelphia: W. B. Saunders.
Lehne, R. (1998). *Pharmacology for nursing care* (3rd ed.). Philadelphia: W. B. Saunders.
Luckmann, J. (1997). *Saunders manual of nursing care.* Philadelphia: W. B. Saunders.
Monahan, F., & Neighbors, M. (1998). *Medical-surgical nursing: Foundations for clinical practice* (2nd ed.). Philadelphia: W. B. Saunders.
National Council of State Boards of Nursing (1998). *National Council Detailed Test Plan for the NCLEX-PN Examination.* Chicago: Author.

CHAPTER 11

Nutritional Components of Care

....

PYRAMID TERMS

Absorption—Passage of digested nutrients through the wall of the stomach or small intestine into the blood or lymph system.

Anorexia—A lack of appetite with no desire to eat.

Central Parenteral Nutrition (CPN)—Parenteral nutrition, administered through the subclavian or internal jugular vein, that is used when feeding must last longer than 7 days; known as total parenteral nutrition (TPN).

Digestion—The breakdown of carbohydrates, fats, and proteins into monosaccharides, fatty acids, and amino acids.

Enteral Nutrition—Administering nutrition with liquefied foods into the gastrointestinal (GI) tract via a tube.

Fat Emulsion—Administered during TPN therapy; provides up to 30% of caloric (energy) needs, provides nonprotein calories, and prevents fatty acid deficiency.

Malnutrition—The deficiency of nutrients resulting from improper diet or from some defect in metabolism that prevents the body from using its food properly.

Metabolism—Ongoing chemical process within the body that converts digested nutrients into energy for the functioning of the body cells.

Nutrients—Include carbohydrates, fats/lipids, proteins, vitamins, minerals, and water and must be supplied in adequate amounts to provide energy, growth, development, and maintenance of the human body.

Peripheral Parenteral Nutrition (PPN)—Parenteral nutrition administered through a peripheral vein; used for short-term therapy (5 to 7 days) and when the client needs only small concentrations of carbohydrates, fats, and proteins; known as total parenteral nutrition (TPN).

◆ PYRAMID TO SUCCESS

Nutrition is a basic need that must be met for all clients. Nurses must have the knowledge to educate and care for healthy clients, as well as clients with nutritional needs or disorders requiring alterations in dietary measures. NCLEX-PN addresses the dietary measures required for basic needs and for particular body system alterations. When presented with a question related to nutrition, consider the client diagnosis and the particular requirement or restriction necessary for treatment of the disorder. Pyramid points focus on the common types of therapeutic diets, nutrients contained in food items, enteral feedings, and caring for the client receiving total parenteral nutrition.

NURSING PROCESS

DATA COLLECTION

Nutritional history, meal patterns
Age
Appetite
Vital signs
Height and weight
Physical problems related to eating

Existing disorders
Food preferences and sociocultural or religious considerations
Elimination schedule
Signs of infection and complications related to TPN
Laboratory data

PLANNING

Client maintains adequate intake and output and consumes proper amounts of foods. Client complies with diet therapy. Client tolerates tube feeding. Client is free of signs and symptoms of infection. Client is free of signs and symptoms of complications related to enteral nutrition and TPN.

IMPLEMENTATION

Perform nutritional assessment including history, physical, and diagnostic data. Incorporate a diet considering nutritional needs, physiological disorders, and sociocultural and religious preferences. Initiate dietary consult as necessary. Monitor food and fluid intake. Inform client of the purpose and importance of prescribed diet, and food requirements or restrictions. Monitor I&O and weight. Encourage client to select foods. Monitor tube feedings if prescribed and client's ability to tolerate feeding. Monitor vital signs and for signs of infection or complications in the client receiving TPN.

EVALUATION

Food and fluid I&O is adequate. Client describes appropriate diet. Client independently selects own foods. Client tolerates tube feedings. Vital signs remain within normal limits. Laboratory values are within normal limits. Target weight is achieved. Client remains free of complications. Client complies with diet prescription.

◆ CLIENT NEEDS

SAFE, EFFECTIVE CARE ENVIRONMENT

Standard (universal) and other precautions
Asepsis
Informed consent
Dietary consultation
Home care referral

HEALTH PROMOTION AND MAINTENANCE

Lifestyle choices
Disease prevention
Health and wellness
Health promotion programs
Collecting physical data
Client and family dietary teaching

PSYCHOSOCIAL INTEGRITY

Religious and cultural influences on health
Lifestyle changes
Role changes
Promoting self-care
Support systems

PHYSIOLOGICAL INTEGRITY

Nutrition and oral hydration
Assistance with care
Rest and sleep
Elimination
Enteral feedings

Laboratory values
Alteration in body systems
Monitoring for potential complications of enteral feedings and TPN
Monitoring for expected effects of treatment
Documentation

I. Nutrients

A. Carbohydrates (Table 11–1)
   1. The preferred source of energy
   2. Includes sugars, starches, and cellulose, and provides 4 kcal/g
   3. Promotes normal fat **metabolism,** spares protein, and enhances lower GI function
   4. Major food sources include milk, grains, fruits, and vegetables
   5. Inadequate carbohydrate intake affects **metabolism**

B. Fats (Table 11–2)
   1. Provide a concentrated source of energy and a stored form of energy
   2. Spare protein, improve satiety and palatability
   3. Protect internal organs and maintain body temperature
   4. Enhance **absorption** of the fat-soluble vitamins
   5. Provide 9 kcal/g
   6. Inadequate fat intake leads to clinical manifestations of sensitivity to cold, skin lesions, increased risk of infection, and amenorrhea in women
   7. Diets high in fat can lead to obesity and increase the risk of cardiac disease and some cancers

C. Proteins (Box 11–1)
   1. Made from amino acids, critical to all aspects of growth and development of body tissues, and provide 4 kcal/g

Table 11–1. Carbohydrate Food Sources

Glucose	Fructose	Cellulose	Lactose
Grapes	Honey	Bran	Milk
Oranges	Fruits	Apples	
Dates		Beans	
Corn		Cabbage	
Carrots			

Sucrose	Starch
Granulated table sugar	Wheat
Molasses	Corn
Apricots	Oats
Peaches	Rye
Plums	Barley
Honeydew and cantaloupe	Potatoes and pasta
Peas and corn	Beets, carrots, and peas

BOX 11–1. Protein Food Sources

Cereal products
Dairy products
Dried beans
Meats

Table 11–2. Fat Food Sources

Saturated Fats	*Cholesterol*
Beef	Animal products
Lunchmeats	Egg yolks
Hard yellow cheeses	Liver and organ meats
Butter	

Polyunsaturated Fats	*Monounsaturated Fats*
Safflower oil	Duck and goose
Corn oil	Eggs
Sunflower oil	Olive and peanut oils

2. Build and repair body tissues, regulate fluid balance, maintain acid-base balance, produce antibodies, provide energy, and produce enzymes and hormones
3. Essential amino acids (EAAs) are required in the diet because the body cannot manufacture them
4. High-quality proteins or complete proteins such as eggs, dairy products, meat, fish, and poultry contain adequate amounts of EAAs
5. Foods that do not contain the EAAs in sufficient amounts are lower quality or incomplete proteins
6. Inadequate protein can cause protein energy **malnutrition** and severe wasting of fat and muscle tissue

D. Vitamins (Box 11–2)
1. Facilitate **metabolism** of proteins, fats, and carbohydrates; act as a catalyst for metabolic functions; promote life and growth processes; and maintain and regulate body functions
2. Fat-soluble vitamins A, D, E, and K can be stored in the body, so an excess can cause toxicity
3. The B vitamins and vitamin C are water soluble, are not stored in the body, and can be excreted in the urine
4. Vitamin K acts as a catalyst for facilitating blood-clotting factors, especially prothrombin
5. Vitamin C produces collagen, a vital component in wound healing
6. Vitamin A maintains eyesight and epithelial linings

E. Minerals (Box 11–3)

BOX 11–2. Food Sources of Vitamins

WATER SOLUBLE

Vitamin C (ascorbic acid): citrus fruits, tomatoes, broccoli, cabbage
Vitamin B_1 (thiamine): pork, nuts, whole grain cereals, legumes
Vitamin B_2 (riboflavin): milk, lean meats, fish, grains
Niacin: meats, poultry, fish, beans, peanuts, grains
Vitamin B_6 (pyridoxine): yeast, corn, meat, poultry, fish
Vitamin B_{12} (cobalamin): meat, liver
Folic acid; green leafy vegetables; liver, beef, and fish; legumes; grapefruit and oranges

FAT SOLUBLE

Vitamin A: liver, egg yolk, whole milk, green and orange vegetables, fruits
Vitamin D: fortified milk, fish oils, cereals
Vitamin E: vegetable oils; green leafy vegetables; cereals; apricots, apples, and peaches
Vitamin K: green leafy vegetables, cauliflower, and cabbage

BOX 11–3. Food Sources of Minerals

CALCIUM

Milk and dairy products
Dark green leafy vegetables
Sardines
Fortified orange juice

CHLORIDE

Salt

MAGNESIUM

Whole-grain products
Nuts and beans
Bananas
Green leafy vegetables

PHOSPHORUS

Meat and dairy products
Meats
Whole grains
Legumes and nuts

POTASSIUM

Dried fruits
Baked potato
Cantaloupe
Bananas
Spinach
Milk
Steak
Beans

SODIUM

Canned foods
Cheeses
Ham, pork, sausages, luncheon meats, hot dogs
Soy sauce
Salt

IRON

Liver, meats
Egg yolk
Dark green vegetables
Breads and cereals

ZINC

Meats
Eggs
Leafy vegetables
Protein-rich foods

1. Components of hormones, cells, tissues, and bones
2. Act as catalysts for chemical reactions and as enhancers of cell function
3. Almost all foods contain some form of minerals
4. A deficiency of minerals can occur in chronically ill or hospitalized clients

II. Food Guide Pyramid (Fig. 11–1)

A. Groups six broad families of foods with similar kinds of **nutrients** together
B. Levels of the pyramid
1. Level one (base of the pyramid)
   a. Bread, cereal, rice, and pasta group
   b. Daily recommendation is 6 to 11 servings
2. Level two
   a. Vegetables and fruit group
   b. Daily recommendation is 3 to 5 servings of vegetables and 2 to 4 servings of fruit
3. Level three
   a. Includes the milk, yogurt, and cheese group and the meats, poultry, fish, dry beans and peas, eggs, and nuts group
   b. Daily recommendation is 2 to 3 servings for each group
   c. The recommendation for the milk group depends on the various life stage of the individual
4. Peak of the pyramid
   a. Includes fats and sweets group
   b. Foods high in fats, sugar, or alcohol and are to be eaten sparingly because they are kilocalorie-dense, nutrient-sparse foods

III. Therapeutic Diets

A. Clear liquid
1. Indications
   a. Serves a primary function of providing fluids and electrolytes to prevent dehydration
   b. Initial feeding after complete bowel rest
   c. Used to feed a malnourished person or a person that has not had any oral intake for some time
   d. Bowel preparation for surgery or tests
   e. Postsurgical diet
   f. Diarrhea
2. Nursing considerations
   a. Is deficient in energy and most **nutrients**
   b. The body digests and absorbs clear liquids easily
   c. Contributes to little or no residue in the GI tract
   d. Can be unappetizing and boring
   e. Client should not stay on a clear liquid diet for more than 1 to 2 days
   f. Consists of foods that are relatively transparent to light, are in liquid form at body temperature, and may be semisolid when cooled
   g. Foods include water, bouillon, clear broth, carbonated beverages, either regular or decaffeinated coffee, fruit drinks or strained fruit juices, gelatin, hard candy, honey, lemonade, Popsicles, and tea
   h. Client may have salt or sugar
   i. Dairy products are not allowed

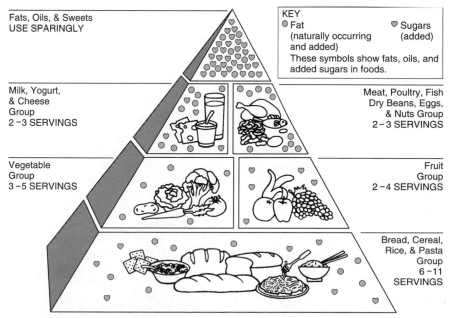

FIGURE 11–1. The food guide pyramid.

B. Full liquid
 1. Indication: may be used as a second diet after clear liquids following surgery, or for the client who is unable to chew or swallow
 2. Nursing considerations
    a. Nutritionally deficient in energy and most **nutrients**
    b. Includes both clear and opaque liquid foods and those that liquefy at body temperature
    c. Foods include all clear liquids, butter, margarine, cream, cooked strained cereals, cream custard, soft cooked or scrambled eggs, plain ice cream, breakfast drinks, milk, mashed potatoes, pudding, sherbet, strained soups, strained vegetables, and fruit juices
C. Soft
 1. Indications
    a. Used in clients with dental problems, clients with poor-fitting dentures, and clients who have difficulty chewing or swallowing
    b. Used for ulcerations of the mouth or gums, oral surgery, broken jaw, plastic surgery of head or neck, dysphagia, stroke, acquired immunodeficiency syndrome (AIDS)
    c. Therapeutic for clients with impaired **digestion** and/or **absorption** due to conditions such as ulcerative colitis and Crohn's disease
 2. Nursing considerations
    a. Clients with mouth sores should be served foods at cooler temperatures
    b. Clients who have difficulty chewing and swallowing due to a reduced flow of saliva can increase salivary flow by sucking on sour candy or chewing gum
    c. Encourage the client to eat a variety of foods; all foods and seasonings are permitted
    d. Provide plenty of fluids with meals to ease chewing and swallowing of foods
    e. Sucking fluids through a straw may be easier than drinking them from a cup or glass
    f. Liquid, chopped, pureed, or regular foods with a soft consistency are best tolerated
    g. Avoid foods that contain nuts or seeds because these can become easily trapped in the mouth and cause discomfort
    h. Avoid raw fruits and vegetables, fried foods, and whole grains
D. Bland
 1. Indication: Used for gastritis, ulcers, reflux esophagitis, congestive heart failure (CHF), and myocardial infarction (MI)
 2. Nursing considerations
    a. Bland foods are less likely to form gas than regular diets
    b. Eliminate foods that stimulate gastric acid secretions
    c. Eliminate foods that are irritating to the gastric mucosa
    d. Foods to be avoided include alcohol, caffeine, and caffeine-containing beverages such as cola, cocoa, coffee, and tea; fried foods; pepper and spicy foods
E. Low residue/low fiber
 1. Indications
    a. Supplies foods that are least likely to form an obstruction when the intestinal tract is narrowed by inflammation or scarring, or when GI motility is slowed
    b. Used for inflammatory bowel disease, ileostomy, colostomy, partial obstructions of the intestinal tract, enteritis, or diarrhea
 2. Nursing considerations
    a. Foods high in carbohydrates are usually low in residue and include white bread, cereals, pasta
    b. Foods to be avoided are raw fruits (except bananas), vegetables, seeds, plant fiber, and whole grains
    c. Dairy products are limited to two servings a day
F. High-fiber diet
 1. Indications
    a. Used in constipation
    b. Used in irritable bowel syndrome and when the primary symptom of irritable bowel syndrome is alternating constipation and diarrhea
    c. Helps regulate blood glucose in clients with diabetes mellitus
    d. Helps control blood cholesterol in clients with heart disease
 2. Nursing considerations
    a. Provides 20 to 25 g of dietary fiber daily
    b. Adds volume and weight to the stool and speeds the movement of undigested materials through the intestine
    c. Consists of fruits and vegetables
G. Fat-controlled diet (Box 11–4)
 1. Indications
    a. Indicated for atherosclerosis, diabetes, hyperlipidemia, hypertension, MI, nephrotic syndrome, and renal failure
    b. Reduces the risk of heart disease
 2. Nursing consideration: Limit the total amount of fats as well as amounts of polyunsaturated, monounsaturated, and saturated fats and cholesterol
H. High-calorie diet
 1. Indications: severe stress, burns, cancer, human immunodeficiency virus (HIV) and AIDS, chronic obstructive pulmonary disease (COPD), respiratory failure
 2. Nursing considerations
    a. High-calorie diets are also high-protein diets because the purpose of the diet is to build or maintain lean body mass
    b. Add fats to foods whenever possible

BOX 11–4. Foods High in Fat

- Canned, cured, salted, or smoked meats
- Lunchmeats
- Sausage, ham, bacon, and hot dogs
- Organ meats
- Caviar
- Whole milk
- Buttermilk
- Ice cream, half-and-half cream
- Eggnog, nondairy coffee creamer, high-fat cheeses
- Fried foods
- Butter rolls, egg bread, bagels, biscuits, muffins, doughnuts, sweet rolls, pancakes, french toast, cheese and butter crackers, cereal containing coconut oil or nuts
- Potato chips, corn chips, other fried snacks
- Grains prepared with eggs, milk, cream, fat, or vegetable shortening
- Butter, lard, margarine, salad dressings, chocolates, palm oil, cashews, pistachios, macadamia nuts

---

    c. Add nuts and dried fruits such as raisins to desserts or cereals

    d. Add sugar to food and encourage high-calorie desserts

    e. Encourage snacks between meals, such as milkshakes and instant breakfasts

I. Sodium-restriction diet (Box 11–5)

    1. Indications: hypertension, CHF, kidney diseases, cardiac diseases, and cirrhosis

    2. Nursing considerations (Box 11–6)

BOX 11–5. Foods High in Sodium

- Highly salted snacks
- Bouillon cubes
- Catsup
- Horseradish
- Meat extracts
- Monosodium glutamate
- Prepared mustard, olives, onion salt, pickles, relishes, saccharin, soy sauce, and other sauces and tenderizers
- Canned foods and commercial foods made with milk; ice cream, sherbert, artichokes, beets, carrots, cabbage, sauerkraut, and spinach
- Maraschino cherries; glazed fruit and dried fruits; grains; kidneys; canned, salted, or smoked meats
- Bacon, lunchmeats, hot dogs, corned beef, kosher meats, shellfish, and cod fish; regular cheeses; egg substitutes; peanut butter
- Salted butter or margarine, saltpork, commercial salad dressing, and salted nuts
- Baking powder and baking soda
- Pudding mixes
- Molasses
- Instant cocoa mixes
- Candy, cakes, cookies, sweetened gelatin mixes, pastry, puddings, and biscuit mix

---

BOX 11–6. Sodium-Free Spices and Flavorings

Allspice, almond extract, bay leaves, caraway seeds, cinnamon, curry powder, garlic powder or garlic, ginger, lemon extract, maple extract, marjoram, mustard powder, and nutmeg

---

    a. The amount of sodium allowed varies from 250 mg to about 4 g daily

    b. A no-added-salt diet includes no salt at the table and lightly salting foods during cooking

    c. Foods allowed on a sodium-restricted diet include dried or instant cereals, puffed wheat, puffed rice, and shredded wheat

J. Protein-restricted diet

    1. Indications: acute renal failure, chronic renal disease, cirrhosis, and hepatic coma

    2. Nursing considerations

       a. Provide enough protein to maintain nutritional status but not enough to allow the build-up of waste products from protein **metabolism** (40 to 60 g of protein daily)

       b. The lower the amount of protein allowed, the more important it becomes that all protein included in the diet be of high quality

       c. An adequate total energy intake is critical for clients on protein-restricted diets because without adequate energy, protein will be used for energy rather than in protein synthesis

       d. To boost energy intake, clients may use fats and concentrated sweets from margarine, creamed butter, hard candy, jelly, and sugar whenever possible

       e. Special low-protein products such as pastas, breads, cookies, wafers, and gelatin made with wheat starch can improve energy intake and add variety to the diet

       f. Carbohydrates in powdered or liquid forms can also provide additional energy

       g. Vegetables and fruits contain some protein, and for very-low-protein diets, these foods must be calculated into the diet

       h. Foods are limited from the milk, meat, bread, and starch exchanges

K. High-protein diet

    1. Indications: tissue building, burns, liver disease, and maternity clients

    2. Nursing considerations

       a. High-protein diets correct protein loss or assist with tissue repair

       b. Increase foods such as meat, fish, fowl, and dairy products

       c. Client may need protein supplements

L. Low-calcium diet

    1. Indication: to prevent renal calculi (Table 11–3)

Table 11–3. **Diets for Renal Calculi**

Alkaline Ash Diet

To increase pH
Milk
Fruits except cranberries, plums, and prunes
Rhubarb
Vegetables
Small amounts of beef, halibut, veal, trout, and salami are allowed

Acid Ash Diet

To decrease pH
Eggs
Meat
Cranberries, plums, prunes
Fish
Poultry
Oysters

2. Nursing considerations
   a. Decrease the total intake of calcium to prevent further stone formation
   b. Avoid whole grains, milk and dairy products, and green leafy vegetables
M. Low-purine diet
   1. Indication: used to treat gout
   2. Nursing considerations
      a. Purine is a precursor for uric acid that forms stones and crystals
      b. Avoid glandular meats and gravies
N. High-iron diet
   1. Indication: used in anemia
   2. Nursing considerations
      a. Replace iron deficit from inadequate intake or loss
      b. Include organ meats, meat, egg yolks, whole wheat products, leafy vegetables, dried fruit, and legumes
O. Diet for diverticular disease
   1. Foods with seeds need to be avoided as they get trapped in the diverticula and cause irritation
   2. Foods to avoid include whole grain breads and cereals, fruits, vegetables, dried beans, peas, and nuts
   3. Gas-forming foods should be avoided in clients with irritable bowel syndrome (Box 11–7)
P. Fluid restriction (Box 11–8)
   1. Indications: Acute renal failure-oliguric phase, chronic renal disease, cirrhosis, CHF, hepatic coma, MI

BOX 11–7. Gas-Forming Foods

Apples, artichokes, barley, beans, bran, broccoli, Brussel sprouts, cabbage, celery, cherries, coconuts, eggplant, figs, honey, melons, milk, molasses, nuts, onions, radishes, soybeans, wheat, and yeast

BOX 11–8. Measures to Relieve Thirst

Chew gum or suck hard candy
Freeze fluids so they take longer to consume
Add lemon juice to water to make it more refreshing
Gargle with refrigerated mouthwash

2. Nursing considerations
   a. Usually this diet restricts those foods that are composed largely of water
   b. Restrict carbonated beverages, coffee, juices, milk, tea, water, frozen yogurt, gelatin, ice cream, ice milk, Popsicles, sherbet, soup, cream, and liquid medications
Q. Carbohydrate-controlled diet
   1. Indications
      a. Helps maintain normal glucose levels in clients with disorders that cause blood glucose levels to rise or fall abnormally, such as diabetes or hypoglycemia
      b. Used for diabetes mellitus, hypoglycemia, lactose intolerance, galactosemia, dumping syndrome, obesity and overweight
   2. Nursing considerations
      a. Adjust energy intake from foods to provide specific amounts and types of carbohydrates
      b. The exchange list system most frequently used to plan carbohydrate-controlled diets
R. Miscellaneous diets
   1. See Box 11–9 for foods high in potassium
   2. See Box 11–10 for foods high in phosphorus

IV. The Exchange System

A. Starches and breads
   1. One bread is equal to 15 g carbohydrate, 3 g protein, trace of fat, and 80 calories
   2. Equal to ¾ cup ready-to-eat cereal, ⅓ cup cooked beans, ½ cup corn
B. Meats
   1. One lean meat is equal to 7 g protein, 3 g fat, and 55 calories

BOX 11–9. High-Potassium Foods

Vegetables: artichokes, asparagus, beets, broccoli, Brussel sprouts, cabbage, dried beans and peas, green beans, kale, mixed vegetables, parsnips, pinto beans, potatoes, pumpkins, spinach, squash, tomatoes, tomato juice, turnip greens, vegetable juice, winter squash, and yams
   Fruits: apricots, avocados, bananas, cantaloupe, dates, figs, grapefruit, honeydew melon, kiwifruit, nectarines, orange juice, papayas, peaches, pears, pineapple, prune juice, prunes, raisins, rhubarb, strawberries, and tangerines
   Chocolate, cocoa, meat, milk, molasses, peanuts, walnuts, wheat germ

2. One meat exchange is equal to 1 ounce
3. One ounce of lean meat is equal to 1 ounce of chicken meat without skin, 1 ounce of any fish, ¼ cup canned tuna, or 1 ounce low-fat cheese
4. Medium-fat meats
   a. One medium-fat meat is equal to 7 g protein, 5 g fat, and about 75 calories
   b. One ounce medium-fat meat is equal to 1 ounce lean meat in protein content but has 5 g of fat
   c. Equal to 1 ounce of pork loin, 1 egg, ¼ cup creamed cottage cheese
5. High-fat meats
   a. One high-fat meat is equal to 7 g protein, 8 g fat, and 100 calories
   b. A hot dog counts as 1 high-fat meat exchange plus 1 fat exchange
   c. One ounce of high-fat meat is equal to 1 ounce lean meat in protein content plus 1 fat exchange
   d. Peanut butter is like a meat in terms of its protein content
   e. One tablespoon of peanut butter is equal to 1 high-fat meat
   f. One tablespoon of peanut butter is equal to 7 g protein, 8 g fat, and 100 calories
C. Vegetables
   1. One vegetable is equal to 5 g of carbohydrate, 2 g of protein, and 25 calories
   2. One half cup of carrots is equal to ½ cup of greens, ½ cup of Brussel sprouts, ½ cup of beets
D. Fruits
   1. One fruit is equal to 15 g of carbohydrate and 60 calories
   2. One half banana is equal to 1 small apple, ½ grapefruit, or ½ cup orange juice
E. Milks
   1. One milk is equal to 12 g of carbohydrate, 8 g of protein, trace of fat, and 90 calories
   2. One cup nonfat milk is equal to 1 cup nonfat plain yogurt, 1 cup nonfat buttermilk, or ½ cup evaporated nonfat milk
F. Fats
   1. One fat is equal to 5 g fat and 45 calories
   2. One teaspoon of butter is equal to 1 teaspoon margarine, 1 teaspoon any oils, 1 tablespoon of salad dressing, 1 strip of bacon, 5 large olives, 10 whole peanuts
G. Legumes
   1. Similar to meats, legumes are rich in protein and iron, and are lower in fat than meat

2. Contain starch
3. One cup of legumes is equal to 1 lean meat plus 2 starches
4. One cup legumes is equal to 30 g of carbohydrate, 13 g of protein, 3 g of fat, and 215 calories

V. Enteral Nutrition

A. Description
   1. Tube feedings that consist of blenderized food or prepared products that provide carbohydrates, fat, protein, and water
   2. Administered through nasogastric or gastrostomy tube
   3. Administered continuously or intermittently
B. Indications
   1. When the gastrointestinal (GI) tract is functional but oral intake is not feasible
   2. Used for clients with swallowing problems, cancer, burns, major trauma, liver failure, or severe **malnutrition**
C. Administering enteral feedings
   1. Keep the head of the bed elevated to prevent aspiration
   2. Warm feeding to room temperature to prevent diarrhea and cramps
   3. Check placement of tube every 4 hours by aspirating gastric contents and measuring the pH (should be 4 or less)
   4. Aspirate all stomach contents (residual), measure the amount, and return contents to the stomach to prevent electrolyte imbalance
   5. Usually, if residual is less than 100 to 150 mL, feeding is administered; if greater than 150 mL, hold the feeding
   6. Check for bowel sounds; hold the feeding if bowel sounds are absent and report the findings
   7. Flush tubing with water following feeding to maintain fluid balance and patency of tube
   8. Use a feeding pump for continuous feedings
   9. Do not allow feeding to hang longer than 8 hours and change feeding bag every 24 hours to avoid contamination
D. Prevention of complications
   1. Diarrhea
      a. Use fiber-containing feedings
      b. Administer feeding slowly and at room temperature
   2. Aspiration
      a. Verify tube placement
      b. Do not administer feeding if residual is greater than 150 mL
      c. Keep the head of the bed elevated
      d. If aspiration occurs, suction as needed, monitor temperature for aspiration pneumonia, monitor for dyspnea, monitor respiratory rate, and prepare the client for a chest radiograph
   3. Clogged tube

a. Flush the tube with 20 to 50 mL of water before and after feeding administration
b. Flush with water every 4 hours for continuous feeding
4. Vomiting
   a. Administer feedings slowly, and for bolus feedings, make feeding last for 30 minutes
   b. Measure abdominal girth
   c. Do not allow feeding to run dry
   d. Do not allow air to enter the tubing
   e. Administer feeding at room temperature
   f. Elevate the head of the bed
   g. Administer antiemetics as prescribed
   h. If client vomits, place in side-lying position

VI. Total Parenteral Nutrition (TPN)

A. Description
   1. Supplies necessary nutrients via veins
   2. Supplies carbohydrates in the form of dextrose, fats in a special emulsified form, proteins in the form of amino acids, vitamins, and minerals
   3. Prevents subcutaneous fat and muscle protein from being catabolized by the body for energy
B. Indications
   1. When the GI tract is severely dysfunctional or nonfunctional
   2. Clients who can take some oral nutrition, but not enough to meet the body's needs
   3. Clients with multiple GI surgeries, GI trauma, severe intolerance to enteral feedings, intestinal obstructions, or when the bowel needs to rest for healing
   4. Clients with AIDS, cancer, or malnutrition
C. Intravenous sites
   1. Peripheral parenteral nutrition (PPN)
      a. Administered through a peripheral vein
      b. Used for short periods (5–7 days) and when the client needs only small concentrations of carbohydrates, fats, and proteins
   2. Central parenteral nutrition (CPN)
      a. Administered through the subclavian or internal jugular vein
      b. Used when feeding must last longer than 7 days
D. Complications (Box 11–11)
E. Precautions
   1. Assist with insertion of catheter; position the client in Trendelenburg position with a towel under the scapula
   2. Ask the client to perform the Valsalva maneuver during insertion to prevent air emboli
   3. When the central line is inserted, placement is confirmed by chest x-ray
   4. TPN catheter is not used for blood draws or the administration of other medications or fluids
   5. TPN is always delivered via an electronic infusion device
   6. Solutions should be stored under refrigeration
   7. TPN solution is changed every 24 hours
F. Nursing interventions
   1. Maintain aseptic technique
   2. Monitor vital signs
   3. Monitor weight and intake and output (I&O) daily
   4. Monitor site for redness, swelling, tenderness, or drainage
   5. Monitor urine for sugar and acetone four times per day
   6. Electrolytes, glucose, and blood urea nitrogen (BUN) are monitored as prescribed
   7. Monitor rate hourly
   8. If sepsis is suspected, a blood culture will be drawn, and the tip of the catheter will be cultured for bacteria
   9. Monitor for signs of fluid overload such as a bounding pulse, jugular vein distention, headache, increased blood pressure, and lung crackles
   10. Keep tubing connections taped
   11. If the intravenous (IV) tubing disconnects, instruct the client to perform the Valsalva maneuver
   12. Monitor for signs of an air embolus such as confusion, pallor, light-headedness, tachycardia, tachypnea, hypotension, anxiety, and unresponsiveness
   13. Place the client in the left side-lying position with the head lower than the feet if air embolism is suspected, and contact the physician
G. Fat emulsion
   1. Assess for allergy to eggs, a contraindication for lipid infusion
   2. Administer slowly for the first 15 to 30 minutes and monitor the client for adverse reactions such as dyspnea, cyanosis, and allergic responses
   3. Monitor for signs and symptoms of fat overload, which include fever, leukocytosis, hyperlipidemia, pruritic urticaria, and possibly focal seizures

---

BOX 11–11. Complications of TPN

Infection
Hyperglycemia
Fluid overload
Air embolism

PRACTICE QUESTIONS

1. An alkaline ash diet is prescribed for the client with renal calculi. Which of the following diet menus does the nurse advise the client to select?
   1 A spinach salad, milk, and a banana
   2 Pasta with shrimp, tossed salad, and a plum
   3 Turkey, rice, and cranberries
   4 Peanut butter sandwich, salad, and prunes

2. A low-sodium diet has been prescribed for the client with hypertension. Following diet teaching, which of the following foods, if selected from the menu by the client, best indicates an understanding of this diet?
   1 Tomato soup
   2 Baked turkey
   3 Chicken gumbo soup
   4 Boiled shrimp

3. The nurse is providing dietary instructions to a client with gout. Which of the following foods does the nurse instruct the client to avoid?
   1 Macaroni products
   2 Cornbread
   3 Scallops
   4 Chocolate

4. A clear liquid diet has been prescribed for the client with gastroenteritis. Which of the following nutritional items is most appropriate to offer to the client?
   1 Orange juice
   2 Strained soup
   3 Fat-free broth
   4 Soft custard

5. A potassium-sparing diuretic is prescribed for the client with CHF. Which of the following foods does the nurse instruct the client to avoid?
   1 Bananas
   2 Cranberry juice
   3 Plums
   4 Cheddar cheese

6. The diabetic client has been instructed in the dietary exchange system. The client asks the nurse if bacon is allowed in the diet. Which of the following responses is most appropriate?
   1 "Bacon is much too high in fat."
   2 "Bacon is not allowed."
   3 "One strip of bacon may be eaten if you eliminate 1 teaspoon of butter."
   4 "Bacon may be eaten if you eliminate one meat item from your diet."

7. The client has been diagnosed with ulcerative colitis. Which of the following diets does the nurse anticipate would be prescribed for the client?
   1 High residue
   2 Low residue
   3 High carbohydrate
   4 Low fat

8. The client with heart disease is instructed regarding a low-fat diet. The nurse evaluates that the client understands the diet if the client states a food item to avoid is
   1 Apples
   2 Oranges

   3 Avocado
   4 Cherries

9. The nurse instructs a client to increase the content of riboflavin in the diet. The nurse tells the client to select which of the following food items that is especially high in riboflavin?
   1 Milk
   2 Liver
   3 Chicken
   4 Eggs

10. The nurse instructs a client to increase the content of thiamine in the diet. The nurse tells the client to select which of the following food items that is especially high in thiamine?
    1 Chicken
    2 Broccoli
    3 Pork
    4 Milk

11. The nurse caring for a client with a neurological disorder is assisting in planning care to maintain nutritional status. The nurse is concerned about the client's swallowing ability. The nurse does not include which of the following food items in this client's diet?
    1 Cheese casserole
    2 Scrambled eggs
    3 Mashed potatoes
    4 Spinach

12. The nurse is assisting in planning a diet for the client with acute renal failure (ARF). The nurse restricts which of the following dietary components from this client's diet?
    1 Carbohydrates
    2 Fats
    3 Vitamins
    4 Potassium

13. The nurse is assisting in preparing a diet plan for the postgastrectomy client with dumping syndrome. The nurse does not include which of the following in the teaching plan?
    1 Lie down after eating
    2 Drink liquids with meals
    3 Eat small meals six times daily
    4 Avoid concentrated sweets

14. The nurse is assisting in preparing a diet plan for the client who is taking warfarin (Coumadin), an anticoagulant, daily. The nurse instructs the client to exclude which of the following foods from the diet?
    1 Pasta
    2 Broccoli
    3 Oranges
    4 Potatoes

15. A client has been diagnosed with pernicious anemia. In planning care for the client, the nurse anticipates that the client will be treated with

1 Thiamine
2 Iron
3 Vitamin B_{12}
4 Folic acid

16. An elderly postoperative client has been tolerating a full liquid diet and the nurse plans to advance the diet to solid food as prescribed. The nurse collects data regarding which of the following most important items before advancing the diet to solids?
    1 Food preferences
    2 Cultural preferences
    3 Presence of bowel sounds
    4 Ability to chew

17. A burned client is transferred to the nursing unit and a regular diet has been prescribed. The nurse encourages the client to eat which dietary item in order to promote wound healing?
    1 Veal, potatoes, Jell-O, orange juice
    2 Peanut butter and jelly sandwich, cantaloupe, tea
    3 Chicken breast, broccoli, strawberries, milk
    4 Spaghetti with tomato sauce, garlic bread, ginger ale

18. The nurse is caring for a postoperative client. The physician has prescribed a clear liquid diet. In planning to initiate this diet, which of the following priority items does the nurse place at the bedside?
    1 Code cart
    2 A straw
    3 Cardiac monitor
    4 Suction equipment

19. The nurse is assisting a client who has had a cerebrovascular accident (CVA) to eat. The nurse implements which of the following that will best promote independence?
    1 Offer only pureed foods
    2 Sit the client in high Fowler's position
    3 Place the food tray on the unaffected side
    4 Encourage the client to eat with other clients who have had CVAs

20. The nurse has completed diet teaching for a client on a low-sodium diet for hypertension. The nurse evaluates that further teaching is necessary when the client makes which of these statements?
    1 "This diet will help to lower my blood pressure."
    2 "The reason I need lower salt intake is to reduce fluid retention."
    3 "This diet is not a replacement for my antihypertensive medications."
    4 "Frozen foods are lowest in sodium."

21. The nurse who is assisting in conducting a weight-loss program prepares to monitor a client's weight loss. The nurse implements which method that would most accurately determine the effectiveness of weight loss?
    1 Daily weights
    2 Serum protein levels
    3 Calorie counts
    4 Daily intake and output

22. The nurse is monitoring a client with anorexia nervosa. Which statement, if made by the client, indicates to the nurse that treatment has been effective?
    1 "I no longer have a weight problem."
    2 "I don't want to starve myself anymore."
    3 "I'll eat until I don't feel hungry."
    4 "My friends and I went out to lunch today."

23. The nurse is preparing to instruct a pregnant client about nutrition. The nurse plans to include which of the following in this client's teaching plan?
    1 The nutritional status of the mother significantly influences fetal growth and development
    2 All mothers are at high risk for nutritional deficiencies
    3 Calcium is not important until the third trimester
    4 Iron supplements are not necessary unless the mother has iron-deficiency anemia

24. A client with lung cancer receiving chemotherapy tells the nurse that the food on the meal tray tastes "funny." Which of the following is the most appropriate nursing intervention?
    1 Keep the client NPO
    2 Administer an antiemetic as prescribed
    3 Provide oral hygiene care frequently
    4 Consult with other health care providers regarding an order for total parenteral nutrition (TPN)

25. A client is on a diet designed to avoid concentrated sugars. The nurse evaluates that the client understands the diet plan if which of these diets is selected by the client?
    1 Strawberry yogurt, lettuce salad, coffee
    2 Chicken salad, tomato, Jell-O, instant iced tea
    3 Peanut butter and jelly sandwich, sherbet, cola
    4 Tuna sandwich, lettuce salad, watermelon, herbal tea

26. A client who has a gastrostomy tube for feeding refuses to participate in the plan of care, will not make eye contact, and does not speak to the family or visitors. The nurse identifies that this client is using which type of coping mechanism?
    1 Self-control
    2 Problem-solving
    3 Accepting responsibility
    4 Distancing

27. A client receiving enteral feedings develops abdominal distention and diarrhea shortly after initiation of the feedings. When reviewing the nursing history for this client, which of these notations indicates the need to notify the primary health care provider?
    1 Prior history of enteral feedings
    2 Difficulty swallowing
    3 History of hemorrhoids
    4 Lactose intolerance since childhood

28. The nurse is assigned to care for a client receiving enteral feedings. The nurse plans care knowing that which of the following is of highest priority for this client?
    1 Altered nutrition
    2 Risk for aspiration
    3 Risk for fluid volume deficit
    4 Risk for diarrhea

29. The nurse is preparing to administer a feeding to the client receiving enteral nutrition through a nasogastric tube. The nurse performs which of the following as the priority nursing action?
    1 Measuring intake and output
    2 Weighing the client
    3 Adding blue food coloring to the formula
    4 Determining tube placement

30. The nurse has reinforced discharge teaching with the family of a client who is to have enteral feedings at home. The nurse uses which method of evaluation to best determine the family's competence in performing the feeding procedure?
    1 A return demonstration of the feeding procedure
    2 Selection of appropriate equipment for the feeding procedure
    3 Written testing on the steps of the feeding procedure
    4 Verbal description of the feeding procedure by each member of the family

31. The nurse is asked to assist in preparing a client who will be receiving total parenteral nutrition (TPN) solution via the central line. The nurse obtains which of the following most essential pieces of equipment for this procedure?
    1 Electronic infusion pump
    2 Blood glucose meter
    3 Urine test strips
    4 Noninvasive blood pressure monitor

32. The client is receiving TPN. The nurse monitors the client for which of the following signs of hyperglycemia, a complication of this therapy?
    1 Nausea, vomiting, and oliguria
    2 Sweating, chills, and abdominal pain
    3 Pallor, weak pulse, and thirst
    4 Nausea, thirst, and increased urine output

33. The client receiving TPN complains of headache. The nurse notes that the client has an increased blood pressure and a bounding pulse. The nurse reports the findings, knowing that these signs are indicative of which complication of TPN therapy?
    1 Hyperglycemia
    2 Air embolism
    3 Sepsis
    4 Fluid overload

34. The client receiving TPN may begin to take small amounts of clear liquids today. The nurse's priority is to collect data regarding which of the following before giving the client anything by mouth?
    1 Client's appetite
    2 Client's weight today
    3 Presence of swallow reflex
    4 Adequate pulse and blood pressure

35. The nurse is assigned to assist in caring for a client who is receiving TPN with fat emulsion. The nurse is instructed to monitor the client for signs of fat overload. The nurse monitors for which of the following signs and symptoms of this complications?
    1 Fever and pruritic urticaria
    2 Hypothermia and muscle weakness
    3 Hypertension and decreased urine output
    4 Bradycardia and chest pain

ANSWERS

1. **1**

RATIONALE: In an alkaline ash diet all fruits are allowed except cranberries, prunes, and plums. Options 2, 3, and 4 represent an acid ash diet.
TEST-TAKING STRATEGY: Use the process of elimination. Remembering that cranberries, prunes, and plums are not allowed in an alkaline ash diet will direct you to the correct option. Review the foods allowed in this diet now if you had difficulty with this question.

LEVEL OF COGNITIVE ABILITY: Application
PHASE OF NURSING PROCESS: Implementation
CLIENT NEEDS: Physiological Integrity
CONTENT AREA: Adult Health/Renal
REFERENCE
Mahan, L., & Escott-Stump, S. (1996). *Krause's food, nutrition, & diet therapy* (9th ed.). Philadelphia: W. B. Saunders. p. 780.

2. **2**

RATIONALE: Regular soup (1 cup) contains 900 mg Na. Fresh shellfish (1 oz) contains 50 mg Na. Poultry (1 oz) contains 25 mg Na.

TEST-TAKING STRATEGY: Eliminate options 1 and 3 first because they are similar. Also recall that canned foods are high in sodium. From the remaining two options, select option 2 over option 4 remembering that shellfish is also high in sodium. Review foods high in sodium now if you had difficulty with this question.
LEVEL OF COGNITIVE ABILITY: Comprehension
PHASE OF NURSING PROCESS: Evaluation
CLIENT NEEDS: Health Promotion and Maintenance
CONTENT AREA: Adult Health/Cardiovascular
REFERENCE
Peckenpaugh, N., & Poleman, C. (1999). *Nutrition essentials and diet therapy* (8th ed.) Philadelphia: W. B. Saunders. p. 147.

3. 3

RATIONALE: Scallops should be omitted from the diet of a client who has gout because of the high purine content. The food items identified in options 1, 2, and 4 contain a negligible purine content and may be consumed daily by the client with gout.
TEST-TAKING STRATEGY: Knowledge regarding high-purine foods is required to answer this question. Review foods high in purine now if you had difficulty with this question.
LEVEL OF COGNITIVE ABILITY: Application
PHASE OF NURSING PROCESS: Implementation
CLIENT NEEDS: Health Promotion and Maintenance
CONTENT AREA: Adult Health/Musculoskeletal
REFERENCE
Peckenpaugh, N., & Poleman, C. (1999). *Nutrition essentials and diet therapy* (8th ed.) Philadelphia: W. B. Saunders. p. 146.

4. 3
RATIONALE: A clear liquid diet consists of foods that are relatively transparent. The food items in options 1, 2, and 4 would be included in a full liquid diet.
TEST-TAKING STRATEGY: Remember that a clear liquid diet consists of foods that are relatively transparent. By the process of elimination you should easily select option 3 because this is the only food item that is transparent. Review food items allowed on a clear liquid and full liquid diet now if you had difficulty with this question.
LEVEL OF COGNITIVE ABILITY: Application
PHASE OF NURSING PROCESS: Implementation
CLIENT NEEDS: Physiological Integrity
CONTENT AREA: Adult Health/Gastrointestinal
REFERENCE
Luckmann, J. (1997). *Saunders manual of nursing care.* Philadelphia. W. B. Saunders. p. 311.

5. 1

RATIONALE: When the client is taking a potassium-sparing diuretic, the client should avoid foods high in potassium. A banana contains 451 mg of K. Cranberry juice (1 cup) contains 61 mg of K. A plum contains 48 mg of K, and 1 oz of cheddar cheese contains 28 mg of K.
TEST-TAKING STRATEGY: Knowledge that the client should avoid foods high in potassium will easily direct you to option 1. If you had difficulty with this question, review foods high in potassium.
LEVEL OF COGNITIVE ABILITY: Application
PHASE OF NURSING PROCESS: Implementation
CLIENT NEEDS: Physiological Integrity
CONTENT AREA: Pharmacology

REFERENCE
Hodgson, B., & Kizior, R. (1999). *Saunders nursing drug handbook 1999.* Philadelphia: W. B. Saunders. pp. 942–944.

6. 3

RATIONALE: Bacon is a component of the fat group in the exchange system. One teaspoon of butter is equal to 1 tsp margarine, 1 tsp of any oil, 1 tbsp of salad dressing, 1 strip of bacon, 5 large olives, or 10 whole peanuts.
TEST-TAKING STRATEGY: Note the key words "most appropriate" in the stem of the question. Eliminate options 1 and 2 because they are similar. Select option 3 over option 4, knowing that bacon is an item of the fat group. Review foods in the exchange system now if you had difficulty with this question.
LEVEL OF COGNITIVE ABILITY: Application
PHASE OF NURSING PROCESS: Implementation
CLIENT NEEDS: Health Promotion and Maintenance
CONTENT AREA: Adult Health/Endocrine
REFERENCE
Monahan, F., & Neighbors, M. (1998). *Medical-surgical nursing: Foundations for clinical practice* (2nd ed.). Philadelphia: W. B. Saunders. p. 1233.

7. 2

RATIONALE: A low-residue (low-fiber) diet places less strain on the intestines because this type of diet is easier to digest. This diet is used for ulcerative colitis, diverticulitis, and irritable bowel syndrome.
TEST-TAKING STRATEGY: Note that the diagnosis in the question refers to an inflammation in the colon. With this in mind, you should easily be directed to option 2, the diet that would place the least strain on the intestinal tract. If you had difficulty with this question, take time now to review the diet prescribed for ulcerative colitis.
LEVEL OF COGNITIVE ABILITY: Comprehension
PHASE OF NURSING PROCESS: Planning
CLIENT NEEDS: Physiological Integrity
CONTENT AREA: Adult Health/Gastrointestinal
REFERENCE
Luckmann, J. (1997). *Saunders manual of nursing care.* Philadelphia. W. B. Saunders. p. 311.

8. 3

RATIONALE: Fruits and vegetables, except avocados, olives, and coconut, contain minimal amounts of fat.
TEST-TAKING STRATEGY: Knowledge regarding the fat content of fruits is required to answer this question. Options 1 and 2 can be easily eliminated. Recalling that avocado is high in fat content will easily direct you to option 3.
LEVEL OF COGNITIVE ABILITY: Comprehension
PHASE OF NURSING PROCESS: Evaluation
CLIENT NEEDS: Health Promotion and Maintenance
CONTENT AREA: Adult Health/Cardiovascular
REFERENCE
Luckmann, J. (1997). *Saunders manual of nursing care.* Philadelphia. W. B. Saunders. p. 311.

9. 2

RATIONALE: Riboflavin is present in a variety of foods of animal and vegetable origin. Good sources are meats, chicken, eggs, and milk. Liver, however, has an especially high riboflavin content.

TEST-TAKING STRATEGY: Note the key words "especially high." This may indicate that more than one option may contain riboflavin. Knowledge regarding food items high in riboflavin is required to answer this question. If you are unfamiliar with these foods, take time now to review.
LEVEL OF COGNITIVE ABILITY: Application
PHASE OF NURSING PROCESS: Implementation
CLIENT NEEDS: Health Promotion and Maintenance
CONTENT AREA: Fundamental Skills
REFERENCE
Lehne, R. (1998). *Pharmacology for nursing care* (3rd ed.). Philadelphia: W. B. Saunders. p. 811.

10. 3

RATIONALE: Thiamine is present in a variety of foods of plant and animal origin. Pork products are especially rich in the vitamin. Other good sources include peanuts, asparagus, and whole grain and enriched cereals.
TEST-TAKING STRATEGY: Note the key words "especially high." This may indicate that more than one option may contain thiamine. Knowledge regarding food items high in thiamine is required to answer this question. If you are unfamiliar with these foods, take time now to review this important content.
LEVEL OF COGNITIVE ABILITY: Application
PHASE OF NURSING PROCESS: Implementation
CLIENT NEEDS: Health Promotion and Maintenance
CONTENT AREA: Fundamental Skills
REFERENCE
Lehne, R. (1998). *Pharmacology for nursing care* (3rd ed.). Philadelphia: W. B. Saunders. p. 811.

11. 4

RATIONALE: Moist pastas, casseroles, egg dishes, and potatoes are usually well tolerated by the client who has difficulty swallowing. Raw vegetables, chunky vegetables such as diced beets, and stringy vegetables such as spinach, corn, and peas are foods commonly excluded from the diet of a client with a poor swallow reflex.
TEST-TAKING STRATEGY: Note the key words "not" and "swallowing ability." Use the process of elimination to select option 4 as the food that would be most difficult to swallow. If you had difficulty with this question, take time now to review feeding measures for a client with an altered swallow reflex.
LEVEL OF COGNITIVE ABILITY: Comprehension
PHASE OF NURSING PROCESS: Planning
CLIENT NEEDS: Physiological Integrity
CONTENT AREA: Adult Health/Neurological
REFERENCE
Peckenpaugh, N., & Poleman, C. (1999). *Nutrition essentials and diet therapy* (8th ed.) Philadelphia: W. B. Saunders. p. 103.

12. 4

RATIONALE: In the client with renal failure, potassium intake must be restricted as much as possible (30–50 mEq/day). The primary mechanism of potassium removal during ARF is dialysis. Options 1, 2, and 3 are not normally restricted in the client with ARF.
TEST-TAKING STRATEGY: Noting the diagnosis of the client in this question will assist in directing you to option 4. Use the process of elimination. The items in options 1, 2, and 3 would least likely promote a workload on the kidneys. Review the therapeutic diet in the client with ARF now if you had difficulty with this question.

LEVEL OF COGNITIVE ABILITY: Application
PHASE OF NURSING PROCESS: Planning
CLIENT NEEDS: Physiological Integrity
CONTENT AREA: Adult Health/Renal
REFERENCE
Peckenpaugh, N., & Poleman, C. (1999). *Nutrition essentials and diet therapy* (8th ed.) Philadelphia: W. B. Saunders. pp. 235–239.

13. 2

RATIONALE: The client with dumping syndrome should be placed on a high-protein, moderate-fat, and high-calorie diet. The client should avoid drinking liquids with meals. Frequent small meals are encouraged and the client should avoid concentrated sweets.
TEST-TAKING STRATEGY: Note the key word "not" in the stem of the question. Use the process of elimination to select option 2 as the item that will contribute to the problems associated with dumping syndrome. If you had difficulty with this question, take time now to review the diet associated with this disorder.
LEVEL OF COGNITIVE ABILITY: Application
PHASE OF NURSING PROCESS: Planning
CLIENT NEEDS: Physiological Integrity
CONTENT AREA: Adult Health/Gastrointestinal
REFERENCE
Peckenpaugh, N., & Poleman, C. (1999). *Nutrition essentials and diet therapy* (8th ed.) Philadelphia: W. B. Saunders. p. 145.

14. 2

RATIONALE: Anticoagulant medications act to prevent coagulation by antagonizing the action of vitamin K. When a client is taking an anticoagulant, foods high in vitamin K are often omitted from the diet. Vitamin K is found in large amounts in green leafy vegetables, especially broccoli, cabbage, turnip greens, and lettuce. Pasta, oranges, and potatoes are very low in vitamin K.
TEST-TAKING STRATEGY: Knowledge regarding the relationship between warfarin and vitamin K is required to answer this question. Note the key word "exclude," and select the food item that is highest in vitamin K. If you had difficulty with this question, take time now to review foods high in vitamin K.
LEVEL OF COGNITIVE ABILITY: Comprehension
PHASE OF NURSING PROCESS: Planning
CLIENT NEEDS: Physiological Integrity
CONTENT AREA: Pharmacology
REFERENCE
Peckenpaugh, N., & Poleman, C. (1999). *Nutrition essentials and diet therapy* (8th ed.) Philadelphia: W. B. Saunders. pp. 162–163.

15. 3

RATIONALE: Pernicious anemia is caused by a deficiency of vitamin B_{12}. Treatment consists of monthly injections of vitamin B_{12}. Thiamine is most often prescribed for the client with alcoholism. Iron is administered for iron deficiency anemia and folic acid for folic acid deficiency.
TEST-TAKING STRATEGY: Knowledge regarding the relationship between pernicious anemia and vitamin B_{12} is required to answer this question. If you are unfamiliar with this disorder, take time now to review.
LEVEL OF COGNITIVE ABILITY: Comprehension
PHASE OF NURSING PROCESS: Planning
CLIENT NEEDS: Physiological Integrity
CONTENT AREA: Adult Health/Gastrointestinal

REFERENCE
Peckenpaugh, N., & Poleman, C. (1999). *Nutrition essentials and diet therapy* (8th ed.) Philadelphia: W. B. Saunders. p. 88.

16. **4**

RATIONALE: It may be necessary to modify a client's diet to a soft or mechanical chopped diet if the client has difficulty chewing. Food and cultural preferences should have been determined on admission. Bowel sounds should be present before introducing any diet.
TEST-TAKING STRATEGY: Note the key word "elderly." Eliminate options 1 and 2 first because they are similar. Eliminate option 3 next because the client has been tolerating a liquid diet; therefore, bowel sounds have been present. The issue relates to consistency of food. Option 4 is the only option that addresses a factor affecting food consistency.
LEVEL OF COGNITIVE ABILITY: Application
PHASE OF NURSING PROCESS: Data Collection
CLIENT NEEDS: Physiological Integrity
CONTENT AREA: Fundamental Skills
REFERENCE
Leahy, J., & Kizilay, P. (1998). *Foundations of nursing practice: A nursing process approach.* Philadelphia: W. B. Saunders. pp. 753, 765.

17. **3**

RATIONALE: Protein and vitamin C are necessary for wound healing. Poultry and milk are good sources of protein. Broccoli and strawberries are good sources of vitamin C. Peanut butter is a source of niacin. Jell-O and jelly have no nutrient value. Spaghetti is a complex carbohydrate.
TEST-TAKING STRATEGY: Knowledge that protein and vitamin C are necessary for wound healing assists in selecting the option that contains those nutrients. Eliminate options 1 and 2 first because jelly and Jell-O have no nutrient value related to healing. From the remaining options, select option 3 over option 4 because of the greater nutrient value in these food items. Review foods high in protein and vitamin C now if you had difficulty with this question.
LEVEL OF COGNITIVE ABILITY: Application
PHASE OF NURSING PROCESS: Implementation
CLIENT NEEDS: Physiological Integrity
CONTENT AREA: Fundamental Skills
REFERENCE
Peckenpaugh, N., & Poleman, C. (1999). *Nutrition essentials and diet therapy* (8th ed.) Philadelphia: W. B. Saunders. p. 89.

18. **4**

RATIONALE: In a postoperative client, a concern related to initiating a diet is aspiration. Suction equipment must be available. A cardiac monitor and a code cart is unnecessary. A straw may help the client sip fluids, but is not necessary.
TEST-TAKING STRATEGY: Note the key words "postoperative" and "priority." Use the ABCs, Airway, Breathing, and Circulation, to answer this question. Option 4 will maintain airway clearance. If you had difficulty with this question, take time now to review care to the postoperative client.
LEVEL OF COGNITIVE ABILITY: Application
PHASE OF NURSING PROCESS: Planning
CLIENT NEEDS: Physiological Integrity
CONTENT AREA: Fundamental Skills
REFERENCE
deWit, S. (1998). *Essentials of medical-surgical nursing* (4th ed.). Philadelphia: W. B. Saunders. p. 82.

19. **3**

RATIONALE: Independence is promoted by allowing the client to have control in a given situation. Placing the client's tray on the unaffected side will facilitate the client's ability to perform the activity of eating. Options 1, 2, and 4 do not offer the client control.
TEST-TAKING STRATEGY: Note the key words "promote independence." With this issue in mind, by the process of elimination, you should easily be directed to option 3. Review measures related to promoting independence now if you had difficulty with this question.
LEVEL OF COGNITIVE ABILITY: Application
PHASE OF NURSING PROCESS: Implementation
CLIENT NEEDS: Physiological Integrity
CONTENT AREA: Adult Health/Neurological
REFERENCE
Monahan, F., & Neighbors, M. (1998). *Medical-surgical nursing: Foundations for clinical practice* (2nd ed.). Philadelphia: W. B. Saunders. p. 813.

20. **4**

RATIONALE: A low-sodium diet is used as an adjunct to antihypertensive medications for treatment of hypertension. Sodium retains fluid that leads to hypertension secondary to increased fluid volume. Frozen foods use salt as a preservative and should not be encouraged as part of a low-sodium diet.
TEST-TAKING STRATEGY: Note the key words "further teaching is necessary." Use the process of elimination. Eliminate options 1, 2 and 3 because these are accurate statements related to hypertension. If you had difficulty with this question, take time now to review the treatment of hypertension and foods high in sodium.
LEVEL OF COGNITIVE ABILITY: Comprehension
PHASE OF NURSING PROCESS: Evaluation
CLIENT NEEDS: Health Promotion and Maintenance
CONTENT AREA: Adult Health/Cardiovascular
REFERENCE
Peckenpaugh, N., & Poleman, C. (1999). *Nutrition essentials and diet therapy* (8th ed.) Philadelphia: W. B. Saunders. pp. 146–147.

21. **1**

RATIONALE: The most accurate measurement of weight loss is daily weighing of the client at the same time, in the same clothes, and using the same scale. Options 2, 3, and 4 assist in measuring nutrition and hydration status rather than actual loss of pounds.
TEST-TAKING STRATEGY: Note the key phrase "most accurately." Also note the similar words in the question and option. If you had difficulty with this question, take time now to review the methods of monitoring weight loss.
LEVEL OF COGNITIVE ABILITY: Application
PHASE OF NURSING PROCESS: Data Collection
CLIENT NEEDS: Physiological Integrity
CONTENT AREA: Fundamental Skills
REFERENCE
Peckenpaugh, N., & Poleman, C. (1999). *Nutrition essentials and diet therapy* (8th ed.) Philadelphia: W. B. Saunders. p. 425.

22. **4**

RATIONALE: In anorexia nervosa, the client tries to establish identity and control by self-imposed starvation. Options 1, 2, and 3 are verbalizations of the client's intentions. Option 4 is a measurable action that can be verified.

TEST-TAKING STRATEGY: Note the key words "that treatment has been effective." With this in mind, use the process of elimination and select the option that is measurable. Option 4 is the only measurable action.
LEVEL OF COGNITIVE ABILITY: Comprehension
PHASE OF NURSING PROCESS: Evaluation
CLIENT NEEDS: Psychosocial Integrity
CONTENT AREA: Mental Health
REFERENCE
Varcarolis, E. (1998). *Foundations of psychiatric mental health nursing* (3rd ed.). Philadelphia: W. B. Saunders. pp. 802–803.

23. **1**

RATIONALE: Poor nutrition during pregnancy can negatively influence fetal growth and development. Although pregnancy poses some nutritional risk for the mother, not all clients are at high risk. Calcium is critical during the third trimester, but must be increased from the onset of pregnancy. Intake of dietary iron is usually insufficient for the majority of pregnant women and iron supplements are routinely encouraged.
TEST-TAKING STRATEGY: Eliminate option 2 because of the absolute term "all." Note the absolute "not" in options 3 and 4. Option 1 is a general statement true for any stage of pregnancy and is the most global statement.
LEVEL OF COGNITIVE ABILITY: Application
PHASE OF NURSING PROCESS: Planning
CLIENT NEEDS: Physiological Integrity
CONTENT AREA: Maternity
REFERENCE
Peckenpaugh, N., & Poleman, C. (1999). *Nutrition essentials and diet therapy* (8th ed.) Philadelphia: W. B. Saunders. p. 338.

24. **3**

RATIONALE: Chemotherapy may cause distortion of taste. Frequent oral hygiene aids in preserving taste function. Keeping a client NPO increases nutritional risks. Antiemetics are used when nausea and vomiting are a problem. TPN is used when oral intake is not possible.
TEST-TAKING STRATEGY: The issue of the question is a change in taste sensation. Eliminate options 1, 2, and 4 because they are unrelated to the issue of the question. Option 3 is the only option that addresses the issue of the question. If you had difficulty with this question, take time now to review interventions related to nutrition in the client receiving chemotherapy.
LEVEL OF COGNITIVE ABILITY: Application
PHASE OF NURSING PROCESS: Implementation
CLIENT NEEDS: Physiological Integrity
CONTENT AREA: Adult Health/Oncology
REFERENCE
Peckenpaugh, N., & Poleman, C. (1999). *Nutrition essentials and diet therapy* (8th ed.) Philadelphia: W. B. Saunders. pp. 282–283.

25. **4**

RATIONALE: Concentrated sugars are found in fruit yogurt, gelatin desserts, prepared drink mixes, jelly, and sherbet.
TEST-TAKING STRATEGY: Use knowledge of foods containing concentrated sugar to answer the question. Note that option 4 is the only option that does not identify a prepackaged food item. Review foods containing concentrated sugar now if you had difficulty with this question.

LEVEL OF COGNITIVE ABILITY: Comprehension
PHASE OF NURSING PROCESS: Evaluation
CLIENT NEEDS: Health Promotion and Maintenance
CONTENT AREA: Fundamental Skills
REFERENCE
Peckenpaugh, N., & Poleman, C. (1999). *Nutrition essentials and diet therapy* (8th ed.) Philadelphia: W. B. Saunders. p. 218.

26. **4**

RATIONALE: Self-control is demonstrated by stoicism and hiding feelings. Problem solving involves making plans and verbalizing what will be done. Accepting responsibility places the responsibility for a situation on one's self. Distancing is an unwillingness or inability to discuss events.
TEST-TAKING STRATEGY: Note the key words "refuses," "will not," and "does not." These words indicate ineffective coping. Option 4, distancing, is indicative of ineffective coping. If you had difficulty with this question, take time now to review coping mechanisms.
LEVEL OF COGNITIVE ABILITY: Comprehension
PHASE OF NURSING PROCESS: Data Collection
CLIENT NEEDS: Psychosocial Integrity
CONTENT AREA: Fundamental Skills
REFERENCE
Luckmann, J. (1997). *Saunders manual of nursing care*. Philadelphia: W. B. Saunders. p. 316.

27. **4**

RATIONALE: A lactose intolerance requires that the client be placed on a lactose-free formula. The primary health care provider needs to be notified to change the prescribed enteral solution. Options 1, 2, and 3 are unrelated to the client's problem.
TEST-TAKING STRATEGY: Option 1 indicates that the client has tolerated this treatment before. Option 2 is an indication for enteral feeding. Option 3 is most commonly associated with constipation, not diarrhea. Option 4 warrants the need to change the enteral solution to a lactose-free formula. If you had difficulty with this question, take time now to review the complications of tube feeding formulas.
LEVEL OF COGNITIVE ABILITY: Comprehension
PHASE OF NURSING PROCESS: Data Collection
CLIENT NEEDS: Physiological Integrity
CONTENT AREA: Fundamental Skills
REFERENCE
Luckmann, J. (1997). *Saunders manual of nursing care*. Philadelphia: W. B. Saunders. p. 319.

28. **2**

RATIONALE: Any condition in which GI motility is slowed or esophageal reflux is possible places a client at risk for aspiration. Options 1 and 4 may be appropriate, but are not of highest priority. Option 3 is not likely to occur in this client.
TEST-TAKING STRATEGY: Note the key words "highest priority." Use the ABCs, Airway, Breathing, and Circulation. Option 2 addresses airway management. Options 1, 3, and 4 are possible problems, but not as high a priority as airway maintenance.
LEVEL OF COGNITIVE ABILITY: Comprehension
PHASE OF NURSING PROCESS: Planning
CLIENT NEEDS: Physiological Integrity
CONTENT AREA: Fundamental Skills

REFERENCE
Luckmann, J. (1997). *Saunders manual of nursing care*. Philadelphia: W. B. Saunders. p. 316

29. **4**

RATIONALE: Initiating a tube feeding prior to checking aspiration. Options 1 and 2 are part of the total plan of care for a client on enteral feedings. Option 3 is instituted for a client who has been identified as a high risk for aspiration. Option 4 is the priority nursing action.
TEST-TAKING STRATEGY: Use the ABCs—Airway, Breathing, and Circulation—and the nursing process to answer the question. Option 4 relates to the risk of aspiration. If you had difficulty with this question, take time now to review nursing interventions when initiating a tube feeding.
LEVEL OF COGNITIVE ABILITY: Application
PHASE OF NURSING PROCESS: Implementation
CLIENT NEEDS: Physiological Integrity
CONTENT AREA: Fundamental Skills
REFERENCE
Luckmann, J. (1997). *Saunders manual of nursing care*. Philadelphia: W. B. Saunders. p. 316.

30. **1**

RATIONALE: Return demonstration is the most reliable evaluation of procedure performance. Selection of equipment is included in a return demonstration. Written testing is not useful for performance testing of procedures. Verbal description does not allow the nurse to observe the psychomotor skill needed to perform the procedure.
TEST-TAKING STRATEGY: Note the similar words in the question and option. "Performing" in the question and "demonstration" in the option indicate action. Review basic teaching/learning principles now if you had difficulty with this question.
LEVEL OF COGNITIVE ABILITY: Comprehension
PHASE OF NURSING PROCESS: Evaluation
CLIENT NEEDS: Health Promotion and Maintenance
CONTENT AREA: Fundamental Skills
REFERENCE
Luckmann, J. (1997). *Saunders manual of nursing care*. Philadelphia: W. B. Saunders. p. 316.

31. **1**

RATIONALE: The nurse obtains an electronic infusion pump in preparation for this procedure. It is necessary to use an infusion pump to ensure that the solution does not infuse too rapidly or fall too far behind. Because the client's blood glucose is monitored every 6 to 8 hours during administration of TPN, a blood glucose meter will also be needed, but this is not the most essential item needed. Urine test strips may be needed to measure glucose. A noninvasive blood pressure cuff is totally unnecessary for this procedure.
TEST-TAKING STRATEGY: Note that the question contains the key words "most essential." Use knowledge of principles of TPN administration to eliminate each of the incorrect options easily. Review these principles now if you had difficulty with this question!
LEVEL OF COGNITIVE ABILITY: Application
PHASE OF NURSING PROCESS: Planning
CLIENT NEEDS: Physiological Integrity
CONTENT AREA: Fundamental Skills
REFERENCE
de Wit, S. (1998). *Essentials of medical-surgical nursing* (4th ed.). Philadelphia: W. B. Saunders. p. 130.

32. **4**

RATIONALE: The high glucose concentration in TPN places the client at risk for hyperglycemia. Signs of hyperglycemia include polyuria, polydipsia, blurred vision, nausea and vomiting, and abdominal pain.
TEST-TAKING STRATEGY: Remember that in order for an option to be correct, all of the parts of that option must be correct. Recalling the signs of hyperglycemia will easily direct you to option 4. Review the signs of hyperglycemia now if you had difficulty with this question.
LEVEL OF COGNITIVE ABILITY: Application
PHASE OF NURSING PROCESS: Data Collection
CLIENT NEEDS: Physiological Integrity
CONTENT AREA: Fundamental Skills
REFERENCE
Monahan, F., & Neighbors, M. (1998). *Medical-surgical nursing: Foundations for clinical practice* (2nd ed.). Philadelphia: W. B. Saunders. p. 1246.

33. **4**

RATIONALE: The client's signs and symptoms are consistent with fluid overload. The increased intravascular volume increases the blood pressure, while the pulse rate increases as the heart tries to pump the extra fluid volume. A fever is present in sepsis. Signs and symptoms of an air embolus include confusion, pallor, light-headedness, tachycardia, tachypnea, hypotension, anxiety, and unresponsiveness. Polyuria, polydipsia, and polyphagia are manifestations of hyperglycemia.
TEST-TAKING STRATEGY: To answer this question accurately, it is necessary to be familiar with the various complications of TPN and their manifestations. If needed, take a few moments to review the signs and symptoms of these complications now.
LEVEL OF COGNITIVE ABILITY: Comprehension
PHASE OF NURSING PROCESS: Data Collection
CLIENT NEEDS: Physiological Integrity
CONTENT AREA: Fundamental Skills
REFERENCE
Leahy, J., & Kizilay, P. (1998). *Foundations of nursing practice: A nursing process approach*. Philadelphia: W. B. Saunders. p. 785.

34. **3**

RATIONALE: The nurse ensures that the client has intact gag and swallow reflexes. The nurse also checks for the presence of bowel sounds. Pulse, blood pressure, and weight require ongoing monitoring but are not the most important, given the wording of the question. The client may be expected to have a poor appetite after being without oral intake for a time.
TEST-TAKING STRATEGY: Focus on the issue of the question, noting the key word "priority." Option 3 is most closely associated with the issue of the question, feeding the client. Review nursing care measures for the client resuming an oral intake if this question was difficult.
LEVEL OF COGNITIVE ABILITY: Application
PHASE OF NURSING PROCESS: Data Collection
CLIENT NEEDS: Physiological Integrity
CONTENT AREA: Fundamental Skills
REFERENCE
Luckmann, J. (1997). *Saunders manual of nursing care*. Philadelphia: W. B. Saunders. p. 321.

35. **1**

RATIONALE: Signs and symptoms of fat overload include fever, leukocytosis, hyperlipidemia, pruritic urticaria and possibly focal seizures. Hepatosplenomegaly may also be present. Options 2, 3, and 4 are not signs of this complication.

TEST-TAKING STRATEGY: To answer this question accurately, it is necessary to be able to recognize signs and symptoms of fat overload. If needed, take a few moments to review these now.
LEVEL OF COGNITIVE ABILITY: Comprehension
PHASE OF NURSING PROCESS: Data Collection
CLIENT NEEDS: Physiological Integrity
CONTENT AREA: Fundamental Skills
REFERENCE
Luckmann, J. (1997). *Saunders manual of nursing care.* Philadelphia: W. B. Saunders. p. 321.

BIBLIOGRAPHY

deWit, S. (1998). *Essentials of medical-surgical nursing* (4th ed.). Philadelphia: W. B. Saunders.

Hodgson, B., & Kizior, R. (1999). *Saunders nursing drug handbook 1999.* Philadelphia: W. B. Saunders.

Leahy, J., & Kizilay, P. (1998). *Foundations of nursing practice: A nursing process approach.* Philadelphia: W. B. Saunders.

Lehne, R. (1998). *Pharmacology for nursing care* (3rd ed.). Philadelphia: W. B. Saunders.

Luckmann, J. (1997). *Saunders manual of nursing care.* Philadelphia: W. B. Saunders.

Mahan, L., & Escott-Stump, S. (1996). *Krause's food, nutrition, & diet therapy* (9th ed.). Philadelphia: W. B. Saunders.

Monahan, F., & Neighbors, M. (1998). *Medical-surgical nursing: Foundations for clinical practice* (2nd ed.). Philadelphia: W. B. Saunders.

National Council of State Boards of Nursing (1998). *National Council Detailed Test Plan for the NCLEX-PN Examination.* Chicago: Author.

Peckenpaugh, N., & Poleman, C. (1999). *Nutrition essentials and diet therapy* (8th ed.) Philadelphia: W. B. Saunders.

Varcarolis, E. (1998). *Foundations of psychiatric mental health nursing* (3rd ed.). Philadelphia: W. B. Saunders.

CHAPTER 12

Intravenous Therapy and Blood Administration

PYRAMID TERMS

ABO—ABO represents a type of antigen system. The ABO type of the donor should be compatible with the recipient's. Type A can match with types A or O; type B can match with types B or O; type O can match only with type O; type AB can match with A, B, or O.

Air Embolism—A bolus of air enters the vein through an inadequately primed IV line, from a loose connection, or during tubing change or removal of the IV.

Circulatory Overload—A complication resulting from the infusion of blood at a rate too rapid for body size, cardiac status, or clinical condition of the recipient.

Compatibility—Determined by two different types of antigen systems, the ABO system antigens and the RH antigen, present on the membrane surface of the red blood cells (RBCs).

Crossmatching—The testing of the donor's blood and the recipient's blood for compatibility.

Infiltration—Seepage of the intravenous fluid out of the vein into the surrounding tissue.

Phlebitis—An inflammation of the vein that can occur from either mechanical or chemical (medication) trauma or a local infection.

Rh—Represents a type of antigen system. Rh-negative blood can be given to an Rh-negative or Rh-positive recipient.

Septicemia—The presence of infective agents or their toxins in the bloodstream. A serious infection that must be treated promptly; otherwise, the infection leads to circulatory collapse, profound shock, and death.

Transfusion Reaction—A hemolytic transfusion reaction is caused by blood type or Rh incompatibility. An allergic transfusion reaction is most often seen in clients with a history of allergy. A febrile transfusion reaction most commonly occurs in clients with antibodies directed against the transfused white blood cells (WBCs). A bacterial transfusion reaction is seen after transfusion of contaminated blood products.

◆ PYRAMID TO SUCCESS

The nurse is responsible for monitoring clients receiving parenteral therapies. Pyramid points focus on the safety related to monitoring an infusion rate, and monitoring for complications related to the IV. Focus on the signs and symptoms of infiltration, phlebitis, circulatory overload, and air embolism and the treatment measures associated with each. Pyramid points also focus on safety related to monitoring a client receiving a blood transfusion, and monitoring for complications related to the transfusion. Focus on the signs and symptoms of a transfusion reaction and the immediate interventions if a transfusion reaction occurs. Documentation of expected and unexpected effects of the therapy is also a pyramid point.

NURSING PROCESS

DATA COLLECTION

Vital signs
Weight and I&O
Informed consent

Previous reactions to blood transfusions
Cardiovascular and respiratory status
Renal status

PLANNING
Client maintains adequate I&O and hydration status. Client will remain free of infection. Client will maintain fluid balance. Client will remain free of injury.

IMPLEMENTATION
Note health history and existing health conditions in client. Maintain body fluid precautions. Monitor vital signs, weight, and I&O. Monitor IV frequently. Monitor for complications related to IV or blood transfusion. Notify primary health care provider if a complication is suspected. Document expected and unexpected client responses to therapy.

EVALUATION
Vital signs remain within normal limits. Fluid balance and electrolyte balance is maintained. Laboratory values return to within normal range. Client tolerates therapy without complications. Client remains free of injury.

◆ CLIENT NEEDS

SAFE, EFFECTIVE CARE ENVIRONMENT

Informed consent for therapy
Continuity of care
Close supervision during IV infusion
Error prevention in monitoring
IVs Handling hazardous or infectious materials
Asepsis
Standard (universal) precautions

HEALTH PROMOTION AND MAINTENANCE

Health and wellness
Lifestyle choices related to transfusion
Techniques of collecting physical data

PSYCHOSOCIAL INTEGRITY

Identifying coping mechanisms
Support systems for the client
Communication regarding the procedure for IV infusion and blood administration
Religious and cultural considerations related to blood administration

PHYSIOLOGICAL INTEGRITY

Safe administration of IV and blood transfusion
Monitoring infusion rates
Monitoring for expected effects
Monitoring for complications related to IV therapy and the administration of blood
Documentation of the effects of therapy

I. Intravenous Therapy (Table 12–1)

A. Used to sustain clients who are unable to take substances orally
B. Replaces water, electrolytes, and nutrients more rapidly than oral administration
C. Provides immediate access to the vascular system for the rapid delivery of specific solutions without the time required for GI tract absorption
D. Provides a vascular route for the administration of medication or blood components

II. Intravenous Devices

A. IV cannulas
   1. Steel needles or butterfly set
      a. Used when the infusion time will be short
      b. **Infiltration** is more common with these devices
      c. The butterfly infusion set may commonly be used in children and elderly clients, whose veins are likely to be small or fragile

2. Plastic cannulas
   a. Used when longer infusion time is expected
   b. Can cause catheter embolism if the tip of the cannula breaks
B. IV gauges
   1. The smaller the gauge number, the larger the outside diameter of the cannula
   2. The size used depends on the solution to be administered and the diameter of the available vein
   3. For rapid emergency fluid administration, blood products, or anesthetics, a large needle such as 14, 16, 18, or 19 gauge is used
   4. For standard IV fluid, a 22 or 24 gauge is used
   5. If the client has very small veins, a 24 to 25 gauge is used

Table 12–1. **Types of Intravenous Solutions**

Type	Description
Isotonic	Solutions with the same osmolality as body fluids
Hypotonic	Solutions that are more dilute or have a lower osmolality than body fluids
Hypertonic	Solutions that are more concentrated or have a higher osmolality than body fluids

Solution	Tonicity
Lactated Ringer's solution (RL)	Isotonic
0.9% saline (NS)	Isotonic
0.45% saline (½ NS)	Hypotonic
0.225% saline (¼ NS)	Hypotonic
0.33% saline (⅓ NS)	Hypotonic
3% saline (3% NS)	Hypertonic
5% saline (5% NS)	Hypertonic
5% dextrose in water (5% D/W)	Isotonic before administration Hypotonic effect in the body after sugar enters cells
10% dextrose in water (10% D/W)	Hypertonic before administration Hypotonic effect in the body after sugar enters cells
5% dextrose in 0.9% saline (5% D/NS)	Hypertonic
5% dextrose in 0.45% saline (5% D/½ NS)	Hypertonic before administration Hypotonic effect in the body after sugar enters cells
5% dextrose in 0.225% saline (5% D/¼ NS)	Isotonic before administration Hypotonic effect in the body after sugar enters cells
5% dextrose in lactated Ringer's solution	Hypertonic

C. IV containers (Fig. 12–1)
1. Container may be glass or plastic
2. Squeeze the plastic bag or check the glass bottle to ensure intactness and check for any small punctures or cracks
3. Do not write on the plastic IV bag with a marking pen because it may be absorbed into the solution
4. Use a label and a ballpoint pen for marking the bag, placing the label onto the bag
D. Intravenous tubing (Fig. 12–2)
1. Contains a spike end for the bag or bottle, a drop chamber, a roller clamp, a Y-site, and an adapter end for attachment to the needle
2. Some tubing contains a vent that allows air to enter the IV container as the fluid leaves
3. Vented tubing is used for glass or rigid plastic containers to allow air to enter and displace the fluid as it leaves; fluid will not flow from a rigid IV container unless it is vented
4. Tubing may be nonvented tubing and is used for flexible containers
5. Extension tubing may be attached to the IV tubing for children, clients who are restless, or clients who have special mobility needs
E. Drip chambers (Fig. 12–3)
1. Microdrip chamber
   a. Normally this has a short vertical metal piece where the drop forms
   b. Delivers between 50 and 60 drops/mL
   c. Read the tubing package to determine how many drops per milliliter are delivered (drop factor)
   d. Used if fluid will be infused at a slow rate (less than 50 mL/hour), if the solution contains medication, and in the pediatric client
2. Macrodrip chamber
   a. Drop factor varies from 8 to 20 drops/mL
   b. Used if the solution is thick or is to infuse rapidly
   c. Read the tubing package to determine how many drops per milliliter are delivered (drop factor)
F. Filters: may be used in IV lines to trap small particles and provide protection by preventing particles from entering the client's veins
G. Needleless systems: includes recessed needles, plastic cannulas, or one-way valves that decrease the exposure to contaminated needles
H. Intermittent infusion sets: used when intravascular accessibility is desired for intermittent administration of medications or solutions

III. Peripheral IV Sites

A. The most frequently used sites are the veins of

INTRAVENOUS CONTAINERS

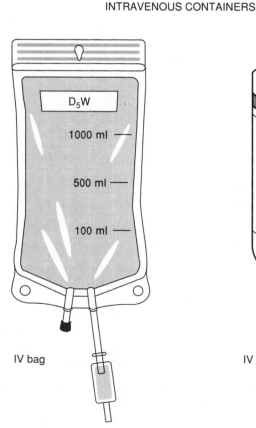

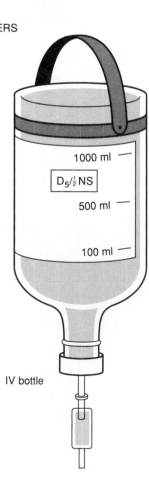

IV bag

IV bottle

FIGURE 12–1. Intravenous containers. (From Kee, J. L., & Marshall, S. M. [1996]. Clinical calculations: With applications to general and specialty areas [2nd ed.]. Philadelphia: W. B. Saunders. p. 166.)

INTRAVENOUS TUBING

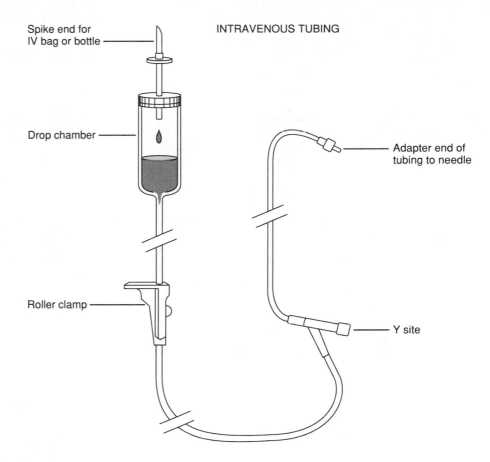

Spike end for IV bag or bottle

Drop chamber

Roller clamp

Adapter end of tubing to needle

Y site

FIGURE 12–2. Intravenous tubing. (From Kee, J. L., & Marshall, S. M. [1996]. Clinical calculations: With applications to general and specialty areas [2nd ed.]. Philadelphia: W. B. Saunders. p. 167.)

MACRODRIP AND MICRODRIP SIZES

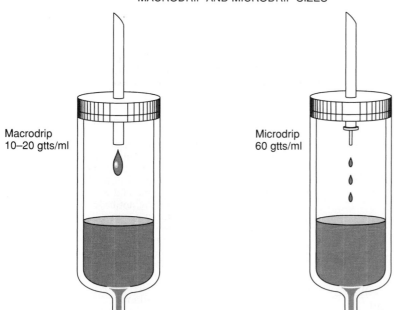

Macrodrip
10–20 gtts/ml

Microdrip
60 gtts/ml

FIGURE 12–3. Macrodrip and microdrip sizes. (From Kee, J. L., & Marshall, S. M. [1996]. Clinical calculations: With applications to general and specialty areas [2nd ed.]. Philadelphia: W. B. Saunders. p. 166.)

the forearm, because the bones of the forearm act as a natural support and splint
B. Veins in the lower extremities are not suitable due to the risk of thrombus formation and possible pooling in areas of decreased venous return
C. Veins in the scalp and feet may be suitable sites for infants
D. Bending the elbow on the arm with an IV may easily obstruct the flow of solution, causing **infiltration** that could lead to thrombophlebitis
E. Avoid checking the blood pressure on the arm receiving the IV infusion
F. Do not place restraints over the venipuncture site
G. An arm board may be prescribed when the venipuncture site is located in an area of flexion

IV. Administering IV Solutions

A. The IV solution should be checked against the physician's orders for the type, amount, percent of solution, and rate of flow
B. Wash hands thoroughly and use sterile technique when working with an IV
C. When preparing a new solution for administration, clamp tubing, attach the spike end of the tubing to the IV bag, and then prime the tubing to remove air from the tubing and IV system
D. Change the IV tubing every 24 to 72 hours depending on agency policy
E. Do not let an IV bag or bottle hang for more than 24 hours
F. Do not allow the IV tubing to touch the floor
G. Change the IV dressing every 72 hours, when the dressing is wet or contaminated, or as specified by the agency policy
H. Label the tubing, dressing, and solution bags clearly, including the date and time when changed

V. IV Precautions

A. Can cause initial pain and discomfort for the client
B. Provides a route of entry for microorganisms into the body
C. Fluid overload or electrolyte imbalances can occur from an excessive or too rapid infusion of fluids
D. Incompatibilities between certain solutions can occur
E. Clients with cardiac, respiratory, renal, or liver diseases, and the elderly and very young persons cannot tolerate an excessive fluid volume, and the risk of fluid overload exists with these clients
F. A client with congestive heart failure is usually not given a saline solution because this type of fluid encourages the retention of water and therefore exacerbates heart failure by increasing the fluid overload

G. A diabetic client does not typically receive dextrose (sugar) solutions

VI. Complications (Table 12–2)

A. Infection
   1. Description
      a. The entry of microorganisms into the body through the venipuncture site
      b. Venipuncture interrupts the integrity of the skin, the first line of defense against infection
      c. The longer the therapy continues, the greater the risk of infection
   2. At-risk clients
      a. Immunocompromised clients from diseases such as cancer or acquired immunodeficiency syndrome (AIDS)
      b. Clients receiving treatments such as chemotherapy that have an altered or lowered WBC count
      c. Elderly clients, because aging alters the effectiveness of the immune system
   3. Prevention and implementation
      a. Maintain strict asepsis when caring for the IV site
      b. Monitor vital signs, particularly temperature
      c. Monitor for local inflammation at the IV site
      d. Check fluid containers for cracks, leaks, or cloudiness or other evidence of contamination
      e. Change the tubing and site dressing every 24 to 72 hours according to agency policy

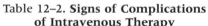

Table 12–2. Signs of Complications of Intravenous Therapy

Complication	Signs
Phlebitis	Heat, redness, tenderness at site Not swollen or hard IV infusion sluggish
Thrombophlebitis	Hard and cordlike vein Heat, redness, tenderness at site IV infusion sluggish
Infiltration	Edema, pain, and coolness at site May or may not have a blood return
Catheter embolism	Decrease in blood pressure (BP) Pain along vein Weak, rapid pulse Cyanosis of nailbeds Loss of consciousness
Fluid overload	Increased BP Rapid breathing Dyspnea Moist cough and crackles
Air embolus	Tachycardia Dyspnea Cyanosis Hypotension Decreased level of consciousness

f. Antimicrobial ointment is used at the IV site

g. Ensure that the IV solution is not hanging for more than 24 hours

h. Monitor for systemic infection, which includes malaise, headache, chills, fever, nausea, vomiting, backache, tachycardia

i. If infection occurs, the IV is discontinued and the physician is notified; blood cultures may be prescribed

B. **Phlebitis** and thrombophlebitis
  1. Description
    a. An inflammation of the vein that can occur from either mechanical or chemical (medication) trauma or a local infection
    b. Phlebitis can cause the development of a clot (thrombophlebitis)
  2. Prevention and implementation
    a. An IV cannula smaller than the vein is used, and very small veins or veins over an area of flexion are avoided
    b. Anchor the cannula and a loop of tubing securely with tape
    c. Use an armboard or a splint as prescribed if the client is restless or active
    d. If **phlebitis** occurs, the IV device is removed immediately
    e. The physician is notified if **phlebitis** is suspected and warm, moist compresses are applied as prescribed

C. **Infiltration**
  1. Description
    a. A form of tissue damage that is also called extravasation
    b. Seepage of the intravenous fluid out of the vein into the surrounding tissues
    c. Occurs when an IV device has become dislodged or perforates the wall of the vein
  2. Prevention and implementation
    a. IV sites over an area of flexion are avoided
    b. Anchor the cannula and a loop of tubing securely with tape
    c. Use an armboard or a splint as prescribed if the client is restless or active
    d. Monitor the IV site for pain, edema, or coolness, comparing it with the opposite extremity
    e. Monitor the IV rate for a decrease or a halt in flow
    f. If **infiltration** has occurred, the IV device is removed immediately and the physician is notified
    g. Do not rub an infiltrated area, which can cause the development of a hematoma
    h. If **infiltration** has occurred, the extremity is elevated and compresses are applied (warm or cool, depending on the physician's order) over the affected area

D. Catheter embolism
  1. Description: the tip of the catheter breaks off during IV insertion or removal resulting in the possibility of an embolus

2. Prevention and implementation
    a. Remove the IV catheter carefully and inspect the catheter when removed
    b. If the catheter tip has broken off, the physician is notified; a tourniquet is placed high on the limb of IV site as prescribed and an x-ray is obtained
    c. The client may require surgery to remove the catheter pieces

E. Fluid (circulatory) overload
  1. Description: results from the administration of fluids too rapidly or in a client at risk for fluid overload
  2. Prevention and implementation
    a. Identify clients at risk for fluid overload
    b. Calculate and monitor the drip rate frequently
    c. An infusion controller device may be used for clients at risk for overload
    d. If fluid overload occurs, the physician is notified

F. Air embolism
  1. Description: a bolus of air enters the vein through an inadequately primed IV line, from a loose connection, or during tubing change or removal of the IV
  2. Prevention and implementation
    a. Prime the tubing with fluid before use and monitor for any air bubbles in the tubing
    b. Secure all connections
    c. Replace IV fluid before the bag or bottle is dry
    d. If an air embolus is suspected, the physician is notified; the tubing is clamped; the client is turned on the left side with the head of the bed lowered to trap the air in the right atrium

VII. Central Venous Catheters

A. Description
  1. Placed in large central veins
  2. Used to infuse TPN, multiple IV infusions, or medications
  3. Catheter position is determined by x-ray following insertion

B. Tunneled central venous catheters
  1. A more permanent type of catheter such as the Hickman, Broviac, or Groshong catheter that is used for long-term IV therapy
  2. Inserted in the operating room; the catheter is threaded into the lower part of the vena cava at the entrance of the right atrium

C. Vascular access ports: surgically implanted under the skin and used for long-term administration of repeated IV therapy

D. Peripherally inserted central catheter (PICC) line
  1. Used for long-term IV therapy, frequently in the home
  2. Threaded so that the catheter tip may terminate in either the axillary or subclavian vein or superior vena cava

3. **Phlebitis** is a common complication
4. Insertion is below the heart level; therefore, **air embolism** is not common

VIII. Blood Administration

A. Types of blood components
   1. Red blood cells (RBCs)
      a. Used to replace erythrocytes
      b. Evaluation of an effective response is based on the resolution of the symptoms of anemia and an increase of the erythrocyte count
   2. Whole blood
      a. Rarely used because treatment with a specific blood component is usually prescribed
      b. Used to resolve hypovolemic shock due to hemorrhage
      c. Contains **RBCs**, plasma, and plasma proteins
      d. Evaluation of an effective response is based on the resolution of the symptoms of hypovolemia
   3. Platelets
      a. Platelets are used to treat thrombocytopenia and platelet dysfunctions
      b. **Crossmatching** is not required but is usually done (platelet concentrates contain few RBCs)
      c. Evaluation of an effective response is based on improvement in the platelet count
   4. Fresh-frozen plasma
      a. Fresh-frozen plasma may be used to provide clotting factors or volume expansion; it contains no platelets
      b. **Rh** and **ABO** compatibility are required for the transfusion of plasma products
      c. Evaluation of an effective response is assessed by monitoring coagulation studies
B. Compatibility
   1. Client blood samples are drawn and labeled at the bedside when drawn; clients are asked to state their name and this is compared to the identification bracelet
   2. The recipient's **ABO** and **Rh** type are identified
   3. An antibody screen is done to determine the presence of antibodies
   4. **Crossmatch** testing is done in which donor RBCs are combined with the recipient's serum and Coombs' serum; a **crossmatch** is compatible if no RBC agglutination has occurred
   5. In an emergency, O-negative RBCs and AB plasma can be safely administered to most clients without serologic testing
C. Implementation
   1. The temperature is checked before beginning a transfusion; a fever may be a cause for delaying the transfusion; in addition, a fever

will mask a possible symptom of an acute transfusion reaction
   2. During the transfusion, the client is monitored for signs and symptoms of a **transfusion reaction**; the first 10 to 15 minutes of the transfusion are the most critical and the nurse must stay with client; if a major **ABO** incompatibility exists or a severe allergic reaction occurs, it is usually evident within the first 50 mL of the transfusion
   3. The client is instructed to report anything unusual immediately
   4. If a reaction occurs, the transfusion is stopped and the physician is notified; the blood bag and tubing are returned to the blood bank
   5. If a reaction occurs, the client is monitored for any life-threatening symptoms and the appropriate blood and urine samples are obtained as prescribed
   6. Document the client's tolerance to the administration of the blood product
D. Transfusion reactions
   1. Immediate **transfusion reaction**
      a. Chills and diaphoresis
      b. Rapid, thready pulse
      c. Pallor and cyanosis
      d. Muscle aches, back pain, or chest pain
      e. Headache
      f. Apprehension
      g. Tingling and numbness
      h. Dyspnea, cough, or wheezing
      i. Nausea, vomiting, abdominal cramping, and diarrhea
      j. Rashes, hives, itching, and swelling
   2. Delayed **transfusion reactions**
      a. Reactions can occur days to years after a transfusion
      b. Signs include fever, mild jaundice, and a decreased hematocrit level

PRACTICE QUESTIONS

1. The client has an order to receive 1000 mL 5% dextrose in 0.45% sodium chloride. After gathering the appropriate equipment, the nurse takes which of the following actions first before spiking the IV bag with the tubing?
   1 Uncap the spike portion of the tubing
   2 Uncap the distal end of the tubing
   3 Close the roller clamp on the IV tubing
   4 Open the roller clamp on the IV tubing

2. The nurse is preparing to hang an IV solution of 1000 mL 5% dextrose in lactated Ringer's to flow at 80 mL/hour. The nurse time-tapes the bag with a start time of 07:00. After making hourly marks on the time tape, the nurse notes that the completion time for the bag is
   1 17:00
   2 17:30
   3 19:30
   4 21:00

3. The nurse is checking the IV dressing of a client with a peripheral intravenous infusion running. The date on the dressing is 2/9 (February 9). The nurse calculates that the dressing should be changed on which of the following dates?
   1 2/10
   2 2/12
   3 2/14
   4 2/16

4. The nurse is doing a routine assessment of a client's peripheral IV site. The nurse notes that the site is cool, pale, and swollen. The IV has stopped running. The nurse interprets that which of the following has probably occurred?
   1 Infiltration
   2 Phlebitis
   3 Thrombosis
   4 Infection

5. The nurse is assigned to care for a client with a peripheral IV infusion. The nurse is providing hygiene care to the client and would avoid which of the following while changing the client's hospital gown?
   1 Using a hospital gown with snaps at the sleeves
   2 Putting the bag and tubing through the sleeve, followed by the client's arm
   3 Disconnecting the IV tubing from the catheter in the vein
   4 Checking the IV flow rate immediately after changing the hospital gown

6. The nurse is making a worksheet and is listing the tasks that need to be done during the shift on assigned clients. The nurse writes on the plan to check the IV of an assigned client receiving fluid replacement therapy every
   1 4 hours
   2 3 hours
   3 2 hours
   4 1 hour

7. The nurse is checking the insertion site of a peripheral intravenous catheter. The nurse notes the site to be reddened, warm, painful, and slightly edematous in the area of the vein that is proximal to the IV catheter. The nurse interprets that this is most likely due to
   1 Infiltration of the IV line
   2 Phlebitis of the vein
   3 Hypersensitivity to the IV solution
   4 Allergic reaction to the IV catheter material

8. The nurse is assigned to reinforce instructions to a client and the family about the management of home IV infusion therapy. The nurse begins the process by first teaching the client and family principles related to
   1 Proper handwashing technique
   2 The handling of equipment

3 Where to obtain supplies
4 How to report signs of infection

9. The nurse has been instructed to discontinue an intravenous line. The nurse removes the catheter by withdrawing the catheter while applying pressure to the site with a(n)
   1 Alcohol swab
   2 Betadine swab
   3 Band-Aid
   4 Sterile 2 × 2 gauze

10. The nurse is asked to regulate the flow rate of an IV solution being administered to the client. The IV bag contains 50 mL of solution and the solution is to be administered over 30 minutes. The administration set has a drop factor of 10 gtts/mL. The nurse regulates the roller clamp on the infusion set to deliver how many drops per minute?
    1 9
    2 17
    3 30
    4 50

11. The nurse is preparing an IV solution and tubing for a client requiring IV fluids. While priming the tubing, the tubing drops and hits the top of the medication cart. The nurse should do which of the following?
    1 Scrub the catheter before attaching the new setup
    2 Change the IV tubing
    3 Wipe the tubing with Betadine
    4 Scrub the tubing with an alcohol swab

12. The nurse is completing a time tape for a 1000 mL IV bag that is scheduled to infuse over 8 hours. The nurse has just placed the 11:00 marking at the 500 mL level. The nurse places the mark for 12:00 at which of the following levels on the time tape?
    1 425 mL
    2 400 mL
    3 375 mL
    4 350 mL

13. The nurse is assisting in caring for a client receiving a unit of packed red blood cells. The nurse tells the client that it is most important to report which of the following signs immediately?
    1 Mild discomfort at the catheter site
    2 Chills, itching, or rash
    3 Unusual sleepiness or fatigue
    4 Headache, nausea, or vomiting

14. The nurse is assisting in caring for a client who will receive a unit of blood. Just prior to the infusion, it is most important for the nurse to assess
    1 Skin color
    2 Oxygen saturation

3 Vital signs
4 Latest hematocrit

15. The client receiving a blood transfusion rings the call bell for the nurse. Upon entering the room, the nurse notes that the client is flushed, dyspneic, and is complaining of generalized itching. The nurse interprets that the client is experiencing
    1 Fluid overload
    2 Bacteremia
    3 Hypovolemic shock
    4 Transfusion reaction

16. The client who was receiving a blood transfusion has experienced a transfusion reaction. The nurse should prepare to send the blood bag used for the client to which of the following areas?
    1 Risk management department
    2 Laboratory
    3 Pharmacy
    4 Blood bank

17. The nurse takes the client's temperature prior to a blood transfusion. The temperature is 100° F orally. The nurse reports the finding to the registered nurse and anticipates that which of the following actions will take place?
    1 The transfusion will begin as prescribed
    2 The blood will be held and the physician will be notified
    3 The transfusion will begin after administering an antihistamine
    4 The transfusion will begin after administering 600 mg acetaminophen (Tylenol)

18. The nurse is assisting in caring for a client who has received a transfusion of platelets. The nurse evaluates that the client is benefiting most from this therapy if the client exhibits which of the following?
    1 Decline of temperature to normal
    2 Decrease in oozing from puncture sites and gums
    3 Increased hemoglobin level
    4 Increased hematocrit level

ANSWERS

1. **3**

RATIONALE: The nurse should first clamp the tubing to prevent the solution from running freely through the tubing once it is attached to the IV bag. The nurse should next uncap the proximal (spike) portion of the tubing and attach it to the IV bag. Then the roller clamp is opened slowly and the fluid is allowed to flow through the tubing in a controlled fashion to prevent air from remaining in parts of the tubing.
TEST-TAKING STRATEGY: This question tests a specific procedure related to intravenous therapy. Attempt to visualize this process in order to answer the question correctly. If this question was difficult, take a few moments to review the key aspects of this procedure at this time.
LEVEL OF COGNITIVE ABILITY: Application
PHASE OF NURSING PROCESS: Implementation
CLIENT NEEDS: Safe, Effective Care Environment
CONTENT AREA: Fundamental Skills
REFERENCE
Leahy, J., & Kizilay, P. (1998). *Foundations of nursing practice: A nursing process approach.* Philadelphia: W. B. Saunders. pp. 489–490.

2. **3**

RATIONALE: At a rate of 80 mL/hour, the 1000 mL bag will be finished infusing in 12.5 hours. This brings the end time to 19:30, using military time.
TEST-TAKING STRATEGY: To answer this question accurately, it is necessary to be familiar with the key points related to time-taping an IV, and also to be familiar with military time. This question is a fundamental and important question related to the client with an intravenous line. If this question was difficult, review either or both of these areas.

LEVEL OF COGNITIVE ABILITY: Application
PHASE OF NURSING PROCESS: Implementation
CLIENT NEEDS: Safe, Effective Care Environment
CONTENT AREA: Fundamental Skills
REFERENCE
Taylor, C., Lillis, C., & LeMone, P. (1997). *Fundamentals of nursing: The art and science of nursing care* (3rd ed.). Philadelphia: Lippincott–Raven. pp. 1414–1415.

3. **2**

RATIONALE: The IV site dressing should be changed every 48 to 72 hours, which is every 2 to 3 days. With an insertion date of 2/9, the due date for change depending on agency policy would be either 2/11 or 2/12. Changing the dressing every 5 to 7 days (options 3 and 4) places the client at risk of infection. Changing the dressing on a daily basis is not necessary unless the dressing becomes wet.
TEST-TAKING STRATEGY: To answer this question accurately, it is necessary to be familiar with the standard accepted guidelines for intravenous site maintenance. If this question was difficult, take a few moments to review these key concepts at this time.
LEVEL OF COGNITIVE ABILITY: Application
PHASE OF NURSING PROCESS: Planning
CLIENT NEEDS: Physiological Integrity
CONTENT AREA: Fundamental Skills
REFERENCE
Leahy, J., & Kizilay, P. (1998). *Foundations of nursing practice: A nursing process approach.* Philadelphia: W. B. Saunders. p. 814.

4. **1**

RATIONALE: An infiltrated IV is one that has dislodged from the vein and is lying in subcutaneous tissue. The pallor, coolness, and swelling are the result of IV fluid being deposited in the subcutaneous tissue. When the pressure in the tissues exceeds the pressure in the tubing, the flow of

the IV solution will stop. The other three options are likely to be accompanied by warmth at the site, not coolness.
TEST-TAKING STRATEGY: To answer this question accurately, it is necessary to be familiar with the signs and symptoms that accompany complications of IV therapy. If this question was difficult, take a few moments to review the signs of infiltration now.
LEVEL OF COGNITIVE ABILITY: Analysis
PHASE OF NURSING PROCESS: Data Collection
CLIENT NEEDS: Physiological Integrity
CONTENT AREA: Fundamental Skills
REFERENCE
Leahy, J., & Kizilay, P. (1998). *Foundations of nursing practice: A nursing process approach.* Philadelphia: W. B. Saunders. p. 822.

5. 3

RATIONALE: The tubing should not be removed from the IV catheter. With each break in the system, there is an increased chance of introducing bacteria into the system, leading to infection. This is poor aseptic technique. Options 1 and 2 are appropriate. The flow rate should be checked immediately after changing the hospital gown because the position of the roller clamp may have been affected during the change.
TEST-TAKING STRATEGY: Visualize this procedure and use knowledge of basic principles related to intravenous therapy and asepsis to direct you to option 3. Review these principles now if you had difficulty with this question.
LEVEL OF COGNITIVE ABILITY: Application
PHASE OF NURSING PROCESS: Implementation
CLIENT NEEDS: Safe, Effective Care Environment
CONTENT AREA: Fundamental Skills
REFERENCE
Leahy, J., & Kizilay, P. (1998). *Foundations of nursing practice: A nursing process approach.* Philadelphia: W. B. Saunders. p. 818.

6. 4

RATIONALE: Safe nursing practice includes monitoring an IV infusion at least once per hour in an adult client. Options 1, 2, and 3 do not provide time frames that are safe or acceptable.
TEST-TAKING STRATEGY: To answer this question accurately, it is necessary to be familiar with the specific time frames indicated in this nursing procedure. In questions similar to this one, it is best to select the most frequent time frame. If this question was difficult, take a few moments now to review the essentials of safe IV administration.
LEVEL OF COGNITIVE ABILITY: Application
PHASE OF NURSING PROCESS: Planning
CLIENT NEEDS: Physiological Integrity
CONTENT AREA: Fundamental Skills
REFERENCE
Leahy, J., & Kizilay, P. (1998). *Foundations of nursing practice: A nursing process approach.* Philadelphia: W. B. Saunders. p. 819.

7. 2

RATIONALE: Phlebitis at an IV site can be distinguished by client discomfort at the site, as well as by redness, warmth, and swelling proximal to the catheter. The line should be discontinued, and a new line should be inserted at a different site. The remaining options are incorrect.
TEST-TAKING STRATEGY: Remember that options that are similar are not likely to be correct. In this case, options

3 and 4 are similar and are therefore eliminated. Choose option 2 over option 1 by knowing the signs and symptoms of common IV complications. Review these signs and symptoms now if you had difficulty with this question.
LEVEL OF COGNITIVE ABILITY: Analysis
PHASE OF NURSING PROCESS: Data Collection
CLIENT NEEDS: Physiological Integrity
CONTENT AREA: Fundamental Skills
REFERENCE
Leahy, J., & Kizilay, P. (1998). *Foundations of nursing practice: A nursing process approach.* Philadelphia: W. B. Saunders. p. 822.

8. 1

RATIONALE: Teaching should begin with an emphasis on proper handwashing technique. This is essential for prevention of infection. The items in options 2, 3, and 4 are components of the instructions, but proper handwashing is primary.
TEST-TAKING STRATEGY: Note the key word "first." This tells you that more than one option may be a correct action, but that one of them is of greater priority, or should be completed before the others. Use knowledge of basic medical asepsis to choose correctly. Remember that handwashing is always the first step.
LEVEL OF COGNITIVE ABILITY: Application
PHASE OF NURSING PROCESS: Implementation
CLIENT NEEDS: Health Promotion and Maintenance
CONTENT AREA: Fundamental Skills
REFERENCE
Leahy, J., & Kizilay, P. (1998). *Foundations of nursing practice: A nursing process approach.* Philadelphia: W. B. Saunders. p. 823.

9. 4

RATIONALE: A dry sterile dressing such as a sterile 2 × 2 is used to apply pressure to the site while the catheter is discontinued and removed. This material is absorbent, sterile, and nonirritating to the site. A Betadine swab or alcohol swab would irritate the opened puncture site and would not stop the blood flow. A Band-Aid may be used to cover the site once hemostasis has occurred.
TEST-TAKING STRATEGY: Visualize this procedure and think about each of the items identified in the options to answer the question. Familiarity with this basic nursing procedure is needed to answer this question correctly. If needed, take a few minutes to review this procedure at this time.
LEVEL OF COGNITIVE ABILITY: Application
PHASE OF NURSING PROCESS: Implementation
CLIENT NEEDS: Safe, Effective Care Environment
CONTENT AREA: Fundamental Skills
REFERENCE
Luckmann, J. (1997). *Saunders manual of nursing care.* Philadelphia: W. B. Saunders. p. 256.

10. 2

RATIONALE: The formula for calculating IV drip rates is:

$$\text{gtts/min} = \frac{\text{volume (mL)} \times \text{drop factor (gtts/mL)}}{\text{time (in minutes)}}$$

$$= \frac{50 \text{ mL} \times 10 \text{ gtts/mL}}{30 \text{ min}} = \frac{500}{30}$$

$$= 16.66 \text{ or } 17 \text{ gtts/min}$$

TEST-TAKING STRATEGY: To calculate the answer to this question correctly, you must be familiar with the standard formula for calculating IV flow rates. If you answered incorrectly, take a few moments to relearn this formula now.
LEVEL OF COGNITIVE ABILITY: Application
PHASE OF NURSING PROCESS: Implementation
CLIENT NEEDS: Physiological Integrity
CONTENT AREA: Fundamental Skills
REFERENCE
Leahy, J., & Kizilay, P. (1998). *Foundations of nursing practice: A nursing process approach*. Philadelphia: W. B. Saunders. p. 813.

11. **2**

RATIONALE: The nurse should change the IV tubing. The tubing has become contaminated and could result in systemic infection to the client. Wiping or scrubbing the port is insufficient to prevent systemic infection.
TEST-TAKING STRATEGY: Use knowledge of basic infection control measures and intravenous therapy concepts to answer this question. Note the similarity between options 1, 3, and 4 and eliminate these options. Review aseptic technique now if you had difficulty with this question.
LEVEL OF COGNITIVE ABILITY: Application
PHASE OF NURSING PROCESS: Planning
CLIENT NEEDS: Safe, Effective Care Environment
CONTENT AREA: Fundamental Skills
REFERENCE
Leahy, J., & Kizilay, P. (1998), *Foundations of nursing practice: A nursing process approach*. Philadelphia: W. B. Saunders. p. 813.

12. **3**

RATIONALE: If the IV is scheduled to run over 8 hours, then the hourly rate is 125 mL/hour. Using 500 mL as the reference point for 11:00, the next hourly marking (12:00) would be at 375 mL, which is 125 mL less than 500.
TEST-TAKING STRATEGY: Use basic principles related to pharmacology calculations and IV administration to answer this question. If this question was difficult, take time to review this essential material.
LEVEL OF COGNITIVE ABILITY: Application
PHASE OF NURSING PROCESS: Implementation
CLIENT NEEDS: Safe, Effective Care Environment
CONTENT AREA: Fundamental Skills
REFERENCE
Leahy, J., & Kizilay, P. (1998). *Foundations of nursing practice: A nursing process approach*. Philadelphia: W. B. Saunders. p. 818.

13. **2**

RATIONALE: The client is told to report chills, itching, or rash immediately. These could possibly be signs of transfusion reaction. Mild discomfort at the catheter site may be indicative of a problem, or could result from the size of the IV catheter required to infuse the blood product. Sleepiness, fatigue, headache, nausea, or vomiting are unrelated to transfusion reaction.
TEST-TAKING STRATEGY: Note the key words "most important" and "immediately." This tells you that more than one or all of the options may be partially or totally correct. Knowing that a transfusion reaction is of most concern to the nurse, you must prioritize your answer to select the option that characterizes this problem. Review the signs of a transfusion reaction now if you had difficulty with this question!

LEVEL OF COGNITIVE ABILITY: Application
PHASE OF NURSING PROCESS: Implementation
CLIENT NEEDS: Physiological Integrity
CONTENT AREA: Fundamental Skills
REFERENCE
Luckmann, J. (1997). *Saunders manual of nursing care*. Philadelphia: W. B. Saunders. p. 1164.

14. **3**

RATIONALE: A change in vital signs may indicate that a transfusion reaction is occurring. This is why the nurse assesses vital signs prior to the procedure, every 15 minutes for the first half hour, and every half hour thereafter.
TEST-TAKING STRATEGY: Note the key words "just prior" and "most important." This tells you that more than one of the options may be partially or totally correct. Use knowledge of blood transfusions and client assessment to prioritize your answer. Additionally, vital signs is the most global response.
LEVEL OF COGNITIVE ABILITY: Application
PHASE OF NURSING PROCESS: Data Collection
CLIENT NEEDS: Physiological Integrity
CONTENT AREA: Fundamental Skills
REFERENCE
deWit, S. (1998). *Essentials of medical-surgical nursing* (4th ed.). Philadelphia: W. B. Saunders. p. 129.

15. **4**

RATIONALE: The signs and symptoms exhibited by the client are consistent with transfusion reaction. With fluid overload, the client would be expected to have crackles in addition to dyspnea. With bacteremia, the client would have a fever, which is not part of the clinical picture presented. There is no correlation between the signs mentioned and hypovolemic shock. The signs are indicative of allergic reaction, which is one type of blood transfusion reaction.
TEST-TAKING STRATEGY: To answer this question correctly, it is necessary to be able to recognize and accurately interpret signs of transfusion reaction. If needed, review the complications of blood administration and this key content area related to transfusion therapy at this time.
LEVEL OF COGNITIVE ABILITY: Analysis
PHASE OF NURSING PROCESS: Data Collection
CLIENT NEEDS: Physiological Integrity
CONTENT AREA: Fundamental Skills
REFERENCE
Monahan, F., & Neighbors, M. (1998). *Medical-surgical nursing: Foundations for clinical practice* (2nd ed.). Philadelphia: W. B. Saunders. p. 458.

16. **4**

RATIONALE: The nurse prepares to return the blood transfusion bag containing any remaining blood to the blood bank. This allows the blood bank to complete any follow-up testing procedures needed once a transfusion reaction has been documented.
TEST-TAKING STRATEGY: Specific knowledge related to routine transfusion-related procedures is needed to answer this question accurately. Knowing that blood is issued from the blood bank may help you to eliminate each of the incorrect options fairly easily. If needed, take a few moments to review this content area now.

LEVEL OF COGNITIVE ABILITY: Application
PHASE OF NURSING PROCESS: Planning
CLIENT NEEDS: Safe, Effective Care Environment
CONTENT AREA: Fundamental Skills
REFERENCE
Monahan, F., & Neighbors, M. (1998). *Medical-surgical nursing: Foundations for clinical practice* (2nd ed.). Philadelphia: W. B. Saunders. p. 457.

17. **2**

RATIONALE: If the client has a temperature equal to or greater than 100°F, the unit of blood should be held until the physician is notified and has the opportunity to give further orders. The other options are incorrect.
TEST-TAKING STRATEGY: Familiarity with basic procedures related to blood administration is needed to answer this question correctly. Eliminate options 1, 3, and 4 because they are similar. Remember that the physician needs to be notified prior to initiating blood, if the temperature is elevated. If needed, take a few moments to review this content at this time.
LEVEL OF COGNITIVE ABILITY: Application
PHASE OF NURSING PROCESS: Planning
CLIENT NEEDS: Safe, Effective Care Environment
CONTENT AREA: Fundamental Skills

REFERENCE
Monahan, F., & Neighbors, M. (1998). *Medical-surgical nursing: Foundations for clinical practice* (2nd ed.). Philadelphia: W. B. Saunders. p. 457.

18. **2**

RATIONALE: Platelets are necessary for proper blood clotting. The client with insufficient platelets may exhibit frank bleeding or oozing of blood from puncture sites, wounds, and mucous membranes. A temperature would decline to normal following infusion of granulocytes if those cells were then instrumental in fighting infection in the body. An increased hemoglobin and hematocrit would be seen when the client has received transfusion of red blood cells.
TEST-TAKING STRATEGY: To answer this question accurately, it is necessary to understand the action of platelets. Recalling that bleeding is a concern when the platelets are low will easily direct you to option 2. Review the action of platelets now if you had difficulty with this question.
LEVEL OF COGNITIVE ABILITY: Analysis
PHASE OF NURSING PROCESS: Evaluation
CLIENT NEEDS: Physiological Integrity
CONTENT AREA: Fundamental Skills
REFERENCE
Leahy, J., & Kizilay, P. (1998). *Foundations of nursing practice: A nursing process approach*. Philadelphia: W. B. Saunders. p. 824.

BIBLIOGRAPHY

deWit, S. (1998). *Essentials of medical-surgical nursing* (4th ed.). Philadelphia: W. B. Saunders.
Leahy, J., & Kizilay, P. (1998). *Foundations of nursing practice: A nursing process approach*. Philadelphia: W. B. Saunders.
Luckmann, J. (1997). *Saunders manual of nursing care*. Philadelphia: W. B. Saunders.

Monahan, F., & Neighbors, M. (1998). *Medical-surgical nursing: Foundations for clinical practice* (2nd ed.). Philadelphia: W. B. Saunders.
National Council of State Boards of Nursing (1998). *National Council detailed test plan for the NCLEX-PN examination*. Chicago: Author.
Taylor, C., Lillis, C., & LeMone, P. (1997). *Fundamentals of nursing: The art and science of nursing care* (3rd ed.). Philadelphia: Lippincott–Raven.

UNIT IV

....

Fundamental Skills

CHAPTER 13

Hygiene and Safety

PYRAMID TERMS

Chemical Restraints—Medications given to inhibit a specific behavior or movement

Hygiene—The activity of providing care or promoting self-care, which includes bathing and grooming

Nosocomial Infections—Infections acquired in the hospital or other health care facility that were not present or incubating at the time of the client's admission; also referred to as hospital-acquired infections

Physical Restraints—Restriction of client movement through the application of a device

Poison—Any substance that impairs health and destroys life when ingested, inhaled, or otherwise absorbed by the body

Standard Precautions—Guidelines used by all health care providers with all clients to reduce the risk of infection for clients and caregivers

Transmission-Based Precautions—Guidelines that are used in addition to standard precautions and are to be used for specific syndromes that are highly suspicious for infections until a diagnosis is confirmed

◆ PYRAMID TO SUCCESS

Safety and infection control is a subcategory of the Client Needs component, Safe, Effective Care Environment, of the test plan for NCLEX-PN. Basic Care and Comfort, which includes personal hygiene measures, is a subcategory of the Client Needs component, Physiological Integrity of the Test Plan. Pyramid points focus on hygiene measures, maintaining environmental safety, preventing accidents, using restraints, and priority nursing actions in the event of an emergency or a disaster. Pyramid points also focus on standard and transmission-based precautions and the measures required to handle hazardous and infectious materials.

NURSING PROCESS

DATA COLLECTION

Age of the client
Lifestyle, cultural, and religious practices and
    preferences
Sensory, perceptual, and mental status alterations

Presence of infections
Risk factors related to injury or infection
History of falls
Home safety

PLANNING

Client will identify factors that increase the potential for injury. Client will implement safety measures that decrease the risk of injury. Client will practice appropriate hygiene measures.

IMPLEMENTATION

Monitor actual and potential risk for injury. Monitor effects of medication on the client. Implement environmental precautions. Use infection control practices. Comply with agency's environmental and safety guidelines. Implement emergency measures during fires or disasters. Document findings, risk potential, and measures implemented to provide safety. Reinforce client education regarding the identification of hazards and health promotion practices. Collaborate with other health care members to ensure client safety.

EVALUATION

Client remains free of preventable injuries. Client remains free of nosocomial infections. Client complies with health promotion and safety measures.

◆ CLIENT NEEDS

SAFE, EFFECTIVE CARE ENVIRONMENT

Maintaining precautions to prevent accidents
Disaster planning
Standard and Transmission-Based Precautions
Handling hazardous and infectious materials
Guidelines regarding the use of restraints

HEALTH PROMOTION AND MAINTENANCE

Health and wellness and disease prevention
Home safety measures
Assisting clients and families to identify environmental hazards in the home
Client and family education regarding accident prevention
Client and family education regarding prevention of the spread of infection
Client and family education regarding measures to be implemented in an emergency

PSYCHOSOCIAL INTEGRITY

Cultural and religious lifestyles
Sensory/perceptual alterations
Support systems

PHYSIOLOGICAL INTEGRITY

Providing comfort and assistance to client
Assisting the client with activities of daily living (ADLs)
Use of assistive devices to prevent injury
Managing and providing care to clients with infectious diseases
Priority nursing actions in an emergency

I. Hygiene

A. Description
   1. The activity of providing care or promoting self-care, which includes bathing and grooming
   2. Includes care of the skin, hair, nails, mouth, teeth, eyes, ears, nasal cavities, and perineal and genital areas
   3. Personal hygiene is the activity of self-care, including bathing and grooming
B. General principles
   1. Wash hands and wear gloves
   2. Ensure privacy
   3. Explain procedures to the client
   4. Determine the client's health status and readiness for hygiene procedures

Table 13–1. Fire Extinguishers

Type of Extinguishers	Class of Fires
TYPE A: water	Wood, draperies, upholstery, paper, and rubbish
TYPES B and C: carbon dioxide or dry chemical	Flammable liquids or gases, grease, and electrical
TYPES A, B, or C: multipurpose, dry chemical	Any fire

   5. Determine the client's routine hygiene practices
   6. Use proper body mechanics during bathing and hygiene activities
   7. Use time spent with the client as an opportunity for communication and teaching
   8. Maintain and encourage independence as much as possible

II. Environmental Safety

A. Fire safety (Box 13–1)
   1. Keep open spaces free of clutter
   2. Clearly mark fire exits
   3. Know the location of all fire alarms, exits, and extinguishers (Table 13–1; Box 13–2)
   4. Know the telephone number for reporting fires
   5. Know the agency's fire drill and evacuation plan
   6. Never use the elevator in the event of a fire
   7. Turn off oxygen and appliances in the vicinity of the fire
   8. In the event of a fire, if the client is on life support, maintain the client's respiratory status manually with an Ambu bag until the client is moved away from the threat of the fire
   9. In the event of a fire, ambulatory clients can be directed to walk by themselves to a safe area; and in some cases they may be able to assist in moving clients in wheelchairs
   10. Bedridden clients are generally moved from the scene of a fire by a stretcher, a bed, or a wheelchair
   11. If a client must be carried from the area of a fire, appropriate transfer techniques need to be used

---

BOX 13–1. Priority Actions in the Event of a Fire

Remember the mnemonic RACE to set priorities in the event of a fire
   R—Rescue: remove all clients from the vicinity of a fire
   A—Alarm: activate the fire alarm; report a fire before attempting to extinguish it
   C—Confine: close doors and windows when a fire is detected
   E—Extinguish: extinguish the fire, using the appropriate fire extinguisher

---

BOX 13–2. Using a Fire Extinguisher

Remember the mnemonic PASS to use a fire extinguisher
   P—Pull the pin
   A—Aim at the base of the fire
   S—Squeeze the handle
   S—Sweep the fire from side to side

12. If fire department personnel are at the scene of the fire, they can help evacuate clients
B. Electrical safety
   1. Electrical equipment must be maintained in good working order and should be grounded
   2. Use a three-pronged electrical cord
   3. In a three-pronged electrical cord, the longer prong of the cord is the ground; the other two prongs carry the power to the piece of electrical equipment
   4. Any electrical equipment that the client brings in to the health care facility must be inspected for safety prior to use
   5. Check electrical cords and outlets for exposed, frayed, and damaged wires
   6. Avoid overloading any circuit
   7. Read warning labels on all equipment; never operate unfamiliar equipment
   8. Use safety extension cords only when absolutely necessary and tape to the floor with electrical tape
   9. Never run electrical wiring under carpets
   10. Never pull a plug using the cord; always grasp the plug itself
   11. Never use electrical appliances near sinks, bathtubs, or other water sources
   12. Always disconnect a plug from the outlet before cleaning equipment or appliances
   13. If a client receives an electrical shock, turn off the electricity before touching the client
C. Radiation safety
   1. Know the health care agency protocols and guidelines
   2. Label potentially radioactive material
   3. To reduce exposure to radiation:
      a. The time spent near the source should be limited
      b. The distance from the source should be as great as possible
      c. A shielding device such as a lead apron should be used
   4. Monitor radiation exposure with a film badge (dosimeter)
   5. Place the client with a radiation implant in a private room
   6. Never touch dislodged implants
   7. Wear gloves when handling body discharges
D. Disposal of infectious wastes
   1. Handle all infectious materials as hazardous
   2. Dispose of all waste in designated areas only, using proper containers for disposal
   3. Ensure that infectious material is properly labeled
   4. Needles should not be recapped, bent, or broken
   5. Dispose of all sharps immediately after use in closed, puncture-resistant disposal containers that are leakproof and labeled or color-coded
E. Falls (Box 13–3)
F. **Restraints**
   1. Protective devices used to limit the physical

BOX 13–3. Measures to Prevent Falls

Assess client's risk for falling
Assign clients at risk for falling to rooms near the nurses' station
Alert all personnel to the client's risk for falling
Orient client to physical surroundings
Instruct client to seek assistance when getting up
Explain use of call bell system
Keep bed in the low position with side rails up if required
Lock all beds, wheelchairs, and stretchers
Keep personal items within reach
Eliminate clutter and obstacles in client's room
Provide adequate lighting
Reduce bathroom hazards
Maintain client's toileting schedule throughout the day

---

activity of a client or to immobilize a client or an extremity
2. **Physical restraints:** restrict client movement through the application of a device
3. **Chemical restraints:** medication given to inhibit a specific behavior or movement
4. Implementation
   a. When **restraints** are necessary, the physician's orders should state the type of restraint and specific client behaviors for which **restraints** are to be used, and identify a limited time frame for use (Box 13–4)
   b. Physician's orders for **restraints** should be renewed within a specific time frame according to the agency's policy
   c. **Restraints** are not to be ordered PRN
   d. The reason for the **restraints** should be given to the client and the family, and their permission should be sought
   e. **Restraints** should not interfere with any treatments or affect the client's health problem
   f. Use a clove hitch knot so that the restraint can be changed and released easily
   g. Ensure that there is enough slack on the straps to allow some movement of the body part

---

BOX 13–4. Documentation Points with Use of a Restraint

Reason for restraint
Method of restraint
Date and time of application of restraint
Duration of use of the restraint and client's response
Release from restraint with periodic exercise and circulatory, neurovascular, and skin assessment
Assessment of continued need for restraint
Evaluation of the client's response

    h. Secure the restraint to the bed frame not the side rails

    i. Monitor skin integrity, neurovascular, and circulatory status every 30 minutes

    j. Release the **restraints** at least every 2 hours to permit muscle exercise and promote circulation

    k. Continually monitor the need for **restraints**

5. Alternatives to **restraints**

    a. Orient the client and family to the surroundings

    b. Explain all procedures and treatments to the client and family

    c. Encourage family and friends to stay with the client and use sitters for clients who need supervision

    d. Assign confused and disoriented clients to rooms near the nurses' station

    e. Provide appropriate visual and auditory stimuli to the client, such as clocks and a radio

    f. Place familiar items near the client's bedside, such as family pictures

    g. Maintain toileting routines

    h. Eliminate bothersome treatments, such as tube feedings, as soon as possible

    i. Evaluate all medications that the client is receiving

    j. Use relaxation techniques with the client

    k. Institute exercise and ambulation schedules as the client's condition allows

G. **Poisons**

1. Any substance that impairs health and can destroy life when ingested, inhaled, or otherwise absorbed by the body

2. Specific antidotes or treatments are available for only some types of **poisons**

3. The capacity of body tissue to recover from the **poison** determines the reversibility of the effect

4. **Poison** can impair the respiratory, circulatory, central nervous, hepatic, gastrointestinal, and renal systems of the body

5. The toddler, preschooler, and the young school-aged child must be protected from accidental **poisoning**

6. In older adults, diminished eyesight and impaired memory may result in accidental ingestion of poisonous substances or an overdose of prescribed medications

7. The Poison Control Center phone number should be visible on the telephone in homes with small children; in all cases of expected **poisoning,** the number should be called immediately

8. Implementation

    a. Remove any obvious materials from the mouth, eyes, or body area immediately

    b. Identify the type and amount of substance ingested

    c. Call the Poison Control Center before attempting an intervention

    d. If victim vomits or vomiting is induced, save vomitus if requested to do so, and deliver to the Poison Control Center

    e. If instructed by the Poison Control Center to take the person to the emergency room, call an ambulance

    f. Vomiting is never induced following ingestion of lye, household cleaners, grease, or petroleum products

    g. Vomiting is never induced in an unconscious victim

III. Disasters

A. Know the agency's disaster plan

B. Internal disasters are those in which the agency is in danger

C. External disasters occur in the community and many victims will be brought to the health care facility for care

D. When the health care agency is notified of a disaster, plans specified in the agency policy must be carried out

IV. Nosocomial Infections

A. Description

1. Also referred to as hospital-acquired infections

2. Infections acquired in the hospital or other health care facility that were not present or incubating at the time of the client's admission

3. Illness impairs the body's normal defense mechanism

4. The hospital environment provides exposure to a variety of virulent organisms that the client has not been exposed to in the past; therefore, the client has not developed resistance to these organisms

5. Infections can be transmitted by health care personnel who fail to practice proper handwashing procedures or fail to change gloves between client contacts

B. Drug-resistant **nosocomial infections**

1. Vancomycin-resistant enterococci (VRE)

2. Methicillin-resistant *Staphylococcus aureus* (MRSA)

3. Multidrug-resistant (MDR) tuberculosis (TB)

V. Standard Precautions

A. Description

1. Combine the major features of universal precautions (UP) and body substance isolation (BSI)

2. Must be practiced with all clients

3. Promote handwashing and the use of gloves, masks, eye protection, and gowns when appropriate for client contact

B. Precautions
  1. Blood
  2. All body fluids, secretions and excretions, and contaminated items regardless of whether or not they contain visible blood
  3. Nonintact skin
  4. Mucous membranes
C. Implementation
  1. Handle all blood and body fluids from all clients as if they are contaminated
  2. Gloves should be removed and hands washed between client care
  3. Masks, eye protection, or face shields are worn if client care activities may generate splashes or sprays of blood or body fluid
  4. Gowns are worn if soiling of clothing is likely from blood or body fluid
  5. Wash hands after removing a gown
  6. Client care equipment is properly cleaned and reprocessed and single-use items are discarded
  7. Contaminated linen is placed in leakproof bags and handled to prevent skin and mucous membrane exposure
  8. Needles are disposed of uncapped, or a mechanical device for recapping is used if necessary
  9. All sharp instruments and needles are discarded in a puncture-resistant container
  10. Clean up spills of blood or body fluids with a solution of bleach and water (diluted 1:10) or agency-approved disinfectant

◆ **VI. Transmission-Based Precautions**

A. Airborne precautions
  1. Diseases
    a. Measles
    b. Chickenpox (varicella)
    c. Disseminated varicella zoster (shingles)
    d. Pulmonary or laryngeal TB
  2. Barrier protection
    a. Private room for client
    b. Negative airflow pressure in room of 6 to 12 exchanges per hour
    c. Discharge of air outdoors or high-efficiency particulate air (HEPA) filtration system if air is recirculated
    d. Keep room door closed
    e. Wear a N95 respirator when entering the room of a client with known or suspected infectious TB, or a client with measles and varicella if not immune to these diseases
B. Droplet precautions
  1. Diseases
    a. Diphtheria (pharyngeal)
    b. Rubella
    c. Streptococcal pharyngitis
    d. Mycoplasma or menigococcal pneumonia
    e. Scarlet fever in infants and younger children
    f. Pertussis
    g. Mumps
  2. Barrier protection
    a. Private room for the client
    b. A mask is required when within 3 feet of the client
    c. Place a mask on the client during transport
C. Contact precautions
  1. Diseases
    a. Respiratory syncytial virus (RSV)
    b. *Shigella* and other enteric pathogens
    c. Major wound infections
    d. Herpes simplex
    e. Scabies
    f. Disseminated varicella zoster (shingles)
    g. Colonization or infection with multidrug-resistant organisms
  2. Barrier protection
    a. Private room for the client
    b. Wear gloves and a gown when in contact with the client

PRACTICE QUESTIONS

1. The nurse enters a client's room and finds that the wastebasket is on fire. The nurse immediately assists the client out of the room. The next nursing action is to
   1 Confine the fire by closing the room door
   2 Activate the fire alarm
   3 Call for help
   4 Extinguish the fire

2. A nurse enters the nursing lounge and discovers that a chair is on fire. The nurse activates the alarm, closes the lounge door, and obtains the fire extinguisher to put out the fire. The nurse pulls the pin on the fire extinguisher. The next appropriate action is to
   1 Squeeze the handle on the extinguisher
   2 Aim at the base of the fire
   3 Sweep the fire from side to side with the extinguisher
   4 Sweep the fire from top to bottom with the extinguisher

3. The nurse conducts a home safety assessment with a client preparing for discharge and the client tells the nurse that a space heater is used to heat the apartment. Which of the following instructions does the nurse provide to the client regarding the use of the space heater?
   1 A space heater should not be used in an apartment
   2 The space heater needs to be placed at least 3 feet from anything that can burn
   3 The space heater should be placed in the hallway at nighttime
   4 The space heater should be kept at a low setting at all times

4. The nurse is preparing to initiate a tube feeding to a client and the physician has prescribed the

use of an electronic food pump. The nurse brings the pump to the bedside and prepares to plug the pump cord into the wall. There is no available plug in the wall socket. Which of the following is the most appropriate nursing action?
1   Use an extension cord from the nurse's lounge for the pump plug
2   Initiate the feeding without the use of a pump
3   Plug in the pump cord in the available plug above the room sink
4   Contact the electrical maintenance department for assistance

5. The nurse obtains an order from the physician to restrain the client using a jacket restraint. The nurse instructs the nursing assistant to apply the restraint to the client. Which of the following observations, if made by the nurse, indicates inappropriate application of the restraint?
1   A clove hitch knot in the restraint strap
2   Restraint straps are safely secured to the side rails
3   The jacket restraint is secure and two fingers can easily slide between the restraint and the client's skin
4   The jacket restraint strap does not tighten when force is applied against it

6. The nurse is giving report to the nursing assistant who will be caring for a client with hand restraints. The nurse instructs the nursing assistant to remove the restraints to permit muscle exercise and promote circulation at least
1   Every 2 hours
2   Every 3 hours
3   Every 4 hours
4   Once during the shift

7. The nurse is planning care for a client with an internal radiation implant. Which of the following is not an appropriate component of this plan of care?

1   Placing the client in a semiprivate room at the end of the hallway
2   Wearing gloves when emptying the client's bedpan
3   Keeping all linens in the room until the implant is removed
4   Wearing a lead apron when providing direct care to the client

8. A mother calls a neighborhood nurse and tells the nurse that her 3-year-old child has just ingested liquid furniture polish. The nurse directs the mother to immediately
1   Administer ipecac to induce vomiting
2   Take the child to the emergency department
3   Call an ambulance
4   Call the poison control center

9. The emergency department nurse receives a telephone call and is informed that a tornado hit a local residential area, resulting in numerous casualties. The victims will be brought to the emergency department. The initial nursing action is which of the following?
1   Prepare the triage rooms
2   Obtain additional supplies from the central supply department
3   Activate the agency disaster plan
4   Obtain additional nursing staff to assist in treating the casualties

10. The nurse is caring for a client with a nosocomial infection caused by methicillin-resistant, *S. aureus* (MRSA). Contact precautions are initiated. The nurse prepares to provide colostomy care to the client. Which of the following protective items is required to perform this procedure?
1   Gloves, gown, and goggles
2   Gloves and goggles
3   Gloves, gown, and shoe protectors
4   Gloves and a gown

ANSWERS

1. **2**

RATIONALE: The order of priority in the event of a fire is to rescue the clients in immediate danger. The next step is to activate the fire alarm. The fire is then confined by closing all doors, and then the fire is extinguished.
TEST-TAKING STRATEGY: Remember the mnemonic RACE to prioritize in the event of a fire. R = Rescue clients in immediate danger; A = Alarm, sound the alarm; C = Confine the fire by closing all doors; E = Extinguish or evacuate. If you had difficulty with this question, take time now to review fire safety.
LEVEL OF COGNITIVE ABILITY: Application
PHASE OF NURSING PROCESS: Implementation
CLIENT NEEDS: Safe, Effective Care Environment

CONTENT AREA: Fundamental Skills
REFERENCE
Leahy, J., & Kizilay, P. (1998). *Foundations of nursing practice: A nursing process approach.* Philadelphia: W. B. Saunders. p. 393.

2. **2**

RATIONALE: A fire can be extinguished by smothering it with a blanket or using a fire extinguisher. To use the extinguisher, the pin is pulled first. The extinguisher should then be aimed at the base of the fire. The handle of the extinguisher is then squeezed and the fire is extinguished by sweeping from side to side to coat the area evenly.
TEST-TAKING STRATEGY: Note the key word "next." Remember the mnemonic PASS to prioritize in the use of a fire extinguisher. P = Pull the pin; A = Aim at the base of the fire; S = Squeeze the handle; S = Sweep from side to

side to coat the area evenly. If you had difficulty with this question, take time now to review the appropriate use of a fire extinguisher.
LEVEL OF COGNITIVE ABILITY: Application
PHASE OF NURSING PROCESS: Implementation
CLIENT NEEDS: Safe, Effective Care Environment
CONTENT AREA: Fundamental Skills
REFERENCE
Leahy, J., & Kizilay, P. (1998). *Foundations of nursing practice: A nursing process approach.* Philadelphia: W. B. Saunders. pp. 392–393.

3. **2**

RATIONALE: Space heaters need to be used appropriately because they present a great risk of fire. A space heater needs to be placed at least 3 feet from anything that can burn. Placing a heater in a hallway does not guarantee that it will be 3 feet from anything flammable. A low setting does not reduce the risk of fire. A space heater can be used in an apartment if there is ample space and safety precautions are followed.
TEST-TAKING STRATEGY: Use the process of elimination keeping in mind the issue related to fire safety. Note that option 2 is the only option that specifically defines a safety measure related to the use of a space heater. Review fire safety prevention measures in the home now if you had difficulty with this question.
LEVEL OF COGNITIVE ABILITY: Application
PHASE OF NURSING PROCESS: Implementation
CLIENT NEEDS: Safe, Effective Care Environment
CONTENT AREA: Fundamental Skills
REFERENCE
Leahy, J., & Kizilay, P. (1998). *Foundations of nursing practice: A nursing process approach.* Philadelphia: W. B. Saunders. p. 392.

4. **4**

RATIONALE: The nurse needs to use hospital resources for assistance. A regular extension cord should not be used because it poses the risk of fire. Using electrical appliances near a sink also presents a hazard. If a pump is prescribed, the nurse must provide the safe means for its use.
TEST-TAKING STRATEGY: Eliminate option 2 because the physician has ordered an electronic pump. Recalling safety issues related to electrical hazards will assist in eliminating options 1 and 3. If you had difficulty with this question, take time to review electrical safety.
LEVEL OF COGNITIVE ABILITY: Application
PHASE OF NURSING PROCESS: Implementation
CLIENT NEEDS: Safe, Effective Care Environment
CONTENT AREA: Fundamental Skills
REFERENCE
Leahy, J., & Kizilay, P. (1998). *Foundations of nursing practice: A nursing process approach.* Philadelphia: W. B. Saunders. p. 389.

5. **2**

RATIONALE: A clove hitch knot should be used for applying a restraint because it does not tighten when force is applied against it and allows quick and easy removal of the restraint in case of an emergency. The restraint strap is secured to the bed frame and never to the side rail to avoid accidental injury in the event that the side rail is released. The jacket restraint should be secure and one to two fingers should easily slide between the restraint and the client's skin.
TEST-TAKING STRATEGY: Note the key word "inappro-

priate." This indicates that you are looking for a response that identifies an inaccurate measure related to the application of restraints. The words "secured to the side rails" in option 2 should direct your attention as an inappropriate action. Review guidelines related to the application of restraints now if you had difficulty with this question.
LEVEL OF COGNITIVE ABILITY: Comprehension
PHASE OF NURSING PROCESS: Evaluation
CLIENT NEEDS: Safe, Effective Care Environment
CONTENT AREA: Fundamental Skills
REFERENCE
deWit, S. (1998). *Essentials of medical-surgical nursing* (4th ed.). Philadelphia: W. B. Saunders. p. 1028.

6. **1**

RATIONALE: The nurse should instruct the nursing assistant to release the restraints at least every 2 hours to permit muscle exercise and promote circulation. Agency guidelines regarding the use of restraints should always be followed.
TEST-TAKING STRATEGY: Knowledge regarding the use of restraints is required to answer this question. In this situation, it is best to select the option that identifies the most frequent time frame. Review guidelines related to the use of restraints now if you had difficulty with this question.
LEVEL OF COGNITIVE ABILITY: Application
PHASE OF NURSING PROCESS: Implementation
CLIENT NEEDS: Physiological Integrity
CONTENT AREA: Fundamental Skills
REFERENCE
deWit, S. (1998). *Essentials of medical-surgical nursing* (4th ed.). Philadelphia: W. B. Saunders. p. 1028.

7. **1**

RATIONALE: A private room with a private bath is essential if a client has an internal radiation implant. This is necessary to prevent accidental exposure of radiation to other clients. Options 2, 3, and 4 are accurate interventions for a client with a radiation implant.
TEST-TAKING STRATEGY: Note the key words "not an appropriate." Option 2 can be eliminated first because this is a component of standard precautions for all clients. Options 3 and 4 can be eliminated next because they directly relate to radiation safety. Review radiation safety principles now if you had difficulty with this question.
LEVEL OF COGNITIVE ABILITY: Application
PHASE OF NURSING PROCESS: Planning
CLIENT NEEDS: Safe, Effective Care Environment
CONTENT AREA: Fundamental Skills
REFERENCE
Monahan, F., & Neighbors, M. (1998). *Medical-surgical nursing: Foundations for clinical practice* (2nd ed.). Philadelphia: W. B Saunders. p. 1519.

8. **4**

RATIONALE: If a poisoning occurs, the poison control center should be contacted immediately. Vomiting should not be induced if the victim is unconscious or if the substance ingested was a strong corrosive or petroleum product. Taking the child to the emergency department and calling an ambulance are not the initial action as this would delay treatment. The poison control center may advise the mother to take the child to the emergency department, and if this is the case, the mother should call an ambulance.

TEST-TAKING STRATEGY: Note the key word "immediately." Eliminate options 2 and 3 because these options will delay treatment. Recalling that vomiting should not be induced if a corrosive substance was ingested will assist in eliminating option 1. Review poison control measures now if you had difficulty with this question.

LEVEL OF COGNITIVE ABILITY: Application
PHASE OF NURSING PROCESS: Implementation
CLIENT NEEDS: Physiological Integrity
CONTENT AREA: Child Health
REFERENCE
deWit, S. (1998). *Essentials of medical-surgical nursing* (4th ed.). Philadelphia: W. B. Saunders. p. 983.

9. **3**

RATIONALE: In an external disaster, many people will be taken to the emergency room for treatment. Although options 1, 2, and 4 may be a component of preparing for the casualties, the initial nursing action must be to activate the disaster plan.

TEST-TAKING STRATEGY: Note the key word "initial." Use the process of elimination to determine the priority action. Note that option 3 is the global response. Review procedures related to management of a disaster now if you had difficulty with this question.

LEVEL OF COGNITIVE ABILITY: Application
PHASE OF NURSING PROCESS: Implementation
CLIENT NEEDS: Safe, Effective Care Environment
CONTENT AREA: Fundamental Skills
REFERENCE
deWit, S. (1998). *Essentials of medical-surgical nursing* (4th ed.). Philadelphia: W. B. Saunders. pp. 988–989.

10. **1**

RATIONALE: Goggles are worn to protect the mucous membranes of the eye during interventions that may produce splashes of blood, body fluids, secretions, and excretions. In addition, contact precautions requires the use of gloves, and a gown should be worn if direct client contact is anticipated. Shoe protectors are not necessary.

TEST-TAKING STRATEGY: Note the key words "contact precautions" and "colostomy." Use the process of elimination in determining the necessary items required caring for this client. If you had difficulty with this question, take time now to review transmission-based precautions.

LEVEL OF COGNITIVE ABILITY: Application
PHASE OF NURSING PROCESS: Implementation
CLIENT NEEDS: Safe, Effective Care Environment
CONTENT AREA: Fundamental Skills
REFERENCE
Leahy, J., & Kizilay, P. (1998). *Foundations of nursing practice: A nursing process approach.* Philadelphia: W. B. Saunders. pp. 1236–1238.

BIBLIOGRAPHY

deWit, S. (1998). *Essentials of medical-surgical nursing* (4th ed.). Philadelphia: W. B. Saunders.

Leahy, J., & Kizilay, P. (1998). *Foundations of nursing practice: A nursing process approach.* Philadelphia: W. B. Saunders.

Luckmann, J. (1997). *Saunders manual of nursing care.* Philadelphia: W. B. Saunders.

Monahan, F., & Neighbors, M. (1998). *Medical-surgical nursing: Foundations for clinical practice* (2nd ed.). Philadelphia: W. B. Saunders.

CHAPTER 14

Medication and Intravenous Administration

....

PYRAMID TERMS

Conversion—The first step in the calculation of a medication problem.

Generic Name—The official accepted name of a medication.

Milliequivalent—Abbreviated as mEq; it is an expression of the number of grams of a medication contained in 1 mL of a normal solution.

Parenteral—Parenteral always means injection route. Injections are administered by intravenous (IV), intramuscular (IM), and subcutaneous (SQ, SC) methods.

Percentage Solutions—Express the number of grams of the medication per 100 mL of solution.

Ratio Solutions—Express the number of grams of the medication per total milliliters of solution.

Reconstitution—Powders must be dissolved with a sterile diluent before use, and usually sterile water or normal saline is used. The dissolving procedure is called reconstitution.

Trade Name—Also called brand name or proprietary name; is followed by the sign ® meaning that the name is a registered trademark.

Unit—Abbreviated as U or u; measures a medication in terms of its action, not its physical weight.

PYRAMID TO SUCCESS

When a medication or intravenous calculation question is presented, the nurse should always use the appropriate formula to calculate the problem. Short cuts should not be used when calculating these problems. The problem and answer should be labeled with the correct measurement. Be careful with decimal points. It is important to place the decimal points in the correct places or the answer will be incorrect. When calculating the problem, the nurse evaluates whether the answer is within reason and makes sense. In the clinical setting, the nurse should always seek assistance if unsure of the accuracy in calculating. On CAT NCLEX-PN, it is important to check the calculation before selecting the answer to the question. REMEMBER, on CAT NCLEX-PN, the correct answer will be on the screen. Following the formula, placing the decimal points in the correct places, and checking the accuracy of the calculation will ensure selection of the correct answer. PRACTICE MAKES PERFECT!

NURSING PROCESS

DATA COLLECTION

Medication order
Five rights: right medication, right dose, right client, right route, and right time
The client's history of allergies
The client's current condition and the purpose for the medication or intravenous solution

The client's understanding of the purpose of the medication
Need for conversion when preparing a dose of medication

141

PLANNING
Client will remain free of injury.

IMPLEMENTATION
Check medication order. Ask client about a history of allergies. Identify client's current condition. Check the five rights. Identify the need for conversion when calculating the correct dose of medication. Prepare and administer medication or intravenous solution once correct dosage is determined.

EVALUATION
Correct dosage is determined and administered to client. Client does not experience any adverse effects.

PLANNING
Client will remain free of infection.

IMPLEMENTATION
Check vital signs. Monitor for signs of infection.

EVALUATION
Vital signs remain within normal limits. Client does not develop an infection.

PLANNING
Client will maintain fluid balance.

IMPLEMENTATION
Monitor for signs of fluid overload.

EVALUATION
Client does not experience fluid overload.

PLANNING
Client will verbalize purpose of medication or intravenous solution.

IMPLEMENTATION
Determine client's understanding regarding the purpose of the prescribed medication. Reinforce teaching about the medication. Document the administration of the prescribed therapy and client's response to the therapy.

EVALUATION
Client verbalizes purpose of prescribed therapy. Effectiveness of the medication is achieved.

◆ CLIENT NEEDS

SAFE, EFFECTIVE CARE ENVIRONMENT

Client rights
Medication calculations
Intravenous fluid and medication calculations
Error prevention
Handling hazardous and infectious materials
Asepsis
Standard (universal) precautions

HEALTH PROMOTION AND MAINTENANCE

Collecting physical data
Reinforcing teaching regarding prescribed medication(s) or IV therapy
Disease prevention

PSYCHOSOCIAL INTEGRITY

Use of support systems
Communication
Caring and providing emotional comfort
Cultural awareness
Use of coping mechanisms

PHYSIOLOGICAL INTEGRITY

Administration of medications and monitoring IV therapy
Expected effects of pharmacological therapy
Actions, side effects, and untoward effects of medications and IV therapy
Unexpected responses to therapy
Alterations in body systems
Laboratory values
Fluid and electrolyte imbalances

I. Drug Measurement Systems

A. Metric system
1. The basic units of metric measures are meter, liter, and gram (Table 14–1)
2. Meter measures length
3. Liter measures volume
4. Gram measures weight

B. Apothecary and household systems (Table 14–2)
1. The apothecary and household systems are the oldest of the medication measurement systems
2. The four apothecary measures sometimes used are the grain, minim, dram, and ounce
3. Grain measures weight
4. Minim, dram, and ounce measure volume
5. The three household measures commonly used are tablespoon, teaspoon, and drop

C. Additional common medication measures
1. Milliequivalent
   a. Abbreviated mEq
   b. It is an expression of the number of grams of a medication contained in 1 mL of a normal solution
   c. Example: potassium
2. Unit
   a. Abbreviated as U or u; measures a medication in terms of its action, not its physical weight
   b. Examples: penicillin, heparin, insulin

II. Conversions

A. Conversion between metric units (Box 14–1)
1. The metric system is a decimal system;

Table 14–1. **Metric System**

Abbreviations	Equivalents
meter—m	1 L = 1000 mL
liter—L	1 mL = 0.001 L or 1 cc
gram—g, gm, Gm	1 mL = 1 cc or 0.001 L
milligram—mg, mgm	1 gm = 1000 mg
microgram—μg, mcg	1 mg = 1000 μg or 0.001 g
kilogram—kg, Kg	1 μg = 0.000001 g
milliliter—mL	1 kg = 1000 g
cubic centimeter—cc	1 kg = 2.2 lb

Table 14–2. Apothecary and Household Systems

Abbreviations	Equivalents
grain—gr	gr 1 = 60 mg
dram—dr	gr 5 = 300 mg
ounce—oz	gr 15 = 1000 mg or 1 gm
minim—min, M or m	gr 1/150 = 0.4 mg
quart—qt	1 oz = 30 mL
pint—pt	1 dr = 4 mL
drop—gtt	1 T = 15 mL or 3 tsp
teaspoon—t or tsp	1 t or tsp = 5 mL
tablespoon—T or tbs	1 min = 1 gtt
pound—lb	15 min = 1 mL
	60 min = 1 dr
	8 dr = 1 oz
	1 qt = 2 pt or 32 oz
	1 qt = 1000 mL or 1 L
	1 pt = 16 oz
	16 oz = 1 lb
	2.2 lb = 1 kg

therefore, conversions between the units in this system can be done by either dividing or multiplying by 1000 or by moving the decimal point three places to the right or three places to the left

2. In the metric system, to convert larger to smaller, multiply by 1000 or move the decimal three places to the right
3. In the metric system, to convert smaller to larger, divide by 1000 or move the decimal three places to the left

B. Conversion between apothecary, household, and metric systems
  1. Conversions between the metric, apothecary, and household measures are equivalent, not equal, measures
  2. Conversion to equivalent measures between systems is necessary when a medication order is written in one system but the medication label is stated in another
  3. Medications are not always ordered and prepared in the same system of measurement;

BOX 14–1. Conversion Between Metric Units

1. PROBLEM

Convert 2 grams to milligrams

Solution
Change a larger unit to a smaller unit
2.000 grams = 2000 mg (moving the decimal three places to the right)

2. PROBLEM

Convert 250 mL to liters

Solution
Change a smaller unit to a larger unit
250 mL = 0.250 L or 0.25 L (moving decimal three places to the left)

BOX 14–2. Calculating Equivalents Between Two Systems

Calculating equivalents between two systems may be done using the method of ratio and proportion

PROBLEM
The physician orders nitroglycerin, gr 1/150. The medication label reads 0.4 mg per tablet. How many tablets will you administer to the client?

gr 1 : 60 mg = gr 1/150 : X mg
60 × 1/150 = X
X = 0.4 mg (1 tablet)

it is therefore necessary to convert units from one system to another
4. Conversion is the first step in the calculation of dosages
5. Calculating equivalents between two systems may be done using the method of ratio and proportion (Box 14–2)

III. Celsius and Fahrenheit Temperature
(Table 14–3)

A. To convert Fahrenheit to Celsius, subtract 32 and divide the result by 1.8
B. To convert Celsius to Fahrenheit, multiply by 1.8 and add 32

IV. Medication Labels

A. A medication label will contain both the **generic** and **trade name** of the medication
B. The **generic name** is the official accepted name of a medication; the **generic name** is not capitalized
C. The **trade name**, also called brand name or proprietary name, is followed by the sign ®, meaning the name is registered; trade names are capitalized or written with the first letter capitalized
D. Each medication has only one official name, but may have several trade names, each for the exclusive use of the company that manufactures the medication
E. Always check expiration dates on medication labels

Table 14–3. Celsius and Fahrenheit Temperature

Fahrenheit to Celsius
To convert Fahrenheit to Celsius, subtract 32 and divide the result by 1.8
Formula: C = (F − 32) ÷ 1.8

Celsius to Fahrenheit
To convert Celsius to Fahrenheit, multiply by 1.8 and add 32
Formula: F = 1.8 C + 32

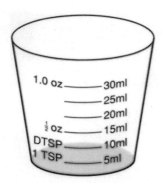

FIGURE 14–1. Calibrated measuring devices. (From Kee, J., & Marshall, S. [1996]. Clinical calculations. With applications to general and specialty area [3rd ed.]. Philadelphia: W. B. Saunders. p. 192.)

V. Medication Orders (Box 14–3)

A. In a medication order, the name of the medication is written first, followed by the dosage, route, and frequency

B. If there are any questions or inconsistencies with the written order, the person who wrote the order must be contacted immediately, and the order must be verified

VI. Oral Medications

A. Scored tablets contain an indented marking to make breakage for partial dosages possible; when necessary, scored tablets (those marked for division) can be divided in halves or quarters

B. Enteric-coated tablets and sustained-released capsules delay absorption until the medication reaches the small intestine; these medications should not be crushed

C. Capsules contain a powered or oily medication in a gelatin cover

D. Oral liquids are supplied in solution form and contain a specific amount of medication in a given amount of solution, as stated on the label

E. The medicine cup (Fig. 14–1)
  1. Has a capacity of 30 mL or 1 ounce
  2. Is used for oral liquids
  3. Is calibrated to measure teaspoons, tablespoons, and drams
  4. To pour accurately, hold the medication cup at eye level, then line up the measure that is needed and pour

F. Volumes of less than 5 mL are measured using a syringe with the needle removed

G. A calibrated dropper is used when giving medicine to children and when adding small

BOX 14–3. Medication Orders

Name of client
Date and time when order was written
Name of medication to be given
Dosage of medication
Route
Time and frequency of administration
Signature of person writing the order

amounts of liquid to water or juice; calibrations are in milliliters, cubic centimeters, drops, or minims

VII. Parenteral Medications

A. **Parenteral** always means injection route, and **parenteral** medications are administered by intravenous (IV), intramuscular (IM), or by subcutaneous (SC) routes

B. **Parenteral** medications are packaged in single-use ampules, single and multiple-use rubber-stoppered vials, and in premeasured syringes and cartridges

C. The nurse should not administer more than 3 mL per IM or SC injection site because volumes larger than 3 mL are difficult for a single injection site to absorb

D. Always question excessively large or small volumes of medication

E. The standard 3 mL (cubic centimeter [cc]) syringe is used to measure most injectable medications; it is calibrated in tenths (0.1) of a mL (Fig. 14–2)

F. The calibrations on a syringe are read from the top black ring on the syringe, not the raised middle section and not the bottom ring

G. Injection cartridges (Fig. 14–3)
  1. Tubex and Carpuject are **trade names** of two widely used injection cartridges
  2. These cartridges slip into plastic injectors that provide a plunger for injection of the medication
  3. The cartridge is prefilled with sterile medication and is labeled with the medication name and dosage
  4. The cartridges contain a volume of 2.5 mL and are calibrated in tenths
  5. The cartridges are routinely overfilled with 0.1 to 0.2 mL of medication to allow for manipulation of the syringe to expel air from the needle prior to injection

THREE MILLILITER SYRINGE

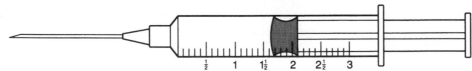

FIGURE 14–2. Three-milliliter syringe. (From Kee, J., & Marshall, S. [1996]. Clinical calculations: With applications to general and specialty areas [3rd ed.]. Philadelphia: W. B. Saunders. p. 125.)

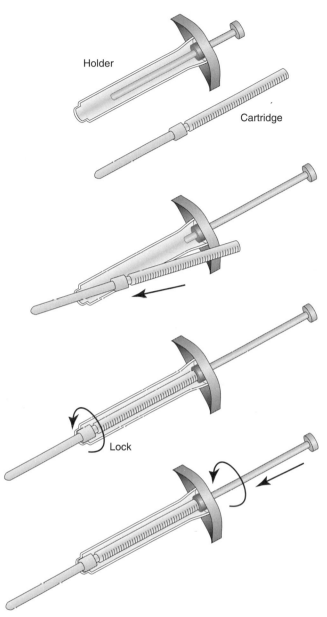

FIGURE 14–3. Cartridge-type syringe, Tubex. (From Leahy, J., & Kizilay, P. [1998]. Foundations of nursing practice: A nursing process approach. Philadelphia: W. B. Saunders. p. 469.)

6. The cartridges are designed to provide sufficient capacity to allow for the addition of a second medication when combined dosages are prescribed
7. The prefilled syringe is to be used once and discarded; if the nurse is to give less than a full single dose provided, the nurse needs to discard the extra amount before injecting the client

H. Standard medication doses are to be rounded to the nearest tenth (0.1) of a mL or cc and measured on the mL scale; for example, 1.25 mL is rounded to 1.3 mL

I. When volumes larger than 3 mL are required, a 5-, 6-, 10-, or 12-mL syringe may be used; these syringes are calibrated in fifths (Fig. 14–4)

J. Syringes larger than 12 mL are calibrated in full mL measures
K. Tuberculin syringe (Fig. 14–5)
   1. Holds a total capacity of 1 mL or cc and is used to measure small or critical amounts of medications such as allergen extract, vaccine, or a child's medication
   2. It is calibrated in hundredths (0.01) of a mL, with each one tenth (0.1) marked on the metric scale
L. Insulin syringe (Fig. 14–6)
   1. The standard U-100 insulin syringe is used to measure U-100 insulin only; it is calibrated for a total of 100 units, or 1 mL (cc)
   2. The Lo-Dose U-100 insulin syringe is used for measuring small amounts of U-100 insulin; it is calibrated for a total of 50 units, or 0.5 mL (cc)
   3. Insulin should not be measured in any other type of syringe
   4. When the insulin order states to combine Regular and NPH insulin, remember to draw the Regular insulin first, and then draw the NPH insulin

VIII. Injectable Medications in Powder Form

A. Some medications become unstable when stored in solution form and are therefore packaged in powder form
B. Powders must be dissolved with a sterile diluent before use, and usually sterile water or normal saline is used. The dissolving procedure is called **reconstitution** (Box 14–4)

IX. Calculating the Correct Dosage (Table 14–4)

A. When calculating oral medications, check the calculation and question an order if the amount is for more than three tablets
B. When calculating parenteral medications, check the calculation and question an order if the amount to be given is too large a dose

---

BOX 14–4. Reconstitution

In reconstituting the medication, locate the instructions on the label or in the vial package insert and read and follow the directions carefully.

Instructions will state the volume of diluent to be used and the resulting volume of the reconstituted medication.

Often the powdered medication adds volume to the solution in addition to the amount of diluent added.

When you reconstitute a multiple-dose vial, label the medication vial with the date and time of preparation, your initials, and the date of expiration.

It is also important to label the strength per volume.

The total volume of the prepared solution will always exceed the volume of the diluent you add.

FIVE MILLILITER SYRINGE

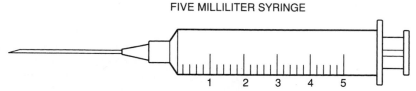

FIGURE 14–4. Five-milliliter syringe. (From Kee, J., & Marshall, S. [1996]. Clinical calculations: With applications to general and specialty areas [3rd ed.]. Philadelphia: W. B. Saunders. p. 125.)

TUBERCULIN SYRINGE

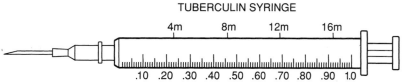

FIGURE 14–5. Tuberculin syringe. (From Kee, J., & Marshall, S. [1996]. Clinical calculations: With applications to general and specialty areas [3rd ed.]. Philadelphia: W. B. Saunders. p. 126.)

INSULIN SYRINGE

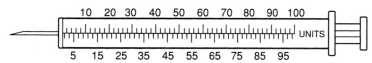

FIGURE 14–6. Insulin syringe. (From Kee, J., & Marshall, S. [1996]. Clinical calculations: With applications to general and specialty areas [3rd ed.]. Philadelphia: W. B. Saunders. p. 126.)

Table 14–4. Formula for Calculating Medication Dosage

$$\frac{D \text{ (desired)}}{A \text{ (available)}} \times Q \text{ (quantity)} = X$$

D (desired) = the dosage that the physician ordered
A (Available) = the dosage strength as stated on the medication label
Q (quantity) = the volume that the dosage strength is available in, such as tablets, capsules, or mL

Table 14–5. Formulas for IV Calculations

Flow Rates
$$\frac{\text{Total volume} \times \text{gtt factor}}{\text{Time in minutes}} = \text{gtt per min}$$

Infusion Time
$$\frac{\text{Total volume to infuse}}{\text{mL per hour being infused}} = \text{Infusion time}$$

C. Regardless of the source of the error, if the nurse gives an incorrect dose, the nurse is legally responsible for the action

D. Be sure that all measures are in the same system, and all units are in the same size, converting when necessary; carefully consider what is the reasonable amount of the medication that should be administered

E. Round standard injection doses to tenths and measure in a 3 mL syringe

F. Round small, critical, or children's doses to hundredths and measure in the 1 mL tuberculin syringe

X. Calculating Dosages Expressed as Ratio or Percent

A. Percentage solutions
1. Express the number of grams of the medication per 100 mL of solution
2. Example: calcium gluconate 10% = 10 g of pure medication per 100 mL of solution

B. Ratio solutions
1. Express the number of grams of the medication per total milliliters of solution
2. Example: epinephrine 1:1000 = 1 g pure medication per 1000 mL solution

XI. Intravenous Flow Rates (Table 14–5)

A. Monitor an IV every 30 minutes for adults and every 15 minutes for children

B. If the IV is running behind schedule, collaborate with the registered nurse and/or the physician to determine the client's ability to tolerate an increased flow rate, particularly those clients with cardiac, pulmonary, renal, and neurological conditions

C. The nurse should never arbitrarily speed up an IV to catch up if the IV is running behind schedule

D. Whenever an IV rate is increased, the nurse should monitor the client for increased heart rate, increased respirations, or increased lung congestion, which could indicate fluid overload

E. IV fluids are most frequently ordered on the basis of mL per hour to be administered

F. The volume ordered is administered by adjusting the rate at which the IV infuses, which is counted in drops (gtt) per minute

G. Most flow rate calculations involve changing mL per hour into gtt per minute

H. IV tubing
1. Calibrated in gtt per milliliter, and this calibration is needed for calculating flow rates
2. A standard or macrodrip set is used for routine adult IV administrations; depending on the manufacturer and type of tubing, it will require 10, 15, or 20 gtt to equal 1 mL
3. A mini- or microdrip set is used when more exact measurements are needed, and in pediatric units
4. In a mini- or microdrip set, 60 gtt are equal to 1 mL
5. The calibration, in gtt per mL, is written on the IV tubing package

XII. Electronic IV Flow Rate Regulators

A. Controller
1. Works on the same principle of gravity as a regular IV drip, with the rate of flow being maintained by rapid compression and decompression of the IV tubing by the machine
2. The desired flow rate is set on the controller in milliliters per hour
3. Because controllers work by gravity, the height of the solution bag is critical and must be maintained at a minimum of 36 inches above the controller
4. The nurse should continue to monitor the amount of IV solution in the IV container and monitor the controller to ensure proper functioning of the machine

B. Pump
1. A pump is different from a controller in that it physically pumps fluids against resistance
2. Gravity is not a factor in the use of a pump, and the height of the IV solution bag is not a critical factor
3. The flow rate on a pump is set in milliliters per hour
4. The nurse should continue to monitor the amount of IV solution in the IV container and monitor the pump to ensure proper functioning of the machine

PRACTICE QUESTIONS

1. The physician orders 1000 mL of 0.9% NS to run over 12 hours. The drop factor is 15 drops per 1 mL. The nurse plans to adjust the flow rate at how many drops per minute?
   1 15 drops per minute
   2 17 drops per minute
   3 21 drops per minute
   4 23 drops per minute

2. The physician orders an IM dose of 400,000 units of penicillin G benzathine (Bicillin). The label on the 10 mL ampule sent from the pharmacy reads penicillin G benzathine (Bicillin) 300,000 units per mL. The nurse prepares to administer how many mL to administer the correct dose?
   1 1.3 mL
   2 13 mL
   3 1.5 mL
   4 10 mL

3. The physician orders 3000 mL of D5W to run over a 24-hour period. The drop factor is 10 drops per 1 mL. The nurse plans to adjust the flow rate at how many drops per minute?
   1 15 drops per minute
   2 17 drops per minute
   3 21 drops per minute
   4 24 drops per minute

4. The physician's order reads phenytoin (Dilantin) 0.2 g PO BID. The medication label states 100-mg capsules. How many capsule(s) will the nurse prepare to administer one dose?
   1 1 capsule
   2 2 capsules
   3 3 capsules
   4 4 capsules

5. The physician orders 1000 mL of 1/2% NS to run over 8 hours. The drop factor is 15 drops per 1 mL. The nurse plans to adjust the flow rate at how many drops per minute?
   1 20 drops per minute
   2 22 drops per minute
   3 28 drops per minute
   4 31 drops per minute

6. The physician orders 2000 mL of D5 1/2% NS to run over 24 hours. The drop factor is 15 drops per 1 mL. The nurse plans to adjust the flow rate at how many drops per minute?
   1 15 drops per minute
   2 17 drops per minute
   3 21 drops per minute
   4 28 drops per minute

7. The physician's order reads cyanocobalamin (vitamin B_{12}) 100 μg IM. The medication label reads cyanocobalamin (vitamin B_{12}), 0.5 mg per mL. The nurse administers how many mL to the client?
   1 0.2 mL
   2 0.5 mL
   3 1 mL
   4 2 mL

8. The physician orders 3000 mL of D5W to be administered over a 24-hour period. The nurse prepares to set the infusion rate knowing that how many mL per hour are to be administered?
   1 50 mL per hour
   2 75 mL per hour
   3 100 mL per hour
   4 125 mL per hour

9. The physician's order reads levothyroxine (Synthroid), 150 μg PO daily. The medication label reads Synthroid 0.1 mg per tablet. The nurse prepares to administer how many tablet(s) to the client?
   1 1 tablet
   2 1.5 tablets

3 2 tablets
4 2.5 tablets

10. The physician orders 1000 mL D5W to run at 125 mL per hour. The nurse calculates the infusion rate knowing that it will take how many hours for 1 liter to infuse?
    1 8 hours
    2 10 hours
    3 12 hours
    4 15 hours

11. The physician orders 500 mL of 0.9% NS to run over 5 hours. The drop factor is 10 drops per 1 mL. The nurse plans to adjust the flow rate at how many drops per minute?
    1 15 drops
    2 17 drops
    3 20 drops
    4 22 drops

12. The physician orders one unit of packed red blood cells to run over 4 hours. The unit of blood contains 250 mL. The drop factor is 10 drops per 1 mL. The registered nurse (RN) asks the licensed practical nurse (LPN) to assist in monitoring the flow rate during the infusion. The LPN monitors the flow rate knowing that how many drops per minute should infuse?
    1 15 drops
    2 17 drops
    3 10 drops
    4 20 drops

13. The physician orders 3000 mL of 0.9% NS to run over 24 hours. The drop factor is 15 drops per 1 mL. The nurse plans to adjust the flow rate at how many drops per minute?
    1 17 drops
    2 20 drops
    3 24 drops
    4 31 drops

14. The physician's order reads quinidine gluconate (Quinaglute), 0.3 g PO BID. The medication label reads quinidine gluconate (Quinaglute), 150-mg tablets. The nurse prepares how many tablet(s) to administer one dose?
    1 0.5 tablet
    2 1 tablet
    3 2 tablets
    4 3 tablets

15. The physician orders tetracycline hydrochloride (Achromycin) 0.5 g PO QID. The medication label on the bottle of medication reads tetracycline hydrochloride (Achromycin) 250 mg tablets. The nurse prepares how many tablet(s) to administer one dose?
    1 0.5 tablet
    2 1 tablet

3 2 tablets
4 3 tablets

16. The physician's order reads triazolam (Halcion), 125 μg PO at HS daily. The medication bottle is labeled triazolam (Halcion), 0.125-mg tablets. The nurse prepares how many tablet(s) to administer one dose?
    1 1 tablet
    2 1.5 tablets
    3 2 tablets
    4 2.5 tablets

17. The physician's order reads atenolol (Tenormin), 0.025 g PO QD. The medication bottle reads atenolol (Tenormin) 50-mg tablets. The nurse prepares how many tablet(s) to administer the dose?
    1 0.5 tablet
    2 1 tablet
    3 2 tablets
    4 3 tablets

18. The physician's order reads hydromorphone hydrochloride (Dilaudid), 3 mg IM q4h PRN. The medication label reads hydromorphone hydrochloride (Dilaudid), 4 mg per 1 mL. The nurse prepares to administer which of the following to the client?
    1 1.5 mg
    2 4 mg
    3 0.8 mL
    4 1.3 mL

19. The physician's order reads digoxin (Lanoxin), 0.25 mg PO daily. The medication label reads digoxin (Lanoxin), 0.125 mg per tablet. The nurse prepares how many tablet(s) to administer the dose?
    1. 0.5 tablet
    2. 1 tablet
    3. 1.5 tablets
    4. 2 tablets

20. The physician orders meperidine hydrochloride (Demerol), 80 mg IM PRN. The medication label reads meperidine hydrochloride (Demerol), 100 mg per mL. The nurse prepares to administer how many mL to the client?
    1 1.25 mL
    2 100 mL
    3 0.8 mL
    4 1 mL

21. The physician orders heparin sodium (Liquaemin), 650 units SC q12h. The medication vial reads heparin sodium (Liquaemin), 1000 units per mL. The nurse prepares how many mL to administer one dose?
    1 1.5 mL
    2 0.7 mL

3 1.3 mL
4 1.0 mL

22. The physician orders trimethobenzamide hydrochloride (Tigan), 250 mg IM PRN. The medication label reads trimethobenzamide hydrochloride (Tigan) 200 mg per 2 mL. The nurse plans to prepare how much medication to administer the dose?
    1 0.4 mL
    2 1.0 mL
    3 1.25 mL
    4 2.5 mL

23. The physician orders meperidine hydrochloride (Demerol), 35 mg IM stat. The medication label states meperidine hydrochloride (Demerol), 50 mg per mL. The nurse plans to prepare how much medication to administer the dose?
    1 0.5 mL
    2 0.6 mL
    3 0.7 mL
    4 1.0 mL

24. The physician orders prochlorperazine (Compazine), 20 mg q4h IM PRN. The medication label states prochlorperazine (Compazine), 10 mg per mL. The nurse prepares how much medication to administer the dose?
    1 0.5 mL
    2 2.0 mL
    3 2.5 mL
    4 2.9 mL

25. The physician orders potassium chloride elixir (KCl) 20 mEq PO BID. The medication label states potassium chloride (KCl), 30 mEq per 15 mL. The nurse prepares to administer the morning dose. How many milliliters will the nurse administer to the client?
    1 10 mL
    2 15 mL
    3 32 mL
    4 40 mL

26. The physician orders atropine sulfate, 0.4 mg IM stat. The medication label states atropine sulfate, 0.3 mg per 0.5 mL. The nurse prepares how much medication to administer the dose?
    1 0.1 mL
    2 0.4 mL
    3 0.5 mL
    4 0.7 mL

27. The physician orders levodopa (Dopar), 1 g PO BID. The medication label states 500 mg tablets. The nurse prepares to administer how many tablets at the evening dose?
    1 2 tablets
    2 3 tablets
    3 4 tablets
    4 5 tablets

28. The physician orders zidovudine (AZT), 0.2 g PO q8h. The medication label states zidovudine (AZT), 100-mg tablets. The nurse prepares to administer how many tablets for one dose?
    1   0.5 tablet
    2   1 tablet
    3   1.5 tablets
    4   2 tablets

29. The physician orders atropine sulfate, gr 1/300 to be administered. The medication label states atropine sulfate, 0.5 mg per 0.5 mL. How many milliliters does the nurse prepare to administer to the client?

    1   0.1 mL
    2   0.2 mL
    3   1 mL
    4   2 mL

30. The physician's order states to administer aspirin (acetylsalicylic acid), 650 mg PO for a temperature above 38°C. The medication bottle states aspirin (acetylsalicylic acid), gr 5 per tablet. The nurse takes the client's temperature and notes that it is 101°F. The nurse plans to take which of the following actions?
    1   Not administer the aspirin at this time
    2   Check the client's temperature in 30 minutes
    3   Administer 2 aspirin tablets
    4   Administer 3 aspirin tablets

ANSWERS

1. **3**

RATIONALE: The prescribed 1000 mL is to be infused over 12 hours. Follow the formula and multiply 1000 mL by 15 (gtt factor). Then, divide the result by 720 minutes (12 hours x 60 minutes). The infusion is to run at 20.8 or 21 drops per minute.
FORMULA:

$$\frac{\text{Total volume in mL} \times \text{drop factor}}{\text{Time in minutes}} =$$

$$\text{Flow rate in drops per minute}$$

$$\frac{1000 \text{ mL} \times 15 \text{ drops}}{720 \text{ minutes}} = \frac{15,000}{720} =$$

$$20.8 \text{ or } 21 \text{ drops per minute}$$

TEST-TAKING STRATEGY: Follow the formula for calculating the infusion rate for an IV. Label the problem and the answer. Make sure that the answer makes sense. Be sure to change 12 hours to minutes. Review the formula for calculating infusion rates now if you had difficulty with this question.
LEVEL OF COGNITIVE ABILITY: Application
PHASE OF NURSING PROCESS: Planning
CLIENT NEEDS: Safe, Effective Care Environment
CONTENT AREA: Fundamental Skills
REFERENCE
Kee, J., & Hayes, E. (1997). *Pharmacology: A nursing process approach* (2nd ed.). Philadelphia: W. B. Saunders. p. 113.

2. **1**

RATIONALE: Follow the formula for dosage calculation.

$$\frac{\text{Desired}}{\text{Available}} \times \text{mL} = \text{mL per dose}$$

$$\frac{400,000 \text{ units}}{300,000 \text{ units}} \times 1 \text{ mL} = 1.3 \text{ mL per dose}$$

TEST-TAKING STRATEGY: Follow the formula for the calculation of the correct dose. Label each figure including the answer. Focus on the key information: 300,000 units per mL. Recheck your work and make sure that the answer makes sense. If you had difficulty with this question, take time now to review medication calculation problems.

LEVEL OF COGNITIVE ABILITY: Application
PHASE OF NURSING PROCESS: Planning
CLIENT NEEDS: Safe, Effective Care Environment
CONTENT AREA: Fundamental Skills
REFERENCE
Kee, J., & Hayes, E. (1997). *Pharmacology: A nursing process approach* (2nd ed.). Philadelphia: W. B. Saunders. p. 53.

3. **3**

RATIONALE: The prescribed 3000 mL is to be infused over 24 hours. Follow the formula and multiply 3000 mL by 10 (gtt factor). Then, divide the result by 1440 minutes (24 hours × 60 minutes). The infusion is to run at 20.8 or 21 drops per minute.
FORMULA:

$$\frac{\text{Total volume in mL} \times \text{drop factor}}{\text{Time in minutes}} =$$

$$\text{Flow rate in drops per minute}$$

$$\frac{3000 \text{ mL} \times 10 \text{ drops}}{1440 \text{ minutes}} = \frac{30,000}{1440} =$$

$$20.8 \text{ or } 21 \text{ drops per minute}$$

TEST-TAKING STRATEGY: Follow the formula for calculating the infusion rate for an IV. Label the problem and the answer. Make sure that the answer makes sense. Be sure to change 24 hours to minutes. Review the formula for calculating infusion rates now if you had difficulty with this question.
LEVEL OF COGNITIVE ABILITY: Application
PHASE OF NURSING PROCESS: Planning
CLIENT NEEDS: Safe, Effective Care Environment
CONTENT AREA: Fundamental Skills
REFERENCE
Kee, J., & Hayes, E. (1997). *Pharmacology: A nursing process approach* (2nd ed.). Philadelphia: W. B. Saunders. p. 113.

4. **2**

RATIONALE: Convert 0.2 g to mg. In the metric system, to convert larger to smaller, multiply by 1000 or move the decimal three places to the right. Therefore, 0.2 g = 200 mg.

FORMULA:

$$\frac{\text{Desired}}{\text{Available}} \times \text{Capsules} = \text{Capsules per dose}$$

$$\frac{200 \text{ mg}}{100 \text{ mg}} \times 1 \text{ capsule} = 2 \text{ capsules}$$

TEST-TAKING STRATEGY: In this medication calculation problem, it is necessary to first convert grams to milligrams. Follow the formula for conversion and read the question carefully. Recheck your work and make sure that the answer makes sense. If you had difficulty with this question, take time now to review conversions and medication calculation problems.
LEVEL OF COGNITIVE ABILITY: Application
PHASE OF NURSING PROCESS: Planning
CLIENT NEEDS: Safe, Effective Care Environment
CONTENT AREA: Fundamental Skills
REFERENCE
Kee, J., & Hayes, E. (1997). *Pharmacology: A nursing process approach* (2nd ed.). Philadelphia: W. B. Saunders. pp. 53–54.

5. 4

RATIONALE: The prescribed 1000 mL is to be infused over 8 hours. Follow the formula and multiply 1000 mL by 15 (gtt factor). Then divide the result by 480 minutes (8 hours × 60 minutes). The infusion is to run at 31.2 or 31 drops per minute.
FORMULA:

$$\frac{\text{Total volume in mL} \times \text{drop factor}}{\text{Time in minutes}} =$$

$$\text{Flow rate in drops per minute}$$

$$\frac{1000 \text{ mL} \times 15 \text{ drops}}{480 \text{ minutes}} = \frac{15,000}{480} =$$

$$31.2 \text{ or } 31 \text{ drops per minute}$$

TEST-TAKING STRATEGY: Follow the formula for calculating the infusion rate for an IV. Label the problem and the answer. Make sure that the answer makes sense. Be sure to change 8 hours to minutes. Review the formula for calculating infusion rates now if you had difficulty with this question.
LEVEL OF COGNITIVE ABILITY: Application
PHASE OF NURSING PROCESS: Planning
CLIENT NEEDS: Safe, Effective Care Environment
CONTENT AREA: Fundamental Skills
REFERENCE
Kee, J., & Hayes, E. (1997). *Pharmacology: A nursing process approach* (2nd ed.). Philadelphia: W. B. Saunders. p. 113.

6. 3

RATIONALE: The prescribed 2000 mL is to be infused over 24 hours. Follow the formula and multiply 2000 mL by 15 (gtt factor). Then divide the result by 1440 minutes (24 hours x 60 minutes). The infusion is to run at 20.8 or 21 drops per minute.
FORMULA:

$$\frac{\text{Total volume in mL} \times \text{drop factor}}{\text{Time in minutes}} =$$

$$\text{Flow rate in drops per minute}$$

$$\frac{2000 \text{ mL} \times 15 \text{ drops}}{1440 \text{ minutes}} = \frac{30,000}{1440} =$$

$$20.8 \text{ or } 21 \text{ drops per minute}$$

TEST-TAKING STRATEGY: Follow the formula for calculating the infusion rate for an IV. Label the problem and the answer. Make sure that the answer makes sense. Be sure to change 24 hours to minutes. Review the formula for calculating infusion rates now if you had difficulty with this question.
LEVEL OF COGNITIVE ABILITY: Application
PHASE OF NURSING PROCESS: Planning
CLIENT NEEDS: Safe, Effective Care Environment
CONTENT AREA: Fundamental Skills
REFERENCE
Kee, J., & Hayes, E. (1997). *Pharmacology: A nursing process approach* (2nd ed.). Philadelphia: W. B. Saunders. p. 113.

7. 1

RATIONALE: Convert 100 μg to mg. In the metric system, to convert smaller to larger, divide by 1000 or move the decimal three places to the left. Therefore, 100 μg = 0.1 mg.
FORMULA:

$$\frac{\text{Desired}}{\text{Available}} \times \text{mL} = \text{mL per dose}$$

$$\frac{0.1 \text{ mg}}{0.5 \text{ mg}} \times 1 \text{ mL} = \frac{0.1}{0.5} = 0.2 \text{ mL}$$

TEST-TAKING STRATEGY: In this medication calculation problem, it is necessary to first convert μg to mg. Follow the formula for conversion and read the question carefully. Focus on the key information, 0.5 mg per mL. Recheck your work and make sure that the answer makes sense. If you had difficulty with this question, take time now to review medication calculation problems.
LEVEL OF COGNITIVE ABILITY: Application
PHASE OF NURSING PROCESS: Implementation
CLIENT NEEDS: Safe, Effective Care Environment
CONTENT AREA: Fundamental Skills
REFERENCE
Kee, J., & Hayes, E. (1997). *Pharmacology: A nursing process approach* (2nd ed.). Philadelphia: W. B. Saunders. pp. 53–54.

8. 4

RATIONALE: To determine how many mL per hour are to be administered, simply divide the total prescribed amount of IV solution by the prescribed time period for infusion.
FORMULA:

$$\frac{\text{Total volume in mL}}{\text{Number of hours}} = \text{amount of mL per hour}$$

$$\frac{3000 \text{ mL}}{24 \text{ hours}} = 125 \text{ mL per hour}$$

TEST-TAKING STRATEGY: Focus on the issue of the question, mL per hour. Following the formula and simply dividing will direct you to the correct option. If you had difficulty with this question, take time now to review calculation of IV infusions.

LEVEL OF COGNITIVE ABILITY: Application
PHASE OF NURSING PROCESS: Planning
CLIENT NEEDS: Safe, Effective Care Environment
CONTENT AREA: Fundamental Skills
REFERENCE
Leahy, J., & Kizilay, P. (1998). *Foundations of nursing practice: A nursing process approach*. Philadelphia: W. B. Saunders. p. 813.

9. **2**

RATIONALE: Convert 150 μg to mg. In the metric system, to convert smaller to larger divide by 1000 or move the decimal three places to the left. Therefore, 150 μg = 0.15 mg.
FORMULA:

$$\frac{\text{Desired}}{\text{Available}} \times \text{tablet(s)} = \text{tablet(s) per dose}$$

$$\frac{0.15 \text{ mg}}{0.1 \text{ mg}} \times 1 \text{ tablet} = 1.5 \text{ tablets}$$

TEST-TAKING STRATEGY: In this medication calculation problem, it is necessary to first convert μg to mg. Follow the formula for conversion and read the question carefully. Recheck your work and make sure that the answer makes sense. If you had difficulty with this question, take time now to review conversions and medication calculation problems.
LEVEL OF COGNITIVE ABILITY: Application
PHASE OF NURSING PROCESS: Planning
CLIENT NEEDS: Safe, Effective Care Environment
CONTENT AREA: Fundamental Skills
REFERENCE
Kee, J., & Hayes, E. (1997). *Pharmacology: A nursing process approach* (2nd ed.). Philadelphia: W. B. Saunders. pp. 53–54.

10. **1**

RATIONALE: To determine how many hours it will take for 1 L to infuse, first recall that 1 liter is equal to 1000 mL. Next, divide the 1000 mL by the amount being delivered in 1 hour.
FORMULA:

$$\frac{\text{Total volume in mL}}{\text{mL per hour}} = \text{Infusion time in hours}$$

$$\frac{1000 \text{ mL}}{125 \text{ mL}} = 8 \text{ hours}$$

TEST-TAKING STRATEGY: Focus on the issue of the question, how many hours it takes for 1 liter to infuse. Following the formula and simply dividing will direct you to the correct option. If you had difficulty with this question, take time now to review calculations related to IV infusions.
LEVEL OF COGNITIVE ABILITY: Application
PHASE OF NURSING PROCESS: Implementation
CLIENT NEEDS: Safe, Effective Care Environment
CONTENT AREA: Fundamental Skills
REFERENCE
Leahy, J., & Kizilay, P. (1998). *Foundations of nursing practice: A nursing process approach*. Philadelphia: W. B. Saunders. p. 813.

11. **2**

RATIONALE: The prescribed 500 mL is to be infused over 5 hours. Follow the formula and multiply 500 mL by 10 (gtt factor). Then, divide the result by 300 minutes (5 hours × 60 minutes). The infusion is to run at 16.6 or 17 drops per minute.
FORMULA:

$$\frac{\text{Total volume in mL} \times \text{drop factor}}{\text{Time in minutes}} =$$

$$\text{Flow rate in drops per minute}$$

$$\frac{500 \text{ mL} \times 10 \text{ gtt}}{300 \text{ minutes}} = \frac{5000}{300} =$$

$$16.6 \text{ or } 17 \text{ drops per minute}$$

TEST-TAKING STRATEGY: Follow the formula for calculating the infusion rate for an IV. Label the problem and the answer. Make sure that the answer makes sense. Be sure to change 5 hours to minutes. Review the formula for calculating infusion rates now if you had difficulty with this question.
LEVEL OF COGNITIVE ABILITY: Application
PHASE OF NURSING PROCESS: Planning
CLIENT NEEDS: Safe, Effective Care Environment
CONTENT AREA: Fundamental Skills
REFERENCE
Kee, J., & Hayes, E. (1997). *Pharmacology: A nursing process approach* (2nd ed.). Philadelphia: W. B. Saunders. p. 113.

12. **3**

RATIONALE: The prescribed 250 mL is to be infused over 4 hours. Follow the formula and multiply 250 mL by 10 (gtt factor). Then, divide the result by 240 minutes (4 hours × 60 minutes). The infusion is to run at 10.4 or 10 drops per minute.
FORMULA:

$$\frac{\text{Total volume in mL} \times \text{drop factor}}{\text{Time in minutes}} =$$

$$\text{Flow rate in drops per minute}$$

$$\frac{250 \text{ mL} \times 10 \text{ drops}}{240 \text{ minutes}} = \frac{2500}{240} =$$

$$10.4 \text{ or } 10 \text{ drops per minute}$$

TEST-TAKING STRATEGY: Follow the formula for calculating the infusion rate for an IV. Label the problem and the answer. Make sure that the answer makes sense. Be sure to change 4 hours to minutes. Review the formula for calculating infusion rates now if you had difficulty with this question.
LEVEL OF COGNITIVE ABILITY: Application
PHASE OF NURSING PROCESS: Implementation
CLIENT NEEDS: Safe, Effective Care Environment
CONTENT AREA: Fundamental Skills
REFERENCE
Kee, J., & Hayes, E. (1997). *Pharmacology: A nursing process approach* (2nd ed.). Philadelphia: W. B. Saunders. p. 113.

13. **4**

RATIONALE: The prescribed 3000 mL is to be infused over 24 hours. Follow the formula and multiply 3000 mL by 15 (gtt factor). Then, divide the result by 1440 minutes (24 hours × 60 minutes). The infusion is to run at 31.2 or 31 drops per minute.
FORMULA:

$$\frac{\text{Total volume in mL} \times \text{drop factor}}{\text{Time in minutes}} =$$

$$\text{Flow rate in drops per minute}$$

$$\frac{3000 \text{ mL} \times 15 \text{ drops}}{1440 \text{ minutes}} = \frac{45,000}{1440} =$$

31.2 or 31 drops per minute

TEST-TAKING STRATEGY: Follow the formula for calculating the infusion rate for an IV. Label the problem and the answer. Make sure that the answer makes sense. Be sure to change 24 hours to minutes. Review the formula for calculating infusion rates now if you had difficulty with this question.
LEVEL OF COGNITIVE ABILITY: Application
PHASE OF NURSING PROCESS: Planning
CLIENT NEEDS: Safe, Effective Care Environment
CONTENT AREA: Fundamental Skills
REFERENCE
Kee, J., & Hayes, E. (1997). *Pharmacology: A nursing process approach* (2nd ed.). Philadelphia: W. B. Saunders. p. 113.

14. **3**

RATIONALE: Convert 0.3 g to mg. In the metric system, to convert larger to smaller, multiply by 1000 or move the decimal three places to the right. Therefore, 0.3 g = 300 mg.
FORMULA:

$$\frac{\text{Desired}}{\text{Available}} \times \text{Tablet} = \text{Number of tablets per dose}$$

$$\frac{300 \text{ mg}}{150 \text{ mg}} \times 1 \text{ tablet} = 2 \text{ tablets}$$

TEST-TAKING STRATEGY: In this medication calculation problem, it is necessary to first convert grams to milligrams. Follow the formula for conversion and read the question carefully. Recheck your work and make sure that the answer makes sense. If you had difficulty with this question, take time now to review conversions and medication calculation problems.
LEVEL OF COGNITIVE ABILITY: Application
PHASE OF NURSING PROCESS: Planning
CLIENT NEEDS: Safe, Effective Care Environment
CONTENT AREA: Fundamental Skills
REFERENCE
Kee, J., & Hayes, E. (1997). *Pharmacology: A nursing process approach* (2nd ed.). Philadelphia: W. B. Saunders. pp. 53–54.

15. **3**

RATIONALE: Convert 0.5 g to mg. In the metric system, to convert larger to smaller, multiply by 1000 or move the decimal three places to the right. Therefore, 0.5 g = 500 mg.
FORMULA:

$$\frac{\text{Desired}}{\text{Available}} \times \text{Tablet} = \text{Number of tablets per dose}$$

$$\frac{500 \text{ mg}}{250 \text{ mg}} \times 1 \text{ tablet} = 2 \text{ tablets}$$

TEST-TAKING STRATEGY: In this medication calculation problem, it is necessary to first convert grams to milligrams. Follow the formula for conversion and read the question carefully. Recheck your work and make sure that the answer makes sense. If you had difficulty with this question, take time now to review medication calculation problems.

LEVEL OF COGNITIVE ABILITY: Application
PHASE OF NURSING PROCESS: Planning
CLIENT NEEDS: Safe, Effective Care Environment
CONTENT AREA: Fundamental Skills
REFERENCE
Kee, J., & Hayes, E. (1997). *Pharmacology: A nursing process approach* (2nd ed.). Philadelphia: W. B. Saunders. pp. 53–54.

16. **1**

RATIONALE: Convert 125 μg to mg. In the metric system, to convert smaller to larger, divide by 1000 or move the decimal 3 places to the left. Therefore, 125 μg = 0.125 mg. One tablet is administered.
TEST-TAKING STRATEGY: In this medication calculation problem, it is necessary to first convert μg to mg. Follow the formula for conversion and read the question carefully. Recheck your work and make sure that the answer makes sense. If you had difficulty with this question, take time now to review conversions and medication calculation problems.
LEVEL OF COGNITIVE ABILITY: Application
PHASE OF NURSING PROCESS: Planning
CLIENT NEEDS: Safe, Effective Care Environment
CONTENT AREA: Fundamental Skills
REFERENCE
Kee, J., & Hayes, E. (1997). *Pharmacology: A nursing process approach* (2nd ed.). Philadelphia: W. B. Saunders. pp. 53–54.

17. **1**

RATIONALE: Convert 0.025 g to mg. In the metric system, to convert larger to smaller, multiply by 1000 or move the decimal three places to the right. Therefore, 0.025 g = 25.0 mg.
FORMULA:

$$\frac{\text{Desired}}{\text{Available}} \times \text{Tablet} = \text{Number of tablets per dose}$$

$$\frac{25.0 \text{ mg}}{50 \text{ mg}} \times 1 \text{ tablet} = 0.5 \text{ tablets}$$

TEST-TAKING STRATEGY: In this medication calculation problem, it is necessary to first convert grams to milligrams. Follow the formula for conversion and read the question carefully. Recheck your work and make sure that the answer makes sense. If you had difficulty with this question, take time now to review conversions and medication calculation problems.
LEVEL OF COGNITIVE ABILITY: Application
PHASE OF NURSING PROCESS: Planning
CLIENT NEEDS: Safe, Effective Care Environment
CONTENT AREA: Fundamental Skills
REFERENCE
Kee, J., & Hayes, E. (1997). *Pharmacology: A nursing process approach* (2nd ed.). Philadelphia: W. B. Saunders. pp. 53–54.

18. **3**

RATIONALE: Follow the formula for dosage calculation.
FORMULA:

$$\frac{\text{Desired}}{\text{Available}} \times \text{mL} = \text{mL per dose}$$

$$\frac{3 \text{ mg}}{4 \text{ mg}} \times 1 \text{ mL} = 0.75 \text{ or } 0.8 \text{ mL}$$

TEST-TAKING STRATEGY: Follow the formula for the calculation of the correct dose. Label each figure including the answer. Focus on the key information, 4 mg per 1 mL. Recheck your work and make sure that the answer makes sense. If you had difficulty with this question, take time now to review medication calculation problems.
LEVEL OF COGNITIVE ABILITY: Application
PHASE OF NURSING PROCESS: Planning
CLIENT NEEDS: Safe, Effective Care Environment
CONTENT AREA: Fundamental Skills
REFERENCE

Kee, J., & Hayes, E. (1997). *Pharmacology: A nursing process approach* (2nd ed.). Philadelphia: W. B. Saunders. p. 53.

19. **4**

RATIONALE: Follow the formula for dosage calculation.
FORMULA:

$$\frac{\text{Desired}}{\text{Available}} \times \text{Tablet} = \text{Number of tablets per dose}$$

$$\frac{0.25 \text{ mg}}{0.125 \text{ mg}} \times 1 \text{ tablet} = 2 \text{ tablets}$$

TEST-TAKING STRATEGY: Follow the formula for the calculation of the correct dose. Label each figure including the answer. Focus on the key information, 0.125 mg per tablet. Recheck your work and make sure that the answer makes sense. If you had difficulty with this question, take time now to review medication calculation problems.
LEVEL OF COGNITIVE ABILITY: Application
PHASE OF NURSING PROCESS: Planning
CLIENT NEEDS: Safe, Effective Care Environment
CONTENT AREA: Fundamental Skills
REFERENCE

Kee, J., & Hayes, E. (1997). *Pharmacology: A nursing process approach* (2nd ed.). Philadelphia: W. B. Saunders. p. 53.

20. **3**

RATIONALE: Follow the formula for dosage calculation.
FORMULA:

$$\frac{\text{Desired}}{\text{Available}} \times \text{mL} = \text{mL per dose}$$

$$\frac{80 \text{ mg}}{100 \text{ mg}} \times 1 \text{ mL} = 0.8 \text{ mL}$$

TEST-TAKING STRATEGY: Follow the formula for the calculation of the correct dose. Label each figure including the answer. Focus on the key information, 100 mg per mL. Recheck your work and make sure that the answer makes sense. If you had difficulty with this question, take time now to review medication calculation problems.
LEVEL OF COGNITIVE ABILITY: Application
PHASE OF NURSING PROCESS: Planning
CLIENT NEEDS: Safe, Effective Care Environment
CONTENT AREA: Fundamental Skills
REFERENCE

Kee, J., & Hayes, E. (1997). *Pharmacology: A nursing process approach* (2nd ed.). Philadelphia: W. B. Saunders. p. 53.

21. **2**

RATIONALE: Follow the formula for dosage calculation.

FORMULA:

$$\frac{\text{Desired}}{\text{Available}} \times \text{mL} = \text{mL per dose}$$

$$\frac{650 \text{ units}}{1000 \text{ units}} \times 1 \text{ mL} = 0.65 \text{ or } 0.7 \text{ mL}$$

TEST-TAKING STRATEGY: Follow the formula for the calculation of the correct dose. Label each figure including the answer. Focus on the key information, 1000 units per mL. Recheck your work and make sure that the answer makes sense. If you had difficulty with this question, take time now to review medication calculation problems.
LEVEL OF COGNITIVE ABILITY: Application
PHASE OF NURSING PROCESS: Planning
CLIENT NEEDS: Safe, Effective Care Environment
CONTENT AREA: Fundamental Skills
REFERENCE

Kee, J., & Hayes, E. (1997). *Pharmacology: A nursing process approach* (2nd ed.). Philadelphia: W. B. Saunders. p. 53.

22. **4**

RATIONALE: Follow the formula for dosage calculation.
FORMULA:

$$\frac{\text{Desired}}{\text{Available}} \times \text{mL} = \text{mL per dose}$$

$$\frac{250 \text{ mg}}{200 \text{ mg}} \times 2 \text{ mL} = 2.5 \text{ mL}$$

TEST-TAKING STRATEGY: Follow the formula for the calculation of the correct dose. Label each figure including the answer. Focus on the key information, 200 mg per 2 mL. Recheck your work and make sure that the answer makes sense. If you had difficulty with this question, take time now to review medication calculation problems.
LEVEL OF COGNITIVE ABILITY: Application
PHASE OF NURSING PROCESS: Planning
CLIENT NEEDS: Safe, Effective Care Environment
CONTENT AREA: Fundamental Skills
REFERENCE

Kee, J., & Hayes, E. (1997). *Pharmacology: A nursing process approach* (2nd ed.). Philadelphia: W. B. Saunders. p. 53.

23. **3**

RATIONALE: Follow the formula for dosage calculation.
FORMULA:

$$\frac{\text{Desired}}{\text{Available}} \times \text{mL} = \text{mL per dose}$$

$$\frac{35 \text{ mg}}{50 \text{ mg}} \times 1 \text{ mL} = 0.7 \text{ mL}$$

TEST-TAKING STRATEGY: Follow the formula for the calculation of the correct dose. Label each figure including the answer. Focus on the key information, 50 mg per mL. Recheck your work and make sure that the answer makes sense. If you had difficulty with this question, take time now to review medication calculation problems.
LEVEL OF COGNITIVE ABILITY: Application
PHASE OF NURSING PROCESS: Planning
CLIENT NEEDS: Safe, Effective Care Environment
CONTENT AREA: Fundamental Skills
REFERENCE

Kee, J., & Hayes, E. (1997). *Pharmacology: A nursing process approach* (2nd ed.). Philadelphia: W. B. Saunders. p. 53.

24. **2**

RATIONALE: Follow the formula for dosage calculation.
FORMULA:

$$\frac{\text{Desired}}{\text{Available}} \times \text{mL} = \text{mL per dose}$$

$$\frac{20 \text{ mg}}{10 \text{ mg}} \times 1 \text{ mL} = 2.0 \text{ mL}$$

TEST-TAKING STRATEGY: Follow the formula for the calculation of the correct dose. Label each figure including the answer. Focus on the key information, 10 mg per mL. Recheck your work and make sure that the answer makes sense. If you had difficulty with this question, take time now to review medication calculation problems.
LEVEL OF COGNITIVE ABILITY: Application
PHASE OF NURSING PROCESS: Planning
CLIENT NEEDS: Safe, Effective Care Environment
CONTENT AREA: Fundamental Skills
REFERENCE
Kee, J., & Hayes, E. (1997). *Pharmacology: A nursing process approach* (2nd ed.). Philadelphia: W. B. Saunders. p. 53.

25. **1**

RATIONALE: Follow the formula for dosage calculation.
FORMULA:

$$\frac{\text{Desired}}{\text{Available}} \times \text{mL} = \text{mL per dose}$$

$$\frac{20 \text{ mEq}}{30 \text{ mEq}} \times 15 \text{ mL} = 10 \text{ mL}$$

TEST-TAKING STRATEGY: Follow the formula for the calculation of the correct dose. Label each figure including the answer. Focus on the key information, 30 mEq per 15 mL. Recheck your work and make sure that the answer makes sense. If you had difficulty with this question, take time now to review medication calculation problems.
LEVEL OF COGNITIVE ABILITY: Application
PHASE OF NURSING PROCESS: Planning
CLIENT NEEDS: Safe, Effective Care Environment
CONTENT AREA: Fundamental Skills
REFERENCE
Kee, J., & Hayes, E. (1997). *Pharmacology: A nursing process approach* (2nd ed.). Philadelphia: W. B. Saunders. p. 53.

26. **4**

RATIONALE: Follow the formula for dosage calculation.
FORMULA:

$$\frac{\text{Desired}}{\text{Available}} \times \text{mL} = \text{mL per dose}$$

$$\frac{0.4 \text{ mg}}{0.3 \text{ mg}} \times 0.5 \text{ mL} = 0.66 \text{ or } 0.7 \text{ mL}$$

TEST-TAKING STRATEGY: Follow the formula for the calculation of the correct dose. Label each figure including the answer. Focus on the key information, 0.3 mg per 0.5 mL. Recheck your work and make sure that the answer makes sense. If you had difficulty with this question, take time now to review medication calculation problems.

LEVEL OF COGNITIVE ABILITY: Application
PHASE OF NURSING PROCESS: Planning
CLIENT NEEDS: Safe, Effective Care Environment
CONTENT AREA: Fundamental Skills
REFERENCE
Kee, J., & Hayes, E. (1997). *Pharmacology: A nursing process approach* (2nd ed.). Philadelphia: W. B. Saunders. p. 53.

27. **1**

RATIONALE: Convert 1 g to mg. In the metric system, to convert larger to smaller, multiply by 1000 or move the decimal three places to the right. Therefore, 1 g = 1000 mg.
FORMULA:

$$\frac{\text{Desired}}{\text{Available}} \times \text{Tablet} = \text{Number of tablets per dose}$$

$$\frac{1000 \text{ mg}}{500 \text{ mg}} \times 1 \text{ tablet} = 2 \text{ tablets}$$

TEST-TAKING STRATEGY: In this medication calculation problem, it is necessary to first convert grams to milligrams. Follow the formula for conversion and read the question carefully. Recheck your work and make sure that the answer makes sense. If you had difficulty with this question, take time now to review conversions and medication calculation problems.
LEVEL OF COGNITIVE ABILITY: Application
PHASE OF NURSING PROCESS: Planning
CLIENT NEEDS: Safe, Effective Care Environment
CONTENT AREA: Fundamental Skills
REFERENCE
Kee, J., & Hayes, E. (1997). *Pharmacology: A nursing process approach* (2nd ed.). Philadelphia: W. B. Saunders. pp. 53–54.

28. **4**

RATIONALE: Convert 0.2 g to mg. In the metric system, to convert larger to smaller, multiply by 1000 or move the decimal three places to the right. Therefore, 0.2 g = 200 mg.
FORMULA:

$$\frac{\text{Desired}}{\text{Available}} \times \text{Tablet} = \text{Number of tablets per dose}$$

$$\frac{200 \text{ mg}}{100 \text{ mg}} \times 1 \text{ tablet} = 2 \text{ tablets}$$

TEST-TAKING STRATEGY: In this medication calculation problem, it is necessary to first convert grams to milligrams. Follow the formula for conversion and read the question carefully. Recheck your work and make sure that the answer makes sense. If you had difficulty with this question, take time now to review conversions and medication calculation problems.
LEVEL OF COGNITIVE ABILITY: Application
PHASE OF NURSING PROCESS: Planning
CLIENT NEEDS: Safe, Effective Care Environment
CONTENT AREA: Fundamental Skills
REFERENCE
Kee, J., & Hayes, E. (1997). *Pharmacology: A nursing process approach* (2nd ed.). Philadelphia: W. B. Saunders. pp. 53–54.

29. **2**

RATIONALE: Convert gr 1/300 to mg using ratio and proportion. Then use the dosage calculation formula.

60 mg : gr 1 :: X mg : gr 1/300
1 X = 1/300 × 60/1
X = 60/300 = 1/5 mg, or 0.2 mg

FORMULA:

$$\frac{\text{Desired}}{\text{Available}} \times \text{mL} = \text{mL per dose}$$

$$\frac{0.2 \text{ mg}}{0.5 \text{ mg}} \times 0.5 \text{ mL} = \frac{0.1 \text{ mg}}{0.5 \text{ mg}} = 0.2 \text{ mL}$$

TEST-TAKING STRATEGY: In this medication calculation problem, it is necessary to first convert grains to milligrams. Follow the formula for conversion and read the question carefully. Focus on the issue, 0.5 mg per 0.5 mL. Recheck your work and make sure that the answer makes sense. If you had difficulty with this question, take time now to review medication calculation problems.
LEVEL OF COGNITIVE ABILITY: Application
PHASE OF NURSING PROCESS: Planning
CLIENT NEEDS: Safe, Effective Care Environment
CONTENT AREA: Fundamental Skills
REFERENCE
Kee, J., & Hayes, E. (1997). *Pharmacology: A nursing process approach* (2nd ed.). Philadelphia: W. B. Saunders. pp. 53–54.

30. **3**

RATIONALE: Calculation of this problem requires more than one step. Convert Fahrenheit to Celsius, convert mg to gr, and then calculate the dose to be administered.

Step 1: Convert Fahrenheit to Celsius
To convert Fahrenheit to Celsius, subtract 32 and divide the result by 1.8.
C = (101 − 32) divided by 1.8; C = (69) divided by 1.8; C = 38.3

Step 2: Convert mg to gr
gr 1 : 60 mg :: X gr : 650 mg
60 X = 650
X = gr 10.8

Step 3: Dosage calculation

$$\frac{\text{Desired}}{\text{Available}} \times \text{Tablet} = \text{Number of tablets per dose}$$

$$\frac{\text{gr } 10.8}{\text{gr } 5} \times 1 \text{ tablet} = 2.16 \text{ or } 2 \text{ tablets}$$

TEST-TAKING STRATEGY: Focus on what the question is asking you to determine. In this medication calculation problem, it is necessary to first convert Fahrenheit to Celsius, then you need to convert mg to gr. Follow the formula for conversion and read the question carefully. Recheck your work and make sure that the answer makes sense. If you had difficulty with this question, take time now to review conversions and medication calculation problems.
LEVEL OF COGNITIVE ABILITY: Application
PHASE OF NURSING PROCESS: Planning
CLIENT NEEDS: Safe, Effective Care Environment
CONTENT AREA: Fundamental Skills
REFERENCE
Kee, J., & Hayes, E. (1997). *Pharmacology: A nursing process approach* (2nd ed.). Philadelphia: W. B. Saunders. pp. 53–54.

REFERENCES

Hodgson, B., & Kizior, R. (1999). *Saunders nursing drug handbook 1999*. Philadelphia: W. B. Saunders.
Kee, J., & Hayes, E. (1997). *Pharmacology: A nursing process approach* (2nd ed.). Philadelphia: W. B. Saunders.
Leahy, J., & Kizilay, P. (1998). *Foundations of nursing practice: A nursing process approach*. Philadelphia: W. B. Saunders.
National Council of State Boards of Nursing (1998). *National Council detailed test plan for the NCLEX-PN examination*. Chicago: Author.

CHAPTER 15

Basic Life Support

....

PYRAMID TERMS

Automated External Defibrillator (AED)— Converts ventricular fibrillation into a perfusing rhythm and allows for early defibrillation by first responders.

Basic Life Support (BLS)—Providing oxygen to the brain, heart, and other vital organs until help arrives.

Cardiopulmonary Resuscitation (CPR)—An interchangeable term for Basic Life Support.

Head Tilt–Chin Lift—Preferred method to open a victim's airway.

Heimlich Maneuver—Method of rescue to remove foreign objects from a choking victim.

Jaw Thrust Maneuver—Method used to open a victim's airway if a neck injury is suspected.

PYRAMID TO SUCCESS

The Pyramid to Success focuses on the emergency measures related to performing **basic life support.** Focus on the points related to the breaths and compression ratio with one-man and two-man adult **CPR** and **CPR** in the infant and child. Pyramid points focus on airway management in **CPR** and in performing the **Heimlich maneuver.** Focus on the correct hand placements for cardiac compressions and the differences between the adult, child, and infant. Remember prior to initiating **CPR,** determining unresponsiveness is the initial action. Remember the ABCs: airway, breathing, and circulation, when performing **CPR.**

NURSING PROCESS

DATA COLLECTION

Responsiveness or consciousness
Airway
Breathing
Circulation

PLANNING
Client maintains a patent airway. Client demonstrates effective breathing pattern. Client maintains adequate gas exchange.

IMPLEMENTATION
Assess airway, breathing, and circulation. Maintain open airway. Provide ventilations to victim as necessary. Perform chest compressions as necessary. Perform Heimlich maneuver if necessary. Evaluate response to interventions continually.

EVALUATION
Airway is patent. Breathing patterns are normal. Adequate circulation is maintained.

CLIENT NEEDS

SAFE, EFFECTIVE CARE ENVIRONMENT

Advanced directives regarding client's documented requests
Advocacy regarding client's wishes
Client rights
Ethical and legal responsibilities
Standard (universal) precautions

HEALTH PROMOTION AND MAINTENANCE

Health promotion programs
Teaching significant other to perform basic life support (BLS)

PSYCHOSOCIAL INTEGRITY

Religious, spiritual, and cultural influences
Communication and emotional support to significant other

PHYSIOLOGICAL INTEGRITY

Alterations in cardiopulmonary system
Assisting in medical emergencies
Administration of medications
Documentation of response to BLS

> **BOX 15–1 The ABCs of Basic Life Support (BLS)**
>
> A—Airway
> B—Breathing
> C—Circulation
> Each step of the ABCs of BLS begins with assessment.

I. Basic Life Support (BLS) (Box 15–1)

A. Providing oxygen to the brain, heart, and other vital organs until help arrives

B. Also known as cardiopulmonary resuscitation **(CPR)**

II. Adult Basic Life Support

A. Description: An adult can be defined as an individual 8 years of age or older

B. Airway
1. Remember that assessment is the first step of **BLS**
2. The first thing to do in assessing a victim of sudden illness or accident is assess unconsciousness or unresponsiveness
3. Assess the victim for 5 to 10 seconds
4. Gently shake the victim's shoulders and ask "Are you okay?" In shaking the victim, be alert to the potential for a head or neck injury
5. Call, "Help! Help!"
6. If the victim is unresponsive, activate the emergency medical system (EMS)
7. Place the victim in a supine position on a firm, flat surface and kneel near the shoulders of the victim
8. Open the airway
9. The **head tilt–chin lift** is the preferred method for opening the airway; if there is a neck injury, the **jaw thrust maneuver** is used to open the airway
10. Look for any foreign material, liquids, or solids in the victim's mouth; wipe out any foreign material with a hooked index or middle finger

C. Breathing
1. Assess breathing
2. Maintain an open airway and place your ear over the victim's nose and mouth
3. Look for the chest to rise and fall; listen for air moving in and out of the lungs and feel for the flow of air on the cheek
4. Breathing victim
   a. Place the victim on his or her side in the recovery position if no cervical trauma is suspected
   b. Roll the victim onto the side as a unit (without twisting) to help maintain an open airway
   c. If trauma or injury is suspected, the victim should not be moved

5. Nonbreathing victim
   a. Pinch the nostrils closed, give two full ventilations (breaths) of 1.5 to 2 seconds per breath
   b. In the adult, give 10 to 12 ventilations (vents) per minute or one every 5 to 6 seconds
   c. If unsuccessful (unable) at giving the breaths or ventilations, reposition the victim's head and try again
   d. Improper chin and head position is the most common cause of difficulty in ventilating the victim
   e. If still unsuccessful, check the victim's mouth for a foreign body or for loose dentures (remove dentures only if they interfere with mouth seal)
   f. Clear the airway and try to ventilate again
   g. Be alert to gastric distention when giving vents

D. Circulation
1. Assess circulation; always check for the absence of a pulse before beginning chest compressions on the victim
2. Maintain an open airway and palpate for a carotid pulse for 5 to 10 seconds
3. If there is a pulse, give 10 to 12 ventilations a minute, or one every 5 to 6 seconds
4. Recheck the pulse after 1 minute; if there is no pulse, start chest compressions on the victim

E. Chest compressions
1. Hand placement
   a. Correct placement of the hands for chest compressions is crucial
   b. Always recheck the landmarks for chest compressions; hand placement is on the lower half of the sternum
   c. With the hand closest to the victim's feet, locate the lower margin of the rib cage
   d. Move your fingertips along the margin to the notch where the ribs meet the sternum
   e. Place the middle finger on the notch and the index finger next to the middle finger
   f. Place the heel of the hand next to the index finger and place the other hand on top
2. Complications of chest compressions
   a. Laceration of internal organs such as the liver, spleen, or stomach
   b. Punctured lungs
   c. Fractured ribs or sternum

III. Adult One-Man BLS

A. The ratio is 15:2; that is, 15 chest compressions to 2 ventilations

B. The rate of compression is 80 to 100 a minute at a depth of 1.5 to 2 inches

C. Perform four complete cycles, then reassess the victim

D. Check the carotid pulse after the first four cycles

of **CPR** and every few minutes thereafter; if no pulse is felt, continue **CPR**

IV. Adult Two-Man BLS

A. One person is at the victim's side performing chest compressions; one person is at the victim's head, maintaining an open airway, monitoring the carotid pulse, and doing the rescue breathing

B. The adult ratio for two-man **BLS** is 5:1 or 5 compressions at a rate of 80 to 100 per minute, and 1 ventilation at 1.5 to 2 seconds per breath

C. When the second rescuer arrives at the scene, he or she must identify himself or herself and tell the first rescuer that he or she knows two-man **CPR**

D. The second rescuer activates EMS if this hasn't been done, and then returns to the scene to help

E. The second rescuer can perform one-man **CPR** if the first rescuer is fatigued; or, the first rescuer finishes 15 compressions, gives 2 ventilations, moves to the head, opens the airway, and checks the carotid pulse

F. If there is no pulse, that first rescuer announces, "No pulse, continue **CPR**"

G. The second rescuer locates the landmark for chest compressions

H. The two rescuers begin **CPR** at a ratio of 5 compressions to 1 ventilation

I. At the end of 1 minute, the ventilator checks for a pulse and checks for breathing; if none, the ventilator says, "No pulse, continue **CPR**"

J. When the compressor becomes tired, the compressor may call for a switch in position, stating, "Switch (change), 2, 3, 4, 5"

K. The ventilator gives a breath and moves to the chest and locates the correct hand placement or landmark for chest compressions

L. The compressor moves to the head and checks for a carotid pulse; if no pulse, the rescuer states, "No pulse, continue **CPR**"

V. Pediatric BLS

A. Description
1. A child can be defined as an individual between the ages of 1 and 8 years of age
2. An infant can be defined as an individual under 1 year old

B. Airway
1. Assess unresponsiveness
2. Gently shake the victim; be alert to the potential for a head or neck injury
3. Call out for help
4. Position the victim
5. Open the airway using the **head tilt–chin lift** or the **jaw thrust** if a neck injury is suspected
6. With infants, place the head in a sniffing or neutral position
7. With a child, tilt the head back slightly farther than for an infant

C. Breathing
1. Assess for breathing
2. Maintain an open airway and place your ear over the victim's nose and mouth
3. Look for the chest to rise and fall, listen for air moving in and out of the lungs, and feel for the flow of air on the cheek
4. Breathing victim: Keep the airway open
5. Nonbreathing victim
   a. Give two ventilations at 1 to 1.5 seconds per breath
   b. If unsuccessful, reposition the victim's head
   c. If still unsuccessful, check for a foreign body in the victim's mouth
   d. With an infant, provide ventilations by mouth to mouth and nose
   e. With a larger child, provide ventilations by mouth to mouth
   f. With an infant and child, give 20 ventilations per minute or 1 every 3 seconds
   g. Provide 1 minute of rescue breathing, then activate EMS

D. Circulation
1. Assess circulation
2. If the victim is older than 1 year, assess circulation via the carotid pulse
3. If the victim is younger than 1 year, assess circulation via the brachial pulse
4. The ratio is 5 compressions to 1 ventilation
5. Reassess the victim after 20 cycles (approximately 1 minute), and activate EMS if not already done
6. Continue to reassess every few minutes
7. Infant chest compressions
   a. The imaginary line between the nipples is located over the breast bone (sternum)
   b. The index finger of the hand farthest from the infant's head is placed just under the intermammary line where it intersects the sternum
   c. The area of compression is one fingerwidth below this intersection, at the location of the middle and ring fingers
   d. Using two to three fingers, the breast bone is compressed 0.5 to 1 inch at 100 times a minute
8. Chest compressions for a child
   a. The location for hand placement is the same as an adult
   b. Depress the chest 1 to 1.5 inches at 100 times a minute with the heel of one hand

VI. The Choking Victim and Heimlich Maneuver

A. Conscious adult
1. Ask the victim, "Are you choking?"
2. The victim won't be able to speak or cough if choking
3. If the victim's airway is partially obstructed,

BOX 15–2 Heimlich Maneuver

Stand behind the victim
 Place arms around the victim's waist
 Make a fist
 Place the thumb side of the fist just above the umbilicus (navel) and well below the xiphoid process
 Perform five quick in and up thrusts (between the umbilicus and xiphoid process)
 Use chest thrusts for the markedly obese or for the advanced pregnancy victim

---

a crowing sound will be heard; encourage the victim to cough

4. Relieve the obstruction by the **Heimlich maneuver** (Box 15–2)
5. Perform the **Heimlich maneuver** until the object is dislodged or the victim becomes unconscious

B. Unconscious adult
1. Assess consciousness by gently shaking the victim; place the victim in a supine position
2. Call for help; activate EMS
3. Open the airway
4. Assess breathing; attempt ventilation
5. Reposition the head if unsuccessful; reattempt ventilation
6. Relieve the obstruction by the **Heimlich maneuver** with five thrusts, then fingersweep the mouth
7. To perform the **Heimlich maneuver,** kneel astride the thighs, place the heel of one hand on top of the other between umbilicus and xiphoid process and give five thrusts in and up with the heel of the bottom hand
8. To open the airway, grasp the tongue and lower jaw between the thumb and fingers, lift the jaw and insert the index finger in a hooking motion to relieve the obstruction
9. Reattempt ventilation
10. Repeat the sequence of breaths, five abdominal thrusts, and fingersweep until successful
11. Be sure to assess the victim's pulse and respirations
12. Perform **CPR** if required

C. Choking child or infant
1. Choking is suspected in infants and children experiencing acute respiratory distress associated with coughing, gagging, or stridor (high-pitched noisy breathing)
2. Allow the victim to continue to cough if the cough is forceful
3. If the cough is ineffective or the victim develops increased respiratory difficulty accompanied by a high-pitched noise while inhaling, help is needed
4. Conscious child
   a. Assess for obstruction by asking the child, "Are you choking?"

b. Relieve the obstruction by the **Heimlich maneuver** until the obstruction is dislodged or the victim becomes unconscious
5. Unconscious child
   a. Assess unconsciousness
   b. Call for help; activate EMS
   c. Open the airway by the **head tilt–chin lift**
   d. Check for breathing; attempt ventilation
   e. If unsuccessful, reposition the head; reattempt ventilation
   f. Relieve the obstruction using the **Heimlich maneuver,** giving five thrusts and fingersweep the mouth only if the object is seen
   g. Reattempt ventilation; repeat the sequence
   h. Assess pulse and respirations
   i. Perform **CPR** if required
6. Conscious infant
   a. Assess for obstruction and note breathing problems
   b. Relieve the obstruction by five back blows and five chest thrusts in the infant
   c. Straddle the infant over your arm, place the infant's head lower than the trunk, and support the head firmly, holding the jaw
   d. Give five back blows with the heel of the hand between the shoulder blades
   e. Turn the infant; place the head lower than the trunk
   f. Give five chest thrusts at the same location as for chest compressions
   g. Check for the object and remove if seen
   h. Blind fingersweeps are avoided in the infant and in small children because the object may be pushed back farther into the airway, causing further obstruction
   i. Continue until the object is removed or the victim becomes unconscious
7. Unconscious infant
   a. Assess consciousness by gentle taps
   b. Call for help; activate EMS
   c. Open the airway by the **head tilt–chin lift** (sniffing or neutral position)
   d. Check for breathing; attempt ventilation
   e. Reposition the head if unsuccessful; reattempt ventilation
   f. Relieve the obstruction by five back blows and five chest thrusts
   g. Fingersweep the mouth only if the object is seen

BOX 15–3 Pyramid Points

Do not interrupt CPR for more than 5 seconds!
Stop CPR *only* IF:
 Pulse and respiration return
 Emergency medical system arrives
 The rescuer becomes exhausted
 A physician declares the victim deceased

h. Reattempt ventilation; repeat the sequence
i. Perform **CPR** if required (Box 15–3)

VII. Automated External Defibrillator (AED)

A. Description
1. Used to convert ventricular fibrillation into a perfusing rhythm
2. Differentiates nonventricular fibrillation rhythms and allows for early defibrillation by first responders
B. Implementation
1. Attach **AED** leads to the victim
2. Turn on the **AED** and push button to activate the analyzer
3. Follow instructions given for the **AED,** usually to "assess," "stand back," "shock," and "reassess"
4. Evaluate for return of the pulse, and if pulseless, repeat defibrillation as directed up to three times, then perform **CPR**

PRACTICE QUESTIONS

1. The nurse is providing instructions to a group of high school students regarding BLS procedures. The nurse tells the students the complications associated with performing chest compressions includes which of the following?
   1 Dislocation of the shoulder
   2 Laceration of the liver
   3 Perforation of the bladder
   4 Fracture of the pelvis

2. The nurse on the day shift walks into a client's room and finds the client unresponsive. The client is not breathing and does not have a pulse. The nurse immediately calls out for help. The next nursing action is which of the following?
   1 Ventilate with a mouth-to-mask device
   2 Start chest compressions
   3 Give the client oxygen
   4 Open the airway

3. The nurse is performing CPR on an adult client. The correct hand placement for chest compressions is which of the following?
   1 Placing the hands on the lower third of the sternum
   2 Placing the hands on the upper half of the sternum
   3 Placing the hands on the upper third of the sternum
   4 Placing the hands on the lower half of the sternum

4. A nurse witnesses a neighbor's husband sustain a fall from the roof of the house. The nurse arrives at the victim and determines the need to open the airway. The nurse plans to use which method to open the airway in this victim?

1 Head tilt–chin lift
2 Neutral or sniffing position
3 Modified head tilt–chin lift
4 Jaw thrust maneuver

5. The nurse is preparing to do the Heimlich maneuver on a 3-year-old conscious child. The correct hand placement to perform this maneuver is which of the following?
   1 Between the umbilicus and the groin
   2 Between the groin and the abdomen
   3 Between the umbilicus and xiphoid process
   4 Between the lower abdomen and chest

6. The nurse is performing CPR on a 7-year-old child. The nurse delivers how many breaths per minute to the child?
   1 12 breaths/minute
   2 16 breaths/minute
   3 18 breaths/minute
   4 20 breaths/minute

7. When performing CPR on an infant, the nurse performs chest compression at a rate of:
   1 At least 60 times/minute
   2 At least 80 times/minute
   3 At least 100 times/minute
   4 At least 160 times/minute

8. A nursing instructor teaches a group of students about BLS. The instructor asks a student to identify the most appropriate location to assess the pulse of an infant. Which of the following, if stated by the student, indicates that the student understands the appropriate procedure?
   1 Brachial
   2 Carotid
   3 Popliteal
   4 Radial

9. The nurse is teaching CPR to a group of community members. The nurse asks a member of the group to describe the reason that blind fingersweeps are avoided in infants. Which of the following responses is accurate?
   1 The object may be forced back farther into the throat
   2 The mouth is too small to see the object
   3 The object may have been swallowed
   4 The infant may bite down on the finger

10. The nurse is performing CPR on an adult client. When performing chest compressions, the sternum should be depressed:
   1 ½ to ¾ inch
   2 ¾ to 1 inch
   3 2½ to 3 inches
   4 1½ to 2 inches

ANSWERS

1. **2**

RATIONALE: Complications associated with performing chest compressions during BLS include pneumothorax, fractured ribs and sternum, and laceration of the liver, spleen, or stomach. Gastric distention can also occur. Options 1, 3, and 4 will not result from performing chest compressions.
TEST-TAKING STRATEGY: Focus on the issue of the question and visualize the anatomical location of the hands when performing chest compressions. Using the process of elimination, you should easily be directed to option 2. Review the complications associated with chest compressions now if you had difficulty with this question.
LEVEL OF COGNITIVE ABILITY: Comprehension
PHASE OF NURSING PROCESS: Implementation
CLIENT NEEDS: Physiological Integrity
CONTENT AREA: Fundamental Skills
REFERENCE
Monahan, F., & Neighbors, M. (1998). *Medical-surgical nursing: Foundations for clinical practice* (2nd ed.). Philadelphia: W. B. Saunders. p. 264.

2. **4**

RATIONALE: The next nursing action is to open the airway. Ventilation cannot be initiated unless the airway is opened. Chest compressions are started after the airway is opened and ventilation is initiated. Oxygen may be helpful at some point, but the airway is opened first.
TEST-TAKING STRATEGY: Visualize the steps of BLS to answer the question. Recalling the ABCs—airway, breathing, and circulation—will assist in directing you to option 4. Review the steps of BLS now if you had difficulty with this question.
LEVEL OF COGNITIVE ABILITY: Application
PHASE OF NURSING PROCESS: Implementation
CLIENT NEEDS: Physiological Integrity
CONTENT AREA: Adult Health/Cardiovascular
REFERENCE
Monahan, F., & Neighbors, M. (1998). *Medical-surgical nursing: Foundations for clinical practice* (2nd ed.). Philadelphia: W. B. Saunders. p. 264.

3. **4**

RATIONALE: If a pulse is not present, chest compressions will need to be initiated. Determine proper hand placement for chest compressions by locating the notch where the rib margin meets the sternum and place the middle finger on this notch and the index finger next to it. Then place the heel of the opposite hand on the lower half of the sternum close to the index finger. Remove the first hand and place it on top of the hand on the sternum, and begin chest compressions. This location is the lower half of the sternum.
TEST-TAKING STRATEGY: Consider the anatomical location of the heart to answer this question. Eliminate options 2 and 3 first because this location is ineffective. The lower half of the sternum is the most effective location for chest compressions. If you had difficulty with this question, take time now to review landmarks for chest compressions.
LEVEL OF COGNITIVE ABILITY: Application
PHASE OF NURSING PROCESS: Implementation
CLIENT NEEDS: Physiological Integrity
CONTENT AREA: Adult Health/Cardiovascular

REFERENCE
Monahan, F., & Neighbors, M. (1998). *Medical-surgical nursing: Foundations for clinical practice* (2nd ed.). Philadelphia: W. B. Saunders. p. 264.

4. **4**

RATIONALE: If a neck injury is suspected, the jaw thrust maneuver is used to open the airway. The head tilt–chin lift produces hyperextension of the neck and could cause complications if a neck injury is present. The neutral or sniffing position is used to open the airway in an infant. There is no such position as a modified head tilt–chin lift.
TEST-TAKING STRATEGY: Eliminate option 2 first because this position is used in an infant. Eliminate options 1 and 3 next because they are similarly stated. Knowledge of BLS will direct you toward option 4. If you had difficulty with this question, review the appropriate methods to open an airway.
LEVEL OF COGNITIVE ABILITY: Application
PHASE OF NURSING PROCESS: Planning
CLIENT NEEDS: Physiological Integrity
CONTENT AREA: Fundamental Skills
REFERENCE
Leahy, J., & Kizilay, P. (1998). *Foundations of nursing practice: A nursing process approach*. Philadelphia: W. B. Saunders. p. 971.

5. **3**

RATIONALE: To perform the Heimlich maneuver, the rescuer stands behind the victim and places his or her arms directly under the victim's axillae and around the victim. The thumb side of one fist is placed against the victim's abdomen in the midline slightly above the navel and well below the tip of the xiphoid process. The fist is grasped with the other hand and a series of upward thrusts are delivered. Care must be taken not to touch the xiphoid process or the lower margins of the rib cage because force applied to these structures may damage internal organs.
TEST-TAKING STRATEGY: Eliminate options 1 and 2 first because they are similar. To select from the remaining options, consider the anatomical location and the effect of the maneuver in dislodging an obstruction. If you had difficulty with this question, take time now to review the correct hand placement for the Heimlich maneuver.
LEVEL OF COGNITIVE ABILITY: Application
PHASE OF NURSING PROCESS: Implementation
CLIENT NEEDS: Physiological Integrity
CONTENT AREA: Child Health
REFERENCE
Ashwill, J., & Droske, S. (1997). *Nursing care of children: Principles and practice*. Philadelphia: W. B. Saunders. p. 325.

6. **4**

RATIONALE: In a child between the ages of 1 and 8 years, 20 breaths per minute are delivered. Initially, the nurse gives the child two breaths at 1 to 1.5 seconds per breath.
TEST-TAKING STRATEGY: Knowledge regarding performing CPR on a child is required to answer this question. Note the age of the child in the question. If you had difficulty with this question, take time now to review BLS in a child.
LEVEL OF COGNITIVE ABILITY: Application
PHASE OF NURSING PROCESS: Implementation
CLIENT NEEDS: Physiological Integrity
CONTENT AREA: Child Health

REFERENCE

Ashwill, J., & Droske, S. (1997). *Nursing care of children: Principles and practice*. Philadelphia: W. B. Saunders. p. 326.

7. **3**

RATIONALE: In an infant, the rate of chest compressions is at least 100 per minute.
TEST-TAKING STRATEGY: Consider the normal heart rate of an infant to answer this question. You can easily eliminate options 1 and 2 because of the low rates identified in the options. Eliminate option 4 because this rate would be much too rapid for an infant. If you had difficulty with this question, take time now to review CPR for an infant.
LEVEL OF COGNITIVE ABILITY: Application
PHASE OF NURSING PROCESS: Implementation
CLIENT NEEDS: Physiological Integrity
CONTENT AREA: Fundamental Skills
REFERENCE
Ashwill, J., & Droske, S. (1997). *Nursing care of children: Principles and practice*. Philadelphia: W. B. Saunders. p. 326.

8. **1**

RATIONALE: When assessing a pulse in an infant (under 1 year of age), the pulse should be checked at the brachial artery. The infant's relatively short, fat neck makes palpation of the carotid artery difficult.
TEST-TAKING STRATEGY: Knowledge regarding circulatory assessment in an infant is required to answer this question. Options 3 and 4 can be easily eliminated. Consider the body structure of an infant to assist in directing you to option 1. Review cardiac assessment and BLS in an infant now if you had difficulty with this question.
LEVEL OF COGNITIVE ABILITY: Comprehension
PHASE OF NURSING PROCESS: Evaluation
CLIENT NEEDS: Physiological Integrity
CONTENT AREA: Child Health
REFERENCE
Ashwill, J., & Droske, S. (1997). *Nursing care of children: Principles and practice*. Philadelphia: W. B. Saunders. p. 323.

9. **1**

RATIONALE: Blind fingersweeps are not recommended for infants and children due to the risk of forcing the object farther down into the airway. Options 2, 3, and 4 are not directly related to the issue of the question.
TEST-TAKING STRATEGY: Use the ABCs—airway, breathing, and circulation—to answer this question. Option 1 addresses the concern of airway patency. If you had difficulty with this question, take time now to review obstructed airway management of an infant or child.
LEVEL OF COGNITIVE ABILITY: Comprehension
PHASE OF NURSING PROCESS: Evaluation
CLIENT NEEDS: Physiological Integrity
CONTENT AREA: Child Health
REFERENCE
Ashwill, J., & Droske, S. (1997). *Nursing care of children: Principles and practice*. Philadelphia: W. B. Saunders. p. 323.

10. **4**

RATIONALE: When performing CPR on an adult client, the sternum should be depressed 1½ to 2 inches.
TEST-TAKING STRATEGY: Knowledge regarding the procedure for performing chest compression on an adult client is required to answer the question. Note the key word "adult" in the question. Consider the normal body structure of an adult to assist in answering the question. If you had difficulty with this question, take time now to review adult CPR.
LEVEL OF COGNITIVE ABILITY: Application
PHASE OF NURSING PROCESS: Implementation
CLIENT NEEDS: Physiological Integrity
CONTENT AREA: Adult Health/Cardiovascular
REFERENCE
Monahan, F., & Neighbors, M. (1998). *Medical-surgical nursing: Foundations for clinical practice* (2nd ed.). Philadelphia: W. B. Saunders. p. 264.

BIBLIOGRAPHY

Ashwill, J., & Droske, S. (1997). *Nursing care of children: Principles and practice*. Philadelphia: W. B. Saunders.

Leahy, J., & Kizilay, P. (1998). *Foundations of nursing practice: A nursing process approach*. Philadelphia: W. B. Saunders.

Luckmann, J. (1997). *Saunders manual of nursing care*. Philadelphia: W. B. Saunders.

Monahan, F., & Neighbors, M. (1998). *Medical-surgical nursing: Foundations for clinical practice* (2nd ed.). Philadelphia: W. B. Saunders.

National Council of State Boards of Nursing. (1998). *National Council detailed test plan for the NCLEX-PN examination*. Chicago: Author.

CHAPTER 16

Perioperative Nursing Care

. . . .

PYRAMID TERMS

Atelectasis—A collapsed or airless state of the lung that may be the result of airway obstruction due to accumulated secretions or failure of the client to deep breathe. It is the most common postoperative complication and usually occurs 1 to 2 days postoperative.

Extended Postoperative Stage—The period of at least 1 to 4 days postoperatively.

Immediate Postoperative Stage—The period of 1 to 4 hours after surgery.

Intermediate Postoperative Stage—The period of 4 to 24 hours after surgery.

Wound Dehiscence—An opening of the wound edges.

Wound Evisceration—Protrusion of internal organs through an opening in wound edges.

PYRAMID TO SUCCESS

Pyramid points focus on reinforcing instructions to the client and family or significant other in the preoperative stage, preparing the client for the operative procedure, ensuring that prescribed preoperative procedures have been performed, and that the results of the procedures are within expected range and are documented. In the postoperative stage, pyramid points focus on monitoring for surgical complications and on the implementation of initial nursing measures if a complication arises. Pyramid points also focus on preparing the client for discharge, reinforcing instructions related to the prescribed treatments, and identifying the need for home care support services.

NURSING PROCESS

DATA COLLECTION

Major complaint
Preexisting conditions that increase the risks of surgery
Allergies
Client's present lifestyle related to diet, exercise, substance abuse, and support systems
Vital signs
Level of consciousness, alertness, and orientation
Circulatory status and capillary refill
Nutritional status

Presence of conditions that may produce nutritional deficiencies
Urinary output
Bowel sounds
Muscular weakness
Laboratory results
Anxiety levels, fears, and emotional issues
Financial concerns

PLANNING
The client maintains an effective airway. The client demonstrates the use of coughing and deep-breathing exercises and the use of an incentive spirometer.

IMPLEMENTATION
Monitor vital signs. Monitor for signs of respiratory distress. Assist with repositioning. Instruct on proper coughing and breathing techniques.

EVALUATION
Vital signs remain within normal limits. The client coughs and deep breathes and uses assistive devices. Encourage client to demonstrate techniques and use of incentive spirometer. Assist client with splinting incision. Encourage ambulation.

PLANNING
The client requests pain medication. The client demonstrates and uses relaxation and noninvasive techniques to control anxiety and postoperative pain.

IMPLEMENTATION
Assess pain level using a 1 to 10 pain scale. Administer pain medication as prescribed, noting time and effect of last dosage of medication. Use noninvasive pain control techniques. Document the effectiveness of pain control measures.

EVALUATION
The client achieves pain control.

PLANNING
The client tolerates intake as prescribed.

IMPLEMENTATION
Monitor I&O. Monitor for signs of dehydration. Monitor IV fluids as prescribed. Assess for nausea and vomiting. Administer antiemetics as prescribed. Resume diet as prescribed. Document I&O and client's ability to tolerate food and fluids.

EVALUATION
Fluid and electrolyte status remains normal. Weight remains normal.

PLANNING
The surgical wound remains clean and dry.

IMPLEMENTATION
Maintain aseptic techniques. Monitor for signs and symptoms of infection. Check the wound area, drains, and dressing frequently for signs of infection.

EVALUATION
The client is free of infection.

PLANNING
The client maintains an adequate urinary output. The client resumes normal bowel patterns.

IMPLEMENTATION
Check bladder for distention. Monitor for urinary output. Monitor for bowel sounds. Encourage ambulation. Monitor for bowel movement and return of normal bowel patterns.

EVALUATION
Normal urinary and bowel patterns return.

PLANNING
The client expresses feelings related to surgery.

IMPLEMENTATION
Allow the client to talk about concerns and fears related to surgery. Teach the client relaxation techniques to deal with preoperative anxiety and postoperative pain. Describe any alterations in body appearance or function, or lifestyle changes that may occur. Assist the client to adapt to any changes resulting from the surgery. Suggest a visit from someone who has undergone the same surgical procedure. Assist the client to set realistic goals regarding any lifestyle changes.

EVALUATION
The client expresses a positive outlook for the impending surgery. The client sets goals and makes decisions regarding care.

PLANNING
The client verbalizes understanding of the events that will occur before, during, and following surgery. The client verbalizes the prescribed treatment plan for discharge. The client expresses feelings of personal control regarding rehabilitation.

IMPLEMENTATION
Reinforce instructions regarding the events of surgery. Reinforce instructions of the prescribed discharge plan. Assist to develop a rehabilitation program that maximizes client control and involvement. Include family members in the rehabilitation process. Suggest appropriate support groups.

EVALUATION
The client describes the rehabilitation process. The client uses support groups. The client participates actively in the rehabilitation process.

◆ CLIENT NEEDS

SAFE, EFFECTIVE CARE ENVIRONMENT

Advance directives
Client rights
Informed consent for the surgical procedure
Informing the client of the surgical process
Providing safety to the medicated client
Surgical asepsis
Standard (universal) precautions

HEALTH PROMOTION AND MAINTENANCE

Expected body image changes
Reinforcing instructions related to the prescribed
  discharge plan
Health and wellness to prevent complications
Promoting lifestyle choices
Suggesting appropriate support services

PSYCHOSOCIAL INTEGRITY

Promoting an environment that will allow the client to
  express concerns
Unexpected body image changes
Assisting the client to develop coping methods
Support systems

PHYSIOLOGICAL INTEGRITY

Safe administration of preoperative and postoperative
  medications
Providing respiratory care
Providing basic care and comfort
Monitoring for surgical complications
Monitoring for unexpected responses to treatments and
  procedures
Initiating nursing interventions when surgical
  complications arise

I. Preoperative Care

A. Obtaining informed consent
   1. The surgeon is responsible for obtaining the
      consent for surgery
   2. No sedation should be administered to the
      client before signing the consent
   3. Minors may need a parent or legal guardian
      to sign the consent form
   4. Older clients may need a legal guardian to
      sign the consent form
   5. The nurse may witness the client signing the
      preoperative consent, but the nurse must be
      sure that the client has understood the
      surgeon's explanation of the surgery
   6. The nurse needs to document the witnessing
      of the signing of the operative consent after
      the client acknowledges understanding the
      procedure
B. Nutrition
   1. Check the physician's orders regarding the
      NPO status prior to surgery
   2. Solid foods and liquids are generally withheld
      for 6 to 8 hours prior to general anesthesia
      and for 3 hours before surgery with local
      anesthesia, to avoid aspiration
   3. Monitor IV fluids if prescribed
   4. Note that total parenteral nutrition (TPN) may

be prescribed for clients who are
malnourished, have protein or metabolic
deficiencies, or cannot ingest foods
C. Elimination
   1. If the client is to have intestinal or abdominal
      surgery, an enema or laxative or both may be
      prescribed the night before surgery
   2. The client should void immediately before
      surgery
   3. Prepare to insert a Foley catheter if prescribed
   4. If there is a Foley catheter in place, it should
      be emptied immediately before surgery and
      the amount and quality of urine output
      documented
D. Surgical site
   1. Prepare to clean the surgical site with a mild
      antiseptic soap the night before surgery, as
      prescribed
   2. Prepare to shave the operative site as
      prescribed
   3. Hair should be shaved only if it will interfere
      with the surgical procedure and only if
      prescribed
   4. Shaving of hair, if prescribed, should be done
      in the direction of hair growth with a sharp
      razor, and caution should be used to prevent
      cuts or epidermal damage
E. Reinforcing preoperative instructions (Boxes
   16–1 and 16–2)
   1. Inform the client about what to expect
      postoperatively
   2. Inform clients to notify the nurse if they
      experience any pain postoperatively and that
      pain medication will be prescribed to be
      given as the client requests
   3. Instruct clients to use the noninvasive pain
      relief techniques before the pain occurs and
      as soon as the pain is noticed
   4. Reinforce instructions about the use of a
      client-controlled analgesia pump if its use is
      prescribed
   5. Inform the client that requesting a narcotic
      after surgery will not make the client a drug
      addict
   6. Clients should be instructed not to smoke for
      at least 12 hours before surgery
   7. Instruct the client in deep-breathing and
      coughing techniques, the use of incentive
      spirometry, and the importance of
      performing the techniques postoperatively to
      prevent the development of pneumonia and
      atelectasis
   8. Instruct the client in leg and foot exercises to
      prevent venous stasis of blood and facilitate
      venous blood return
   9. Instruct clients how to splint an incision and
      to turn and reposition
  10. Inform clients of any invasive devices that
      may be needed following surgery
  11. Inform the client not to pull on any of the
      invasive devices, as they will be removed as
      soon as possible

BOX 16-1. Preoperative Instructions

LEG AND HIP EXERCISES

Instruct the client to press the back of the knees against the bed, and then to relax the knees.

This contracts and relaxes the thigh and calf muscles to prevent thrombus formation.

Instruct the client to rotate each foot in a circle at least 10 times an hour.

Have the client flex the knee and thigh, straighten the leg up in the air, and hold for 5 seconds before lowering, performing the exercise 10 times per day.

COUGHING AND DEEP-BREATHING EXERCISES

Instruct the client that a sitting position gives the best lung expansion for coughing and deep-breathing exercises.

Instruct the client to breath deeply three times, inhaling through the nostrils and exhaling through the mouth.

Instruct the client that the third breath should be held for 3 seconds, then the client should forcefully cough out three times.

The client should perform this exercise every 2 hours.

SPLINTING INCISION

If the surgical incision is abdominal or thoracic, instruct the client to place a pillow, or one hand with the other hand on top, over the incisional area.

During deep breathing and coughing, the client presses gently against the incisional area to splint or support it.

INCENTIVE SPIROMETRY

Instruct the client to assume a sitting position

Instruct the client that lips need to cover the mouthpiece completely.

Instruct the client to inhale slowly and maintain a constant flow through the unit.

When maximal inspiration is reached, the client should hold the breath for 2 or 3 seconds and then exhale slowly.

Instruct the client that the number of breaths should not exceed more than 12 breaths/minute.

F. Psychosocial preparation
   1. Be alert to the client's anxiety level
   2. Ask the client about questions or concerns the client may have regarding surgery
   3. Allow time for privacy for the client to prepare for surgery psychologically
   4. Provide support and assistance as needed
G. Preoperative checklist
   1. Ensure that the client has an identification bracelet on
   2. Check for client allergies
   3. Review the preoperative check list to be sure that each item is addressed before the client is transported to surgery
   4. Ensure that consent forms were signed for the operative procedure, for any blood transfusions, for disposal of a limb, or for surgical sterilization procedures
   5. Ensure that a history and physical exam were completed and documented in the client's record
   6. Ensure that consultations prescribed were

BOX 16-2. Medications That Can Affect the Surgical Client

ANTIBIOTICS

Potentiate the action of anesthetic agents.

If taken for 2 weeks before surgery, aminoglycosides such as gentamicin (Garamycin), tobramycin (Nebcin), and neomycin (Mycifradin) may cause mild respiratory depression from depressed neuromuscular transmission.

ANTIDYSRHYTHMICS

Reduce cardiac contractility and impair cardiac conduction during anesthesia.

ANTICOAGULANTS

Alter normal clotting factors and increase the risk of hemorrhaging.

Aspirin (acetylsalicylic acid, ASA) and ibuprofen (Motrin, Advil) are commonly used medications that can alter clotting mechanisms.

They should be discontinued at least 48 hours before surgery.

ANTICONVULSANTS

Long-term use of certain anticonvulsants can alter the metabolism of anesthetic agents.

ANTIHYPERTENSIVES

Can interact with anesthetic agents and cause bradycardia, hypotension, and impaired circulation.

CORTICOSTEROIDS

Cause adrenal atrophy and reduce the body's ability to withstand stress.

Before and during surgery, dosages may be temporarily increased.

INSULIN

The need for insulin after surgery in a diabetic is reduced because the client's nutritional intake is decreased.

Stress response and IV administration of glucose solutions can increase dosage requirements after surgery.

DIURETICS

Potentiate electrolyte imbalances after surgery.

ANTIDEPRESSANTS

May lower the blood pressure during anesthesia.

ANTICHOLINERGICS

Medications with anticholinergic effects increase the potential for confusion.

completed and documented in the client's record

7. Ensure that the prescribed laboratory results are documented in the client's record
8. Ensure that ECG and chest radiograph reports are noted in the client's record
9. Ensure that blood type and screen or type and cross match is noted in the client's record
10. Document that the client has voided prior to surgery
11. Remove jewelry, makeup, dentures, hairpins, nail polish, glasses, and any prosthesis
12. Document that valuables were given to the client's family members or locked in the hospital safe
13. Document that the prescribed preoperative medication was given
14. Monitor and document the client's vital signs
15. Document the last time the client ate or drank

H. Preoperative medications
1. Prepare to administer preoperative medication as prescribed, or on call to the operating room immediately before the surgery
2. Instruct clients that they will feel drowsy after the medications are given
3. After administering the preoperative medications, keep the client in bed with the side rails up
4. Place the call bell next to the client, instruct the client not to get out of bed and to call for assistance if needed

I. Arrival at the operating room
1. When the client arrives at the operating room, the operating room nurse will verify the identification bracelet with the client's verbal response and will review the client's chart
2. The operating room nurse will confirm the operative procedure and site to be operated on
3. The client's chart will be checked for completeness
4. The client's chart will be reviewed for consent forms, history and physical examination, and allergic reaction information
5. The physician's orders will be reviewed and verified that they were carried out
6. The IV line may be initiated at this time if prescribed
7. The anesthesia team will administer the prescribed anesthesia

II. Postoperative Care

A. Immediate stage
1. Description: The period of 1 to 4 hours after surgery
2. Respiratory system
   a. Monitor vital signs
   b. Monitor airway patency and adequate ventilation, since prolonged mechanical ventilation during anesthesia may affect postoperative lung function
   c. Remember that extubated clients who are lethargic may not be able to maintain an airway
   d. Monitor for secretions and remove by suctioning if the client is unable to clear the airway by coughing
   e. Observe chest movement for symmetry and the use of accessory muscles
   f. Monitor oxygen administration if prescribed
   g. Monitor pulse oximetry as prescribed
   h. Encourage coughing and deep-breathing exercises as soon as possible
   i. Note the rate, depth, and quality of respirations: the respiratory rate should be greater than 10 and less than 30
   j. Monitor client for signs of **atelectasis,** pneumonia, and pulmonary embolism
3. Cardiovascular system
   a. Check the client's color
   b. Observe capillary refill, mucous membranes, and sclera
   c. Check peripheral pulses and for peripheral edema
   d. Monitor for bleeding
   e. Check pulse for rate and rhythm; a bounding pulse may indicate hypertension, fluid overload, or excitement
   f. Monitor for signs of hypertension and hypotension
   g. Monitor for cardiac irregularities
   h. Check for Homans' sign, particularly in clients in lithotomy position during surgery, as these clients may be predisposed to developing deep vein thrombosis
4. Musculoskeletal system
   a. Check the client for moving extremities
   b. Check the physician's orders regarding client positioning or restrictions
   c. Unless contraindicated, place clients in a low Fowler's position after surgery to increase the size of the thorax
   d. Avoid positioning clients in a supine position until pharyngeal reflexes have returned
   e. If the client is comatose or semicomatose, position on the side unless contraindicated
5. Neurological system
   a. Check level of consciousness
   b. Closely monitor the client who may be drowsy or unconscious
   c. Periodic frequent attempts to awaken the client should continue until the client awakens
   d. Orient the client to the environment
   e. Speak in a soft tone and filter out extraneous noises in the environment
   f. Maintain body temperature and prevent

heat loss by providing clients with warm blankets and raising the room temperature as necessary
6. Temperature control
   a. Monitor temperature
   b. Monitor for signs of hypothermia that may result from anesthesia, a cool operating room, and exposure of the skin and internal organs during surgery
   c. Apply warm blankets and continue oxygen as prescribed if the client is shivering
7. Integumentary system
   a. Check surgical site, drains, and wound dressings
   b. Monitor for and document any drainage or bleeding from surgical site
   c. Check skin for redness, abrasions, or breakdown that may have resulted from surgical positioning
8. Fluid and electrolyte balance
   a. Monitor IV administration as prescribed
   b. Accurately record I&O
9. Gastrointestinal system
   a. Monitor for nausea and vomiting
   b. Maintain patency of nasogastric tube, if present, as prescribed
   c. Monitor for abdominal distention
   d. Monitor for return of bowel sounds
10. Renal system
    a. Check bladder for distention
    b. Monitor color, quantity, and quality of urine output if a Foley catheter is present
    c. Expect the client to void 6 to 8 hours following the surgical procedure, depending on the type of anesthesia administered
11. Pain management
    a. Check for pain
    b. Note the type of anesthetic used and preoperative medication that the client received, and note if the client received any pain medications in the postanesthesia period
    c. Ask the client to rate the degree of pain on a scale of 1 to 10, with 10 being the most severe
    d. Monitor such objective data as facial expressions, body gestures, pulse rate, blood pressure, and respirations
    e. Inquire about the effectiveness of the last pain medication
    f. If a narcotic has been prescribed, during the initial administration check the client every 30 minutes for respiratory rate and pain relief
    g. Use noninvasive measures to relieve postoperative pain including distraction, comfort measures, positioning, backrubs, and providing a quiet and restful environment
    h. Document effectiveness of pain medication

B. Intermediate stage
1. Description
   a. The period of 4 to 24 hours after surgery
   b. Nursing care implemented during the immediate stage is continued
2. Respiratory system: Encourage coughing and deep breathing
3. Cardiovascular system: Encourage the use of antiembolism stockings if prescribed to promote venous return, strengthen muscle tone, and prevent pooling of secretions in the lungs
4. Musculoskeletal system
   a. Before ambulation, instruct the client to sit at the edge of the bed with the feet supported
   b. If the client is unable to walk, turn the client every 1 to 2 hours
5. Neurological system: Check level of consciousness
6. Integumentary system
   a. Monitor the wound for signs of infection
   b. Maintain a dry and intact dressing
   c. Reinforce with a sterile dressing if necessary and notify the primary health care provider if bleeding occurs from the site
   d. Change dressings as prescribed, noting the amount of bleeding or drainage, odor, and intactness of sutures or staples
   e. Use an abdominal binder for obese and debilitated individuals to prevent rupture of the incision
   f. Drains should be patent and there should be minimal bleeding or drainage
   g. Prepare to assist with the removal of drains as prescribed by the physician when the drainage amount becomes insignificant
7. Gastrointestinal system
   a. Turn the unconscious client to a side-lying position if vomiting occurs, and have suctioning equipment available and ready to use
   b. Administer frequent mouth care
   c. Maintain the NPO status until the gag reflex returns and peristalsis returns
   d. Assess for bowel sounds in all four quadrants
   e. When oral fluids are permitted, start with ice chips and water
   f. Monitor the client for gas pains and encourage ambulation, positioning, and a rectal tube as prescribed
8. Renal system
   a. Monitor urinary output (should be greater than 30 mL/hour)
   b. If the client does not have a Foley catheter, client is expected to void within 6 to 8 hours postoperatively and ensure that the amount is at least 200 mL
9. Pain management
   a. Use noninvasive measures to relieve postoperative pain

b. Administer pain medication as prescribed
c. Document effectiveness of pain medication

C. Extended stage
1. Description: The period of at least 1 to 4 days postoperatively
2. Implementation
a. Continue to check and observe the client's body systems during this stage
b. Monitor for signs of infection such as redness, swelling and tenderness at the surgical site, fever, and leukocytosis
c. Encourage active range of motion every 2 hours
d. Continue to encourage ambulation that will promote peristalsis and the passage of fluid and flatus
e. Increase ambulation every day to increase muscle strength
f. Encourage the client to perform as many activities of daily living as possible
g. Instruct clients to eat foods that are high in protein and vitamin C to promote wound healing

III. Pneumonia and Atelectasis (Box 16–3)

A. Description
1. Pneumonia, an inflammation of the alveoli caused by infectious process, may develop 3 to 5 days postoperatively because of infection, aspiration, or immobility
2. **Atelectasis,** a collapse of the alveoli with retained mucus secretions, is the most common postoperative complication and usually occurs 1 to 2 days postoperatively
B. Data collection
1. Dyspnea
2. Increased respiratory rate
3. Elevated temperature
4. Productive cough
5. Chest pain
6. Crackles over involved lung area
C. Implementation
1. Monitor temperature
2. Encourage ambulation
3. Reposition the client every 1 to 2 hours
4. Encourage the client to use incentive spirometer, coughing, and deep breathing

---

BOX 16–3. Postoperative Complications

Pneumonia and atelectasis	Urinary retention
Hypoxia	Constipation
Pulmonary embolism	Paralytic ileus
Hemorrhage	Wound infection
Shock	Wound dehiscence
Thrombophlebitis	Wound evisceration

 The nurse always notifies the RN and/or physician if signs of complications are noted.

---

5. Suction to clear secretions if the client is unable to cough
6. Encourage fluid intake

IV. Hypoxia

A. Description: An inadequate concentration of oxygen in arterial blood
B. Data collection
1. Restlessness
2. Dyspnea
3. Diaphoresis
4. Increased heart rate and blood pressure
5. Cyanosis
C. Implementation
1. Eliminate cause of hypoxia
2. Encourage coughing and deep breathing and use of incentive spirometry
3. Turn and reposition the client frequently
4. Monitor pulse oximetry
5. Administer oxygen as prescribed

V. Pulmonary Embolism

A. Description: An embolus blocking the pulmonary artery and disrupting blood flow to one or more lobes of the lung
B. Data collection
1. Dyspnea
2. Sudden sharp chest or upper abdominal pain
3. Increased heart rate and a decrease in blood pressure
4. Cyanosis
C. Implementation
1. Notify the registered nurse and/or physician immediately
2. Monitor vital signs

VI. Hemorrhage

A. Description: The loss of a large amount of blood externally or internally in a short period of time
B. Data collection
1. Restlessness
2. Weak, rapid pulse and hypotension
3. Cool, clammy skin
4. Rapid breathing
5. Decreased urine output
C. Implementation
1. Provide pressure to the site of bleeding
2. Notify the registered nurse and/or physician immediately

VII. Shock

A. Description: Loss of circulatory fluid volume that is usually caused by hemorrhage
B. Data collection
1. Restlessness
2. Weak, rapid pulse and hypotension
3. Cool, clammy skin
4. Rapid breathing

5. Decreased urine output
6. Disorientation
C. Implementation
  1. If shock develops, elevate the legs
  2. If the client had spinal anesthesia, do not elevate the legs any higher than placing them on the pillow, otherwise diaphragm muscles could be impaired
  3. Notify the registered nurse and/or physician immediately

VIII. Thrombophlebitis

A. Description
  1. Inflammation of a vein, often accompanied by a clot formation
  2. Veins in legs are most commonly affected
B. Data collection
  1. Aching or cramping leg pain
  2. Vein feels hard and cordlike and is tender to touch
  3. Elevated temperature
  4. Positive Homans' sign
C. Implementation
  1. Monitor legs for swelling, inflammation, cyanosis, pain, tenderness, and venous distention
  2. Elevate the extremity 30 degrees without allowing any pressure on the popliteal area
  3. Encourage coughing and deep breathing
  4. Encourage the use of antiembolism stockings as prescribed, removing them twice a day to wash and inspect the legs
  5. Use intermittent pneumatic compression stockings as prescribed
  6. Perform passive range of motion every 2 hours if the client is on bed rest
  7. Do not allow the client to dangle
  8. Instruct the client not to sit in one position for an extended period of time
  9. Heparin or warfarin (Coumadin) may be prescribed

IX. Urinary Retention

A. Description
  1. Involuntary accumulation of urine in the bladder from loss of muscle tone
  2. Due to the effects of anesthetics and narcotic analgesics
  3. Appears 6 to 8 hours after surgery
B. Data collection
  1. Restlessness
  2. Inability to void and a distended bladder
  3. Lower abdominal pain
  4. Elevated blood pressure
  5. Diaphoresis
  6. On percussion, the bladder sounds like a drum
C. Implementation
  1. Check for distended bladder
  2. Encourage ambulation when prescribed

3. Encourage fluid intake unless contraindicated
4. Provide privacy when attempting to void
5. Assist the client to void by helping to stand
6. Pour warm water over the perineum
7. Allow the client to hear running water
8. Catheterize the client as prescribed after all noninvasive techniques have been attempted

X. Constipation

A. Description
  1. Infrequent passage of stool
  2. When the client resumes a solid diet postoperatively, failure to pass stool within 48 hours is a cause for concern
B. Data collection
  1. Abdominal distention
  2. Absence of bowel movements
C. Implementation
  1. Check bowel sounds
  2. Encourage fluid intake up to 3000 mL/day unless contraindicated
  3. Encourage early ambulation
  4. Encourage consumption of fiber and roughage
  5. Administer stool softeners and laxatives as prescribed
  6. Provide privacy and adequate time for bowel elimination

XI. Ileus

A. Description
  1. Failure of appropriate forward movement of bowel contents
  2. May occur as a result of anesthetic medications or manipulation of the bowel during the surgical procedure
B. Data collection
  1. Nausea and vomiting postoperatively
  2. Abdominal distention
  3. Absence of bowel sounds, bowel movement, or flatus
C. Implementation
  1. Maintain NPO status until bowel sounds return
  2. Maintain patency of NG tube
  3. Encourage ambulation
  4. Monitor IV fluids as prescribed
  5. Administer medications as prescribed to increase GI motility and secretions

XII. Wound Infection

A. Description
  1. Caused by poor aseptic technique or a contaminated wound before surgical exploration
  2. Usually occurs 3 to 6 days after surgery
  3. Purulent material may exit from the drains or separated wound edges
B. Data collection
  1. Fever and chills

2. Warm, tender, painful, and inflamed incision site
3. Edematous skin at incision and tight skin sutures
4. Elevated white blood cell count

C. Implementation
1. Monitor temperature
2. Monitor incision site for approximation of suture line, edema or bleeding, and signs of infection
3. Maintain patency of drains and keep drain and tubes away from incision line
4. Monitor drains and assess drainage amount, color, and consistency
5. Change dressing as prescribed
6. Administer antibiotics as prescribed

XIII. Wound Dehiscence

A. Description
1. Separation of the wound edges at the suture line
2. Usually occurs 6 to 8 days after surgery

B. Data collection
1. Increased drainage
2. Opened wound edges
3. Appearance of underlying tissues through the wound

C. Implementation
1. Notify the registered nurse and/or physician immediately
2. Cover the wound with a sterile normal saline dressing
3. Place the client in low Fowler's position with knees bent to prevent abdominal tension on abdominal wounds
4. Prevent wound infection
5. Administer antiemetics as prescribed to prevent vomiting and further strain on the incision
6. Instruct the client to splint the incision when coughing

XIV. Wound Evisceration

A. Description
1. Protrusion of the internal organs through an opening in wound edges
2. Most common among obese clients, clients who had abdominal surgery, or those who have poor wound healing ability
3. Usually occurs 6 to 8 days after surgery
4. **Wound evisceration** is an emergency

B. Data collection
1. Discharge of serosanguineous fluid from a previously dry wound
2. The appearance of loops of bowel or other wound contents through the wound
3. The client may report feeling a popping sensation after coughing or turning

C. Implementation
1. Notify the registered nurse and/or physician immediately

2. Cover the wound with a sterile normal saline dressing
3. Place the client in low Fowler's position with knees bent to prevent abdominal tension
4. Prevent wound infection
5. Administer antiemetics as prescribed to prevent vomiting and further strain on the incision
6. Instruct the client to splint the incision when coughing

XV. Ambulatory Surgery

A. Criteria for client discharge
1. Is alert and oriented
2. Has voided
3. Has no respiratory distress
4. Is able to ambulate, swallow, and cough
5. Has minimal pain
6. Is not vomiting
7. Has minimal, if any, bleeding from incision site
8. A responsible adult is available to drive the client home
9. The surgeon has signed a release form

B. Reinforcing discharge instructions (Box 16–4)

BOX 16–4. Reinforcing Discharge Instructions

Demonstrate care to the incision and how to change the dressing

Instruct the client to cover the incision with plastic if showering is allowed

Be sure the client is provided with a 48-hour supply of dressings for home use

Instruct the client on the importance of returning to the physician's office for a checkup

Instruct the client that sutures are usually removed in the physician's office 7 to 10 days after surgery

Inform the client that staples are removed 7 to 14 days after surgery and that they may become slightly reddened when they are ready to be removed

Steri-strips may be applied to provide extra support after the sutures are removed

Instruct the client on the use of medications, the purpose, doses, administration, and side effects

Instruct the client on diet

Instruct the client to drink 6 to 8 glasses of liquid a day unless contraindicated

Instruct the client on activity levels

Clients should be instructed to resume normal activities gradually

Instruct the client to avoid lifting for 6 weeks if a major surgical procedure was performed

Instruct the client to not lift anything weighing 10 pounds or more and not engage in any activities that involve pushing or pulling with abdominal incisions

Clients usually can return to work in 6 to 8 weeks as prescribed by the physician

Instruct the client on the signs and symptoms of complications and when to call a physician

1. Should be performed prior to the date of the scheduled procedure
2. Provide written instructions to the client and family regarding the specifics of care
3. Instruct the client and family of postoperative complications that can occur
4. Suggest appropriate resources for home care support
5. Instruct clients that they should not drive for 24 hours if they had general anesthesia
6. Inform the client to call the surgeon, ambulatory center, or emergency department if postoperative problems occur
7. Instruct the client to keep follow-up appointments with the surgeon

PRACTICE QUESTIONS

1. The nurse is reviewing the laboratory results of a client scheduled for surgery. Which of these laboratory results indicates to the nurse that the surgery may be postponed?
   1 Sodium (Na$^+$) 140 mEq/L
   2 Hemoglobin (Hgb) 9.2 g/dL
   3 Platelets 200,000/mm$^+$
   4 Serum creatinine 0.9 mg/100 mL

2. The nurse is preparing a client for surgery. The nurse plans to implement which of the following on the day of surgery?
   1 Remove colored nail polish
   2 Immediately report an increase in blood pressure of 120/72 to 128/84 mmHg
   3 Verify that the client has not eaten for the last 24 hours
   4 Avoid oral hygiene and rinsing with mouthwash

3. Emergency surgery is scheduled for a client with a bowel obstruction. The licensed practical nurse (LPN) tells the registered nurse (RN) that he or she is unable to obtain informed consent from the client because the client has received narcotic analgesics and is very sedated. The LPN understands that the most appropriate action is which of the following?
   1 Perform the surgery without an informed consent
   2 Call the family and tell them that they must come to the hospital immediately to sign the informed consent
   3 Obtain a telephone consent from the family member ensuring that the oral consent is witnessed by two people
   4 Have the client sign the consent form because this is an emergency situation

4. The nurse is caring for a client scheduled for surgery. The client is concerned about the surgical procedure. To alleviate the client's fears and misconceptions about surgery, the nurse should first

   1 Provide explanations about procedures involved in the planned surgery
   2 Explain all nursing care and possible discomfort that may result
   3 Tell the client that preoperative fear is normal
   4 Ask the client to discuss information known about planned surgery

5. The nurse is reinforcing instructions to a client regarding the use of the incentive spirometer. Which of the following statements indicates that the client does <u>not</u> clearly understand the procedure?
   1 "My lips should cover the mouthpiece completely."
   2 "I should inhale slowly to maintain a constant flow through the unit."
   3 "After maximum inspiration, I should hold my breath for 2 or 3 seconds then exhale slowly."
   4 "I can use the incentive spirometer in any position to achieve optimal lung expansion."

6. The nurse is collecting data from a client who is scheduled for surgery in 1 week in the ambulatory care surgical center. The nurse notes that the client has a history of arthritis and has been taking aspirin (acetylsalicylic acid, ASA). The nurse reports the information to the physician and anticipates that the physician will prescribe which of the following?
   1 Continue to take the aspirin as prescribed
   2 Decrease the dose of the aspirin to half of what is normally taken
   3 Discontinue the aspirin immediately
   4 Discontinue the aspirin 48 hours before the scheduled surgery

7. A nursing instructor asks a nursing student about the reason for the reduction of anesthetic medication dosage in the older person. The nursing student appropriately responds by stating
   1 "The increase of fatty tissue allows anesthetic agents, which have an affinity for fatty tissue, to concentrate in body fat."
   2 "The decrease in liver size increases the rate at which the liver can inactivate many anesthetics."
   3 "The decrease in plasma proteins causes fewer of the anesthetic agents to remain free or unbound."
   4 "An increase in the function of kidney cells increases the excretion of waste products and anesthetics."

8. The nurse preparing a client for surgery reviews the client's medication record. The client is to be NPO after midnight. Which of the following medications, if noted on the client's record, does the nurse question?
   1 Cyclobenzaprine (Flexeril)
   2 Fentanyl (Duragesic)

3 Allopurinol (Zyloprim)
4 Prednisone (Deltasone)

9. When applying the safety strap across the client's legs on the operating table, the nurse should avoid pressure on the popliteal nerve. Which of the following nursing actions is most appropriate to avoid this pressure?
   1 Apply the safety strap 2 inches above the knees
   2 Apply the safety strap 2 inches below the knees
   3 Apply the safety strap 6 inches above the knees
   4 Apply the safety strap over the ankles

10. During a surgical procedure, the nurse prevents the client's extremities from dangling over the sides of the table, knowing that this action may cause
   1 An increase in pulse rate
   2 Nerve and muscle damage
   3 A drop in blood pressure
   4 The extremities to get tired

11. The nurse obtains the vital signs on a postoperative client. The client's blood pressure (BP) is 100/60 mmHg, pulse is 90 beats/minute, and respiration rate is 20 breaths/minute. Based on these findings, which of the following nursing actions should be performed?
   1 Cover the client with a warm blanket
   2 Shake gently to arouse
   3 Continue to monitor the vital signs
   4 Call the surgeon immediately

12. The client arrives at the surgical nursing unit after surgery. The initial nursing action is to check the
   1 Dressing for bleeding
   2 Tubes or drains for patency
   3 Patency of the airway
   4 Vital signs to compare with preoperative measurements

13. The nurse is monitoring the adult client for postoperative complications. Which of the following is most indicative of a potential postoperative complication that requires further observation?
   1 Urinary output of 20 mL/hour
   2 Temperature of 37.6°C (99.6°F)
   3 Serous drainage on the surgical dressing
   4 Blood pressure of 100/70 mmHg

14. The nurse monitors the postoperative client frequently for the presence of secretions in the lungs, knowing that accumulated secretions can lead to
   1 Pulmonary edema
   2 Pneumonia
   3 Fluid imbalance
   4 Carbon dioxide retention

15. The nurse is caring for a postoperative client who has a drain inserted in the surgical wound. Which of the following nursing actions is inappropriate in the care of the drain?
   1 Maintain aseptic technique when emptying
   2 Observe for bright red bloody drainage
   3 Check the drain for patency
   4 Secure by curling or folding and taping firmly to body

16. The nurse is caring for a postoperative client who is being monitored by pulse oximetry. Which of the following is an expected measurement determined by the pulse oximeter?
   1 Oxygen saturation 95% to 100%
   2 Blood pressure 120/80 to 130/80 mmHg
   3 Respiration rate 18 to 22 breaths/minute
   4 Temperature 36.7° to 37.2°C (98° to 99°F)

17. The nurse checks the client's surgical incision for signs of infection. Which of the following is not indicative of a potential infection?
   1 The presence of serous drainage
   2 Warm, red, tender skin around the incision
   3 Chills and fever
   4 The presence of purulent drainage

18. The nurse is checking a client's surgical incision and notes an increase in the amount of drainage, a separation of the incision line, and the appearance of underlying tissue. Which of the following is the most appropriate initial action?
   1 Clean the wound using aseptic technique and apply a sterile dry dressing
   2 Apply a sterile dressing soaked with normal saline to the wound
   3 Leave the incision open to the air to assist in drying the drainage
   4 Cover the wound with a Betadine-soaked dressing

19. The nurse monitors the postoperative client for signs of complications. Which of the following does the nurse determine to be indicative of a sign of a potential complication?
   1 Faint bowel sounds heard in all four quadrants
   2 A negative Homans' sign
   3 A blood pressure of 120/70 mmHg with a pulse of 90 beats/minute
   4 Increasing restlessness

20. The nurse is assisting in planning discharge instructions for a postoperative client. Which of the following instructions is least appropriate to include in the postoperative discharge plan of care?
   1 Wound care
   2 Activity restrictions
   3 Personal hygiene
   4 Turning and deep breathing

ANSWERS

1. 2

RATIONALE: Routine screening tests include a complete blood count, serum electrolyte analysis, coagulation studies, and serum creatinine tests. The complete blood count includes the hemoglobin analysis. All of these values are within normal range except the hemoglobin. If a client has a low hemoglobin level, the surgery may be postponed.
TEST-TAKING STRATEGY: Knowledge of the normal values for serum sodium, hemoglobin, platelets, and creatinine is required to answer this question. If you know the normal values for these tests, use the process of elimination. Take time now to review these laboratory values if you had difficulty answering this question.
LEVEL OF COGNITIVE ABILITY: Analysis
PHASE OF NURSING PROCESS: Evaluation
CLIENT NEEDS: Physiological Integrity
CONTENT AREA: Fundamental Skills
REFERENCE
Potter, P., & Perry, A. (1997). *Fundamentals of nursing: Concepts, process, and practice* (4th ed.). St. Louis: Mosby–Year Book. pp. 1389–1390.

2. 1

RATIONALE: Nail polish should be removed from at least one nail for the pulse oximeter to check oxygen saturation. Some increase in blood pressure is common because of anxiety. The client usually has a restriction of food and fluids for 8 hours prior to surgery instead of 24 hours. Oral hygiene is allowed, but the client should not swallow any water.
TEST-TAKING STRATEGY: Use the principles associated with prioritization when answering this question. Remember the ABCs of airway, breathing, and circulation. Monitoring the oxygen saturation level through the nails assesses airway, breathing, and circulation. Review general preoperative care now if you had difficulty with this question.
LEVEL OF COGNITIVE ABILITY: Application
PHASE OF NURSING PROCESS: Planning
CLIENT NEEDS: Physiological Integrity
CONTENT AREA: Fundamental Skills
REFERENCE
Leahy, J., & Kizilay, P. (1998). *Foundations of nursing practice: A nursing process approach.* Philadelphia: W. B. Saunders. p. 1183.

3. 3

RATIONALE: Every effort must be made to obtain permission from a responsible family member to perform surgery if the client is unable to sign the consent form. A telephone consent must be witnessed by two people who hear the family member's oral consent. The two witnesses then sign the consent with the name of the family member, noting that an oral consent was obtained. In emergencies, the client may be unable to sign and family members may not be available. In this type of situation, the physician is legally permitted to perform surgery without consent. Consent is not informed if it is obtained from the client who is confused, unconscious, mentally incompetent, or under the influence of sedatives.
TEST-TAKING STRATEGY: Knowledge regarding the implications related to informed consent is required to answer this question. Note the key words "most appropriate." Eliminate options 1 and 4 first. For the remaining two options, select option 3 because it is legally acceptable to obtain a telephone permission from a family member if it is witnessed by two people. Take time now to review the implications surrounding informed consent if you had difficulty with this question.
LEVEL OF COGNITIVE ABILITY: Application
PHASE OF NURSING PROCESS: Implementation
CLIENT NEEDS: Safe, Effective Care Environment
CONTENT AREA: Fundamental Skills
REFERENCE
Potter, P. & Perry, A. (1997). *Fundamentals of nursing: Concepts, process, and practice* (4th ed.). St. Louis: Mosby–Year Book. p. 1393.

4. 4

RATIONALE: Explanations should begin with the information that the client knows. Option 3 is a block to communication. Options 1 and 2 may produce additional anxiety in the client.
TEST-TAKING STRATEGY: Note the key word "first." Remember to always focus on the client's feelings and knowledge first, such as option 4. Additionally, option 4 is the only option that addresses data collection, the first step of the nursing process.
LEVEL OF COGNITIVE ABILITY: Application
PHASE OF NURSING PROCESS: Implementation
CLIENT NEEDS: Psychosocial Integrity
CONTENT AREA: Fundamental Skills
REFERENCE
deWit, S. (1998). *Essentials of medical-surgical nursing* (4th ed.). Philadelphia: W. B. Saunders. pp. 59–60.

5. 4

RATIONALE: For optimal lung expansion with incentive spirometer, the client should assume the semi-Fowler's or high Fowler's position. The mouthpiece should be covered completely while the client inhales slowly with a constant flow through the unit. The breath should be held for 2 or 3 seconds before exhaling slowly.
TEST-TAKING STRATEGY: Knowledge of the procedure for using the incentive spirometer is required to answer the question. Remember that for optimal lung expansion, the head should be elevated to decrease the pressure of the internal organs on the diaphragm and to increase the expansion of the diaphragm. If you had difficulty with this question, take time now to review the correct procedure related to the use of an incentive spirometer.
LEVEL OF COGNITIVE ABILITY: Analysis
PHASE OF NURSING PROCESS: Evaluation
CLIENT NEEDS: Health Promotion and Maintenance
CONTENT AREA: Fundamental Skills
REFERENCE
Leahy, J., & Kizilay, P. (1998). *Foundations of nursing practice: A nursing process approach.* Philadelphia: W. B. Saunders. p. 868.

6. 4

RATIONALE: Anticoagulants alter normal clotting factors and increase the risk of hemorrhage. Aspirin has properties that can alter the clotting mechanism and should be discontinued at least 48 hours before surgery.
TEST-TAKING STRATEGY: Knowledge regarding the medications that affect the surgical client is required to answer this question. Remembering that aspirin has properties that can alter normal clotting factors and that it should be discontinued at least 48 hours before surgery will assist in directing you to option 4. If you had difficulty with this

question, take time now to review medications that affect the client preparing for surgery.
LEVEL OF COGNITIVE ABILITY: Comprehension
PHASE OF NURSING PROCESS: Planning
CLIENT NEEDS: Physiological Integrity
CONTENT AREA: Pharmacology
REFERENCE
Potter, P. & Perry, A. (1997). *Fundamentals of nursing: Concepts, process, and practice* (4th ed.). St. Louis: Mosby–Year Book. p. 1384.

7. **1**

RATIONALE: An older person needs fewer anesthetic agents to produce anesthesia, and it takes longer for the older person to eliminate anesthetic agents. One reason for the reduction of dosage is that the percentage of fatty tissue increases as people age. Anesthetic agents that have an affinity for fatty tissue concentrate in body fat and the brain. Another reason is that older clients may have low plasma proteins, particularly when malnourished. With decreased plasma proteins, more of the anesthetic agent remains free or unbound, which results in a more potent action. Reduction in liver size decreases the rate at which the liver can inactivate many anesthetic agents. The decreased functioning of kidney cells reduces excretion of waste products and anesthetic agents.
TEST-TAKING STRATEGY: Knowledge of the action of anesthetic agents and their effects on the body of an older person is required to answer this question. Read each option carefully. Through the process of elimination, you should select option 1 as the best explanation for a reduction of anesthetic agents for the older person. If you had difficulty with this question, take time now to review the effects of medications on the older person.
LEVEL OF COGNITIVE ABILITY: Comprehension
PHASE OF NURSING PROCESS: Implementation
CLIENT NEEDS: Physiological Integrity
CONTENT AREA: Fundamental Skills
REFERENCE
Tyson, S. (1999). *Gerontological nursing care.* Philadelphia: W. B. Saunders. p. 248.

8. **4**

RATIONALE: Prednisone is a corticosteroid that can cause adrenal atrophy, which reduces the body's ability to withstand stress. Before and during surgery, dosages may be temporarily increased. Cyclobenzaprine is a skeletal muscle relaxant. Fentanyl is an opioid analgesic. Allopurinol is an antigout medication.
TEST-TAKING STRATEGY: Knowledge regarding medications that may have special implications for the surgical client is required to answer this question. Corticosteroids are extremely important medications to be familiar with. Take time now to review corticosteroids if you had difficulty with this question.
LEVEL OF COGNITIVE ABILITY: Comprehension
PHASE OF NURSING PROCESS: Implementation
CLIENT NEEDS: Physiological Integrity
CONTENT AREA: Pharmacology
REFERENCES
Potter, P., & Perry, A. (1997). *Fundamentals of nursing: Concepts, process, and practice* (4th ed.). St. Louis: Mosby–Year Book. p. 1384.
Hodgson, B., & Kizior, R. (1999). *Saunders nursing drug handbook 1999.* Philadelphia: W. B. Saunders. pp. 24, 269, 405.

9. **1**

RATIONALE: The safety strap is applied to prevent the client from falling off the surgery table. The strap should be applied 2 inches above the knees to avoid pressure on the popliteal nerve. Options 2, 3, and 4 are inappropriate and unsafe.
TEST-TAKING STRATEGY: Knowledge regarding the anatomy related to the location of the popliteal nerve is helpful to answer this question. Use the process of elimination and identify the key words "most appropriate." Take time now to review the anatomical location of the popliteal nerve if you had difficulty with this question.
LEVEL OF COGNITIVE ABILITY: Application
PHASE OF NURSING PROCESS: Implementation
CLIENT NEEDS: Physiological Integrity
CONTENT AREA: Fundamental Skills
REFERENCE
Leahy, J., & Kizilay, P. (1998). *Foundations of nursing practice: A nursing process approach.* Philadelphia: W. B. Saunders. p. 1191.

10. **2**

RATIONALE: The client's extremities should not be allowed to dangle over the sides of the table because this may impair circulation or cause nerve and muscle damage. Options 1, 3, and 4 are not associated with the issue of the question.
TEST-TAKING STRATEGY: Note the key word "cause," which indicates an effect. Focus on the issue of the question. Use the process of elimination. The client is anesthetized; therefore, the sense of position or tiredness is absent. The vital signs would not be affected significantly either. Review care to the perioperative client now if you had difficulty with this question.
LEVEL OF COGNITIVE ABILITY: Comprehension
PHASE OF NURSING PROCESS: Implementation
CLIENT NEEDS: Physiological Integrity
CONTENT AREA: Fundamental Skills
REFERENCE
Black, J., & Matassarin-Jacobs, E. (1997). *Medical-surgical nursing: Clinical management for continuity of care* (5th ed.). Philadelphia: W. B. Saunders. p. 477.

11. **3**

RATIONALE: A slightly lower than normal BP and an increased pulse rate are common after surgery. Warm blankets are applied to maintain the client's body temperature. Level of consciousness can be determined by checking the client's response to light touch and verbal stimuli, rather than by shaking the client. There is no reason to contact the surgeon.
TEST-TAKING STRATEGY: The principles of prioritizing should be used to answer this question. Use the ABCs of airway, breathing, and circulation. Monitoring vital signs takes priority over warming and arousing the client. The vital signs are within normal limits following the surgical procedure; therefore, the surgeon does not need to be notified immediately. Review postoperative findings now if you had difficulty with this question.
LEVEL OF COGNITIVE ABILITY: Application
PHASE OF NURSING PROCESS: Implementation
CLIENT NEEDS: Physiological Integrity
CONTENT AREA: Fundamental Skills

REFERENCE
Black, J., & Matassarin-Jacobs, E. (1997). *Medical-surgical nursing: Clinical management for continuity of care* (5th ed.). Philadelphia: W. B. Saunders. pp. 481–483.

12. 3

RATIONALE: If the airway is not patent, immediate measures must be taken for the survival of the client. After checking the client's airway, the nurse then checks the client's vital signs, followed by checking the dressing, tubes, and drains.
TEST-TAKING STRATEGY: Use the principles of prioritization when answering this question. Remember the ABCs of airway, breathing, and circulation. Airway patency is the first action to be taken. Options 1, 2, and 4 are all nursing actions that should be performed after a patent airway has been established.
LEVEL OF COGNITIVE ABILITY: Application
PHASE OF NURSING PROCESS: Implementation
CLIENT NEEDS: Physiological Integrity
CONTENT AREA: Fundamental Skills
REFERENCE
Monahan, F., & Neighbors, M. (1998). *Medical-surgical nursing: Foundations for clinical practice* (2nd ed.). Philadelphia: W. B. Saunders. p. 145.

13. 1

RATIONALE: Urine output is maintained at a minimum of at least 30 mL/hour for an adult. An output of less than 30 mL for each of 2 consecutive hours should be reported to the physician. A temperature above 37.7°C (100°F) or below 36.1°C (97°F) and a falling systolic blood pressure under 90 mmHg are usually considered reportable at once. The client's preoperative or baseline blood pressure is used to make informed postoperative comparisons. Moderate or light serous drainage from the surgical site is considered normal.
TEST-TAKING STRATEGY: Knowledge of the normal ranges for temperature, blood pressure, urinary output, and wound drainage is necessary to determine the correct answer. Through the process of elimination, you can determine that the urinary output is the only observation that is not within the normal range. Take time now to review normal postoperative findings if you had difficulty with this question.
LEVEL OF COGNITIVE ABILITY: Analysis
PHASE OF NURSING PROCESS: Evaluation
CLIENT NEEDS: Physiological Integrity
CONTENT AREA: Fundamental Skills
REFERENCE
Black, J., & Matassarin-Jacobs, E. (1997). *Medical-surgical nursing: Clinical management for continuity of care* (5th ed.). Philadelphia: W. B. Saunders. p. 484.

14. 2

RATIONALE: The most common postoperative respiratory problems are atelectasis, pneumonia, and pulmonary emboli. Pneumonia is the inflammation of lung tissue that causes productive cough, dyspnea, and crackles. Pulmonary edema usually results from left-sided heart failure and can be caused by medications, fluid overload, and smoke inhalation. Carbon dioxide retention results from inability to exhale carbon dioxide in conditions such as chronic obstructive pulmonary disease. Fluid imbalance can be a deficit or excess related to fluid loss or overload.

TEST-TAKING STRATEGY: Knowledge of the common postoperative respiratory complications is necessary to answer this question. Use the process of elimination, focusing on the issue of the question, the postoperative client. Options 1, 3, and 4 most commonly occur with other conditions. Take time now to review the common postoperative complications if you had difficulty with this question.
LEVEL OF COGNITIVE ABILITY: Comprehension
PHASE OF NURSING PROCESS: Data Collection
CLIENT NEEDS: Physiological Integrity
CONTENT AREA: Fundamental Skills
REFERENCE
Leahy, J., & Kizilay, P. (1998). *Foundations of nursing practice: A nursing process approach.* Philadelphia: W. B. Saunders. p. 1208.

15. 4

RATIONALE: Aseptic technique must be used when emptying the drainage container or changing the dressing to avoid contamination of the wound. Usually the drainage from the wound is pale, red, and watery. Active bleeding will be bright red. The drain should be checked for patency to provide an exit for the fluid or blood to promote healing. Ensure that drainage flows freely and that there are no kinks in the drains. Curling or folding the drain prevents the flow of the drainage.
TEST-TAKING STRATEGY: Knowledge of the care of a drain is necessary to answer this question. Note the key word "inappropriate." Use the process of elimination. Options 1, 2, and 3 are appropriate nursing actions in the care of a drain. If you had difficulty with this question, take time now to review nursing care for the client with a surgical drain.
LEVEL OF COGNITIVE ABILITY: Application
PHASE OF NURSING PROCESS: Implementation
CLIENT NEEDS: Physiological Integrity
CONTENT AREA: Fundamental Skills
REFERENCE
Potter, P. & Perry, A. (1997). *Fundamentals of nursing: Concepts, process, and practice* (4th ed.). St. Louis: Mosby–Year Book. pp. 1436–1437.

16. 1

RATIONALE: Pulse oximetry is a noninvasive method of continuously monitoring the oxygen saturation of hemoglobin (SaO_2). The pulse oximeter does not replace arterial blood gases, but it is an effective tool to monitor the client for subtle or sudden changes in oxygen saturation. It does not measure temperature, blood pressure, or respiratory rate.
TEST-TAKING STRATEGY: Knowledge of the purpose of the pulse oximeter is necessary to answer this question. Use the process of elimination. Options 2, 3, and 4 can be eliminated because these responses do not measure oxygen saturation. If you had difficulty with this question, take time now to review the purpose and expected results of pulse oximetry.
LEVEL OF COGNITIVE ABILITY: Comprehension
PHASE OF NURSING PROCESS: Evaluation
CLIENT NEEDS: Physiological Integrity
CONTENT AREA: Fundamental Skills
REFERENCE
Leahy, J., & Kizilay, P. (1998). *Foundations of nursing practice: A nursing process approach.* Philadelphia: W. B. Saunders. p. 850.

17. **1**

RATIONALE: Wound infection is an invasion of deep or superficial wound tissues by pathogenic microorganisms. Signs and symptoms include warm, red, and tender skin around the incision. The client may have fever and chills. Purulent material may exit from drains or from separated wound edges. It may be caused by poor aseptic technique and a contaminated wound before surgical exploration. It appears 3 to 6 days after surgery.

TEST-TAKING STRATEGY: Note the key word "not." Use the process of elimination. Options 2, 3, and 4 indicate signs of infection. Serous drainage is sometimes normally noted at a surgical incision. Remember, however, that an increased flow of serosanguineous drainage from a surgical incision may be a sign of dehiscence. Review the signs of a wound infection now if you had difficulty with this question.

LEVEL OF COGNITIVE ABILITY: Comprehension
PHASE OF NURSING PROCESS: Data Collection
CLIENT NEEDS: Physiological Integrity
CONTENT AREA: Fundamental Skills
REFERENCE
Potter, P., & Perry, A. (1997). *Fundamentals of nursing: Concepts, process, and practice* (4th ed.) St. Louis: Mosby–Year Book. p. 1422.

18. **2**

RATIONALE: Wound dehiscence is the separation of wound edges at the suture line. Signs and symptoms include increased drainage and the appearance of underlying tissues. It usually occurs 6 to 8 days after surgery. The client should be instructed to remain quiet and to avoid coughing or straining. The client should be positioned to prevent further stress on the wound. Sterile dressings soaked with sterile normal saline should be used to cover the wound. The physician needs to be notified.

TEST-TAKING STRATEGY: Knowledge regarding care to the wound when dehiscence occurs is required to answer this question. Use the process of elimination. Eliminate option 3 first as this action would only expose the open wound and underlying tissues to infection. Eliminate options 1 and 4 next. A dry dressing and a dressing soaked with Betadine will irritate the exposed body tissues. Take time now to review emergency care when dehiscence or evisceration occurs if you had difficulty with this question.

LEVEL OF COGNITIVE ABILITY: Application
PHASE OF NURSING PROCESS: Implementation
CLIENT NEEDS: Physiological Integrity
CONTENT AREA: Fundamental Skills
REFERENCE
Potter, P., & Perry, A. (1997). *Fundamentals of nursing: Concepts, process, and practice* (4th ed.). St. Louis: Mosby–Year Book. p. 1422.

19. **4**

RATIONALE: Increasing restlessness noted in a client is a sign that requires continuous and close monitoring, as it could be indicative of a complication such as hemorrhage or shock. Faint bowel sound heard in all four quadrants is a normal occurrence. A negative Homans' sign is also normal. A positive Homans' sign, however, may be indicative of thrombophlebitis. A blood pressure of 120/70 mmHg with a pulse of 90 is a relatively normal sign.

TEST-TAKING STRATEGY: Use the process of elimination. Eliminate options 1, 2, and 3 as these are normal expected findings. If you had difficulty with this question, take time now to review the normal expected postoperative findings and the signs and symptoms of postoperative complications.

LEVEL OF COGNITIVE ABILITY: Comprehension
PHASE OF NURSING PROCESS: Data Collection
CLIENT NEEDS: Physiological Integrity
CONTENT AREA: Fundamental Skills
REFERENCE
Potter, P., & Perry, A. (1997). *Fundamentals of nursing: Concepts, process, and practice* (4th ed.). St. Louis: Mosby–Year Book. pp. 1421–1422.

20. **4**

RATIONALE: The type of planning and instruction required varies with each individual and type of surgery. Specific instructions that the client needs to receive prior to discharge should include wound care, activity restrictions, dietary instructions, postoperative medication instructions, personal hygiene, and follow-up appointments. Turning and deep breathing are taught in the preoperative period.

TEST-TAKING STRATEGY: Use the strategy of selecting the response that is different. Options 1, 2, and 3 refer to information that needs to be taught postoperatively. Option 4 refers to information that should be taught preoperatively. Take time now to review instructions related to discharge teaching both preoperatively and postoperatively if you had difficulty with this question.

LEVEL OF COGNITIVE ABILITY: Application
PHASE OF NURSING PROCESS: Planning
CLIENT NEEDS: Health Promotion and Maintenance
CONTENT AREA: Fundamental Skills
REFERENCE
deWit, S. (1998). *Essentials of medical-surgical nursing* (4th ed.). Philadelphia: W. B. Saunders. pp. 59–60.

BIBLIOGRAPHY

Black, J., & Matassarin-Jacobs, E. (1997). *Medical-surgical nursing: Clinical management for continuity of care* (5th ed.). Philadelphia: W. B. Saunders.

deWit, S. (1998). *Essentials of medical-surgical nursing* (4th ed.). Philadelphia: W. B. Saunders.

Hodgson, B., & Kizior, R. (1999). *Saunders nursing drug handbook 1999.* Philadelphia: W. B. Saunders.

Leahy, J., & Kizilay, P. (1998). *Foundations of nursing practice: A nursing process approach.* Philadelphia: W. B. Saunders.

Luckmann, J. (1997). *Saunders manual of nursing care.* Philadelphia: W. B. Saunders.

Monahan, F., & Neighbors, M. (1998). *Medical-surgical nursing: Foundations for clinical practice* (2nd ed.). Philadelphia: W. B. Saunders.

National Council of State Boards of Nursing (1998). *National Council detailed test plan for the NCLEX-PN examination.* Chicago: Author.

Potter, P., & Perry, A. (1997). *Fundamentals of nursing: Concepts, process, and practice* (4th ed.). St. Louis: Mosby–Year Book.

Tyson, S. (1999). *Gerontological nursing care.* Philadelphia: W. B. Saunders.

CHAPTER 17

Positioning Clients

. . . .

PYRAMID TERMS

Fowler's Position—The client is supine and the head of the bed is elevated to 45 degrees.

Low Fowler's Position (Semi-Fowler's)—The client is supine and the head of the bed is elevated to 30 degrees.

High Fowler's Position—The client is supine and the head of the bed is elevated to 90 degrees.

Lateral (Side-Lying) Position—The client is lying on the side and the head and shoulders are aligned with the hips and the spine and are parallel to the edge of the mattress. The head, neck, and upper arm are supported by a pillow. The lower shoulder is pulled forward slightly and, along with the elbow, flexed at 90 degrees. The legs are flexed or extended. A pillow is placed to support the back.

Lithotomy Position—The client is lying on the back with the hips and knees flexed at right angles and the feet in stirrups.

Prone Position—The client is lying on the abdomen with head turned to the side. The shoulders are abducted and rotated 90 degrees, with arms flexed at the elbows and palms facing downward along the side of the head. The legs are extended and slightly separated. The feet should extend over the bottom of the mattress with the ankles at a 90-degree angle, or be supported at a 90-degree angle with sandbags.

Supine (Dorsal Recumbent) Position—The client is lying on the back. The head and shoulders are usually slightly elevated with a small pillow. The arms and legs are extended, and the legs are slightly abducted.

Sims' Position (Semiprone)—The client is lying on the side with the body turned prone at 45 degrees. The spine is parallel with the mattress, and shoulders and hips are aligned. The face is supported by a small pillow. The lower arm is behind the body, with the shoulder retracted and hyperextended, and the elbow is slightly flexed. The lower leg is extended, with the upper leg flexed at the hip and knee to a 45- to 90-degree angle. The ankles are supported at 90 degrees.

PYRAMID TO SUCCESS

Nursing responsibility includes positioning clients in a safe and appropriate manner to provide safety and comfort. Knowledge regarding the client position required for a certain procedure or condition is important (Fig. 17–1). It is the nurse's responsibility to assist in preventing the development of complications related to an existing condition, prescribed treatment, or medical and surgical procedure. The nurse must review the physician's orders following treatments and procedures regarding client positioning and mobility.

NURSING PROCESS

DATA COLLECTION

Current client condition and prescribed treatments or procedures

General and specific protective measures for the prescribed procedure or treatment

Need for informed consent

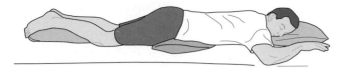
Prone position

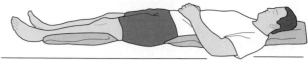
Supine position

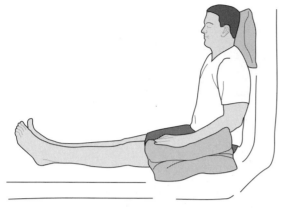
Fowler's position

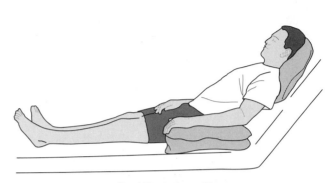
Semi-Fowler's position

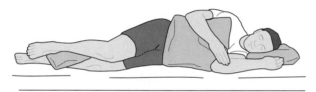
Side-lying position

FIGURE 17–1. Basic positions for patients in bed. (From Lindenman, C. A., & McAthie, M. [1999]. *Fundamentals of contemporary nursing practice*. Philadelphia: W. B. Saunders. p. 507.)

PLANNING
Client will remain free from injury. Client will verbalize comfort control measures. Protective function of the client's skin will be maintained. Client will demonstrate a gradual return to previous level of mobility.

IMPLEMENTATION
Determine status and need for informed consent. Monitor vital signs. Maintain safety measures. Place side rails up and place client's call bell within reach. Turn and reposition client as indicated based on restrictions related to condition. Initiate measures to provide comfort. Provide adequate rest, hydration, and intake as prescribed. Observe dressings and insertion sites for bleeding or signs of infection. Document client status.

EVALUATION
Client remains free of injury. Vital signs remain within normal limits. Interventions employed to provide comfort are effective. Skin integrity remains intact. Prescribed level of activity is maintained.

◆ CLIENT NEEDS

SAFE, EFFECTIVE CARE ENVIRONMENT

Informed consent
Appropriate positioning
Environmental and personal safety
Protective measures
Medical and surgical asepsis

HEALTH PROMOTION AND MAINTENANCE

Techniques of collecting physical data
Instructions regarding the need for prescribed therapies

PSYCHOSOCIAL INTEGRITY

Providing comfort and support to the client
Assisting the client to use coping mechanisms
Keeping the family informed of client progress

PHYSIOLOGICAL INTEGRITY

Using assistive devices
Immobility
Comfort measures for rest and sleep
Providing nutrition and oral intake
Providing personal hygiene as needed
Preventing complications

I. Integumentary System

A. Autograft: following surgery, the site is immobilized for 3 to 7 days to provide the time needed for the graft to adhere and attach to the wound bed

B. Burns of the face and head: elevate the head of the bed to prevent or reduce facial and tracheal edema

C. Circumferential burns of the extremities: elevate the extremities above the level of the heart to prevent or reduce dependent edema

D. Skin graft: elevate and immobilize the graft site to prevent movement and shearing of the graft and disruption of tissue

II. Reproductive System

A. Mastectomy
1. Position the client with the head of the bed elevated at least 30 degrees **(semi-Fowler's)**, with the affected arm elevated on a pillow to promote lymphatic fluid return following the removal of axillary lymph nodes
2. Turn the client only to the back and unaffected side

B. Perineal and vaginal procedures: place the client in the **lithotomy** position

III. Endocrine System

A. Hypophysectomy: elevate the head of the bed to prevent increased intracranial pressure

B. Thyroidectomy
1. Place in the **semi-Fowler's** position to reduce swelling and edema in the neck area
2. Sandbags or pillows may be used to support the client's head or neck

IV. Gastrointestinal System

A. Hemorrhoidectomy: assist the client to a **lateral (side-lying position)** to prevent pain and bleeding

B. Liver biopsy
1. During the procedure: to provide for maximal exposure of the right intercostal space, position the client **supine** with the right side of upper abdomen exposed; the client's right arm is raised and extended over the left shoulder behind the head
2. After the procedure: assist the client into a right **(lateral) side-lying position**; place a small pillow or folded towel under the puncture site for at least 3 hours

C. Intestinal tubes (Miller-Abbott, Cantor, and Harris tubes): following insertion, place the client on the right side to facilitate passage of the tube into the duodenum

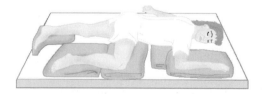

FIGURE 17–2. Sims' position (posterior view). (From Black, J. M., & Matassarin-Jacobs, E. (1997). *Medical-surgical nursing: Clinical management for continuity of care* [5th ed.]. Philadelphia: W. B. Saunders. p. 232.)

D. Nasogastric tube irrigations and tube feedings: elevate the head of the bed 30 degrees **(semi-Fowler's)** to prevent aspiration; maintain head elevation for continuous feedings and for 1 hour after an intermittent feeding

E. Rectal enemas/irrigations: place client in left **Sims'** position to allow the solution to flow by gravity in the natural direction of the colon (Fig. 17–2)

V. Respiratory System

A. Chronic obstructive pulmonary disease: in advanced disease, positioning in a sitting position, leaning forward, with the client's arms over several pillows or an overbed table will assist the client to breathe easier

B. Laryngectomy (radical neck dissection): position the client in the **semi-Fowler's** or **Fowler's position** to maintain a patent airway and minimize edema

C. Pneumonectomy: avoid turning the client onto the operative side. Positioning on the operative side can place increased stress on the bronchial stump and risk disruption of the suture line.

D. Bronchoscopy postprocedure: position the client in a **semi-Fowler's position** to prevent choking or aspiration due to an impaired ability to swallow

E. Postural drainage: the lung segment to be drained should be in the uppermost position

F. Thoracentesis: during the procedure, to facilitate removal of fluid from the chest wall, position the client sitting on the edge of bed leaning over the bedside table, with the feet supported on a stool, or lying in bed on the unaffected side with the head of the bed elevated 45 degrees **(Fowler's)**

VI. Cardiovascular System

A. Abdominal aneurysm resection: following surgery, limit elevation of the head of the bed to 45 degrees **(Fowler's)** to avoid flexion of the graft

B. Amputation of the lower extremity
1. During the first 24 hours after amputation, elevate the foot of the bed (but not the stump itself) to reduce edema, then keep the bed flat to prevent hip flexion contractures
2. When prescribed, the client may be positioned **prone** every 3 to 4 hours for a 20- to 30-minute period to stretch muscles and prevent flexion contractures of the hip
3. In the **prone** position, keep the legs close together to prevent abduction
4. Teach the client to contract the gluteal muscles of the buttocks

C. Arterial vascular grafting of an extremity: to promote graft patency following the procedure, bed rest is maintained for at least 24 hours and the affected extremity is kept straight; limit movement and avoid flexion of the hip and knee

D. Cardiac catheterization
1. Maintain strict bed rest as prescribed, keeping the affected leg straight to prevent arterial occlusion
2. Do not elevate the head of the bed more than 15 degrees
E. Congestive heart failure and pulmonary edema: position the client in **high Fowler's** position to maximize chest expansion and improve oxygenation
F. Peripheral arterial disease: because swelling can prevent arterial blood flow, clients may be advised to elevate their feet at rest, but they should not raise their legs above the level of the heart because extreme elevation slows arterial blood flow to the heart
G. Thrombophlebitis: the client is on bed rest with elevation of the affected extremity; avoid placing a pillow under the knees
H. Vein ligation and stripping: elevate the feet above the level of the heart and instruct the client to avoid leg dangling and chair sitting

VII. Sensory System

A. Cataract surgery
1. Elevate the head of the bed 30 to 45 degrees **(semi-Fowler's** to **Fowler's)**
2. Turn the client to the back or the nonoperative side to prevent the development of edema at the operative site
B. Retinal reattachment
1. If gas or oil has been used to promote retinal reattachment, the client is positioned to allow the gas to float against the retina
2. Most often, the client is positioned on the abdomen, with the head turned to the operative eye so that the client lies with the unaffected eye down
3. This position is maintained for several days until the gas has been absorbed.

VIII. Neurological System

A. Autonomic dysreflexia: elevate the head of the bed to a **high Fowler's** position to assist with adequate ventilation and assist in the prevention of hypertensive stroke
B. Cerebral aneurysm: complete bed rest with the head of the bed elevated 30 to 45 degrees **(semi-Fowler's** to **Fowler's)** to prevent pressure on the aneurysm site
C. Cerebral angiography: maintain bed rest as prescribed; the extremity into which the contrast medium was injected is kept straight and immobilized for approximately the length of the bed rest
D. Cerebrovascular accident (CVA)
1. In clients with hemorrhagic strokes, the head of the bed is elevated to 30 degrees to reduce intracranial pressure (ICP) and to facilitate venous drainage

2. For clients with ischemic strokes, the head of the bed is kept flat
3. Maintain the head in a midline, neutral position to facilitate venous drainage from the head
4. Avoid extreme hip and neck flexion because extreme hip flexion may increase intrathoracic pressure, whereas extreme neck flexion prohibits venous drainage from the brain
E. Craniotomy
1. The client should not be positioned on the operative site, especially if the bone flap has been removed, because the brain has no bony covering on the affected site
2. Elevate the head of the bed 30 to 45 degrees **(semi-Fowler's** to **Fowler's)** and maintain head in a midline, neutral position to facilitate venous drainage from the head
3. Avoid extreme hip and neck flexion
F. Laminectomy
1. Log roll the client by turning the client all at once to keep the back as straight as possible
2. When the client is out of bed, the client's back is kept straight and the client is placed in a straight-backed chair, with the feet resting comfortably on the floor
G. Intracranial pressure
1. Elevate the head of the bed 30 to 45 degrees **(semi-Fowler's** to **Fowler's)** and maintain head in a midline, neutral position to facilitate venous drainage from the head
2. Avoid extreme hip and neck flexion
H. Lumbar puncture
1. During the procedure: assist the client to the **lateral (side-lying) position** with the back bowed at the edge of the examining table, with the knees flexed up to the abdomen, and the head bent so that the chin is resting on the chest
2. After the procedure: place the client in a **prone** position for 4 to 12 hours as prescribed
I. Myelogram postprocedure
1. If water-based iodine solution is used, a sitting position with the head of the bed elevated 30 to 45 **(semi-Fowler's** to **Fowler's)** degrees for an 8- to 16-hour period is maintained to prevent the contrast medium from ascending into the brain; this may be followed by an 8-hour period of a flat-lying **supine** position
2. If an oil-based iodine solution is used, the client is positioned in a flat **supine** position for at least 8 hours to prevent leakage of cerebrospinal fluid (CSF)
J. Spinal cord injury
1. The client is immobilized on a spinal backboard, with the head in a neutral position, to prevent incomplete injury from becoming complete
2. Prevent head flexion, rotation, or extension
3. Maintain traction and alignment of the head by placing the hand on either side of the head near the ears

4. Log roll the client; no part of the body should be twisted or turned nor should the client be allowed to assume a sitting position
5. The head is immobilized with a firm, padded cervical collar

IX. Musculoskeletal System

A. Hip surgery
1. Avoid extreme positions and acute flexion of the operative hip and keep the affected leg abducted
2. Place a pillow between the client's legs to maintain abduction; instruct the client not to cross the legs
3. The physician's orders are checked regarding elevation of the head of the bed
4. Prevent external rotation of the operative leg by placing a trochanter roll beside the external aspect of the thigh, and elevate the heels
5. Turn the client only after checking the physician's orders, because many clients are permitted to turn to the nonoperative side and to the back only

PRACTICE QUESTIONS

1. The client returns to the nursing unit following an above-the-knee amputation of the right leg. The nurse places the client in which of the following most appropriate positions?
   1 Maintains the stump flat on the bed
   2 Elevates the foot of the bed
   3 Reverse Trendelenburg
   4 Prone

2. The nurse is assigned to assist in caring for a client who had an autograft placed on the lower extremity. The nurse plans to
   1 Maintain the surgical extremity in a flat position
   2 Keep the surgical extremity covered with a blanket
   3 Maintain the client in a prone position
   4 Elevate and immobilize the surgical extremity

3. The nurse is assigned to assist in caring for a client following cardiac catheterization. The nurse plans to maintain bed rest with
   1 Head elevation at 45 degrees
   2 Head elevation no greater than 15 degrees
   3 Bathroom privileges only
   4 In semi-Fowler's position

4. The nurse is reinforcing home care instructions to a client and family regarding care following right eye cataract removal. Which of the following statements, if made by the client, indicates effective teaching?
   1 "I will not sleep on my right side."
   2 "I will not sleep on my left side."
   3 "I will take aspirin if I have any pain."
   4 "I will not wear my glasses until my physician says it is OK."

5. Following a liver biopsy, the nurse plans to place the client in which of the following positions?
   1 Supine
   2 Prone
   3 A left side-lying position with a small pillow or folded towel under the puncture site
   4 A right side-lying position with a small pillow or folded towel under the puncture site

6. The nurse is administering a cleansing enema to a client with a fecal impaction. Prior to administering the enema, the nurse positions the client in which of the following positions?
   1 On the left side of the body, with the head of the bed elevated 45 degrees
   2 On the right side of the body, with the head of the bed elevated 45 degrees
   3 Left Sims' position
   4 Right Sims' position

7. The client is being prepared for a thoracentesis. The nurse assigned to care for the client assists the client to which of the following positions for the procedure?
   1 Lying in bed on the affected side, with the head of the bed elevated 45 degrees
   2 Lying in bed on the unaffected side, with the head of the bed elevated 45 degrees
   3 Prone, with the head turned to the side supported by a pillow
   4 Sims' position, with the head of the bed flat

8. The nurse assists the physician with the insertion of a Miller-Abbott tube in a client with a bowel obstruction. Following insertion of the tube, the nurse assigned to care for the client assists the client to which of the following positions?
   1 Prone
   2 Supine
   3 Right side
   4 Left side

9. The client is diagnosed with thrombophlebitis. The nurse tells the client that which of the following is necessary?
   1 Bed rest, with the affected extremity in a dependent position
   2 Bed rest, with bathroom privileges
   3 Bed rest, keeping the affected extremity flat
   4 Bed rest, with elevation of the affected extremity

10. The nurse is assisting in caring for a client following a supratentorial craniotomy. The nurse plans to position the client
    1 Prone
    2 Supine
    3 Semi-Fowler's position
    4 Dorsal recumbent

ANSWERS

1. **2**

RATIONALE: Edema is controlled by elevating the foot of the bed for the first 24 hours after surgery. Following the first 24 hours, the stump is placed flat on the bed to reduce hip contracture.

TEST-TAKING STRATEGY: Note the key words "returns to the nursing unit following." Knowledge regarding positioning of the stump during the first 24 hours and thereafter is required to answer this question. If you had difficulty with this question take time now to review postoperative positioning following amputation.

LEVEL OF COGNITIVE ABILITY: Application
PHASE OF NURSING PROCESS: Implementation
CLIENT NEEDS: Physiological Integrity
CONTENT AREA: Adult Health/Cardiovascular
REFERENCE
deWit, S. (1998). *Essentials of medical surgical nursing* (4th ed.). Philadelphia: W. B. Saunders. pp. 703–704.

2. **4**

RATIONALE: Autografts placed over joints or on lower extremities are often elevated and immobilized following surgery for 3 to 7 days. This period of immobilization allows the autograft time to adhere and attach to the wound bed.

TEST-TAKING STRATEGY: Use the process of elimination. Options 2 and 3 can be eliminated first because both a blanket or a prone position can easily disrupt a graft. Note that option 4 specifically addresses immobilization of the extremity. Review care following an autograft now if you had difficulty with this question.

LEVEL OF COGNITIVE ABILITY: Application
PHASE OF NURSING PROCESS: Planning
CLIENT NEEDS: Physiological Integrity
CONTENT AREA: Adult Health/Integumentary
REFERENCE
deWit, S. (1998). *Essentials of medical-surgical nursing* (4th ed.). Philadelphia: W. B. Saunders. p. 918.

3. **2**

RATIONALE: Following cardiac catheterization, the extremity in which the catheter was inserted is kept straight for the time period as prescribed. The client may turn from side to side. Do not elevate the head of the bed more than 15 degrees, to keep the affected leg straight at the groin and prevent arterial occlusion. Bathroom privileges are not allowed in the immediate postcatheterization period. In the semi-Fowler's position the head of the bed is elevated 30 degrees.

TEST-TAKING STRATEGY: Use the process of elimination. Knowing that the head of the bed should not be elevated greater than 15 degrees will assist in directing you to the correct option. If you had difficulty with this question, take time now to review postcardiac catheterization care.

LEVEL OF COGNITIVE ABILITY: Application
PHASE OF NURSING PROCESS: Planning
CLIENT NEEDS: Physiological Integrity
CONTENT AREA: Adult Health/Cardiovascular
REFERENCE
deWit, S. (1998). *Essentials of medical-surgical nursing* (4th ed.). Philadelphia: W. B. Saunders. p. 543.

4. **1**

RATIONALE: Following cataract surgery, the client should not sleep on the side of the body that was operated on. Clients should be instructed not to take aspirin or medications containing aspirin. Acetaminophen (Tylenol) can be taken as needed for pain. Clients may wear their glasses.

TEST-TAKING STRATEGY: Knowledge regarding postoperative instructions to the client following cataract surgery is required to answer this question. If you can remember to instruct clients to stay off the operative side, this will assist you with answering questions related to cataract surgery. Review care following this type of surgery now if you had difficulty with this question.

LEVEL OF COGNITIVE ABILITY: Comprehension
PHASE OF NURSING PROCESS: Evaluation
CLIENT NEEDS: Health Promotion and Maintenance
CONTENT AREA: Adult Health/Eye
REFERENCE
deWit, S. (1998). *Essentials of medical-surgical nursing* (4th ed.). Philadelphia: W. B. Saunders. pp. 941–942.

5. **4**

RATIONALE: Following a liver biopsy, the client is assisted to assume a right side-lying position with a small pillow or folded towel under the puncture site for at least 3 hours.

TEST-TAKING STRATEGY: Knowledge regarding the anatomy of the body will assist in answering this question. Remember that the liver is on the right side of the body, and that the application of pressure on the right side will minimize the escape of blood or bile through the puncture site. Review care following a liver biopsy now if you had difficulty with this question.

LEVEL OF COGNITIVE ABILITY: Application
PHASE OF NURSING PROCESS: Planning
CLIENT NEEDS: Physiological Integrity
CONTENT AREA: Fundamental Skills
REFERENCE
deWit, S. (1998). *Essentials of medical-surgical nursing* (4th ed.). Philadelphia: W. B. Saunders. p. 646.

6. **3**

RATIONALE: When administering an enema, the client is placed in a left Sims' position so that the enema solution can flow by gravity in the natural direction of the colon. The head of the bed is not elevated.

TEST-TAKING STRATEGY: Knowledge regarding the anatomy of the bowel will assist in answering this question. From this point, you can eliminate options 2 and 4. Option 1 can be eliminated because the head of the bed should be flat during enema administration. Review the procedure for enema administration now if you had difficulty with this question.

LEVEL OF COGNITIVE ABILITY: Application
PHASE OF NURSING PROCESS: Implementation
CLIENT NEEDS: Physiological Integrity
CONTENT AREA: Fundamental Skills
REFERENCE
Leahy, J., & Kizilay, P. (1998). *Foundations of nursing practice: A nursing process approach.* Philadelphia: W. B. Saunders. p. 950.

7. **2**

RATIONALE: To facilitate removal of fluid from the chest wall, position the client sitting on the edge of bed leaning over the bedside table with the feet supported on a stool, or lying in bed on the unaffected side with the head of the bed elevated 45 degrees (Fowler's).
TEST-TAKING STRATEGY: Attempt to visualize this procedure. Option 1 can be eliminated because if the client is lying on the affected side it would be very difficult to perform the procedure. Option 4 can be eliminated because the Sims' position is primarily used for rectal enemas or irrigations. In the prone position, the client is lying on the abdomen, which is not an appropriate position for this procedure. Review this procedure now if you had difficulty with this question.
LEVEL OF COGNITIVE ABILITY: Application
PHASE OF NURSING PROCESS: Implementation
CLIENT NEEDS: Physiological Integrity
CONTENT AREA: Fundamental Skills
REFERENCE
deWit, S. (1998). *Essentials of medical-surgical nursing* (4th ed.). Philadelphia: W. B. Saunders. p. 416.

8. **3**

RATIONALE: The Miller-Abbott tube is a mercury-weighted tube. The weight of the mercury tube carries the tube by gravity. When inserted, it is sometimes difficult to get this intestinal tube to pass through the pylorus. To accomplish this, the client is instructed to lie on the right side.
TEST-TAKING STRATEGY: Knowledge of the anatomy of the gastrointestinal tract and the Miller-Abbott tube will assist in answering this question. Use the process of elimination based on this knowledge. If you had difficulty with this question, take time now to review nursing care related to the client with a Miller-Abbott tube.
LEVEL OF COGNITIVE ABILITY: Application
PHASE OF NURSING PROCESS: Implementation
CLIENT NEEDS: Physiological Integrity
CONTENT AREA: Adult Health/Gastrointestinal
REFERENCE
deWit, S. (1998). *Essentials of medical-surgical nursing* (4th ed.). Philadelphia: W. B. Saunders. p. 623.

9. **4**

RATIONALE: Elevation of the affected leg facilitates blood flow by the force of gravity and also decreases venous pressure that in turn relieves edema and pain. The foot of the bed is elevated and bed rest is indicated to prevent emboli and to prevent pressure fluctuations in the venous system that occur with walking.
TEST-TAKING STRATEGY: Knowledge regarding the pathophysiology related to the venous system will assist in answering this question. Use the process of elimination along with your nursing knowledge. If you had difficulty with this question, take time now to review nursing care for clients with venous disorders.
LEVEL OF COGNITIVE ABILITY: Application
PHASE OF NURSING PROCESS: Implementation
CLIENT NEEDS: Physiological Integrity
CONTENT AREA: Fundamental Skills
REFERENCE
deWit, S. (1998) *Essentials of medical-surgical nursing* (4th ed.). Philadelphia: W. B. Saunders. p. 528.

10. **3**

RATIONALE: In supratentorial surgery (surgery above the brain's tentorium), the client's head is usually elevated 30 degrees to promote venous outflow through the jugular veins. Do not lower the client's head or the head of the bed in the acute phase of care after supratentorial surgery. An exception to this position is the client who has undergone evacuation of a chronic subdural hematoma, but a physician's order is required for an other than head elevation.
TEST-TAKING STRATEGY: This is a difficult question. Knowledge regarding supratentorial surgery and craniotomy is required to answer this question. A pyramid hint: supra, above the brain's tentorium, head up. If you had difficulty with this question, take time now to review positioning following craniotomy surgery.
LEVEL OF COGNITIVE ABILITY: Application
PHASE OF NURSING PROCESS: Planning
CLIENT NEEDS: Physiological Integrity
CONTENT AREA: Adult Health/Neurological
REFERENCE
Monahan, F., & Neighbors, M. (1998). *Medical-surgical nursing: Foundations for clinical practice* (2nd ed.). Philadelphia: W. B Saunders. p. 759.

BIBLIOGRAPHY

deWit, S. (1998). *Essentials of medical-surgical nursing* (4th ed.). Philadelphia: W. B. Saunders.
Leahy, J., & Kizilay, P. (1998). *Foundations of nursing practice: A nursing process approach*. Philadelphia: W. B. Saunders.

Monahan, F., & Neighbors, M. (1998). *Medical-surgical, nursing: Foundations for clinical practice* (2nd ed.). Philadelphia: W. B. Saunders.
National Council of State Boards of Nursing (1998). *National Council detailed test plan for the NCLEX-PN examination*. Chicago: Author.

CHAPTER 18

Care of a Client with a Tube

PYRAMID TERMS

Chest Tube—Returns negative pressure to the intrapleural space; used to remove abnormal accumulations of air and fluids from the pleural space.

Gastrointestinal (GI) Intubation—Refers to the insertion of a tube into the stomach or intestine.

Endotracheal Tube—Used to maintain a patent airway and is indicated when the client needs mechanical ventilation.

Intestinal Tubes—Passed nasally and designed to enter the small intestine through the pyloric sphincter because of the weight of a small bag of mercury at the end of the tube; used to decompress the bowel or to remove intestinal contents.

Miller-Abbott Tube—A double lumen tube passed nasally into the small intestine that is used to decompress the bowel or to remove intestinal contents.

Sengstaken-Blakemore Tube—Triple lumen gastric tube with an inflatable esophageal balloon, an inflatable gastric balloon, and a gastric aspiration lumen; used as a treatment modality for the client with esophageal varices.

Tracheostomy—Artificial opening created into the trachea to establish an airway.

PYRAMID TO SUCCESS

The Pyramid to Success focuses on the common types of tubes used in the clinical setting. NCLEX-PN is likely to address content areas related to the appropriate care of certain tubes, and the immediate interventions required if a complication arises. Focus on the specific data collection points related to the specific type of tube. Review procedures for verifying correct placement of a tube, and procedures for administering medications or feedings through a tube, if appropriate. Pyramid points also focus on interventions associated with complications or emergencies that may occur.

NURSING PROCESS

DATA COLLECTION

Current client condition and prescribed procedures
Status of informed consent as appropriate
Vital signs and respiratory status
Ability to swallow
Skin integrity
Elimination patterns
Mobility restrictions
Level of comfort
Ability to verbally communicate

PLANNING

Client will maintain effective breathing patterns. Client will verbalize any difficulty related to swallowing. Client will be free of infection. Protective function of client's skin will be maintained. Elimination patterns will remain normal. Client will remain free from injury. Client will participate in range of motion exercises. Client will be able to communicate. Client will communicate pain control measures.

IMPLEMENTATION

Determine status of informed consent. Monitor client condition as determined by specific condition and restrictions. Monitor vital signs and respiratory patterns. Monitor ability to swallow. Provide adequate rest, hydration, and intake as determined by condition. Identify the general and specific protective measures for the prescribed procedure or therapy. Observe dressings and insertion sites for bleeding or signs of infection. Monitor skin for redness and signs of breakdown. Monitor elimination patterns. Maintain safety measures as necessary. Place side rails up as required and place client call bell within reach. Turn and reposition client as indicated based on restrictions related to condition. Initiate active and passive range of motion exercises. Initiate measures to provide comfort. Provide the client with methods to communicate. Document status of client's condition.

EVALUATION

Respiratory status remains normal. Vital signs remain within normal limits. Insertion sites on the skin remain free of infection. Skin integrity remains intact. Elimination patterns remain normal. Client remains free of injury. Prescribed level of activity is maintained. Interventions employed to provide comfort are effective. Communication methods are effective.

◆ CLIENT NEEDS

SAFE, EFFECTIVE CARE ENVIRONMENT

Advance directives
Advocacy related to client's concerns
Informed consent for invasive procedure
Client rights
Consultations and referrals as prescribed
Asepsis in administering care
Standard (universal) precautions
Handling infectious materials

HEALTH PROMOTION AND MAINTENANCE

Techniques of collecting physical data
Disease prevention
Lifestyle changes
Client/family instructions regarding care at home

PSYCHOSOCIAL INTEGRITY

Unexpected body image changes
Situational role changes
Support systems

PHYSIOLOGICAL INTEGRITY

Measures to assure basic care and comfort
Nutrition and hydration
Administering medications through a GI tube
Diagnostic tests to confirm accurate placement of tube
Laboratory values
Potential complications associated with the tube
Assisting with emergency interventions for complications

I. Nasogastric (NG) Tubes (Fig. 18–1)

A. Description
   1. Short tubes used to intubate the stomach
   2. Inserted from nose to stomach
B. Types of tubes
   1. Levine
      a. Single-lumen nasogastric tube
      b. Used to remove gastric contents via intermittent suction, or to provide tube feedings

   2. Salem sump
      a. Double-lumen nasogastric tube with an air vent
      b. Used for decompression with continuous suction
      c. Air vent is not to be clamped and is to be kept above the level of the stomach
      d. If leakage occurs through the air vent, instill 30 mL of air into the air vent and irrigate the main lumen with normal saline (NS)
C. Determining placement
   1. Note that the most reliable method to

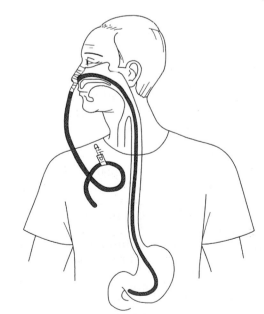

A nasogastric tube is used to aspirate gastric contents or to deliver liquids to the stomach.

FIGURE 18–1. A nasogastric tube is used to aspirate gastric contents or to deliver liquids to the stomach. (From deWit, S. C. [1998]. *Essentials of medical-surgical nursing* [4th ed.]. Philadelphia: W. B. Saunders. p. 622.)

determine placement is by x-ray, which should be performed after initial placement

2. Determine tube placement every 4 hours and before administering feedings or medications

3. Determine tube placement by aspirating gastric contents and measuring the pH, which should be 4 or less (pH values greater than 6 indicate intestinal placement)

4. Inserting 5 to 10 mL of air into the NG tube and listening for the rush of air over stomach with the stethoscope is an alternative method for determining placement, but is not as reliable as an x-ray or checking gastric pH

D. Checking residual

1. Check residual volumes every 4 hours, before each feeding, or before giving medications

2. Aspirate all stomach contents (residual) and measure amount

3. Reinstill residual feeding to prevent excessive fluid and electrolyte losses unless the residual volume appears abnormal

4. Usually if residual is less than 100 to 150 mL, feeding, if prescribed, is administered; if greater than 150 mL, hold the feeding

E. Irrigating

1. Check patency of the tube every 4 hours

2. Check placement before irrigating

3. Gently instill 30 to 50 mL water or NS (depending on agency policy) with irrigation syringe

4. Pull back on syringe plunger to withdraw the fluid to check patency; repeat if the tube remains sluggish

F. Removal of an NG tube: the client is instructed to exhale and the tube is removed with one very smooth continuous pull

II. GI Tube Feedings

A. Tubes
  1. Nasogastric: nose to stomach
  2. Gastrostomy: stomach
  3. Jejunostomy: jejunum

B. Types of administration
  1. Bolus
    a. Resembles normal meal feeding patterns
    b. Approximately 300 to 400 mL of formula is administered over a 30- to 60-minute period every 3 to 6 hours
  2. Continuous
    a. Administered continuously for 24 hours
    b. An infusion pump regulates the flow
  3. Cyclical
    a. Administered either in the daytime or nighttime for 8 to 16 hours
    b. An infusion pump regulates the flow
    c. Feedings at night allow for more freedom during the day

C. Administering feedings
  1. If feedings are prescribed, x-ray confirmation should be done prior to initiating feedings

2. Position the client in high Fowler's or at 30 degrees, and on the right side if comatose

3. Warm the feeding to room temperature to prevent diarrhea and cramps

4. Aspirate all stomach contents (residual), measure amount, and return the contents to the stomach to prevent electrolyte imbalances (unless the residual appears abnormal)

5. Usually if residual is less than 100 to 150 mL, feeding is administered; if greater than 150 mL, hold the feeding

6. Check tube placement by aspirating gastric contents and measuring the pH (should be 4 or less)

7. Check bowel sounds; feeding is held and the physician is notified if bowel sounds are absent

8. Use a feeding pump for continuous or cyclic feedings

9. Flush tubing with water following feeding to maintain fluid balance and patency of tube

10. For bolus feeding, leave client in a high Fowler's position for 30 minutes after feeding

11. For a continuous feeding, keep client in a 30-degree Fowler's position at all times

D. Precautions

1. Change the feeding container and tubing every 24 hours

2. Do not hang more solution than will be required for a 4-hour period to prevent bacterial growth

3. Check the expiration date on the formula prior to administering

4. Shake the formula well prior to inserting it into the container

5. Always check placement of tube prior to feeding

6. Always check bowel sounds, and do not administer any feedings if bowel sounds are absent

7. If an obstruction occurs, try flushing with water, saline, cranberry juice, ginger ale, or cola, if not contraindicated, after checking placement

8. Add a drop of blue food coloring to the feeding as prescribed, particularly with clients who have endotracheal or tracheal tubes

9. Suspect tracheoesophageal fistula when blue gastric contents appear in tracheal excretion, and, if this occurs, the physician is notified immediately

10. Administer the feeding at a prescribed rate, or via gravity flow (intermittent, bolus feedings) with a 60 mL syringe with the plunger removed

11. Gently flush with 30 to 50 mL water or NS (depending on agency policy) with irrigation syringe after feeding

III. Medications Via NG or Gastrostomy Tube

A. Crush medications or use elixir forms of medications

B. Ensure that medication ordered can be crushed or that capsule can be opened

C. Dissolve in 5 to 10 mL of water

D. Check placement and residual prior to instilling medications

E. Draw up the medication into a catheter tip syringe, clear excess air, and insert the medication into the tube

F. Flush with 30 mL of water (depending on agency policy)

G. Clamp the tube for 30 to 60 minutes (depending on medication and agency policy)

IV. Intestinal Tubes

A. Description
1. Passed nasally into the small intestine
2. Used to decompress the bowel or to remove intestinal contents
3. Designed to enter the small intestine through the pyloric sphincter because of the weight of a small bag of mercury at the end

B. Types of tubes
1. Cantor: single-lumen tube with a reservoir for 5 to 10 mL of mercury located at its tip, below the level of the drainage holes
2. **Miller-Abbott tube** (Fig. 18–2)
   a. Double-lumen tube
   b. One lumen is for the instillation of mercury once the tube is in the stomach, and the other for irrigation or drainage

C. Implementation
1. Position the client on the right side to allow the mercury weights within the tube to facilitate passage through the pylorus of the stomach and into the small intestine
2. Do not secure the tube to the client's face with tape until it has reached final placement in the intestines
3. Allow the tube to advance over several hours
4. An x-ray is performed to verify desired placement
5. Monitor drainage from the tube
6. If the tube becomes blocked, the physician is notified (a small amount of air injected into the lumen may be prescribed to clear the tube)
7. Check the abdomen and measure abdominal girth
8. When the tube is removed, dispose the mercury in the appropriate manner per agency policy

V. Esophageal and Gastric Tubes

A. Description
1. Used to apply pressure against esophageal veins to control bleeding
2. Not used if the client has ulceration or necrosis of the esophagus or had previous esophageal surgery

B. **Sengstaken-Blakemore** tube (Fig. 18–3)
1. Triple-lumen gastric tube with an inflatable esophageal balloon, an inflatable gastric balloon, and a gastric aspiration lumen
2. The gastric balloon applies pressure at the cardioesophageal junction to decrease blood flow to esophageal varices, and directly compresses gastric varices; traction is applied to maintain the gastric balloon in place
3. The esophageal balloon directly compresses esophageal varices

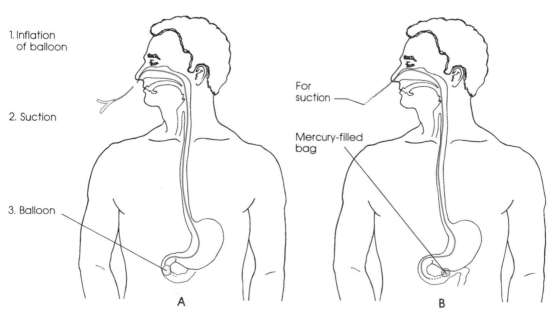

FIGURE 18–2. *A.* Miller-Abbott tube in place. It is advanced through the intestines to the prescribed point. The Miller-Abbott tube has a double lumen. 1, Portion of the metal tip leading to the balloon. 2, Portion of the metal tip leading to the lumen that can be suctioned. 3, Balloon inflated with air. *B,* Cantor tube in place. Intestinal tubes are not taped in place until they have advanced fully. (From deWit, S. C. [1998]. *Essentials of medical-surgical nursing* [4th ed.]. Philadelphia: W. B. Saunders. p. 623.)

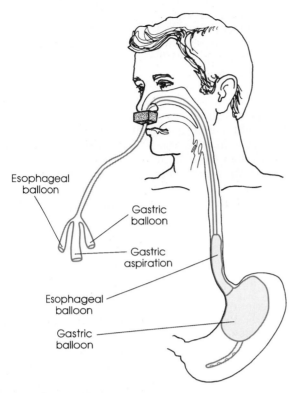

Esophageal
balloon

Gastric
balloon

Gastric
aspiration

Esophageal
balloon

Gastric
balloon

FIGURE 18–3. Sengstaken-Blakemore tube. (From deWit, S. C. [1998]. *Essentials of medical-surgical nursing* [4th ed.]. Philadelphia: W. B. Saunders. p. 606.)

4. An x-ray of upper abdomen and chest confirms placement
5. Gastric contents are aspirated by gastric lavage or intermittent suction via the gastric aspiration port
6. With the **Sengstaken-Blakemore** tube, a nasogastric tube is also inserted in the opposite nares to collect secretions that accumulate above the esophageal balloon
C. Implementation
   1. The patency and integrity of all balloons are checked prior to insertion, and each lumen is labeled
   2. The client is placed in the left lateral or semi-Fowler's position for insertion

3. Prepare the client for an x-ray immediately after insertion to verify placement
4. Maintain head elevation once the tube is in place
5. The balloon ports are double clamped to prevent air leaks
6. Scissors are keep at the bedside at all times
7. The client is monitored for respiratory distress; if it occurs, notify the registered nurse immediately; the tubes will be cut to deflate balloons
8. Monitor for increased bloody drainage that may indicate persistent bleeding
9. Monitor for signs of esophageal rupture that includes a drop in blood pressure, increased heart rate, and back and upper abdominal pain (esophageal rupture is an emergency and must be reported immediately)

VI. Urinary and Renal Tubes (Fig. 18–4)

A. Routine urinary catheter care
   1. Use gloves and wash the perineal area with warm soapy water
   2. With the nondominant hand, pull back the labia or foreskin to expose the meatus (return the foreskin to its normal position)
   3. Cleanse along the catheter with soap and water
   4. Anchor the catheter to the thigh
   5. Maintain the catheter bag below the level of the bladder
B. Ureteral and nephrostomy tubes
   1. Never clamp
   2. Maintain patency
   3. Monitor output closely
   4. Urine output of less than 30 mL/hour or lack of output for more than 15 minutes should be reported immediately

VII. Respiratory System Tubes (Fig. 18–5)

A. Endotracheal tubes
   1. Description
      a. Used to maintain a patent airway
      b. Indicated when the client needs mechanical ventilation

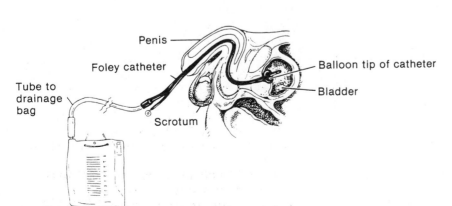

Penis

Foley catheter

Tube to drainage bag

Scrotum

Balloon tip of catheter

Bladder

Drain for emptying container

FIGURE 18–4. Foley (indwelling) catheter drainage system shown in male patient. (From deWit, S. C. [1994]. *Rambo's nursing skills for clinical practice* [4th ed.]. Philadelphia: W. B. Saunders. p.646.)

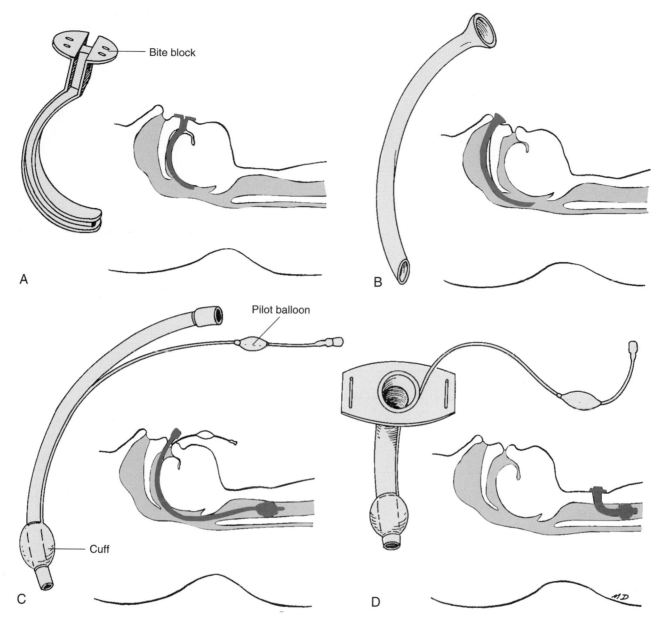

FIGURE 18–5. Artificial airways. *A,* Oral airway; *B,* nasal airway; *C,* endotracheal tube; *D,* tracheostomy tube. Endotracheal tubes have several parts: 15-mm adapter on the proximal end, pilot balloon, radiopaque pilot line, and cuff. All respiratory therapy and anesthesiology equipment is designed to connect with a 15-mm adapter. Consequently, a patient can easily be manually ventilated, mechanically ventilated, or anesthetized via the same endotracheal tube. (From Black, J. M., & Matassarin-Jacobs, E. [eds]. [1993]. *Luckmann and Sorensen's Medical-Surgical Nursing: A Psychophysiologic Approach* [4th ed.]. Philadelphia: W. B. Saunders. p. 963.)

2. Orotracheal
   a. Allows use of a larger-diameter tube and reduces the work of breathing
   b. Indicated when the client has a nasal obstruction or a predisposition to epistaxis
   c. Uncomfortable and can be manipulated by the tongue, causing airway obstruction
3. Nasotracheal
   a. Smaller-sized tube increases resistance and increases the client's work of breathing
   b. Discouraged in clients with bleeding disorders
   c. More comfortable for the client; the client is unable to manipulate with the tongue

4. Implementation
   a. Placement is confirmed by chest x-ray (correct placement is 1 to 2 cm above the carina) and by auscultating both sides of chest while manually ventilating with resuscitation bag
   b. The tube is secured immediately after intubation with adhesive tape
   c. Monitor position of the tube at the lip or nose
   d. Monitor skin and mucous membranes
   e. Suction only when needed
   f. Keep a resuscitation (Ambu) bag at the bedside at all times

g. Cuff inflation is maintained to create a seal and allow for complete mechanical control of respiration

B. **Tracheostomy**
   1. Description: artificial opening created in the trachea to establish an airway
   2. Single cannula tube: has an outer but no inner cannula and is used for clients with a thick neck or on the client when a standard tube will not enter the trachea
   3. Cuffed tube: has an outer and inner cannula, obturator, and cuff
   4. Cuffless tube
      a. Has an outer cannula, an open and a plugged inner cannula, and an obturator
      b. Used for the long term, for evaluating the client's ability to breathe through the upper airway, and for the client no longer at risk for aspiration
   5. Fenestrated tube
      a. Has an opening along the posterior wall of the outer cannula
      b. When the tube is capped, the client can breathe through the upper airway and speak
      c. Cannot be used when the cuff is inflated; the cuff is always deflated before capping the tube
   6. Foam cuffed tube
      a. Cuff is larger than the standard cuffed tube
      b. Is filled with foam, which may apply less pressure to the tracheal mucosa
   7. Jackson metal tube
      a. Has an outer and inner cannula and can be reused after sterilization
      b. Does not have a cuff and is most often used following a permanent **tracheostomy** or laryngectomy
   8. Implementation
      a. Monitor respirations
      b. Monitor pulse oximetry
      c. Encourage coughing and deep breathing
      d. Maintain a semi- to high Fowler's position
      e. Monitor for bleeding, difficulty breathing, and crepitus, which are indications of hemorrhage, pneumothorax, and subcutaneous emphysema
      f. Provide respiratory treatments as prescribed
      g. Suction PRN; hyperoxygenate the client before suctioning
      h. If the client is allowed to eat, sit the client up for meals and for 30 minutes after meals and ensure that the cuff is inflated for meals if the tube is not capped
      i. Assess the stoma and secretions for blood or purulent drainage
      j. Follow the physician's orders and agency policy for cleaning the **tracheostomy** site and inner cannula; usually half-strength hydrogen peroxide is used
      k. Administer humidified oxygen as prescribed, because the normal humidification process is bypassed in a client with a **tracheostomy**
      l. Obtain assistance in changing tracheostomy ties; cut and remove old ties holding the tracheostomy in place
      m. Keep a resuscitation (Ambu) bag, obturator, clamps, and a tracheotomy set at the bedside

VIII. **Chest Tube Drainage System**
   A. Description (Fig. 18–6)
      1. Returns negative pressure to the intrapleural space
      2. Used to remove abnormal accumulations of air and fluids from the pleural space
   B. Collection chamber (Fig. 18–7)
      1. Where the **chest tube** from the client connects to the system
      2. Drainage from the tube drains into and collects in a series of calibrated columns in this chamber
   C. Water seal chamber
      1. Establishes 2 cm of water pressure
      2. If positive pressure is greater than 2 cm, air or fluid is expelled into the drainage system
      3. Allows for air to move from the pleural space into the drainage system but not back into the chest
      4. Water oscillates (moves up as the client inhales and moves down as the client exhales)
      5. Bubbling indicates an air leak from the lung or bronchus
   D. Suction control chamber
      1. Provides the suction, which can be controlled to provide negative pressure to the chest
      2. This chamber is filled with various levels of water to achieve the desired level of suction;

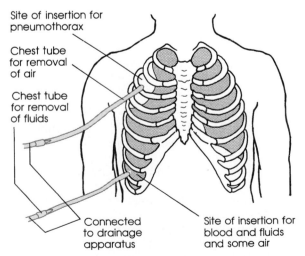

Site of insertion for pneumothorax

Chest tube for removal of air

Chest tube for removal of fluids

Connected to drainage apparatus

Site of insertion for blood and fluids and some air

FIGURE 18–6. Location of sites for insertion of chest tubes for drainage of air and fluids. (From deWit, S. C. [1998]. *Essentials of medical surgical nursing* [4th ed.]. Philadelphia: W. B. Saunders. p. 445.)

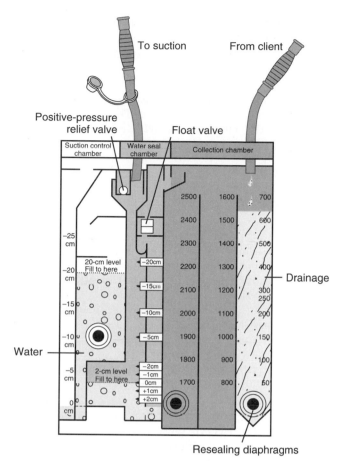

FIGURE 18–7. A commonly used disposable chest drainage system that combines the three bottles into a single device. (Courtesy of Genzyme Surgical Products, Fall River, MA.)

without this control, lung tissue could be sucked into the **chest tube**

3. Bubbling in this chamber indicates that there is suction, and it does not indicate that air is escaping from the pleural space

E. Implementation
   1. An occlusive sterile dressing is maintained at the insertion site
   2. A chest x-ray determines the position of the tube and determines whether the lung has reexpanded
   3. The apparatus and all connections must remain airtight at all times, and all connections must be taped
   4. Keep the drainage system below the level of the chest, free of kinks, dependent loops, or other obstructions
   5. Never pin the tubing to the bedclothes
   6. Do not empty the drainage containers
   7. Keep a clamp and a sterile occlusive dressing at the bedside at all times
   8. Monitor the respiratory status
   9. Monitor for client ease in breathing, pain, level of consciousness and orientation, and anxiety and restlessness
   10. Monitor the entry site for unusual drainage

and the presence of subcutaneous emphysema (crepitus)
   11. Encourage coughing and deep breathing
   12. Change the client's position frequently to promote drainage and ventilation
   13. If the **chest tube** is accidentally removed, immediately cover the opening in the chest with an occlusive petrolatum gauze dressing; notify the physician immediately

F. Conditions requiring immediate attention
   1. Respiratory distress
   2. Persistent bubbling in the underwater seal
   3. Fluid drainage accumulating at a rate of more than 100 mL per hour
   4. The presence of crepitus
   5. Leakage of air around the junctions in the chest tube and drainage tube and disposable drainage device

G. **Chest tube** removal
   1. Medicate the client 30 to 60 minutes before chest tube removal
   2. When the **chest tube** is removed, the physician will ask the client to perform the Valsalva maneuver; an airtight dressing is taped in place after removal of the **chest tube**

PRACTICE QUESTIONS

1. The registered nurse is preparing to insert an NG tube in a client and asks the licensed practical nurse (LPN) to obtain supplies needed for the procedure. Which of the following supplies is not used for this procedure?
   1 One-half-inch tape
   2 Oil-soluble lubricant
   3 A straw
   4 50 mL catheter tip syringe

2. The nurse is checking for correct placement of an NG tube. The nurse aspirates the stomach contents and checks the contents for pH. Which of the following pH values indicates correct placement of the tube?
   1 pH of 7.5
   2 pH of 7.35
   3 pH of 7.0
   4 pH of 4.0

3. The LPN is preparing to assist the RN in removing an NG tube from the client. The LPN plans to instruct the client to do which of the following?
   1 To perform the Valsalva maneuver
   2 To hold the breath
   3 To exhale
   4 To inhale

4. The nurse is preparing to administer medication through an NG tube that is connected to suction. Which of the following indicates the accurate procedure related to the medication administration?

1. Aspirate the NG tube following medication administration to maintain patency
2. Position the client supine to assist in medication absorption
3. Clamp the NG tube for 30 minutes following administration of the medication
4. Change the suction setting to low intermittent suction for 30 minutes after medication administration

5. The nurse assists the physician with the insertion of a Miller-Abbott tube. Following insertion of the tube, the nurse assists the client to which of the following positions?
   1. On the right side
   2. On the left side
   3. Prone
   4. Left lateral Sims'

6. The nurse is assigned to assist in caring for a client with esophageal varices who has a Sengstaken-Blakemore tube inserted. The nurse checks the client's room to ensure that which of the following priority items is at the bedside?
   1. An irrigation set
   2. A pair of scissors
   3. A Kelly clamp
   4. An obturator

7. The nurse is inserting an indwelling urinary catheter into the urethra of a male client. As the nurse inflates the balloon, the client complains of discomfort. The most appropriate nursing action is
   1. Remove the syringe from the balloon; discomfort is normal and temporary
   2. Aspirate the fluid, advance the catheter farther, reinflate the balloon
   3. Aspirate the fluid, withdraw the catheter slightly, reinflate the balloon
   4. Aspirate the fluid, remove the catheter, and insert a new catheter

8. The nurse is inserting an indwelling urinary catheter into a male client. As the catheter is inserted into the urethra, urine begins to flow into the tubing. At this point, the nurse
   1. Immediately inflates the balloon
   2. Withdraws the catheter approximately 1 inch and inflates the balloon
   3. Inserts the catheter until resistance is met and inflates the balloon
   4. Inserts the catheter 2.5 to 5 cm and inflates the balloon

9. The nurse is assigned to assist in caring for a client who has a chest tube. The nurse notes fluctuation of the fluid level in the water seal chamber. Based on this observation, which of the following actions is most appropriate?
   1. Empty the drainage
   2. Encourage the client to deep breathe

3. Continue to monitor as this is an expected finding
4. Encourage the client to periodically hold the breath

10. A nurse is assigned to assist the physician with the removal of a chest tube. The nurse prepares to tell the client to do which of the following during the removal of the chest tube?
    1. Take a deep breath
    2. Hold the breath
    3. Exhale
    4. Perform the Valsalva maneuver

11. A nurse is preparing to change the neck ties on a tracheostomy tube. To perform this procedure, the nurse most appropriately plans to
    1. Remove the old ties, clean the site, and then apply the new ties
    2. Obtain a second health care team member to assist
    3. Call the physician for assistance in changing the ties
    4. Call the respiratory therapy department for assistance in changing the ties

12. The nurse is preparing to begin a continuous tube feeding on a client with a nasogastric tube. The nurse plans to position the client
    1. Supine
    2. Supine on the right side
    3. With the head elevated 15 degrees
    4. With the head elevated 45 degrees

13. The nurse is preparing to administer an intermittent tube feeding to a client with a nasogastric tube. The nurse checks the residual and obtains an amount of 200 mL. The nurse plans to
    1. Administer the feeding
    2. Flush the tubing with 30 mL of water
    3. Hold the feeding
    4. Elevate the head of the bed to 90 degrees and administer the feeding

14. The nurse is preparing to administer a continuous tube feeding to a client with a nasogastric tube. The physician has prescribed an amount of 100 mL per hour. The nurse plans to fill the feeding bag with
    1. 400 mL of formula
    2. 600 mL of formula
    3. 800 mL of formula
    4. Enough formula to last for 8 hours

15. The nurse is preparing to suction a client through a tracheostomy tube. Which of the following is not a component of the plan when performing this procedure?
    1. Moistening the catheter tip in sterile saline solution prior to suctioning

2 Preoxygenating the client prior to suctioning

3 Introducing the catheter into the tracheostomy tube using a sterile gloved hand

4 Placing suction on the catheter while introducing the catheter into the tracheostomy tube

16. The nurse is suctioning a client through a tracheostomy tube. The nurse plans to apply suction during the withdrawal of the catheter for no longer than

1 10 seconds

2 15 seconds

3 20 seconds

4 25 seconds

17. The nurse is told that an assigned client will have a fenestrated tracheostomy tube inserted. The nurse prepares the client for the procedure, knowing that this type of tube

1 Is necessary for mechanical ventilation

2 Enables the client to speak

3 Prevents air from being inhaled through the tracheostomy opening

4 Prevents the client from speaking

18. The nurse is told that an assigned client will have chest tubes removed. In preparation for the procedure, the nurse plans to

1 Clamp the chest tubes

2 Disconnect the drainage system

3 Empty the drainage system

4 Administer pain medication 30 minutes before the procedure

19. The nurse is assisting in developing a plan of care for a client with a chest tube. Which of the following is not a component of the plan?

1 Be sure all connections remain airtight

2 Be sure all connections are taped

3 Pin the tubing to the bedclothes

4 Do not allow the tubing to become kinked or obstructed by the weight of the client

20. The nurse is assigned to care for a client who has a chest tube. The nurse is told to monitor the client for subcutaneous emphysema. The nurse monitors the client for this complication by

1 Monitoring respirations hourly

2 Palpating for leakage of air into the subcutaneous tissues

3 Monitoring for pain

4 Checking the blood pressure every 2 hours

ANSWERS

1. **2**

RATIONALE: Water-soluble lubricant is used to lubricate 3 inches of the tube at the insertion end. An oil lubricant is not used because if the tube accidentally goes into the bronchus, pneumonia can develop. One-half-inch tape is used to secure the tube after correct placement is verified. A 50 mL catheter tip syringe is used to aspirate gastric contents to confirm placement. The client will be asked to take a sip of water through a straw to help with the passage of the tube.

TEST-TAKING STRATEGY: Note the key word "not" in the stem of the question. Remember that water-soluble lubricant must be used to lubricate the tube. If you had difficulty with this question, take time now to review the supplies needed when assisting with inserting an NG tube.

LEVEL OF COGNITIVE ABILITY: Comprehension
PHASE OF NURSING PROCESS: Planning
CLIENT NEEDS: Safe, Effective Care Environment
CONTENT AREA: Adult Health/Gastrointestinal
REFERENCE
Luckmann, J. (1997). *Saunders manual of nursing care.* Philadelphia: W. B. Saunders. p. 1262.

2. **4**

RATIONALE: If the NG tube is in the stomach, the pH of the contents will be acidic. Option 1 indicates an alkaline pH; option 2 indicates a neutral pH; option 3 indicates a slightly acidic pH.

TEST-TAKING STRATEGY: Note the key word "ensure" in the stem of the question. Recalling that gastric contents are acidic will easily direct you to option 4. If you had difficulty with this question, take time now to review the procedure for checking NG tube placement.

LEVEL OF COGNITIVE ABILITY: Comprehension
PHASE OF NURSING PROCESS: Data Collection
CLIENT NEEDS: Physiological Integrity
CONTENT AREA: Adult Health/Gastrointestinal
REFERENCE
deWit, S. (1998). *Essentials of medical-surgical nursing* (4th ed.). Philadelphia: W. B. Saunders. p. 113.

3. **3**

RATIONALE: When a nasogastric tube is removed, the client is instructed to exhale. This will close the epiglottis and allow for easy withdrawal through the esophagus into the nose. The RN removes the tube with one very smooth continuous pull.

TEST-TAKING STRATEGY: Visualize the procedure as a guide in selecting the correct option. Using the process of elimination, consider what each client action identified in the options would produce. Review the procedure for assisting with the removal of an NG tube now if you had difficulty with this question.

LEVEL OF COGNITIVE ABILITY: Application
PHASE OF NURSING PROCESS: Planning
CLIENT NEEDS: Physiological Integrity
CONTENT AREA: Adult Health/Gastrointestinal
REFERENCE
Luckmann, J. (1997). *Saunders manual of nursing care.* Philadelphia: W. B. Saunders. p. 1263.

4. **3**

RATIONALE: If a client has an NG tube connected to suction, the nurse should wait up to 30 minutes before reconnecting the tube to the suction apparatus to allow adequate time for medication absorption. Aspirating the NG tube will remove the medication just administered. Low intermittent suction will also remove the medication just administered. The client should not be placed in the supine position because of the risk for aspiration.
TEST-TAKING STRATEGY: Eliminate options 1 and 4 first because these actions are similar and will produce the same effect. Recalling that the client should not be placed in a supine position will assist in eliminating option 2. If you had difficulty with this question, review the procedure for administering medications through an NG tube.
LEVEL OF COGNITIVE ABILITY: Application
PHASE OF NURSING PROCESS: Implementation
CLIENT NEEDS: Physiological Integrity
CONTENT AREA: Adult Health/Gastrointestinal
REFERENCE
Leahy, J., & Kizilay, P. (1998). *Foundations of nursing practice: A nursing process approach*. Philadelphia: W. B. Saunders. p. 464.

5. **1**

RATIONALE: A Miller-Abbott tube is an intestinal tube that has a double lumen, one for a mercury balloon, and the other for suction or drainage. Following insertion of the tube, the tube is allowed to advance over several hours. The client is positioned on the right side to facilitate passage through the pylorus of the stomach and into the small intestine.
TEST-TAKING STRATEGY: Eliminate options 2 and 4 because they are similar. From the remaining options, recalling the purpose of this tube and the anatomy of the body will assist in directing you to option 1. If you had difficulty with this question, take time now to review care to the client with a Miller-Abbott tube.
LEVEL OF COGNITIVE ABILITY: Application
PHASE OF NURSING PROCESS: Implementation
CLIENT NEEDS: Physiological Integrity
CONTENT AREA: Adult Health/Gastrointestinal
REFERENCE
Luckmann, J. (1997). *Saunders manual of nursing care*. Philadelphia: W. B. Saunders. p. 1263.

6. **2**

RATIONALE: When client has a Sengstaken-Blakemore tube, a pair of scissors must be kept at the client's bedside at all times. The client needs to be observed for sudden respiratory distress, which occurs if the gastric balloon ruptures and the entire tube moves upward. If this occurs, the RN is notified immediately and the balloon lumens will be cut. An obturator and a Kelly clamp is kept at the bedside of a client with a tracheostomy. An irrigation set may be kept at the bedside, but it is not the priority item.
TEST-TAKING STRATEGY: Use knowledge regarding the structure, function, and placement of a Sengstaken-Blakemore tube to answer this question. Note the key word "priority" in the stem of the question. This should assist in eliminating options 1, 3, and 4. If you had difficulty with this question, take time now to review nursing care of a client with a Sengstaken-Blakemore tube.

LEVEL OF COGNITIVE ABILITY: Application
PHASE OF NURSING PROCESS: Implementation
CLIENT NEEDS: Safe, Effective Care Environment
CONTENT AREA: Adult Health/Gastrointestinal
REFERENCE
Monahan, F., & Neighbors, M. (1998). *Medical-surgical nursing: Foundations for clinical practice* (2nd ed.). Philadelphia: W. B. Saunders. p. 1193.

7. **2**

RATIONALE: If the balloon is malpositioned in the urethra, inflating the balloon could produce trauma, and pain will occur. If pain occurs, the fluid should be aspirated and the catheter inserted a little farther in order to provide sufficient space to inflate the balloon. The catheter's balloon is behind the opening at the insertion tip. Inserting the catheter the extra distance will ensure that the balloon is inflated inside the bladder and not in the urethra. There is no need to remove the catheter and insert a new one. Pain when the balloon is inflated is not normal and will not go away.
TEST-TAKING STRATEGY: Visualize the procedure to answer the question. Option 1 is different from the other three options, but can be eliminated since discomfort is neither normal nor temporary when caused by the balloon being inflated. It is not necessary to withdraw the catheter and insert a new catheter. Option 3 will not properly position the balloon in the bladder for safe balloon inflation. Review the procedure for inserting a urinary catheter now if you had difficulty with this question.
LEVEL OF COGNITIVE ABILITY: Application
PHASE OF NURSING PROCESS: Implementation
CLIENT NEEDS: Safe, Effective Care Environment
CONTENT AREA: Adult Health/Renal
REFERENCE
Kozier, B., Erb, G., & Blais, K. (1998). *Fundamentals of nursing: Concepts, process, and practice* (5th ed.). New York: Addison-Wesley. pp. 1256–1257.

8. **4**

RATIONALE: The catheter's balloon is behind the opening at the insertion tip. The catheter is inserted 2.5 to 5 cm after urine begins to flow in order to provide sufficient space to inflate the balloon. Inserting the catheter the extra distance will ensure that the balloon is inflated inside the bladder and not in the urethra. Inflating the balloon in the urethra could produce trauma.
TEST-TAKING STRATEGY: Knowledge of the proper procedure for inserting an indwelling urinary catheter will assist you in answering this question. Note the key phrase "urine begins to flow." Options 2 and 3 can easily be eliminated. Eliminate option 1 next because of the word "immediately." If you had difficulty with this question, take time now to review the procedure for bladder catheterization.
LEVEL OF COGNITIVE ABILITY: Application
PHASE OF NURSING PROCESS: Implementation
CLIENT NEEDS: Safe, Effective Care Environment
CONTENT AREA: Adult Health/Renal
REFERENCE
Kozier, B., Erb, G., & Blais, K. (1998). *Fundamentals of nursing: Concepts, process, and practice* (5th ed.). New York: Addison-Wesley. pp. 1256–1257.

9. **3**

RATIONALE: The presence of fluctuation of the fluid level in the water seal chamber indicates a patent drainage system. With normal breathing, the water level rises with inspiration and falls with expiration. The apparatus and all connections must remain airtight at all times, and the drainage is never emptied. Encouraging the client to deep breathe is unrelated to this observation. The client is not told to hold the breath.

TEST-TAKING STRATEGY: Focusing on the issue of the question, fluctuation of the fluid level in the water seal chamber, will assist in eliminating options 1,2, and 4. If you had difficulty with this question, take time now to review expected and unexpected findings when caring for a client with a chest tube.

LEVEL OF COGNITIVE ABILITY: Comprehension
PHASE OF NURSING PROCESS: Implementation
CLIENT NEEDS: Physiological Integrity
CONTENT AREA: Adult Health/Respiratory
REFERENCE
Monahan, F., & Neighbors, M. (1998). *Medical-surgical nursing: Foundations for clinical practice* (2nd ed.). Philadelphia: W. B. Saunders. p. 578.

10. **4**

RATIONALE: When the chest tube is removed, the client is asked to perform the Valsalva maneuver (take a deep breath, exhale, and bear down), the tube is quickly withdrawn by the physician, and an airtight dressing is taped in place. The pleura seals itself off and the wound heals in less than a week.

TEST-TAKING STRATEGY: Attempt to visualize this procedure to answer the question. Also, note that option 4 is the most global option. If you had difficulty with this question, take time now to review this procedure.

LEVEL OF COGNITIVE ABILITY: Application
PHASE OF NURSING PROCESS: Planning
CLIENT NEEDS: Physiological Integrity
CONTENT AREA: Adult Health/Respiratory
REFERENCE
Monahan, F., & Neighbors, M. (1998). *Medical-surgical nursing: Foundations for clinical practice* (2nd ed.). Philadelphia: W. B. Saunders. p. 579.

11. **2**

RATIONALE: It is best to have two people help change the ties at the tracheostomy. The movement of the tube can easily cause the client to cough and expel the tube from the stoma. Removing the old ties, cleaning the site, then applying the new ties is not appropriate because if the client coughs, the tube could be expelled. This procedure is a nursing procedure; therefore, it is not appropriate to call the physician. The respiratory therapist can assist in changing the ties, but it is not necessary to specifically call the therapist for the procedure.

TEST-TAKING STRATEGY: Visualize this procedure. Eliminate option 1, knowing that this action can present the risk of the tube being expelled if the client coughs. Eliminate option 3 next, knowing that this is a nursing procedure. For the remaining options, select option 2 because it is most global. If you had difficulty with this ques-

tion, take time now to review care to the client with a tracheostomy.

LEVEL OF COGNITIVE ABILITY: Application
PHASE OF NURSING PROCESS: Planning
CLIENT NEEDS: Safe, Effective Care Environment
CONTENT AREA: Adult Health/Respiratory
REFERENCE
Monahan, F., & Neighbors, M. (1998). *Medical-surgical nursing: Foundations for clinical practice* (2nd ed.). Philadelphia: W. B. Saunders. p. 566.

12. **4**

RATIONALE: When a tube feeding is administered, the head of the bed is elevated 30 to 45 degrees to allow gravity to help the flow of formula, to prevent reflux, and to prevent aspiration. Options 1, 2, and 3 are inappropriate positions during a tube feeding.

TEST-TAKING STRATEGY: Use the process of elimination. Eliminate options 1 and 2 first because they are similar. Recalling the risks associated with administering a tube feeding will easily direct you to option 4. If you had difficulty with this question, take time now to review the procedure for administering tube feedings.

LEVEL OF COGNITIVE ABILITY: Application
PHASE OF NURSING PROCESS: Planning
CLIENT NEEDS: Physiological Integrity
CONTENT AREA: Adult Health/Gastrointestinal
REFERENCE
deWit, S. (1998). *Essentials of medical-surgical nursing* (4th ed.). Philadelphia: W. B. Saunders. p. 625.

13. **3**

RATIONALE: When more than 150 mL of residual formula is obtained, the feeding is held and the physician is notified because it is an indication that the feeding is not well tolerated. Elevating the head of the bed to 90 degrees and flushing the tubing are not appropriate actions.

TEST-TAKING STRATEGY: Use knowledge regarding the administration of tube feedings and the process of elimination to answer the question. Eliminate options 1 and 4 first because they are similar. Recalling that the feeding is held when more than 150 mL of residual is obtained will easily direct you to option 3. Review this procedure now if you had difficulty with this question.

LEVEL OF COGNITIVE ABILITY: Application
PHASE OF NURSING PROCESS: Planning
CLIENT NEEDS: Physiological Integrity
CONTENT AREA: Adult Health/Gastrointestinal
REFERENCE
deWit, S. (1998). *Essentials of medical-surgical nursing* (4th ed.). Philadelphia: W. B. Saunders. p. 625.

14. **1**

RATIONALE: Feeding can be hung at room temperature for a period of 4 hours. If 100 mL per hour is prescribed, the nurse fills the feeding bag with a maximum amount of 400 mL. Feedings hung longer than 4 hours at room temperature create the risk of bacterial invasion in the formula.

TEST-TAKING STRATEGY: Recalling that feeding can be hung at room temperature for 4 hours will easily direct you

to option 1. If you had difficulty with this question, take time now to review the procedure for administering tube feedings.
LEVEL OF COGNITIVE ABILITY: Application
PHASE OF NURSING PROCESS: Planning
CLIENT NEEDS: Safe, Effective Care Environment
CONTENT AREA: Adult Health/Gastrointestinal
REFERENCE
dWit, S. (1998). *Essentials of medical-surgical nursing* (4th ed.). Philadelphia: W. B. Saunders. p. 625.

15. **4**

RATIONALE: Suction is not placed on the catheter when the catheter is introduced into the tracheostomy tube. Suction draws out oxygen, and placing suction on the catheter at this time could traumatize tracheal tissue. Options 1, 2, and 3 are appropriate components of the plan of care for suctioning.
TEST-TAKING STRATEGY: Note the key word "not." Attempt to visualize the procedure, recalling the risks associated with this procedure. Review the procedure for suctioning now if you had difficulty with this question.
LEVEL OF COGNITIVE ABILITY: Application
PHASE OF NURSING PROCESS: Planning
CLIENT NEEDS: Physiological Integrity
CONTENT AREA: Adult Health/Respiratory
REFERENCE
deWit, S. (1998). *Essentials of medical-surgical nursing* (4th ed.). Philadelphia: W. B. Saunders. p. 423.

16. **1**

RATIONALE: During suctioning the nurse applies suction during the withdrawal of the catheter for 5 to 10 seconds. Suction applied longer than this can cause hypoxia in the client.
TEST-TAKING STRATEGY: Attempt to visualize this procedure and recall the complications associated with suctioning. Note the key words "no greater than." It is best to select the option that identifies the least amount of time. Review the procedure for suctioning now if you had difficulty with this question.
LEVEL OF COGNITIVE ABILITY: Application
PHASE OF NURSING PROCESS: Planning
CLIENT NEEDS: Physiological Integrity
CONTENT AREA: Adult Health/Respiratory
REFERENCE
deWit, S. (1998). *Essentials of medical-surgical nursing* (4th ed.). Philadelphia: W. B. Saunders. p. 424.

17. **2**

RATIONALE: Fenestrated tubes have a small opening in the outer cannula that allows some air to escape through the larynx. This helps prepare the client for the time when the tracheostomy tube will be removed. A one-way tracheostomy valve box can be fitted into the tube opening. It allows air to be inhaled through the tracheostomy opening, but the valve closes when the client exhales. This diverts the exhaled air through the larynx and enables the client to speak.
TEST-TAKING STRATEGY: Knowledge regarding the design and purpose of a fenestrated tracheostomy tube will easily direct you to option 2. If you are unfamiliar with this type of tube, take time now to review.
LEVEL OF COGNITIVE ABILITY: Comprehension

PHASE OF NURSING PROCESS: Planning
CLIENT NEEDS: Physiological Integrity
CONTENT AREA: Adult Health/Respiratory
REFERENCE
deWit, S. (1998). *Essentials of medical-surgical nursing* (4th ed.). Philadelphia: W. B. Saunders. pp. 456–457.

18. **4**

RATIONALE: Removal of chest tubes can be uncomfortable for a client. The nurse should medicate the client 30 to 60 minutes before the chest tube is removed. Options 1, 2, and 3 are inappropriate actions and are not performed by the nurse.
TEST-TAKING STRATEGY: Use the process of elimination and Maslow's hierarchy of needs theory to answer the question. Option 4 is the only client-centered nursing action and this option addresses physiological integrity. Review care to the client in preparation for chest tube removal now if you had difficulty with this question.
LEVEL OF COGNITIVE ABILITY: Application
PHASE OF NURSING PROCESS: Planning
CLIENT NEEDS: Physiological Integrity
CONTENT AREA: Adult Health/Respiratory
REFERENCE
deWit, S. (1998). *Essentials of medical-surgical nursing* (4th ed.). Philadelphia: W. B. Saunders. p. 446.

19. **3**

RATIONALE: Chest tube tubing is never pinned to bedclothing because is presents the risk of accidental dislodgment of the tube when the client moves. Options 1, 2, and 4 are appropriate interventions in the plan of care for a client with a chest tube.
TEST-TAKING STRATEGY: Note the key word "not" in the stem of the question. Using the process of elimination, recall the complications associated with a chest tube. Review care to the client with a chest tube now if you had difficulty with this question.
LEVEL OF COGNITIVE ABILITY: Application
PHASE OF NURSING PROCESS: Planning
CLIENT NEEDS: Physiological Integrity
CONTENT AREA: Adult Health/Respiratory
REFERENCE
deWit, S. (1998). *Essentials of medical-surgical nursing* (4th ed.). Philadelphia: W. B. Saunders. p. 446.

20. **2**

RATIONALE: Subcutaneous emphysema is also known as crepitus. It presents as a "puffed-up" appearance caused by leakage of air into the subcutaneous tissues. It is monitored by palpating and feels like bubble wrap when palpated. Although options 1, 3, and 4 may be a component of the plan of care for a client with a chest tube, these actions will not identify subcutaneous emphysema.
TEST-TAKING STRATEGY: Note the similarity between the words "subcutaneous emphysema" in the question and "subcutaneous tissues" in the correct option. If you are unfamiliar with this complication, take time now to review.
LEVEL OF COGNITIVE ABILITY: Application
PHASE OF NURSING PROCESS: Implementation
CLIENT NEEDS: Physiological Integrity
CONTENT AREA: Adult Health/Respiratory
REFERENCE
deWit, S. (1998). *Essentials of medical-surgical nursing* (4th ed.). Philadelphia: W. B. Saunders. p. 446.

BIBLIOGRAPHY

deWit, S. (1998). *Essentials of medical-surgical nursing* (4th ed.). Philadelphia: W. B. Saunders.

Kozier, B., Erb, G., & Blais, K. (1998). *Fundamentals of nursing: Concepts, process, and practice* (5th ed.). New York: Addison-Wesley.

Leahy, J., & Kizilay, P. (1998). *Foundations of nursing practice: A nursing process approach*. Philadelphia: W. B. Saunders.

Luckmann, J. (1997). *Saunders manual of nursing care*. Philadelphia: W. B. Saunders.

Monahan, F., & Neighbors, M. (1998). *Medical-surgical nursing: Foundations for clinical practice* (2nd ed.). Philadelphia: W. B. Saunders.

National Council of State Boards of Nursing (1998). *National Council detailed test plan for the NCLEX-PN examination*. Chicago: Author.

UNIT V

··

Growth and Development Across the Life Span

PYRAMID TERMS

Conscious—Includes all experiences that are within an individual's awareness and that the individual is able to control

Ego—One's "sense of self"; provides such functions as problem solving, mobilization of defense mechanisms, reality testing and the capability of functioning independently. The mediator between the id and the superego.

Id—Source of all primitive drives and instincts and is thought of as a reservoir of all psychic energy.

Subconscious—Often called the preconscious and includes experiences, thoughts, feelings, or desires that might not be in the immediate awareness but can be recalled to consciousness; helps repress unpleasant thoughts or feelings.

Superego—Representative of the values, ideals, and moral standards of society.

Unconscious—Memories, feelings, thoughts, or wishes are repressed and are not available to the conscious mind.

PYRAMID TO SUCCESS

Normal growth and development proceeds in an orderly, systematic, and predictable pattern. It provides a basis for identifying an individual's abilities. Understanding the path of growth and development across the life span assists the nurse in identifying appropriate expected human behavior. The Pyramid to Success focuses on the basic concepts of Sigmund Freud's theory of psychosexual development, Jean Piaget's theory of cognitive development, Erik Erikson's psychosocial theory, and Lawrence Kohlberg's theory of moral development.

NURSING PROCESS

DATA COLLECTION

Age
Cultural, religious, and health care beliefs
Family roles and social networks and supports
Development and cognitive levels
Psychosocial and psychosexual behaviors
Moral characteristics

PLANNING

Assist with developing the plan of care based on the unique characteristics of the client, considering the identified stage of development. Include the client and family in the plan of care as appropriate.

IMPLEMENTATION

Identify age-appropriate or altered development of normal skills. Incorporate interventions that are compatible with the client's cultural, religious, and health care beliefs; educational level; and language. Provide care using a nonjudgmental approach. Respect client and family needs based on their preferences.

EVALUATION

Determine compatibility of plan with client and family in meeting needs. Adjust plan of care as appropriate based on meeting expectations and needs.

CLIENT NEEDS

SAFE, EFFECTIVE CARE ENVIRONMENT

Caring
Advocacy
Client rights
Confidentiality
Ethical practice and legal responsibilities
Consultations and referrals

HEALTH PROMOTION AND MAINTENANCE

Aging process
Developmental stages and transitions
Communication
Family planning

Health and wellness
Health care beliefs
Lifestyle choices

PSYCHOSOCIAL INTEGRITY

Communication
Mental health concepts
Coping mechanisms
Cultural heritage
Religious and spiritual influences on health
Support systems

PHYSIOLOGICAL INTEGRITY

Health care preferences
Practices or restrictions related to procedures and
    treatments

BIBLIOGRAPHY

Burroughs, A. (1997). *Maternity nursing: An introductory text* (7th ed.). Philadelphia: W. B. Saunders.

Hill, S., & Howlett, H. (1997). *Success in practical nursing: Personal and vocational issues* (3rd ed.). Philadelphia: W. B. Saunders.

Leahy, J., & Kizilay, P. (1998). *Foundations of nursing practice: A nursing process approach*. Philadelphia: W. B. Saunders.

Leifer, G. (1999). *Thompson's introduction to maternity and pediatric nursing* (3rd ed.). Philadelphia: W. B. Saunders.

Luckmann, J. (1997). *Saunders manual of nursing care*. Philadelphia: W. B. Saunders.

National Council of State Boards of Nursing (1998). *National Council detailed test plan for the NCLEX-PN examination*. Chicago: Author.

O'Toole, M. (1997). *Miller-Keane encyclopedia & dictionary of medicine, nursing, & allied health* (6th ed.). Philadelphia: W. B. Saunders.

Schulte, E., Price, D., & James, S. (1997). *Thompson's pediatric nursing: An introductory text* (7th ed.). Philadelphia: W. B. Saunders.

Varcarolis, E. (1998). *Foundations of psychiatric mental health nursing* (3rd ed.). Philadelphia: W. B. Saunders.

CHAPTER 19

Theories of Growth and Development

I. Psychosocial Development and Erik Erikson

A. The theory
   1. Describes the human life cycle as a series of eight **ego** developmental stages spanning from birth to death
   2. Each stage presents a psychosocial crisis the goal of which is to integrate physical, maturation, and societal demands
   3. Focuses on psychosocial tasks that are accomplished throughout the life cycle
   4. **Ego** development is influenced by family, social, and developmental factors

B. Psychosocial development
   1. A lifelong series of conflicts affected by social and cultural factors
   2. Each conflict must be resolved for the child or adult to progress emotionally
   3. Unsuccessful resolution leaves the individual emotionally handicapped

C. Stages of psychosocial development (Table 19–1)

II. Cognitive Development and Jean Piaget

A. The theory: defines cognitive acts as ways in which the mind organizes and adapts to its environment

B. Stages of cognitive development
   1. Sensorimotor stage
      a. 0 to 2 Years
      b. Development proceeds from reflex activity to imagining and solving problems through the senses and movement
   2. Preoperational stage
      a. 2 to 7 Years
      b. Learning to think in terms of the past, present, and future
      c. The child moves from knowing the world through sensation and movement to prelogical thinking and finding solutions to problems
   3. Concrete operational
      a. 7 to 11 Years
      b. Able to classify, order, and sort facts
      c. The child moves from prelogical thought to solving concrete problems through logic
   4. Formal operations
      a. 11 years to adulthood
      b. Able to think abstractly and logically
      c. Logical thinking is expanded to include solving abstract and concrete problems

III. Moral Development and Lawrence Kohlberg

A. Moral development
   1. A complicated process involving the acceptance of the values and rules of society in a way that shapes behavior
   2. Classified in a series of levels and behaviors

B. Levels of moral development (Box 19–1)

IV. Psychosexual Development and Sigmund Freud

A. Components of the theory
   1. Levels of awareness
   2. Agencies of the mind (**id, ego, superego**)
   3. Concept of anxiety and defense mechanisms
   4. Psychosexual stages of development

B. Levels of awareness
   1. **Conscious** level of awareness
      a. Includes all experiences that are within an individual's awareness and that the individual is able to control
      b. Includes all information that is easily remembered and immediately available to an individual
   2. Preconscious level of awareness
      a. Called the **subconscious**
      b. Includes experiences, thoughts, feelings, or desires that might not be in the immediate awareness but can be recalled to consciousness

Table 19–1. Erik Erikson's Stages of Psychosocial Development

Age	Psychosocial Crisis	Task
Infancy (0–18 months)	Trust versus mistrust	Attachment to the mother

Resolution of Crisis
Trust in people; faith and hope about the environment and the future
Unsuccessful Resolution of Crisis
General difficulties relating to people effectively; suspicion; trust-fear conflict, fear of the future

Age	Psychosocial Crisis	Task
Early childhood (18 months–3 years)	Autonomy versus shame and doubt	Gaining some basic control over self and environment

Resolution of Crisis
Sense of self-control and adequacy; will power
Unsuccessful Resolution of Crisis
Independence-fear conflict; severe feelings of self-doubt

Age	Psychosocial Crisis	Task
Late childhood (3–6 years)	Initiative versus guilt	Becoming purposeful and directive

Resolution of Crisis
Ability to initiate one's own activities; sense of purpose
Unsuccessful Resolution of Crisis
Aggression-fear conflict; sense of inadequacy or guilt

Age	Psychosocial Crisis	Task
School age (6–12 years)	Industry versus inferiority	Developing social, physical, and school skills

Resolution of Crisis
Competence; ability to learn and work
Unsuccessful Resolution of Crisis
Sense of inferiority; difficulty learning and working

Age	Psychosocial Crisis	Task
Adolescence (12–20 years)	Identity versus role confusion	Developing sense of identity

Resolution of Crisis
Sense of personal identity
Unsuccessful Resolution of Crisis
Confusion about who one is; identity submerged in relationships or group memberships

Age	Psychosocial Crisis	Task
Early adulthood (20–35 years)	Intimacy versus isolation	Establishing intimate bonds of love and friendship

Resolution of Crisis
Ability to love deeply and commit oneself
Unsuccessful Resolution of Crisis
Emotional isolation, egocentricity

Age	Psychosocial Crisis	Task
Middle adulthood (35–65 years)	Generativity versus stagnation	Fulfilling life goals that involve family, career, and society

Resolution of Crisis
Ability to give and care for others
Unsuccessful Resolution of Crisis
Self-absorption; inability to grow as a person

Age	Psychosocial Crisis	Task
Later years (65 years to death)	Integrity versus despair	Looking back over one's life and accepting its meaning

Resolution of Crisis
Sense of integrity and fulfillment
Unsuccessful Resolution of Crisis
Dissatisfaction with life

BOX 19-1. Moral Development and Lawrence Kohlberg

LEVEL ONE—PRECONVENTIONAL

Stage 0 (0–2 years)
The infant has no awareness of right or wrong.

Stage 1 (2–3 years)
At this stage children cannot reason as mature members of society.

Children view the world in a selfish way, with no real understanding of right or wrong.

The child obeys rules and demonstrates acceptable behavior to avoid punishment, to avoid displeasing those who are in power, and because he or she fears punishment from a superior force such as a parent.

A toddler typically is at the first substage of the preconventional stage; the toddler makes judgments on the basis of avoiding punishment or obtaining a reward.

Physical punishment and withholding privileges tend to give the toddler a negative view of morals.

Withdrawing love and affection as punishment leads to feelings of guilt in the toddler.

Appropriate discipline includes providing simple explanations of why certain behaviors are unacceptable, praising appropriate behavior, and using distractions when the toddler is headed for danger.

Stage 2 (4–7 years)
The child conforms to rules to obtain rewards or have favors returned.

A preschooler is in the preconventional stage of moral development.

In this stage, conscience emerges and the emphasis is on external control.

LEVEL TWO—CONVENTIONAL
The child conforms to rules to please others.

The child has increased awareness of others' feelings.

A concern for social order begins to emerge.

A child views good behavior as that which those in authority will approve.

If the behavior is not acceptable, the child feels guilty.

Stage 3 (7–10 years)
Conformity occurs to avoid disapproval or dislike by others.

This stage involves living up to what is expected by individuals close to you or what individuals generally expect of others in their role as son, brother, friend, and so on.

Stage 4 (10–12 years)
Child has more concern with society as a whole.

Emphasis is on obeying laws to maintain social order.

The school-aged child is at the conventional level of the role conformity stage and has an increased desire to please others.

The child observes and to some extent internalizes the standards of others.

The child wants to be considered "good" by those individuals whose opinions matter to the child.

LEVEL THREE—POSTCONVENTIONAL
The individual focuses on individual rights and principles of conscience.

The focus is a concern regarding what is best for all.

Stage 5
Being aware that people hold a variety of values and opinions and that most values and rules are relative to the group.

The adolescent in this stage gives as well as takes, and does not expect to get something without paying for it.

Stage 6
This stage involves following self-chosen ethical principles.

The development of the postconventional level of morality occurs in the adolescent at about age 13, marked by the development of an individual conscience and a defined set of moral values.

The adolescent can now acknowledge a conflict between two socially accepted standards and try to decide between them.

---

   c. The **subconscious** can help repress unpleasant thoughts or feelings and can examine and censor certain wishes and thinking
3. **Unconscious** level of awareness
   a. Memories, feelings, thoughts, or wishes are repressed and are not available to the **conscious** mind
   b. These repressed memories, thoughts, or feelings, if made prematurely **conscious,** can cause anxiety
C. Agencies of the mind
  1. **Id, ego** and **superego**
   a. The three systems of personality
   b. In a mature and well-adjusted personality, they work together as a team under the leadership of the **ego**
  2. The **id**
   a. Source of all drives
   b. Is present at birth

   c. Includes genetic inheritance, reflexes, capacities to respond, instincts, basic drives, needs, and wishes that motivate an individual
   d. The **id** does not tolerate uncomfortable states and seeks to discharge the tension and return to a more comfortable constant level of energy
   e. The **id** acts immediately in an impulsive, irrational way and pays no attention to the consequences of its actions, and therefore often behaves in ways harmful to self and others
   f. The "primary" process is a psychological activity in which the **id** attempts to reduce tension
   g. The "primary" process can include hallucinating or forming an image of the object that will satisfy its needs and remove the tension

---

BOX 19–2. Freud's Psychosexual Stages of Development

ORAL STAGE (0–1 years)

During this stage the infant is concerned with his or her own gratification.

The infant is all id, and striving for immediate gratification of needs.

When the infant experiences gratification of basic needs, a sense of trust and security begins.

The ego begins to emerge as the infant begins to see self as separate from the mother; this marks the beginning of the development of a sense of self.

ANAL STAGE (1–3 years)

Toilet training occurs during this period, and the child gains pleasure both from the elimination of the feces and from their retention.

The conflict of this stage is between those demands from society and the parents and the sensations of pleasure associated with the anus.

The child begins to gain a sense of control over instinctive drives and learns to delay immediate gratification to gain a future goal.

PHALLIC STAGE (3–6 years)

The child experiences both pleasurable and conflicting feelings associated with the genital organs.

The pleasures of masturbation and the fantasy life of children set the stage for the Oedipus complex.

The child's unconscious sexual attraction to and wish to possess the parent of the opposite sex, the hostility and desire to remove the parent of the same sex, and the subsequent guilt for these wishes is the conflict the child faces.

The conflict is resolved when the child identifies with the parent of the same sex.

The emergence of the superego is both the solution to and the result of these intense impulses.

LATENCY STAGE (6–12 years)

A tapering off of conscious biological and sexual urges.

The sexual impulses are channeled and elevated into a more culturally accepted level of activity.

Growth of ego functions and the ability to care about and relate to others outside the home is the task of this stage of development.

GENITAL STAGE (12 years and beyond)

Emerges at adolescence with the onset of puberty when the genital organs mature.

The individual gains gratification from his or her own body.

During this stage, the individual develops satisfying sexual and emotional relationships with members of the opposite sex.

The individual plans life goals and gains a strong sense of personal identity.

---

h. The "primary" process by itself is not capable of reducing tension; therefore, a "secondary" psychological process must develop if the individual is to survive; when this occurs, the structure of the second system of the personality, the **ego,** begins to take form

3. The **ego**
   a. The functions of the **ego** include reality testing and problem solving
   b. Begins its development during the fourth or fifth month of life
   c. The **ego** merges out of the **id** and acts as an intermediary between the **id** and the external world
   d. Emerges because the needs, wishes, and demands of the **id** require appropriate exchanges with the outside world of reality
   e. Reality testing is a function of the **ego,** and the **ego** uses realistic thinking

4. The **superego**
   a. A necessary part of socialization that develops during the phallic stage during 3 to 5 years of age
   b. It develops from the interactions with one's parents during the extended period of childhood dependency
   c. It includes the internalization of the values, ideals, and moral standards of society
   d. The **superego** consists of the conscience and the **ego** ideal
   e. The conscience refers to the capacity for self-evaluation and criticism; when moral codes are violated, the conscience punishes the individual by instilling guilt
   f. The **superego** strives for perfection rather than pleasure and represents the ideal rather than the real

D. Anxiety and defense mechanisms
   1. The **ego** develops defenses or defense mechanisms to fight off anxiety
   2. Defense mechanisms operate on an **unconscious** level, except for suppression, so the individual is not aware of their operation
   3. Defense mechanisms deny, falsify, or distort reality to make it less threatening
   4. An individual cannot survive without defense mechanisms; however, if they become too extreme in distorting reality, then interference in healthy adjustment and personal growth may occur

E. Psychosexual stages of development (Box 19–2)
   1. Each stage is associated with a particular conflict that must be resolved before the child can move successfully to the next stage
   2. Experiences during the early stages determines an individual's adjustment patterns and the personality traits that an individual has as an adult

PRACTICE QUESTIONS

1. The nurse is reinforcing instructions to a new mother regarding the psychosocial development of the infant. Using Erikson's psychosocial development theory, the nurse would instruct the mother to
   1 Allow the infant to signal a need
   2 Anticipate all of the needs of the infant
   3 Avoid the infant during the first 10 minutes of crying
   4 Attend to the infant immediately when crying

2. A mother of a 3-year-old tells the nurse that the child is constantly rebelling and having temper tantrums. The most appropriate instruction to the mother is
   1 Punish the child every time the child says "no," to change the behavior
   2 Allow the behavior, because this is normal at this age period
   3 Set limits on the child's behavior
   4 Ignore the child when this behavior occurs

3. The nurse employed in a long-term care facility is caring for a 70-year-old woman. The client reminisces about life experiences in a positive way. The nurse interprets this behavior as
   1 A normal psychosocial response
   2 Requiring a psychiatric consultation
   3 A mental status alteration
   4 A sensory deficit requiring social activities

4. The mother of an 8-year-old child tells the nurse that she is concerned about the child because the child seems to be more attentive to friends than anything else. The most appropriate nursing response is which of the following?
   1 "You need to be concerned."
   2 "You need to monitor the child's behavior closely."
   3 "At this age, the child is developing his or her own personality."
   4 "You need to provide more praise to the child to stop this behavior."

5. The mother of a 4-year-old child tells the nurse that she is concerned because the child has been masturbating. The most appropriate response by the nurse is which of the following?
   1 "The child is very young to begin this behavior and should be brought to the mental health clinic."
   2 "This is not normal behavior and the child should be brought to the mental health clinic."
   3 "This is a normal behavior at this age."
   4 "Children usually begin this behavior at age 8 years."

6. The nursing instructor asks a nursing student to present a clinical conference to peers regarding Freud's psychosexual stages of development, specifically the anal stage. The nursing student prepares for the conference knowing that which of the following most appropriately relates to this stage of development?
   1 This stage is associated with toilet training
   2 This stage is associated with pleasurable and conflicting feelings about the genital organs
   3 This stage is characterized by a tapering-off of conscious biological and sexual urges
   4 This stage is characterized by the gratification of self

7. A mother of a 5-year-old child tells the nurse that the child scolds the floor or a table if the child hurts herself on the object. According to Piaget's theory of cognitive development, this behavior is identified as
   1 Object permanence
   2 Egocentric speech
   3 Animism
   4 Global organization

8. A nursing instructor asks the nursing student to describe the formal operations stage of Piaget's cognitive developmental theory. The most appropriate response by the nursing student is
   1 "The child has the ability to think abstractly."
   2 "The child develops logical thought patterns."
   3 "The child has difficulty separating fantasy from reality."
   4 "The child begins to understand the environment."

9. According to Kohlberg's theory of moral development, in the preconventional level, moral development is thought to be motivated by which of the following?
   1 The parent's behavior
   2 Peer pressure
   3 Social pressures
   4 Punishment and reward

10. The nursing instructor asks the nursing student about the theories of growth and development. The student responds knowing that which of the following is not a component of Kohlberg's theory of moral development?
   1 Moral development progresses in relationship to cognitive development
   2 Individuals move through all six stages in a sequential fashion
   3 It provides a framework for understanding how individuals determine a moral code to guide their behavior
   4 A person's ability to make moral judgments develops over time

ANSWERS

1. 1

RATIONALE: According to Erikson, the caregiver should not try to anticipate the infant's needs at all times but must allow the infant to signal needs. If an infant is not allowed to signal a need, he or she will not learn how to control the environment. Erikson believed that a delayed or prolonged response to an infant's signal would inhibit the development of trust and lead to mistrust of others.

TEST-TAKING STRATEGY: Eliminate options 3 and 4 first because of the words "avoid" and "immediately." Additionally, option 2 can be eliminated because of the absolute term "all."

LEVEL OF COGNITIVE ABILITY: Application
PHASE OF NURSING PROCESS: Implementation
CLIENT NEEDS: Psychosocial Integrity
CONTENT AREA: Child Health
REFERENCE

Leahy, J., & Kizilay, P. (1998). *Foundations of nursing practice: A nursing process approach.* Philadelphia: W. B. Saunders. p. 264.

2. 3

RATIONALE: According to Erikson, the child focuses on independence between ages 1 and 3 years. Gaining independence often means that the child has to rebel against the parents' wishes. Saying things like "no" or "mine" and having temper tantrums are common during this period of development. Being consistent and setting limits on the child's behavior are necessary elements.

TEST-TAKING STRATEGY: Options 2 and 4 can be eliminated first because they are similar. Eliminate option 1 because this action is likely to produce a negative response during this normal developmental pattern. Review psychosocial development of the toddler according to Erikson now if you had difficulty with this question.

LEVEL OF COGNITIVE ABILITY: Application
PHASE OF NURSING PROCESS: Implementation
CLIENT NEEDS: Psychosocial Integrity
CONTENT AREA: Child Health
REFERENCE

Leahy, J., & Kizilay, P. (1998). *Foundations of nursing practice: A nursing process approach.* Philadelphia: W. B. Saunders. p. 264.

3. 1

RATIONALE: According to Erikson, the later years are 65 years to death. The adult reminisces about life experiences, viewing them in a positive way. The adult needs to feel good about accomplishments, see successes in life, and feel that he or she has made a contribution to society.

TEST-TAKING STRATEGY: Use knowledge regarding Erikson's theory of psychosocial development of late adulthood to answer the question. Note the similarity in options 2, 3, and 4. Review psychosocial development now if you had difficulty with this question.

LEVEL OF COGNITIVE ABILITY: Comprehension
PHASE OF NURSING PROCESS: Data Collection
CLIENT NEEDS: Psychosocial Integrity
CONTENT AREA: Fundamental Skills
REFERENCE

Varcarolis, E. (1998). *Foundations of psychiatric mental health nursing* (3rd ed.). Philadelphia: W. B. Saunders. p. 44.

4. 3

RATIONALE: According to Erikson, during middle childhood (ages 7–12 years), the child begins to move for support toward peers and friends and away from the parents. The child also begins to develop special interests that reflect his or her own developing personality instead of the parents'.

TEST-TAKING STRATEGY: Use Erikson's psychosocial development theory related to middle childhood to answer the question. Options 1 and 2 can be easily eliminated first. Eliminate option 4 next because, although praising the child for accomplishments is important at this age, the behavior that the child is exhibiting is normal.

LEVEL OF COGNITIVE ABILITY: Comprehension
PHASE OF NURSING PROCESS: Implementation
CLIENT NEEDS: Psychosocial Integrity
CONTENT AREA: Child Health
REFERENCE

Varcarolis, E. (1998). *Foundations of psychiatric mental health nursing* (3rd ed.). Philadelphia: W. B. Saunders, p. 44.

5. 3

RATIONALE: According to Freud's psychosexual stages of development, between the ages of 3 and 6 years the child is in the phallic stage. At this time, the child devotes much energy to examining the genitalia, masturbating, and expressing interest in sexual concerns.

TEST-TAKING STRATEGY: Eliminate options 1 and 2 because they are similar. Using Freud's psychosexual stages of development will easily direct you to option 3. If you had difficulty with this question, take time now to review Freud's psychosocial stages of development.

LEVEL OF COGNITIVE ABILITY: Comprehension
PHASE OF NURSING PROCESS: Implementation
CLIENT NEEDS: Psychosocial Integrity
CONTENT AREA: Child Health
REFERENCE

Varcarolis, E. (1998). *Foundations of psychiatric mental health nursing* (3rd ed.). Philadelphia: W. B. Saunders. p. 40.

6. 1

RATIONALE: Generally, toilet training occurs during this period. According to Freud, the child gains pleasure both from the elimination of feces and from their retention. Option 2 relates to the phallic stage. Option 3 relates to the latency period. Option 4 relates to the oral stage.

TEST-TAKING STRATEGY: Note the relationship between the words "anal" in the question and "toilet training" in the correct option. If you had difficulty with this question, take time now to review Freud's psychosocial stages of development.

LEVEL OF COGNITIVE ABILITY: Comprehension
PHASE OF NURSING PROCESS: Planning
CLIENT NEEDS: Psychosocial Integrity
CONTENT AREA: Child Health
REFERENCE

Varcarolis, E. (1998). *Foundations of psychiatric mental health nursing* (3rd ed.). Philadelphia: W. B. Saunders, pp. 40–42.

7. 3

RATIONALE: Animism means that all inanimate objects are given living meaning. Object permanence, the realization that something out of sight still exists, occurs in the later stages of the sensorimotor stage of development. Egocentric speech occurs when the child talks just for fun and cannot see another's point of view. Global organization means that if any part of an object or situation changes, the whole thing has changed. Options 2 and 4 occur during the preoperational stage.

TEST-TAKING STRATEGY: This is a difficult question. Attempt to make a relationship with the behavior identified in the question and the correct option. This will easily direct you to option 3. If you had difficulty with this question, take time to review the concepts of Piaget's theory of cognitive development.

LEVEL OF COGNITIVE ABILITY: Analysis
PHASE OF NURSING PROCESS: Data Collection
CLIENT NEEDS: Psychosocial Integrity
CONTENT AREA: Child Health
REFERENCE

Leahy, J., & Kizilay, P. (1998). *Foundations of nursing practice: A nursing process approach.* Philadelphia: W. B. Saunders. pp. 266–267.

8. 1

RATIONALE: In the formal operation stage, the child has the ability to think abstractly and solve hypotheses. Option 2 identifies the concrete operations stage. Option 3 identifies the preoperational stage. Option 4 identifies the sensorimotor stage.

TEST-TAKING STRATEGY: Knowledge regarding the characteristics of Piaget's cognitive developmental theory is required to answer this question. If you had difficulty with this question, review these concepts.

LEVEL OF COGNITIVE ABILITY: Comprehension
PHASE OF NURSING PROCESS: Implementation
CLIENT NEEDS: Psychosocial Integrity
CONTENT AREA: Child Health
REFERENCE

Leahy, J., & Kizilay, P. (1998). *Foundations of nursing practice: A nursing process approach.* Philadelphia: W. B. Saunders, p. 268.

9. 4

RATIONALE: In the preconventional stage, morals are thought to be motivated by punishment and reward. If the child is obedient and is not punished, then he or she is being moral. The child sees actions as either good or bad. If the child's actions are good, the child is praised. If the child's actions are bad, the child is punished.

TEST-TAKING STRATEGY: Eliminate options 2 and 3 because they are similar. Knowledge that the preconventional stage occurs between the ages of 2 and 7 years will assist in directing you to option 4. If you had difficulty with this question, take time now to review Kohlberg's theory of moral development.

LEVEL OF COGNITIVE ABILITY: Comprehension
PHASE OF NURSING PROCESS: Data Collection
CLIENT NEEDS: Psychosocial Integrity
CONTENT AREA: Child Health
REFERENCE

Leahy, J., & Kizilay, P. (1998). *Foundations of nursing practice: A nursing process approach.* Philadelphia: W. B. Saunders. p. 268.

10. 2

RATIONALE: Kohlberg's theory states that individuals move through the stages of development in a sequential fashion but that not everyone reaches stages 5 and 6 in their development of personal morality. Options 1, 3, and 4 are correct statements regarding Kohlberg's theory.

TEST-TAKING STRATEGY: Note the key word "not." Also, note the absolute word "all" in option 2. If you had difficulty with this question, take time now to review Kohlberg's theory.

LEVEL OF COGNITIVE ABILITY: Comprehension
PHASE OF NURSING PROCESS: Implementation
CLIENT NEEDS: Psychosocial Integrity
CONTENT AREA: Fundamental Skills
REFERENCE

Leahy, J., & Kizilay, P. (1998). *Foundations of nursing practice: A nursing process approach.* Philadelphia: W. B. Saunders. p. 268.

BIBLIOGRAPHY

Burroughs, A. (1997). *Maternity nursing: An introductory text* (7th ed.). Philadelphia: W. B. Saunders.

Leahy, J., & Kizilay, P. (1998). *Foundations of nursing practice: A nursing process approach.* Philadelphia: W. B. Saunders.

Leifer, G. (1999). *Thompson's introduction to maternity and pediatric nursing* (3rd ed.). Philadelphia: W. B. Saunders.

Luckmann, J. (1997). *Saunders manual of nursing care.* Philadelphia: W. B. Saunders.

O'Toole, M. (1997). *Miller-Keane encyclopedia & dictionary of medicine, nursing, & allied health* (6th ed.). Philadelphia: W. B. Saunders.

Schulte, E., Price, D., & James, S. (1997). *Thompson's pediatric nursing: An introductory text* (7th ed.). Philadelphia: W. B. Saunders.

Varcarolis, E. (1998). *Foundations of psychiatric mental health nursing* (3rd ed.). Philadelphia: W. B. Saunders.

UNIT VI

....

Maternity Nursing

PYRAMID TERMS

Amniotic Fluid—Fluid that surrounds and protects the fetus; consists of 500 to 1000 mL in amount by the end of pregnancy. The fetus floats in the amniotic fluid, which serves as a cushion against injury from sudden blows or movements and helps maintain a constant body temperature for the fetus.

Ballottement—Rebounding of the fetus against the examiner's finger on palpation. When the cervix is tapped, the fetus floats upward in the amniotic fluid. A rebound is felt by the examiner when the fetus falls back.

Chadwick's Sign—Bluish coloration of the mucous membranes of cervix, vagina, and vulva.

Delivery—Actual event of birth; the expulsion or extraction of the neonate and fetal membranes at birth.

Fertilization—Takes place when sperm and ovum unite. Occurs within 12 hours of ovulation and within 2 to 3 days of insemination, the average duration of viability for the ovum and sperm.

Goodell's Sign—Softening of the cervix; occurs at the beginning of the second month of gestation and is a probable sign of pregnancy.

Gravida—A pregnant woman; called gravida I (primigravida) during the first pregnancy, gravida II (secundigravida) during the second, and so on.

Hegar's Sign—Compressibility and softening of the lower uterine segment; occurs at about week 6 of gestation; a probable sign of pregnancy.

Implantation—Zygote propels toward the uterus and implants in the uterine wall 6 to 8 days after ovulation.

Infant—A baby born alive; also from 28 days of age until the first birthday.

Labor—Coordinated sequence of involuntary uterine contractions resulting in effacement and dilation of the cervix, followed by expulsion of the products of conception.

Lochia—Discharge from the uterus that consists of blood from the vessels of the placental site and debris from the decidua.

Nagele's Rule—Determines the estimated date of confinement (EDC). Add 7 days to the first day of last menstrual period (LMP). Subtract 3 months and add 1 year.

Neonate—A human offspring from the time of birth to the 28th day of life; also called a newborn.

Newborn—A human offspring from the time of birth to the 28th day of life; also called a neonate.

Parity—The number of pregnancies that have been carried to viability.

Placenta—Provides for the exchange of nutrients and waste products between the fetus and mother. Develops by the third month of gestation; also called afterbirth.

Quickening—First perception of fetal movement appearing usually in the 16th to 18th week of pregnancy.

◆ PYRAMID TO SUCCESS

The Pyramid to Success focuses on the physiological and psychosocial aspects related to the experience of pregnancy. Pyramid points begin with instructing the pregnant client in measures that will promote a healthy environment for both the mother and fetus. Focus on the importance of antenatal follow-up, nutrition, and the interventions for common discomforts that occur during pregnancy. Review the purpose of the commonly prescribed diagnostic tests and procedures in the antenatal period. Focus on disorders that can occur during pregnancy, particularly pregnancy-induced hypertension (PIH) and diabetes. Review the labor and delivery process and the immediate interventions when the mother or fetal status is compromised, such as a prolapsed cord or an altered fetal heart rate. Review fetal effects from the mother with AIDS or the substance abuse mother. Focus on the normal expectations of the postpartum period and the complications that can occur. Pyramid points also focus on the normal physical assessment findings in the newborn and the early identification of disorders in the newborn.

NURSING PROCESS

DATA COLLECTION

- Vital signs, weight, and height
- Nutritional status
- Gestation status
- Gravidity and parity
- Signs of pregnancy
- Physiological changes associated with the pregnancy
- Psychological changes associated with the pregnancy
- Risk factors or concerns related to the pregnancy
- Laboratory and diagnostic studies
- Available support systems
- Need for support and referral to community agencies

PLANNING	IMPLEMENTATION	EVALUATION
Client verbalizes nutritional requirements of pregnancy. Client gains weight appropriate for size and pregnancy.	Instruct client on nutritional needs and requirements. Monitor weight. Monitor nutritional status and weight at each prenatal visit. Consider religious and cultural considerations when planning care.	Client maintains adequate nutritional status during pregnancy.
Client verbalizes the physiological and psychological changes that may occur. Client verbalizes the discomforts that may occur and the appropriate treatments.	Inform client of the physiological and psychological changes that may occur. Monitor for physiological and psychological changes. Inform client of the discomforts that may occur and the treatments. Inquire regarding existing discomforts.	Client obtains relief from treatments implemented for discomforts. Vital signs remain within normal limits.
Client identifies risks associated with pregnancy and the conditions necessitating notifying the physician. Client verbalizes the need for and the procedure for any scheduled diagnostic tests or procedures. Client verbalizes the need for community resources if necessary.	Instruct client on the need for and plan for prenatal visits. Instruct client about any scheduled diagnostic tests or procedures. Instruct client regarding the need to and when to notify the physician. Support and encourage the use of community resources.	Client verbalizes the schedule for prenatal visits. Client complies with schedule for prenatal visits. Client notifies the physician appropriately. Client prepares adequately for scheduled diagnostic tests or procedures. Client uses community resources as necessary.
Parent(s) verbalize confidence in the care of the newborn and the parenting role. Parent(s) demonstrate nurturing behaviors toward the newborn.	Assist client to identify parenting skills. Encourage expression of feelings regarding parenting role. Plan to assist parents in developing parenting skills. Encourage bonding and frequent opportunities for newborn-parent interaction. Reinforce instructions and demonstrate care measures for the newborn. Allow ample opportunity for the parents to demonstrate care to the newborn. Assist with follow-up via a telephone call after discharge or assist with initiating support services for home as appropriate.	Parent(s) demonstrate bonding with the newborn. Parent(s) demonstrate appropriate infant care techniques. Parent(s) use support services as needed.

PLANNING	IMPLEMENTATION	EVALUATION
Parent(s) verbalize coping patterns. Parent(s) verbalize expected changes in family role.	Encourage parental interaction with the newborn. Encourage parent(s) to verbalize feelings related to entry of new family member into the home. Note status of feelings of siblings, if appropriate, regarding potential role changes.	Parent(s) identify role changes. Parent(s) and family members acknowledge change in family roles.

◤ CLIENT NEEDS

SAFE, EFFECTIVE CARE ENVIRONMENT

Parent rights
Confidentiality
Informed consent for procedures
Continuity of care
Handling infectious materials
Standard (universal) precautions when delivering care
Asepsis

HEALTH PROMOTION AND MAINTENANCE

Reproduction and human sexuality
Antenatal, intrapartum, and postpartum care
Expected body image changes
Family interaction patterns
Family planning
Health and wellness
Growth and development and health care screening
Lifestyle choices

PSYCHOSOCIAL INTEGRITY

Communication
Cultural and religious influences regarding birth and motherhood
Coping mechanisms
Role changes
Support systems

PHYSIOLOGICAL INTEGRITY

Alterations in body systems
Normal expectations during pregnancy
Physiological changes that occur during pregnancy
Nutrition
Labor and delivery process
Commonly prescribed diagnostic tests and procedures
Risk identification during the pregnancy
Interventions for unexpected events during the pregnancy

BIBLIOGRAPHY

Burroughs, A. (1997). *Maternity nursing: An introductory text* (7th ed.). Philadelphia: W. B. Saunders.

Cox, H., Hinz, M., & Lubno, M., et al. (1997). *Clinical applications of nursing diagnosis: Adult, child, women's, psychiatric, gerontic, and home health considerations* (3rd ed.). Philadelphia: F. A. Davis.

Hill, S., & Howlett, H. (1997). *Success in practical nursing: Personal and vocational issues* (3rd ed.). Philadelphia: W. B. Saunders.

Leifer, G. (1999). *Thompson's introduction to maternity and pediatric nursing* (3rd ed.). Philadelphia: W. B. Saunders.

Luckmann, J. (1997). *Saunders manual of nursing care*. Philadelphia: W. B. Saunders.

National Council of State Boards of Nursing (1997). *National Council detailed test plan for the NCLEX-PN examination*. Chicago: Author.

O'Toole, M. (ed.). (1997). *Miller-Keane encyclopedia & dictionary of medicine, nursing, & allied health* (6th ed.). Philadelphia: W. B. Saunders.

Schulte, E., Price, D., & James, S. (1997). *Thompson's pediatric nursing: An introductory text* (7th ed.). Philadelphia: W. B. Saunders.

CHAPTER 20

Female Reproductive System

. . . .

I. Organs

A. Ovaries
   1. Formation and expulsion of ova
   2. Secrete estrogen and progesterone
B. Fallopian Tube
   1. Muscular tubes (oviducts) approximate to the ovaries and connect to the uterus
   2. Propel the ova from the ovaries to the uterus
C. Uterus
   1. Organ in which the fetus develops
   2. Organ from which menstruation occurs
D. Cervix
   1. Internal os opens into the body of the uterine cavity
   2. Cervical canal is located between internal os and external os
   3. External os opens into the vagina
E. Vagina
   1. Passageway for menstrual blood
   2. Organ of copulation
   3. Passageway for fetus

II. Menstrual Cycle (Table 20–1)

A. Ovarian hormones
   1. Includes the follicle-stimulating hormone (FSH) and luteinizing hormone (LH)
   2. Released by the anterior pituitary gland
   3. Produce changes in the ovaries
   4. Secretion of ovarian hormones leads to changes in the endometrium
   5. Menstrual cycle—the regularly recurring physiological changes in the endometrium that culminate in its shedding—may vary in length, with the average length of approximately 28 days
B. Ovarian changes
   1. Preovulatory phase
   2. Luteal phase
C. Uterine changes
   1. Menstrual phase

2. Proliferative phase
3. Secretory phase

III. Female Pelvis and Measurements

A. True pelvis
   1. Lies below the pelvic brim
   2. Consists of pelvic inlet, midpelvis, and pelvic outlet
B. False pelvis
   1. Shallow portion above the pelvic brim
   2. Supports the abdominal viscera
C. Types of pelvis (Fig. 20–1)
   1. Gynecoid
      a. Normal female pelvis
      b. Transversely rounded or blunt
      c. Most favorable for successful labor and birth
   2. Android
      a. Wedge-shaped or angulated
      b. Seen in males
      c. Not favorable for labor
      d. Narrow pelvic planes can cause slow descent and midpelvis arrest
   3. Anthropoid
      a. Oval-shaped
      b. The outlet is adequate, with a normal or moderately narrow pubic arch
   4. Platypelloid
      a. Flat-shaped with an oval inlet
      b. Transverse diameter is wide but anteroposterior diameter is short, making the outlet inadequate
D. Pelvic measurements
   1. Diagonal conjugate
      a. Distance between sacral promontory and lower margin of symphysis pubis
      b. Greater than 11.5 cm is adequate
   2. True conjugate, or conjugate vera
      a. Distance from upper margin of symphysis to sacral promontory

Table 20–1. **Menstrual Cycle**

Ovarian Changes	
Pre-Ovulatory Phase	*Luteal Phase*
The hypothalamus releases gonadotropin-releasing hormone (GnRH) through the portal system to the anterior pituitary system Secretion of FSH by the anterior lobe of the pituitary gland stimulates growth of follicles Most follicles die, leaving one to mature into a large graafian follicle Estrogen produced by the follicle stimulates increased secretions of LH by the anterior lobe of the pituitary gland The follicle ruptures and releases an ovum into the peritoneal cavity	Begins with ovulation Body temperature drops and then rises by 0.5° to 1°F around the time of ovulation Corpus luteum is formed from follicle cells that remain in the ovary following ovulation Corpus luteum secretes estrogen and progesterone during remaining 14 days of the cycle Corpus luteum degenerates if the ovum is not fertilized, and secretion of estrogen and progesterone declines Estrogen and progesterone inhibit secretions of FSH and LH Once corpus luteum degenerates pituitary secretion of estrogen and progesterone decreases and ovarian cycle begins again

Uterine Changes		
Menstrual Phase	*Proliferative Phase*	*Secretory Phase*
Consists of 4 to 6 days of bleeding as the endometrium breaks down owing to the decreased amount of estrogen and progesterone FSH rises, enabling the beginning of a new cycle	Estrogen stimulates proliferation and growth of the endometrium This phase lasts about 9 days As estrogen increases it suppresses secretion of FSH and increases the secretion of LH LH stimulates ovulation and the development of the corpus luteum Ovulation occurs between day 12 and day 16 Estrogen is high and progesterone is low	This phase lasts about 12 days Follows ovulation Initiated in response to the increase of LH Graafian follicle replaced by corpus luteum Corpus luteum secretes progesterone and estrogen Progesterone prepares the endometrium for pregnancy should a fertilized ovum be implanted

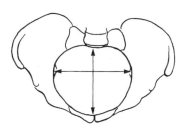

Gynecoid

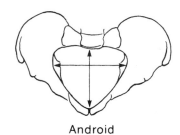

Android

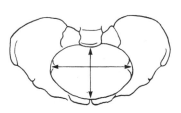

Anthropoid   Platypelloid

FIGURE 20–1. Four basic types of pelves (Caldwell-Moloy classification). (From Burroughs, A. [1997]. *Maternity nursing: An introductory text* [7th ed.]. Philadelphia: W. B. Saunders. p. 22.)

b. Greater than 11 cm is adequate
3. Intertuberous diameter
   a. Transverse diameter of outlet between the ischial tuberosities
   b. Greater than 8 cm is adequate

IV. Fertilization and Implantation

A. **Fertilization**
   1. Occurs in the upper region of the fallopian tubes
   2. Occurs within 12 hours of ovulation and within 2 to 3 days of insemination, the average duration of viability for the ovum and sperm
   3. Takes place when sperm and ovum unite
   4. Once **fertilized**, the membrane of the ovum undergoes changes that prevent the entry of other sperm
   5. Each reproductive cell carries 23 chromosomes
   6. Sperm carry an X and Y chromosome
   7. When united with female X chromosome, determines the sex of the child; XY: male, XX: female

B. **Implantation**
   1. Zygote propelled toward the uterus
   2. Implants 6 to 8 days after ovulation
   3. Blastocyst secretes chorionic gonadotropin to ensure that the corpus luteum remains viable and secretes estrogen and progesterone for the first 2 to 3 months of gestation

V. Fetal Development (Table 20–2)

A. Embryonic stage from conception to 12 weeks
B. Fetal period from third month to gestation

VI. Fetal Environment

A. Amnion
   1. Encloses the amniotic cavity
   2. Inner membrane that forms about the second week of embryonic development
   3. Forms a fluid-filled sac that surrounds the embryo and later the fetus
B. Chorion
   1. Outer membrane
   2. Becomes vascularized and forms the fetal part of the placenta
C. **Amniotic Fluid**
   1. Consists of 500 to 1000 mL by the end of pregnancy
   2. Surrounds, cushions, and protects the fetus and allows for fetal movement
   3. Maintains the body temperature of the fetus
D. **Placenta**
   1. Provides for exchange of nutrients and waste products between the fetus and mother
   2. Develops by the third month
   3. Dependent upon maternal circulation
   4. Large particles such as bacteria cannot pass through the **placenta**
   5. In addition to nutrients, drugs, antibodies, and viruses can pass through the placenta
   6. In the third trimester, transfer of maternal immunoglobulin provides fetus passive immunity to certain diseases for the first few months after birth
   7. By week 8, genetic testing can be done

VII. Fetal Circulation

A. Umbilical cord
   1. Contains two arteries and one vein
   2. Arteries carry deoxygenated blood and waste products from the fetus
   3. The vein carries oxygenated blood and provides oxygen and nutrients to the fetus
B. Fetal heart rate
   1. 120 to 160 beats per minute
   2. Approximately twice the maternal heart rate
C. Fetal circulation bypass
   1. Present due to nonfunctioning lungs
   2. Bypasses must close following birth to allow blood to flow through the lungs and liver
   3. Ductus arteriosus connects the pulmonary artery to aorta, bypassing the lungs
   4. Ductus venosus connects the umbilical vein and inferior vena cava, bypassing the liver
   5. Foramen ovale is the opening between the right and left atria of the heart, bypassing the lungs

PRACTICE QUESTIONS

1. A pregnant client asks the nurse about the hormone that causes milk production. The nurse tells the client that the primary hormone that stimulates the secretion of milk is
   1 Testosterone
   2 Oxytocin
   3 Prolactin
   4 Progesterone

2. The licensed practical nurse (LPN) is assisting a high school nurse in conducting a session with female adolescents regarding the menstrual cycle. The LPN tells the adolescents that the normal duration of the menstrual cycle is about
   1 14 days
   2 28 days
   3 30 days
   4 45 days

3. A maternity nursing instructor asks a nursing student to identify the hormones that are produced by the ovaries. Which of the following responses if made by the student indicates an understanding of the hormones produced by this endocrine gland?
   1 Estrogen and progesterone
   2 Follicle-stimulating hormone (FSH)

Table 20–2. **Fetal Development**

Embryonic Stage	Fetal Period
Week 1 Free-floating blastocyst	**Week 16** ▲ Active movements are present Fetal skin is transparent Lanugo hair begins to develop Skeletal ossification occurs
Week 2 to 3 Two mm in length Groove formed along middle of back Beginning of blood circulation Heart tubular in shape	**Week 20** 19 cm in length 465 g in weight Lanugo covers the entire body Fetus has nails Muscles are developed Enamel and dentin depositing ▲ Heartbeat detected by fetoscope
Week 4 4–6 mm in length 0.4 g in weight ▲ Double heart chambers visible ▲ Heart beginning to beat Limb buds	**Week 24** 28 cm in length 780 g in weight Hair on head well formed Skin reddish and wrinkled Reflex hand grasp Vernix caseosa covers entire body Has ability to hear

Week 8
3 cm in length
2 g in weight
Eyelids begin to fuse
Circulatory system through umbilical cord
  well established
Every organ system present
	Week 28
	38 cm in length
	1200 g in weight
	Limbs are well flexed
	Brain develops rapidly
	Eyelids open and close
	▲ Lungs sufficiently developed to provide gas exchange
	  (lecithin forming)
	If born, neonate can breathe at this time

Week 12 8 cm in length 45 g in weight Face well formed Limbs long and slender Kidneys begin to form urine Spontaneous movements occur ▲ Heart tones detected by electronic devices between 8–12 weeks ▲ Sex recognizable and can be determined at this time	**Week 32** 30 cm in length 2000 g (5.5 lbs) in weight Bones are fully developed Subcutaneous fat collected L/S (lecithin/sphingomyelin) ratio switching to 1.2:1
	Week 36 42 to 48 cm in length 2500 g in weight Skin pink, body rounded Less wrinkled Lanugo disappearing L/S (lecithin/sphingomyelin) ratio $\geq$2:1
	Week 40 48 to 52 cm in length 3000 to 3600 g in weight Skin pinkish and smooth Lanugo present in upper arms and shoulders Vernix caseosa decreases Fingernails extend beyond fingertips Sole (plantar) creases down to heel Testes in scrotum Labia majora well developed

3 Luteinizing hormone (LH)
4 Oxytocin

4. A nurse midwife is conducting a session on the process of fertilization with a group of nursing students. The nurse midwife asks a student to identify the structure where fertilization of an ovum takes place. Which of the following responses if made by a nursing student indicates an understanding of this process?
   1 Fallopian tube
   2 Fundus of the uterus
   3 In the ovary
   4 In the corpus of the uterus

5. The nurse is reviewing the health record of a female client who is suspected of having Mittelschmerz. Which of the following does the nurse expect to note documented in the client's record?
   1 Client complaints of pain at the beginning of menstruation
   2 Profuse vaginal bleeding
   3 Sharp pain located on the right side of the pelvis
   4 Pain that occurs during intercourse

6. A client has been seen in the clinic and has been diagnosed with endometriosis. The client asks the nurse to describe this condition. The nurse responds that it is which of the following?
   1 It is the presence of tissue outside the uterus that resembles the endometrium
   2 It is pain that occurs during ovulation
   3 It is also known as primary dysmenorrhea
   4 It causes the cessation of menstruation

7. A client calls the physician's office to schedule an appointment because a home pregnancy test was performed and the results were positive. The nurse determines that the home pregnancy test identified the presence of which of the following in the urine?
   1 Estrogen
   2 Progesterone
   3 Human chorionic gonadotropin (hCG)
   4 Follicle-stimulating hormone (FSH)

8. A nursing student is conducting a clinical conference regarding the hormones that are related to pregnancy. The instructor asks the student about the function of progesterone. Which of the following responses if made by the student indicates an understanding of the function of this hormone?
   1 "It softens the muscles and joints of the pelvis."
   2 "It is the primary hormone of milk production."
   3 "It increases during pregnancy to stimulate the basal metabolic rate."
   4 "It maintains the uterine lining for implanta-

tion and relaxes all smooth muscles including the uterus."

9. The nurse is reinforcing teaching to a pregnant woman about the physiological effects and hormone changes that occur in pregnancy. The woman asks the nurse about the purpose of estrogen. The nurse bases the response on which of the following purposes of estrogen?
   1 It maintains the uterine lining for implantation
   2 It stimulates metabolism of glucose and converts the glucose to fat
   3 It prevents the involution of the corpus luteum and maintains the production of progesterone until the placenta is formed
   4 It stimulates uterine development to provide an environment for the fetus, and stimulates the breasts to prepare for lactation

10. A pregnant client is seen in the health care clinic and asks the nurse what causes the breasts to change in size and appearance during pregnancy. The nurse bases the response on which of the following?
    1 The breast changes are due to the secretion of estrogen and progesterone
    2 The breasts become stretched because of the weight gain
    3 The increased metabolic rate causes the breasts to become larger
    4 Cortisol secreted by the adrenals plays a factor in increasing the size and appearance of the breasts

11. The nurse is reviewing the record of a pregnant client and notes that the physician has documented the presence of Chadwick's sign. The nurse understands that the hormone responsible for the development of this sign is which of the following?
    1 Human chorionic gonadotropin (hCG)
    2 Estrogen
    3 Progesterone
    4 Prolactin

12. The nursing instructor asks the nursing student about the physiology related to the cessation of ovulation that occurs during pregnancy. Which of the following responses if made by the student indicates an understanding of this physiological process?
    1 Ovulation ceases during pregnancy because the circulating levels of estrogen and progesterone are high
    2 Ovulation ceases during pregnancy because the circulating levels of estrogen and progesterone are low
    3 The low levels of estrogen and progesterone increase the release of the follicle-stimulating hormone and the luteinizing hormone
    4 The high levels of estrogen and progesterone

promote the release of the follicle-stimulating hormone and luteinizing hormone

13. The maternity nurse is describing the ovarian cycle to a group of nursing students. The instructor asks a nursing student to identify the phases of the cycle. Which of the following if stated by the nursing student indicates a need to further research this area?
    1 Follicular phase
    2 Ovulatory phase
    3 Luteal phase
    4 Proliferative phase

14. A client is seen in the health care clinic with a diagnosis of mild anemia. The anemia is believed to be a result of the menstrual period. The woman asks the nurse how much blood is lost during a menstrual period. The nurse bases the response on which of the following amounts of blood lost during this time?
    1 40 mL
    2 60 mL
    3 80 mL
    4 100 mL

15. The nursing instructor asks the nursing student to describe Montgomery's tubercles of the breast. Which of the following responses if made by the student indicates an understanding of this anatomical structure?
    1 "These are sebaceous glands that are located in the areola."
    2 "These are lobes of glandular tissue that secrete milk."
    3 "These are small sacs that contain acinar cells to secrete milk."
    4 "These are ducts containing milk from all areas of the breast."

16. A nursing student is asked to describe the size of the uterus in a nonpregnant client. Which of the following responses if made by the student indicates an understanding of the anatomy of this structure?
    1 "The uterus weighs about 2 ounces."
    2 "The uterus weighs about 2.2 pounds."
    3 "The uterus has a capacity of about 50 mL."
    4 "The uterus is round and weighs approximately 1000 grams."

17. The nurse is reviewing the health record of a pregnant client at 16 weeks' gestation. The nurse expects to note documentation that the fundus of the uterus is located at which of the following areas?
    1 Midway between the symphysis pubis and the umbilicus
    2 Located at the umbilicus
    3 Just above the symphysis pubis
    4 At the level of the xiphoid process

18. The maternity nurse is providing an inservice educational session to nursing students regarding the process of conception. The nurse determines that a nursing student understands this process if the student states that fertilization of a mature ovum occurs in which of the following areas?
    1 In the uterus
    2 In the ovary
    3 In the distal third of the fallopian tube
    4 In the wall of the myometrium

19. The nursing student is asked to describe the corpus of the uterus. Which of the following responses if made by the student indicates an understanding of the anatomy of the uterus?
    1 It is the lower portion of the uterus
    2 It is the uppermost part of the uterus
    3 It is the area where the cervix meets the external os
    4 It is the area where the vagina meets the uterus

20. The nurse is collecting data from a client during the first prenatal visit. The client is anxious to know the sex of the fetus and asks the nurse when she will be able to know. The nurse responds to the client by telling the client that the sex of the fetus can be determined by
    1 Weeks 6 to 8
    2 Weeks 8 to 10
    3 Weeks 12 to 16
    4 Weeks 20 to 22

21. The nurse is collecting data from a pregnant client. The client asks the nurse about the purpose of the fallopian tubes. The nurse responds to the client that the fallopian tubes
    1 Secrete estrogen and progesterone
    2 Are the organ of copulation
    3 Are where the fetus develops
    4 Are where fertilization occurs

22. The nursing student is assigned to care for an adolescent female client in the health care clinic. The instructor reviews the menstrual cycle with the student. The instructor evaluates that the student understands the process of secretion of the follicle-stimulating hormone (FSH) and the luteinizing hormone (LH) if the student states
    1 "FSH and LH are released from the anterior pituitary gland."
    2 "FSH and LH are secreted by the corpus luteum of the ovary."
    3 "FSH and LH are secreted by the adrenal glands."
    4 "FSH and LH stimulate the formation of milk during pregnancy."

23. The nurse, working in a prenatal clinic, reviews a client's chart and notes that the physician documents that the client has a gynecoid pelvis. Based

on this documentation, the nurse determines that this type of pelvis is
1 Not favorable for labor
2 Seen in 25% of women
3 A wide pelvis with a short diameter
4 The most favorable for labor and birth

24. The client asks the nurse about the purpose of the placenta. The nurse plans to respond that the placenta
1 Prevents antibodies and viruses from passing to the fetus
2 Cushions and protects the fetus
3 Provides an exchange of nutrients and waste products between the mother and fetus
4 Maintains the body temperature of the fetus

25. The nurse is describing the process of fetal circulation to a client during a prenatal visit. The nurse tells the client that fetal circulation consists of
1 Two umbilical veins and one umbilical artery
2 Two umbilical arteries and one umbilical vein
3 Arteries carrying oxygenated blood to the fetus
4 Veins carrying deoxygenated blood to the fetus

26. The nursing student is assigned to a client in labor. The nursing instructor asks the student to describe fetal circulation, specifically the ductus venosus. The instructor determines that the student understands the structure of the ductus venosus if the student states that it
1 Connects the pulmonary artery to the aorta
2 Is an opening between the right and left atria
3 Connects the umbilical artery to the inferior vena cava
4 Connects the umbilical vein to the inferior vena cava

27. The nurse is caring for a client during the prenatal period. The client tells that nurse that she wants to know the sex of the fetus as soon as it can be determined. The nurse responds that the sex of the fetus can be determined as early as
1 Week 6
2 Week 8
3 Week 12
4 Week 20

28. The nursing instructor instructs the nursing students that surfactant is a substance needed to facilitate neonatal breathing. The instructor asks a nursing student to identify when this substance is produced. The nursing student responds correctly by stating that this substance is produced at approximately which gestational week?
1 Week 12
2 Week 18
3 Week 28
4 Week 32

29. The nurse is preparing to monitor the fetal heart rate (FHR). The nurse knows that the fetal heart rate can first be heard with a fetoscope at
1 Gestational week 5
2 Gestational week 10
3 Gestational week 16
4 Gestational week 20

30. During the prenatal visit, the nurse checks the fetal heart rate (FHR) using a fetoscope. The nurse determines that the FHR is normal if which of the following heart rates is noted?
1 80 to 100 beats/minute
2 90 to 120 beats/minute
3 120 to 160 beats/minute
4 160 to 180 beats/minute

ANSWERS

1. **3**

RATIONALE: Prolactin stimulates the secretion of milk, called lactogenesis. Oxytocin stimulates contractions during birth and stimulates postpartum contractions to compress uterine vessels and control bleeding. Testosterone is produced by the adrenal glands in the female and induces the growth of pubic and axillary hair at puberty. Progesterone stimulates the secretions of the endometrial glands and causes the endometrial vessels to become dilated and tortuous in preparation for possible embryo implantation.
TEST-TAKING STRATEGY: Knowledge regarding the functions of the various hormones in the female reproductive system is required to answer this question. Note the relationship between secretion of milk and the hormone prolactin in the correct option. If you had difficulty with this question, take time now to review the functions of the various hormones of the female reproductive system.

LEVEL OF COGNITIVE ABILITY: Application
PHASE OF NURSING PROCESS: Implementation
CLIENT NEEDS: Physiological Integrity
CONTENT AREA: Maternity
REFERENCE
Gorrie, T., McKinney, E., & Murray, S. (1998). *Foundations of maternal-newborn nursing* (2nd ed.). Philadelphia: W. B. Saunders. p. 57.

2. **2**

RATIONALE: The normal duration of the menstrual cycle is about 28 days, although it may range from 20 to 45 days. The first day of the menstrual period is counted as day 1 of the woman's cycle.
TEST-TAKING STRATEGY: Knowledge regarding the duration of the menstrual cycle is required to answer this question. Note the key words "normal duration" in the question. This will assist in eliminating options 1, 3, and 4. If you had difficulty with this question, take time now to review the menstrual cycle.

LEVEL OF COGNITIVE ABILITY: Application
PHASE OF NURSING PROCESS: Implementation
CLIENT NEEDS: Physiological Integrity
CONTENT AREA: Maternity
REFERENCE
Gorrie, T., McKinney, E., & Murray, S. (1998). *Foundations of maternal-newborn nursing* (2nd ed.). Philadelphia: W. B. Saunders. p. 67.

3. 1

RATIONALE: The ovaries are the endocrine glands that produce estrogen and progesterone. The FSH and LH are produced by the anterior pituitary gland. Oxytocin is produced by the posterior pituitary gland and stimulates the uterus to produce contractions during birth.
TEST-TAKING STRATEGY: Knowledge regarding the various hormones and the production and secretion of the hormones is required to answer this question. If you had difficulty with this question or are unfamiliar with these hormones, take time now to review.
LEVEL OF COGNITIVE ABILITY: Comprehension
PHASE OF NURSING PROCESS: Evaluation
CLIENT NEEDS: Physiological Integrity
CONTENT AREA: Maternity
REFERENCE
Gorrie, T., McKinney, E., & Murray, S. (1998). *Foundations of maternal-newborn nursing* (2nd ed.). Philadelphia: W. B. Saunders. pp. 56, 60.

4. 1

RATIONALE: Fallopian tubes also called oviducts and are 8 to 14 cm long and are quite narrow. The fallopian tubes are a pathway for the ovum between the ovary and the uterus. Fertilization occurs in the fallopian tube. Options 2, 3, and 4 are incorrect.
TEST-TAKING STRATEGY: Knowledge regarding the process of fertilization and the area in which fertilization occurs is required to answer this question. If you had difficulty with this question, take time now to review the function and structure of the fallopian tube.
LEVEL OF COGNITIVE ABILITY: Comprehension
PHASE OF NURSING PROCESS: Evaluation
CLIENT NEEDS: Physiological Integrity
CONTENT AREA: Maternity
REFERENCE
Gorrie, T., McKinney, E., & Murray, S. (1998). *Foundations of maternal-newborn nursing* (2nd ed.). Philadelphia: W. B. Saunders. p. 63.

5. 3

RATIONALE: Mittelschmerz (middle pain) refers to pelvic pain that occurs midway between menstrual periods or at the time of ovulation. The pain is due to growth of the dominant follicle within the ovary, or rupture of follicle and subsequent spillage of follicular fluid and blood into the peritoneal space. The pain is fairly sharp and is felt on the right or left side of the pelvis. It generally lasts a few hours to 2 days, and slight vaginal bleeding may accompany the discomfort.
TEST-TAKING STRATEGY: Knowledge that Mittelschmerz is "middle pain" will assist in eliminating option 1. Knowing that this occurs due to growth of the follicle, or rupture of the follicle will assist in eliminating options 2 and 4. If you are unfamiliar with this disorder, take time now to review.

LEVEL OF COGNITIVE ABILITY: Comprehension
PHASE OF NURSING PROCESS: Data Collection
CLIENT NEEDS: Physiological Integrity
CONTENT AREA: Maternity
REFERENCE
Gorrie, T., McKinney, E., & Murray, S. (1998). *Foundations of maternal-newborn nursing* (2nd ed.). Philadelphia: W. B. Saunders. p. 938.

6. 1

RATIONALE: Endometriosis is defined as the presence of tissue outside the uterus that resembles the endometrium in both structure and function. The response of this tissue to the stimulation of estrogen and progesterone during the menstrual cycle is identical to that of the endometrium. Primary dysmenorrhea refers to menstrual pain without identified pathology. Mittelschmerz refers to pelvic pain that occurs midway between menstrual periods, and amenorrhea is the cessation of menstruation for a period of at least three cycles or 6 months in a woman who has established a pattern of menstruation, and can be due to a variety of causes.
TEST-TAKING STRATEGY: Knowledge regarding the pathophysiology associated with endometriosis is required to answer this question. If you had difficulty with this question and are unfamiliar with this disorder, take time now to review.
LEVEL OF COGNITIVE ABILITY: Comprehension
PHASE OF NURSING PROCESS: Implementation
CLIENT NEEDS: Physiological Integrity
CONTENT AREA: Maternity
REFERENCE
Gorrie, T., McKinney, E., & Murray, S. (1998). *Foundations of maternal-newborn nursing* (2nd ed.). Philadelphia: W. B. Saunders. pp. 937–938.

7. 3

RATIONALE: In early pregnancy, hCG is produced by trophoblastic cells that surround the developing embryo. This hormone is responsible for positive pregnancy tests. Options 1, 2, and 4 are incorrect.
TEST-TAKING STRATEGY: Knowledge regarding the changes caused by placental hormones in early pregnancy is required to answer this question. If you are unfamiliar with this pregnancy test, take time now to review.
LEVEL OF COGNITIVE ABILITY: Comprehension
PHASE OF NURSING PROCESS: Data Collection
CLIENT NEEDS: Physiological Integrity
CONTENT AREA: Maternity
REFERENCE
Gorrie, T., McKinney, E., & Murray, S. (1998). *Foundations of maternal-newborn nursing* (2nd ed.). Philadelphia: W. B. Saunders. p. 132.

8. 4

RATIONALE: Progesterone maintains uterine lining for implantation and relaxes all smooth muscle including the uterus. Relaxin is the hormone that softens the muscles and joints of the pelvis. Thyroxine increases during pregnancy to stimulate basal metabolic rates, and prolactin is the primary hormone of milk production.
TEST-TAKING STRATEGY: Knowledge regarding the function of the various hormones related to pregnancy is required to answer this question. If you are unfamiliar with these hormones, take time now to review.

LEVEL OF COGNITIVE ABILITY: Comprehension
PHASE OF NURSING PROCESS: Evaluation
CLIENT NEEDS: Physiological Integrity
CONTENT AREA: Maternity
REFERENCE
Gorrie, T., McKinney, E., & Murray, S. (1998). *Foundations of maternal-newborn nursing* (2nd ed.). Philadelphia: W. B. Saunders. p. 131.

9. **4**

RATIONALE: Estrogen stimulates uterine development to provide an environment for the fetus, and stimulates the breasts to prepare for lactation. Progesterone maintains uterine lining for implantation and relaxes all smooth muscle. Human placental lactogen stimulates the metabolism of glucose and converts the glucose to fat. Human chorionic gonadotropin prevents involution of the corpus luteum and maintains the production of progesterone until the placenta is formed.
TEST-TAKING STRATEGY: Knowledge regarding the functions of various hormones related to pregnancy is required to answer this question. If you had difficulty with this question or are unfamiliar with these hormones, take time now to review.
LEVEL OF COGNITIVE ABILITY: Comprehension
PHASE OF NURSING PROCESS: Planning
CLIENT NEEDS: Physiological Integrity
CONTENT AREA: Maternity
REFERENCE
Gorrie, T., McKinney, E., & Murray, S. (1998). *Foundations of maternal-newborn nursing* (2nd ed.). Philadelphia: W. B. Saunders. p. 131.

10. **1**

RATIONALE: During pregnancy the breasts change in both size and appearance. The increase in size is due to the effects of estrogen and progesterone. Estrogen stimulates the growth of mammary ductal tissue, and progesterone promotes the growth of lobes, lobules, and alveoli. A delicate network of veins is often visible just beneath the surface of the skin. Options 2, 3, and 4 are incorrect.
TEST-TAKING STRATEGY: Knowledge regarding the physiological changes that occur during pregnancy is required to answer this question. If you are unfamiliar with the effects of hormones and the changes that occur, take time now to review.
LEVEL OF COGNITIVE ABILITY: Comprehension
PHASE OF NURSING PROCESS: Planning
CLIENT NEEDS: Physiological Integrity
CONTENT AREA: Maternity
REFERENCE
Gorrie, T., McKinney, E., & Murray, S. (1998). *Foundations of maternal-newborn nursing* (2nd ed.). Philadelphia: W. B. Saunders. p. 124.

11. **2**

RATIONALE: The cervix undergoes significant changes following conception. The most obvious changes occur in color and consistency. In response to the increasing levels of estrogen, the cervix becomes congested with blood resulting in the characteristic bluish color that extends to include the vagina and labia. This discoloration, referred to as Chadwick's sign, is one of the earliest signs of pregnancy. Options 1, 3, and 4 are incorrect.

TEST-TAKING STRATEGY: Knowledge regarding physiological changes and the hormones responsible for these changes is required to answer this question. If you are unfamiliar with the physiological changes, take time now to review.
LEVEL OF COGNITIVE ABILITY: Comprehension
PHASE OF NURSING PROCESS: Data Collection
CLIENT NEEDS: Physiological Integrity
CONTENT AREA: Maternity
REFERENCE
Gorrie, T., McKinney, E., & Murray, S. (1998). *Foundations of maternal-newborn nursing* (2nd ed.). Philadelphia: W. B. Saunders. p. 123.

12. **1**

RATIONALE: Ovulation ceases during pregnancy because the circulating levels of estrogen and progesterone are high, inhibiting the release of follicle stimulating hormones and luteinizing hormones which are necessary for ovulation. Options 2, 3, and 4 are incorrect.
TEST-TAKING STRATEGY: Knowledge regarding the hormonal changes that occur during the menstrual cycle and during pregnancy is required to answer this question. If you are unfamiliar with these physiological changes, take time now to review.
LEVEL OF COGNITIVE ABILITY: Comprehension
PHASE OF NURSING PROCESS: Evaluation
CLIENT NEEDS: Physiological Integrity
CONTENT AREA: Maternity
REFERENCE
Gorrie, T., McKinney, E., & Murray, S. (1998). *Foundations of maternal-newborn nursing* (2nd ed.). Philadelphia: W. B. Saunders. pp. 123–124.

13. **4**

RATIONALE: The ovarian cycle consists of three phases, the follicular, ovulatory, and luteal phase. The proliferative phase is a phase of the endometrial cycle.
TEST-TAKING STRATEGY: Note the key words "indicates a need to further research." Knowledge regarding the ovarian cycle and the phases included in the cycle is required to answer this question. If you are unfamiliar with the ovarian cycle, take time now to review.
LEVEL OF COGNITIVE ABILITY: Comprehension
PHASE OF NURSING PROCESS: Evaluation
CLIENT NEEDS: Physiological Integrity
CONTENT AREA: Maternity
REFERENCE
Gorrie, T., McKinney, E., & Murray, S. (1998). *Foundations of maternal-newborn nursing* (2nd ed.). Philadelphia: W. B. Saunders. p. 67.

14. **1**

RATIONALE: During a menstrual period, a woman loses about 40 mL of blood. Because of the recurrent loss of blood, many women are mildly anemic during their reproductive years, especially if their diets are low in iron. Options 2, 3, and 4 are incorrect.
TEST-TAKING STRATEGY: Knowledge regarding the menstrual phase of the menstrual cycle and the amount of blood lost during a menstrual period is required to answer this question. If you are unfamiliar with the menstrual phase, take time now to review.
LEVEL OF COGNITIVE ABILITY: Comprehension

PHASE OF NURSING PROCESS: Planning
CLIENT NEEDS: Physiological Integrity
CONTENT AREA: Maternity
REFERENCE
Gorrie, T., McKinney, E., & Murray, S. (1998). *Foundations of maternal-newborn nursing* (2nd ed.). Philadelphia: W. B. Saunders. p. 68.

15. 1

RATIONALE: Montgomery's tubercles are sebaceous glands in the areola. They are inactive and not obvious except during pregnancy and lactation, when they enlarge and secrete a substance that keeps the nipple soft. Within each breast are lobes of glandular tissue that secrete milk. Alveoli are small sacs that contain acinar cells to secrete milk. The alveoli drain into lactiferous ducts, which connect to drain milk from all areas of the breast.
TEST-TAKING STRATEGY: Knowledge regarding the anatomy and physiology of the breast is required to answer this question. If you are unfamiliar with the structures of the female breast, take time now to review.
LEVEL OF COGNITIVE ABILITY: Comprehension
PHASE OF NURSING PROCESS: Evaluation
CLIENT NEEDS: Physiological Integrity
CONTENT AREA: Maternity
REFERENCE
Gorrie, T., McKinney, E., & Murray, S. (1998). *Foundations of maternal-newborn nursing* (2nd ed.). Philadelphia: W. B. Saunders. p. 68.

16. 1

RATIONALE: Prior to conception, the uterus is a small pear-shaped organ contained entirely in the pelvic cavity. Before pregnancy, the uterus weighs approximately 60 g (2 oz) and has a capacity of about 10 mL (one-third of an ounce). At the end of pregnancy, the uterus weighs approximately 1000 g (2.2 lb) and has a sufficient capacity for the fetus, placenta, and amniotic fluid, a total of about 5000 mL.
TEST-TAKING STRATEGY: Knowledge regarding the structure of the uterus is required to answer this question. Note the key word "nonpregnant" to assist in directing you to the correct option. Attempt to visualize each of the items identified in the options. Take time now to review the anatomical structure of the uterus if you had difficulty with this question!
LEVEL OF COGNITIVE ABILITY: Comprehension
PHASE OF NURSING PROCESS: Evaluation
CLIENT NEEDS: Physiological Integrity
CONTENT AREA: Maternity
REFERENCE
Gorrie, T., McKinney, E., & Murray, S. (1998). *Foundations of maternal-newborn nursing* (2nd ed.). Philadelphia: W. B. Saunders. p. 122.

17. 1

RATIONALE: At 12 weeks' gestation, the uterus extends out of the maternal pelvis and can be palpated above the symphysis pubis. At 16 weeks, the fundus reaches midway between the symphysis pubis and the umbilicus. At 20 weeks, the fundus is located at the umbilicus. By 36 weeks, the fundus reaches its highest level at the xiphoid process.
TEST-TAKING STRATEGY: Knowledge regarding the patterns of uterine growth is required to answer this question. Focus on the weeks of gestation identified in the

question to assist in directing you to the correct option. If you are unfamiliar with the patterns of uterine growth during pregnancy, take time now to review.
LEVEL OF COGNITIVE ABILITY: Comprehension
PHASE OF NURSING PROCESS: Data Collection
CLIENT NEEDS: Physiological Integrity
CONTENT AREA: Maternity
REFERENCE
Gorrie, T., McKinney, E., & Murray, S. (1998). *Foundations of maternal-newborn nursing* (2nd ed.). Philadelphia: W. B. Saunders. p. 122.

18. 3

RATIONALE: The mature ovum is transported through the fallopian tube by the muscular action of the tube and the movement of the cilia within the tube. Fertilization normally occurs in the distal third of the fallopian tube near the ovaries. The ovum, fertilized or not, enters the uterus about 3 days after its release from the ovary. The other options are incorrect.
TEST-TAKING STRATEGY: Knowledge regarding the process of fertilization is required to answer this question. If you are unfamiliar with this process, take time now to review.
LEVEL OF COGNITIVE ABILITY: Comprehension
PHASE OF NURSING PROCESS: Evaluation
CLIENT NEEDS: Physiological Integrity
CONTENT AREA: Maternity
REFERENCE
Gorrie, T., McKinney, E., & Murray, S. (1998). *Foundations of maternal-newborn nursing* (2nd ed.). Philadelphia: W. B. Saunders. p. 100.

19. 2

RATIONALE: The uterus has three divisions, the corpus, the isthmus, and the cervix. The upper division is the corpus or the body of the uterus. The uppermost part of the uterine corpus, above the area where the fallopian tubes enter the uterus, is the fundus of the uterus.
TEST-TAKING STRATEGY: Knowledge regarding the divisions of the uterus is required to answer this question. Note the similarity related to anatomical location in options 1, 3, and 4. If you had difficulty with this question, take time now to review the anatomical structure of the uterus.
LEVEL OF COGNITIVE ABILITY: Comprehension
PHASE OF NURSING PROCESS: Evaluation
CLIENT NEEDS: Physiological Integrity
CONTENT AREA: Maternity
REFERENCE
Gorrie, T., McKinney, E., & Murray, S. (1998). *Foundations of maternal-newborn nursing* (2nd ed.). Philadelphia: W. B. Saunders. p. 61.

20. 3

RATIONALE: By the end of the 12th week, the fetal sex can be determined by the appearance of the external genitalia of the fetus.
TEST-TAKING STRATEGY: Knowledge regarding fetal development is required to answer this question. If you had difficulty with this question, take time now to review fetal development.
LEVEL OF COGNITIVE ABILITY: Application
PHASE OF NURSING PROCESS: Implementation
CLIENT NEEDS: Physiological Integrity
CONTENT AREA: Maternity

REFERENCE
Gorrie, T., McKinney. E., & Murray., S. (1998). *Foundations of maternal-newborn nursing* (2nd ed.). Philadelphia: W. B. Saunders. p. 108.

21. 4

RATIONALE: Each fallopian tube is a hollow muscular tube that transports a mature oocyte for final maturation and fertilization. Fertilization typically occurs near the boundary between the ampulla and isthmus of the tube. Estrogen is a hormone produced by the ovarian follicles, corpus luteum, adrenal cortex, and placenta during pregnancy. Progesterone is a hormone secreted by the corpus luteum of the ovary, adrenal glands, and placenta during pregnancy. The vagina is the organ of copulation, and the fetus develops in the uterus.
TEST-TAKING STRATEGY: Knowledge of the anatomy and physiology of the female reproductive system is required to answer this question. Use the process of elimination to answer the question. If you had difficulty with this question, take time now to review anatomy and physiology.
LEVEL OF COGNITIVE ABILITY: Comprehension
PHASE OF NURSING PROCESS: Implementation
CLIENT NEEDS: Physiological Integrity
CONTENT AREA: Maternity
REFERENCE
Leifer, G. (1999). *Thompson's introduction to maternity and pediatric nursing* (3rd ed.). Philadelphia: W. B. Saunders. pp. 29–30.

22. 1

RATIONALE: FSH and LH, when stimulated by GnRH from the hypothalamus, are released from the anterior pituitary gland to stimulate follicular growth and development, growth of the graafian follicle, and the production of progesterone. Options 2, 3, and 4 are incorrect.
TEST-TAKING STRATEGY: Knowledge of the hormones associated with the menstrual cycle is required to answer the question. Use the process of elimination to answer the question. Option 4 can be eliminated because the case of the question does not address pregnancy. From this point, use your knowledge related to the menstrual cycle to select the correct option. If you had difficulty with this question, review the menstrual cycle now.
LEVEL OF COGNITIVE ABILITY: Comprehension
PHASE OF NURSING PROCESS: Evaluation
CLIENT NEEDS: Physiological Integrity
CONTENT AREA: Maternity
REFERENCE
Leifer, G. (1999). *Thompson's introduction to maternity and pediatric nursing* (3rd ed.). Philadelphia: W. B. Saunders. pp. 33–34.

23. 4

RATIONALE: A gynecoid pelvis is a normal female pelvis and is the most favorable for successful labor and birth. An android pelvis, seen in 20% of women, would not be favorable for labor because of the narrow pelvic planes. An anthropoid pelvis has an outlet that is adequate, with a normal or moderately narrow pubic arch, and is seen in 25% of women. The platypelloid pelvis, seen in 5% of women, has a wide transverse diameter, but the anteroposterior diameter is short, making the outlet inadequate.
TEST-TAKING STRATEGY: Knowledge regarding pelvic types is required to answer this question. Remember that the gynecoid pelvis is the normal female pelvis. Review pelvic types now if you had difficulty with this question.

LEVEL OF COGNITIVE ABILITY: Comprehension
PHASE OF NURSING PROCESS: Data Collection
CLIENT NEEDS: Physiological Integrity
CONTENT AREA: Maternity
REFERENCE
Leifer, G. (1999). *Thompson's introduction to maternity and pediatric nursing* (3rd ed.). Philadelphia: W. B. Saunders. p. 32.

24. 3

RATIONALE: The placenta provides an exchange of nutrients and waste products between the mother and fetus. The amniotic fluid surrounds, cushions, protects and maintains the body temperature of the fetus. Nutrients, drugs, antibodies, and viruses can pass through the placenta.
TEST-TAKING STRATEGY: Knowledge regarding the purpose of the placenta and amniotic fluid is required to answer this question. Remember that the placenta provides nutrients. If you had difficulty with this question, take time now to review the structure and function of the placenta and amniotic fluid.
LEVEL OF COGNITIVE ABILITY: Comprehension
PHASE OF NURSING PROCESS: Planning
CLIENT NEEDS: Physiological Integrity
CONTENT AREA: Maternity
REFERENCE
Leifer, G. (1999). *Thompson's introduction to maternity and pediatric nursing* (3rd ed.). Philadelphia: W. B. Saunders. p. 42.

25. 2

RATIONALE: Blood pumped by the fetus's heart leaves the fetus through two umbilical arteries. Once oxygenated, the blood is then returned by one umbilical vein. Arteries carry deoxygenated blood and waste products from the fetus and veins carry oxygenated blood and provide oxygen and nutrients to the fetus.
TEST-TAKING STRATEGY: Knowledge regarding fetal circulation is required to answer this question. Remember that there are three umbilical vessels within an umbilical cord (two arteries and one vein). If you had difficulty with this question, take time now to review fetal circulation.
LEVEL OF COGNITIVE ABILITY: Application
PHASE OF NURSING PROCESS: Implementation
CLIENT NEEDS: Physiological Integrity
CONTENT AREA: Maternity
REFERENCE
Nichols, F., & Zwelling, E. (1997). *Maternal-newborn nursing: Theory and practice.* Philadelphia: W. B. Saunders. p. 385.

26. 4

RATIONALE: The ductus venosus connects the umbilical vein to the inferior vena cava. The foramen ovale is a temporary opening between the right and left atria. The ductus arteriosus joins the aorta and the pulmonary artery.
TEST-TAKING STRATEGY: Knowledge regarding fetal circulation is required to answer this question. Review fetal circulation now if you had difficulty with this question.
LEVEL OF COGNITIVE ABILITY: Comprehension
PHASE OF NURSING PROCESS: Evaluation
CLIENT NEEDS: Physiological Integrity
CONTENT AREA: Maternity
REFERENCE
O'Toole, M. (ed.). (1997). *Miller-Keane encyclopedia & dictionary of medicine, nursing, & allied health* (6th ed.). Philadelphia: W. B. Saunders. p. 486.

27. **3**

RATIONALE: The sex of the fetus is clearly identifiable by gestational week 12.
TEST-TAKING STRATEGY: Knowledge regarding fetal development is required to answer this question. It is important to remember that the sex of the fetus can be determined by gestational week 12. If you had difficulty with this question, take time now to review fetal development.
LEVEL OF COGNITIVE ABILITY: Comprehension
PHASE OF NURSING PROCESS: Data Collection
CLIENT NEEDS: Physiological Integrity
CONTENT AREA: Maternity
REFERENCE
Leifer, G. (1999). *Thompson's introduction to maternity and pediatric nursing* (3rd ed.). Philadelphia: W. B. Saunders. p. 46.

28. **3**

RATIONALE: Surfactant, a substance needed to facilitate neonatal breathing, begins to be produced at approximately week 28.
TEST-TAKING STRATEGY: Knowledge regarding neonatal development in relation to the development of surfactant is needed to answer this question. If you had difficulty with this question, take time now to review information related to surfactant development.
LEVEL OF COGNITIVE ABILITY: Comprehension
PHASE OF NURSING PROCESS: Evaluation
CLIENT NEEDS: Physiological Integrity
CONTENT AREA: Maternity
REFERENCE
Nichols, F., & Zwelling, E. (1997). *Maternal-newborn nursing: Theory and practice.* Philadelphia: W. B. Saunders. p. 379.

29. **4**

RATIONALE: The fetal heart rate can first be heard with a fetoscope at 18 to 20 weeks' gestation. If a Doppler ultrasound device is used, the fetal heart rate can be detected as early as 10 weeks' gestation.
TEST-TAKING STRATEGY: Knowledge regarding assessment of the fetal heart rate is required to answer this question. It is important that you are familiar with detecting fetal heart sounds. If you had difficulty with this question, take time now to review fetal heart monitoring.
LEVEL OF COGNITIVE ABILITY: Knowledge
PHASE OF NURSING PROCESS: Data Collection
CLIENT NEEDS: Physiological Integrity
CONTENT AREA: Maternity
REFERENCE
Leifer, G. (1999). *Thompson's introduction to maternity and pediatric nursing* (3rd ed.). Philadelphia: W. B. Saunders. p. 59.

30. **3**

RATIONALE: The normal fetal heart rate is 120 to 160 beats/minute. If the fetal heart rate is less than 100 or more than 160 beats/minute with the uterus at rest, the fetus may be in distress.
TEST-TAKING STRATEGY: Knowledge regarding normal fetal heart rate is required to answer this question. Review fetal heart rate now if you had difficulty with this question.
LEVEL OF COGNITIVE ABILITY: Comprehension
PHASE OF NURSING PROCESS: Data Collection
CLIENT NEEDS: Physiological Integrity
CONTENT AREA: Maternity
REFERENCE
Leifer, G. (1999). *Thompson's introduction to maternity and pediatric nursing* (3rd ed.). Philadelphia: W. B. Saunders. p. 46.

BIBLIOGRAPHY

Gorrie, T., McKinney, E., & Murray, S. (1998). *Foundations of maternal-newborn nursing* (2nd ed.). Philadelphia: W. B. Saunders.

Leifer, G. (1999). *Thompson's introduction to maternity and pediatric nursing* (3rd ed.). Philadelphia: W. B. Saunders.

Nichols, F., & Zwelling, E. (1997). *Maternal-newborn nursing: Theory and practice.* Philadelphia: W. B. Saunders.

O'Toole, M. (ed.). (1997). *Miller-Keane encyclopedia & dictionary of medicine, nursing, & allied health* (6th ed.). Philadelphia: W. B. Saunders.

CHAPTER 21

Obstetrical Assessment

I. Gestation

A. Estimated date of confinement (EDC)
B. Lasts approximately 280 days
C. **Nägele's rule** for estimating EDC (Box 21–1)
   1. For **Nägele's rule** to be accurate requires that the woman have a regular 28-day menstrual cycle
   2. Add 7 days to the first day of the last menstrual period (LMP), subtract 3 months, and then add 1 year to that date

II. Gravidity and Parity

A. **Gravidity**
   1. **Gravida** refers to a pregnant woman
   2. **Gravidity** refers to the number of pregnancies
   3. **Nulligravida** is a woman who has never been pregnant
   4. **Primigravida** is a woman who is pregnant for the first time
   5. **Multigravida** is a woman in at least her second pregnancy
B. **Parity**
   1. **Parity** is the number of births (not the number of fetuses, e.g., twins) past 20 weeks' gestation, whether the fetus was born alive or not
   2. **Nullipara** is a woman who has not had a birth at more than 20 weeks of gestation
   3. **Primipara** is a woman who has had one birth that occurs after the 20th week of gestation

---

BOX 21–1. Nägele's Rule for Estimating EDC

First day of LMP: September 11, 1999
Add 7 days: September 18, 1999
Subtract 3 months: June 18, 1999
Add 1 year: June 18, 2000
EDC: June 18, 2000

---

   4. **Multipara** is a woman who has had two or more pregnancies resulting in viable offspring

III. Pregnancy Signs

A. Presumptive signs
   1. Amenorrhea
   2. Nausea and vomiting
   3. Increased size and increased feeling of fullness in the breasts
   4. Pronounced nipples
   5. Urinary frequency
   6. **Quickening**: first perception of fetal movement in the 16th to 18th week
   7. Fatigue
   8. Discoloration and thickening of vaginal mucosa
B. Probable signs
   1. Uterine enlargement
   2. **Hegar's sign**: softening of the uterus that occurs about week 6
   3. **Goodell's sign**: softening of the cervix that occurs at the beginning of the second month
   4. **Chadwick's sign**: bluish coloration of the mucous membranes of cervix, vagina, and vulva
   5. **Ballottement**: rebounding of the fetus against the examiner's fingers on palpation
   6. Braxton Hicks contractions
   7. Positive pregnancy test measuring for human chorionic gonadotropin (hCG)
C. Positive signs
   1. Fetal heart rate by Doppler at 10 to 12 weeks and by fetoscope at 18 to 20 weeks
   2. Active fetal movements palpable
   3. Outline of fetus via ultrasound

IV. Fundal Height (Box 21–2)

A. Performed to evaluate fetus's gestational age
B. Between 18 and 32 weeks, fundal height in centimeters equals the fetus's age in weeks
C. At 16 weeks, the fundus can be found halfway between the symphysis pubis and the umbilicus

> **BOX 21–2. Measuring Fundal Height**
>
> 1. Place the client in a supine position
> 2. Place the end of a tape measure at the level of the symphysis pubis
> 3. Stretch the tape to the top of the uterine fundus
> 4. Note and record measurement

D. At 20 to 22 weeks, the fundus is at the umbilicus
E. At 36 weeks, the fundus is at the xiphoid process

V. Maternal Risk Factors

A. German measles (rubella)
   1. The risk of maternal and fetal or congenital infection is related to trimester of placental infection
   2. Maternal infection during the first 8 weeks of gestation carries the highest rate of maternal and fetal infection
B. Sexually transmitted diseases
   1. Syphilis
      a. May cross the **placenta**
      b. Usually leads to spontaneous abortion
      c. Increases the incidence of mental subnormality and physical deformities in the fetus
   2. Genital herpes
      a. May cross the **placenta**
      b. The fetus is contaminated after membranes rupture or with vaginal **delivery**
   3. Gonorrhea
      a. The fetus is contaminated at the time of **delivery**
      b. May result in postpartum infection
      c. Risks to the neonate include ophthalmia neonatorum, pneumonia, and sepsis
C. Human immunodeficiency virus (HIV)
   1. The virus is transmitted through blood, blood products, and other bodily fluids such as urine, semen, and vaginal fluid
   2. Repeated exposure to HIV during pregnancy through unsafe sex practices or intravenous drug use can increase the risk of transmission to the fetus
D. Substance abuse
   1. Many substances cross the **placenta**; therefore, no drugs, including over-the-counter medications, should be taken unless prescribed by a physician
   2. Substances commonly abused include alcohol, cocaine, crack, marijuana, amphetamines, barbiturates, and heroin
   3. Substance abuse threatens normal fetal growth and successful term completion of the pregnancy
   4. Substance abuse places the pregnancy at risk for fetal growth retardation, **abruptio placentae**, and fetal bradycardia
   5. Physical signs of drug abuse may include

dilated or contracted pupils, fatigue, track marks, skin abscesses, inflamed nasal mucosa, and inappropriate behavior by the mother
   6. Alcohol during pregnancy may lead to fetal alcohol syndrome and can cause jitteriness, physical abnormalities, congenital anomalies, and growth deficits
   7. Smoking leads to low birthweights, a higher incidence of birth defects, and stillbirths
E. Adolescent pregnancy
   1. Factors that result in adolescent pregnancy include the early onset of menarche, changing sexual behaviors in this age group, faulty family development, poverty, and the lack of knowledge of reproduction and birth control
   2. The major concerns related to adolescent pregnancy include poor nutritional status, emotional and behavioral difficulties, the lack of support systems, increased risk of stillbirth, low-birthweight newborns, fetal mortality, cephalopelvic disproportion, and the increased risks of maternal complications such as hypertension, anemia, prolonged **labor**, and infections

PRACTICE QUESTIONS

1. The client arrives at the prenatal clinic for the first prenatal assessment. The client tells the nurse that the first day of her last menstrual period was September 19, 1999. Using Nägele's rule, the nurse determines the estimated date of confinement as
   1 July 26, 2000
   2 June 12, 2000
   3 June 26, 2000
   4 July 12, 2000

2. The client is in her second trimester of pregnancy. During her routine prenatal visit, she tells the primary health care provider that she frequently has calf pain when she walks. The nurse reviews the health record to note documentation of which of the following that will differentiate the origin of the discomfort?
   1 Chadwick's sign
   2 Leopold's sign
   3 Homans' sign
   4 Kernig's sign

3. The nurse is collecting data during an admission assessment on a client, pregnant with twins. The client also has a 5-year-old. The nurse documents which gravida and para status on this client?
   1 Gravida III, para II
   2 Gravida II, para II
   3 Gravida I, para I
   4 Gravida II, para I

4. A primipara is being evaluated in the clinic during her second trimester of pregnancy. Which of the following indicates an abnormal physical finding necessitating further testing?

1 Consistent increase in fundal height
2 Fetal heart rate of 180 beats/minute
3 Braxton Hicks contractions
4 Quickening

5. In planning the care of a pregnant client with herpes genitalis, the nurse in the clinic prepares to include which of the following when reinforcing teaching measures for this disorder?
   1 Daily administration of acyclovir (Zovirax)
   2 Total abstinence from sexual intercourse
   3 Sitzbath every 4 hours while awake
   4 Preparation for a Cesarean section if vaginal lesions are present at the time of labor

6. The client has tested positive for gonorrhea. The nurse reviews the physician's orders and expects to note that which of the following medications will be prescribed?
   1 Ceftriaxone sodium (Rocephin) IM
   2 Penicillin G potassium (Pfizerpen) IM
   3 Metronidazole (Flagyl) PO
   4 Clindamycin phosphate (Cleocin) IV

7. A pregnant client tests positive for hepatitis B virus (HBV). The nurse determines that the client understands about this infection when the client says
   1 "I know my baby will be immune from hepatitis for the first 2 months of life."
   2 "I feel sad that my baby is going to be isolated in the nursery after my delivery."
   3 "Hepatitis B will cause a severe eye infection in my baby."
   4 "I am so glad that I can breast-feed my baby after it has been vaccinated with immune serum globulin."

8. In the prenatal clinic, the nurse is gathering data from a new client for the health history information. What is the best way for the nurse to elicit correct responses to questions that refer to sexually transmitted diseases?
   1 Establish a therapeutic relationship between the nurse and pregnant client
   2 Use specific closed-ended questions
   3 Omit this area of questions because they are highly personal
   4 Apologize for the embarrassment that these questions will cause the client

9. The pregnant client is positive for the human immunodeficiency virus (HIV). Based on this information, the nurse determines that
   1 The client has the herpes simplex virus
   2 HIV antibodies are detected on the ELISA test
   3 The newborn infant will develop this disease after birth
   4 This client has contacted an airborne disease

10. The nurse is gathering data from a 16-year-old during her initial prenatal clinic visit. She is beginning week 18 of her first pregnancy. Which of the following statements made by the client indicates an immediate need for further investigation?
   1 "I don't like my face anymore. I always look like I have been crying."
   2 "I don't like my breasts anymore. These silver lines are ugly."
   3 "I don't like my stomach anymore. That brown line is disgusting."
   4 "I don't like my figure anymore. My clothes are all too tight."

ANSWERS

1. **3**

RATIONALE: Accurate use of Nägele's rule requires that the woman have a regular 28-day menstrual cycle. Add 7 days to the first day of the LMP, subtract 3 months, and then add 1 year to that date. First day of the LMP: September 19, 1999; add 7 days: September 26, 1999; subtract 3 months: June 26, 1999; add 1 year: June 26, 2000.
TEST-TAKING STRATEGY: Knowledge regarding the use of Nägele's rule is required to answer this question. Use caution when following steps to determine the EDC. Avoid taking shortcuts, particularly when math is involved. Review Nägele's rule now if you had difficulty with this question.
LEVEL OF COGNITIVE ABILITY: Comprehension
PHASE OF NURSING PROCESS: Data Collection
CLIENT NEEDS: Physiological Integrity
CONTENT AREA: Maternity
REFERENCE
Leifer, G. (1999). *Thompson's introduction to maternity and pediatric nursing* (3rd ed.). Philadelphia: W. B. Saunders. pp. 56–57.

2. **3**

RATIONALE: Chadwick's sign is a cervical change and is a probable sign of pregnancy. Leopold's sign is a fictitious term. Leopold's maneuvers are a series of abdominal palpation maneuvers that provide information regarding fetal presentation, position, presenting part, attitude, and descent. Kernig's sign tests for meningeal irritability. Homans' sign tests for venous thrombosis of the lower extremity. Pain in the calf during walking could indicate venous thrombosis.
TEST-TAKING STRATEGY: Knowledge of the signs related to pregnancy and signs indicating a potential problem are required to answer this question. Review the signs identified in the options 1, 3, and 4 now if you had difficulty with this question.
LEVEL OF COGNITIVE ABILITY: Comprehension
PHASE OF NURSING PROCESS: Data Collection
CLIENT NEEDS: Physiological Integrity
CONTENT AREA: Maternity
REFERENCE
Gorrie, T., McKinney, E., & Murray, S. (1998). *Foundations of maternal-newborn nursing* (2nd ed.). Philadelphia: W. B. Saunders. p. 793.

3. 4

RATIONALE: Gravida is a term that refers to a woman who is or has been pregnant regardless of the duration of the pregnancy. Para is a term that means the number of pregnancies that have progressed past 20 weeks' gestation. Parity does not reflect the number of fetuses or infants. Options 1, 2, and 3 are incorrect based on the above definition.

TEST-TAKING STRATEGY: Knowledge of the terms gravida and para is necessary in order to answer this question correctly. If you had difficulty answering this question, review these definitions now.

LEVEL OF COGNITIVE ABILITY: Application
PHASE OF NURSING PROCESS: Data Collection
CLIENT NEEDS: Physiological Integrity
CONTENT AREA: Maternity
REFERENCE
Gorrie, T., McKinney, E., & Murray, S. (1998). *Foundations of maternal-newborn nursing* (2nd ed.). Philadelphia: W. B. Saunders. p. 296.

4. 2

RATIONALE: The fetal heart rate should be 120 to 160 beats/minute throughout pregnancy. Options 1, 3, and 4 are normal expected findings. An important factor to assess regarding uterine growth is its constant, steady, predictable increase in size. Uterine contractions begin early in pregnancy and are present throughout the rest of the pregnancy, becoming stronger and harder as the pregnancy advances. These are termed Braxton Hicks contractions. Fetal movement can be felt by the mother (quickening) beginning at 18 to 20 weeks of pregnancy and reaches a peak at 29 to 38 weeks.

TEST-TAKING STRATEGY: This question asks you to select the option that would indicate that the client needs further testing. Use the process of elimination. Knowledge regarding the normal fetal growth and development is essential in answering this question. Review normal assessment findings in pregnancy now if you had difficulty with this question.

LEVEL OF COGNITIVE ABILITY: Comprehension
PHASE OF NURSING PROCESS: Data Collection
CLIENT NEEDS: Physiological Integrity
CONTENT AREA: Maternity
REFERENCE
Burroughs, A. (1997). *Maternity nursing: An introductory text* (7th ed.). Philadelphia: W. B. Saunders. p. 144.

5. 4

RATIONALE: For women with active lesions, either recurrent or primary, at the time of labor, delivery should be by cesarean section. The safety of acyclovir has not been established during pregnancy and should be used only when there is a life-threatening infection. Clients should be advised to abstain from sexual contact while the lesions are present. If it is an initial infection, they should continue to abstain until they become culture negative because prolonged viral shedding may occur in such cases. Keeping the genital area clean and dry will promote healing.

TEST-TAKING STRATEGY: It is necessary to understand the physiology and the treatment plan for the client to answer this question. If you had difficulty with this question, review content related to herpes as a maternal risk factor now.

LEVEL OF COGNITIVE ABILITY: Application
PHASE OF NURSING PROCESS: Planning
CLIENT NEEDS: Health Promotion and Maintenance
CONTENT AREA: Maternity
REFERENCE
Nichols, F., & Zwelling, E. (1997). *Maternal-newborn nursing: Theory and practice*. Philadelphia: W. B. Saunders. p. 1496.

6. 1

RATIONALE: Treatment for gonorrhea consists of antibiotic therapy with ceftriaxone IM or oral amoxicillin plus oral doxycycline for 7 days; therefore, option 1 is correct. Option 2 is the treatment for syphilis, option 3 is the treatment for trichomoniasis, and option 4 is the treatment for bacterial vaginosis.

TEST-TAKING STRATEGY: Focus on the issue of the question. In this case, the issue is the specific medication required to treat gonorrhea. Review content regarding gonorrhea and the medication used to treat this sexually transmitted disease now if you had difficulty with this question.

LEVEL OF COGNITIVE ABILITY: Comprehension
PHASE OF NURSING PROCESS: Data Collection
CLIENT NEEDS: Physiological Integrity
CONTENT AREA: Maternity
REFERENCE
Gorrie, T., McKinney, E., & Murray, S. (1998). *Foundations of maternal-newborn nursing* (2nd ed.). Philadelphia: W. B. Saunders. p. 954.

7. 4

RATIONALE: Although HBV is transmitted in breast milk, once serum immune globulin has been administered, women may breast-feed without risk to the newborn. Option 1 is incorrect. To reduce the possibility of hepatitis B virus being spread to the newborn, neonates are now routinely vaccinated at birth. Options 2 and 3 are inaccurate.

TEST-TAKING STRATEGY: This question requires an understanding of hepatitis B virus and its effects on the fetus and newborn. If you had difficulty with this question, review the content related to HBV.

LEVEL OF COGNITIVE ABILITY: Analysis
PHASE OF NURSING PROCESS: Evaluation
CLIENT NEEDS: Health Promotion and Maintenance
CONTENT AREA: Maternity
REFERENCE
Leifer, G. (1999). *Thompson's introduction to maternity and pediatric nursing* (3rd ed.). Philadelphia: W. B. Saunders. pp. 56–57.

8. 1

RATIONALE: The initial data collection interview establishes the therapeutic relationship between the nurse and the pregnant woman. It is planned, purposeful communication that focuses on specific content. Options 2, 3, and 4 are incorrect and do not lend themselves to eliciting correct responses.

TEST-TAKING STRATEGY: Focus on the issue of the question. Look for the option that focuses on the client as a worthy human being. Remember, establishing a therapeutic relationship is most meaningful.

LEVEL OF COGNITIVE ABILITY: Comprehension
PHASE OF NURSING PROCESS: Data Collection
CLIENT NEEDS: Psychosocial Integrity
CONTENT AREA: Maternity
REFERENCE
Nichols, F., & Zwelling, E. (1997). *Maternal-newborn nursing: Theory and practice*. Philadelphia: W. B. Saunders. p. 1497.

9. **2**

RATIONALE: Diagnosis depends on serological studies to detect HIV antibodies. The most commonly used test is the enzyme-linked immunosorbent assay (ELISA) test. Options 1 and 4 are incorrect because HIV stands for human immunodeficiency virus and it occurs primarily through the exchange of body fluids. Option 3 is incorrect. A neonate born to an HIV-positive mother has a 20% to 40% risk of developing this disease.
TEST-TAKING STRATEGY: Knowledge related to HIV is required to answer this question. Use the process of elimination. Review this content now if you had difficulty with this question.
LEVEL OF COGNITIVE ABILITY: Comprehension
PHASE OF NURSING PROCESS: Evaluation
CLIENT NEEDS: Physiological Integrity
CONTENT AREA: Maternity
REFERENCE
Nichols, F., & Zwelling, E. (1997). *Maternal-newborn nursing: Theory and practice.* Philadelphia: W. B. Saunders. p. 1498.

10. **1**

RATIONALE: Options 2, 3, and 4 are dealing with body image. Although these comments should not be ignored, the need for follow-up is not urgent. In option 1, there is an implication of periorbital and facial edema, which could be indicative of pregnancy-induced hypertension (PIH). Since this is an adolescent who has not sought early prenatal care, she is at higher risk for the development of PIH.
TEST-TAKING STRATEGY: Note the key words "immediate need." Note the week of the first prenatal visit (week 18). Review complications associated with pregnancy and the associated clinical manifestations now if you had difficulty with this question.
LEVEL OF COGNITIVE ABILITY: Analysis
PHASE OF NURSING PROCESS: Data Collection
CLIENT NEEDS: Physiological Integrity
CONTENT AREA: Maternity
REFERENCE
Gorrie, T., McKinney, E., & Murray, S. (1998). *Foundations of maternal-newborn nursing* (2nd ed.). Philadelphia: W. B. Saunders. p. 703.

BIBLIOGRAPHY

Burroughs, A. (1997). *Maternity nursing: An introductory text* (7th ed.). Philadelphia: W. B. Saunders.
Gorrie, T., McKinney, E., & Murray, S. (1998). *Foundations of maternal-newborn nursing* (2nd ed.). Philadelphia: W. B. Saunders.

Leifer, G. (1999). *Thompson's introduction to maternity and pediatric nursing* (3rd ed.). Philadelphia: W. B. Saunders.
Nichols, F., & Zwelling, E. (1997). *Maternal-newborn nursing: Theory and practice.* Philadelphia: W. B. Saunders.

CHAPTER 22

Prenatal Period and Risk Conditions

....

I. Physiological Maternal Changes

A. Cardiovascular system
1. Circulating blood volume increases
2. Heart is elevated upward and to the left due to displacement of the diaphragm as the uterus enlarges
3. Pulse may increase about 10 beats/minute; blood pressure may decline in the second trimester
4. Iron requirements are increased

B. Respiratory system
1. Oxygen consumption increases
2. Diaphragm is elevated due to the enlarged uterus
3. Respiratory rate remains unchanged
4. Shortness of breath may be experienced

C. Gastrointestinal system
1. Nausea and vomiting may occur due to the secretion of human chorionic gonadotropin (hCG), which subsides by the third month
2. Constipation due to decreased GI motility or pressure of the uterus
3. Flatulence and heartburn due to decreased motility and slow emptying of the stomach
4. Hemorrhoids due to increased venous pressure

D. Renal system
1. Decreased bladder tone is caused by hormonal changes
2. Renal threshold for glucose may be reduced

E. Endocrine system: basal metabolic rate rises

F. Reproductive system
1. Uterus
   a. Uterus increases from 60 g to 1000 g
   b. Irregular contractions occur
2. Cervix
   a. Becomes shorter, more elastic, and larger in diameter
   b. Endocervical glands secrete a thick mucus plug, which is expelled from the canal when dilation begins
   c. Increased vascularization causes a softening and blue-purple discoloration (**Chadwick's sign**)
3. Ovaries: the ovaries cease ovum production
4. Vagina
   a. Hypertrophy and thickening of muscle
   b. Increase in vaginal secretions, and secretions are usually thick, white, and acidic
5. Breast
   a. Breast size increases
   b. Nipples become more pronounced and areola becomes darker in color
   c. Colostrum may appear from the breast

G. Skin
1. A dark streak down the midline of the abdomen may appear (linea nigra)
2. Melasma (chloasma), or mask of pregnancy, may occur over the forehead, cheeks, and nose
3. Reddish purple stretch marks (striae) may occur on the abdomen, breasts, thighs, and upper arms

H. Skeletal system: postural changes occur as the increased weight of the uterus causes a forward pull of the bony pelvis

I. Metabolism
1. The average expected weight gain during pregnancy is 2 to 4 pounds in the first trimester, and approximately 1 pound per week in the second and third trimesters
2. Water retention occurs, which can contribute to weight gain

II. Psychological Maternal Changes

A. Ambivalence
1. Occurs early in pregnancy even when the pregnancy is planned
2. Mother may experience dependence-independence conflict and ambivalence related to role changes

3. Father may experience ambivalence related to the new role he is assuming, the increased financial responsibilities, and sharing the wife's attention with the child

B. Acceptance
1. Factors that may be related to acceptance of the pregnancy are the woman's readiness for the experience and her identification with the motherhood role
2. When the mother plans and expects the pregnancy, she tends to display pleasure and experience fewer physical discomforts

C. Emotional lability
1. May be manifested by frequency in the change of emotional states or extremes in emotional states
2. These emotional changes are common, but the mother may feel that these changes are abnormal

D. Body image changes: The changes in a woman's perception of her image during pregnancy occurs gradually and may be either positive or negative

III. Discomforts of Pregnancy

A. Nausea and vomiting
1. Occurs in the first trimester
2. Due to elevated hCG levels and changes in carbohydrate metabolism
3. Implementation
   a. Eating dry crackers before arising
   b. Eating small, frequent, low-fat meals during the day
   c. Drinking liquids between meals

B. Syncope
1. Usually occurs in the first trimester
2. May be hormonally triggered or caused by the increased blood volume, anemia, fatigue, or sudden position changes
3. Implementation
   a. Sitting with the feet up
   b. Changing positions slowly
   c. Changing the position to the left side to relieve the pressure of the uterus on the inferior vena cava

C. Urinary urgency and frequency
1. Usually occurs in first and third trimesters due to pressure of the uterus on the bladder
2. Implementation
   a. Drinking 2 quarts of fluid per day, limiting fluid intake in the evening
   b. Voiding at regular intervals
   c. Wearing perineal pads if necessary

D. Breast tenderness
1. Can occur from the first through the third trimesters
2. Due to increased levels of estrogen and progesterone
3. Implementation
   a. Encouraging the use of a supportive bra with nonelastic straps
   b. Avoiding the use of soap on the nipples and areola area to prevent drying

E. Increased vaginal discharge
1. Can occur from the first through the third trimesters
2. Due to hyperplasia of vaginal mucosa and increased mucus production
3. Implementation
   a. Wearing cotton underwear
   b. Avoiding douching
   c. Proper cleansing and hygiene
   d. Advising the client to consult the physician or health care provider if infection is suspected

F. Nasal stuffiness
1. Occurs during the first through the third trimesters
2. Occurs due to increased estrogen that causes swelling of the nasal tissues and dryness
3. Implementation
   a. Encouraging the use of a humidifier
   b. Avoiding the use of nasal sprays or antihistamines

G. Fatigue
1. Occurs usually in the first and third trimesters
2. Is usually due to hormonal changes
3. Implementation
   a. Arranging frequent rest periods throughout the day
   b. Obtaining regular exercise

H. Heartburn
1. Occurs in the second and third trimesters
2. Results from increased progesterone levels, decreased GI motility and esophageal reflux, and displacement of the stomach by the enlarging uterus
3. Implementation
   a. Eating small, frequent meals, and avoiding fatty and spicy foods
   b. Sitting upright for 30 minutes following a meal
   c. Drinking milk between meals
   d. Taking Maalox or Mylanta only when recommended by the physician

I. Ankle edema
1. Usually occurs in second and third trimesters
2. Occurs due to vasodilation, venous stasis, and increased venous pressure below the uterus
3. Implementation
   a. Elevating the legs during the day
   b. Sleeping on the left side
   c. Avoiding sitting or standing in one position for long periods

J. Varicose veins
1. Usually occur in the second and third trimesters
2. Occurs due to weakening walls of the veins or valves and venous congestion
3. Implementation
   a. Wearing support hose
   b. Sitting or lying with feet and hips elevated

c. Avoiding leg-crossing
d. Avoiding long periods of standing or sitting
e. Avoiding constricting articles of clothing

K. Headaches
1. Usually occur in the second and third trimesters
2. Occur due to changes in blood volume and vascular tone
3. Implementation
   a. Changing positions slowly
   b. Applying a cool cloth to the forehead
   c. Using acetaminophen (Tylenol) sparingly only if prescribed by the physician

L. Hemorrhoids
1. Usually occur in second and third trimesters
2. Occur due to increased venous pressure and/or constipation
3. Implementation
   a. Soaking in a warm sitz bath
   b. Eating a high-fiber diet, drinking sufficient fluids, and avoiding constipation
   c. Increasing exercise such as walking
   d. Applying ointments, suppositories, or compresses as prescribed

M. Constipation
1. Usually occurs in the second and third trimesters
2. Occurs due to decreased intestinal motility, the displacement of the intestines, and from taking iron supplements
3. Implementation
   a. Eating high-fiber foods such as fresh fruits, vegetables, and bran
   b. Drinking sufficient fluids
   c. Exercising regularly
   d. Avoiding mineral oil or castor oil laxatives and using psyllium (Metamucil), senna (Senokot), or 1 teaspoon of milk of magnesia at bedtime only as prescribed by the physician

N. Backache
1. Usually occurs in the second and third trimesters
2. Occurs from an exaggerated lumbosacral curve due to the enlarged uterus
3. Implementation
   a. Encouraging rest and sleeping on a firm mattress
   b. Using good body mechanics
   c. Wearing low-heeled shoes
   d. Performing pelvic tilt exercises and exercises such as squatting, sitting, and pelvic rocking

O. Leg cramps
1. Usually occur in second and third trimesters
2. Occur due to an altered calcium-phosphorus balance and pressure of the uterus on nerves, or from fatigue
3. Implementation
   a. Getting regular exercise, especially walking

b. Elevating the feet and dorsiflexing the feet when resting
c. Increasing calcium intake

P. Shortness of breath
1. Can occur in the second and third trimesters
2. Occurs due to pressure on the diaphragm
3. Implementation
   a. Allowing frequent rest periods and avoid overexertion
   b. Sleeping with the head elevated or on the side

IV. Laboratory Tests (Box 22–1)

A. Blood type and Rh factor
1. ABO typing is performed to determine the woman's blood type
2. Rh typing is done to determine the presence or absence of Rh antigen (Rh positive or Rh negative)
3. If the client is Rh negative and has a negative antibody screen, the client will need repeat antibody screens and should receive Rh immune globulin at 28 weeks' gestation

B. Rubella titer
1. If the client has a negative titer, indicating susceptibility to the rubella virus, the client should receive the appropriate immunization postpartum
2. The client must be using effective birth control at the time of the immunization and counseled not to become pregnant for 3 months following immunization

C. Hemoglobin and hematocrit levels
1. Hemoglobin and hematocrit levels will drop during gestation as a result of increased plasma volume
2. An increase in the hematocrit level may indicate the development of pregnancy-induced hypertension (PIH); a decrease indicates anemia

D. Papanicolaou smear: done during initial prenatal exam to screen for cervical neoplasia

E. Gonorrhea culture: done during initial prenatal exam and may be repeated during the third trimester in high-risk clients

F. Syphilis screening: done during initial prenatal exam and may be repeated during the third trimester in high-risk clients

G. Herpes cultures
1. Indicated for clients with a positive history or those with suspected active lesions
2. Performed to determine the route of **delivery**
3. Weekly cultures may be done beginning at

BOX 22–1. Prenatal Visits

Every 4 weeks first 28–32 weeks
Every 2 weeks from 32–36 weeks
Every week from 36–40 weeks

the 35th or 36th week of pregnancy until delivery

H. Chlamydia culture: indicated if the client is in a high-risk group or if infants from previous pregnancies have developed neonatal conjunctivitis or chlamydial infection

I. Sickle cell screening: indicated for clients at risk for sickle cell disease

J. Tuberculin skin test
1. Indicated only if all past skin tests have been negative; may not be done until after delivery
2. A positive skin test indicates the need for chest x-ray (using an abdominal lead shield) to rule out active disease
3. Converters to positive may be referred for treatment with medication following **delivery**

K. Hepatitis B surface antigens: recommended for all women because of the prevalence of the disease in the general population

L. Urinalysis and urine culture
1. A urine specimen for glucose and protein should be obtained at every prenatal visit
2. Glycosuria is a common result of decreased renal threshold in pregnancy
3. If glycosuria persists, this may indicate diabetes
4. White blood cells in the urine may indicate infection
5. Ketonuria may result from insufficient food intake or vomiting
6. Levels of 2+ to 4+ protein in the urine may indicate infection or PIH

V. Diagnostic Tests

A. Ultrasound
1. Description: outlines and identifies fetal and maternal structures and assists to confirm estimated date of **delivery**
2. Implementation
   a. Instruct the client to drink six to eight glasses of water before the test and not to void because the test is done with a full bladder
   b. Inform the client that the test presents no known risks to client or fetus

B. Alpha-fetoprotein screening (AFP)
1. Assesses the quantity of fetal serum proteins; if elevated, is associated with open neural tube and abdominal wall defects
2. Can detect spina bifida and Down's syndrome
3. Implementation
   a. Explain that the level is determined by a single maternal blood sample drawn at 15 to 18 weeks' gestation
   b. If the level is elevated and the gestation is less than 18 weeks, a second sample is drawn
   c. An ultrasound is performed for elevated levels to rule out fetal abnormalities or multiple gestation

C. Chorionic villus sampling (CVS)
1. Aspiration of a small sample of chorionic villus tissue at 8 to 12 weeks' gestation
2. Test is performed for the purpose of detecting genetic abnormalities
3. Implementation
   a. Instruct the client to drink water to fill the bladder before the procedure to aid in the position of the uterus for catheter insertion
   b. Instruct the client to report bleeding, infection, or leakage of fluid at insertion site after the procedure
   c. Rh-negative women may be given RhoGam for risks related to the procedure

D. Kick test (fetal movement counting)
1. The mother lies down on her left side for 1 hour after meals and counts fetal kicks for 30 minutes
2. Instruct the client to notify the physician or health care provider if there are fewer than 5 kicks in 1 hour

E. Amniocentesis
1. Aspiration of **amniotic fluid**; done from 14 weeks of pregnancy and on
2. Performed to determine genetic disorders, the sex of the fetus, and fetal lung maturity
3. Implementation
   a. Instruct the client to empty the bladder before the procedure
   b. Prepare the client for an ultrasound, which is performed to locate the **placenta**
   c. Obtain baseline vital signs and FHR, and monitor every 15 minutes
   d. Position the client supine
   e. Instruct the client that if chills, fever, leakage of fluid at the needle insertion site, decreased fetal movement, or uterine contractions occur, to notify the physician or health care provider

F. Fern test
1. A microscopic slide test to determine the presence of **amniotic fluid** leakage
2. Specimen is obtained from the external os of the cervix and vaginal pool
3. Fluid is examined on a slide under a microscope and a fernlike pattern indicates the presence of **amniotic fluid**
4. Implementation
   a. Position client in the dorsal lithotomy position
   b. Instruct the client to cough to cause the fluid to leak from the uterus if the membranes are ruptured

G. Nitrazine test
1. Use of Nitrazine test strip or cotton swab to detect the presence of **amniotic fluid** in vaginal secretions
2. Amniotic fluid turns the yellow Nitrazine blue
3. Implementation
   a. Position the client in the dorsal lithotomy position
   b. Touch the test tape to the fluid

  c. Check the test tape for a blue-green, blue-gray, or deep blue color, which indicates that the membranes are probably ruptured
H. Nonstress test (NST) and contraction stress test (Box 22–2 and Box 22–3)

◆ VI. Nutrition

◆ A. General guidelines
  1. Choose foods from the four basic food groups or food guide pyramid
  2. An increase of about 300 calories per day is needed during pregnancy
  3. Calorie needs are greater in the last two trimesters than in the first
  4. An increase of about 500 calories per day is needed during lactation
  5. Encourage a diet high in folic acid with folic acid supplements

---

BOX 22–2. Nonstress Test (NST)

DESCRIPTION

Performed to assess placental function and oxygenation and fetal well-being
Evaluates fetal heart rate (FHR) in response to fetal movement

IMPLEMENTATION

External ultrasound transducer and the tocodynamometer (toco) are applied to the mother, and a tracing of at least 20 minutes' duration is obtained so that the FHR and the uterine activity can be observed
Obtain baseline blood pressure and monitor BP frequently
Position mother in the left lateral position to avoid vena cava compression
Ask mother to press a button every time she feels fetal movement
The monitor records a mark at each occurrence of fetal movement, which is used as a reference point to assess FHR response

RESULTS

Reactive Nonstress Test (Normal/Negative)
An increase in FHR is expected with fetal activity and indicates a healthy fetus with adequate fetal oxygenation, a functioning placenta, and an intact central nervous system

Nonreactive Nonstress Test (Abnormal)
If the fetal heart does not increase with movement, the fetus may be suffering with anoxia due to diminished placental blood flow
Lack of FHR acceleration with movement is called a nonreactive fetus
Lack of fetal movement during a 20-minute test may indicate fetal sleep

Unsatisfactory
Cannot be interpreted because of the poor quality of the FHR

BOX 22–3. Contraction Stress Test

DESCRIPTION

Assesses placental oxygenation and function
Determines fetal ability to tolerate labor and determines fetal well-being
Fetus is exposed to the stressor of contractions to assess the adequacy of placental perfusion under simulated labor conditions
Performed if nonstress test is abnormal

IMPLEMENTATION

The external fetal monitor is applied to the mother, and a 20- to 30-minute baseline strip is recorded
The uterus is stimulated to contract either by the administration of a dilute dose of oxytocin (Pitocin) or by having the mother use nipple stimulation until three palpable contractions with a duration of 40 seconds or more in a 10-minute period have been achieved
Frequent maternal BP readings are done, and the client is monitored closely while increasing doses of oxytocin are given

RESULTS

Negative Contraction Stress Test
No change in FHR occurs during three uterine contractions lasting more than 30 seconds each within a 10-minute period

Positive Contraction Stress Test (Abnormal)
Repetitive late FHR decelerations occur, demonstrating the stress of uterine contractions on FHR

Hyperstimulation
Occurs when contractions occur more frequently than every 2 minutes or last longer than 90 seconds each

Suspicious
When there are inconsistent but definite late decelerations in FHR

---

  6. A diet rich in folic acid is necessary for all women of childbearing age to prevent neural tube defect
  7. Drink at least eight glasses of water a day
B. Vegetarianism
  1. During pregnancy, it is necessary to obtain ample and complete proteins from dairy products and eggs
  2. An adequate pure vegetarian diet contains protein from unrefined grains such as brown rice and whole wheat, legumes such as beans, split peas, and lentils; nuts in large quantities, and a variety of cooked and fresh vegetables and fruits
C. Lactose intolerance
  1. Lactose consumed by an individual with intolerance can cause abdominal distention, discomfort, nausea, vomiting, loose stool, and cramps

2. Milk may be tolerated in cooked form, as in custards or fermented dairy products
3. Cheese and yogurt are sometimes tolerated
4. Lactase, an enzyme, may be prescribed and is available as a tablet to be chewed before ingesting milk or milk products, or as a liquid to add to milk itself
5. Lactase-treated milk or lactose-free products are also available commercially

D. Pica
1. Defined as eating substances that are not ordinarily considered edible or to have nutritive value such as dirt, clay, starch, and freezer frost
2. Practiced in poverty-stricken areas where diets tend to be inadequate, but pica may also be found at other socioeconomic levels
3. Iron deficiency anemia occurs as a result of pica

VII. Abortion

A. Description: termination of pregnancy before the fetus is viable (20 weeks or a weight of 500 g)
B. Data collection
1. Spontaneous vaginal bleeding
2. Passage of clots and tissue through vagina
3. Low uterine cramping and contractions
C. Implementation
1. Maintain bed rest and vital signs
2. Count perineal pads to evaluate blood loss
3. Save expelled tissues and clots
4. Monitor IV fluids as prescribed to prevent shock
5. Prepare client for dilatation and curettage as prescribed for incomplete abortion

VIII. Acquired Immunodeficiency Syndrome (AIDS)

A. Description: women infected with the AIDS virus may first demonstrate symptoms at the time of pregnancy or possibly develop life-threatening infections because normal pregnancy involves some suppression of the maternal immune system
B. Transmission in pregnancy
1. All body fluids from an infected host, except perspiration, have been shown to contain the virus

2. Blood, semen, and breast milk have higher concentrations of the virus than urine, saliva, vomitus, and stool
3. The virus can cross some membranes such as the **placental** barrier, blood-brain barrier, and vaginal mucosa, and (in the neonate) the walls of the gastrointestinal tract
4. Perinatal transmission from infected mother to fetus or newborn infant via transplacental transmission, contamination with maternal blood during birth, or through breast milk

C. Risks to the mother
1. The mother with HIV is managed as high risk
2. Frequent complaints of fatigue, shortness of breath, nausea, back pain, urinary frequency, and headaches
3. More vulnerable to postpartum infections
4. May need longer courses of antibiotics for infection
5. AZT (zidovudine), starting in the 14th week of pregnancy may be prescribed to minimize teratogenicity and may be administered to the woman with HIV infection to prevent transmission to the fetus; it may also be necessary to add a second medication to decrease the risk of transmission to the fetus

D. Diagnosis
1. Client may be infected with the virus but not yet have produced antibodies, thereby testing negative but being capable of infecting others
2. Clients who by history may be at risk for possible HIV but test negative for the HIV antibody should be retested; it usually takes 6 to 12 weeks for a host to manufacture detectable HIV antibodies
3. Enzyme-linked immunosorbent assay (ELISA) screening test for AIDS antibody is a very sensitive test but not highly specific; a positive ELISA test indicates the need for further testing using the Western blot

E. Data collection (Table 22–1)
F. Implementation
1. Prenatal period
   a. Prevention of opportunistic infections
   b. Instruct the client on good handwashing procedures
   c. Avoid people who are ill
   d. Avoid exposure to cat feces, cat or dog litter, or fish tanks

Table 22–1. **The Stages of AIDS**

Stage 1	Stage 2	Stage 3	Stage 4
Fever	Active but asymptomatic and may	Symptomatic	Advanced HIV infection
Myalgia	remain so for years	Evidence of immune dysfunction	Vulnerable to common bacterial
Lymphadenopathy	May experience an outbreak of	All body systems can present	infections
Headache	herpes zoster (shingles)	with signs of immune	Development of opportunistic
	May experience a transient	dysfunction	infections
	thrombocytopenia	Integumentary and gynecological	Serious immune compromise
		problems are common	

e. Avoid undercooked meats, raw eggs, and unpasteurized milk
f. Prevent further exposure to HIV through sexual contact or use of needles
g. Avoid procedures that increase the risk of perinatal transmission, such as amniocentesis and fetal scalp sampling

2. Intrapartal period
   a. Note that if the fetus has not been exposed to HIV in utero, the highest risk exists during **delivery** through the birth canal
   b. Scalp electrodes are never used
   c. Episiotomy is avoided to decrease the amount of maternal blood in and around the birth canal
   d. The administration of oxytocin is avoided since oxytocin contractions can be strong, inducing vaginal tears or necessitating the need for episiotomy
   e. Minimize the infant's exposure to maternal blood and body fluids
   f. Place heavy absorbent pads under the mother's hips to absorb **amniotic fluid** and maternal blood during **delivery**
   g. Promptly remove newborn from mother's blood after **delivery**
   h. Suction infant promptly after **delivery**
   i. Intravenous AZT (zidovudine) may be administered during **delivery**

3. Postpartum period
   a. Monitor for signs of infection such as increased temperature and WBC count
   b. Place the client in protective isolation to prevent client infection if she is experiencing a suppressed immune response
   c. Restrict breast-feeding
   d. Instruct the client how to take her temperature and to identify symptoms necessitating immediate follow-up care

G. The neonate and HIV
   1. Description
      a. The fetus of an HIV antibody–positive woman should be monitored closely throughout the pregnancy
      b. Serial ultrasound screenings should be done to identify intrauterine growth restriction
      c. Weekly nonstress testing after 32 weeks of gestation may be necessary
      d. Infants born to HIV-positive clients may test positive because the mother's positive antibodies may persist for as long as 18 months after birth
      e. The use of antiviral medication, reduction of infant exposure to maternal blood and body fluids, and the early identification of HIV in pregnancy reduce the risk of transmission to the infant
      f. The infant will acquire maternal antibody to HIV infection, but not all infants acquire the infection

   2. Transmission to the neonate
      a. Across the **placental** barrier
      b. During the process of **labor** and **delivery**
      c. Via breast milk

   3. Implementation
      a. Bathe the infant carefully before any invasive procedure such as the administration of vitamin K, heel sticks, or venipunctures
      b. The infant can room with the mother
      c. AZT (zidovudine) may be prescribed for the first 6 weeks of life
      d. All HIV-exposed infants should be treated with medication to prevent infection by *Pneumocystis carinii*
      e. Note that an HIV culture is recommended at age 1 month and after 4 months of age; infants at risk for HIV infection should be seen by the physician at birth, 1 week, 2 weeks, 1 month, and 2 months of life
      f. Infants at risk for HIV infection need to receive all recommended immunizations at the regular schedule
      g. No live immunizations should be administered; inactivated polio vaccine by injection rather than oral polio vaccine should be administered because the oral polio vaccine causes a shedding of polio virus in the stool, which may be a risk to the immunocompromised family
      h. Note that the neonate may be asymptomatic for the first several years of life; monitor for early signs of immune deficiency, such as enlarged spleen or liver, lymphadenopathy, and impairment in growth and development

IX. Anemia

A. Description
   1. A condition that can develop as a result of iron deficiency with a hemoglobin below 10 g/dL or a hematocrit level below 30g/dL
   2. Anemia predisposes the client to postpartum infection and hemorrhage

B. Data collection
   1. Fatigue
   2. Headache
   3. Pallor
   4. Tachycardia

C. Implementation
   1. Hemoglobin and hematocrit levels may be monitored every 2 weeks
   2. Instruct the client about iron and folic acid supplements
   3. Instruct the client to take iron with a source of vitamin C and to avoid taking iron with tea
   4. Instruct the client to eat foods high in iron, folic acid, and protein

X. Cardiac Disease

A. Description: the inability to cope with the added plasma volume and the increased cardiac output
B. Data collection
  1. Dyspnea and fatigue
  2. Cough
  3. Peripheral edema
  4. Anginal-type pain
  5. Palpitations and tachycardia
C. Implementation
  1. Monitor vital signs, fetal heart rate, and condition of fetus
  2. Plan activity level and stress the need for sufficient rest
  3. Encourage adequate nutrition to prevent anemia
  4. Maintain bed rest for the client as prescribed during the last weeks of pregnancy
  5. During **labor**
    a. Monitor vital signs frequently
    b. Place the client on a cardiac monitor and on an external fetal monitor
    c. Maintain bed rest with the mother lying on her side or in semirecumbent position
    d. Administer oxygen as prescribed
    e. Monitor for signs of pulmonary edema and heart failure
    f. Provide emotional support

XI. Chronic Hypertension

A. Description
  1. Hypertension that occurs before pregnancy, is diagnosed before the 20th week of gestation, or is diagnosed for the first time during pregnancy and persists beyond the 42nd day postpartum
  2. The condition predisposes the client to PIH
  3. Can cause abruptio **placentac** and intrauterine growth retardation
B. Data collection
  1. Headaches
  2. Visual changes
  3. BP of 140/90 mmHg or greater
C. Implementation
  1. Monitor blood pressure
  2. Monitor fetal activity and fetal growth
  3. Encourage frequent rest periods, instructing the client to lie in the left lateral position
  4. Administer antihypertensive medications as prescribed for diastolic pressures greater than 100 mmHg
  5. Monitor intake and output (I&O)

XII. Diabetes Mellitus

A. Description: pregnancy places demands on carbohydrate metabolism and causes insulin requirements to increase
B. Insulin-dependent diabetes
  1. Maternal glucose crosses the **placenta** but insulin does not
  2. During the first trimester, maternal insulin needs decrease
  3. The fetus produces its own insulin and pulls glucose from the mother, which predisposes the mother to hypoglycemic reactions
  4. During the second and third trimesters, increases in **placental** hormones cause an insulin-resistant state requiring an increase in the client's insulin dose
  5. After **placental delivery, placental** hormone levels drop abruptly and insulin requirements decrease
C. Diabetes in pregnancy
  1. Diabetes is more difficult to control during pregnancy
  2. Premature **delivery** is more frequent
  3. The infant of a diabetic mother may be large in size but will have functions related to gestational age rather than size
  4. The infant of a diabetic mother is subject to hypoglycemia, hyperbilirubinemia, respiratory distress syndrome, and congenital anomalies
  5. Stillborn and neonatal mortality rates are higher in pregnancies of a diabetic woman
D. Gestational diabetes
  1. Occurs during the second or third trimester
  2. Occurs in pregnancy in clients not previously diagnosed as diabetic and occurs when the pancreas cannot respond to the demand for more insulin
  3. Pregnant women should be screened for glucose levels at the 26th week of gestation
  4. Glucose levels should remain at 105 mg/dL except for brief periods after meals
  5. A 3-hour glucose tolerance test will confirm diabetes when two or more values are above normal
  6. Oral hypoglycemic agents are never used during pregnancy
  7. Frequently can be treated by diet alone; however, insulin may be needed for some clients
  8. Most gestational diabetics convert to normal after **delivery**; however, these individuals have an increased risk of developing diabetes in their lifetime
E. Predisposing conditions to gestational diabetes
  1. Over age 35
  2. Obesity
  3. Multiple gestation
  4. Family history of diabetes
F. Data collection
  1. Excessive thirst and hunger
  2. Weight loss
  3. Blurred vision
  4. Frequent urination
  5. Recurrent urinary tract infections and vaginal yeast infections
  6. Glycosuria and ketonuria
  7. Signs of pregnancy-induced hypertension
  8. The fetus is large for gestational age

G. Implementation
1. Clients are screened between the 24th and 28th weeks of pregnancy
2. Prenatal visits bimonthly for 6 months and weekly thereafter
3. Monitor for signs of hypoglycemia and give the client 8 oz skim milk for hypoglycemic reactions to elevate blood glucose levels gradually
4. Observe for signs of hyperglycemia and for glycosuria and ketonuria
5. Monitor weight
6. Monitor for signs of preeclampsia, which include hypertension, proteinuria, and edema
7. Check for increased temperature and signs of infection
8. Instruct the client to report burning and pain on urination or vaginal discharge or itching
9. Monitor fetal status
10. Monitor for signs of premature **labor**
H. Implementation during **labor**
1. Monitor fetal status continuously for signs of distress, and if noted, the client may be prepared for immediate cesarean section
2. Insulin and IV glucose are carefully regulated as prescribed because **labor** depletes glycogen
I. Implementation during the postpartum period
1. Observe the client closely for an insulin reaction, since a precipitous drop in insulin requirements is usual
2. The client may not require insulin for the first 24 hours
3. Monitor for signs of infection or postpartum hemorrhage

XIII. Disseminated Intravascular Coagulation (DIC)

A. Description
1. A condition in the mother's body that results in an exaggerated clotting process, which increases the formation of clots in the microcirculation
2. The rapid and extensive formation of clots results in bleeding and the potential vascular occlusion of organs from thromboembolus formation
B. Predisposing conditions
1. Abruptio placentae
2. Intrauterine fetal death
3. **Amniotic fluid** embolism
4. PIH
5. Liver disease
6. Sepsis
C. Data collection
1. Uncontrolled bleeding
2. Bruising, purpura, petechiae, and ecchymosis
3. Hematuria, hematemesis, or vaginal bleeding
D. Implementation
1. Monitor vital signs
2. Administer oxygen as prescribed
3. Monitor for signs of shock

4. Heparin may be prescribed to prevent clot formation

XIV. Ectopic Pregnancy

A. Description: a pregnancy that occurs in an other than uterine area, with **implantation** usually occurring in the fallopian tubes
B. Data collection
1. Pain unilaterally, with cramping and tenderness
2. Mass in the adnexa or cul-de-sac
3. Slight, dark vaginal bleeding
4. Fever
5. Low hemoglobin and hematocrit, elevated erythrocyte sedimentation rate
6. Profound shock if rupture occurs
C. Implementation
1. Obtain vital signs
2. Monitor bleeding
3. Obtain blood for type and cross-match
4. Prepare the client for the administration of methotrexate if prescribed, for masses smaller than 4 cm, to induce abortion and preserve the fallopian tube
5. Prepare the client for laparotomy and removal of pregnancy and tube, if necessary, or repair of tube

XV. Fetal Death In Utero (FDIU)

A. Description
1. The death of a fetus after the 20th week of gestation and before birth
2. DIC can develop if the dead fetus is retained in the uterus for 3 to 4 weeks or more
B. Data collection
1. Absence of fetal movement
2. Absence of fetal heart tones
3. Maternal weight loss
4. Lack of fetal growth or decrease in fundal height
5. Lack of cardiac activity and other characteristics suggestive of fetal death noted on the ultrasound
C. Implementation
1. Prepare for the **delivery** of the fetus
2. Support the client's decision about **labor,** birth, and the postpartum period
3. Facilitate the grieving process
4. Allow the parents to hold the infant after birth
5. Allow the parents to name the infant
6. Accept behaviors such as anger and hostility from the parents
7. Refer parents to an appropriate support group

XVI. Hepatitis B

A. Description: an inflammation of the liver caused by the hepatitis B virus
B. Transmission to the fetus and neonate

1. Transplacental
2. Intrapartum exposure to infected blood, **amniotic fluid,** or vaginal secretions
3. Through postpartum exposure
4. Through breast-feeding

C. Risks to the mother
   1. Maternal fetal risk in uncomplicated hepatitis B is not generally increased unless infection occurs in the third trimester or in the immediate postpartum period
   2. Intrapartum risks include increased risk for prematurity, premature **delivery,** and fetal transmission
   3. Postpartum risk for transmission is by contact, by oral transmission through saliva exchange and kissing, food preparation, and utensils/fomites

D. Risk to the fetus and neonate
   1. The infant is identified as an HBsAg carrier
   2. Infections in early life are usually asymptomatic
   3. Chronic hepatitis
   4. Associated with glomerulonephritis and nephritis

E. Implementation
   1. Minimize the number of vaginal exams
   2. Minimize the risk for intrapartum ascending infections
   3. Double-glove for extended periods of blood contact with the client
   4. Antibiotics may be administered as prescribed during labor to decrease the risk of transmission to the infant especially if the membranes are ruptured
   5. Remove maternal blood from the newborn immediately after birth
   6. Protect the newborn's scalp integrity
   7. Suction the newborn immediately after birth
   8. Cut the cord with new sterile scissors, not the scissors used on the perineum
   9. Bathe the newborn prior to invasive procedures
   10. Clean and dry the face and eyes before instilling eye prophylaxis
   11. Discourage kissing until mother and infant have been treated
   12. Support breast-feeding after maternal and newborn treatment; breast-feeding is not contraindicated if an infected mother and infant are treated
   13. Immune globulin and vaccine are given to all HbsAg-positive newborns within 2 to 12 hours of **delivery,** at least before 24 hours and not more than 7 days after birth
   14. Inform the mother that HBV vaccine will be administered to the neonate, with the first dose given before the infant leaves the hospital; the second dose at 1 month; and the third dose at 6 months
   15. If the mother is identified positive more than 1 month after **delivery,** her HbsAg-negative infant should be treated
   16. Discourage sharing razors, toothbrushes, and engaging in unprotected intercourse

XVII. Hydatidiform Mole

A. Description
   1. A developmental anomaly of the **placenta** that changes chorionic villi into a mass of clear vesicles
   2. Presents as an edematous grapelike cluster that may be nonmalignant or may develop into choriocarcinoma

B. Data collection
   1. Fetal heart rate not detectable
   2. Vaginal bleeding, which usually occurs by week 12, bright red or dark brown that may be slight, profuse, or intermittent
   3. Symptoms of PIH such as elevated blood pressure, edema, and proteinuria, which may be present before week 20
   4. Fundal height is greater than expected for date
   5. Elevated hCG levels
   6. Ultrasound shows a characteristic snowstorm pattern

C. Implementation
   1. Monitor vital signs
   2. Monitor fetal heart rate and fetal activity
   3. Prepare the mother for uterine evacuation or induced abortion
   4. Prepare for hysterectomy if necessary
   5. Monitor for postprocedure hemorrhage and infection

XVIII. Hyperemesis Gravidarum

A. Description: intractable nausea and vomiting that persists beyond the first trimester and causes disturbances in nutrition, electrolytes, and fluid balance

B. Data collection
   1. Nausea most pronounced on arising; however, can occur at other times of the day
   2. Persistent vomiting
   3. Signs of dehydration

C. Implementation
   1. Monitor vital signs
   2. Monitor fetal heart rate and fetal activity
   3. Monitor for signs of dehydration
   4. Monitor daily weight
   5. Monitor I&O and calorie count
   6. Restrict PO intake until vomiting subsides
   7. Begin on a dry diet, alternating liquids and solids in small quantities, and advance diet slowly

XIX. Incompetent Cervix

A. Description
   1. Premature dilatation of cervix, which occurs in the fourth or fifth month of pregnancy
   2. Associated with cervical trauma as a result of previous surgery or birth

3. Treatment is surgical
B. Data collection
  1. Vaginal bleeding at 18 to 28 weeks of gestation
  2. Fetal membranes visible through cervix
C. Implementation
  1. Monitor vital signs
  2. Monitor fetal heart rate
  3. Provide bed rest
  4. Prepare the client for surgery as prescribed

XX. Infections

A. Toxoplasmosis (protozoa)
  1. Produces symptoms of acute, flulike infection in the mother
  2. Transmitted through raw meat or handling cat litter of infected cats
  3. Organism passes through **placenta**
  4. Spontaneous abortion likely to occur early in pregnancy
B. Rubella
  1. Organism transmitted across the **placenta**
  2. Extremely teratogenic in the first trimester
  3. Causes congenital defects of eyes, heart, ears, and brain
  4. Women with low titers should be vaccinated at least 3 months before becoming pregnant or following a delivery
C. Cytomegalovirus (CMV)
  1. Produces flulike or mononucleosis-like symptoms in the mother
  2. Transmitted through the respiratory or sexual route
  3. Organism crosses the **placenta,** or the fetus may be infected through the birth canal
  4. May cause fetal death, retardation, heart defects, and deafness
  5. No effective treatment available
D. Genital herpes
  1. Affects the external genitalia, vagina, and cervix
  2. Causes draining, painful vesicles
  3. Virus can be lethal to the fetus if contracted during vaginal **delivery**
  4. **Delivery** of the fetus is usually by cesarean section if active lesions are present
  5. Maintain precautions during the vaginal examination
  6. Maintain isolation procedures during hospitalization if the disease is active
  7. Infant and mother may be separated during the active period, or other special precautionary measures may be used to avoid transmission to neonate

XXI. Multiple Gestation

A. Description: caused by double ovulation (fraternal or dizygotic) or a splitting of the fertilized egg (identical or monozygotic)
B. Data collection
  1. Excessive fetal activity

  2. Uterus large for gestational age
  3. Palpation of three or four large parts in the uterus
  4. Auscultation of more than one fetal heart rate
C. Implementation
  1. Monitor vital signs
  2. Monitor fetal heart rate and fetal activity
  3. Monitor for cervical changes
  4. Assess fetal growth
  5. Administer supplemental iron and vitamins as prescribed for anemia
  6. Monitor for preterm **labor**
  7. Prepare the client for ultrasound as prescribed
  8. Prepare the client for cesarean section for abnormal presentation as prescribed
  9. Oxytoxic medications may be prescribed after **delivery** to prevent postpartum hemorrhage from uterine overdistension

XXII. Pregnancy-Induced Hypertension (PIH)

A. Description
  1. An acute hypertensive state that develops after the 20th week of gestation
  2. The condition can be mild or severe and can progress to seizures (eclampsia) (Box 22–4)
B. Predisposing conditions
  1. Primigravida
  2. Teenagers and women over 35 years of age
  3. Poor nutrition
  4. Low socioeconomic status
  5. Chronic hypertension
  6. Diabetes
  7. Chronic renal disease
  8. History of PIH
C. Complications of PIH
  1. Abruptio placentae
  2. Disseminated intravascular coagulation (DIC)
  3. Thrombocytopenia
  4. **Placental** insufficiency
  5. Intrauterine fetal death
D. Mild preeclampsia
  1. Data collection
    a. Hypertension of 15 to 30 mmHg above baseline
    b. Weight gain of 1 lb or more per week in last trimester
    c. Mild, generalized edema
    d. Proteinuria of 1+
  2. Implementation
    a. Provide bed rest and position client in the left lateral position

BOX 22–4. Signs of Worsening PIH or Impending Seizures	
BP 160/110 mmHg or above	Visual changes
Epigastric pain	Headache
Decreased urinary output	Excessive proteinuria

b. Monitor blood pressure and weight
c. Monitor neurological status because changes can indicate cerebral hypoxia or impending seizure
d. Deep tendon reflexes are monitored and for the presence of clonus as hyperreflexia indicates increased central nervous system irritability (Box 22–5)
e. Provide adequate fluids
f. Monitor I&O; a urinary output of 30 mL/hour indicates adequate renal perfusion
g. Increase dietary protein and carbohydrates with no added salt as prescribed
h. Administer medications as prescribed to lower blood pressure to prevent a cerebrovascular accident; however, blood pressure should not be lowered drastically because **placental** perfusion can be compromised

E. Severe preeclampsia
   1. Data collection
      a. Severe hypertension, 30 to 40 mmHg above baseline while on bed rest
      b. Massive, generalized edema and weight gain
      c. Proteinuria 4+

BOX 22–5. Reflexes

PATELLAR
Client is positioned with legs dangling over the edge of the examining table or lying on back with legs slightly flexed
Strike patellar tendon just below the kneecap with the percussion hammer
Normal response: extension or kicking out of leg

BICEPS
The thumb is positioned over the client's biceps tendon supporting the client's elbow with the palm of the hand
Strike a downward blow over the examiner's thumb with the percussion hammer
Normal response: flexion of the arm at the elbow

CLONUS
Position the client with legs dangling over the edge of the examining table
The leg is supported with one hand; sharply dorsiflex the client's foot with the other hand
A dorsiflexed position is maintained for a few seconds, then release foot
Normal response: (negative clonus response)
Foot will remain steady in the dorsiflexed position
No rhythmic oscillations or jerking of the foot will be felt
When released, the foot will drop to a plantar flexed position with no oscillations
Abnormal response: (positive clonus response)
Rhythmic oscillations when the foot is dorsiflexed
Similar oscillations when the foot drops to the plantar flexed position

---

d. Less than 400 mL urine output in 24 hours
e. Severe headache
f. Dizziness
g. Blurred vision and spots before eyes
h. Nausea and vomiting
i. Epigastric pain
j. Central nervous system irritability
   2. Implementation
      a. Magnesium sulfate may be prescribed
      b. Antihypertensives may be prescribed to prevent cerebrovascular accident
      c. Prepare the client for the induction of **labor**
      d. Plan for the administration of magnesium sulfate for 24 to 48 hours postpartum as prescribed

F. Eclampsia
   1. Data collection
      a. Severe edema
      b. Proteinuria 4+
      c. Sudden large increase in weight
      d. BP greater than 160/110 mmHg
      e. Cyanosis
      f. Fetal distress
      g. Seizures
      h. Coma
   2. Implementation
      a. Protect the client from injury
      b. Administer oxygen as prescribed
      c. Monitor fetal heart rate and contractions
      d. Initiate seizure precautions
      e. Anticonvulsants may be prescribed
      f. Prepare for **delivery** after stabilization of client

XXIII. Sexually Transmitted Diseases (STDs)

A. *Chlamydia*
   1. Description
      a. Common, sexually transmitted pathogen associated with an increased risk for premature births, stillborn, neonatal conjunctivitis, and newborn chlamydial pneumonia
      b. In the nonpregnant state, it can cause salpingitis, pelvic abscesses, and chronic pelvic pain and infertility
      c. Incubation period is 5 to 10 days or longer, up to 28 days
      d. Diagnostic test is *Chlamydia* culture for *Chlamydia trachomatis*
   2. Data collection
      a. Increased vaginal discharge and itching
      b. Low-grade temperature
      c. Right upper quadrant abdominal pain
      d. Bleeding between periods
      e. Pain with coitus
      f. Dysuria
      g. Rectal pain or discharge
      h. Mucopurulent cervicitis
      i. Cervix that bleeds easy

j. In the newborn, conjunctivitis and pneumonia
3. Implementation
  a. Screen the client to determine if high risk
  b. Instruct the nonpregnant client about medication therapy, such as antibiotics
  c. Instruct the client regarding prescribed medication therapy for self and newborn
  d. Instruct the client in the importance of rescreening, because reinfection can occur as the client nears term
  e. Administer appropriate eye prophylaxis to the newborn as prescribed
  f. Monitor newborn for signs and symptoms of pneumonia if at risk
  g. Ensure that the sexual partner is treated
B. Syphilis
  1. Description
    a. A chronic infectious disease caused by the organism *Treponema pallidum*
    b. Transmission is by intimate physical contact with syphilitic lesions, which are usually found on the skin or mucous membranes of the mouth and genitals
    c. The incubation period is 2 to 6 weeks following exposure
    d. The infection may cause abortion or premature **labor** and is passed to the fetus after the fourth month of pregnancy as congenital syphilis
  2. Data collection (Table 22–2)
  3. Implementation
    a. Obtain serum test for syphilis on first prenatal visit
    b. Prepare to repeat serum test for syphilis just before the fourth month as the disease may be acquired after initial visit
    c. Instruct the client that treatment of the partner is necessary if infection occurs
    d. Prepare to administer procaine penicillin G to the mother as prescribed
    e. All cases are reported to health authorities for treatment of contacts
C. Gonorrhea
  1. Description
    a. Infection from *Neisseria gonorrhoeae* that causes inflammation of the mucous membranes of the genital and urinary tract
    b. Transmission of organism is by sexual intercourse

c. Infection may be transmitted to the baby's eyes during **delivery** causing blindness (ophthalmia neonatorum)
  2. Data collection
    a. Female: usually asymptomatic; vaginal discharge, urinary frequency, and pain
    b. Male: fever, painful urination, pelvic pain, epididymitis with pain, tenderness, and swelling
  3. Implementation
    a. Obtain culture for gonorrhea on the first prenatal visit
    b. Prepare to repeat culture for gonorrhea as infection may occur during pregnancy
    c. Administer prophylactic antibiotics to the newborn as prescribed
    d. Instruct the client that treatment of the partner is necessary if infection occurs
D. Genital warts
  1. Description
    a. Caused by human papillomavirus (HPV) and affects the cervix, urethra, penis, scrotum, and anus
    b. Appears 1 to 2 months after exposure
    c. Transmitted through sexual contact
    d. There is no cure for HPV
  2. Data collection
    a. Small to large wartlike growths on the genitals
    b. Cervical cell changes noted because HPV is associated with cervical malignancies
  3. Implementation
    a. Encourage yearly Papanicolaou (Pap) smear
    b. Limit sexual contacts and use condoms
    c. Instruct the client regarding potential treatment, including cytotoxic, cryotherapy, electrocautery, and surgical excision to remove lesions

XXIV. Tuberculosis

A. Description
  1. A highly communicable disease caused by *Mycobacterium tuberculosis*
  2. It is transmitted by the airborne route
  3. Tuberculosis has an insidious onset, and many clients are not aware of symptoms until the disease is well advanced
  4. A multidrug-resistant strain (MDR-TB) of TB

Table 22–2. The Stages of Syphilis

Primary Stage	Secondary Stage	Tertiary Stage
Most infectious stage Appearance of ulcerative, painless lesions produced by spirochetes at the point of entry into the body	Highly infectious stage Lesions appear about 3 weeks after the primary stage and may occur anywhere on the skin and mucous membranes Generalized lymphadenopathy occurs	Spirochetes enter the internal organs and cause permanent damage; symptoms may occur 10–30 years following the occurrence of an untreated primary lesion Invades the CNS, causing meningitis, ataxia, general paresis, and progressive mental deterioration Affects the aortic valve and aorta

can exist as a result of improper use or noncompliance with treatment programs and the development of mutations in the tubercle bacilli

B. Transmission
   1. Transplacental transmission is rare
   2. Can occur during birth through aspiration of infected **amniotic fluid**
   3. Neonate can become infected from contact with infected individuals
C. Risk to mother: active disease during pregnancy has been associated with an increase in hypertensive disorders of pregnancy
D. Diagnosis
   1. If a chest x-ray is required for the mother, a lead shield to the abdomen is required
   2. TB skin testing is safe during pregnancy
E. Data collection
   1. Maternal
      a. May be asymptomatic
      b. Fever and chills
      c. Night sweats
      d. Weight loss
      e. Fatigue
      f. Cough
      g. Green or yellow sputum
      h. Hemoptysis
      i. Dyspnea
      j. Pleural pain
   2. Neonate
      a. Fever
      b. Lethargy
      c. Poor feeding
      d. Failure to thrive
      e. Respiratory distress
      f. Hepatosplenomegaly
      g. Meningitis
      h. Disease may spread to all major organs
F. Implementation
   1. Mother
      a. Administration of isoniazid (INH), ethambutol (Myambutol), and rifampin (Rifadin) for 6 to 12 months during and after pregnacy
      b. Pyridoxine should be administered with INH to pregnant women to prevent the development of peripheral neuropathy due to INH
      c. Note that teratogenicity is unknown with rifampin
      d. Promote breast-feeding only if the mother is noninfectious
      e. Breast-feeding is not contraindicated with INH, ethambutol, and rifampin
      f. Note that pregnancy and immunosuppression are contraindications to bacille Calmette-Guerín (BCG) administration
   2. Neonate
      a. If born to a mother with active TB, treat with INH for 3 months

   b. Neonates born to infected mothers with active disease can be vaccinated with BCG
   c. Isolate and separate the infant from the mother during active disease until the mother is known to be noninfectious after a minimum of 3 weeks of medication therapy
   d. Administer BCG vaccine to the infant as prescribed
   e. Note that a Mantoux's test turns positive after a BCG is given

PRACTICE QUESTIONS

1. The client is in her second trimester of pregnancy. She complains of frequent low back pain and ankle edema at the end of the day. Which of the following measures can be recommended by the nurse to help relieve both discomforts?
   1 Lie on the floor with legs elevated on a couch or padded chair, hips and knees at right angles
   2 Lie on the left side with the feet dorsiflexed
   3 Soak the feet in hot water after performing 10 pelvic tilt exercises
   4 Lie on the right side with feet elevated on a pillow and a heating pad to the back

2. The client is beginning week 30 of gestation. She has come to the clinic for a routine visit. She is wearing hose and flat shoes. Which of the following observations by the nurse indicates a need for teaching?
   1 The client is wearing panty hose
   2 The client is wearing shoes with arch supports
   3 The client is wearing nonslip shoes
   4 The client is wearing knee-high hose

3. The plan of care for the pregnant teen should include teaching regarding which of the following concerning dental care?
   1 Use toothpaste with baking soda to decrease plaque build-up
   2 Avoid the use of local anesthetics during dental work
   3 Expect to lose at least one tooth due to calcium and phosphorus needed to nourish the fetus
   4 Tell the dentist office staff that she is pregnant

4. A pregnant woman complains of being frequently awakened by leg cramps. The nurse reinforces instructions to the client's partner and tells the partner to
   1 Dorsiflex the client's foot while flexing the knee
   2 Dorsiflex the client's foot while extending the knee
   3 Plantarflex the client's foot while flexing the knee
   4 Plantarflex the client's foot while extending the knee

5. The nurse is providing instructions to a pregnant client with heartburn regarding measures that will alleviate the discomfort. The nurse instructs the client to
   1. Lie down for 30 minutes after eating
   2. Drink decaffeinated coffee and tea
   3. Substitute salt in cooking with other spices
   4. Eliminate between-meal snacks

6. The nurse is reinforcing instructions to a pregnant woman who is complaining of low back pain. The nurse instructs the mother
   1. To wear an adbominal support
   2. In the technique of pelvic tilt
   3. To relax abdominal muscles when standing
   4. To wear at least a 2-inch heel on her shoes

7. The client of 28 weeks' gestation is Rh negative and Coombs' antibody negative. The nurse determines that the client understands what the nurse has taught her about Rh sensitization when the client states
   1. "I know I can never have another child."
   2. "I will have to have an injection once per month until the baby is born."
   3. "I will tell the nurse at the hospital that I had RhoGAM during pregnancy."
   4. "I am glad I won't have to have these shots if I have another child."

8. While assisting with the measurement of fundal height, the client (36 weeks' gestation) states she is feeling light-headed. Based on the nurse's knowledge of pregnancy, the nurse determines that this is most likely due to
   1. Emotional instability
   2. Compression of the vena cava
   3. A full bladder
   4. Insufficient iron intake

9. The nurse is providing information to the pregnant woman about food items high in folic acid. Which of the following midafternoon snacks is recommended to supply folic acid?
   1. 1 medium banana
   2. ½ banana, nuts, green leafy vegetables
   3. 1 cup milk with 2 graham crackers
   4. 1 cup yogurt

10. A contraction stress test is scheduled for the client. The woman asks the nurse about the test. The most accurate description of the test includes which of the following?
    1. "Small amounts of oxytocin are administered during internal fetal monitoring to stimulate uterine contractions."
    2. "An external fetal monitor is attached and you ambulate on a treadmill until contractions begin."
    3. "The uterus is stimulated to contract by either small amounts of oxytocin or by nipple stimulation."
    4. "Uterine contractions are stimulated by Leopold's maneuvers."

11. The client at 38 weeks of pregnancy is admitted to the birthing center in early labor. The client is carrying twins and one of the fetuses is a breech presentation. The nurse assists in planning care for the client and lists which of the following as the lowest priority in the care of this client?
    1. Attach electronic fetal monitoring
    2. Prepare the client for a possible cesarean section
    3. Measure fundal height
    4. Gather equipment for starting an IV

12. A stillborn was delivered in the birthing suite a few hours ago. After the birth, the family has remained together, holding and touching the baby. Which statement by the nurse further assists the family in their initial period of grief?
    1. "Don't worry, there is nothing you could do to prevent this from happening."
    2. "We need to take the baby from you now so that you can get some sleep."
    3. "What have you named your lovely baby?"
    4. "We will see to it that you have an early discharge so that you don't have to be reminded of this experience."

13. The nurse is collecting data from a prenatal client. The nurse determines that which of the following places the prenatal client into the high-risk category for contracting human immunodeficiency virus (HIV)?
    1. Living in an area where HIV infections are minimal
    2. A history of IV drug use in the past year
    3. A history of one sexual partner within the past 10 years
    4. A spouse who is heterosexual and had only one sexual partner in the past 10 years

14. A perinatal client is admitted to the obstetric unit during an exacerbation of a heart condition. When planning for the nutritional requirements of the client, the nurse consults with the dietitian to ensure which of the following?
    1. A low-calorie diet to ensure no weight gain
    2. A diet low in fluids and fiber to decrease blood volume
    3. A diet high in fluids and fiber to decrease constipation
    4. Unlimited sodium intake to increase circulating blood volume

15. The perinatal client is at risk for toxoplasmosis. The nurse teaches the client which of the following to prevent exposure to this disease?
    1. Wash hands only before meals
    2. Eat raw meats
    3. Avoid exposure to litter boxes used by cats
    4. Use topical steroid treatments prophylactically

16. A client in labor has an underlying diagnosis of sickle cell anemia. During labor, the client is at high risk for sickling crisis. Which of the following is the priority action by the nurse to assist in preventing a crisis from occurring during labor?
    1 Reassure the client
    2 Administer oxygen as prescribed throughout labor
    3 Maintain strict asepsis
    4 Prevent bearing down

17. The nurse has a teaching session with a malnourished client regarding iron supplementation to prevent anemia during pregnancy. Which of the following statements if made by the client indicates successful learning?
    1 "The iron is needed to make red blood cells to supply my baby with food."
    2 "Meat does not provide iron and should be avoided."
    3 "Iron supplements will give me diarrhea."
    4 "My body has all the iron it needs and I don't need to take supplements."

18. During a prenatal visit, the nurse is explaining dietary management to a client with diabetes. The nurse determines that the teaching has been effective when the client states
    1 "I can eat more sweets now because I need more calories."
    2 "I need more fat in my diet so the baby can gain enough weight."
    3 "I need to eat a high-protein, low-carbohydrate diet now in order to control my blood sugar."
    4 "I need to increase the fiber in my diet to control my blood glucose and prevent constipation."

19. The nurse is assigned to assist in caring for a client at risk for eclampsia. When a client progresses from preeclampsia to eclampsia, the nurse's first action is to
    1 Prepare for the administration of IV magnesium sulfate
    2 Check the blood pressure and fetal heart tones
    3 Clear and maintain an open airway
    4 Administer oxygen by face mask

20. The nurse is doing a 48-hour postpartum check on a client with mild pregnancy-induced hypertension (PIH). Which of the following data indicates that the PIH is not resolving?
    1 Blood pressure reading has returned to the prenatal baseline
    2 Urinary output has increased
    3 The client complains of a daily headache and developed blurred vision this morning
    4 There is no evidence of dependent edema

ANSWERS

1. **1**

RATIONALE: The position described in option 1 will produce the posture of the pelvic tilt while countering gravity as the force that leads to edema of the lower extremities. Although the other options might seem useful, options 3 and 4 identify heat, which should be prescribed by the physician. Option 2 might be helpful for the reduction of hemorrhoids.
TEST-TAKING STRATEGY: Focus on the issue of the question, back pain and ankle edema. Eliminate options 3 and 4 because the application of heat needs to be prescribed by the physician. Review measures that will reduce these discomforts now if you had difficulty with this question.
LEVEL OF COGNITIVE ABILITY: Comprehension
PHASE OF NURSING PROCESS: Implementation
CLIENT NEEDS: Physiological Integrity
CONTENT AREA: Maternity
REFERENCE
Leifer, G. (1999). *Thompson's introduction to maternity and pediatric nursing* (3rd ed.). Philadelphia: W. B. Saunders. p. 62.

2. **4**

RATIONALE: Varicose veins often develop in the lower extremities during pregnancy. Any constricting clothing such as knee-high hose impedes venous return from the lower legs and thus places the client at higher risk for developing varicosities. Clients should be encouraged to wear support hose. Flat, nonslip shoes with proper support are important to assist the pregnant woman to maintain proper posture, balance, and minimize falls.
TEST-TAKING STRATEGY: Note the key words "need for teaching." Use the process of elimination to find the option that will cause complications. Recalling that knee-high hose impedes venous return from the lower legs will easily direct you to option 4.
LEVEL OF COGNITIVE ABILITY: Comprehension
PHASE OF NURSING PROCESS: Evaluation
CLIENT NEEDS: Health Promotion and Maintenance
CONTENT AREA: Maternity
REFERENCE
Burroughs, A. (1997). *Maternity nursing: An introductory text* (7th ed.). Philadelphia: W. B. Saunders. p. 89.

3. **4**

RATIONALE: Baking soda may irritate gums, which are more likely to bleed due to hormonal changes of pregnancy. Local anesthetics for minor dentalwork should not have adverse effects on the fetus. Option 3 is inaccurate information. The dental staff needs to know about the pregnancy so that care is taken during examinations and x-rays are avoided.
TEST-TAKING STRATEGY: Use the process of elimination. Focus on the safety of the unseen client (fetus). Option 4 is the most global option.
LEVEL OF COGNITIVE ABILITY: Application
PHASE OF NURSING PROCESS: Planning
CLIENT NEEDS: Safe, Effective Care Environment
CONTENT AREA: Maternity

REFERENCE
Burroughs, A. (1997). *Maternity nursing: An introductory text* (7th ed.). Philadelphia: W. B. Saunders. p. 95.

4. 2

RATIONALE: Leg cramps often occur when the pregnant woman stretches the leg and plantarflexes the foot. Dorsiflexion of the foot while extending the knee stretches the gastrocnemius muscle, prevents the muscle from contracting, and halts the cramping.
TEST-TAKING STRATEGY: Knowledge regarding the actions that will alleviate muscle cramps will assist you in answering the question. Attempt to visualize each of the descriptions in the options to assist in directing you to the correct option. Review these measures now if you had difficulty with this question.
LEVEL OF COGNITIVE ABILITY: Application
PHASE OF NURSING PROCESS: Implementation
CLIENT NEEDS: Health Promotion and Maintenance
CONTENT AREA: Maternity
REFERENCE
Gorrie, T., McKinney, E., & Murray, S. (1998). *Foundations of maternal-newborn nursing* (2nd ed.). Philadelphia: W. B. Saunders. p. 151.

5. 2

RATIONALE: Lying down after meals is likely to lead to reflux of stomach contents. Spices tend to trigger heartburn. Eating smaller, more frequent portions is preferred over eating three large meals to control heartburn. Caffeine, like spices, may cause heartburn.
TEST-TAKING STRATEGY: Use the process of elimination recalling those items that will cause heartburn. Review measures to alleviate heartburn now if you had difficulty with this question.
LEVEL OF COGNITIVE ABILITY: Application
PHASE OF NURSING PROCESS: Implementation
CLIENT NEEDS: Health Promotion and Maintenance
CONTENT AREA: Maternity
REFERENCE
Burroughs, A. (1997). *Maternity nursing: An introductory text* (7th ed.). Philadelphia: W. B. Saunders. p. 89.

6. 2

RATIONALE: Pelvic tilt exercises decrease strain to the muscles of the abdomen and lower back caused by the added weight of the abdomen and the shift in the center of gravity. An abdominal support should only be worn if recommended by the physician. Relaxing abdominal muscles will add to the problem. Wearing 2-inch heels on shoes will add to the strain on the muscles and will exaggerate the shift in the center of gravity.
TEST-TAKING STRATEGY: Focus on the issue and use the process of elimination. If you had difficulty with this question, review the measures that will alleviate back pain.
LEVEL OF COGNITIVE ABILITY: Application
PHASE OF NURSING PROCESS: Implementation
CLIENT NEEDS: Health Promotion and Maintenance
CONTENT AREA: Maternity
REFERENCE
Leifer, G. (1999). *Thompson's introduction to maternity and pediatric nursing* (3rd ed.). Philadelphia: W. B. Saunders. p. 166.

7. 3

RATIONALE: It is accepted practice to administer Rho-GAM at 28 weeks of gestation to a woman as described, with a second injection within 72 hours of delivery. This prevents sensitization that could jeopardize a future pregnancy. For subsequent pregnancies or abortions, the injections must be repeated because immunity is passive. Options 1, 2, and 4 are inaccurate information.
TEST-TAKING STRATEGY: Knowledge regarding the administration of RhoGAM is required to answer the question. Note the key words "that the client understands." From this point, use the process of elimination. Review RhoGAM administration now if you had difficulty with this question.
LEVEL OF COGNITIVE ABILITY: Comprehension
PHASE OF NURSING PROCESS: Evaluation
CLIENT NEEDS: Health Promotion and Maintenance
CONTENT AREA: Maternity
REFERENCE
Gorrie, T., McKinney, E., & Murray, S. (1998). *Foundations of maternal-newborn nursing* (2nd ed.). Philadelphia: W. B. Saunders. pp. 695–696.

8. 2

RATIONALE: Compression of the inferior vena cava and aorta by the uterus may cause supine hypotension syndrome late in pregnancy. Having the woman turn onto her left side or elevating the left buttock during fundal height measurement will correct or prevent the problem. Options 1, 3, and 4 are not the cause of the client's problem described in the question.
TEST-TAKING STRATEGY: Focus on physiological integrity. Use the ABCs, airway, breathing, and circulation, to answer the question. Review vena cava syndrome now if you had difficulty with this question.
LEVEL OF COGNITIVE ABILITY: Comprehension
PHASE OF NURSING PROCESS: Data Collection
CLIENT NEEDS: Physiological Integrity
CONTENT AREA: Maternity
REFERENCE
Gorrie, T., McKinney, E., & Murray, S. (1998). *Foundations of maternal-newborn nursing* (2nd ed.). Philadelphia: W. B. Saunders. p. 126.

9. 2

RATIONALE: Folic acid is needed during pregnancy for healthy cell growth and repair. A pregnant woman should have at least four servings of folic acid–rich foods per day. All three food items in option 2 contain folic acid. Bananas provide potassium. Milk and yogurt supply calcium.
TEST-TAKING STRATEGY: Knowledge regarding food sources high in folic acid is required to answer the question. Review these food sources now if you had difficulty with this question.
LEVEL OF COGNITIVE ABILITY: Application
PHASE OF NURSING PROCESS: Implementation
CLIENT NEEDS: Physiological Integrity
CONTENT AREA: Maternity
REFERENCE
Burroughs, A. (1997). *Maternity nursing: An introductory text* (7th ed.). Philadelphia: W. B. Saunders. p. 99.

10. 3

RATIONALE: A contraction stress test assesses placental oxygenation and function, determines fetal ability to tolerate labor, determines fetal well-being and is performed if the nonstress test is abnormal. The fetus is exposed to the stressor of contractions to assess the adequacy of placental perfusion under simulated labor conditions. An external

fetal monitor is applied to the mother and a 20- to 30-minute baseline strip is recorded. The uterus is stimulated to contract either by the administration of a dilute dose of oxytocin (Pitocin) or by having the mother use nipple stimulation until three palpable contractions with a duration of 40 seconds or more in a 10-minute period have been achieved. Frequent maternal BP readings are done and the client is monitored closely while increasing doses of oxytocin are given.
TEST-TAKING STRATEGY: Knowledge regarding the contraction stress test is required to answer the question. Read each option carefully. Remember that in both the nonstress test and the contraction stress test, external monitoring is performed. If you had difficulty answering this question, take time now to review the contraction stress test.
LEVEL OF COGNITIVE ABILITY: Comprehension
PHASE OF NURSING PROCESS: Implementation
CLIENT NEEDS: Physiological Integrity
CONTENT AREA: Maternity
REFERENCE
Gorrie, T., McKinney, E., & Murray, S. (1998). *Foundations of maternal-newborn nursing* (2nd ed.). Philadelphia: W. B. Saunders. p. 223.

11. **3**

RATIONALE: Option 3 is a low priority because fundal height should be measured at each antepartal clinic visit and not as a priority of care in the intrapartum period. Options 1, 2, and 4 are all high priorities. The twins should be monitored by dual electronic fetal monitoring and in so doing, any signs of distress need to be reported to the obstetrician. Because most breech presentations are born by cesarean, many physicians choose cesarean birth if either of the twins is breech. The mother should have an IV in place in case fluid or blood replacement is required.
TEST-TAKING STRATEGY: Note the key words "lowest priority." Use Maslow's hierarchy of needs theory and the ABCs, airway, breathing, and circulation, to prioritize.
LEVEL OF COGNITIVE ABILITY: Comprehension
PHASE OF NURSING PROCESS: Planning
CLIENT NEEDS: Physiological Integrity
CONTENT AREA: Maternity
REFERENCE
Leifer, G. (1999). *Thompson's introduction to maternity and pediatric nursing* (3rd ed.). Philadelphia: W. B. Saunders. p. 129.

12. **3**

RATIONALE: Nurses should explore measures that assist the family to create memories of an infant so that the existence of the child is confirmed and so that the parents can complete the grieving process. Option 3 meets this goal and also demonstrates a caring and empathic response. Options 1, 2, and 4 are blocks to communication and devalue the parents' feelings.
TEST-TAKING STRATEGY: Use therapeutic communication techniques. Always focus on the client's feelings first. Choose an option that demonstrates a caring and empathic response by the nurse, that meets the psychosocial needs of the client/family, and that focuses on the client as a worthy human being, not one that devalues feelings.
LEVEL OF COGNITIVE ABILITY: Application
PHASE OF NURSING PROCESS: Implementation
CLIENT NEEDS: Psychosocial Integrity
CONTENT AREA: Maternity

REFERENCE
Gorrie, T., McKinney, E., & Murray, S. (1998). *Foundations of maternal-newborn nursing* (2nd ed.). Philadelphia: W. B. Saunders. p. 648.

13. **2**

RATIONALE: HIV is transmitted by intimate sexual contact and the exchange of body fluids, exposure to infected blood, and transmission from an infected woman to her fetus. Women who fall into the high-risk category for HIV infection include those with persistent and recurrent sexually transmitted diseases or a history of multiple sexual partners, and those who use or have used IV drugs. Options 1, 3, and 4 are not situations that contribute to the incidence of contracting HIV.
TEST-TAKING STRATEGY: Knowledge regarding risk factors for HIV is necessary to answer the question. Use the process of elimination, recalling that IV drug use places the client at high risk for contracting the disease. Review these risk factors now if you had difficulty with this question.
LEVEL OF COGNITIVE ABILITY: Comprehension
PHASE OF NURSING PROCESS: Data Collection
CLIENT NEEDS: Health Promotion and Maintenance
CONTENT AREA: Maternity
REFERENCE
Leifer, G. (1999). *Thompson's introduction to maternity and pediatric nursing* (3rd ed.). Philadelphia: W. B. Saunders. p. 284.

14. **3**

RATIONALE: Constipation causes the client to use the Valsalva maneuver. This causes blood to rush to the heart and overload the cardiac system. Absence of weight gain is not recommended during pregnancy. Diets low in fluid and fiber would cause a decrease in blood volume, which in turn deprives the fetus of nutrients. Too much sodium could cause an overload to the circulating blood volume and contribute to the cardiac condition.
TEST-TAKING STRATEGY: Try to relate the situation to something you are familiar with. Look for the option that applies to any heart condition, then use the process of elimination. Review dietary measures for the client with cardiac disease now if you had difficulty with this question.
LEVEL OF COGNITIVE ABILITY: Application
PHASE OF NURSING PROCESS: Planning
CLIENT NEEDS: Physiological Integrity
CONTENT AREA: Maternity
REFERENCE
Gorrie, T., McKinney, E., & Murray, S. (1998). *Foundation of maternal-newborn nursing* (2nd ed.). Philadelphia: W. B. Saunders. p. 455.

15. **3**

RATIONALE: Infected house cats transmit the disease through feces. Handling litter boxes can transmit the disease to the maternity client. Meats that are undercooked can harbor microorganisms that can cause infection. Hands should be washed throughout the day when handling items that could be contaminated. Topical steroids are not the pharmacological treatment of choice for toxoplasmosis.
TEST-TAKING STRATEGY: Avoid option 1, which uses the absolute word "only." Option 2 also represents an extreme statement. Knowledge regarding the transmission and treatment of the organism is required to discriminate between options 3 and 4. Review the causes of toxoplasmosis now if you had difficulty with this question.

LEVEL OF COGNITIVE ABILITY: Application
PHASE OF NURSING PROCESS: Implementation
CLIENT NEEDS: Health Promotion and Maintenance
CONTENT AREA: Maternity
REFERENCE
Gorrie, T., McKinney, E., & Murray, S. (1998). *Foundations of maternal-newborn nursing* (2nd ed.). Philadelphia: W. B. Saunders. pp. 737–738.

16. **2**

RATIONALE: During the labor process, the client is at high risk for being unable to meet the oxygen demands of labor and unable to prevent sickling. An intervention to prevent sickle cell crisis during labor includes administering oxygen as needed. Options 1, 3, and 4 are accurate information but not for the situation described in the question.
TEST-TAKING STRATEGY: Use the ABCs, airway, breathing, and circulation, to answer the question. Option 2 addresses airway. Review sickle cell crisis now if you had difficulty with this question.
LEVEL OF COGNITIVE ABILITY: Application
PHASE OF NURSING PROCESS: Implementation
CLIENT NEEDS: Physiological Integrity
CONTENT AREA: Maternity
REFERENCE
Leifer, G. (1999). *Thompson's introduction to maternity and pediatric nursing* (3rd ed.). Philadelphia: W. B. Saunders. p. 110.

17. **1**

RATIONALE: The nutritional supplement most commonly needed during pregnancy is iron. Anemia of pregnancy is primarily caused by iron deficiency. Iron supplements usually cause constipation. Meats are an excellent source of iron. Iron for the fetus comes from the maternal serum.
TEST-TAKING STRATEGY: Note the key word "malnourished." Eliminate options 2 and 4 because of absolute terminology as "not" and "all." Knowledge regarding the effects of iron supplements assists in eliminating option 3. Review the relationship of nutrition to anemia now if you had difficulty with this question.
LEVEL OF COGNITIVE ABILITY: Comprehension
PHASE OF NURSING PROCESS: Evaluation
CLIENT NEEDS: Physiological Integrity
CONTENT AREA: Maternity
REFERENCE
Leifer, G. (1999). *Thompson's introduction to maternity and pediatric nursing* (3rd ed.). Philadelphia: W. B. Saunders. p. 109.

18. **4**

RATIONALE: An increase in calories is needed with pregnancy, but concentrated sugars should be avoided because they may cause hyperglycemia. The fat intake should remain at 30% of the total calories. The fetus of a diabetic mother is prone to macrosomia. The diabetic client needs about 40% to 50% of the diet from carbohydrates and about 20% to 25% of the diet from protein. High-fiber foods will cause blood glucose levels to rise more slowly by delaying gastrointestinal absorption.
TEST-TAKING STRATEGY: Note the key words "teaching has been effective." Use the process of elimination and knowledge regarding diet therapy to direct you to the correct option. Review the key components of the diabetic diet now if you had difficulty with this question.
LEVEL OF COGNITIVE ABILITY: Comprehension
PHASE OF NURSING PROCESS: Evaluation
CLIENT NEEDS: Health Promotion and Maintenance
CONTENT AREA: Maternity
REFERENCE
Leifer, G. (1999). *Thompson's introduction to maternity and pediatric nursing* (3rd ed.). Philadelphia: W. B. Saunders. p. 71.

19. **3**

RATIONALE: The first action is to keep an open airway and prevent injuries to the client. Options 1, 2, and 4 may be components of care but are not the first action.
TEST-TAKING STRATEGY: Note the key word "first." Use the ABCs, airway, breathing, and circulation, to answer the question. Airway is the first priority.
LEVEL OF COGNITIVE ABILITY: Application
PHASE OF NURSING PROCESS: Implementation
CLIENT NEEDS: Physiological Integrity
CONTENT AREA: Maternity
REFERENCE
Leifer, G. (1999). *Thompson's introduction to maternity and pediatric nursing* (3rd ed.). Philadelphia: W. B. Saunders. p. 94.

20. **3**

RATIONALE: Options 1, 2, and 4 are all signs that the PIH is being resolved. Option 3 is a symptom of worsening of the PIH.
TEST-TAKING STRATEGY: Note the key word "not." Use the process of elimination to direct you to the correct option. If you had difficulty with this question, review PIH now.
LEVEL OF COGNITIVE ABILITY: Comprehension
PHASE OF NURSING PROCESS: Evaluation
CLIENT NEEDS: Physiological Integrity
CONTENT AREA: Maternity
REFERENCE
Leifer, G. (1999). *Thompson's introduction to maternity and pediatric nursing* (3rd ed.). Philadelphia: W. B. Saunders. p. 101.

BIBLIOGRAPHY

Burroughs, A. (1997). *Maternity nursing: An introductory text* (7th ed.). Philadelphia: W. B. Saunders.

deWit, S. (1998). *Essentials of medical-surgical nursing* (4th ed.). Philadelphia: W. B. Saunders.

Gorrie, T., McKinney, E., & Murray, S. (1998). *Foundations of maternal-newborn nursing* (2nd ed.). Philadelphia: W. B. Saunders.

Leahy, J., & Kizilay, P. (1998). *Foundations of nursing practice: A nursing process approach.* Philadelphia: W. B. Saunders.

Leifer, G. (1999). *Thompson's introduction to maternity and pediatric nursing* (3rd ed.). Philadelphia: W. B. Saunders.

Schulte, E., Price, D., & James, S. (1997). *Thompson's pediatric nursing: An introductory text* (7th ed.). Philadelphia: W. B. Saunders.

CHAPTER 23

Labor and Delivery and Associated Complications

. . . .

I. The Process of Labor

A. Labor
   1. Coordinated sequence of involuntary uterine contractions
   2. Results in effacement and dilation of the cervix, followed by expulsion of products of conception
B. Delivery: actual event of birth
C. Passenger: the fetus
D. Attitude
   1. The relationship of the fetal body parts to one another
   2. Normal intrauterine attitude is flexion, in which the fetal back is rounded, the head is forward on the chest, and the arms and legs are folded in against the body
E. Lie
   1. Relationship of the spine of the fetus to the spine of the mother
   2. Longitudinal or vertical: Fetal spine is parallel with the mother's spine; fetus is either cephalic or breech presentation
   3. Transverse or horizontal
      a. Fetal spine is at a right angle or perpendicular to the mother's spine
      b. Presenting part is the shoulder
      c. **Delivery** by cesarean section
   4. Oblique
      a. Fetal spine is at a slight angle from a true horizontal lie
      b. **Delivery** is by cesarean section if uncorrectable
F. Presentation
   1. Presenting part: portion of the fetus that enters the pelvis first
   2. Cephalic
      a. The most common presentation
      b. Fetal head presents first
   3. Breech
      a. Buttocks present first

b. **Delivery** by cesarean section may be required, although it is often possible to deliver vaginally
   4. Shoulder
      a. The fetus is in a transverse lie, or the arm, back, abdomen or side could present
      b. If the fetus does not spontaneously rotate or if it is not possible to manually turn the fetus, a cesarean section may be performed
G. Position: relationship of the assigned area of the presenting part or landmark to the maternal pelvis (Box 23-1)
H. Station
   1. The measurement of the progress of descent in centimeters above or below the midplane from the presenting part to the ischial spines
   2. Station 0—at ischial spine
   3. Minus station—above ischial spine
   4. Plus station—below ischial spine
I. Powers
   1. The forces acting to expel the fetus
   2. Effacement: shortening and thinning of the cervix during the first stage of **labor**
   3. Dilation: enlargement of cervical os and cervical canal during the first stage

---

BOX 23-1. Fetal Positions

ROA—right occiput anterior
LOA—left occiput anterior
ROP—right occiput posterior
LOP—left occiput posterior
ROT—right occiput transverse
LOT—left occiput transverse
RMA—right mentum anterior
LMA—left mentum anterior
RMP—right mentum posterior
LSA—left sacrum anterior
LSP—left sacrum posterior

II. Mechanisms of Labor (Table 23–1)

A. Data collection
1. Lightening or dropping: the fetus descends into the pelvis about 2 weeks prior to delivery
2. Braxton Hicks contractions increase
3. Show
4. Vaginal mucosa congested and vaginal mucus increases
5. Brownish or blood-tinged cervical mucus is passed
6. Cervix ripens, becomes soft and partly effaced, and may begin to dilate
7. Sudden burst of energy
8. Loss of 1 to 3 lb from water loss resulting from fluid shifts produced by changes in progesterone and estrogen levels
9. Spontaneous rupture of membranes

B. False **labor**
1. Exaggeration of normal contractions
2. Does not produce dilation, effacement, or descent
3. Contractions are irregular without progression
4. Walking has no effect on contractions and often relieves false **labor**

Table 23–1. Mechanisms of Labor

Engagement

Mechanism by which the fetus nestles into the pelvis
Also termed lightening or dropping

Descent

The process that the fetal head undergoes as it begins its journey through the pelvis
A continuous process from the time of engagement until birth and is assessed by the measurement called station

Flexion

Process of the fetal head's nodding forward toward the fetal chest

Internal Rotation

Internal rotation of the fetus, most commonly from the occiput transverse position assumed at engagement into the pelvis, to the occiput anterior position while continuously descending

Extension

Enables the head to be born when the fetus is in a cephalic position
Begins after the head is crowned
Is complete when the head passes under the symphysis pubis and the occiput, and the anterior fontanel, brow, face, and chin pass over the sacrum and coccyx and are over the perineum

Restitution

Realignment of the fetal head with the body after the head emerges

External Rotation

The shoulders externally rotate after the head is born and restitution occurs, so that the shoulders are in the anteroposterior diameter of the pelvis

Expulsion

The birth of the entire body

C. True **labor**
1. Contractions increase in duration and intensity
2. Cervical dilation and effacement are progressive

III. Leopold's Maneuvers

A. Description: to determine position, presentation, and engagement
B. Preparation
1. Ask the mother to empty her bladder
2. Hands are warmed and applied to the abdomen with firm and gentle pressure
C. First maneuver
1. Determines which part of the fetus is in the fundus
2. The palms are placed on each side of the upper abdomen and palpation around the fundus is done
3. If the head is in fundus, the examiner feels a hard, round, movable object
4. The buttocks will feel soft and have an irregular shape and are more difficult to move
D. Second maneuver
1. The hands are moved downward over each side of the abdomen, applying firm, even pressure
2. The fetus's back, which is a smooth, hard surface, should be felt on one side of the abdomen
3. Irregular knobs and lumps—the hands, feet, elbows, and knees—will be felt on the opposite side of the abdomen
E. Third maneuver
1. To confirm fetal position
2. A hand is placed above the symphysis pubis
3. The thumb and fingers are brought together and grasp the part of fetus between them, either the head or buttocks
F. Fourth maneuver
1. Used in the late stage to determine how far the fetus has descended into the pelvic inlet
2. Hands are placed on the sides of the lower abdomen, close to the midline
3. Hands are slid downward and pressed inward
4. If it has been determined that the buttocks are in the fundus, then the head is felt for
5. If the head cannot be felt, it has probably descended

IV. Breathing Techniques

A. Abdominal breathing
1. Used until **labor** is more advanced
2. The abdomen moves outward during inhalation and downward during exhalation
3. The rate remains slow, with approximately 6 to 9 breaths/minute
B. Pant-pant-blow
1. Used in advanced **labor**
2. A more rapid pattern, consisting of two short

pants from the mouth followed by a longer blow
3. All exhalations are a blowing motion

V. Fetal Monitoring

A. Description
1. Displays the fetal heart rate (FHR)
2. Monitors uterine activity, frequency, duration, and intensity of contractions
3. Monitors the fetal heart rate in relation to maternal contractions
4. Baseline FHR is measured between contractions
5. The normal fetal heart rate is 120 to 160 beats/minute

B. External fetal monitoring
1. Noninvasive and performed by the use of a tocotransducer or ultrasonic transducer
2. Leopold's maneuvers are performed to determine on which side the fetal back is located; the ultrasonic transducer is placed over this area
3. Place tocotransducer over the fundus of the uterus
4. Fasten the transducer to the abdomen
5. Allow the client to assume a comfortable position, avoiding vena cava compression

C. Internal fetal monitoring
1. Invasive and requires rupturing of the membranes and attaching an electrode to the presenting part of the fetus
2. The mother must be dilated 2 to 3 cm to perform internal monitoring

D. Patterns
1. Fetal bradycardia
   a. Less than 120 beats/minute
   b. Change position of the mother and administer oxygen as prescribed
   c. Notify the physician
2. Fetal tachycardia
   a. Fetal heart rate is greater than 160 beats/minute
   b. Change position of the mother and administer oxygen as prescribed
   c. Notify the physician
3. Variability
   a. A change in the baseline FHR in response to fetal sleep, wake states, medications, and hypoxia
   b. A FHR that fluctuates 6 to 25 beats/minute at the baseline indicates a well-oxygenated functioning central nervous system (CNS)
4. Acceleration
   a. A transient rise in the FHR of more than 15 beats/minute for more than 15 seconds
   b. May or may not be related to uterine contractions
   c. Marked acceleration (more than 180 beats/minute) may be related to

prematurity, maternal fever, hypoxia, fetal infection, or medications
5. Decelerations: a transient decrease in the FHR
6. Early deceleration
   a. Decrease in the FHR below baseline
   b. Can be due to head compression
7. Variable deceleration
   a. An abrupt decrease in FHR that is variable in duration, intensity, and timing
   b. Can be due to cord compression
8. Late deceleration
   a. Decrease in FHR below baseline
   b. Due to uteroplacental insufficiency
9. Hyperstimulation: increasing resting tone or peak contraction pressures
10. Implementation for altered patterns
    a. The physician is notified
    b. Check for cord prolapse
    c. Maintain the client in a left lateral position
    d. Administer oxygen as prescribed
    e. Oxytocin infusion is discontinued as prescribed
    f. Fetal scalp pH is done to determine a blood pH value
    g. IV fluids are increased as prescribed
    h. Monitor and maintain blood pressure if hypotension occurs
    i. Prepare the client for cesarean delivery as prescribed

VI. Stages of Labor

A. Stage I latent phase
1. Data collection
   a. Cervical dilation of 1 to 4 cm
   b. Uterine contractions every 15 to 30 minutes; 15 to 30 seconds' duration of mild intensity
   c. The mother is talkative and eager to be in **labor**
2. Implementation
   a. Encourage the mother and partner to participate in care
   b. Assist with comfort measures, changes of position, and ambulation
   c. Keep the mother and partner informed of progress
   d. Offer fluids and ice chips
   e. Encourage voiding every 1 to 2 hours

B. Stage I active phase
1. Data collection
   a. Cervical dilation of 4 to 7 cm
   b. Uterine contractions every 3 to 5 minutes, 30 to 60 seconds' duration of moderate intensity
   c. The mother may experience feelings of helplessness
   d. The mother becomes restless and anxious as contractions become stronger
2. Implementation

a. Encourage maintenance of effective breathing patterns
b. Provide a quiet environment
c. Keep the mother and partner informed of progress
d. Promote comfort with backrubs, sacral pressure, pillow support, and position changes
e. Instruct the partner in effleurage
f. Offer ointment for dry lips
g. Offer fluids and ice chips
h. Encourage voiding every 1 to 2 hours

C. Stage I transition phase
  1. Data collection
    a. Cervical dilation of 8 to 10 cm
    b. Uterine contractions every 2 to 3 minutes, 45 to 90 seconds' duration of strong intensity
    c. The mother becomes tired, is restless and irritable, and feels out of control
  2. Implementation
    a. Encourage rest between contractions
    b. Wake the mother at beginning of contraction so she can begin breathing pattern
    c. Keep the mother and partner informed of progress
    d. Provide privacy
    e. Offer ointment for dry lips
    f. Offer fluids and ice chips
    g. Encourage voiding every 1 to 2 hours

D. Implementation throughout stage I
  1. Monitor maternal vital signs
  2. Monitor FHR before, during, and after a contraction, noting that the normal FHR is 120 to 160 beats/minute
  3. Monitor uterine contractions by palpation or monitor, determining frequency, duration, and intensity
  4. Assist with monitoring the status of cervical dilation and effacement
  5. Assist with monitoring the fetal station presentation and position by Leopold's maneuvers
  6. Assist with the pelvic exam and prepare for a Nitrazine test and a fern test
  7. Monitor the color of the **amniotic fluid** if the membranes have ruptured, because meconium-stained fluid can indicate fetal distress

E. Stage 2
  1. Data collection
    a. Cervical dilation is complete
    b. Progressive **labor** continues, with cervical dilation of 1 cm/hour for primigravidas and 1.5 cm/hour for multigravidas
    c. Fetal descent occurring and demonstrated by change in fetal station
    d. Uterine contractions occur every 2 to 3 minutes lasting 60 to 75 seconds, and the intensity is strong
    e. Increase in bloody show occurs

f. The mother may feel out of control, helpless, and panicky
g. The mother feels the urge to bear down; assist her in pushing efforts

  2. Implementation
    a. Monitor maternal vital signs
    b. Monitor the FHR before, during, and after a contraction
    c. Monitor uterine contractions by palpation or monitor, determining frequency, duration, and intensity
    d. Provide the mother with encouragement and praise
    e. Keep the mother and partner informed of progress
    f. Maintain privacy
    g. Provide ice chips
    h. Assist the mother into a position that promotes comfort and assists pushing efforts such as lithotomy, semisitting, kneeling, side-lying, or squatting
    i. Monitor for signs of approaching birth, such as perineal bulging or visualization of the fetal head
    j. Prepare for birth

F. Stage 3
  1. Data collection
    a. Contractions occur until **placenta** is born
    b. **Placental** separation and expulsion occurs
    c. Birth of **placenta** occurs 5 to 30 minutes after birth of the baby
    d. Schultze's mechanism: center portion of the **placenta** separates first and its shiny fetal surface emerges from the vagina
    e. Duncan's mechanism: margin of the **placenta** separates, and a dull, red, rough maternal surface emerges from the vagina first
  2. Implementation
    a. Monitor maternal vital signs and uterine status
    b. Following birth of the **placenta**, the uterine fundus remains firm and is located two fingerbreadths below the umbilicus
    c. Examine the **placenta** for cotyledons and membranes
    d. Monitor the mother for shivering and provide warmth
    e. Promote parent-newborn attachment
    f. Initial newborn assessment
    g. Assess newborn's Apgar score

G. Stage 4
  1. Description: the period from 1 to 4 hours after **delivery**
  2. Data collection
    a. Blood pressure returns to the prelabor level
    b. Pulse is slightly lower than it is during **labor**
    c. The fundus remains contracted, in midline, one to two fingerbreadths below the umbilicus

    d. **Lochia** is moderate or scant and is red

3. Implementation
   a. Monitor maternal vital signs frequently
   b. Provide warm blankets
   c. Provide ice packs to the perineum
   d. Massage the uterus if needed as prescribed

VII. Anesthesia

A. Local anesthetic
   1. Used for blocking pain during the episiotomy
   2. Administered just before the birth of the baby
   3. No effect on the fetus
B. Paracervical block
   1. Used in the first stage of labor
   2. Provides a rapid block of uterine pain
   3. No effect on the perineal area
   4. No effect on the ability to bear down
   5. May cause fetal bradycardia
C. Pudendal block
   1. Administered just before the birth of the baby
   2. Injection site is at the pudendal nerve through a transvaginal route
   3. Blocks the perineal area for episiotomy
   4. Effects last about 30 minutes
   5. No effects on contractions or the fetus
D. Epidural
   1. Injection site in epidural space at L3–L4
   2. Administered during the first stage of **labor**, after 5 to 6 cm dilation or during the second stage
   3. Relieves pain from contractions and numbs the vagina and perineum
   4. May cause hypotension
   5. Does not cause headache because the dura mater is not penetrated
   6. Monitor maternal blood pressure
   7. Maintain mother in side-lying position
   8. IV fluids are administered and increased as prescribed if hypotension occurs
E. Spinal block
   1. Injection site in spinal subarachnoid space at L3–L5
   2. Administered just before the birth of the baby
   3. Relieves uterine and perineal pain and numbs the vagina, perineum, and lower extremities
   4. May cause maternal hypotension
   5. May cause postpartum headache
   6. Client must lie flat 8 to 12 hours following a spinal block
   7. Place a rolled blanket under right hip to displace the uterus from the vena cava
   8. IV fluids are administered as prescribed
F. General anesthetic
   1. May be used for some surgical interventions
   2. The client is not awake and the danger of respiratory depression and vomiting is present

VIII. Obstetric Procedures

A. Bishop score (Box 23–2)
   1. Used to determine maternal readiness for **labor**

BOX 23–2. Factors of the Bishop Score

Dilation of cervix
Effacement of cervix
Consistency of cervix
Position of cervix
Station of presenting part

---

   2. Evaluates cervical status and fetal position
   3. Indicated before the induction of **labor**
   4. The five factors are assigned a score of 0 to 3, and the total score is calculated
   5. A score of 6 or more indicates a success rate for **labor** induction
B. Induction
   1. A deliberate initiation of uterine contractions that stimulates **labor**
   2. Elective induction may be accomplished by oxytocin (Pitocin) infusion
   3. IV dosage of oxytocin is increased as prescribed only after assessing contractions, FHR, and maternal blood pressure and pulse
   4. The rate of oxytocin is not increased once the desired contraction pattern is obtained (contraction frequency of 2 to 3 minutes lasting 60 seconds)
   5. Oxytocin infusion is discontinued as prescribed if contraction frequency is less than 2 minutes or duration is more than 90 seconds or if fetal distress is noted
C. Amniotomy
   1. Artificial rupture of membranes (AROM) to stimulate **labor**
   2. Increases risk of prolapsed cord and infection
   3. Monitor FHR before and after AROM
   4. Record the time of AROM, FHR, and characteristics of fluid
   5. Meconium-stained fluid may be associated with fetal distress
   6. Bloody fluid may indicate **abruptio placentae** or fetal trauma
   7. An unpleasant odor is associated with infection
D. External version
   1. External manipulation of the fetus from an abnormal position into a normal presentation
   2. Indicated for an abnormal presentation that exists after the 34th week
   3. If mother is Rh negative, ensure Rh immune globulin was given at 28 weeks' gestation
   4. Nonstress test may be performed to evaluate fetal well-being
   5. IV fluids and tocolytic therapy may be administered to relax the uterus and permit easier manipulation of the fetus
   6. Ultrasound is used during the procedure to evaluate fetal position and **placental** placement and guide direction of the fetus

7. Abdominal wall is manipulated to direct fetus into a cephalic presentation if possible
8. Monitor blood pressure to identify vena cava compression
9. Monitor for unusual pain
10. After the procedure
    a. A nonstress test is performed to evaluate fetal well-being
    b. Monitor for uterine activity, bleeding, ruptured membranes, and decreased fetal activity
    c. With Rh-negative clients, a Kleihauer-Betke test is performed as prescribed to detect the presence and amount of fetal blood in the maternal circulation and to identify clients who need additional Rh immune globulin

E. Episiotomy
1. Incision made into perineum to enlarge vaginal outlet and facilitate **delivery**
2. Check episiotomy site
3. Institute measures to relieve pain
4. Provide ice pack during the first 24 hours
5. Instruct the client in the use of sitz baths
6. Apply analgesic spray or ointment as prescribed
7. Provide perineal care using clean technique
8. Instruct the client in the proper care of the incision
9. Instruct the client to dry the perineal area from front to back and to blot the area rather than wiping it
10. Instruct the client to shower rather than tub bathe
11. Apply a perineal pad without touching the inside surface of the pad
12. Report any bleeding or discharge

F. Forceps **delivery**
1. Two double-crossed, spoonlike articulated blades that are used to assist in **delivery** of the fetal head
2. Reassure the client and explain the need for forceps
3. Check the newborn and mother after **delivery** for any possible injury
4. Assist with repair of any lacerations

G. Vacuum extraction
1. A caplike suction device applied to the fetal head to facilitate extraction
2. Suction is used to assist in **delivery** of the fetal head
3. Traction is applied during uterine contractions until descent of the fetal head is achieved
4. Suction device should not be kept in place any longer than 25 minutes
5. Monitor FHR every 5 minutes if external fetal monitoring is not used
6. Monitor the newborn at birth and throughout postpartum for signs of cerebral trauma
7. Caput succedaneum is normal and will resolve in 24 hours

H. Cesarean **delivery**
1. **Delivery** of the fetus through a transabdominal, low-segment incision of the uterus
2. Preoperative
    a. If planned, prepare the client and partner
    b. If an emergency, quickly explain the need and procedure to the client and partner
    c. Obtain a signed informed consent
    d. Make sure that the preoperative diagnostic tests are done, including the Rh factor
    e. Prepare the client for insertion of an IV line and Foley catheter
    f. Prepare the abdomen as prescribed
    g. Monitor the client and fetus continuously for vital signs and signs of **labor**
    h. Provide emotional support
    i. Administer preoperative medications as prescribed
3. Postoperative
    a. Monitor vital signs
    b. Provide pain relief
    c. Encourage turning, coughing, and deep breathing
    d. Encourage ambulation
    e. Monitor for signs of infection and bleeding
    f. Burning and pain on urination may indicate bladder infection
    g. A tender uterus and foul-smelling **lochia** may indicate endometritis
    h. A productive cough or chills may indicate pneumonia
    i. A positive Homans' sign, pain, or edema of an extremity may indicate thrombophlebitis

IX. Dystocia

A. Description
1. Difficult **labor** that is prolonged or more painful
2. Occurs because of problems caused by uterine contractions, the fetus, or the bones and tissues of the maternal pelvis
3. Contractions may be hypotonic or hypertonic
4. Fetus may be excessively large, malpositioned, or in an abnormal presentation

B. Data collection
1. Excessive abdominal pain
2. Abnormal contraction pattern
3. Fetal distress
4. Elevated maternal temperature
5. Maternal or fetal tachycardia
6. Lack of progress in **labor**
7. Ketonuria
8. Decreased urine output

C. Implementation
1. Monitor FHR and for fetal distress
2. Monitor uterine contractions, maternal temperature, and heart rate
3. Assist with pelvic examination,

measurements, ultrasound, and other procedures
4. Oxytocin infusion may be prescribed; prophylactic antibiotics may be prescribed to prevent infection
5. Monitor IV fluids, I&O, and for signs of dehydration
6. Instruct client in breathing techniques and relaxation exercises
7. Monitor color of **amniotic fluid**
8. Provide comfort as with a normal **delivery** such as backrubs and position changes
9. Monitor the client's fatigue and pain and administer sedatives and pain medication as prescribed
10. Monitor for prolapse of the cord after rupture of the membranes
11. If prolapse occurs
   a. Place the client in Trendelenburg's or knee-chest position to minimize pressure on the cord
   b. Administer oxygen as prescribed
   c. The physician is notified
   d. Prepare client for emergency cesarean section

X. Precipitate Labor and Delivery

A. Description: **labor** lasts less than 3 hours
B. Implementation
   1. Stay with the client at all times
   2. Provide emotional support and keep the client calm
   3. Encourage the mother to pant between contractions
   4. Prepare the client for rupturing membranes when head crowns if not already ruptured
   5. Do not try to keep the fetus from being delivered
   6. Gentle pressure is applied to the fetal head upward toward the vagina to prevent damage to the head and vaginal lacerations
   7. Fetus is delivered between contractions, checking for the cord around the neck
   8. If outside the hospital, the cord is clamped in two places and cut between with a clean knife or scissors after the cord stops pulsating, the **placenta** is allowed to separate naturally, and the newborn is placed on mother's abdomen or breast to induce uterine contractions

XI. Preterm Labor

A. Description
   1. **Labor** occurring after the 20th week but before the 37th week
   2. Contractions occurring at least once every 10 minutes and lasting 30 seconds or longer
   3. Documented cervical change or cervical effacement of 80% or dilation of 2 cm
B. Data collection
   1. Increased or bloody discharge

2. Backache, pressure, and cramping
3. Palpable uterine contractions
4. Diarrhea
C. Implementation
   1. Maintain bed rest, a quiet environment, and a lateral recumbent position
   2. Tocolytic medications may be prescribed to suppress **labor**
   3. Betamethasone (Celestone) may be administered to stimulate fetal lung maturity when preterm **delivery** appears inevitable
   4. When magnesium sulfate is administered
      a. Monitor effects of medications on **labor** and fetus; monitor the FHR
      b. Monitor reflexes
      c. Have antidote (calcium gluconate) available at the bedside
      d. Monitor vital signs and for signs of maternal hypotension
      e. Monitor for increased respiratory rate, which may indicate pulmonary edema
      f. Monitor for signs of fluid overload

XII. Rupture of the Uterus

A. Description: complete or incomplete separation of the uterine tissue due to rupture of the uterus from the stress of **labor**
B. Complete rupture of the uterus
   1. Pain, which is shearing, excruciating, diffuse, or localized
   2. Contractions may stop or fail to progress
   3. Relaxation between contractions is incomplete
   4. Rigid abdomen
   5. Signs of maternal shock
   6. Absent FHR
   7. Fetus palpated outside the uterus
C. Incomplete rupture of the uterus
   1. Abdominal pain that occurs during contractions
   2. Cervix fails to dilate
   3. Slight vaginal bleeding
   4. FHR absent
D. Implementation
   1. Monitor maternal and fetal vital signs
   2. Prepare client for cesarean section or hysterotomy with hysterectomy
   3. Provide emotional support for the client and partner
   4. Monitor for and treat signs of shock as prescribed

XIII. Placenta Previa

A. Description
   1. Improperly implanted **placenta** in the lower uterine segment near or over the internal os of the cervix
   2. Complete, total, or central: internal os covered by **placenta** when the cervix is fully dilated
   3. Partial: incomplete coverage of os, marginal or

low-lying with only the edge of the **placenta** approaching the internal os

B. Data collection
1. Painless bleeding as early as 7 months
2. Bleeding may range from mild to hemorrhage
3. Soft uterus
4. Abnormal fetal position of breech or transverse lie
5. High presenting part
6. Uterine contractions

C. Implementation
1. Monitor maternal vital signs, FHR, and fetal activity
2. Monitor bleeding, including amount and quality
3. Maintain bed rest and position the client in left lateral position
4. Monitor IV fluids as prescribed and for signs of shock
5. Avoid a vaginal examination if bleeding is occurring
6. Prepare for ultrasound for **placental** localization
7. Prepare to administer Rh immune globulin if the mother is Rh negative and has not been given the injection at 28 weeks' gestation
8. Prepare for premature birth or cesarean section

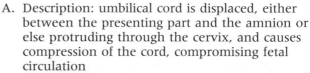

XIV. Abruptio Placentae

A. Description: premature separation of the **placenta** from the uterine wall after the 20th week of gestation and before the fetus is delivered

B. Data collection
1. Painful vaginal bleeding
2. Hypertonic to tetanic, enlarged uterus
3. Board-like rigidity of abdomen
4. Abnormal or absent fetal heart tones
5. Bloody **amniotic fluid**
6. Rising fundal height from blood trapped behind the **placenta**
7. Signs of shock

C. Implementation
1. Monitor maternal vital signs and FHR
2. Monitor for vaginal bleeding, abdominal pain, and an increase in fundal height
3. Maintain bed rest
4. Administer oxygen as prescribed
5. Monitor and report any uterine activity
6. Monitor IV fluids as prescribed
7. Monitor I&O, because a urine output of less than 30 mL/hour indicates decreased renal perfusion
8. Prepare for the **delivery** of the fetus as quickly as possible with vaginal **delivery** preferable if the fetus is healthy and stable, and the presenting part is in the pelvis
9. Prepare for emergency cesarean section if the fetus is alive but shows signs of distress

10. Monitor for signs of DIC particularly in the postpartum period

XV. Prolapsed Cord

A. Description: umbilical cord is displaced, either between the presenting part and the amnion or else protruding through the cervix, and causes compression of the cord, compromising fetal circulation

B. Data collection
1. A feeling that something is coming through the vagina
2. Umbilical cord is seen or palpated
3. FHR is irregular and slow
4. If fetal hypoxia is severe, violent fetal activity may occur and then cease

C. Implementation
1. Relieve cord pressure immediately
2. Place the mother in knee-chest or Trendelenburg's position
3. Elevate the fetal presenting part that is lying on the cord by applying finger pressure with a sterile gloved hand
4. Do not attempt to push the cord into the uterus
5. Monitor FHR and for signs of fetal hypoxia
6. Administer oxygen by face mask to the mother as prescribed
7. Prepare for cesarean birth

XVI. Inverted Uterus

A. Description: uterus turns inside out usually during **delivery** of the **placenta**

B. Data collection
1. Hemorrhage
2. Severe pain
3. Signs of shock

C. Implementation
1. Monitor vital signs
2. Monitor for signs of shock
3. Prepare the client for a return of the uterus to the correct position via the vagina

XVII. Amniotic Fluid Embolism

A. Description
1. The escape of **amniotic fluid** into the maternal circulation
2. The debris containing **amniotic fluid** deposits in the pulmonary arterioles and is usually fatal to the mother

B. Data collection
1. Dyspnea
2. Sudden chest pain
3. Cyanosis
4. Pulmonary edema

C. Implementation
1. Institute emergency measures to maintain life
2. Monitor vital signs
3. Administer oxygen as prescribed

4. Monitor for uncontrolled hemorrhage
5. Assist with the administration of medications as prescribed
6. Prepare for forceps **delivery** if the cervix is dilated

XVIII. Vena Cava Syndrome (Supine Hypotensive Syndrome) (Fig. 23–1)

A. Description
  1. Occurs when the venous return to the heart is impaired by the weight of the uterus
  2. Results in partial occlusion of the vena cava
B. Data collection
  1. Signs of shock
  2. Hypotension
  3. Tachycardia
  4. Sweating
  5. Nausea and vomiting
  6. Fetal distress
C. Implementation
  1. Monitor vital signs
  2. Monitor the FHR
  3. Administer oxygen as prescribed
  4. Position the client by turning her to her left side to shift the weight of the fetus off the inferior vena cava
  5. Monitor for signs of shock caused by reduced cardiac output

XIX. Hematoma

A. Description
  1. The formation of a hematoma following the escape of blood into the tissues of the reproductive sac after the **delivery**
  2. Predisposing conditions include operative **delivery** with forceps or injury to a blood vessel
  3. A life-threatening condition
B. Data collection

1. Abnormal severe pain and pressure in the perineal area
2. Sensitive, palpable tumor in the perineal area with discolored skin
3. Inability to void
4. Decreased hemoglobin and hematocrit (H&H)
5. Signs of shock such as pallor, tachycardia, and hypotension if significant blood loss has occurred
C. Implementation
  1. Monitor vital signs
  2. Monitor the client for abnormal pain, especially when forceps **delivery** has occurred
  3. Place ice to the hematoma site
  4. Administer analgesics as prescribed
  5. Monitor I&O
  6. Encourage fluids
  7. Encourage voiding
  8. Prepare for urinary catheterization if the client is unable to void
  9. Monitor for signs of infection such as increased temperature, pulse rate, and WBC count
  10. Prepare for incision and evacuation of hematoma if necessary

XX. Fetal Distress

A. Data collection
  1. Fetal heart rate above 160 or below 120 beats/minute
  2. Meconium-stained fluid
  3. Fetal hyperactivity
  4. Fetal pH below 7.2
B. Implementation
  1. Monitor vital signs
  2. Oxytocin infusion is discontinued as prescribed
  3. Position the mother by turning her to the left side

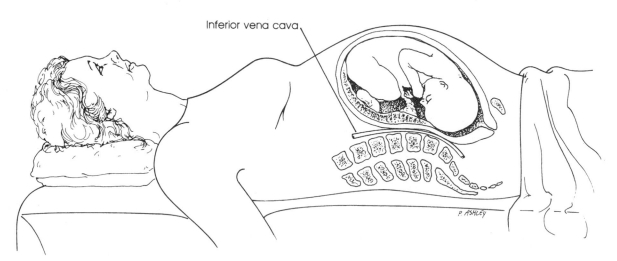

Inferior vena cava

P. ASHLEY

FIGURE 23–1. Supine hypotensive syndrome (vena caval syndrome). Gravid uterus compresses vena cava when the woman is in a supine position. The blood flow returning to the heart is decreased, and maternal hypotension may result. (From Burroughs A. [1997]. Maternity Nursing: An Introductory Text [7th ed.]. Philadelphia: W. B. Saunders, p. 71.)

4. Administer oxygen via face mask as prescribed
5. Elevate legs
6. IV may be increased to treat hypotension
7. Prepare for emergency cesarean section

PRACTICE QUESTIONS

1. The nurse is assigned to assist in caring for a client admitted to the labor unit. The client is 9 cm dilated and is experiencing precipitate labor. A priority nursing action is to
   1 Prepare for an oxytocin infusion
   2 Keep the client in a side-lying position
   3 Prepare the client for an epidural anesthesia
   4 Encourage the client to start pushing with the contractions

2. A client is admitted to the labor suite complaining of painless vaginal bleeding. The nurse assists with the examination of the client knowing that a routine labor procedure contraindicated with this client's situation is
   1 Leopold's maneuvers
   2 External electronic fetal heart rate monitoring
   3 Manual pelvic exam
   4 Hemoglobin and hematocrit evaluation

3. The nurse is assigned to assist in caring for a client with abruptio placentae who is experiencing vaginal bleeding. The nurse collects data from the client knowing that abruptio placentae is accompanied by which of the following additional findings?
   1 Abdomen soft upon palpation
   2 No complaint of abdominal pain
   3 Lack of uterine irritability or tetanic contractions
   4 Uterine tenderness upon palpation

4. The nurse is assigned to work in the delivery room and is assisting in caring for a client who has just delivered a baby. The nurse is monitoring for signs of placental separation knowing that which of the following indicates that the placenta has separated?
   1 Shortening of the umbilical cord
   2 Decrease in blood loss from the vagina
   3 Change in the uterine contour
   4 Sudden, sharp abdominal pain

5. A woman at 20 weeks of gestation calls the physician's office and speaks to a nurse. The client states that she is having subtle but persistent changes in her vaginal discharge, menstrual-like cramps, and diarrhea. Which of the following is the least helpful response to the client?
   1 "This is an emergency; you should come to the clinic within the hour."
   2 "Drink three glasses of water and lie on your left side for 1 hour."
   3 "Palpate for contractions and if 4 or more are felt within 1 hour, you need to be seen by the physician."

4 "Tell me about your activity, food, fluid, and medication intake for the past 24 hours."

6. The nurse is assisting in caring for a client who has a placenta previa. The nurse understands that a cervical examination will not be performed on the client primarily because it could
   1 Increase the chance of infection
   2 Initiate premature labor
   3 Cause profound hemorrhage
   4 Rupture the fetal membranes

7. The nurse caring for a client with abruptio placentae is monitoring the client for signs of disseminated intravascular coagulopathy (DIC). The nurse suspects DIC if the nurse observes
   1 Pain and swelling of the calf of one leg
   2 Rapid clotting times
   3 Lab values indicating increased platelets
   4 Petechiae, oozing from injection sites, and hematuria

8. The nurse is assisting in caring for a client with abruptio placentae. While caring for the client, the nurse notes that the client begins to develop signs of shock. A first priority nursing action is to
   1 Turn the client onto her side
   2 Monitor maternal pulse
   3 Monitor urinary output
   4 Monitor maternal blood pressure

9. A client being prepared for a cesarean delivery is brought to the delivery room. In order to maintain optimal perfusion of oxygenated blood to the fetus, the nurse plans to place the client in a
   1 Trendelenburg's position
   2 Semi-Fowler's position
   3 Supine position with a wedge under the right hip
   4 Prone position

10. The nurse is reinforcing instructions to the postpartum cesarean delivery client who is preparing for discharge. Which statement made by the client indicates a need for more information?
    1 "I can start doing abdominal exercises as soon as I get home."
    2 "I will lift nothing heavier than the baby for 2 weeks."
    3 "If I develop a fever, I will call my doctor."
    4 "When getting out of bed, I will turn on my side and push up with my arms."

11. The nurse is asked to assist the primary health care provider in performing Leopold's maneuvers on a client. Which priority nursing intervention should be implemented before this procedure is performed?
    1 Locate fetal heart tones
    2 Have the client drink 8 oz of water
    3 Warm the sonogram gel
    4 Have the client empty her bladder

12. A woman in active labor has contractions every 2 to 3 minutes lasting 45 seconds. The fetal heart rate between contractions is 100 beats/minute. Based on these findings, the priority nursing intervention is to
    1 Notify the registered nurse (RN) immediately
    2 Encourage relaxation and breathing techniques between contractions
    3 Continue monitoring labor and fetal heart rate
    4 Monitor maternal vital signs

13. The nurse is assigned to assist in caring for a client being admitted to the birthing center in early labor. On admission, the nurse plans to
    1 Check pelvic adequacy
    2 Administer an analgesic
    3 Estimate fetal size
    4 Determine maternal and fetal vital signs

14. Leopold's maneuvers will be performed on a pregnant client. The client asks the nurse about this procedure. The nurse responds that this procedure
    1 Determines the "lie" and "attitude" of the fetus
    2 Is a systematic method for palpating the fetus through the maternal back
    3 Is a systematic method for palpating the fetus through the maternal abdominal wall
    4 Measures the height of the maternal fundus

15. The nurse reviews the client's health record and notes that based on Leopold's maneuvers, the fetus is a cephalic presentation. The nurse understands that this is
    1 An abnormal presentation
    2 The least favorable presentation
    3 A presentation associated with prolonged labor
    4 The most common presentation

16. The nurse is assigned to care for a client who is in early labor. When collecting data from the client, it is most important for the nurse to first determine which of the following?

    1 Intensity of contractions
    2 Frequency of contractions
    3 Baseline fetal heart rate
    4 Maternal blood pressure

17. The nurse is caring for a client in labor. The nurse rechecks the client's blood pressure and determines it has dropped. To decrease the incidence of supine hypotension, the nurse should encourage the client to remain in which position?
    1 Left lateral
    2 Semi-Fowler's
    3 Squatting
    4 Tailor sitting

18. The nurse instructs the client in active relaxation techniques to help her cope with the discomfort of contractions. The nurse determines teaching has been effective when the client tells the nurse that active relaxation includes
    1 Assuming a state of mind that is open to suggestions from a coach
    2 Believing that a supreme power can help relieve the discomfort of contractions
    3 Relaxing uninvolved muscles while the uterus contracts
    4 Understanding the origin of contraction discomfort to be more psychological than physical

19. A primigravida's membranes rupture spontaneouly. The nurse's first action is to
    1 Monitor contraction pattern
    2 Determine the fetal heart rate
    3 Note the amount, color, and odor of the amniotic fluid
    4 Prepare for immediate delivery

20. After a client vaginally delivers a viable newborn, the nurse observes the umbilical cord lengthen and a spurt of blood from the vagina. The nurse recognizes these findings as signs of
    1 Abruptio placentae
    2 Placenta previa
    3 Placental separation
    4 Uterine atony

ANSWERS

1. **2**

RATIONALE: Priority care of this client includes promotion of fetal oxygenation. Precipitate labor progresses quickly with frequent contractions and short periods of relaxation between contractions. This does not allow for maximal reperfusion of the placenta with oxygenated blood. A side-lying position can assist in blood flow to the uterus by preventing vena cava and abdominal aorta compression. Further stimulation with oxytocin is contraindicated. There may not be enough time to administer an epidural anesthesia prior to delivery with such quick progression. The chance of an unattended birth is possible. Pushing with contractions is not indicated, especially with this type of labor. Controlled delivery of the baby is essential to prevent maternal and fetal injury.
TEST-TAKING STRATEGY: Note the key words "precipitate" and "priority." Using Maslow's hierarchy of needs theory, physiological integrity needs to be dealt with first. Also, use the ABCs when prioritizing, including the baby's needs as well as the client's.
LEVEL OF COGNITIVE ABILITY: Application
PHASE OF NURSING PROCESS: Implementation

CLIENT NEEDS: Physiological Integrity
CONTENT AREA: Maternity
REFERENCE

Gorrie, T., McKinney, E., & Murray, S. (1998). *Foundations of maternal-newborn nursing* (2nd ed.). Philadelphia: W. B. Saunders. p. 755.

2. **3**

RATIONALE: Painless vaginal bleeding is a sign of a possible placenta previa. Digital examination of the cervix can lead to maternal and fetal hemorrhage. Leopold's maneuvers can reveal a nonengaged presenting part or malpresentation, both of which often accompany placenta previa due to the placenta filling the lower uterine segment. Hemoglobin and hematocrit values help to estimate the amount of blood loss. Electronic fetal monitoring (external) is crucial in evaluating the status of the fetus who is at risk for severe hypoxia. Options 1, 2, and 4 are procedures that would not place the client at further risk.
TEST-TAKING STRATEGY: Knowledge of the risks associated with placenta previa is required to answer this question. Use the process of elimination. Option 3 is the only procedure that is invasive to the pregnancy and endangers the physiological safety of the client and fetus. Review this content now if you had difficulty with this question.
LEVEL OF COGNITIVE ABILITY: Comprehension
PHASE OF NURSING PROCESS: Data Collection
CLIENT NEEDS: Physiological Integrity
CONTENT AREA: Maternity
REFERENCE

Burroughs, A. (1997). *Maternity nursing: An introductory text* (7th ed.). Philadelphia: W. B. Saunders. p. 385.

3. **4**

RATIONALE: Vaginal bleeding in a pregnant client most often is caused by placenta previa or a placental abruption. Uterine tenderness accompanies abruptio placentae, especially with a central abruption and trapped blood behind the placenta. The abdomen will feel hard and board-like upon palpation as the blood penetrates the myometrium and causes uterine irritability. A sustained tetanic contraction can occur if the client is in labor and the uterine muscle cannot relax.
TEST-TAKING STRATEGY: Note the issue of the question, abruptio placentae. It can be easy to confuse a placenta previa and abruption. Remember, the difference involves the presence of uterine pain and tenderness with an abruptio placentae as opposed to painless bleeding with a placenta previa. Options 1, 2, and 3 describe the absence of a sign or symptom of abruptio placentae, while option 4 is the only option that describes a sign. Review this content now if you had difficulty with this question.
LEVEL OF COGNITIVE ABILITY: Comprehension
PHASE OF NURSING PROCESS: Data Collection
CLIENT NEEDS: Physiological Integrity
CONTENT AREA: Maternity
REFERENCE

Burroughs, A. (1997). *Maternity nursing: An introductory text* (7th ed.). Philadelphia: W. B. Saunders. p. 385.

4. **3**

RATIONALE: Signs of placental separation include lengthening of the umbilical cord, a sudden gush of dark blood from the vagina, a firmly contracted uterus, and the uterus changing from a discoid to globular shape. The client may experience vaginal fullness, but not sudden and sharp abdominal pain.
TEST-TAKING STRATEGY: Use the process of elimination. Thinking about what one would expect to occur when the placenta separates will assist in eliminating options 1 and 2. Option 4 is eliminated because of the words "sudden, sharp." Review the signs of placental separation now if you had difficulty with this question.
LEVEL OF COGNITIVE ABILITY: Comprehension
PHASE OF NURSING PROCESS: Data Collection
CLIENT NEEDS: Physiological Integrity
CONTENT AREA: Maternity
REFERENCE

Burroughs, A. (1997). *Maternity nursing: An introductory text* (7th ed.). Philadelphia: W. B. Saunders. p. 171.

5. **1**

RATIONALE: If the woman is active it may be helpful for her to lie on her side, drink fluids, and keep her bladder empty to eliminate uterine hypoxia and thereby decrease uterine activity. If the woman continues to have persistent uterine activity after 1 hour or counts four or more contractions in less than 1 hour, she should be seen for further evaluation. Option 4 addresses the process of data collection and is an important initial component of care.
TEST-TAKING STRATEGY: Note the key words "least helpful." Eliminate option 4 first because it addresses the process of data collection. For the remaining options, note that option 1 contains language that would alarm the client. This statement is least helpful to the client.
LEVEL OF COGNITIVE ABILITY: Application
PHASE OF NURSING PROCESS: Implementation
CLIENT NEEDS: Psychosocial Integrity
CONTENT AREA: Maternity
REFERENCE

Burroughs, A. (1997). *Maternity nursing: An introductory text* (7th ed.). Philadelphia: W. B. Saunders. p. 89.

6. **3**

RATIONALE: Since the placenta is implanted low in the uterus, cervical examination could cause the disruption of the placenta and initiate profound hemorrhage. The other options are also correct, but the profound hemorrhage is of the greatest concern in this instance.
TEST-TAKING STRATEGY: Note the key word "primarily." Recalling that bleeding is a primary concern will easily direct you to option 3. Review the care of the client with placenta previa now if you had difficulty with this question.
LEVEL OF COGNITIVE ABILITY: Comprehension
PHASE OF NURSING PROCESS: Planning
CLIENT NEEDS: Physiological Integrity
CONTENT AREA: Maternity
REFERENCE

Leifer, G. (1999). *Thompson's introduction to maternity and pediatric nursing* (3rd ed.). Philadelphia: W. B. Saunders. p. 90.

7. **4**

RATIONALE: DIC is a state of diffuse clotting in which clotting factors are consumed. This leads to widespread bleeding. Platelets are decreased because they are consumed by the process; coagulation studies show no clot formation (and are thus prolonged); and fibrin plugs may clog the microvasculature diffusely, rather than in an isolated area.
TEST-TAKING STRATEGY: Use the process of elimination. Eliminate option 1 based on the knowledge that DIC

is a widespread problem, not a localized one. Eliminate options 2 and 3 next because they are similar. Review the signs related to DIC now if you had difficulty with this question.
LEVEL OF COGNITIVE ABILITY: Comprehension
PHASE OF NURSING PROCESS: Data Collection
CLIENT NEEDS: Physiological Integrity
CONTENT AREA: Maternity
REFERENCE
Burroughs, A. (1997). *Maternity nursing: An introductory text* (7th ed.). Philadelphia: W. B. Saunders. p. 387.

8. **1**

RATIONALE: With a client in shock, the nurse increases perfusion to the placenta. A simple way, requiring no equipment, is to turn the mother on her side. This increases blood flow to the placenta by relieving pressure from the gravid uterus on the great vessels. The nurse immediately contacts the registered nurse, who then contacts the physician. The other options follow quickly.
TEST-TAKING STRATEGY: Note the key word "first." Eliminate options 2 and 4 because they are similar. Recalling that positioning will affect the status of blood flow will assist in directing you to option 1. Review care to the client in shock now if you had difficulty with this question.
LEVEL OF COGNITIVE ABILITY: Application
PHASE OF NURSING PROCESS: Implementation
CLIENT NEEDS: Physiological Integrity
CONTENT AREA: Maternity
REFERENCE
Leifer, G. (1999). *Thompson's introduction to maternity and pediatric nursing* (3rd ed.). Philadelphia: W. B. Saunders. p. 90.

9. **3**

RATIONALE: Vena cava and descending aorta compression by the pregnant uterus impedes blood return from the lower trunk and extremities, thereby decreasing cardiac return, cardiac output, and blood flow to the uterus and subsequently the fetus. The best position to prevent this is side-lying with the uterus displaced off the abdominal vessels. Positioning for abdominal surgery necessitates a supine position; however, a wedge placed under the right hip provides displacement of the uterus. Trendelenburg positioning places pressure from the pregnant uterus on the diaphragm and lungs, decreasing respiratory capacity and oxygenation. A semi-Fowler's or prone position is not practical for this type of abdominal surgery.
TEST-TAKING STRATEGY: Note the key words "maintain optimal perfusion." Use the process of elimination and visualize each of the positions and their effect on the fetus. Review client positioning now if you had difficulty with this question.
LEVEL OF COGNITIVE ABILITY: Application
PHASE OF NURSING PROCESS: Planning
CLIENT NEEDS: Physiological Integrity
CONTENT AREA: Maternity
REFERENCE
Gorrie, T., McKinney, E., & Murray, S. (1998). *Foundations of maternal-newborn nursing* (2nd ed.). Philadelphia: W. B. Saunders. p. 413.

10. **1**

RATIONALE: Abdominal exercises should not start following abdominal surgery until 3 to 4 weeks postoperatively to allow for healing of the incision. Options 2, 3, and 4 reflect proper understanding of self-care after discharge.

TEST-TAKING STRATEGY: Note the key words "cesarean delivery" and "need for more information." Use general principles related to abdominal surgery to assist in directing you to option 1. Review client teaching points following cesarean delivery now if you had difficulty with this question.
LEVEL OF COGNITIVE ABILITY: Comprehension
PHASE OF NURSING PROCESS: Evaluation
CLIENT NEEDS: Health Promotion and Maintenance
CONTENT AREA: Maternity
REFERENCE
Burroughs, A. (1997). *Maternity nursing: An introductory text* (7th ed.). Philadelphia: W. B. Saunders. p. 422.

11. **4**

RATIONALE: An empty bladder contributes to a woman's comfort during the examination. Drinking water to fill the bladder and warming the sonogram gel may be performed prior to a sonogram. Often Leopold's maneuvers are performed to aid the examiner in locating the fetal heart tones.
TEST-TAKING STRATEGY: Use the process of elimination. Eliminate option 1 because Leopold's maneuvers are often used to help locate fetal heart tones. Eliminate options 2 and 3 because sonogram gel is not used during Leopold's maneuvers and often the client is requested to have a full bladder before ultrasonography. Review the preparation of a client for this procedure now if you had difficulty with this question.
LEVEL OF COGNITIVE ABILITY: Application
PHASE OF NURSING PROCESS: Planning
CLIENT NEEDS: Physiological Integrity
CONTENT AREA: Maternity
REFERENCE
Burroughs, A. (1997). *Maternity nursing: An introductory text* (7th ed.). Philadelphia: W.B. Saunders. p. 180.

12. **1**

RATIONALE: Fetal bradycardia between contractions may indicate the need for immediate medical management. The nurse immediately contacts the RN, who in turn contacts the physician. Options 2, 3, and 4 will delay necessary and immediate interventions.
TEST-TAKING STRATEGY: Use the ABCs, airway, breathing, and circulation. Note that the woman is in active labor and that the fetal heart rate is below normal. It is imperative that the circulation in the fetus be restored to normal limits.
LEVEL OF COGNITIVE ABILITY: Application
PHASE OF NURSING PROCESS: Implementation
CLIENT NEEDS: Physiological Integrity
CONTENT AREA: Maternity
REFERENCE
Burroughs, A. (1997). *Maternity nursing: An introductory text* (7th ed.). Philadelphia: W. B. Saunders. p. 144.

13. **4**

RATIONALE: To evaluate a woman's physical well-being, assess the temperature, pulse, respirations and blood pressure, as well as the fetal heartbeat in order to determine the level of risk. Option 2 is incorrect because it would be too premature for an analgesic. Medication given too early tends to slow or stop labor contractions. Options 1 and 3 are incorrect. These assessments should be done by the physician or a nurse midwife during prenatal visits.

TEST-TAKING STRATEGY: Use the ABCs, airway, breathing, and circulation. This will easily direct you to option 4. Remember, measuring vital signs is the priority.
LEVEL OF COGNITIVE ABILITY: Application
PHASE OF NURSING PROCESS: Planning
CLIENT NEEDS: Physiological Integrity
CONTENT AREA: Maternity
REFERENCE
Burroughs, A. (1997). *Maternity nursing: An introductory text* (7th ed.). Philadelphia: W. B. Saunders. p. 179.

14. **3**

RATIONALE: Leopold's maneuvers is a systematic method for palpating the fetus through the maternal abdominal wall. Options 1, 2, and 4 are incorrect.
TEST-TAKING STRATEGY: Knowledge of Leopard's maneuvers is required to answer this question. If you are unfamiliar with this procedure, take the time to review it now.
LEVEL OF COGNITIVE ABILITY: Comprehension
PHASE OF NURSING PROCESS: Implementation
CLIENT NEEDS: Physiological Integrity
CONTENT AREA: Maternity
REFERENCE
Gorrie, T., McKinney, E., & Murray, S. (1998). *Foundations of maternal-newborn nursing* (2nd ed.). Philadelphia: W. B. Saunders. p. 146.

15. **4**

RATIONALE: The cephalic presentation is more favorable than others and is the most common. Other presentations are associated with prolonged labor or other abnormalities and are more likely to necessitate a cesarean birth.
TEST-TAKING STRATEGY: Knowledge regarding the types of fetal presentation is required to assist in selecting the correct option. Review this content now if you had difficulty with this question.
LEVEL OF COGNITIVE ABILITY: Comprehension
PHASE OF NURSING PROCESS: Data Collection
CLIENT NEEDS: Physiological Integrity
CONTENT AREA: Maternity
REFERENCE
Gorrie, T., McKinney, E., & Murray, S. (1998). *Foundations of maternal-newborn nursing* (2nd ed.). Philadelphia: W. B. Saunders. p. 277.

16. **3**

RATIONALE: The nurse should first determine the baseline fetal heart rate. Although options 1, 2, and 4 are components of the data collection process, the fetal heart rate is the priority.
TEST-TAKING STRATEGY: Note the key word "first." Utilize Maslow's hierarchy of needs theory to prioritize. Physiological needs come first, so select an answer that addresses physiological needs. Also utilize the ABCs when selecting an answer. Remember the order of priority of airway, breathing, and circulation. Fetal heart rate reflects ABCs.
LEVEL OF COGNITIVE ABILITY: Comprehension
PHASE OF NURSING PROCESS: Data Collection
CLIENT NEEDS: Physiological Integrity
CONTENT AREA: Maternity
REFERENCE
Burroughs, A. (1997). *Maternity nursing: An introductory text* (7th ed.). Philadelphia: W. B. Saunders. p. 169.

17. **1**

RATIONALE: Pressure from the enlarged uterus and the aorta and vena cava when the woman is supine can result in hypotension, which can be relieved by having the woman lie on her left side. Options 2, 3, and 4 are incorrect.
TEST-TAKING STRATEGY: This question requires an understanding of the anatomy of the pregnant uterus and the physiological response caused by pressure on the large abdominal vessels. Note that options 2, 3, and 4 are all similar in that the client is upright. Review nursing measures when the pregnant client becomes hypotensive if you had difficulty with this question.
LEVEL OF COGNITIVE ABILITY: Application
PHASE OF NURSING PROCESS: Implementation
CLIENT NEEDS: Physiological Integrity
CONTENT AREA: Maternity
REFERENCE
Gorrie, T., McKinney, E., & Murray, S. (1998). *Foundations of maternal-newborn nursing* (2nd ed.). Philadelphia: W. B. Saunders. p. 270.

18. **3**

RATIONALE: Active relaxation techniques include specific relaxation exercises and conditioned responses such as distraction from the discomfort of labor. The woman is an active participant in the use of the technique that focuses on relaxing uninvolved muscles while the uterus contracts.
TEST-TAKING STRATEGY: Note the key words "active relaxation techniques." Use the process of elimination, noting that option 3 contains an active verb and is different from the others. Review the purpose of active relaxation techniques now if you had difficulty with this question.
LEVEL OF COGNITIVE ABILITY: Comprehension
PHASE OF NURSING PROCESS: Evaluation
CLIENT NEEDS: Physiological Integrity
CONTENT AREA: Maternity
REFERENCE
Gorrie, T., McKinney, E., & Murray, S. (1998). *Foundations of maternal-newborn nursing* (2nd ed.). Philadelphia: W. B. Saunders. p. 371.

19. **2**

RATIONALE: When the membranes rupture, the nurse immediately assesses the fetal heart rate to detect changes associated with prolapse or compression of the umbilical cord. Monitoring the contraction pattern and noting the amount, color, and odor of the amniotic fluid may be performed but is not the first action. There are no data in the question that indicate the necessity to prepare the client for immediate delivery.
TEST-TAKING STRATEGY: Note the key word "first." Use the ABCs, airway, breathing, and circulation. Fetal heart rate is associated with fetal breathing and circulation.
LEVEL OF COGNITIVE ABILITY: Application
PHASE OF NURSING PROCESS: Implementation
CLIENT NEEDS: Physiological Integrity
CONTENT AREA: Maternity
REFERENCE
Gorrie, T., McKinney, E., & Murray, S. (1998). *Foundations of maternal-newborn nursing* (2nd ed.). Philadelphia: W. B. Saunders. p. 269.

20. **3**

RATIONALE: As the placenta separates, it settles downward into the lower uterine segment, the umbilical cord lengthens, and a sudden trickle or spurt of blood appears. The clinical manifestations identified in the question are not related to options 1, 2, and 4.

TEST-TAKING STRATEGY: Note the similarity between options 1, 2, and 4 in that they represent complications associated with pregnancy. Option 3 indicates a normal finding following vaginal delivery of the newborn. Review this stage of labor now if you had difficulty with this question.

LEVEL OF COGNITIVE ABILITY: Comprehension
PHASE OF NURSING PROCESS: Data Collection
CLIENT NEEDS: Physiological Integrity
CONTENT AREA: Maternity
REFERENCE
Gorrie, T., McKinney, E., & Murray, S. (1998). *Foundations of maternal-newborn nursing* (2nd ed.). Philadelphia: W. B. Saunders. pp. 288–289.

BIBLIOGRAPHY

Gorrie, T., McKinney, E., & Murray, S. (1998). *Foundations of maternal-newborn nursing* (2nd ed.). Philadelphia: W. B. Saunders.

Burroughs, A. (1997). *Maternity nursing: An introductory text* (7th ed.). Philadelphia: W. B. Saunders.

Leifer, G. (1999). *Thompson's introduction to maternity and pediatric nursing* (3rd ed.). Philadelphia: W. B. Saunders.

CHAPTER 24

The Postpartum Period and Associated Complications

I. Postpartum

A. Description: period when the reproductive tract returns to the normal, nonpregnant state

B. Postpartum period: starts immediately after **delivery** and is completed usually by week 6 following **delivery**

II. Physiological Maternal Changes

A. Involution (Fig. 24–1)
   1. Description

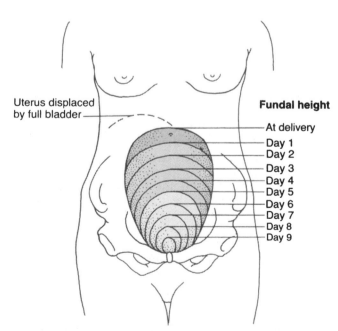

Uterus displaced by full bladder

Fundal height

At delivery
Day 1
Day 2
Day 3
Day 4
Day 5
Day 6
Day 7
Day 8
Day 9

FIGURE 24–1. Changes in the height of the uterine fundus each day as involution progresses. (From Leifer, G. [1999]. *Thompson's introduction to maternity and pediatric nursing* [3rd ed.]. Philadelphia: W. B. Saunders. p. 224.)

     a. The rapid decrease in the size of the uterus as it returns to the nonpregnant state
     b. Clients who breast-feed may experience a more rapid involution
  2. Data collection
     a. Weight of the uterus decreases from 2 lb to 2 oz in 6 weeks
     b. Fundus steadily descends into the pelvis; the fundal height decreases about 1 fingerbreadth (1 cm) per day
     c. By 10 days' postpartum, the uterus cannot be palpated abdominally
     d. A flaccid fundus indicates uterine atony
     e. A tender fundus indicates an infection

B. **Lochia** (Fig. 24–2)
  1. Description: discharge from the uterus that consists of blood from the vessels of the **placental** site and debris from the decidua
  2. Data collection
     a. Rubra: bright red discharge that occurs from **delivery** day to day 3
     b. Serosa: brownish pink discharge that occurs from days 4 to 10
     c. Alba: white discharge that occurs from days 10 to 14
     d. Normally, the discharge has a fleshy odor
     e. Discharge decreases daily in amount
     f. Discharge increases with ambulation

C. Cervix: cervical involution; after 1 week the muscle begins to regenerate

D. Vagina: vaginal distention decreases, although muscle tone is never restored completely to the pregravid state

E. Ovarian function and menstruation
  1. Menstrual flow resumes within 8 weeks in nonbreast-feeding mothers
  2. Menstrual flow usually resumes within 3 to 4 months in breast-feeding mothers

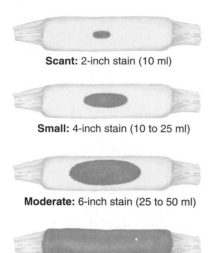

Scant: 2-inch stain (10 ml)

Small: 4-inch stain (10 to 25 ml)

Moderate: 6-inch stain (25 to 50 ml)

Large: >6-inch stain (50 to 80 ml)

FIGURE 24–2. Guidelines for assessing the volume of lochia based on amount of stain on the perineal pad. (From Gorrie, T., McKinney, E., & Murray, S. [1998]. *Foundations of maternal-newborn nursing* [2nd ed.]. Philadelphia: W. B. Saunders. p. 429.)

3. Breast-feeding mothers may experience amenorrhea during the entire period of lactation
4. A woman may ovulate without menstruating, so breast-feeding should not be considered a form of birth control

F. Breasts
1. A decrease of estrogen and progesterone levels after **delivery** stimulates increased prolactin levels, which promotes breast milk production
2. Breasts become distended with milk on the third day
3. Engorgement occurs in 48 to 72 hours in nonbreast-feeding mothers; breast-feeding will relieve engorgement

G. Urinary tract
1. May have urinary retention due to loss of elasticity and tone and loss of sensation in the bladder from trauma, medications, anesthesia, and lack of privacy
2. Diuresis usually begins within first 12 hours after **delivery**

H. Gastrointestinal tract
1. Women are usually very hungry after **delivery**
2. Constipation can occur
3. Hemorrhoids are common

I. Vital signs
1. Temperature may be elevated during the first 24 hours due to dehydration
2. Bradycardia is common during the first week, with a range of 50 to 70 beats per minute
3. Blood pressure remains unchanged

III. Postpartum Implementation

A. Data collection
1. Monitor vital signs

2. Monitor height, consistency, and location of the fundus
3. Monitor color, amount, and odor of **lochia**
4. Check breasts for engorgement
5. Monitor perineum for swelling or discoloration; episiotomy for healing
6. Check incisions or dressings of cesarean birth client
7. Monitor I&O
8. Monitor bowel status
9. Encourage frequent voiding
10. Encourage ambulation
11. RhoGam is prescribed to be administered within 72 hours' postpartum to the Rh-negative client who is not sensitized
12. Monitor parent-**newborn** bonding
13. Monitor emotional status

B. Client teaching
1. Demonstrate **newborn** care skills as necessary
2. Provide the opportunity for the mother to bathe the newborn
3. Instruct on feeding technique
4. Instruct the mother to avoid heavy lifting for at least 3 weeks
5. Instruct the mother to plan at least one rest period per day
6. Instruct the mother that contraception should begin after **delivery** or with the initiation of intercourse
7. Instruct the mother on the importance of follow-up, which should be scheduled at 4 to 6 weeks
8. Instruct the mother to report any signs of chills, fever, increased **lochia**, or depressed feelings to the physician immediately

IV. Postpartum Discomforts

A. Afterbirth pains
1. Occur due to contractions of the uterus
2. Are more common in multiparas, breast-feeding mothers, clients treated with oxytocin (Pitocin), and clients who had an overdistended uterus during pregnancy

B. Perineal discomfort
1. Apply ice packs to the perineum as prescribed during the first 24 hours to reduce swelling
2. After the first 24 hours, apply warmth by sitzbaths as prescribed

C. Episiotomy
1. Instruct the client to administer perineal care after each voiding
2. Encourage the use of analgesic spray as prescribed
3. Administer analgesics as prescribed if comfort measures are unsuccessful

D. Breast discomfort from engorgement
1. Encourage wearing a support bra at all times, even while sleeping
2. Encourage the use of ice packs if not breast-feeding

3. Encourage the use of warm soaks before feeding for a breast-feeding mother
4. Administer analgesics as prescribed if comfort measures are unsuccessful

E. Postpartum blues
1. The condition may be caused by physiological or emotional stress
2. Weepiness, mood changes, anxiety, and irritability in the first few days following childbirth
3. Verbalization should be encouraged
4. If unresolved, postpartum blues may progress to postpartum depression

V. Nutrition

A. Nutritional needs depend on prepregnancy weight, ideal weight for height, and whether the mother is breast-feeding
B. If the mother is breast-feeding, calorie needs increase by approximately 500 calories per day, and the mother may require increased fluids and the continuance of prenatal vitamins and minerals

VI. Breast-feeding

A. General principles
1. Put the baby to breast as soon as the mother and baby's condition is stable; on **delivery** table if possible
2. Stay with the mother each time she nurses until she feels secure or confident with the baby and her feelings
3. Uterine cramping may occur the first day after **delivery** while nursing, when oxytocin stimulation causes the uterus to contract
4. Use general hygiene and wash the breasts once daily
5. Do not use soap on the breasts because it tends to remove natural oils and increases the chances of cracking
6. Bra should be well fitted and supporting
7. Breasts may leak between feedings or during coitus; place a breast pad in bra
8. Calories are increased by 500 per day, and the diet should include additional fluids; prenatal vitamins should be taken as prescribed
9. Baby's stools will be light yellow, watery, and frequent
10. Medications should be avoided unless prescribed
11. Gas-producing foods and caffeine should be avoided
12. Birth control pills should not be taken
13. **Newborns** should be put to the breast as soon as possible after **delivery**
14. The baby will develop his or her own feeding schedule

B. Breast-feeding procedure for mother
1. Wash the hands and assume a comfortable position
2. Start with the breast that the last feeding ended with (baby sucks more vigorously at the beginning of feeding)
3. Brush the **newborn's** lower lip with the nipple
4. Tickle lips to have the baby open the mouth wide
5. Guide the nipple and surrounding areola into the baby's mouth
6. After the baby has nursed, release suction by depressing the **newborn's** chin or inserting a clean finger into the baby's mouth
7. Burp the baby after the first breast
8. Repeat the procedure on the second breast until the baby stops nursing
9. Burp the baby again
10. Instruct the mother to listen for audible sucking and swallowing

C. Engorgement
1. Breast-feed frequently
2. Apply warm packs before feeding
3. Apply ice packs between feedings

D. Cracked nipples
1. Expose nipples to air for 10 to 20 minutes after feeding
2. Rotate the position of the baby for each feeding

VII. Cystitis

A. Description: an infection of the bladder
B. Data collection
1. Burning and pain on urination
2. Lower abdominal pain
3. Increased frequency of urination
4. Fever
5. Proteinuria, hematuria, bacteriuria, WBCs in urine
C. Implementation
1. Palpate the bladder for distention
2. Palpate the fundus for position
3. Obtain a urine specimen for culture and sensitivity if prescribed
4. Institute measures to assist the client to void
5. Encourage frequent and complete emptying of the bladder
6. Force fluids to 3000 mL per day
7. Administer antibiotics as prescribed after the urine culture is obtained

VIII. Hematoma

A. Description
1. Occurs following the escape of blood into the tissues of the reproductive sac after the **delivery**
2. Predisposing conditions include operative **delivery** with forceps or injury to a blood vessel
3. Can be a life-threatening condition
B. Data collection
1. Abnormal, severe pain and pressure in perineal area

2. Inability to void
3. Palpable tumor
4. Decreased hemoglobin and hematocrit (H&H)
5. Signs of shock such as pallor, tachycardia, and hypotension if significant blood loss has occurred

C. Implementation
1. Monitor vital signs
2. Monitor the client for abnormal pain especially when forceps **delivery** has occurred
3. Place ice to the hematoma site
4. Administer analgesics as prescribed
5. Monitor intake and output (I&O); encourage fluids
6. Monitor for signs of infection such as increased temperature, pulse rate, and WBC count
7. Prepare the client for incision and evacuation of hematoma if necessary

IX. Hemorrhage

A. Description: bleeding of 500 mL or more following **delivery**
B. Data collection
1. Early
   a. Hemorrhage occurs during first 24 hours after **delivery**
   b. Caused by uterine atony, lacerations, or inversion of the uterus
2. Late
   a. Hemorrhage occurs after the first 24 hours following **delivery**
   b. Caused by retained **placental** fragments
C. Implementation
1. Monitor vital signs and fundus every 5 to 15 minutes
2. Monitor and estimate blood loss by pad count
3. Massage fundus, with care not to overmassage
4. Notify the physician or health care provider if hemorrhage occurs
5. Maintain asepsis because hemorrhage predisposes to infection
6. Monitor level of consciousness
7. Oxytocin (Pitocin) may be administered
8. H&H is monitored; blood transfusions may be administered

X. Infection

A. Description: any infection of the reproductive organs that occurs within 28 days of **delivery** or abortion
B. Data collection
1. Fever and chills
2. Pelvic discomfort or pain
3. Vaginal discharge
4. Elevated WBC count
C. Implementation
1. Monitor vital signs and temperature every 2 to 4 hours

2. Make the client as comfortable as possible; position for comfort and to promote drainage
3. Keep the mother warmed if chilled
4. Isolate the baby from the mother only if the mother is infected
5. Provide nutritious high-calorie protein diet
6. Monitor I&O
7. Force fluids to 3000 mL a day, if not contraindicated
8. Encourage frequent voiding
9. Administer antibiotics as prescribed

XI. Mastitis

A. Description
1. Inflammation of the breast as a result of infection
2. Primarily seen in breast-feeding mothers 2 to 3 weeks after **delivery**
B. Data collection
1. Localized heat and swelling
2. Pain
3. Elevated temperature
4. Complaints of flulike symptoms
C. Implementation
1. Instruct the mother in good handwashing and breast hygiene
2. Apply heat or cold to the site as prescribed
3. Maintain lactation in breast-feeding mothers
4. Encourage manual expression of breast milk or use of a breast pump every 4 hours
5. Encourage the mother to wear a supportive bra to support her breasts
6. Administer analgesics or antibiotics as prescribed

XII. Pulmonary Embolism

A. Description: the passage of thrombus, often originating in one of the uterine or other pelvic veins, into the lungs, where it disrupts the circulation of blood
B. Data collection
1. Dyspnea and cough
2. Tachypnea and tachycardia
3. Hemoptysis
4. Pleuritic chest pain
C. Implementation
1. Administer oxygen as prescribed
2. Position the client with the head of the bed elevated to promote comfort
3. Monitor vital signs frequently
4. Frequently monitor respiratory rate
5. Monitor for signs of respiratory distress and hypoxemia such as tachypnea, tachycardia, restlessness, cool and clammy skin, cyanosis, and the use of accessory muscles
6. Increased IV fluids may be prescribed
7. Anticoagulants may be prescribed

XIII. Subinvolution

A. Description: incomplete involution or failure of the uterus to return to its normal size and condition
B. Data collection
  1. Uterine pain on palpation
  2. Uterus is larger than expected
  3. Greater than normal vaginal bleeding
C. Implementation
  1. Monitor vital signs
  2. Monitor the uterus and fundus and for vaginal bleeding
  3. Elevate the legs to promote venous return
  4. Encourage frequent voiding
  5. H&H is monitored
  6. Methylergonovine maleate (Methergine) or ergonovine maleate (Ergotrate) may be prescribed

XIV. Thrombophlebitis

A. Description
  1. A condition in which a clot forms in a vessel wall secondary to the inflammation of the vessel wall
  2. A partial obstruction of the vessel can occur
  3. Increased blood-clotting factors in the postpartum period place the client at risk
B. Data collection (Table 24–1)
  1. Superficial thrombophlebitis
  2. Femoral thrombophlebitis
  3. Pelvic thrombophlebitis
C. Implementation
  1. Assess lower extremities for edema, tenderness, varices, and increased skin temperature
  2. Maintain bed rest; elevate the affected leg
  3. Apply a bed cradle and keep bedclothes off affected leg
  4. Never massage the leg
  5. Apply hot packs to the affected site as prescribed
  6. Apply elastic stockings to the legs as prescribed

BOX 24–1. Client Education for Thrombophlebitis
Avoid pressure behind the knees
Avoid prolonged sitting
Avoid constrictive clothing
Avoid crossing the legs
Never massage the leg
Know how to apply support hose if prescribed
Understand the importance of anticoagulant therapy as prescribed
Understand the importance of follow-up with the health care provider

  7. Monitor for signs of pulmonary embolism
  8. Administer analgesics and antibiotics as prescribed
  9. Intravenous heparin may be prescribed to prevent further thrombus formation
D. Client teaching (Box 24–1)

PRACTICE QUESTIONS

1. A postpartum client that delivered at 32 weeks' gestation would like to breast-feed her preterm infant. At this time, the infant is receiving tube feedings only. What is the nurse's best response to the mother?
  1 "There is no need to prepare for breast-feeding now because the infant is receiving tube feedings."
  2 "You can prepare your breast by pinching and rolling the nipples and hand-expressing colostrum."
  3 "You can begin pumping as soon as possible after delivery with an electric breast pump."
  4 "You need to pump your breasts every 6 hours to establish a good milk supply."

2. The nurse is assisting in developing a plan of care for a client preparing to breast-feed. In planning care, which of the following factors is the most significant in teaching a client to breast-feed?
  1 Brief separation of infant and mother after birth to allow the mother to rest
  2 A client with previous breast-feeding experience
  3 A physician that encourages clients to breast-feed
  4 A positive nurse-client relationship

3. The nurse palpates the fundus and checks the character of the lochia of a postpartum client in the fourth stage of labor. The nurse expects the lochia to be
  1 White
  2 Pink
  3 Serosanguineous
  4 Red

4. Following episiotomy and delivery of a newborn, the nurse performs a perineal check on the

Table 24–1. Data Collection: The Types of Thrombophlebitis

Superficial	Femoral	Pelvic
Tenderness and pain in the affected lower extremity	Chills and fever	Severe chills
	Malaise	Dramatic body temperature changes
Warm and pinkish red color over thrombus area	Pain, stiffness, and swelling of the affected leg	Occurrence of pulmonary embolism may be the first sign
Palpable thrombus that feels bumpy and hard	Shiny, white skin over the affected area	
Slightly elevated pulse rate	Positive Homans' sign	
	Diminished peripheral pulses	

mother. The nurse notes a trickle of bright red blood coming from the perineum. The nurse checks the fundus and notes that it is firm. The nurse determines that

1 This is a normal expectation following episiotomy
2 The perineal assessment should be performed more frequently
3 The bright red bleeding is abnormal and should be reported
4 The mother should be allowed bathroom privileges only

5. A nurse is assigned to care for a client in the postpartum period. The client asks the nurse what the term involution means. The nurse responds to the client knowing that involution is

1 A progressive descent of the uterus into the pelvic cavity occurring approximately 1 cm per day
2 The gradual reversal of the uterine muscle into the abdominal cavity
3 The descent of the uterus into the pelvic cavity occurring at a rate of 2 cm daily
4 The inverted uterus returning to normal

6. A mother is breast-feeding her newborn. The mother complains to the nurse that she is experiencing nipple soreness. The nurse provides which of the following suggestions to the client?

1 Avoid rotating breast-feeding positions so that the nipple will toughen
2 Stop nursing during the period of nipple soreness to allow the nipples to heal
3 Nurse the newborn infant less frequently and substitute a bottle-feeding until the nipples become less sore
4 Position the newborn infant with the ear, shoulder, and hip in straight alignment and with the baby's stomach against the mother's

7. The mother is breast-feeding her newborn baby and experiences breast engorgement. The nurse encourages the mother to do which of the following measures to provide comfort for the engorgement?

1 Breast-feed only during the daytime hours
2 Apply cold compresses to the breast
3 Massage the breasts before feeding to stimulate let-down
4 Avoid the use of a bra while the breasts are engorged

8. The nurse is assisting in developing a plan of care for a client in the fourth stage of labor. Which of the following problems is most likely to occur during this stage?

1 Pain because of the process of labor or birth
2 Anxiety related to childbirth
3 Fatigue owing to physical exertion during labor

4 Urinary retention caused by the loss of sensation to void and rapid bladder filling

9. Following delivery, the nurse checks the height of the uterine fundus. The nurse expects that the position of the fundus is most likely noted

1 At the level of the umbilicus
2 Above the level of the umbilicus
3 One fingerbreadth above the symphysis pubis
4 To the right of the abdomen

10. The nurse is caring for a postpartum client. Four hours' postpartum, the client's temperature is 101°F. The most appropriate nursing action is

1 Continue to monitor the temperature
2 Notify the registered nurse, who will then contact the physician
3 Apply cool packs to the abdomen
4 Remove the blanket from the client's bed

11. The nurse is assigned to care for a client in the immediate postpartum period who received epidural anesthesia for delivery. The nurse monitors the client for complications. Which of the following best identifies an indicator of a hematoma?

1 Complaints of a tearing sensation
2 Complaints of intense pressure
3 Changes in vital signs
4 Signs of heavy bruising

12. The nurse is assisting in planning care for the postpartum woman who has small vulvar hematomas. To assist in reducing the swelling, the nurse suggests

1 Checking vital signs every 4 hours
2 Preparing a heat pack for application to the area
3 Measuring fundal height every 4 hours
4 Preparing an ice pack for application to the area

13. The client received epidural anesthesia during labor and had a forceps delivery after pushing for 2 hours. At 6 hours' postpartum, the client's systolic blood pressure (BP) drops 20 points, the diastolic BP drops 10 points, and the pulse is 120 bpm. The client is very anxious and restless. The nurse is told that the client has a vulvar hematoma. Based on this diagnosis, the nurse most appropriately plans to

1 Monitor fundal height
2 Apply perineal pressure
3 Prepare the client for surgery
4 Reassure the client

14. After surgical evacuation and repair of a vaginal hematoma, the 3-day postpartum mother is discharged. The nurse knows that the new mother needs further discharge instructions when the new mother states:

1 "Because I am so sore, I will nurse the baby while lying on my side."

2 "I will probably need my mother to help me with housekeeping."

3 "My husband and I will not have intercourse until the stitches are healed."

4 "The only medications I will take are prenatal vitamins and stool softeners."

15. A 45-year-old woman delivered her first baby by cesarean section 5 days ago. The postpartum recovery has been complicated by thrombophlebitis in her left leg. She cries frequently and requests to have her newborn infant stay in the nursery. The nurse recognizes that the mother may have intensified postpartum blues because she is
    1 An older first-time mother
    2 Considering giving the baby up for adoption
    3 Required to stay on bed rest
    4 Unable to nurse the baby

16. The nurse is assigned to care for a client following cesarean section. To prevent thrombophlebitis, the nurse encourages the woman to
    1 Ambulate frequently
    2 Apply warm moist packs to the legs
    3 Remain on bed rest with legs elevated
    4 Wear support stockings

17. A postpartum client has developed thrombophlebitis. The nurse knows that the affected extremity should be elevated by
    1 Elevating the affected extremity on a pillow
    2 Elevating the foot of the bed
    3 Placing the bed in reverse Trendelenburg position
    4 Placing the bed in the Trendelenburg position

18. The nurse is caring for a postpartum client who is being treated for thrombophlebitis. The client is receiving an anticoagulant by intravenous infusion. The nurse understands that the client is experiencing an adverse response to treatment if she exhibits
    1 Dysuria
    2 Epistaxis, hematuria, and dysuria
    3 Hematuria, ecchymosis, and epistaxis
    4 Hematuria, ecchymosis, and vertigo

19. The nurse is caring for a postpartum client with a diagnosis of thrombophlebitis. The client suddenly complains of chest pain and dyspnea. The nurse initially checks
    1 Level of consciousness (LOC)
    2 Fundal height
    3 Presence of Homans' sign
    4 Vital signs

20. The goal for the postpartum client with thromboembolic disease is to prevent the complication of pulmonary embolism. In planning care to assist in meeting this goal, the nurse should
    1 Administer anticoagulants as prescribed

2 Check respirations every hour
3 Check heart rate every hour
4 Check blood pressure every hour

21. The nurse suspects the client has a pulmonary embolism. The most important nursing action is to
    1 Administer oxygen by face mask as prescribed
    2 Elevate the head of the bed
    3 Increase the IV rate
    4 Monitor vital signs

22. The postpartum client with pulmonary embolism has been separated from her newborn infant for 2 days. Which observation by the nurse indicates a potential client need?
    1 The client is nursing her newborn infant
    2 The client is breast-feeding her newborn infant
    3 The newborn infant prefers the bottle over breast milk
    4 The newborn infant is receiving adequate nutrition from breast-feeding

23. The nurse notes that the 4-hour postpartum client has cool, clammy skin, and is restless and excessively thirsty. The nurse immediately notifies the primary health care provider and then
    1 Encourages ambulation
    2 Checks vital signs
    3 Begins fundal massage
    4 Encourages the client to drink fluids

24. The nurse is assisting in caring for a postpartum client experiencing uterine hemorrhage. In planning to meet the psychosocial needs of the client, the nurse
    1 Keeps the client and her family members informed of progress
    2 Monitors vital signs every 2 hours
    3 Maintains strict bed rest
    4 Performs firm fundal massage every 2 hours

25. The nurse is assigned to assist in preparing a woman who is gravida 6 for delivery. In planning care for this client, the nurse places which of the following at the client's bedside?
    1 Code cart
    2 Suction machine
    3 IV supplies
    4 Nasogastric tube

26. The postpartum client has lost 700 mL of blood. The vital signs indicate hypovolemia and the uterus remains atonic in spite of treatment. The nurse assisting in caring for the client understands the treatment that is necessary in this situation and prepares the client for
    1 A blood transfusion
    2 An infusion of oxytocin (Pitocin)
    3 Emergency surgery
    4 Fundal massage

27. The new mother attempting breast-feeding for the first time has developed mastitis. She states, "My breasts look terrible and I think that I will stop breast-feeding." The nurse plans care knowing that the client's problem relates to
    1 Body image
    2 Newborn nutrition
    3 Inadequacy
    4 Infection

28. Breast-feeding instructions for the postpartum mother should include avoidance of soaps on the nipples, frequent changing of breast pads, intermittent exposure of nipples to air, and hand-washing before handling the breast and before breast-feeding. The nurse understands that these measures are specific to the prevention of
    1 Engorgement
    2 Newborn colic
    3 Let-down reflex
    4 Mastitis

29. The nurse is caring for the woman who is being treated with antibiotics for mastitis. The nurse reinforces instructions and tells the woman to
    1 Stop breast-feeding
    2 Complete the entire antibiotic regimen
    3 Avoid wearing a bra
    4 Avoid taking analgesics

30. The new breast-feeding mother is being discharged from the hospital after being treated for mastitis. The nurse knows that the mother needs further teaching when the mother states
    1 "I need to change my breast pads when they are wet."
    2 "I will wash my breasts gently with plain water."
    3 "My left breast is sore, so I will offer the right breast frequently for breast-feeding."
    4 "When my breasts feel engorged, I will use an ice pack for the pain."

ANSWERS

1. 3

RATIONALE: Prematurity usually causes a delay before the baby can be fed at the breast. Mothers must initiate and maintain their milk supply with an electric breast pump. Milk expression by electric pump needs to begin as soon as possible after delivery and continue eight or more times each 24 hours. Hand expression is not as effective as using an electric pump.
TEST-TAKING STRATEGY: Use the process of elimination and knowledge related to the principles associated with breast-feeding to answer the question. Review these principles now if you had difficulty with this question.
LEVEL OF COGNITIVE ABILITY: Application
PHASE OF NURSING PROCESS: Implementation
CLIENT NEEDS: Psychosocial Integrity
CONTENT AREA: Maternity
REFERENCE
Nichols, F., & Zwelling, E. (1997). *Maternal newborn nursing: Theory and practice.* Philadelphia: W. B. Saunders. pp. 1238–1239.

2. 4

RATIONALE: The nurse-client relationship is most significant. Option 1 is exactly opposite of what needs to happen. Brief separation decreases the chance of correct latch and suck in the immediate postpartum period. Infants should be placed at the breast immediately after delivery. Previous breast-feeding experience and a physician that encourages clients to breast-feed are not the most significant factors.
TEST-TAKING STRATEGY: Use the process of elimination. Recalling the importance and significance of a positive nurse-client relationship will easily direct you to option 4. Review the importance of a nurse-client relationship now if you had difficulty with this question.

LEVEL OF COGNITIVE ABILITY: Comprehension
PHASE OF NURSING PROCESS: Planning
CLIENT NEEDS: Psychosocial Integrity
CONTENT AREA: Maternity
REFERENCE
Nichols, F., & Zwelling, E. (1997). *Maternal newborn nursing: Theory and practice.* Philadelphia: W. B. Saunders. pp. 1238–1239.

3. 4

RATIONALE: The color of the lochia during the fourth stage of labor is bright red. This may last from 1 to 3 days. The lochia then changes to a pinkish brown and lasts 4 to 10 days. Finally, the lochia changes to a creamy white that lasts approximately 2 weeks.
TEST-TAKING STRATEGY: Knowledge regarding the color, amount, and consistency of lochia following delivery is required to answer the question. Focus on the key words "fourth stage of labor." Review postpartum expected findings now if you had difficulty with this question.
LEVEL OF COGNITIVE ABILITY: Comprehension
PHASE OF NURSING PROCESS: Data Collection
CLIENT NEEDS: Physiological Integrity
CONTENT AREA: Maternity
REFERENCE
Burroughs, A. (1997). *Maternity nursing: An introductory text* (7th ed.). Philadelphia: W. B. Saunders. p. 317.

4. 3

RATIONALE: Lochial flow should be distinguished from bleeding originating from a laceration or episiotomy, which is usually brighter red than lochia and presents as a continuous trickle of bleeding even though the fundus of the uterus is firm. This bright red bleeding is abnormal and needs to be reported.
TEST-TAKING STRATEGY: Knowledge regarding lochial flow and complications associated with episiotomy are required to answer the question. Note the key words "bright red." This should be an indication that the flow is not

normal. Review lochial flow and complications associated with episiotomy now if you had difficulty with this question.
LEVEL OF COGNITIVE ABILITY: Comprehension
PHASE OF NURSING PROCESS: Evaluation
CLIENT NEEDS: Physiological Integrity
CONTENT AREA: Maternity
REFERENCE
Nichols, F., & Zwelling, E. (1997). *Maternal newborn nursing: Theory and practice*. Philadelphia: W. B. Saunders. p. 768.

5. **1**

RATIONALE: Involution is a progressive descent of the uterus into the pelvic cavity. After birth, descent occurs approximately 1 fingerbreadth, or approximately 1 cm per day.
TEST-TAKING STRATEGY: Knowledge regarding the definition and process of involution is required to answer this question. Use medical terminology to assist you in defining the word "involution." This will assist in directing you to the correct option. If you had difficulty with this question, take time now to review the process of involution.
LEVEL OF COGNITIVE ABILITY: Comprehension
PHASE OF NURSING PROCESS: Implementation
CLIENT NEEDS: Physiological Integrity
CONTENT AREA: Maternity
REFERENCE
Leifer, G. (1999). *Thompson's introduction to maternity and pediatric nursing* (3rd ed.). Philadelphia: W. B. Saunders. p. 221.

6. **4**

RATIONALE: Comfort measures for nipple soreness include positioning the newborn with the ear, shoulder, and hip in straight alignment and with the baby's stomach against the mother's. Options 1, 2, and 3 do not identify measures that will alleviate the nipple soreness.
TEST-TAKING STRATEGY: Use the process of elimination to answer the question. Knowledge regarding the self-care measures to promote comfort to the mother with nipple soreness is required to answer the question. If you had difficulty answering the question, take time now to review these measures.
LEVEL OF COGNITIVE ABILITY: Application
PHASE OF NURSING PROCESS: Implementation
CLIENT NEEDS: Health Promotion and Maintenance
CONTENT AREA: Maternity
REFERENCE
Luckmann, J. (1997). *Saunders manual of nursing care*. Philadelphia: W. B. Saunders. p. 463.

7. **3**

RATIONALE: Comfort measures for breast engorgement include massaging the breasts before feeding to stimulate let-down; wearing a supportive well-fitting bra at all times; taking a warm shower or applying warm compresses just before feeding; alternating breasts during feeding.
TEST-TAKING STRATEGY: Use the process of elimination to answer the question. Eliminate option 1 because of the absolute word "only." Knowledge regarding the self-care measures to promote comfort to the mother with breast engorgement will assist in directing you to option 3. If you had difficulty answering the question, take time now to review these measures.
LEVEL OF COGNITIVE ABILITY: Application

PHASE OF NURSING PROCESS: Implementation
CLIENT NEEDS: Health Promotion and Maintenance
CONTENT AREA: Maternity
REFERENCE
Luckmann, J. (1997). *Saunders manual of nursing care*. Philadelphia: W. B. Saunders. p. 463.

8. **4**

RATIONALE: The fourth stage of labor is composed of the first hour postpartum when the woman's body begins to readjust and relax. Options 1 and 2 relate to the first stage of labor. Option 3 relates to the second stage of labor. Option 4 is related to the third and fourth stages of labor.
TEST-TAKING STRATEGY: Focus on the key words "fourth stage of labor." Remembering that the fourth stage of labor is the last stage will direct you toward the correct option. Review the stages of labor now if you had difficulty with this question.
LEVEL OF COGNITIVE ABILITY: Analysis
PHASE OF NURSING PROCESS: Planning
CLIENT NEEDS: Physiological Integrity
CONTENT AREA: Maternity
REFERENCE
Nichols, F., & Zwelling, E. (1997). *Maternal-newborn nursing: Theory and practice*. Philadelphia: W. B. Saunders. p. 769.

9. **1**

RATIONALE: Immediately after delivery, the uterine fundus should be at the level of the umbilicus or 1 to 3 fingerbreadths below it and in the midline of the abdomen. If the fundus is above the umbilicus, this may indicate that there are blood clots in the uterus that need to be expelled by fundal massage.
TEST-TAKING STRATEGY: Knowledge regarding normal postdelivery findings in the mother and normal anatomy is required to answer this question. If you had difficulty with this question, take time now to review postdelivery findings.
LEVEL OF COGNITIVE ABILITY: Comprehension
PHASE OF NURSING PROCESS: Data Collection
CLIENT NEEDS: Physiological Integrity
CONTENT AREA: Maternity
REFERENCE
Nichols, F., & Zwelling, E. (1997). *Maternal-newborn nursing: Theory and practice*. Philadelphia: W. B. Saunders. p. 768.

10. **2**

RATIONALE: Vital signs return to normal within the first hour postpartum if no complications arise. If the temperature is greater than 2° F above normal, this may indicate infection and the physician will need to be notified.
TEST-TAKING STRATEGY: Knowledge regarding the expected vital signs following delivery is required to answer this question. Focus on the key words "four hours" and "101° F." Review the expected findings in the postpartum period now if you had difficulty with this question.
LEVEL OF COGNITIVE ABILITY: Application
PHASE OF NURSING PROCESS: Implementation
CLIENT NEEDS: Physiological Integrity
CONTENT AREA: Maternity
REFERENCE
Nichols, F., & Zwelling, E. (1997). *Maternal-newborn nursing: Theory and practice*. Philadelphia: W. B. Saunders. p. 767.

11. **3**

RATIONALE: Changes in vital signs indicate hypovolemia in the anesthetized postpartum woman with vulvar hematoma. Options 1 and 2 are inaccurate for a client who is anesthetized. Heavy bruising may be noted but VS changes are most likely to indicate the presence of a hematoma.
TEST-TAKING STRATEGY: Use the process of elimination. Eliminate options 1 and 2 first. Because the woman is anesthetized, she cannot feel pain or pressure. Option 4 (heavy bruising) may be visualized, but vital sign changes indicate hematoma caused by blood collection in the perineal tissues. Review the signs of a hematoma now if you had difficulty with this question.
LEVEL OF COGNITIVE ABILITY: Comprehension
PHASE OF NURSING PROCESS: Data Collection
CLIENT NEEDS: Physiological Integrity
CONTENT AREA: Maternity
REFERENCE
Nichols, F., & Zwelling, E. (1997). *Maternal-newborn nursing: Theory and practice*. Philadelphia: W. B. Saunders. p. 1287.

12. **4**

RATIONALE: Application of ice will reduce swelling caused by hematoma formation in the vulvar area. Options 1, 2, and 3 will not reduce the swelling.
TEST-TAKING STRATEGY: Focus on the issue of the question "reducing the swelling." This will assist in eliminating options 1 and 3. Recalling the principles related to heat and cold will easily direct you to option 4. Review nursing care to the client with a hematoma now if you had difficulty with this question.
LEVEL OF COGNITIVE ABILITY: Application
PHASE OF NURSING PROCESS: Planning
CLIENT NEEDS: Physiological Integrity
CONTENT AREA: Maternity
REFERENCE
Leifer, G. (1999). *Thompson's introduction to maternity and pediatric nursing* (3rd ed.). Philadelphia: W. B. Saunders. p. 263.

13. **3**

RATIONALE: The data provided in the question indicate that the client is experiencing blood loss. Surgery is indicated for this complication to stop the bleeding. Options 1, 2, and 4 do not assist in controlling the bleeding in this emergency situation.
TEST-TAKING STRATEGY: Focus on the data provided in the question. Noting the signs and symptoms in the question will indicate the presence of bleeding. This should easily direct you to option 3. Review nursing content related to vulvar hematomas now if you had difficulty with this question.
LEVEL OF COGNITIVE ABILITY: Analysis
PHASE OF NURSING PROCESS: Planning
CLIENT NEEDS: Physiological Integrity
CONTENT AREA: Maternity
REFERENCE
Leifer, G. (1999). *Thompson's introduction to maternity and pediatric nursing* (3rd ed.). Philadelphia: W. B. Saunders. p. 263.

14. **4**

RATIONALE: The postoperative client will need an antibiotic because she is at increased risk for infection due to the break in skin integrity and collection of blood at the hematoma site. The client statements in options 1, 2, and 3 indicate that the client understands the necessary home care measures.
TEST-TAKING STRATEGY: Focus on the key words "needs further discharge instructions." Knowledge of the need for an antibiotic following this surgical procedure is required to answer this question. Review treatment plans associated with hematoma now if you had difficulty with this question.
LEVEL OF COGNITIVE ABILITY: Analysis
PHASE OF NURSING PROCESS: Evaluation
CLIENT NEEDS: Health Promotion and Maintenance
CONTENT AREA: Maternity
REFERENCE
Nichols, F., & Zwelling, E. (1997). *Maternal-newborn nursing: Theory and practice*. Philadelphia: W. B. Saunders. p. 1288.

15. **3**

RATIONALE: Clients with thrombophlebitis are placed on bed rest with elevation of the affected extremity. Bedrest restricts normal newborn care, feeding, and parenting and will require interventions which promote attachment. Options 1, 2, and 4 are unrelated to the issue of the question.
TEST-TAKING STRATEGY: Note the diagnosis of the client and focus on the issue of the question. Recalling that the client with thrombophlebitis will require bed rest will easily direct you to option 3. Review interventions related to thrombophlebitis now if you had difficulty answering this question.
LEVEL OF COGNITIVE ABILITY: Comprehension
PHASE OF NURSING PROCESS: Data Collection
CLIENT NEEDS: Psychosocial Integrity
CONTENT AREA: Maternity
REFERENCE
Nichols, F., & Zwelling, E. (1997). *Maternal-newborn nursing: Theory and practice*. Philadelphia: W. B. Saunders. p. 1293.

16. **1**

RATIONALE: Stasis is believed to be a major predisposing factor in the development of thrombophlebitis. Because cesarean delivery poses a risk factor, the client should ambulate early and frequently to promote circulation and prevent stasis. Options 2, 3, and 4 are implemented if thrombophlebitis occurs.
TEST-TAKING STRATEGY: Focus on the issue of the question, prevention of thrombophlebitis. Use the process of elimination. Options 2, 3, and 4 are implemented if thrombophlebitis occurs. Ambulating frequently (option 1) is a preventative measure. Review content related to the prevention of thrombophlebitis in the postoperative period now if you had difficulty with this question.
LEVEL OF COGNITIVE ABILITY: Application
PHASE OF NURSING PROCESS: Implementation
CLIENT NEEDS: Health Promotion and Maintenance
CONTENT AREA: Maternity
REFERENCE
Nichols, F., & Zwelling, E. (1997). *Maternal-newborn nursing: Theory and practice*. Philadelphia: W. B. Saunders. p. 1291.

17. **4**

RATIONALE: Placing the bed in the Trendelenburg position rather than flexing the leg at the hip promotes venous drainage. The reverse Trendelenburg position will not aid in promoting venous return. Elevating the extremity by

using a pillow, or elevating the foot of the bed will cause flexion at the hip, thus impeding venous drainage.
TEST-TAKING STRATEGY: Focus on the issue of the question and use the process of elimination. Recalling that flexion at the hip area restricts venous flow will easily direct you to option 4. Review these concepts now if you had difficulty answering this question.
LEVEL OF COGNITIVE ABILITY: Comprehension
PHASE OF NURSING PROCESS: Implementation
CLIENT NEEDS: Physiological Integrity
CONTENT AREA: Maternity
REFERENCE
Leifer, G. (1999). *Thompson's introduction to maternity and pediatric nursing* (3rd ed.). Philadelphia: W. B. Saunders. p. 265.

18. **3**

RATIONALE: The treatment for thrombophlebitis is anti-coagulant therapy. Adverse effects of anticoagulants include bleeding and are recognized by the presence of hematuria, ecchymosis, and epistaxis.
TEST-TAKING STRATEGY: Remember that when an option contains more than one part, all parts need to be correct for the option to be correct. Recall that bleeding is the major concern with the use of anticoagulants. Note that option 3 is the only option that addresses bleeding in all of its components. Review the treatment for thrombophlebitis now if you had difficulty with this question.
LEVEL OF COGNITIVE ABILITY: Comprehension
PHASE OF NURSING PROCESS: Data Collection
CLIENT NEEDS: Physiological Integrity
CONTENT AREA: Maternity
REFERENCE
Leifer, G. (1999). *Thompson's introduction to maternity and pediatric nursing* (3rd ed.). Philadelphia: W. B. Saunders. p. 264.

19. **4**

RATIONALE: Pulmonary embolism is a complication of thrombophlebitis. Vital signs will be one of the first changes to occur with pulmonary embolism as pulmonary blood flow is compromised. LOC may change as the condition worsens and would indicate hypoxia. Homans' sign is an indicator of thrombophlebitis. Fundal height is unrelated to the issue of the question.
TEST-TAKING STRATEGY: Note the key word "initially." Use the ABCs, airway, breathing, and circulation, to assist in directing you to option 4. Review the complications of thrombophlebitis now if you had difficulty with this question.
LEVEL OF COGNITIVE ABILITY: Application
PHASE OF NURSING PROCESS: Data Collection
CLIENT NEEDS: Physiological Integrity
CONTENT AREA: Maternity
REFERENCE
Leifer, G. (1999). *Thompson's introduction to maternity and pediatric nursing* (3rd ed.). Philadelphia: W. B. Saunders. p. 264.

20. **1**

RATIONALE: The purpose of anticoagulant therapy is to prevent the clot from moving to another area. Options 2, 3, and 4 will not prevent pulmonary embolism.
TEST-TAKING STRATEGY: Focus on the issue, "prevent pulmonary embolism," and use the process of elimination. Review treatment for thromboembolic disease now if you had difficulty with this question.

LEVEL OF COGNITIVE ABILITY: Application
PHASE OF NURSING PROCESS: Planning
CLIENT NEEDS: Physiological Integrity
CONTENT AREA: Maternity
REFERENCE
Leifer, G. (1999). *Thompson's introduction to maternity and pediatric nursing* (3rd ed.). Philadelphia: W. B. Saunders. p. 264.

21. **1**

RATIONALE: Because pulmonary circulation is compromised in the presence of an embolus, cardiorespiratory support is initiated by oxygen administration. Options 2 and 4 may be a component of the plan of care but are not the most important action. The nurse does not increase the IV rate.
TEST-TAKING STRATEGY: Note the key words "most important" and use the ABCs, airway, breathing, and circulation. This will easily direct you to option 1. Review care to the client in the event of a pulmonary embolism now if you had difficulty with this question.
LEVEL OF COGNITIVE ABILITY: Application
PHASE OF NURSING PROCESS: Implementation
CLIENT NEEDS: Physiological Integrity
CONTENT AREA: Maternity
REFERENCE
Gorrie, T., McKinney, E., & Murray, S. (1998). *Foundations of maternal-newborn nursing* (2nd ed.). Philadelphia: W. B. Saunders. p. 796.

22. **3**

RATIONALE: Breast-feeding will be compromised and the newborn infant may begin to prefer the bottle over the breast if the mother and newborn are separated for an extended period. When the mother's condition is stable after being separated, reestablishing breast-feeding should be a nursing priority. Options 1, 2, and 4 do not indicate the need for intervention.
TEST-TAKING STRATEGY: Use the process of elimination focusing on the key words "separated from her newborn infant for 2 days." This should easily direct you to option 3. Review the concepts related to maternal-infant bonding now if you had difficulty with this question.
LEVEL OF COGNITIVE ABILITY: Comprehension
PHASE OF NURSING PROCESS: Data Collection
CLIENT NEEDS: Psychosocial Integrity
CONTENT AREA: Maternity
REFERENCE
Nichols, F., & Zwelling, E. (1997). *Maternal-newborn nursing: Theory and practice.* Philadelphia: W. B. Saunders. p. 1295.

23. **2**

RATIONALE: Symptoms of hypovolemia include cool, clammy, pale skin, sensations of anxiety, restlessness, and thirst. The nurse should check the vital signs. The nurse should not ambulate the client or encourage fluids until specific orders are given to do so. There are no data in the question indicating the need for fundal massage.
TEST-TAKING STRATEGY: Focus on the symptoms in the question. Use the ABCs, airway, breathing, and circulation, to assist in directing you to option 2. Review nursing care for the client with hypovolemia now if you had difficulty with this question.
LEVEL OF COGNITIVE ABILITY: Application
PHASE OF NURSING PROCESS: Implementation

CLIENT NEEDS: Physiological Integrity
CONTENT AREA: Maternity
REFERENCE

Gorrie, T., McKinney, E., & Murray, S. (1998). *Foundations of maternal-newborn nursing* (2nd ed.). Philadelphia: W. B. Saunders. p. 790.

24. **1**

RATIONALE: Keeping the client and her family informed of her condition will help minimize fear and apprehension. Options 2, 3, and 4 identify physiological interventions.
TEST-TAKING STRATEGY: Focus on the key words "meet the psychosocial needs." Option 1 is the only option that addresses psychosocial needs.
LEVEL OF COGNITIVE ABILITY: Application
PHASE OF NURSING PROCESS: Planning
CLIENT NEEDS: Psychosocial Integrity
CONTENT AREA: Maternity
REFERENCE

Gorrie, T., McKinney, E., & Murray, S. (1998). *Foundations of maternal-newborn nursing* (2nd ed.). Philadelphia: W. B. Saunders. p. 791.

25. **3**

RATIONALE: The client who is a gravida 6 is at risk for possible uterine atony. An IV access is needed so that blood and medication can be administered if necessary. Options 1, 2, and 4 are unnecessary items.
TEST-TAKING STRATEGY: Use the process of elimination, focusing on the client described in the question. Knowledge that uterine atony is a risk associated with this client will assist in directing you to option 3. Review care to the client at risk for uterine atony now if you had difficulty with this question.
LEVEL OF COGNITIVE ABILITY: Application
PHASE OF NURSING PROCESS: Planning
CLIENT NEEDS: Physiological Integrity
CONTENT AREA: Maternity
REFERENCE

Nichols, F., & Zwelling, E. (1997). *Maternal-newborn nursing: Theory and practice.* Philadelphia: W. B. Saunders. p. 1287.

26. **3**

RATIONALE: When uterine atony cannot be reversed, surgery is required. Options 1, 2, and 4 are treatments for uterine atony.
TEST-TAKING STRATEGY: Focus on the data provided in the question and note the key words "in spite of treatment." If you had difficulty with this question, take time now to review the treatment for uterine atony.
LEVEL OF COGNITIVE ABILITY: Comprehension
PHASE OF NURSING PROCESS: Planning
CLIENT NEEDS: Physiological Integrity
CONTENT AREA: Maternity
REFERENCE

Nichols, F., & Zwelling, E. (1997). *Maternal-newborn nursing: Theory and practice.* Philadelphia: W. B. Saunders. p. 1287.

27. **1**

RATIONALE: Inflammation and engorgement are major symptoms of mastitis that may alter the new breast-feeding mother's body image. There is no information in the question that indicates a problem with newborn nutrition, inadequacy, or infection.
TEST-TAKING STRATEGY: Focus on the information in

the question and use the process of elimination. Noting the key words "My breasts look terrible" will easily direct you to option 1.
LEVEL OF COGNITIVE ABILITY: Comprehension
PHASE OF NURSING PROCESS: Planning
CLIENT NEEDS: Psychosocial Integrity
CONTENT AREA: Maternity
REFERENCE

Nichols, F., & Zwelling, E. (1997). *Maternal-newborn nursing: Theory and practice.* Philadelphia: W. B. Saunders. p. 1302.

28. **4**

RATIONALE: Mastitis is an infection frequently associated with a break in the skin surface of the nipple. The measures described are personal hygiene measures to help prevent mastitis.
TEST-TAKING STRATEGY: Use the process of elimination. Knowledge of the cause and prevention of mastitis is required to answer this question. If you had difficulty with this question, review content related to mastitis now.
LEVEL OF COGNITIVE ABILITY: Application
PHASE OF NURSING PROCESS: Planning
CLIENT NEEDS: Health Promotion and Maintenance
CONTENT AREA: Maternity
REFERENCE

Gorrie, T., McKinney, E., & Murray, S. (1998). *Foundations of maternal-newborn nursing* (2nd ed.). Philadelphia: W. B. Saunders. p. 801.

29. **2**

RATIONALE: If antibiotics are prescribed, it is essential that the client complete the regime even though symptoms will be reduced in 24 to 48 hours. Options 1, 3, and 4 are inappropriate treatment measures for mastitis.
TEST-TAKING STRATEGY: Focus on the information in the question. Note the key word "antibiotics." Option 2 is the only option that relates to the information in the question. Additionally, options 1, 3, and 4 are inappropriate treatment measures for mastitis. Review treatment measures for mastitis now if you had difficulty with this question.
LEVEL OF COGNITIVE ABILITY: Application
PHASE OF NURSING PROCESS: Implementation
CLIENT NEEDS: Health Promotion and Maintenance
CONTENT AREA: Maternity
REFERENCE

Nichols, F., & Zwelling, E. (1997). *Maternal-newborn nursing: Theory and practice.* Philadelphia: W. B. Saunders. p. 1301.

30. **3**

RATIONALE: Failure to nurse equally on both sides will decrease the flow of milk through the breasts, causing engorgement of the breast offered less frequently. Options 1, 2, and 4 are appropriate measures.
TEST-TAKING STRATEGY: Note the key words "needs further teaching." Use knowledge regarding the treatment for mastitis and the process of elimination to select the correct option. If you had difficulty with this question, review the concepts related to mastitis and breast-feeding now.
LEVEL OF COGNITIVE ABILITY: Comprehension
PHASE OF NURSING PROCESS: Evaluation
CLIENT NEEDS: Health Promotion and Maintenance
CONTENT AREA: Maternity
REFERENCE

Gorrie, T., McKinney, E., & Murray, S. (1998). *Foundations of maternal-newborn nursing* (2nd ed.). Philadelphia: W. B. Saunders. p. 801.

BIBLIOGRAPHY

Burroughs, A. (1997). *Maternity nursing: An introductory text* (7th ed.). Philadelphia: W. B. Saunders.

Gorrie, T., McKinney, E., & Murray, S. (1998). *Foundations of maternal-newborn nursing* (2nd ed.). Philadelphia: W. B. Saunders.

Leifer, G. (1999). *Thompson's introduction to maternity and pediatric nursing* (3rd ed.). Philadelphia: W. B. Saunders.

Luckmann, J. (1997). *Saunders manual of nursing care*. Philadelphia: W. B. Saunders.

Nichols, F., & Zwelling, E. (1997). *Maternal-newborn nursing: Theory and practice*. Philadelphia: W. B. Saunders.

O'Toole, M. (ed.). (1997). *Miller-Keane encyclopedia & dictionary of medicine, nursing, & allied health* (6th ed.). Philadelphia: W. B. Saunders.

CHAPTER 25

Care of the Newborn

....

◆ I. Initial Care of the Newborn

A. Data collection
1. Observe or assist with initiation of respirations
2. Assess Apgar score
3. Note characteristics of cry
4. Obtain vital signs
5. Monitor for nasal flaring, grunting, retractions, and abnormal respirations
6. Observe the **newborn** for signs of hypothermia or hyperthermia
7. Monitor for gross anomalies

B. Implementation
1. Suction the mouth then nares with a bulb syringe
2. Dry the **newborn** and stimulate crying by rubbing
3. Maintain temperature stability
4. Wrap the **newborn** in warm blankets
5. Place a stockinette cap on the **newborn's** head
6. Keep the **newborn** with the mother to facilitate bonding
7. Place the **newborn** at mother's breast if breast-feeding is planned or place on the mother's abdomen
8. Place the **newborn** in a warmer
9. Position the **newborn** on the side or abdomen or modified Trendelenburg position to facilitate drainage of mucus
10. Ensure the **newborn's** proper identification
11. Footprint the **newborn** and fingerprint the mother on the identification sheet
12. Place matching identification bracelets on the mother and **newborn**

C. Apgar scoring system
1. Perform and record Apgar score at 1 minute and 5 minutes
2. If the score is less than 7 at 5 minutes, the Apgar score should be performed at 10 minutes
3. Assess each of the five items to be scored and assign a value of 0 (very poor) to 2 (excellent) for each item
4. Add the points to determine the **newborn's** total score
   a. A score of 7 to 10 indicates a healthy **newborn**
   b. A score of 3 to 6 is considered moderately depressed
   c. A score of 0 to 2 is severely depressed
5. Five vital indicators (Table 25–1)
   a. Heart rate
   b. Respiratory rate
   c. Muscle tone
   d. Reflex irritability
   e. Skin color
6. Implementation (Table 25–2)

◆ II. Initial Physical Examination

A. General guidelines
1. Keep the **newborn** warm during the examination
2. Begin with general observations and proceed to detailed findings

Table 25–1. **Apgar Scoring**

Indicator	0 Points	1 Point	2 Points
Heart rate	Absent	Less than 100	More than 100
Respiratory rate	Absent	Slow, irregular weak cry	Good, vigorous cry
Muscle tone	Flaccid, limp	Some flexion of extremities	Good flexion, active motion
Reflex irritability	No response	Weak cry and grimace	Vigorous cry, cough, sneeze
Skin color	Blue	Body skin normal, extremities blue	Body and extremity skin color normal

Table 25–2. **Apgar Score Implementation**

Score	Implementation
7 to 10	Rarely need resuscitation
3 to 6	Require resuscitation
	Suction
	Dry quickly
	Maintain warmth
	Ventilate 30 to 50 times a minute until heart rate is above 100, color is pink, and spontaneous respirations begin.
	Provide oxygen
	Careful observation during the first few days of life
0 to 2	Require intensive resuscitation
	Clear airway
	Insert endotracheal tube
	Use Ambu bag if necessary
	Ventilate with 100% oxygen at 40 to 60 breaths/minute
	Initiate full CPR as needed at 1:5 (breaths to chest compressions) ratio
	Maintain body temperature
	Support parents

3. Perform assessments that are least disturbing to the **newborn** first
4. Initiate nursing interventions for abnormal findings
5. Document all abnormal findings

B. Vital signs
   1. Heart rate: 120 to 160 beats/minute (apical); assess for a full minute due to irregularities after birth
   2. Respirations: 30 to 60 breaths/minute; assess for a full minute
   3. Axillary temperature: 36.4°C to 37°C (97.6°F to 98.6°F)
   4. Blood pressure: 60/40 to 80/50 mm Hg

C. Body measurements
   1. Length: 45 to 55 cm (18 to 22 inches)
   2. Weight: 2500 to 4300 g (5.5 to 9.5 lb)
   3. Head circumference: 33 to 35.5 cm (13 to 14 inches)
   4. Chest circumference: 30 to 33 cm (12 to 13 inches) and should be equal to or 2 to 3 cm less than the head circumference

D. Head
   1. 25% of the body length (cephalocaudal development)
   2. Bones of the skull are not fused
   3. Palpable sutures (connective tissue between the skull bones)

4. Fontanels: unossified membranous tissue at the junction of the sutures (Table 25–3)
   5. Molding
      a. Asymmetry of head due to pressure in birth canal
      b. Disappears in about 72 hours
   6. Masses from birth trauma
      a. Caput succedaneum: edema of the soft tissue over bone (crosses over suture line); subsides within a few days
      b. Cephalohematoma: swelling caused by bleeding into an area between the bone and its periosteum (does not cross over suture line); usually absorbed within 6 weeks with no treatment
   7. Head lag
      a. Common when pulling the **newborn** to a sitting position
      b. When prone, the **newborn** should be able to lift the head slightly and turn from side to side

E. Eyes
   1. Slate gray (light skin) or brown-gray (dark skin)
   2. Symmetrical and clear
   3. Pupils equal, round, react to light by accommodation
   4. Blink reflex present
   5. Eyes cross due to weak extraocular muscles
   6. Able to track and fixate momentarily
   7. Red reflex present
   8. Eyelids often edematous due to pressure during the birth process and the effects of eye medication

F. Ears
   1. Symmetrical
   2. Firm cartilage with recoil
   3. Pinna should be on or above line drawn from the canthus of the eye
   4. Low-set ears associated with Down's syndrome

G. Nose
   1. Flat, broad, and in the center of the face
   2. Obligatory nose breathing
   3. Occasional sneezing to remove obstructions

H. Mouth
   1. Pink moist gums
   2. Soft and hard palate intact
   3. Epstein's pearls (small, white cysts) may be present on hard palate
   4. Uvula in midline

Table 25–3. **Fontaneles**

Fontanele	Characteristics	Closure
Anterior	Soft, flat, diamond-shaped 3 to 4 cm wide by 2 to 3 cm long	Closes between 12 and 18 months
Posterior	Triangular 0.5 to 1 cm wide Located between occipital and parietal bones	Closes between birth and 8 and 12 weeks of age

5. Tongue moves freely, is symmetrical, and has a short frenulum
6. Sucking and crying movements are symmetrical
7. Able to swallow
8. Gag reflex is present

I. Neck
1. Short and thick
2. Head held in midline
3. Trachea on midline
4. Raises head momentarily when prone
5. Good range of motion and is able to flex and extend

J. Chest
1. Appears circular since anteroposterior and lateral diameters are about equal
2. Respirations appear diaphragmatic
3. Bronchial sounds heard on auscultation
4. Nipples prominent and often edematous
5. Milky secretion (witch's milk) common
6. Breast tissue present
7. Clavicles need to be palpated to assess for fractures

K. Skin
1. Pinkish red (light-skinned **newborn**) to pinkish brown or pinkish yellow (dark-skinned **newborn**)
2. Vernix caseosa
3. Lanugo
4. Milia
5. Dry, peeling skin
6. Dark red color common in premature **newborns**
7. Cyanosis common with hypothermia, infection, and hypoglycemia and with cardiac, respiratory, or neurological abnormalities
8. Acrocyanosis is not uncommon and may be due to immature peripheral circulation
9. Assess for ecchymosis and petechiae due to trauma of birth
10. Assess skin turgor over the abdomen to determine hydration status
11. Observe for forceps marks
12. Harlequin sign
   a. Deep red color develops over one side of the **newborn's** body, whereas the other side remains pale due to vasomotor disturbance
   b. Skin resembles a clown's suit
13. Birthmarks (Table 25–4)

L. Abdomen
1. Umbilical cord
   a. Three vessels, two arteries, and one vein in cord; if less than three vessels are noted, notify the physician
   b. Small, thin cord may be associated with poor fetal growth
   c. Assess for intact cord and ensure that the clamp is secured
   d. Cord should be clamped for at least the first 24 hours after birth; clamp can be

removed when the cord is dried and occluded
   e. Note any bleeding or drainage from the cord
   f. Triple dye may be applied for initial cord care because it minimizes microorganisms and promotes drying; use a cotton-tipped applicator to paint the dye, one time, on the cord and on 1 inch of the surrounding skin
   g. Application of 70% isopropyl alcohol to the cord minimizes microorganisms and promotes drying
   h. If symptoms of infection such as moistness, oozing, discharge, and a reddened base occur, antibiotic treatment is prescribed
2. Gastrointestinal
   a. Monitor the cord for meconium staining
   b. Assess for umbilical hernia
   c. Note abdominal depression associated with diaphragmatic hernia
   d. Monitor for abdominal distention associated with obstruction, mass, or sepsis
   e. Monitor bowel sounds, which should occur within 1 to 2 hours after birth
3. Anus
   a. Anal opening patent
   b. First stool meconium should pass within first 24 hours

M. Genitals
1. Female
   a. Labia edematous and clitoris enlarged
   b. Smegma present (thick white mucous discharge)

Table 25–4. Birthmarks

Birthmark	Characteristics
Telangiectatic nevi (stork bites)	Pale pink or red, flat dilated capillaries
	On eyelids, nose, lower occipital bone, and nape of neck
	Blanch easily
	More noticeable during crying periods
	Disappear by age 2
Nevus flammeus (portwine stain)	Capillary angioma directly below epidermis
	Nonelevated sharply demarcated, red to purple dense areas of capillaries
	Commonly appears on face
	Does not fade with time
	May require surgery in the future
Nevus vasculosus (strawberry mark)	Capillary hemangioma
	Raised, clearly delineated, dark red with a rough surface
	Common in head region
	Disappear by age 7 to 9 years
Mongolian spots	Bluish black pigmentation
	On lumbar dorsal area and buttock
	Gradually fade during first and second year of life
	Common in Asian and dark-skinned races

c. Pseudomenstruation possible (blood-tinged mucus)

d. Hymen tag may be visible

e. First voiding should occur within 24 hours

2. Male

a. Prepuce (foreskin) covers glans penis

b. Scrotum edematous

c. Meatus at tip of penis

d. Testes descended but may retract on cold

e. Assess for hernia or hydrocele

f. First voiding should occur within 24 hours

N. Spine

1. Straight

2. Posture flexed

3. Supports head momentarily when prone

4. Arms and legs flexed

5. Chin flexed on upper chest

6. Sporadic movements that are well coordinated

7. Degree of hypotonicity or hypertonicity is indicative of central nervous system (CNS) damage

O. Extremities

1. Flexed

2. Full range of motion (ROM)

3. Movements symmetrical

4. Fists clenched

5. Fingers and toes should be 10 each in number and separate

6. Legs bowed

7. Major gluteal folds even

8. Creases on soles of feet

9. Assess for hip dysplasia

10. When thighs are rotated outward, no clicks should be heard

11. Pulses (radial, brachial, femoral) palpable

12. Assess for fractures (especially clavicle) or dislocations (hip)

13. Slight tremors are common but may be a sign of hypoglycemia or drug withdrawal

III. Body Systems

A. Cardiovascular

1. Keep **newborn** warm

2. Take the apical heart rate for 1 full minute

3. Listen for murmurs

4. Palpate pulses

5. Assess for cyanosis

6. Blanch skin on trunk and extremities to assess circulation

7. Observe cord stump for bleeding

8. Document inability to feed without cardiac distress

B. Respiratory

1. Position **newborn** on the side

2. Suction as necessary

a. Use a bulb syringe for upper airway suctioning (compress bulb before insertion)

b. Use a French catheter for deeper suctioning

3. Observe for respiratory distress and hypoxemia

a. Nasal flaring

b. Increasingly severe retractions

c. Grunting

d. Cyanosis

e. Bradycardia

f. Low body temperature

g. Periods of apnea lasting longer than 15 seconds

4. Administer oxygen per hood if necessary as prescribed

C. Hepatic

1. Normal or physiological jaundice appears after the first 24 hours in full-term babies and after the first 48 hours in premature babies; jaundice occurring prior to this time (pathological jaundice) may indicate early hemolysis of RBCs and must be reported to the physician

2. Physiological jaundice peaks about the fifth day of life

3. Monitor serum bilirubin levels; bilirubin levels should not exceed 12 mg/dL

4. Feed early to stimulate intestinal activity and to keep bilirubin level low

5. For babies with jaundice on breast milk, feed early and every 2 hours to stimulate intestinal activity and keep bilirubin level low

6. Temporarily discontinue breast-feeding for 48 hours if bilirubin levels exceed 15 to 20 mg/dL

7. Prevent chilling because hypothermia can cause acidosis, which interferes with bilirubin conjugation and excretion

8. Liver stores iron passed from the mother for 5 to 6 months

9. Glycogen storage occurs in the liver

10. The **newborn** is at risk for hemorrhagic disorders; coagulation factors synthesized in the liver are dependent on vitamin K, which is not synthesized until intestinal bacteria are present

11. Handle the **newborn** carefully and monitor for any bruising or bleeding episodes

12. Watch for meconium passage and subsequent stools

13. Administer one dose of vitamin K (AquaMEPHYTON) 0.5 to 1.0 mg IM to the **neonate** in the vastus lateralis muscle as prescribed to aid in blood coagulation

14. Assess the **newborn's** hemoglobin and blood glucose levels

D. Renal

1. The immature kidneys are unable to concentrate urine

2. A weight loss of 5% to 15% during the first week of life occurs due to voiding and limited intake

3. Weigh the **newborn** daily

4. Monitor I&O

5. Weigh the diapers if necessary

6. Measure specific gravity if necessary

7. Monitor for signs of dehydration
   a. Dry mucous membranes
   b. Sunken eyeballs
   c. Poor skin turgor
   d. Sunken fontanels
E. Immune
   1. Passive immunity via the **placenta** (IgG)
   2. Passive immunity from colostrum (IgA)
   3. Elevations in IgM indicate infection in utero
   4. Use aseptic technique when caring for the **newborn**
   5. Observe universal precautions when handling the **newborn**
   6. Ensure meticulous handwashing
   7. Wear gowns when caring for the **newborn**
   8. Ensure that an infection-free staff cares for the **newborn**
   9. Monitor the **newborn's** temperature
   10. Observe for any cracks or openings in the skin
   11. Administer eye medication within 1 hour after birth to prevent ophthalmia neonatorum
       a. Erythromycin (0.5%) ophthalmic ointment or drops; also prevents *Chlamydia trachomatis*
       b. Tetracycline (1%) ophthalmic ointment or drops
       c. Silver nitrate (1%) solution; causes chemical conjunctivitis
   12. Provide cord care
       a. Umbilical clamp can be removed after 24 hours
       b. Keep the cord clean and dry by wiping with alcohol
       c. Keep the diaper from covering the cord; fold the diaper below the cord
       d. Assess for odor, swelling, or discharge from the cord
       e. Teach the mother how to perform cord care
   13. Provide circumcision care
       a. Apply petroleum jelly gauze to the penis except when a Plastibell is used
       b. Remove petroleum jelly gauze if applied, after first voiding following circumcision
       c. Observe for swelling, infection, or bleeding from the circumcision site
       d. Monitor for urinary retention
       e. Teach the mother care of circumcision site
F. Metabolic and gastrointestinal
   1. **Newborns** are able to digest simple carbohydrates but unable to digest fats due to the lack of lipase
   2. Proteins may be only partially broken down, so may serve as antigens and provoke an allergic reaction
   3. The **newborn** has a small stomach capacity (about 90 mL) with rapid intestinal peristalsis (bowel emptying time is 2.5 to 3 hours)

4. Most breast-fed babies are put to breast soon after birth
5. Feedings are initiated when readiness is determined and vital signs are stable
6. Start with a feeding of 10 to 15 mL sterile water to assess patency of swallowing and integrity of the GI tract; once a small amount is fed to the **newborn,** the remainder of the feeding is finished with either formula or breast milk
7. Observe feeding reflexes such as rooting, sucking, and swallowing
8. Assist the mother with breast-feeding or formula feeding
9. Burp the **newborn** during and after feeding
10. Assess for regurgitation or vomiting
11. Position the **newborn** on the right side after feeding
12. Observe for the passage of meconium
13. Observe for normal stool
    a. Soft, yellow stools for breast-fed **newborns**
    b. Seedy, yellow stools for formula-fed **newborns**
14. Perform a **newborn** phenylketonuria (PKU) screening test before discharge or as an outpatient after sufficient protein intake occurs; the **newborn** should be on formula or breast milk for 24 hours before screening, and screening must be repeated in 7 to 14 days
G. Neurological
   1. **Newborn** head size is proportionally larger than adults due to cephalocaudal development
   2. Myelinization of nerve fibers is incomplete, so primitive reflexes are present
   3. Fontanels open to allow for brain growth
   4. Assess for an abnormal size and bulging or depressed anterior fontanel
   5. Measure and graph head circumference in relation to chest circumference and length
   6. Assess the **newborn's** movements, noting symmetry, posture, and abnormal movements
   7. Observe for jitteriness, marked tremors, and seizures
   8. Test the **newborn's** reflexes
   9. Assess for lethargy
   10. Assess pitch of cry
H. Thermoregulatory
   1. **Newborns** do not shiver to produce heat
   2. **Newborns** have brown fat deposits that produce heat
   3. Heat is dissipated through vasodilation
   4. Prevent heat loss due to evaporation by keeping the **newborn** dry and well wrapped
   5. Prevent heat loss due to radiation by keeping the **newborn** away from cold objects and outside walls
   6. Prevent heat loss due to convection by shielding the **newborn** from drafts

7. Prevent heat loss due to conduction by performing all treatments on a warm, padded surface
8. Keep the temperature in the room warm
9. Take the **newborn's** axillary temperature every hour for the first 4 hours of life, every 4 hours for the remainder of the first 24 hours, and then every shift

I. Reflexes
1. Sucking and rooting
   a. Touch the **newborn's** lip, cheek, or corner of the mouth with a nipple
   b. The **newborn** turns the head toward the nipple, opens the mouth, takes hold of the nipple, and sucks
   c. Usually disappears after 3 to 4 months but may persist for up to 1 year
2. Swallowing
   a. Occurs spontaneously after sucking and obtaining fluids
   b. The **newborn** swallows in coordination with sucking without gagging, coughing, or vomiting
3. Tonic neck or fencing
   a. While the **newborn** is falling asleep or sleeping, gently and quickly turn the head to one side
   b. As the **newborn** faces the left side, the left arm and leg extend outward while the right arm and leg flex
   c. When turned to the right side, the right arm and leg extend while the left arm and leg flex
   d. Usually disappears within 3 to 4 months
4. Palmar-plantar grasp
   a. Place a finger in the palm of the **newborn's** hand then place a finger at the base of the toes
   b. The **newborn's** fingers curl around the examiner's fingers and the **newborn's** toes curl downward
   c. Palmar response lessens within 3 to 4 months
   d. Plantar response lessens within 8 months
5. Moro reflex
   a. Hold the newborn in a semisitting position then allow the head and trunk to fall backward to at least a 30-degree angle, or place the **newborn** on a flat surface and strike the flat surface to startle the **newborn**
   b. The **newborn** symmetrically abducts and extends the arms
   c. The **newborn** fans the fingers out and forms a C with the thumb and the forefinger
   d. The **newborn** adducts the arms to an embracing position and returns to a relaxed flexion state
   e. Present at birth; a complete response may occur up to 8 weeks

f. A body jerk motion occurs from 8 to 18 weeks
g. No response may be noted by 6 months as long as neurological maturation has not been delayed
h. A persistent response lasting more than 6 months may indicate the occurrence of brain damage during pregnancy
6. Startle reflex
   a. The response is best elicited if the **newborn** is a least 24 hours old
   b. Make a loud noise or clap hands to elicit the response
   c. The **newborn's** arms adduct while the elbows flex
   d. The hands stay clenched
   e. The reflex should disappear within 4 months
7. Pull-to-sit
   a. Pull the **newborn** up from the wrist while the **newborn** is in the prone position
   b. The head will lag until the **newborn** is in an upright position, then the head will be level with the chest and shoulders momentarily before falling forward
   c. The head will then lift for a few minutes
   d. The response depends on the **newborn's** general muscle tone and condition as well as maturity level
8. Babinski's sign—plantar
   a. Beginning at the heel of the foot, gently stroke upward along the lateral aspect of the sole, then move your finger along the ball of the foot
   b. The **newborn's** toes hyperextend while the big toe dorsiflexes
   c. Reflex disappears after the **newborn** is 1 year old
   d. Absence of this reflex indicates the need for a neurological examination
9. Stepping or walking
   a. Hold the **newborn** in a vertical position allowing one foot to touch a table surface
   b. The **newborn** simulates walking alternately flexing and extending the feet
   c. The reflex is usually present for 3 to 4 months
10. Crawling
    a. Place the **newborn** on the abdomen
    b. The **newborn** begins making crawling movements with the arms and legs
    c. The reflex usually disappears after about 6 weeks

IV. Parent Teaching

A. Formula feeding
1. Teach sterilization techniques if the water supply is located in areas where the purification process of the water is questionable

2. Remind the mother not to heat the bottle of formula in a microwave oven
3. Teach the mother that formula is a sufficient diet for the first 4 to 6 months
4. Assess the mother's ability to burp the **newborn**

B. Breast-feeding
1. Assess the **newborn's** ability to attach to the mother's breast and suck
2. Teach the mother about engorgement
3. Teach the mother how to pump her breasts and properly store breast milk
4. Teach the mother that breast milk is a sufficient diet for the first 4 to 6 months
5. Give the mother the phone number of local organizations that offer support to breast-feeding mothers

C. Bathing
1. Bathe the **newborn** in a warm room before feeding
2. Have all the equipment for bathing available
3. Use a mild soap (not on the face)
4. Proceed from the cleanest area to the dirtiest
5. Clean eyes from the inner canthus outward
6. Special care should be taken to clean under the folds of the neck, underarms, groin, and genitals
7. Make bathtime enjoyable for both the **newborn** and mother

D. Clothing
1. Assess diaper and clothing needs for the **newborn** with the mother
2. Instruct the mother that the **newborn's** head should be covered in cold weather to prevent heat loss
3. Instruct the mother to layer the **newborn's** clothing in cooler weather

E. Cord care
1. Clean the cord with alcohol after each diaper change and at least two to three times daily
2. Keep the diaper folded below the cord
3. Sponge bathe **newborn** until the cord falls off
4. The cord should fall off within 2 weeks

F. Circumcision
1. Remove petroleum jelly gauze if applied after the first voiding following circumcision
2. Cleanse the penis after each voiding by squeezing warm water over it
3. Observe for swelling, infection, drainage, or bleeding from the circumcision site
4. A milky covering over the glans penis is normal and should not be disrupted

V. Preterm Newborn

A. Description
1. A **neonate** born before 37 weeks' gestation
2. The primary concern relates to immaturity of all body systems

B. Data collection
1. Respirations irregular with periods of apnea
2. Body temperature is below normal

3. The **newborn** has poor suck and swallow reflexes
4. Bowel sounds are diminished
5. Increased or decreased urinary output
6. Extremities are thin with minimal creasing on soles and palms
7. The **newborn** extends extremities and does not maintain flexion
8. Lanugo, on skin and on the **newborn's** head, is present in woolly patches
9. Skin is thin with visible blood vessels and minimal subcutaneous fat pads
10. Skin may appear jaundiced
11. Testes are undescended in males
12. The labia are narrow in females

C. Implementation
1. Monitor vital signs every 2 to 4 hours
2. Maintain cardiopulmonary functions
3. Administer oxygen and humidification as prescribed
4. Monitor I&O and electrolyte balance
5. Monitor intake closely
6. Monitor daily weight
7. Maintain the **newborn** in warming device
8. Position every 1 to 2 hours, and handle the **newborn** carefully
9. Avoid exposure to infections
10. Provide the **newborn** with appropriate stimulation such as touch

VI. Post-Term Newborn

A. Description: a **newborn** born after 42 weeks of gestation

B. Data collection
1. Hypoglycemia
2. Parchment-like skin without lanugo
3. Dry and cracked skin
4. Fingernails long and extended over the ends of the fingers
5. Profuse scalp hair
6. Body is long and thin
7. Extremities show wasting of fat and muscle
8. Meconium staining may be present on nails and umbilical cord

C. Implementation
1. Provide normal **newborn** care
2. Monitor for hypoglycemia
3. Maintain the **newborn's** temperature
4. Monitor for meconium aspiration
5. Initiate seizure precautions

VII. Small for Gestational Age

A. Description: a **newborn** who is plotted at or below the 10th percentile on the intrauterine growth curve

B. Data collection
1. Fetal distress
2. Gestational age and physical maturity
3. Lowered or elevated body temperature
4. Physical abnormalities

5. Hypoglycemia
6. Signs of polycythemia
    a. Ruddy appearance
    b. Cyanosis
    c. Jaundice
7. Signs of infection
8. Signs of aspiration of meconium
C. Implementation
    1. Maintain airway
    2. Maintain temperature
    3. Observe for signs of respiratory distress
    4. Monitor for signs of infection
    5. Monitor glucose levels
    6. Monitor for signs of hypoglycemia
    7. Initiate feedings and monitor for signs of aspiration
    8. Provide stimulation such as touch and cuddling

VIII. Large for Gestational Age

A. Description: a newborn who is plotted at or above the 90th percentile on the intrauterine growth curve
B. Data collection
    1. Gestational age
    2. Birth trauma or injury
    3. Respiratory distress
    4. Hypoglycemia
C. Implementation
    1. Monitor vital signs
    2. Monitor glucose levels
    3. Observe for signs of hypoglycemia
    4. Initiate early feedings
    5. Monitor for infection and initiate measures to prevent sepsis
    6. Provide touch and cuddling for the **newborn**

◆ IX. Respiratory Distress Syndrome (RDS)

A. Description: a serious lung disorder caused by immaturity and inability to produce surfactant resulting in hypoxia and acidosis
B. Data collection
    1. Tachypnea
    2. Flaring nares
    3. Expiratory grunting
    4. Retractions
    5. Decreased breath sounds
    6. Apnea
    7. Pallor and cyanosis
    8. Hypothermia
    9. Poor muscle tone
C. Implementation
    1. Monitor color, respiratory rate, and degree of effort in breathing
    2. Support respirations as prescribed
    3. Monitor blood gases and oxygen saturation levels (blood gases from umbilical artery)
    4. Monitor blood gases so oxygen administered to the **newborn** is at the lowest possible concentration necessary to maintain adequate arterial oxygenation
    5. Schedule any premature **newborn** who required oxygen support for an eye examination before discharge
    6. Suction every 2 hours or more often as necessary
    7. Position the **newborn** on the side or back with the neck slightly extended
    8. Administer respiratory therapy (percussion and vibration) as prescribed; use a padded small plastic cup or small oxygen mask for percussion; use an electric toothbrush for vibration
    9. Provide nutrition
    10. Support bonding
    11. Prepare parents for short- to long-term period of oxygen dependency if necessary
    12. Encourage the mother to pump her breasts for future breast-feeding if she so desires
    13. Encourage maternal participation in the **newborn's** care as condition allows

X. Hyperbilirubinemia

A. Description
    1. At any serum bilirubin level, the appearance of jaundice during the first day of life indicates a pathological process
    2. Evaluation is indicated when serum levels are over 12 mg/dL in the term **newborn**
    3. Therapy is aimed at preventing kernicterus, which results in permanent neurological damage from the deposition of bilirubin in the brain cells
B. Data collection
    1. Jaundice
    2. Elevated serum bilirubin levels
    3. Enlarged liver
    4. Poor muscle tone
    5. Lethargy
    6. Poor sucking reflex
C. Implementation
    1. Monitor for presence of jaundice
        a. Examine the baby's skin color in natural light
        b. Press a finger over a bony prominence or the tip of the **newborn's** nose to press out capillary blood from the tissues
        c. Note that jaundice starts at the head first, spreads to the chest, and then the abdomen; the arms and legs, followed by the hands and feet, are the last to be jaundiced
    2. Keep the **newborn** well hydrated to maintain blood volume and encourage excretion of bilirubin
    3. Facilitate early, frequent feeding to hasten passage of meconium
    4. Report any signs of jaundice in the first 24 hours and any abnormal signs and symptoms to the physician

5. Prepare for phototherapy and monitor the **newborn** closely during the treatment

D. Phototherapy
1. Description
   a. Use of intense fluorescent lights to reduce serum bilirubin levels in the **newborn**
   b. Injury from treatment such as eye damage, dehydration, or sensory deprivation can occur
2. Implementation
   a. Expose as much of the **newborn's** skin as possible
   b. Cover the genital area and monitor the area for skin irritation or breakdown
   c. Cover the **newborn's** eyes with eye shields
   d. Make sure eyelids are closed when eye shields are applied
   e. Remove the shields at least once per shift to inspect the eyes for infection or irritation and to allow eye contact
   f. Measure the quantity of light every 8 hours
   g. Monitor skin temperature closely
   h. Increase fluids to compensate for water loss
   i. Expect loose, green stools and green urine
   j. Monitor the **newborn's** skin color with the light turned off every 4 to 8 hours
   k. Monitor the skin for bronze baby syndrome, a grayish brown discoloration of the skin
   l. Reposition the **newborn** every 2 hours
   m. Provide stimulation
   n. After treatment, continue monitoring for signs of hyperbilirubinemia because rebound elevations are normal after therapy is discontinued

XI. Erythroblastosis Fetalis

A. Description
1. Destruction of RBCs that results from an antigen antibody reaction
2. Characterized by hemolytic anemia or hyperbilirubinemia
3. Exchange of fetal and maternal blood takes place primarily when the **placenta** separates at birth
4. Rh antigens from the baby's blood enter the maternal bloodstream
5. The mother's blood does not contain Rh factor so the mother produces anti-Rh antibodies
6. Antibodies are harmless to the mother but attach to the erythrocytes in the fetus and cause hemolysis
7. Sensitization is rare with the first pregnancy
8. ABO incompatibility is usually less severe
B. Data collection
1. Anemia
2. Jaundice, which develops rapidly after birth and before 24 hours

3. Edema
C. Implementation
1. Administer RhoGAM to the mother during the first 72 hours after **delivery** if the Rh-negative mother delivers an Rh-positive fetus but remains unsensitized
2. Assist with exchange transfusion after birth or intrauterine transfusion as prescribed
3. The baby's blood is replaced with Rh-negative blood to stop the destruction of the baby's red cells; the Rh-negative blood is replaced with the baby's own blood gradually
4. Reassure the mother that the **newborn** will suffer no untoward effects from the condition

XII. Sepsis

A. Description: generalized infection resulting from the presence of bacteria in the blood
B. Data collection
1. Pallor
2. Tachypnea
3. Tachycardia
4. Poor feeding
5. Abdominal distention
C. Implementation
1. Monitor for periods of apnea or irregular respirations
2. Stimulate if apnea is present by gently rubbing the chest or foot
3. Administer oxygen as prescribed
4. Monitor vital signs
5. Maintain warmth in an isolette
6. Provide isolation as necessary
7. Monitor for low-grade fever
8. Monitor I&O
9. Monitor daily weight
10. Monitor for diarrhea
11. Monitor feeding, which may be poor
12. Monitor the sucking reflex, which may be poor
13. Monitor for jaundice
14. Monitor for irritability and lethargy
15. Administer antibiotics as prescribed and observe carefully for toxicity because the **newborn's** liver and kidney are immature

XIII. TORCH Syndrome

A. Description
1. Refers to infections of the fetus or **newborn**
2. Caused by one of the following
   a. **T**oxoplasmosis
   b. **O**ther viruses
   c. **R**ubella
   d. **C**ytomegalovirus
   e. **H**erpes simplex
B. Infections (Table 25–5)

Table 25–5. Infections

Infection	Characteristics
Toxoplasmosis	Protozoan infection
	Produces no serius effects in the mother
	Can be transmitted to the fetus
	Can result in severe physical and developmental abnormalities
	Common carriers include cat feces and raw beef
Other infections	Syphilis
Rubella	Systemic viral infection
	Causes congenital rubella syndrome, which includes congenital heart disease, cataracts, growth retardation, and pneumonia if the mother becomes infected with the first trimester
	Deafness and some learning disabilities can occur if the mother becomes infected during the first trimester.
Cytomegalovirus	A viral infection that persists in the body indefinitely with periods of reactivation without symptoms
	Can infect the fetus or infant during delivery or after birth through breast milk, blood transfusions, or contact with infected secretions
	May cause microcephaly, blindness, deafness, and mental and motor retardation
Herpes simplex	Sexually transmitted disease caused by a virus
	Periods of reactivation
	Newborn is commonly infected during delivery by direct contact with lesions in the genital tract
	Can cause neurologic impairment or death

XIV. Syphilis

A. Description
1. Sexually transmitted disease
2. Congenital syphilis can result in premature **delivery,** skin lesions, or abnormal skeletal development
3. The organism *Treponema pallidum,* a spirochete, is able to cross the **placenta** throughout pregnancy and infect the fetus usually after 18 weeks' gestation
4. Risks include preterm birth, stillbirth, and low birth weight
5. Congenital effects are irreversible and may include CNS damage and hearing loss
B. Data collection
1. Hepatosplenomegaly
2. Joint swelling
3. Rash
4. Anemia
5. Jaundice
6. Snuffles
7. Ascites
8. Pneumonitis
9. Cerebrospinal fluid changes

C. Implementation
1. Monitor the **newborn** for signs of syphilis
2. Monitor for rash and snuffles
3. Prepare the **newborn** for serological testing if prescribed
4. Administer antibiotic therapy as prescribed
5. Use drainage/secretion precautions with suspected congenital syphilis
6. Wear gloves when handling the **neonate** until 24 hours of antibiotic therapy have been administered
7. Provide psychological support to the mother and provide instructions regarding follow-up care to the **newborn**

XV. The Addicted Newborn

A. Description: **newborn** who has become passively addicted to drugs that have passed through the **placenta**
B. Addicting drugs
1. Heroin
   a. The **newborn** may appear normal at birth with a low birth weight
   b. Withdrawal occurs within 12 to 24 hours and may last 5 to 7 days
2. Methadone
   a. Withdrawal occurs within 1 to 2 days to 1 week or more, is most evident at 48 to 72 hours, and may last 6 days to 8 weeks
   b. The **newborn** appears very ill
   c. May develop jaundice due to prematurity
3. Cocaine
   a. Causes decreased interactive behavior
   b. Feeding problems are present
   c. Irregular sleep patterns and diarrhea occur
   d. Major deformities will occur, especially in the renal system
C. Data collection
1. Irritability
2. Tremors
3. Hyperactivity
4. Hypertonicity
5. Respiratory distress
6. Vomiting
7. High-pitched cry
8. Sneezing
9. Fever
10. Diarrhea
11. Excessive sweating
12. Poor feeding
13. Extreme sucking of the fists
14. Seizures
D. Implementation
1. Monitor respiratory and cardiac rates frequently
2. Monitor temperature and vital signs
3. Hold the **newborn** firmly and close to the body during feeding and when giving care
4. Initiate seizure precautions
5. Pad the sides of the crib

6. Provide small, frequent feedings and allow a longer period for feeding
7. Monitor I&O
8. Administer IV hydration if prescribed
9. Protect the **neonate's** skin from injury that can be caused by the constant rubbing from hyperactive jitters
10. Swaddle the **newborn**
11. Place the **newborn** in a quiet room and reduce stimulation
12. Allow the mother to ventilate feelings of anxiety and guilt
13. Refer the mother for treatment of substance abuse problem

XVI. Fetal Alcohol Syndrome

A. Description
   1. Caused by maternal alcohol use during pregnancy
   2. Most serious cause of teratogenesis
   3. Causes mental and physical retardation
B. Data collection
   1. Facial changes
      a. Short palpebral fissures
      b. Hypoplastic philtrum
      c. Short upturned nose
      d. Flat midface
      e. Thin upper lip
      f. Low nasal bridge
   2. Abnormal palmar creases
   3. Congenital heart disorders
   4. Respiratory distress
   5. Apnea
   6. Cyanosis
   7. Irritability
   8. Tremors
   9. Poor feeding
   10. Hypersensitivity to stimuli
   11. Seizures
C. Implementation
   1. Monitor for respiratory distress
   2. Position the **newborn** on the side to facilitate drainage of secretions
   3. Keep resuscitation equipment at the bedside
   4. Monitor for hypoglycemia
   5. Monitor suck and swallow reflex
   6. Administer small feedings and burp well
   7. Suction as necessary, especially following feedings
   8. Monitor I&O
   9. Monitor weight and head circumference
   10. Decrease environmental stimuli

XVII. Newborn at Risk for Acquired Immunodeficiency Syndrome (AIDS)

A. Description
   1. The fetus of an HIV antibody–positive woman should be monitored closely throughout the pregnancy
   2. Serial ultrasound screenings should be done to identify intrauterine growth restriction
   3. Weekly nonstress testing after 32 weeks of gestation and biophysical profiles may be necessary
   4. **Neonates** born to HIV-positive clients may test positive because the mother's positive antibodies may persist for as long as 18 months after birth
   5. The use of antiviral medication, the reduction of **neonate** exposure to maternal blood and body fluids, and the early identification of HIV in pregnancy reduce the risk of transmission to the **newborn**
   6. All **neonates** acquire maternal antibody to HIV infection, but not all acquire the infection
   7. The **neonate** may be asymptomatic for the first several years of life
B. Transmission
   1. Across the **placental** barrier
   2. During **labor** and **delivery**
   3. Breast milk
C. Data collection
   1. May have no outward signs for the first several months of life
   2. Signs of immune deficiency
   3. Hepatomegaly
   4. Splenomegaly
   5. Lymphadenopathy
   6. Impairment in growth and development
D. Implementation
   1. Cleanse the **newborn's** skin carefully before any invasive procedure such as the administration of vitamin K, heel sticks, or venipunctures
   2. Circumcisions are not done on **newborns** with HIV-positive mothers until the **newborn's** status is determined
   3. The **newborn** can room with the mother
   4. All HIV-exposed **newborns** should be treated with medication to prevent infection by *Pneumocystis carinii*
   5. Administer zidovudine (AZT) as prescribed for the first 6 weeks of life
   6. Monitor for early signs of immune deficiency such as enlarged spleen or liver, lymphadenopathy, and impairment in growth and development
   7. **Newborns** at risk for HIV infection should be seen by the physician at birth, 1 week, 2 weeks, 1 month, and 2 months of life
   8. Inform the mother that an HIV culture is recommended at age 1 month and after 4 months of age
E. Immunizations
   1. **Newborns** at risk for HIV infection need to receive all recommended immunizations at the regular schedule
   2. Inactivated polio vaccine by injection rather than oral polio vaccine should be administered because the oral polio vaccine causes a shedding of polio virus in the stool,

which may be a risk to the immunocompromised family
3. Immunizations with live vaccines such as oral polio, measles-mumps-rubella (MMR), should not be done until the **newborn, infant,** or child's status is confirmed
4. If a child is infected, live vaccine will not be given

XVIII. Newborn of a Diabetic Mother

A. Description
1. A **neonate** born to an insulin-dependent mother or gestational diabetic mother
2. High incidence of congenital anomalies
3. High incidence of hypoglycemia, respiratory distress, hypocalcemia, and hyperbilirubinemia
B. Data collection
1. Excessive size and weight due to excess fat and glycogen in tissues
2. Edema or puffiness in the face and cheeks
3. Signs of hypoglycemia such as twitching, difficulty feeding, lethargy, apnea, seizures, and cyanosis
4. Hyperbilirubinemia
5. Signs of respiratory distress, tachypnea, cyanosis, retractions, grunting, and nasal flaring
C. Implementation
1. Monitor for signs of respiratory distress
2. Monitor bilirubin and blood glucose levels
3. Monitor weight
4. Feed early, with 10% glucose water, breast milk, or formula
5. IV glucose is administered if necessary
6. Monitor for edema
7. Monitor for tremors, seizures, apnea, and acidosis

XIX. Hypoglycemia

A. Description
1. Abnormal low level of glucose in the blood
2. Normal blood glucose level is 40 to 60 mg/dL in a 1-day-old neonate and 50 to 90 mg/dL in a neonate older than 1 day
B. Data collection
1. Increased respiratory rate
2. Twitching, nervousness, or tremors
3. Unstable temperature
4. Cyanosis
C. Implementation
1. Prevent low blood glucose through early feedings
2. Glucose is administered orally or IV as prescribed
3. Monitor blood glucose values as prescribed
4. Monitor for feeding problems
5. Evaluate apneic periods
6. Monitor for shrill or intermittent cries
7. Evaluate lethargy and poor muscle tone

PRACTICE QUESTIONS

1. The nurse is reinforcing measures regarding the care of the newborn. To bathe a newborn, a mother should be taught to
   1 Start with the dirtiest area first
   2 Begin with the eyes and face
   3 Begin with the feet and work upward
   4 Wash only the diaper area, since this is the only part of the baby that gets soiled

2. Following birth, the nurse should plan to prevent hypothermia due to evaporation in the neonate by
   1 Warming the crib pad
   2 Turning on the overhead radiant warmer
   3 Closing the doors to the room
   4 Drying the baby with a warm blanket

3. The nurse is planning to teach cord care to a new mother. The nurse understands that which of the following principles is of greatest importance?
   1 Cord care is done only at birth to control bleeding
   2 Alcohol is the best agent used to clean the cord
   3 The process of keeping the cord clean and dry will decrease bacterial growth
   4 It takes 21 days for the cord to dry up and fall off

4. A male neonate has just been circumcised. The nurse expects the surgical site to appear
   1 Pink, without drainage
   2 Reddened, with a small amount of bloody drainage
   3 Reddened with a large amount of bloody drainage that requires a dressing change every 30 minutes
   4 Reddened with a small amount of yellow exudate on the glans

5. The parents of a male neonate who is not circumcised request information on how to clean the newborn's penis. The best response to the parent's is
   1 "Retract the foreskin and cleanse the glans when bathing the neonate."
   2 "Do not retract the foreskin to cleanse as this may cause adhesions."
   3 "Retract the foreskin no farther than it will easily go and replace over the glans after cleaning."
   4 "Retract the foreskin and cleanse with every diaper change."

6. A new mother is attempting to breast-feed for the first time. The nurse notices that the client has inverted nipples. What nursing action can the nurse take to assist the client in breast-feeding the newborn?
   1 Provide breast shells and assist the mother

with using a breast pump before each feeding to make the nipples easier for the newborn to grasp
2 Have the mother grasp the nipples between the thumb and forefinger and tug firmly to get the nipple to protrude
3 Massage the breast, applying gentle pressure on the areola
4 Take a cool shower, allowing the water to run over the breasts as this will encourage the nipples to protrude

7. Preterm newborns are at risk for developing respiratory distress syndrome (RDS). The nurse monitors for the clinical signs associated with RDS knowing that these signs include
1 Cyanosis, tachypnea, retractions, and expiratory grunt
2 Acrocyanosis, apnea, pnuemothorax, and grunting
3 Barrel-shaped chest, hypotension, and bradycardia
4 Acrocyanosis, emphysema, and interstitial edema

8. A 4-day-old infant will be receiving phototherapy at home for a bilirubin level of 14 mg/dL. The nurse plans to include which of the following in the instructions to the parents regarding the newborn?
1 Having minimal contact with the neonate to prevent stimulation
2 Advising parents to limit newborn PO intake during phototherapy
3 Applying lotions to exposed newborn skin
4 Assessing skin integrity, and fluid status of the neonate

9. The nurse is collecting data on a newborn whose mother had an elevated temperature during a prolonged labor. Which intervention(s) is important to include and document in the newborn's plan of care?
1 Maintain routine vital signs assessment
2 Promote early maternal-newborn interaction
3 Delay feeding the newborn for 4 hours
4 Observe vital signs and central nervous system status frequently during the first 2 days

10. The nurse notes hypotonia, irritability, and a poor sucking reflex in a full-term neonate upon admission to the nursery. The nurse interprets that which of the following additional sign(s) is consistent with fetal alcohol syndrome (FAS)?
1 Head circumference appropriate for gestational age
2 Birth weight 6 pounds 14 ounces
3 Length 19 inches
4 Microcephaly and increased respiratory effort

11. The nurse is caring for the neonate with fetal alcohol syndrome (FAS). The nurse plans to include which of the following priority interventions in the care of this newborn?
1 Monitor neonate response to feedings and weight gain pattern
2 Encourage frequent handling of the neonate by staff and parents
3 Maintain the newborn in a brightly lighted area of the nursery
4 Allow the newborn to establish its own sleep-rest pattern.

12. An HIV-positive woman delivers a baby. The nurse provides guidance to help the client in decision making regarding newborn care. Which statement is not included in the teaching plan for this client?
1 Be sure to wash hands prior to and following bathroom use
2 Launder newborn clothing separately
3 Breast-feeding is encouraged, especially for the first 6 weeks' postpartum
4 The newborn should be on antiviral drugs for the first 6 weeks after delivery

13. A pregnant woman in her second trimester calls the prenatal clinic nurse to report a recent exposure to a child with rubella. Which of the following responses by the nurse is most appropriate?
1 "There is no need to be concerned if you don't have a fever or rash within the next 2 days."
2 "Be sure to tell the doctor on your next prenatal visit, but there is little risk in the second trimester."
3 "You should avoid all school-aged children during pregnancy."
4 "You were wise to call. I will check your rubella titer screening results and we can identify immediately if future interventions are needed."

14. A pregnant woman has a positive history of genital herpes, but has not had lesions during this pregnancy. The nurse plans to provide which of the following information to the client?
1 "You will be isolated from your newborn following delivery."
2 "You will be evaluated at the time of delivery for herpetic genital tract lesions; if present, a cesarean delivery will be needed."
3 "There is little risk to your neonate during this pregnancy, birth, and following delivery."
4 "Vaginal deliveries can reduce neonatal infection risks even if you have an active lesion at birth."

15. The nurse administers erythromycin ointment (0.5%) to the eyes of the newborn. The mother asks the nurse why this is performed. The nurse tells the client that this is routinely done to
1 Minimize spread of microorganisms to the neonate from invasive procedures during labor

2 Protect the neonate's eyes from possible infections acquired while hospitalized

3 Prevent ophthalmia neonatorum from occurring postdelivery to the neonate born to a woman with an untreated gonococcal infection

4 Prevent cataracts in the newborn born to a woman who is rubella susceptible

16. The client asks the nurse why her newborn baby needs an injection of vitamin K. The best response by the nurse is
    1 "Your baby needs vitamin K to develop immunity."
    2 "The vitamin K will protect your baby from being jaundiced."
    3 "Newborns are deficient in vitamin K. This injection prevents your baby from abnormal bleeding."
    4 "Newborns have sterile bowels. Vitamin K will help the bowel become colonized with the necessary bacteria."

17. The nurse is assigned to assist in caring for a newborn with AIDS. The nurse understands that the management of a newborn with AIDS should include which nursing goal?
    1 Instruct breast-feeding mothers regarding the treatment of their nipples with nystatin
    2 Monitor the newborn's vital signs routinely
    3 Maintain universal standards at all times while caring for the newborn
    4 Initiate referral to evaluate for blindness, deafness, and learning or behavioral problems

18. Which specific instruction should be included in the teaching plan for a mother whose infant is HIV positive?
    1 Instruct the mother and family to provide meticulous skin care to the infant and to change the infant's diaper after each voiding or stool
    2 Instruct the mother to feed the infant in an upright position with the head and chest tilted slightly back to avoid aspiration
    3 Instruct the mother to feed the infant with a special nipple and burp the infant frequently to decrease the tendency to swallow air
    4 Instruct the mother to check the anterior fontanel for bulging and sutures for widening each day

19. Which statement by a pregnant client with AIDS indicates her understanding of the risk to her newborn during delivery?
    1 There is a risk of transmission from the mother to the newborn, although the newborn may be asymptomatic at birth
    2 There is no risk to the newborn from an AIDS-infected mother during delivery
    3 Newborns who contract AIDS during delivery will show immediate symptoms

4 Newborns who are HIV positive after delivery will remain HIV positive for life

20. The nurse in the newborn nursery prepares for admission of a 43-week-gestation neonate with Apgar scores of 1 and 4. In planning for admission of this newborn, the nurse's highest priority is to
    1 Connect the resuscitation bag to the oxygen outlet
    2 Turn on the apnea and cardiorespiratory monitor
    3 Set up the intravenous line with dextrose in 5% water
    4 Set up the radiant warmer control temperature at 36.5°C (97.6°F)

21. The nurse is caring for a post-term small for gestational age (SGA) neonate immediately after admission to the nursery. The priority nursing action is to monitor
    1 Urinary output
    2 Total bilirubin levels
    3 Blood glucose levels
    4 Hemoglobin and hematocrit

22. The nurse receives a report that a large for gestational age (LGA) newborn will be admitted to the nursery. Which of the following neonate descriptions does the nurse anticipate seeing in an LGA newborn?
    1 Weight 3600 g, 42 weeks' gestation with absent vernix, cracked thin skin, with yellow staining of the nailbeds and umbilical cord
    2 Weight 3800 g, 40 weeks' gestation with a flexed posture, and pendulous testes with deep rugae
    3 Weight 3200 g, 34 weeks' gestation with smooth pink skin, visible veins, abundant lanugo, and an anterior plantar crease
    4 Weight 3400 g, 38 weeks' gestation with pink skin, rare visible veins, and raised areola with a 4 mm breast bud

23. The nurse is caring for a newborn with respiratory distress syndrome (RDS). Which of the following data obtained by the nurse indicates a potential complication associated with this disorder?
    1 No visible bowel loops; abdomen soft with active bowel sounds
    2 No seizure activity; anterior fontanel soft and flat
    3 No audible murmur; pulse rate between 135 and 145 bpm
    4 No audible breath sounds in the left lung, heart sounds louder in the right side of the chest

24. The nurse is assisting in caring for a newborn whose mother is Rh negative. In planning the newborn's care it is most important for the nurse to
    1 Prepare for an exchange transfusion
    2 Set up a phototherapy unit
    3 Request the newborn's blood type and direct Coombs'
    4 Administer an injection of vitamin K to prevent isoimmunization

25. The nurse is reinforcing instructions to the new mother about cord care and how to monitor for infection. The nurse tells the mother that which of the following is a sign of infection?
    1 A darkened, drying stump
    2 A moist cord with discharge
    3 A purple stump that shows pinkness around the base
    4 A purple stump that shows some moistness at the base

ANSWERS

1. 2

RATIONALE: Bathing should start at the eyes and face, usually the cleanest area. Next, the external ears and behind the ears are cleansed. The newborn's neck should be washed because formula, lint, or breast milk will often accumulate in the folds of the neck. Hands and arms are then washed. The baby's legs are washed, and the diaper area is washed last.
TEST-TAKING STRATEGY: Remember the basic techniques of bathing a client. Remember when bathing an adult or baby, start with the cleanest part of the body and proceed to the dirtiest part. Options 1, 3, and 4 are incorrect.
LEVEL OF COGNITIVE ABILITY: Application
PHASE OF NURSING PROCESS: Implementation
CLIENT NEEDS: Physiological Integrity
CONTENT AREA: Maternity
REFERENCE
Nichols, F., & Zwelling, E. (1997). *Maternal-newborn nursing: Theory and practice.* Philadelphia: W. B. Saunders. pp. 1159–1161.

2. 4

RATIONALE: Evaporation of moisture from wet body surfaces dissipates heat along with the moisture. By keeping the baby dry (by drying the wet baby at birth), evaporation is prevented.
TEST-TAKING STRATEGY: There are four methods of heat loss. Conduction occurs when the baby is on a cold surface, such as a pad. Convection occurs as air moves across the baby's skin from an open door and heat is transferred to the air. Radiation occurs when heat from the body radiates to a colder surface. Evaporation occurs when moisture from the newborn's wet body surface dissipates heat along with moisture. Preventing heat loss in a newborn is an important nursing intervention. Review these concepts now if you had difficulty with this question.
LEVEL OF COGNITIVE ABILITY: Application
PHASE OF NURSING PROCESS: Planning
CLIENT NEEDS: Physiological Integrity
CONTENT AREA: Maternity
REFERENCE
Nichols, F., & Zwelling, E. (1997). *Maternal-newborn nursing: Theory and practice.* Philadelphia: W. B. Saunders. pp. 1072–1073.

3. 3

RATIONALE: The cord should be kept clean and dry to decrease bacterial growth. This includes keeping the diaper folded below the cord to keep urine away from the cord. The cord should be cleansed two to three times a day. It usually falls off within 7 to 14 days.
TEST-TAKING STRATEGY: Utilize the process of elimination in answering the question. Option 1 is incorrect. Cord care is required until the cord dries up and falls off between 7 and 14 days. Agents other than alcohol may be used on the cord. Option 4 is incorrect: the cord should fall off between 7 and 14 days. Option 3 is the most global and correct answer. Review the concepts of cord care now if you had difficulty answering the question.
LEVEL OF COGNITIVE ABILITY: Comprehension
PHASE OF NURSING PROCESS: Planning
CLIENT NEEDS: Physiological Integrity
CONTENT AREA: Maternity
REFERENCE
Gorrie, L., McKinney, E., & Murray, S. (1998). *Foundations of maternal-newborn nursing* (2nd ed.). Philadelphia: W. B. Saunders. p. 568.

4. 2

RATIONALE: The glans penis is normally dark red. During the healing process, the glans become covered with a yellow exudate in 24 hours. This is a part of normal healing. If excessive bleeding is noted from the circumcision, the nurse applies gentle pressure to the site of bleeding with a sterile folded 4×4. If bleeding is not controlled, a blood vessel may need to be ligated. The nurse notifies the physician.
TEST-TAKING STRATEGY: Read the question carefully. The question asks for an expected appearance. Use the process of elimination. A small amount of bloody drainage is expected. Option 1 indicates the appearance of a healed circumcision. Option 3 is incorrect, as there should be only a slight amount of bleeding. Option 4 indicates how the site should appear 24 hours after the circumcision. If a large amount of bleeding occurs, the physician should be notified. Review the procedure related to circumcision now if you had difficulty with this question.
LEVEL OF COGNITIVE ABILITY: Comprehension
PHASE OF NURSING PROCESS: Data Collection
CLIENT NEEDS: Physiological Integrity
CONTENT AREA: Maternity
REFERENCE
Lowdermilk, D., Perry, S., & Bobak, I. (1997). *Maternity & women's health care* (6th ed.). St. Louis: Mosby–Year Book. p. 585.

5. 2

RATIONALE: In newborn males, the prepuce is continuous with the epidermis of the glans and is nonretractable. Forced retraction may cause adhesions to develop. Current recommendations are to allow separation to occur naturally, which will occur between 3 years and puberty. Most

foreskins are retractable by 3 years of age and should be pushed back gently for cleaning once a week.
TEST-TAKING STRATEGY: Look for the option that is different. Options 1, 3, and 4 are incorrect because retracting the foreskin is not recommended in an uncircumcised male. Option 2 is the only different option stating that the foreskin should not be retracted.
LEVEL OF COGNITIVE ABILITY: Application
PHASE OF NURSING PROCESS: Implementation
CLIENT NEEDS: Physiological Integrity
CONTENT AREA: Maternity
REFERENCE
Gorrie, L., McKinney, E., & Murray, S. (1998). *Foundations of maternal-newborn nursing* (2nd ed.). Philadelphia: W. B. Saunders. p. 564.

6. **1**

RATIONALE: Wearing breast shells and using a breast pump before each feeding will make it easier for the newborn to grasp the nipple. True inverted nipples will retract if the areola is pressed between the thumb and forefinger, making option 2 incorrect. Option 3 is good advice for mothers suffering from engorgement. Option 4 will only make the mother cold; it has no effect on inverted nipples.
TEST-TAKING STRATEGY: Use the process of elimination and knowledge regarding breastfeeding to assist with answering this question. Review the concepts related to breast-feeding if you had difficulty with this question.
LEVEL OF COGNITIVE ABILITY: Application
PHASE OF NURSING PROCESS: Implementation
CLIENT NEEDS: Health Promotion and Maintenance
CONTENT AREA: Maternity
REFERENCE
Gorrie, L., McKinney, E., & Murray, S. (1998). *Foundations of maternal-newborn nursing* (2nd ed.). Philadelphia: W. B. Saunders. p. 453.

7. **1**

RATIONALE: The neonate with RDS may present with clinical signs of cyanosis, tachypnea, or apnea, nasal flaring, chest wall retractions, or audible expiratory grunt. Acrocyanosis is not uncommon in a newborn in the first few hours of life. It is the bluish discoloration of the hands or feet.
TEST-TAKING STRATEGY: Read all of the components of each option carefully. Remembering that acrocyanosis is not uncommon in a newborn will assist in eliminating options 2 and 4. Option 1 is the best choice because all of the signs present in this option are related to the respiratory system.
LEVEL OF COGNITIVE ABILITY: Application
PHASE OF NURSING PROCESS: Data Collection
CLIENT NEEDS: Physiological Integrity
CONTENT AREA: Maternity
REFERENCE
Nichols, F., & Zwelling, E. (1997). *Maternal-newborn nursing: Theory and practice*. Philadelphia: W. B. Saunders. pp. 1102, 1342.

8. **4**

RATIONALE: Safe care for the newborn during phototherapy requires shielding the eyes using a soft eye shield to prevent retinal damage, keeping the newborn skin exposed except for a diaper, and changing position frequently. Lotions are not used on the exposed skin. Adequate oral fluids are essential to prevent dehydration because diarrhea is a

common side effect of therapy. Contact with the neonate is important.
TEST-TAKING STRATEGY: Use the process of elimination in answering this question. The nursing care plan for safe home therapy of the newborn is guided by the principles of maintaining adequate skin integrity, parental bonding, and neonatal fluid balance. Recalling these principles allows you to eliminate each of the incorrect options successfully. If you had difficulty with this question, take time now to review the content related to phototherapy.
LEVEL OF COGNITIVE ABILITY: Application
PHASE OF NURSING PROCESS: Planning
CLIENT NEEDS: Safe, Effective Care Environment
CONTENT AREA: Maternity
REFERENCE
Gorrie, L., McKinney, E., & Murray, S. (1998). *Foundations of maternal-newborn nursing* (2nd ed.). Philadelphia: W. B. Saunders. p. 853.

9. **4**

RATIONALE: Clinical signs of sepsis in the newborn include temperature instability, tachycardia, respiratory changes and central nervous symptoms as lethargy, irritability or hypotonia. If sepsis is a potential risk, the nurse would monitor vital signs and central nervous system status frequently.
TEST-TAKING STRATEGY: To answer this question correctly, you need to know the early neonatal signs of sepsis. Note that the question addresses a mother who had an elevated temperature during a prolonged labor. This provides a clue that neonate assessments need to be more frequent than routine. This would eliminate option 1. Promoting early maternal-newborn interaction is always important but is not directly related to answering this question. Delaying a feeding is not appropriate. Frequent monitoring of vital signs and central nervous system adaptation assures recognition of signs early, to prevent further compromise to the airway, breathing and circulatory status of a newborn. Option 4 is the most specific and thorough option.
LEVEL OF COGNITIVE ABILITY: Application
PHASE OF NURSING PROCESS: Planning
CLIENT NEEDS: Physiological Integrity
CONTENT AREA: Maternity
REFERENCE
Lowdermilk, D., Perry, S., & Bobak, I. (1997). *Maternity and women's health care* (6th ed.). St. Louis: Mosby–Year Book. p. 1084.

10. **4**

RATIONALE: Features of neonates at birth who are eventually diagnosed with FAS include craniofacial abnormalities, cleft lip or palate, intrauterine growth retardation (IUGR), cardiac abnormalities, abnormal palmar creases, and irregular hair distribution. Microcephaly, limb anomalies, and increased respiratory effort during the transition to extrauterine life are also frequently noted by caregivers.
TEST-TAKING STRATEGY: Knowledge regarding normal findings in the full-term newborn and FAS is required to answer this question. This question asks the nurse to analyze the characteristics observed by the neonate and continue to collect data based upon the knowledge of the physiological changes that can occur in the neonate exposed to alcohol during pregnancy. Use the process of elimination in answering this question. Options 1, 2, and 3 identify normal findings in the full-term newborn and can be eliminated. If you had difficulty with this question, take

the time now to review the content related to normal newborn findings and FAS.
LEVEL OF COGNITIVE ABILITY: Comprehension
PHASE OF NURSING PROCESS: Data Collection
CLIENT NEEDS: Physiological Integrity
CONTENT AREA: Maternity
REFERENCE
Lowdermilk, D., Perry, S., & Bobak, I. (1997). *Maternity and women's health care* (6th ed.). St. Louis: Mosby–Year Book. pp. 1094–1096.

11. **1**

RATIONALE: A primary nursing goal for the neonate diagnosed with FAS is to establish nutritional balance following delivery. These neonates may exhibit hyperirritability, vomiting, diarrhea, or an uncoordinated sucking and swallowing ability. A quiet environment with minimal stimuli and handling will help establish appropriate sleep-rest cycles in the neonate as well.
TEST-TAKING STRATEGY: Use Maslow's hierarchy of needs theory to assist in answering this question. Option 1 addresses physiological needs most directly, ensures the safest environment for the newborn, and minimizes potential side effects from aspiration or vomiting.
LEVEL OF COGNITIVE ABILITY: Application
PHASE OF NURSING PROCESS: Planning
CLIENT NEEDS: Physiological Integrity
CONTENT AREA: Maternity
REFERENCE
Nichols, F., & Zwelling, E. (1997). *Maternal-newborn nursing: Theory and practice.* Philadelphia: W. B. Saunders. pp. 1359–1361.

12. **3**

RATIONALE: Though more than 50% of all HIV transmission to babies is believed to take place during the intrapartal period, HIV acquisition can occur during breast-feeding; thus, HIV-positive clients should be encouraged to bottle feed their neonates. Neonates of HIV-positive clients are recommended to receive a dose of zidovudine (AZT) every 6 hours for the first 6 weeks of life. Handwashing is critical to prevent the transmission of disease, and the mother should be instructed to launder the newborn clothing separately.
TEST-TAKING STRATEGY: Note the key work "not." The correct response to this question requires that the nurse apply appropriate knowledge of the transmission of HIV and universal precautions to the postpartum guidance of an HIV-infected mother. Use the process of elimination in answering the question. Review these important measures now if you had difficulty with this question.
LEVEL OF COGNITIVE ABILITY: Application
PHASE OF NURSING PROCESS: Planning
CLIENT NEEDS: Safe, Effective Care Environment
CONTENT AREA: Maternity
REFERENCE
Nichols, F., & Zwelling, E. (1997). *Maternal-newborn nursing: Theory and practice.* Philadelphia: W. B. Saunders. pp. 1500–1501.

13. **4**

RATIONALE: Rubella virus is spread by aerosol droplet transmission through the upper respiratory tract and has an incubation period of 14 to 21 days. Rubella can be asymptomatic in up to 50% of cases. The risk of maternal and subsequent fetal infection during the second trimester includes hearing loss and congenital anomalies. An estimated 15% to 20% of the young adult population of the United States, including women of childbearing age, are not vaccinated and are susceptible to infection. Rubella titer determination is a standard antenatal test for childbearing women during their initial screening and entry into the health care delivery system.
TEST-TAKING STRATEGY: Knowledge regarding the transmission of rubella virus to the fetus is required to answer this question. Option 4 reconfirms maternal behavior and helps to clarify maternal concerns with accurate information based upon the acquisition of rubella infection and potential fetal side effects. Use the process of elimination. The remaining options are incorrect and are systematically eliminated as possible choices.
LEVEL OF COGNITIVE ABILIITY: Application
PHASE OF NURSING PROCESS: Implementation
CLIENT NEEDS: Physiological Integrity
CONTENT AREA: Maternity
REFERENCE
Nichols, F., & Zwelling, E. (1997). *Maternal-newborn nursing: Theory and practice.* Philadelphia: W. B. Saunders. pp. 1509–1510.

14. **2**

RATIONALE: The following recommendations have been endorsed by the Infectious Disease Society for Obstetrics–Gynecology for women with a positive history of genital herpes during childbearing. In the absence of genital lesions, vaginal delivery is indicated unless there are other indications for cesarean delivery. With herpetic genital lesions in labor or with ruptured membranes, cesarean delivery can reduce neonatal infection risks. Maternal isolation is not necessary, but potentially exposed neonates should be cultured on the day of delivery.
TEST-TAKING STRATEGY: The nurse's appropriate response is based upon applying the knowledge of the course of transmission of the herpesvirus from an infected mother to the neonate during the childbearing period. Use the process of elimination and this knowledge to answer the question. If you had difficulty with this question, take the time to review this content now.
LEVEL OF COGNITIVE ABILITY: Application
PHASE OF NURSING PROCESS: Planning
CLIENT NEEDS: Health Promotion and Maintenance
CONTENT AREA: Maternity
REFERENCE
Nichols, F., & Zwelling, E. (1997). *Maternal-newborn nursing: Theory and practice.* Philadelphia: W. B. Saunders. pp. 1495–1496.

15. **3**

RATIONALE: During the labor of a woman with a gonococcal infection, ascending infection can occur following the rupture of membranes. Contamination can also occur as the neonate passes through the birth canal. The organism may invade fetal mucosal surfaces such as conjunctiva, rectal mucosa, and pharynx. Erythromycin ophthalmic ointment (0.5%) is an acceptable prophylactic treatment following delivery (1% silver nitrate may also be administered). Options 1, 2, and 4 are incorrect.
TEST-TAKING STRATEGY: This question tests your knowledge of standard nursing protocols of care for all newborns following delivery. The application of knowledge related to the spread of gonococcal infection during the childbearing period is also needed. Knowledge of these areas guides you to eliminate each of the incorrect options. If

you had difficulty with this question, take the time now to review initial care to the newborn.

LEVEL OF COGNITIVE ABILITY: Application
PHASE OF NURSING PROCESS: Implementation
CLIENT NEEDS: Physiological integrity
CONTENT AREA: Maternity
REFERENCE
Lowdermilk, D., Perry S., & Bobak, I. (1997). *Maternity and women's health care* (6th ed.). St. Louis: Mosby–Year Book. p. 1086.

16. **3**

RATIONALE: Vitamin K is administered to the neonate to prevent abnormal bleeding. Newborns are vitamin K deficient because their bowels are sterile. The normal flora in the intestinal tract produces vitamin K. The neonate's bowel does not support the normal production of vitamin K until bacteria adequately colonize it. The bowel becomes colonized by bacteria as food is ingested. Vitamin K is necessary for the body to synthesize coagulation factors. Parenteral administration of vitamin K is a well-substantiated measure to correct the neonate's lag in vitamin K production and prevent hemorrhagic disease of the newborn caused by vitamin K deficiency.
TEST TAKING STRATEGY: A knowledge of the action of vitamin K and the physiology of the gastrointestinal tract is necessary to answer this question. Use the process of elimination. Because jaundice and immunity are not related to the action of vitamin K, options 1 and 2 should be eliminated. Then reread the stem and identify specifically what the question is asking. The issue of the question is about the action of a medication. Note the words "injection" in the question and in the correct option. If you had difficulty with this question, review the purpose of vitamin K injection in the neonate now.
LEVEL OF COGNITIVE ABILITY: Application
PHASE OF NURSING PROCESS: Implementation
CLIENT NEEDS: Physiological Integrity
CONTENT AREA: Maternity
REFERENCE:
Nichols, F., & Zwelling, E. (1997). *Maternal-newborn nursing: Theory and practice.* Philadelphia: W. B. Saunders. pp. 1152, 1141–1142.

17. **3**

RATIONALE: The AIDS infected newborn must be cared for with strict attention to universal standards (precautions). This prevents the transmission of AIDS from the newborn to others and of other infectious agents to the immunocompromised newborn.
TEST-TAKING STRATEGY: Use the process of elimination to answer this question. The client of the question is the newborn; therefore, option 1 can be eliminated because it addresses care to the mother. For the remaining options, note that option 3 is the global option.
LEVEL OF COGNITIVE ABILITY: Comprehension
PHASE OF NURSING PROCESS: Planning
CLIENT NEEDS: Physiological Integrity
CONTENT AREA: Maternity
REFERENCE:
Gorrie, L., McKinney, E., & Murray, S. (1998). *Foundations of maternal-newborn nursing* (2nd ed.). Philadelphia: W. B. Saunders. p. 737.

18. **1**

RATIONALE: Meticulous skin care helps protect the HIV-positive infant from secondary infections. Feeding the in-

fant in an upright position, using a special nipple, and bulging fontanels are unrelated to the pathology associated with HIV.
TEST-TAKING STRATEGY: Read the question carefully. The question specifically asks for instructions to be given to the mother regarding HIV. Although options 2, 3, and 4 may be correct or partially correct in substance, the content does not specifically relate to care to the infant with AIDS.
LEVEL OF COGNITIVE ABILITY: Application
PHASE OF NURSING PROCESS: Planning
CLIENT NEEDS: Safe Effective Care Environment
CONTENT AREA: Maternity
REFERENCE:
Gorrie, L., McKinney, E., & Murray, S. (1998). *Foundations of maternal-newborn nursing* (2nd ed.). Philadelphia: W. B. Saunders. p. 737.

19. **1**

RATIONALE: There is a risk of transmission of AIDS to newborns at delivery when the pregnant woman has AIDS. Newborns may not exhibit symptoms for 18 months or more. Options 2, 3, and 4 are not accurate.
TEST-TAKING STRATEGY: Knowledge regarding the risk of transmission of AIDS to newborns at delivery is necessary to answer this question. Understanding the risk of transmission is an extremely important issue. If you had difficulty answering this question or are unsure of this content area, take the time now to review this material.
LEVEL OF COGNITIVE ABILITY: Comprehension
PHASE OF NURSING PROCESS: Evaluation
CLIENT NEEDS: Health Promotion and Maintenance
CONTENT AREA: Maternity
REFERENCE
Gorrie, L., McKinney, E., & Murray, S. (1998). *Foundations of maternal-newborn nursing* (2nd ed.). Philadelphia: W. B. Saunders. p. 737.

20. **1**

RATIONALE: First priority on admission to the nursery for a newborn with low Apgar scores is airway, which involves preparing respiratory resuscitation equipment. The remaining options are important, although they are of lower priority. Setting up an IV with dextrose in 5% water provides circulatory support. The radiant warmer provides an external heat source that is necessary to prevent further respiratory distress.
TEST-TAKING STRATEGY: Note the key words "highest priority." Remember the ABCs (airway, breathing, and circulation). A method of planning for airway support is to have the resuscitation bag connected to an oxygen source.
LEVEL OF COGNITIVE ABILITY: Application
PHASE OF NURSING PROCESS: Planning
CLIENT NEEDS: Physiological Integrity
CONTENT AREA: Maternity
REFERENCE
Gorrie, L., McKinney, E., & Murray, S. (1998). *Foundations of maternal-newborn nursing* (2nd ed.). Philadelphia: W. B. Saunders. p. 328.

21. **3**

RATIONALE: The most common metabolic complication in the SGA newborn is hypoglycemia, which can produce central nervous system abnormalities and mental retardation if not corrected immediately. Urinary output, although important, is not the highest priority action because the post-term SGA neonate is typically dehydrated due to placental dysfunction. Hemoglobin and hematocrit levels are monitored because the post-term SGA neonate exhibits polycythemia, although this also does not require immediate attention. The polycythemia contributes to increased bilirubin levels, usually beginning on the second day after delivery.

TEST-TAKING STRATEGY: This question asks you to identify the priority nursing action. Knowledge of initial problem in the post-term SGA newborn is also needed to answer this question. Review the SGA newborn content now if you had difficulty with this question.

LEVEL OF COGNITIVE ABILITY: Application
PHASE OF NURSING PROCESS: Planning
CLIENT NEEDS: Physiological Integrity
CONTENT AREA: Maternity
REFERENCE

Gorrie, L., McKinney, E., & Murray, S. (1998). *Foundations of maternal-newborn nursing* (2nd ed.). Philadelphia: W. B. Saunders. p. 837.

22. **3**

RATIONALE: Option 3 describes the characteristics of a preterm (34 weeks) LGA newborn. The weight of 3200 g is above the 90th percentile on an intrauterine growth chart, which is the definitive criterion for the LGA newborn. Option 1 describes a post-term newborn whose weight is within the 10th and 90th percentiles. Options 2 and 4 describe term newborns whose weights are within the 10th and 90th percentiles.

TEST-TAKING STRATEGY: This question asks you to recognize the LGA newborn by weight, gestational age, and description. Options 1, 2, and 4 can be grouped together as not meeting LGA criteria because of the closeness in gestational age and weights. Option 3 can also be compared to option 4, noting that the 200 g weight difference does not equate to a 4-week gestation time span. Use the process of elimination and look at each component in each option to answer the question.

LEVEL OF COGNITIVE ABILITY: Analysis
PHASE OF NURSING PROCESS: Data Collection
CLIENT NEEDS: Physiological Integrity
CONTENT AREA: Maternity
REFERENCE

Reeder, S., Martin, L., & Koniak-Griffin, D. (1997). *Maternity nursing: Family, newborn, and women's health care* (18th ed.). Philadelphia: Lippincott-Raven. pp. 716, 1121–1122.

23. **4**

RATIONALE: Pneumothorax, intraventricular hemorrhage (IVH), patent ductus arteriosus (PDA), and necrotizing enterocolitis (NEC) are complications associated with RDS. Clinical signs of pneumothorax include a sudden rapid deterioration in condition, tachypnea, grunting, pallor, cyanosis, decreased breath sounds in the affected lung, shifting of the cardiac apex away from the affected lung, bradycardia, and hypertension. In IVH the newborn may exhibit a dramatic change in condition, exhibiting apnea, bradycardia, hypotension, seizures, decerebrate posturing, bulging anterior fontanel, and temperature instability. PDA usually presents with a murmur, wide pulse pressures, tachycardia, bounding pulses, signs and symptoms of pulmonary edema, retractions, and rales. Signs found in NEC include lethargy, abdominal distention, temperature instability, retention of feedings, and visible bowel loops.

TEST-TAKING STRATEGY: This question asks you to identify signs and symptoms of potential complications of RDS. Knowledge is required of these complications. Three of the options (1, 2, and 3) can also be grouped together because they each contain normal assessment findings, which leaves option 4 as the correct answer. Additionally, option 4 is the one that identifies respiratory signs.

LEVEL OF COGNITIVE ABILITY: Analysis
PHASE OF NURSING PROCESS: Data Collection
CLIENT NEEDS: Physiological Integrity
CONTENT AREA: Maternity
REFERENCE

Reeder, S., Martin, L., & Koniak-Griffin, D. (1997). *Maternity nursing: Family, newborn, and women's health care* (18th ed.). Philadelphia: Lippincott-Raven. p. 1169.

24. **3**

RATIONALE: To further assess and plan for the newborn's care, the newborn's blood type and direct Coombs' must be known. If the newborn's blood type is Rh negative, or if the newborn's blood type is Rh positive with a negative direct Coombs' test, then there is no concern for Rh incompatibility. If the newborn's blood type is Rh positive and the direct Coombs' is positive, then Rh incompatibility exists. Options 1 and 2 are inappropriate at this time because additional data are needed. Option 4 is incorrect because vitamin K is given to prevent hemorrhagic disease of the newborn.

TEST-TAKING STRATEGY: This question asks you to select the most important plan based on the mother's Rh blood type. Use the nursing process to prioritize and remember data collection is the first step. Additional data are required before any additional nursing plans can be formalized.

LEVEL OF COGNITIVE ABILITY: Application
PHASE OF NURSING PROCESS: Planning
CLIENT NEEDS: Health Promotion and Maintenance
CONTENT AREA: Maternity
REFERENCE

Gorrie, L., McKinney, E., & Murray, S. (1998). *Foundations of maternal-newborn nursing* (2nd ed.). Philadelphia: W. B. Saunders. p. 853.

25. **2**

RATIONALE: Symptoms of infection are moistness, oozing, discharge, and a reddened base. If symptoms of infection occur, the health care provider is notified. Antibiotic treatment is necessary.

TEST-TAKING STRATEGY: Use the process of elimination in answering the question. The word "discharge" in option 2 is the key to indicating infection. Options 1 and 3 are normal signs. Option 4 may suggest signs of infection, but option 2 signifies definite signs of infection. Review the signs and symptoms of infection now if you had difficulty with this question!

LEVEL OF COGNITIVE ABILITY: Application
PHASE OF NURSING PROCESS: Implementation
CLIENT NEEDS: Health Promotion and Maintenance
CONTENT AREA: Maternity
REFERENCE

Nichols, F., & Zwelling, E. (1997). *Maternal-newborn nursing: Theory and practice*. Philadelphia: W. B. Saunders. p. 1147.

BIBLIOGRAPHY

Gorrie, L., McKinney, E., & Murray, S. (1998). *Foundations of maternal-newborn nursing* (2nd ed.). Philadelphia: W. B. Saunders.

Lowdermilk, D., Perry, S., & Bobak, I. (1997). *Maternity & women's health care* (6th ed.). St. Louis: Mosby–Year Book.

Luckmann, J. (1997). *Saunders manual of nursing care.* Philadelphia: W. B. Saunders.

Nichols, F., & Zwelling, E. (1997). *Maternal-newborn nursing: Theory and practice.* Philadelphia: W. B. Saunders.

O'Toole, M. (1997). Miller-Keane *encyclopedia & dictionary of medicine, nursing, & allied health* (6th ed.). Philadelphia: W. B. Saunders.

Reeder, S., Martin, L., & Koniak-Griffin, D. (1997). *Maternity nursing: Family, newborn, and women's health care* (18th ed.). Philadelphia: Lippincott-Raven.

Shulte, E., Price, D., & James, S. (1997). *Thompson's pediatric nursing: An introductory text* (7th ed.). Philadelphia: W. B. Saunders.

CHAPTER 26

Maternity and Newborn Medications

I. Terbutaline sulfate (Brethine)

A. Description
1. Delays premature labor in pregnancies between 20 and 34 weeks
2. Hypokalemia, pulmonary edema, or hypoglycemia may occur if given during labor
3. Hypoglycemia may be noted in the **neonate**

B. Implementation
1. Monitor maternal heart rate, blood pressure, glucose, and fluid status
2. Monitor fetal heart rate (FHR)
3. Monitor uterine contractions for intensity, frequency, and duration
4. Note that contractions may resume when the client is on oral therapy
5. Instruct the client to contact the physician if 4 to 6 contractions/hour occur

II. Ritodrine (Yutopar)

A. Description
1. Uterine relaxant
2. Relaxes uterine muscle and suppresses uterine contractions
3. Used to prolong gestation by inhibiting uterine contractions in preterm **labor**
4. Contraindicated before week 20 of gestation

B. Implementation
1. Monitor vital signs and FHR every 15 minutes
2. Monitor uterine contractions every 15 minutes
3. Monitor for signs of pulmonary edema
4. Potassium and glucose levels are monitored

III. Beractant (Survanta)

A. Description
1. Replenishes surfactant and restores surface activity to the lungs
2. Used to prevent or treat respiratory distress syndrome

B. Implementation
1. Monitor for bradycardia and decreased oxygen saturation during administration
2. Monitor respiratory status and for the presence of rales and moist breath sounds

IV. Betamethasone (Celestone)

A. Description
1. Corticosteroid
2. Used for the client in preterm **labor** to accelerate fetal lung maturity

B. Implementation
1. Decreases mother's resistance to infection
2. Monitor mother for infection
3. Monitor mother's white blood cell (WBC) count
4. Breast-feeding is contraindicated during medication administration
5. Chronic use of the medication during the first trimester may cause cleft palate

V. Ergonovine Maleate (Ergotrate)

A. Description
1. Uterine stimulant—directly stimulates uterine muscle and increases the force and frequency of contractions
2. Produces a firm, tetanic contraction of the uterus
3. Used to prevent or treat postpartum and postabortal hemorrhage due to uterine atony or involution
4. Contraindicated during pregnancy

B. Implementation
1. Not to be used before the **delivery** of the **newborn**
2. Monitor uterine contractions (frequency, strength, and duration) frequently
3. Monitor blood pressure (BP) closely as the medication produces vasoconstriction; if a rise

in BP is noted, the medication is held and the physician is notified
4. Monitor for chest pain, and if it occurs, the physician is notified
5. Assess extremities for color, warmth, movement, or pain
6. Analgesics may be required because the medication produces painful uterine contractions

VI. Methylergonovine (Methergine)

A. Description
   1. Oxytocic
   2. Directly stimulates uterine muscle
   3. Increases strength and frequency of contractions and decreases uterine bleeding
   4. Used to prevent and treat postpartum and postabortal hemorrhage due to uterine atony or involution
   5. Contraindicated during pregnancy
B. Implementation
   1. Monitor maternal vital signs
   2. Assess for uterine bleeding prior to administration
   3. Monitor uterine tone
   4. Assess extremities for color, warmth, movement, or pain
   5. Monitor for chest pain
   6. Monitor for increased cramping or foul-smelling lochia

VII. Oxytocin (Pitocin)

A. Description
   1. Stimulates the smooth muscle of the uterus
   2. Increases the force and frequency of contractions
   3. Enhances milk ejection from the breasts
B. Implementation
   1. Administered by intravenous infusion via an infusion pump to carefully control the rate of flow
   2. Monitor maternal vital signs every 15 to 30 minutes
   3. An internal fetal scalp electrode should be used to monitor for FHR changes
   4. Monitor FHR and uterine activity (frequency, duration, and intensity) every 15 minutes
   5. Administer oxygen if prescribed
   6. Monitor intake and output (I&O) hourly
   7. Monitor for water intoxication as evidenced by nausea, vomiting, or tachycardia
   8. Monitor for hypertonic contractions by palpating uterine contractions that could cause fetal hypoxia, uterine rupture, or abruptio placentae
   9. Use may increase the risk of postpartum hemorrhage owing to hypersensitivity, and the uterus may become atonic when the medication wears off

10. Minimal cervical change is usually noted until the active phase is achieved
11. The physician is notified if contractions last less than 1 minute, occur more frequently than every 2 minutes, or stop
12. The medication is stopped if uterine hyperstimulation or nonreassuring FHR occurs; the client is turned on her side, the IV flow rate is increased, and oxygen via face mask is administered
13. Document the client's response to the medication
14. Keep the family informed of the client's progress
15. Terbutaline or magnesium sulfate should be readily available in case hyperstimulation occurs
16. Breast-feeding is not recommended while the mother is on the medication

VIII. Magnesium Sulfate

A. Description
   1. Anticonvulsant, central nervous system (CNS) depressant, smooth muscle relaxant
   2. Used to prevent and control seizures in preeclamptic and eclamptic client
   3. Used to treat preterm **labor**
B. Implementation
   1. Medication is administered intravenously (IV)
   2. Continuous infusion pump must be used
   3. Deep tendon reflexes are monitored hourly for signs of developing toxicity, because suppressed reflexes may be a sign of impending respiratory arrest
   4. Patellar reflex must be present, and respiratory rate must be greater than 16 breaths/minute during the administration of the medication
   5. Monitor I&O hourly; output should be maintained at 30 mL/hour because the medication is eliminated through the kidneys
   6. The client may complain of flushing, sensation of warmth, or sweating
   7. Monitor vital signs every 30 to 60 minutes, especially respirations
   8. The physician is notified if respirations are less than 12, because this indicates respiratory depression
   9. Magnesium levels are monitored; therapeutic level is 4 to 7 mEq/L
   10. The physician is notified if a rise in the magnesium level occurs (confusion, irregular heartbeat, cramping, unusual tiredness or weakness, light-headedness, or dizziness)
   11. Calcium gluconate (antidote) needs to be available in case of a magnesium sulfate overdose
   12. Continuous IV infusion increases the risk of magnesium toxicity in the **neonate**, and IV

administration should not be used 2 hours preceding delivery
13. Magnesium sulfate is continued for the first 12 to 24 hours postpartum if it is used for preeclampsia

IX. Butorphanol Tartrate (Stadol)

A. Description
1. Exerts an analgesic effect
2. Used to relieve moderate to severe pain associated with **labor**
B. Implementation
1. Used cautiously in clients delivering preterm **infants**
2. Not administered during advanced **labor** if the **neonate** is expected to be delivered before the medication is adequately removed from fetal circulation, because respiratory depression can occur
3. If the woman has a preexisting narcotic dependency, the antagonist effect of the medication will cause her to immediately exhibit symptoms of narcotic withdrawal
4. Monitor fetal heart tones and uterine contractions
5. Not recommended if the client is breast-feeding

X. Meperidine Hydrochloride (Demerol)

A. Description
1. Narcotic analgesic
2. Used to relieve moderate to severe pain associated with **labor**
B. Implementation
1. Used cautiously in clients delivering preterm **infants**
2. Not administered in early **labor** because it may slow the **labor** process
3. Not administered in advanced **labor** if the **neonate** is to be delivered before the medication is adequately removed from the fetal circulation; may cause respiratory depression
4. Should not be administered within 1 hour of delivery because it is circulated to the fetus
5. May cause maternal hypotension; monitor BP
6. Monitor respiratory status; not administered if maternal respirations are depressed
7. May produce nausea when administered alone; therefore, it may be given with promethazine (Phenergan)

XI. Naloxone Hydrochloride (Narcan)

A. Description
1. Narcotic antagonist
2. Prevents or reverses the effects of opioids, including respiratory depression
3. Used to reverse narcotic depression

B. Implementation
1. Maintain patent airway
2. Monitor the heart rate and the depth and rhythm of respirations until the effects of the narcotics wear off
3. Administered cautiously in **newborns** of clients who are known or are suspected to be physically dependent on opioid medications

XII. RhoGAM

A. Description
1. Prevents isoimmunization in Rh-negative clients who are exposed or potentially exposed to Rh-positive red blood cells by transfusion, termination of pregnancy, amniocentesis, chorionic villus sampling (CVS), abdominal trauma, or bleeding during pregnancy or the birth process
2. Prevention of anti-Rh (D) antibody formation is most successful if the medication is administered twice: at 28 weeks of gestation and again within 72 hours after **delivery**
3. Should be administered within 72 hours after potential or actual exposure to Rh-positive blood
4. Must be given with each subsequent exposure or potential exposure to Rh-positive blood
5. Of no benefit once the client has developed a positive antibody titer to the Rh antigen
B. Implementation
1. Side effects are uncommon and mild
2. Temperature may rise slightly
3. Tenderness may occur at the injection site
4. Contraindicated for Rh-positive women
5. Not to be administered to a **newborn**
6. Administered by intramuscular (IM) injection (never administered by IV) within 72 hours after delivery

XIII. Rubella Virus Vaccine

A. Description
1. Induces the production of rubella antibodies to achieve active immunity
2. Used for postpartum clients not immune to rubella
3. Contraindicated in pregnant women
4. Contraindicated in immunosuppressed clients
B. Implementation
1. Monitor the client's prenatal record for rubella status
2. Vaccine will need to be prescribed for clients not demonstrating immunity
3. Educate client about avoiding becoming pregnant for 3 months after receiving vaccine
4. Administration of blood or blood products, including RhoGam, may alter the body's response to vaccine; postpone vaccination until three months after the administration of blood products

5. Obtain documentation of immunity 6 to 8 weeks after vaccination
6. Breast-feeding mothers can be vaccinated

XIV. Silver Nitrate Ophthalmic Solution 1%

A. Description
  1. Used to prevent gonorrheal ophthalmia neonatorum
  2. Does not destroy chlamydia
B. Implementation
  1. Instill 2 drops of 1% solution into each of the **newborn's** eyes within 1 hour after **delivery** if prescribed
  2. Separate the **newborn's** upper and lower lids and place a pool of solution between them
  3. Allow the solution to pool at least 30 seconds, making sure it comes in contact with all areas of the conjunctiva
  4. Remove excess medication to prevent skin discoloration
  5. Use a separate ampule for each eye
  6. Do not irrigate eyes after instilling silver nitrate
  7. Can cause chemical conjunctivitis

XV. Erythromycin Ophthalmic Ointment (0.5% Ilotycin)

A. Description: used prophylactically against gonococcal and chlamydial conjunctivitis in **neonates**
B. Implementation
  1. Instill into each of the neonate's conjunctival sacs within 1 hour after **delivery**
  2. Cleanse the **neonate's** eyes before instilling ointment
  3. Do not flush the eyes after instillation

XVI. Hepatitis B Vaccine

A. Description
  1. Administered at birth, between 1 to 4 months of age, and between 6 to 18 months of age
  2. Contraindicated if sensitivity to vaccine exists, and for those with an allergy to yeast, a severely compromised cardiopulmonary status, a moderate to severe illness, or an immune deficiency condition
B. Implementation
  1. Monitor for fever, and for signs suggesting discomfort or lethargy
  2. Monitor for soreness, induration, redness, swelling, or itching at the injection site

XVII. Vitamin K (AquaMEPHYTON)

A. Description
  1. Used for prophylaxis and to treat hemorrhagic disease of the newborn
  2. Necessary for aiding in the production of active prothrombin

3. **Newborns** are deficient in vitamin K for the first 5 to 8 days of life because of the lack of intestinal flora that are necessary to absorb vitamin K
B. Implementation
  1. Administer during the early neonatal period
  2. Protect the medication from light
  3. Monitor for jaundice, and monitor bilirubin level because the medication can cause hyperbilirubinemia in the **newborn**
  4. Monitor for bruising at the injection site and for bleeding from the cord
  5. Administer in the vastus lateralis muscle of the thigh, in the lateral aspect of the anterior portion

PRACTICE QUESTIONS

1. Butorphanol tartrate (Stadol) is prescribed for the client. The nurse may safely administer this medication to the laboring woman
   1 Anytime during labor
   2 Up to 15 minutes before anticipated delivery
   3 Up to 30 minutes before anticipated delivery
   4 Up to 2 to 3 hours before anticipated delivery

2. When epidural analgesia is given to a woman for pain relief after a cesarean birth, the nurse plans to have which of the following medications readily available for the immediate reversal of respiratory depression?
   1 Betamethasone (Celestone)
   2 Morphine sulfate
   3 Meperidine hydrochloride (Demerol)
   4 Naloxone hydrochloride (Narcan)

3. After delivery, a woman is determined to be a candidate for a RhoGAM [anti-Rh$_o$(D) gamma globulin] injection. The nurse determines that the teaching the client received about the purpose of RhoGAM was effective, when the client states that RhoGAM will protect her next baby from which of the following?
   1 Being affected by Rh incompatibility
   2 Having Rh-positive blood
   3 Developing a rubella infection
   4 Developing physiological jaundice

4. A woman is to receive ergonovine maleate (Methergine) by mouth during the first and second postpartum days. Before administering ergonovine, it is most important to check the woman's
   1 Lochia
   2 Blood pressure
   3 Deep tendon reflexes
   4 Uterine tone

5. A woman was admitted to the hospital in preterm labor at 32 weeks' gestation. The expectant parents are very anxious and fearful about giving birth to a premature infant. The nurse realizes

that the couple's coping may be assisted by explaining to them that upon admission the expectant mother received an injection of betamethasone (Celestone) that will

1 Stop the premature uterine contractions
2 Delay delivery for at least 48 hours
3 Enhance fetal lung maturity
4 Prevent premature closure of the ductus arteriosus

6. A client is to receive a rubella vaccine on the second postpartum day. Included in the teaching plan are the potential risks of the vaccine. Based on these risks, the nurse reinforces teaching and cautions the client to avoid

1 Sunlight for 3 days
2 Scratching the injection site
3 Pregnancy for 2 to 3 months after the vaccination
4 Sexual intercourse for 2 to 3 months after the vaccination

7. The nurse is assisting in caring for a client receiving oxytocin (Pitocin) for the induction of labor. The nurse monitors the client, knowing that the medication will be immediately discontinued if which one of the following occurs?

1 Severe drowsiness
2 Uterine atony
3 Fetal heart rate (FHR) of 140 bpm
4 Uterine hyperstimulation

8. A pregnant teenager is receiving magnesium sulfate therapy for the management of preeclampsia. The nurse assisting in caring for the client identifies that the client has developed an unwanted outcome of magnesium toxicity when which of the following is noted?

1 Deep tendon reflexes $+^{3/4}$
2 Serum magnesium level of 6 mEq/L
3 Proteinuria of + 3
4 Respirations of 10/minute

9. A new mother tells the nurse that the hepatitis B vaccine was administered to her newborn. The mother asks the nurse about the immunization schedule for this vaccine. The nurse responds, knowing that the vaccine will

1 Not be required once the initial dose is given
2 Be administered between 1 and 4 months of age, and between 6 and 18 months of age
3 Be administered at the onset of puberty
4 Be administered at 1 year of age

10. A preeclamptic woman is receiving magnesium sulfate intravenously. The nurse assisting in caring for the client determines that the magnesium sulfate therapy is effective if

1 Ankle clonus is noted
2 Blood pressure is decreased
3 Eclampsia is prevented
4 Scotomas are present

ANSWERS

1. **4**

RATIONALE: Parenteral analgesics can be administered during the first stage of labor, up to 2 to 3 hours before the anticipated delivery. If given after this point in labor, the neonate may be born with respiratory depression because of placental exchange of the medication.
TEST-TAKING STRATEGY: Knowledge of the stage of labor, placental exchange of medication, and the effect on the neonate is necessary to answer the question. Recall that many medications are administered according to stages of labor and estimated delivery time. Review this medication now if you had difficulty with this question.
LEVEL OF COGNITIVE ABILITY: Application
PHASE OF NURSING PROCESS: Implementation
CLIENT NEEDS: Physiological Integrity
CONTENT AREA: Maternity
REFERENCE
Burroughs, A. (1997). *Maternity nursing: An introductory text* (7th ed.). Philadelphia: W. B. Saunders. p. 214.

2. **4**

RATIONALE: Naloxone hydrochloride is a narcotic antagonist that reverses the effects of narcotics and is administered to the client if prescribed if respirations fall below 6 to 8 per minute. Morphine and Demerol are narcotics.

Celestone is a steroid that may be administered to enhance fetal lung maturity.
TEST-TAKING STRATEGY: Knowledge of the action and use of naloxone hydrochloride is required to answer this question. Review this medication now if you had difficulty with this question.
LEVEL OF COGNITIVE ABILITY: Comprehension
PHASE OF NURSING PROCESS: Planning
CLIENT NEEDS: Physiological Integrity
CONTENT AREA: Maternity
REFERENCE
Hodgson, B., & Kizior, R. (1999). *Saunders nursing drug handbook 1999*. Philadelphia: W. B. Saunders. pp. 719–721.

3. **1**

RATIONALE: Rh incompatibility can occur when an Rh-negative mother becomes sensitized to the Rh antigen. Sensitization may develop when an Rh-negative woman becomes pregnant with a fetus who is Rh positive. During pregnancy and at delivery, some of the baby's Rh-positive blood can enter the maternal circulation, causing the woman's immune system to form antibodies against Rh-positive blood. Administration of RhoGAM prevents the woman from developing antibodies against Rh-positive blood by providing passive antibody protection against the Rh antigen.
TEST-TAKING STRATEGY: A knowledge of Rh incompatibility will assist in answering this question. If the words "anti-Rh$_o$(D) gamma globulin" are unfamiliar, try to figure out the meaning by breaking down the words using medical

terminology. Select a response that has similarity to a thought in the question. In this case "anti-$Rh_o(D)$ gamma globulin" indicates an immune response which is similar to "Rh incompatibility" found in option 1. Review this medication now if you had difficulty with this question.
LEVEL OF COGNITIVE ABILITY: Comprehension
PHASE OF NURSING PROCESS: Evaluation
CLIENT NEEDS: Health Promotion and Maintenance
CONTENT AREA: Maternity
REFERENCE
Burroughs, A. (1997). *Maternity nursing: An introductory text* (7th ed.). Philadelphia: W. B. Saunders. p. 375.

4. 2

RATIONALE: Ergonovine is a medication that is used to prevent or control postpartum hemorrhage by contracting the uterus. It causes constant uterine contractions and may elevate blood pressure. Although uterine contractions and bleeding are monitored, a priority action before the administration of ergonovine, and during administration is to check the blood pressure.
TEST-TAKING STRATEGY: Use the ABCs, airway, breathing, and circulation. Blood pressure is a method of determining circulation. Lochia and uterine tone are similar distracters because they are directly related to one another. Deep tendon reflexes are monitored when magnesium sulfate is administered. Review this medication now if you had difficulty with this question.
LEVEL OF COGNITIVE ABILITY: Application
PHASE OF NURSING PROCESS: Data Collection
CLIENT NEEDS: Physiological Integrity
CONTENT AREA: Maternity
REFERENCE
Hodgson, B., & Kizior, R. (1999). *Saunders nursing drug handbook 1999.* Philadelphia: W. B. Saunders. p. 664.

5. 3

RATIONALE: Betamethasone, a corticosteroid, is given to increase the surfactant level and increase lung maturity reducing the incidence of respiratory distress syndrome. Surfactant production does not become stable until after 32 weeks' gestation and if adequate amounts of surfactant are not present in the lungs, respiratory distress and death are a possible consequence. Delivery of the baby needs to be delayed for at least 48 hours after administration of betamethasone in order to allow time for the lungs to mature. By discussing betamethasone with the parents, the nurse may alleviate some of their anxieties and fears.
TEST-TAKING STRATEGY: Recalling that respiratory distress syndrome caused by immature lungs is a major problem of prematurity, and therefore a major concern for the expectant parents, will assist in directing you to the correct option. Review the action of this medication now if you had difficulty with this question.
LEVEL OF COGNITIVE ABILITY: Comprehension
PHASE OF NURSING PROCESS: Implementation
CLIENT NEEDS: Psychosocial Integrity
CONTENT AREA: Maternity
REFERENCE
Burroughs, A. (1997). *Maternity nursing: An introductory text* (7th ed). Philadelphia: W. B. Saunders. p. 404.

6. 3

RATIONALE: Because rubella vaccine is a live vaccine, it will act as the virus and is potentially teratogenic to the fetus. The client needs to be informed about the potential effects that this vaccine may have and the need to avoid becoming pregnant for a period of 2 to 3 months afterward. Abstinence from sexual intercourse is not necessary, unless another form of effective contraception is not being used. The vaccine may cause local or systemic reactions, but all are mild and short lived. Sunlight has no effect on the person who is vaccinated.
TEST-TAKING STRATEGY: Recalling that most vaccinations are either contraindicated or given with caution during pregnancy will assist in directing you to the correct option. Review the contraindications and cautions associated with this vaccine now if you had difficulty with this question.
LEVEL OF COGNITIVE ABILITY: Application
PHASE OF NURSING PROCESS: Implementation
CLIENT NEEDS: Physiological Integrity
CONTENT AREA: Maternity
REFERENCE
Eckler, J., & Fair, J. (1996). *Pharmacology essentials.* Philadelphia: W. B. Saunders. p. 149.

7. 4

RATIONALE: Oxytocin is a synthetic hormone that stimulates uterine contractions and is one of the common pharmacological methods to induce labor. A major danger associated with oxytocin induction of labor is hyperstimulation of uterine contractions. Fetal distress may occur when the uterus is hyperstimulated due to decreased placental perfusion. Therefore, oxytocin infusion must be stopped when there are any signs of uterine hyperstimulation. Options 1, 2, and 3 are not indications of the need to discontinue the infusion. The normal FHR is 120 to 160 bpm.
TEST-TAKING STRATEGY: Focus on the action of the medication and the key words "immediately discontinued" to assist in directing you to option 4. If you had difficulty with this question, take time now to review this medication.
LEVEL OF COGNITIVE ABILITY: Comprehension
PHASE OF NURSING PROCESS: Data Collection
CLIENT NEEDS: Physiological Integrity
CONTENT AREA: Maternity
REFERENCE
Burroughs, A. (1997). *Maternity nursing: An introductory text* (7th ed). Philadelphia: W. B. Saunders. pp. 144, 412.

8. 4

RATIONALE: Magnesium toxicity is a danger of magnesium sulfate therapy. Signs of magnesium sulfate toxicity are related to the central nervous system (CNS) depressant effects of the medication and include respiratory depression, loss of deep tendon reflexes, sudden drop in FHR, and/or maternal heart rate and blood pressure. Proteinuria is associated with pregnancy-induced hypertension. Therapeutic serum levels of magnesium are 4 to 7 mEq/L.
TEST-TAKING STRATEGY: Use the process of elimination. Recalling that magnesium sulfate is a CNS depressant will easily direct you to option 4. Review this medication now if you had difficulty with this question.
LEVEL OF COGNITIVE ABILITY: Comprehension
PHASE OF NURSING PROCESS: Data Collection
CLIENT NEEDS: Physiological Integrity
CONTENT AREA: Maternity
REFERENCE
Burroughs, A. (1997). *Maternity nursing: An introductory text* (7th ed.). Philadelphia: W. B. Saunders. p. 360.

9. 2

RATIONALE: Hepatitis B vaccine is administered in three doses. The first dose is administered at birth, the second dose is administered between 1 and 4 months of age, and the third dose is administered between 6 and 18 months of age.
TEST-TAKING STRATEGY: Recalling that the hepatitis B vaccine is administered in three doses will easily direct you to option 2. If you are unfamiliar with the schedule for the administration of this vaccine, take time now to review.
LEVEL OF COGNITIVE ABILITY: Comprehension
PHASE OF NURSING PROCESS: Implementation
CLIENT NEEDS: Health Promotion and Maintenance
CONTENT AREA: Maternity
REFERENCE
Hodgson, B., & Kizior, R. (1999). *Saunders nursing drug handbook 1999*. Philadelphia: W. B. Saunders. p. 1157.

10. 3

RATIONALE: When caring for a client with preeclampsia, the goal of care is directed at preventing eclampsia (sei-zures). Magnesium sulfate is an anticonvulsant; it is not an antihypertensive agent. Although a decrease in blood pressure may be noted initially, this effect is usually transient. Ankle clonus indicates hyperreflexia and may precede the onset of eclampsia. Scotomas are areas of complete or partial blindness. Visual disturbances, such as scotomas, often precede an eclamptic convulsion.
TEST-TAKING STRATEGY: Focus on the issue of the question, that the magnesium sulfate therapy is effective. Knowing that magnesium sulfate is an anticonvulsant or that avoiding eclamptic seizures is a desired outcome of therapy will direct you to the correct option. Review this medication now if you had difficulty with this question.
LEVEL OF COGNITIVE ABILITY: Analysis
PHASE OF NURSING PROCESS: Evaluation
CLIENT NEEDS: Physiological Integrity
CONTENT AREA: Maternity
REFERENCE
Burroughs, A. (1997). *Maternity nursing: An introductory text* (7th ed.). Philadelphia: W. B. Saunders. p. 360.

BIBLIOGRAPHY

Burroughs, A. (1997). *Maternity nursing: An introductory text* (7th ed.). Philadelphia: W. B. Saunders.
Eckler, J., & Fair, J. (1996). *Pharmacology essentials*. Philadelphia: W. B. Saunders.
Hodgson, B., & Kizior, R. (1999). *Saunders nursing drug handbook 1999*. Philadelphia: W. B. Saunders.
Lehne, R. (1998). *Pharmacology for nursing care* (3rd ed.). Philadelphia: W. B. Saunders.
Leifer, G. (1999). *Thompson's introduction to maternity and pediatric nursing* (3rd ed.). Philadelphia: W. B. Saunders.
O'Toole, M. (Ed.). (1997). *Miller-Keane encyclopedia & dictionary of medicine, nursing, & allied health* (6th ed.). Philadelphia: W. B. Saunders.

UNIT VII

....

Pediatric Nursing

PYRAMID TERMS

Abuse—Includes nonaccidental physical injury or the nonaccidental act of omission by a parent or person responsible for the care of the child.

Active Immunity—The protection that can last months, years, or even a lifetime that forms in response to exposure to antigens in nature or vaccines.

Atresia—Congenital absence or closure of a body orifice.

Attenuated Vaccines—Vaccines derived from microorganisms or viruses whose virulence has been weakened due to passage through another host.

Cephalocaudal—Growth and development that proceeds from head to toe.

Chronological Age—Age in years.

Developmental Age—Age based on functional behavior and ability to adapt to the environment. It does not necessarily correspond to chronological age.

Functional Age—The age equivalent at which the child is actually able to perform specific self-care or related tasks.

Growth—Measurable physical and physiological changes that occur over time.

Growth Spurts—Brief periods of rapid increase in growth rate.

Hereditary—The transmission of genetic characteristics from parent to offspring.

Inactivated Vaccines—Vaccines that contain killed microorganisms.

Intelligence—What an individual can do relative to learning, thinking, and problem solving.

Learning—Behavior changes that occur as a result of both maturation and experience with the environment.

Nasal Flaring—A serious sign of air hunger. A widening of the nares to enable the child to take in more oxygen.

Passive Immunity—Antibody transfer from a person with active immunity to a person who does not have that antibody.

Puberty—The period of time during which the adolescent experiences a growth spurt, develops secondary sex characteristics, and achieves reproductive maturity.

Regression—Behavior that is more appropriate to an earlier stage of development and is often used to cope with stress or anxiety.

Regurgitation—An abnormal backward flow of body fluid.

Retractions—An abnormal movement of the chest wall during inspiration.

Separation Anxiety—Distress and apprehension caused by being removed from parents, home, or familiar surroundings.

Shunt—Abnormal blood flow from one side of the heart to the other.

Stenosis—The narrowing or constriction of an opening.

Stridor—A shrill harsh sound heard during inspiration or expiration, or both, that is produced by the flow of air through a narrowed segment of the respiratory tract.

Wheezing—High-pitched musical whistles heard with or without a stethoscope.

◆ PYRAMID TO SUCCESS

Pyramid points focus on the stages of growth and development. Growth and development includes physical characteristics, nutritional behaviors, skills, play, and specific safety measures relevant to a particular age group. Pyramid points focus on safety and the age-appropriate measures to ensure a safe and hazard-free environment for the child. Additional pyramid points focus on acute disorders that can occur in children. Focus on specific feeding techniques, positioning techniques, and interventions that will provide and maintain adequate airway, breathing, and circulation patterns in the child. On NCLEX-PN, be alert to the age of the child, if the age is presented in a question.

NURSING PROCESS

DATA COLLECTION

- Vital signs
- Age and developmental status
- Routines and rituals
- Family process and unit
- Cultural and religious patterns
- Nutritional intake
- Feeding patterns
- Patterns of urinary and bowel elimination
- Sleep patterns
- Diversional activities

PLANNING	IMPLEMENTATION	EVALUATION
The child's nutritional intake will meet the metabolic needs for the age group.	Identify current nutritional status and compare to age-appropriate requirements. Obtain height and weight. Identify cultural and religious dietary needs. Identify favorite foods and eating rituals. Allow child to select food if appropriate. Offer frequent snacks and small meal portions using small utensils. Allow the child to eat with other children if parents are not present. Encourage the parents to bring food in from home if appropriate.	The child maintains appropriate nutritional intake. The child maintains body weight during hospitalization.
PLANNING	IMPLEMENTATION	EVALUATION
The child will participate in age-appropriate feeding, dressing, toileting, and bathing.	Offer choices and involve the child in care when appropriate.	The child performs activities that maintain independence as much as possible.
PLANNING	IMPLEMENTATION	EVALUATION
The child will maintain a balance of sleep and activity.	Determine the child's usual sleep routines. Plan care to allow time for periods of sleep.	The child takes naps and sleeps an appropriate amount of time based on age requirements.
PLANNING	IMPLEMENTATION	EVALUATION
Parents participate in the care of the child.	Prepare for all procedures and encourage parents to stay with the child as much as possible. Provide the parents with information about support systems. Teach the child, if appropriate, or parents about prescribed medications or other treatments required after discharge.	Family support is available and parents seek resources when necessary.
PLANNING	IMPLEMENTATION	EVALUATION
The child will maintain current level of development.	Follow home routines as much as possible. Identify normal urinary and bowel elimination patterns. Follow home routines of elimination if possible. Do not scold the child if incontinent.	The child maintains the appropriate level of growth and development. The child maintains age-appropriate and condition-appropriate self-care.
PLANNING	IMPLEMENTATION	EVALUATION
The child becomes involved in play activities.	Provide a safe environment for the child. Provide play activities based on the child's developmental level. Encourage the parents to bring in a favorite toy. Introduce the child to other children on the unit. Encourage peer contact if appropriate.	The child plays and communicates with others.

PLANNING	IMPLEMENTATION	EVALUATION
The child will display decreased signs of distress if any are present.	Orient the child and parents to the hospital and routines. Provide opportunities for the child to express his or her feelings. Provide a consistent caregiver as much as possible.	The child separates from the parents in an appropriate manner during hospitalization.

◣ CLIENT NEEDS

SAFE, EFFECTIVE CARE ENVIRONMENT

Parent and child rights
Confidentiality
Informed consent in regard to minors
Continuity of care
Protective measures
Accident prevention
Environmental and personal safety related to the developmental age of the child
Spread and control of infectious agents, particularly with regard to communicable diseases

HEALTH PROMOTION AND MAINTENANCE

Developmental stages
Family interaction patterns
Disease prevention
Health promotion programs
Immunizations
Communicable diseases
Instructions to the child and parents regarding care at home
Protection of the child and other contacts to prevent illness

PSYCHOSOCIAL INTEGRITY

Play
Communication
Cultural, religious, and spiritual differences
Family and support systems
Child abuse and neglect

PHYSIOLOGICAL INTEGRITY

Age-appropriate normal body structure and function
Elimination
Nutrition
Rest and sleep
Medication administration
Comfort measures
Intrusive procedures
Responses to therapies

BIBLIOGRAPHY

Ashwill, J., & Droske, S. (1997). *Nursing care of children: Principles and practice*. Philadelphia: W. B. Saunders.

Burroughs, A. (1997). *Maternity nursing: An introductory text* (7th ed.). Philadelphia: W. B. Saunders.

Hill, S., & Howlett, H. (1997). *Success in practical nursing: Personal and vocational issues* (3rd ed.). Philadelphia: W. B. Saunders.

Leifer, G. (1999). *Thompson's introduction to maternity and pediatric nursing* (3rd ed.). Philadelphia: W. B. Saunders.

Luckmann, J. (1997). *Saunders manual of nursing care*. Philadelphia: W. B. Saunders.

National Council of State Boards of Nursing (1998). *National Council detailed test plan for the NCLEX-PN examination*. Chicago: Author.

Nichols, F., & Zwelling, E. (1997). *Maternal-newborn nursing: Theory and practice*. Philadelphia: W. B. Saunders.

O'Toole, M. (ed.). (1997). *Miller-Keane encyclopedia & dictionary of medicine, nursing, & allied health* (6th ed.). Philadelphia: W. B. Saunders.

Schulte, E., Price, D., & James, S. (1997). *Thompson's pediatric nursing: An introductory text* (7th ed.). Philadelphia: W. B. Saunders.

CHAPTER 27

Growth and Development

I. The Hospitalized Infant and Toddler

A. Separation anxiety
   1. Protest
      a. Cries, screams, searches for parent, and avoids and rejects contact with strangers
      b. Physical fighting; kicks, fights, hits, and pinches
   2. Despair
      a. Withdrawn, depressed, and disinterested in the environment
      b. Loss of newly learned skills
   3. Detachment
      a. If the separation from the parent continues, the child enters the detachment phase
      b. During the detachment phase, the child again becomes interested in the environment and begins to play
      c. If the parents return during this stage, the child may ignore them and the parents may think that the child does not want to see them
      d. This reaction is a coping mechanism that the child uses to protect self from further emotional pain related to separation
B. Fear of injury and pain: Affected by previous experiences, separation from parents, and preparation for the experience
C. Loss of control
   1. Hospitalization with its own set of rituals and routines can severely disrupt the life of a toddler
   2. The lack of control is often exhibited in behaviors related to feeding, toileting, playing, and bedtime
   3. The toddler may demonstrate **regression**
D. Implementation
   1. Provide swaddling and talk softly to the infant
   2. Provide opportunities for sucking and oral stimulation for the infant using a pacifier if the infant is NPO
   3. Provide stimulation if appropriate for the infant using contrasting colors and textures
   4. Provide routines and rituals as close as possible to what the toddler is used to at home
   5. Provide choices as much as possible to the toddler to provide some control
   6. Approach the toddler with a positive attitude
   7. Allow the toddler to express feelings of protest
   8. Encourage toddlers to talk about parents or others in their lives
   9. Accept regressive behavior without ridiculing the toddler
   10. Provide the toddler with favorite and comforting objects
   11. Allow toddlers as much mobility as possible
   12. Anticipate temper tantrums and maintain a safe environment for physical acting out
   13. Employ pain-reduction techniques as appropriate

II. The Hospitalized Preschooler

A. Separation anxiety
   1. Generally less obvious and less serious than in the toddler
   2. As stress increases, the preschooler's ability to separate from the parents decreases
   3. Protest
      a. Less direct and aggressive than the toddler
      b. May displace feelings on others
   4. Despair
      a. Similar to the toddler
      b. Quietly withdrawn, depressed, and disinterested in the environment
      c. Loss of newly learned skills

     d. The child becomes generally uncooperative, refusing to eat or take medication

     e. The child repeatedly asks when the parents will be visiting

  5. Detachment: same response as seen with the hospitalized toddler

B. Fear of injury and pain
  1. The preschooler has a general lack of understanding of body integrity
  2. Fears invasive procedures and mutilation
  3. Imagine things to be much worse than they are
  4. Preschoolers believe that they are ill because of something they did or thought

C. Loss of control
  1. Likes familiar routines and rituals and may show **regression** if not allowed to maintain some control
  2. Has attained a good deal of independence and self-care at home and may expect that to continue in the hospital

D. Implementation
  1. Provide a safe and secure environment
  2. Take time for communication
  3. Allow the child to express anger
  4. Acknowledge fears and anxieties
  5. Accept regressive behavior
  6. Assist the child in moving from regressive to appropriate behaviors according to age
  7. Encourage rooming-in or leave favorite toy
  8. Allow mobility
  9. Provide play and diversional activities
  10. Place the child with other children of the same age if possible
  11. Encourage the child to be independent
  12. Explain procedures simply on the child's level
  13. Avoid intrusive procedures when possible
  14. Allow the child to wear underpants
  15. Employ appropriate interventions to relieve pain

III. The Hospitalized School-Aged Child

A. Separation anxiety
  1. Accustomed to periods of separation from the parents but as stressors are added the separation becomes more difficult
  2. More concerned with missing school and the fear that their friends will forget them
  3. The stages of behavior of protest, despair, and detachment are not usually evident in the school-aged child

B. Fear of injury and pain
  1. Fear bodily injury and pain
  2. Fear of illness itself, disability, death, and intrusive procedures in genital areas
  3. Uncomfortable with any type of sexual exam
  4. Groans or whines, holds rigidly still, communicates about pain

C. Loss of control
  1. Usually highly social, independent, and involved with activities
  2. Seek information
  3. Ask relevant questions about tests and procedures and their illness
  4. Associate their actions as the cause of the illness
  5. May feel helpless and dependent if physical limitations occur

D. Implementation
  1. Encourage rooming-in
  2. Focus on the child's abilities and needs
  3. Encourage the child to become involved with own care
  4. Accept regression but encourage independence
  5. Provide choices to the child
  6. Allow expression of feelings both verbally and nonverbally
  7. Acknowledge fears and concerns and allow for discussion
  8. Explain all procedures using body diagrams or outlines
  9. Provide privacy
  10. Avoid intrusive procedures if possible
  11. Allow the child to wear underpants
  12. Involve the child in activities appropriate to developmental level and physical condition
  13. Provide individualized recreation
  14. Encourage the child to contact friends
  15. Provide for educational needs
  16. Employ appropriate interventions to relieve pain

IV. The Hospitalized Adolescent

A. Separation anxiety
  1. Not sure whether they want their parents with them when they are hospitalized
  2. Separation from friends is a source of anxiety
  3. Become upset if friends go on with their lives, excluding them

B. Fear of injury and pain
  1. Fear of being different from others and their peers
  2. May give the impression that they are not afraid even though they are terrified
  3. Become guarded when any areas related to sexual development are examined

C. Loss of control
  1. Behaviors exhibited include anger, withdrawal, and uncooperativeness
  2. Seek help and then reject it

D. Implementation
  1. Encourage questions about appearance and effects of illness on future
  2. Explore feelings about the hospital and significance the illness might have on relationships
  3. Encourage to wear own clothes and perform normal grooming

4. Allow favorite foods to be brought in if possible
5. Provide privacy
6. Use medical terminology and body diagrams to prepare for procedures
7. Introduce to other adolescents on the unit
8. Encourage maintaining contact with peer groups
9. Provide for educational needs
10. Help develop positive coping mechanisms
11. Employ appropriate interventions to relieve pain

V. Communication Approaches

A. General guidelines
1. Allow the child to feel comfortable with you
2. Communicate through the use of objects
3. Allow the child to express fears and concerns
4. Speak clearly in a quiet, unhurried voice
5. Offer choices when possible
6. Be honest with the child
7. Set limits with the child as appropriate
8. Communicate with the child based on the child's level of growth and development
B. Infants
1. Infants respond to nonverbal communication behaviors of adults such as holding, rocking, patting, and touch
2. Use a slow approach and allow the infant to get to know you
3. Use a calm, soft, soothing voice
4. Be responsive to cries
5. Talk and read to infants
6. Allow security objects such as blankets and pacifiers if the infant has them
C. Toddlers
1. Approach the toddler cautiously
2. Remember that toddlers accept verbal communications of others literally
3. Learn the toddler's words for common items and use them in conversations
4. Use short, concrete terms
5. Prepare toddlers for procedures immediately prior to the event
6. Repeat explanations and descriptions
7. Use play and visual aids such as picture books, puppets, and dolls for demonstrations
8. Allow the toddler to handle instruments
9. Explain what the instrument does and how it feels
10. Encourage the use of comfort objects
D. Preschooler
1. Seek opportunities to offer choices
2. Speak in simple sentences
3. Be concise and limit the length of explanations
4. Allow to ask questions
5. Describe procedures as they are about to be performed
6. Use play to explain procedures and activities

7. Allow to handle the equipment, which will ease fear and help to answer questions
8. Reinforce that procedures are not a form of punishment
E. School-aged child
1. Establish limits
2. Provide reassurance to help in alleviating fears and anxieties
3. Engage in conversations that encourage thinking
4. Use medical play techniques
5. Use photographs, books, teaching dolls, and videos to explain procedures
6. Explain in clear terms
7. Allow time for composure and privacy
F. The adolescent
1. Remember that the adolescent may be preoccupied with body image
2. Encourage and support independence
3. Provide privacy and confidentiality
4. Use photographs, book, and videos to explain procedures
5. Engage in conversations about adolescent interests
6. Avoid becoming too abstract, too detailed, and too technical
7. Avoid responding to less than desirable social behaviors by prying, confrontation, or judgmental attitudes

VI. Developmental Characteristics

A. The infant
1. Physical
   a. Height increases by 3/4 inch per month
   b. Weight is doubled at 5 to 6 months and tripled at 12 months
   c. At birth, the head circumference is 2 cm greater than the chest circumference
   d. Posterior fontanel closes by 2 to 3 months
   e. Lower central incisors present by 6 to 8 months
   f. Reflexes such as rooting, tonic neck, palmar grasp, moro, and stepping disappear by 4 months of age, with sucking lasting through infancy
   g. Sleeps most of the time
2. Vital signs (Table 27–1)

Table 27–1. **Vital Signs**

Infant	1 Year Old
Temperature: axillary 96.8°–99°F	Temperature: axillary 96.8°–99°F
Apical rate: 120–160 beats/minute	Apical rate: 80–160 beats/minute
Respirations: 30–60 breaths/minute	Respirations: 20–40 breaths/minute
Blood pressure: 46–92/38–71 mmHg	Blood pressure: 96/65 mmHg

3. Nutrition
   a. The infant may breast- or bottle-feed depending on the mother's choice
   b. Calorie requirements are 650 kcal/day (1–6 months) and 850 kcal/day (6–12 months)
   c. Give no more than 30 oz of formula per day
   d. Iron stores from birth are depleted by 4 months
   e. Do not give skim milk; fatty acids are required
   f. Introduce solids at approximately 4 to 6 months of age
   g. Introduction of foods should be one at a time, with the sequence as follows: rice cereal; fruits and vegetables starting with yellow and then green; meats; and then egg yolks, avoiding egg whites
   h. Avoid nuts, foods with seeds, raisins, and popcorn
   i. Never mix food and/or medications with formula
   j. Avoid honey or syrup in milk or water to prevent botulism
   k. By 12 to 14 months, the child should drink from a cup
4. Skills (Table 27–2)
5. Play
   a. Solitary
   b. Birth to 3 months: verbal, visual, and tactile stimuli
   c. 4 to 6 months: initiates actions and recognizes new experiences
   d. 6 to 12 months: aware of self, imitates, repeats pleasurable actions
   e. Enjoys soft stuffed animals, crib mobiles with contrasting colors, squeeze toys, rattles, musical toys, water toys during the bath, large picture books, and push toys after beginning to walk
6. Safety
   a. Baby-proof home
   b. Infants who weigh up to 20 lb should be restrained in a car seat in the middle backseat in a semireclined, rear-facing position
   c. Use safety straps for infant seats
   d. Guard the infant when on the bed or changing table
   e. Use gates to protect the infant from stairs
   f. Never shake or vigorously jiggle a baby's head
   g. Be sure that bath water is not hot
   h. Do not leave unattended in bath
   i. Do not hold the infant while drinking or working near hot liquids
   j. Cool vaporizers should be used instead of steam to prevent burn injuries
   k. Avoid food that is round and similar to the size of the airway to prevent choking
   l. Be sure toys have no small pieces
   m. Hanging toys or mobiles over the crib should be well out of reach to prevent strangulation
   n. Avoid placing large toys in the crib as an older infant may use them as steps to climb
   o. Cribs should be positioned away from curtain and blind cords
   p. Cover electrical outlets
   q. Remove hazardous objects from low places
   r. Remove chemicals, poisons, and plants from the infant's reach
   s. Keep syrup of ipecac and poison control telephone number available
B. The toddler
1. Physical
   a. Height and weight increase in a steplike fashion reflecting **growth spurts** and lags
   b. Head circumference increases about 1 inch between ages 1 and 2; thereafter, head circumference increases about ½ inch per year until age 5
   c. By 1 to 2 years of age, measurement of head circumference and chest circumference is equal
   d. Anterior fontanel closes between 12 to 18 months
   e. Ten upper and 10 lower deciduous teeth by 1 to 2 years of age
   f. Weight changes are slower than in infancy by about 4 to 6 lb per year; by age 2, the average weight is 27 lb
   g. Normal height changes include a **growth** of about 3 inches per year; the average height of the toddler is 34 inches at age 2 years
   h. Lordosis is evident with a "potbelly"

Table 27–2. Infant Skills

2–3 Months	8–9 Months
Smiles	Sits steadily unsupported
Turns head side to side	Crawls
Cries	May stand while holding on
Follows objects	Begins to stand without help
Holds head in midline	**10–11 Months**
4–5 Months	Can change from prone to sitting position
Grasps objects	Walks holding on to furniture
Switches objects from hands	Stands securely
Rolls over for the first time	Entertains self for periods of time
Enjoys social interaction	**12–13 Months**
Begins to show memory	Walks with one hand held
Aware of unfamiliar surroundings	Can take a few steps without falling
6–7 Months	**14–15 Months**
Creeps	Walks alone
Sits with support	Can crawl upstairs
Imitates	Shows emotions as anger and affection
Exhibits fear of strangers	Will explore away from mother in familiar surroundings
Holds arms out	
Frequent mood swings	
Waves bye-bye	

i. Should begin brushing teeth with a small soft-bristle toothbrush around age 2, with dentist visits beginning around age 2½

j. Typically sleeps through the night and has one daytime nap and discontinues the daytime nap at about age 3

k. A consistent bedtime ritual helps prepare the toddler for sleep

l. Security objects at bedtime may assist in sleep

2. Vital signs (Box 27–1)
3. Nutrition
   a. Calorie requirements are 1300 kcal/day
   b. Most toddlers prefer to feed themselves
   c. The toddler generally does best by eating several small nutritious meals each day rather than three large meals
   d. Offer a limited number of foods at any one time
   e. Limit concentrated sweets and empty calories
   f. At risk for aspiration of small foods that are not easily chewed, such as peanuts and popcorn
   g. Physiological anorexia is normal owing to the alternating periods of fast and slow **growth**
   h. Sit the toddler in a highchair at the family table
   i. Allow sufficient time to eat but remove the food when the toddler begins playing with it
   j. The toddler drinks well from a cup held with both hands
   k. The toddler is skillful at handling finger foods
   l. Avoid using food as a reward or punishment

4. Skills
   a. The toddler begins to walk by age 12 to 15 months
   b. Runs by age 2 and walks backward and hops on one foot by age 3
   c. The toddler usually cannot alternate feet when climbing stairs
   d. The toddler begins to master fine-motor skills for building, undressing, and drawing lines
   e. Often uses "no" even when the toddler means "yes" to assert independence
   f. Begins to use short sentences and has a vocabulary of about 300 words by age 2
   g. Tends to ask many "why" questions

5. Bowel and bladder control
   a. Signs that a toddler is ready for toilet-training include muscle coordination with walking, communicating with parents, awareness of a wet or soiled diaper, ability to hold urine for 2 hours, and interest in pleasing parents
   b. Bowel control develops before bladder control
   c. By age 3, the toddler achieves fairly good bowel and bladder control
   d. The toddler may stay dry during the day but may need a diaper at night until age 4

6. Play
   a. The major socializing mechanism is parallel play, and therapeutic play can begin at this age
   b. Short attention span causes the toddler to change toys often
   c. Explores body parts of self and others
   d. Typical toys include push/pull toys, blocks, sand, fingerpaints and bubbles, large balls, crayons, trucks and dolls, containers, Play-Doh, toy telephones, cloth books, and wooden puzzles

7. Safety
   a. Toddlers are eager to explore the world around them
   b. Toddlers should be supervised at play
   c. Once toddlers are able to sit up alone they should be restrained in an upright, forward-facing position in a car seat until they weigh 40 lb
   d. Lock car doors
   e. Use back burners on stove to prepare a meal, and turn pot handles inward and toward the middle of the stove
   f. Keep dangling cords from small appliances away from toddlers
   g. Place inaccessible locks on windows and doors, and keep furniture away from windows
   h. Secure screens on all windows
   i. Place gates at stairways
   j. Do not permit a toddler to sleep or play in an upper bunk bed
   k. Never leave the toddler alone near a bathtub, pail of water, swimming pool, or any other body of water
   l. Keep toilet lids closed
   m. Keep all medicines, poisons, household plants, and toxic products high and locked out of reach
   n. Keep syrup of ipecac and poison control telephone number available

C. The preschooler
   1. Physical
      a. Grows 2½ to 3 inches per year
      b. Average height of 37 inches at age 3; is 40½ inches at age 4, and 43 inches at age 5

BOX 27–1. The Toddler's Vital Signs

Temperature: axillary 97.5°–98.6°F
Apical rate: 80–125 beats/minute
Respirations: 25–35 breaths/minute
Blood pressure: average 72–110/40–73 mmHg

c. Gains 5 lb per year; average weight of 32 lb at age 5
d. Requires about 12 hours of sleep each day
e. A security object and nightlight assist with sleeping
f. Can use a toothbrush properly and should brush twice a day

2. Vital signs (Box 27–2)
3. Nutrition
   a. Daily calorie requirement is about 1800 kcal/day
   b. Exhibits food fads and strong taste preferences
   c. By 5 years old, tends to focus on social aspects of eating, table conversations, manners, and willingness to try new foods
4. Skills
   a. Has good posture
   b. Develops fine-motor coordination
   c. Can hop, skip, and run more smoothly
   d. Athletic abilities begin to develop
   e. Demonstrates increased skills in balancing
   f. Alternates feet when climbing stairs
   g. Can tie shoelaces
   h. May talk continuously and ask many "why" questions
   i. Vocabulary increases to about 900 words by age 3 and 2100 words by age 5
   j. By age 3 usually talks in three- or four-word sentences and speaks in short phrases
   k. By age 4 speaks five- or six-word sentences and by age 5 speaks in longer sentences that contain all parts of speech
   l. Can be readily understood by others and can clearly understand what others are saying
5. Bowel and bladder control
   a. By age 4, the child has daytime bowel and bladder control but may experience bed-wetting accidents at night
   b. By age 5, the preschooler achieves both bowel and bladder control, although accidents may occur in stressful situations
6. Play
   a. Cooperative
   b. Imaginary playmates
   c. Likes to build and create things, and play is simple and imaginative
   d. Understands sharing and is able to interact with peers
   e. Requires regular socialization with age mates

f. Play activities include a large space for running and jumping
g. Dress-up clothes, paints, paper, and crayons for creative expressions
h. Swimming and sports for **growth** development
i. Puzzles and toys aid with fine development

7. Safety
   a. Preschoolers are active and inquisitive
   b. Because of their magical thinking, they may believe that daring feats seen in cartoons are possible and they may attempt them
   c. Can learn simple safety practices because they can follow simple and verbal directions; their attention span is lengthened
   d. Once the child has outgrown the car safety seat (weight more than 40 lb), the child should be placed and restrained in a booster seat high enough to allow car seat belts to be correctly positioned over the child's chest and pelvis
   e. Teach the child basic safety rules to ensure safety when playing in a playground near swings and ladders
   f. Never allow the child to play with matches or lighters
   g. The child should be taught what to do in the event of a fire or if the clothes catch fire
   h. Fire drills should be practiced with the child
   i. Guns should be stored unloaded and secured under lock and key
   j. The child should be taught to leave an area immediately if a gun is seen, and to tell an adult
   k. A child should be taught never to point a toy gun at another person
   l. Teach the child that if another person touches their body in an inappropriate way they should tell an adult
   m. Teach the child to avoid speaking to strangers and never to accept a ride, toys, or gifts from a stranger
   n. Teach the child their full name, address, parents' names, and telephone number
   o. Keep syrup of ipecac and the poison control telephone number available
   p. Teach the child how to dial 911 in an emergency situation

D. The school-aged child
   1. Physical
      a. Girls usually grow faster than boys
      b. **Growth** of about 2 inches per year between ages 6 and 12
      c. Height ranges from 45 inches at age 6 to 59 inches at age 12
      d. Weight gain of 4½ to 6½ lb per year; average weight of 46 lb at age 6 and 88 lb at age 12

BOX 27–2. The Preschooler's Vital Signs

Temperature: axillary 97.5°–98.6°F
Apical rate: 90–100 beats/minute
Respirations: 25 breaths/minute
Blood pressure: average 85–60/90–70 mmHg

  e. Permanent teeth erupt around age 6, and deciduous teeth are gradually lost
  f. Brush teeth at least twice a day; regular dentist visits should be stressed
  g. Sleep requirements range from 10 to 12 hours a night
2. Vital signs (Box 27–3)
3. Nutrition
  a. Increased **growth** needs
  b. Balanced diet from basic four food groups
  c. May still be a picky eater but willing to try new foods
4. Skills
  a. Refinement of fine-motor skills
  b. Continued development of gross motor skills
  c. Increase in strength and endurance
5. Play
  a. Play is more competitive
  b. Rules and rituals are important aspects of play and games
  c. Enjoys drawing, collecting items, dolls, pets, guessing games, board games, listening to the radio, TV, reading, and video and computer games
  d. Participation in team sports
  e. Participates in secret clubs, gang activities, scout organizations
6. Safety
  a. Experiences less fear in play activities and frequently imitates real life by using tools and household items
  b. Adjust car seat belts so that the lap belt fits snugly over the bony pelvis and the shoulder harness is positioned across the chest; place the shoulder harness of the seat belt behind the shoulder if it crosses the face or soft tissue of the neck
  c. Major causes of injuries include bicycles, skateboards, and team sports as the child increases motor abilities and independence
  d. Children should always wear a helmet when riding a bike, using inline skates or skateboards
  e. Teach the child water safety rules
  f. Instruct the child to avoid teasing or playing roughly with animals
  g. Never allow the child to play with matches or lighters
  h. Teach the school-aged child about fire safety and gun safety
  i. Teach the child that if another person touches their body in an inappropriate way they should tell an adult
  j. Teach the child to avoid speaking to strangers and never to accept a ride, toys, or gifts from a stranger
  k. Teach traffic safety rules
  l. Teach the child how to dial 911 in an emergency situation
  m. Keep syrup of ipecac and the poison control telephone number available
E. The adolescent
1. Physical
  a. In girls, **puberty** begins between ages 8 and 14
  b. In boys, **puberty** begins between the ages of 9 and 16
  c. Body mass increases to adult size
  d. Sebaceous and sweat glands become active and fully functional
  e. Body hair distribution occurs
  f. Increase in height, weight, breast development, and pelvic girth in girls
  g. Menstrual periods occur about 2½ years after the onset of **puberty**
  h. In boys, increase in height, weight, muscle mass, and penis and testicle size
  i. Voice deepens in boys
  j. Normal weight gain during puberty: girls gain 15 to 55 lb; boys gain 15 to 65 lb
  k. Careful brushing and care of the teeth are important, and many adolescents must wear braces
  l. Sleep patterns include a tendency to stay up late; therefore, in an attempt to catch up on missed sleep, adolescents sleep late at every opportunity
2. Vital signs (Box 27–4)
3. Nutrition
  a. Average daily requirements in girls 38 to 47 kcal/kg/day
  b. Average daily requirements in boys 40 to 55 kcal/kg/day
  c. Basic four food groups are important
  d. Typically eat whenever they have a break in activities
  e. Calcium and protein are needed to aid in bone and muscle growth
4. Skills
  a. Gross and fine-motor skills are well developed
  b. Strength and endurance increase

5. Play
   a. Games and athletics are the most common forms of play
   b. Competition is important
   c. Strict rules are important
   d. Enjoy activities such as sports, videos, movies, reading, parties, hobbies, computer games, music, and experimenting with makeup and hair styles
6. Safety
   a. Risk takers
   b. Have a natural urge to experiment and be independent
   c. Instruct in the dangers related to drugs and alcohol
   d. Help to recognize that there are choices when difficult or potentially dangerous situations arise
   e. Advocate the use of seat belts
   f. Instruct in the injuries that motor vehicle accidents can cause
   g. Instruct in water safety and emphasize that they should enter the water feet first as opposed to diving, especially when the depth of the water is unknown
   h. Instruct about the dangers associated with violence and gangs

PRACTICE QUESTIONS

1. The parents of a 2-year-old arrive at the hospital to visit the child. The child is in the play room and ignores the parents during the visit. This 2-year-old behavior indicates
   1 The child is withdrawn
   2 The child is more interested in playing with other children
   3 The child has adjusted to the hospitalized setting
   4 A normal pattern

2. The most appropriate toy to provide to a 3-year-old is which of the following?
   1 A farm set
   2 A golf set
   3 A puzzle
   4 A wagon

3. The nurse reinforces instructions to the parents of a newborn regarding car travel and safety seats. Which of the following is the most appropriate information related to the safety of the infant?
   1 Restrain in a car seat in the front seat in a semireclined, rear-facing position
   2 Restrain in a car seat in the front seat in a semireclined, face-forward position
   3 Restrain in a car seat in the middle backseat in a semireclined, rear-facing position
   4 Restrain in a car seat in the middle backseat in a semireclined, face-forward position

4. The nurse is assigned to monitor a 3-month-old infant for increased intracranial pressure. On palpation of the fontanels, the nurse notes that the anterior fontanel has not closed and is soft and flat. Which of the following actions should the nurse take?
   1 Elevate the head of the bed 90 degrees
   2 Notify the RN
   3 Increase oral fluids
   4 Document the findings

5. The nurse is caring for a 5-year-old who has been placed in traction following a fracture to the femur. Which of the following is the most appropriate activity for this child?
   1 Large picture books
   2 A radio
   3 A sports video
   4 Fingerpaints

6. The mother of a 16-year-old tells the nurse that she is concerned because the child sleeps until noon every weekend, and whenever the child has a day off from school. The most appropriate nursing response is which of the following?
   1 "The child should have a blood test to check for anemia."
   2 "Adolescents love to sleep late in the morning."
   3 "The child shouldn't be staying up so late at night."
   4 "If the child eats properly, that shouldn't be happening."

7. A 16-year-old is admitted to the hospital for acute appendicitis and an appendectomy is performed. Which of the following interventions is most appropriate to facilitate normal growth and development?
   1 Allow the family to bring in favorite computer games
   2 Encourage the parents to room-in with the child
   3 Encourage the child to rest and read
   4 Allow the child to participate in activities with other individuals in the same age group when the condition permits

8. A 2-year-old is treated in the emergency room for a burn to the chest and abdomen. The child sustained the burn from grabbing a cup of hot coffee that was left on the kitchen counter. The nurse reinforces safety principles with the parents prior to discharge. Which of the following statements, if made by the parents, indicates an understanding of the measures to provide safety in the home?
   1 "I guess my children need to understand what the word 'hot' means."
   2 "We will install a safety gate as soon as we get home so the children can't get into the kitchen."

3 "We will be sure that the children stay in their rooms when we work in the kitchen."
4 "We will be sure not to leave hot liquids unattended."

9. A mother of a 4-year-old expresses concern because her hospitalized child began thumb sucking. The mother states that this behavior began 2 days after hospital admission. The most appropriate nursing response is which of the following?
   1 "A 4-year-old is too old for this type of behavior."
   2 "Your child is acting like a baby."

3 "The doctor will need to be notified."
4 "It is best to ignore the behavior."

10. The mother of a toddler asks the nurse when it is safe to place the car safety seat in a face-forward position. The best nursing response is which of the following?
   1 Once the toddler is able to sit up alone
   2 The seat should not be placed forward unless there are safety locks in the car
   3 The seat should never be placed in a face-forward position because of the risk of the child unbuckling the harness
   4 When the height of the toddler is 27 inches

ANSWERS

1. **4**

RATIONALE: The toddler is particularly vunerable to separation. A toddler often shows anger at being left by ignoring the parent or by pretending to be more interested in play than in going home. Parents of hospitalized toddlers are frequently distressed by such behavior. The toddler engages in parallel play and plays alongside but not with other children.
TEST-TAKING STRATEGY: Use the concepts of growth and development. Option 3 can be easily eliminated first. There are no data in the question to support option 1. From the remaining options, knowledge regarding separation anxiety in the toddler will direct you to option 4. Review these concepts now if you had difficulty with this question.
LEVEL OF COGNITIVE ABILITY: Comprehension
PHASE OF NURSING PROCESS: Data Collection
CLIENT NEEDS: Psychosocial Integrity
CONTENT AREA: Child Health
REFERENCE
Schulte, E., Price, D., & James, S. (1997). *Thompson's pediatric nursing: An introductory text* (7th ed.). Philadelphia: W. B. Saunders. p. 219.

2. **4**

RATIONALE: Toys for the toddler must be strong, safe, and too large to swallow or place in the ear or nose. Toddlers need supervision at all times. Push/pull toys, large balls, large crayons, trucks, and dolls are some of the appropriate toys. A farm set and a golf set may contain items that the child could swallow. A large puzzle only is appropriate.
TEST-TAKING STRATEGY: Options 1 and 2 can be easily eliminated because they contain items that could be swallowed by the child. From the remaining options, the most appropriate toy is a wagon. Remember that large and strong toys are safest for the toddler.
LEVEL OF COGNITIVE ABILITY: Comprehension
PHASE OF NURSING PROCESS: Implementation
CLIENT NEEDS: Physiological Integrity
CONTENT AREA: Child Health
REFERENCE
Schulte, E., Price, D., & James, S. (1997). *Thompson's pediatric nursing: An introductory text* (7th ed.). Philadelphia: W. B. Saunders. p. 196.

3. **3**

RATIONALE: Infants should be placed in a bucket-type car seat that faces backward in the backseat until they weigh 18 to 20 lb. An infant should never face forward or ride in the front seat.
TEST-TAKING STRATEGY: Visualize each of the descriptions in the options with a focus of safety in mind. This should easily direct you to option 3. If you had difficulty with this question, take time now to review safety measures for the infant.
LEVEL OF COGNITIVE ABILITY: Application
PHASE OF NURSING PROCESS: Implementation
CLIENT NEEDS: Health Promotion and Maintenance
CONTENT AREA: Child Health
REFERENCE
Schulte, E., Price, D., & James, S. (1997). *Thompson's pediatric nursing: An introductory text* (7th ed.). Philadelphia: W. B. Saunders. p. 209.

4. **4**

RATIONALE: The anterior fontanel is diamond-shaped and located on the top of the head. It should be soft and flat in a normal infant and it normally closes by 18 to 24 months of age. The posterior fontanel closes by 2 to 3 months of age.
TEST-TAKING STRATEGY: Note the key phrase "soft and flat." This should provide you with the clue that this is a normal finding. A bulging or tense fontanel may result from crying or increased ICP. If you had difficulty with this question, review normal assessment findings in an infant.
LEVEL OF COGNITIVE ABILITY: Comprehension
PHASE OF NURSING PROCESS: Implementation
CLIENT NEEDS: Physiological Integrity
CONTENT AREA: Child Health
REFERENCE
Leifer, G. (1999). *Thompson's introduction to maternity and pediatric nursing* (3rd ed.). Philadelphia: W. B. Saunders. pp. 309–310.

5. **4**

RATIONALE: In the preschooler, play is simple and imaginative, and includes activities such as dressing up, fingerpaints, clay, pasting, and simple board and card games. Large picture books are most appropriate for the infant. A radio and sports video is most appropriate for the adolescent.

TEST-TAKING STRATEGY: Note the age of the child and think about the age-related activity that is most appropriate. Eliminate options 2 and 3, knowing that they are most appropriate for the adolescent. From the remaining options, the word "large" in option 1 should provide you with the clue that this activity is more appropriate for a child younger than age 5. If you had difficulty with this question, review the appropriate activities for a preschooler.
LEVEL OF COGNITIVE ABILITY: Comprehension
PHASE OF NURSING PROCESS: Planning
CLIENT NEEDS: Psychosocial Integrity
CONTENT AREA: Child Health
REFERENCE

Schulte, E., Price, D., & James, S. (1997). *Thompson's pediatric nursing: An introductory text* (7th ed.). Philadelphia: W. B. Saunders. p. 248.

6. **2**

RATIONALE: Sleep patterns in the adolescent vary according to individual need. Adolescents love to sleep late in the morning, but they should be encouraged to be responsible for waking themselves, particularly in time to get ready for school. Options 1, 3, and 4 are incorrect.
TEST-TAKING STRATEGY: The question asks for the most appropriate nursing response. Options 3 and 4 can be eliminated first. From the remaining options, there is no indication that a physiological alteration is present; therefore, option 2 is most appropriate. Review adolescent sleep patterns now if you had difficulty with this question.
LEVEL OF COGNITIVE ABILITY: Comprehension
PHASE OF NURSING PROCESS: Implementation
CLIENT NEEDS: Physiological Integrity
CONTENT AREA: Child Health
REFERENCE

Luckmann, J. (1997). *Saunders manual of nursing care*. Philadelphia: W. B. Saunders. p. 509.

7. **4**

RATIONALE: Adolescents often are not sure whether they want their parents with them when they are hospitalized. Because of the importance of the peer group, separation from friends is a source of anxiety. Ideally, the peer group will support their ill friend. Options 1, 2, and 3 isolate the child from the peer group.
TEST-TAKING STRATEGY: Consider the psychosocial needs of the adolescent when answering the question. Options 1, 2, and 3 are similar in that they isolate the child from their own peer group. If you had difficulty with this question, take time now to review the psychosocial needs of the adolescent.
LEVEL OF COGNITIVE ABILITY: Comprehension
PHASE OF NURSING PROCESS: Implementation
CLIENT NEEDS: Psychosocial Integrity
CONTENT AREA: Child Health
REFERENCE

Schulte, E., Price, D., & James, S. (1997). *Thompson's pediatric nursing: An introductory text* (7th ed.). Philadelphia: W. B. Saunders. p. 387.

8. **4**

RATIONALE: Toddlers, with their increased mobility and developing motor skills, can reach hot water, open fires, or hot objects placed on counters and stoves above their eye level. Parents should be encouraged to remain in the kitchen when preparing a meal and reminded to use the back burners on the stove, and to turn pot handles inward and toward the middle of the stove. Hot liquids should never be left unattended, and the toddler should always be supervised. Options 1, 2, and 3 do not reflect an adequate understanding of the principles of safety.
TEST-TAKING STRATEGY: Option 1 can be easily eliminated. Options 2 and 3 are similar in that they isolate the child from the environment. Review safety principles now if you had difficulty with this question.
LEVEL OF COGNITIVE ABILITY: Comprehension
PHASE OF NURSING PROCESS: Evaluation
CLIENT NEEDS: Health Promotion and Maintenance
CONTENT AREA: Child Health
REFERENCE

Schulte, E., Price, D., & James, S. (1997). *Thompson's pediatric nursing: An introductory text* (7th ed.). Philadelphia: W. B. Saunders. p. 208.

9. **4**

RATIONALE: In the hospitalized preschooler, it is best to accept regression if it occurs. Regression is most often due to the stress of the hospitalization. Parents may be overly concerned about regression and should be told that their child may continue the behavior at home. There is no need to call the physician. Options 1 and 2 are inappropriate.
TEST-TAKING STRATEGY: Note the key words "most appropriate." Options 1, 2, and 3 will cause additional stress and concern in the parent. If you had difficulty with this question, review the psychosocial issues related to the hospitalized preschool child.
LEVEL OF COGNITIVE ABILITY: Comprehension
PHASE OF NURSING PROCESS: Implementation
CLIENT NEEDS: Psychosocial Integrity
CONTENT AREA: Child Health
REFERENCE

Schulte, E., Price, D., & James, S. (1997). *Thompson's pediatric nursing: An introductory text* (7th ed.). Philadelphia: W. B. Saunders. p. 203.

10. **1**

RATIONALE: Once a toddler is able to sit up alone, car safety seats can be adjusted to face forward in an upright position. The car safety seat is suitable for the growing toddler until the toddler reaches the weight of 40 lb. Options 2, 3, and 4 are incorrect.
TEST-TAKING STRATEGY: Knowledge regarding car safety and the toddler is required to answer this question. Review these safety principles now if you had difficulty with this question.
LEVEL OF COGNITIVE ABILITY: Comprehension
PHASE OF NURSING PROCESS: Implementation
CLIENT NEEDS: Health Promotion and Maintenance
CONTENT AREA: Child Health
REFERENCE

Schulte, E., Price, D., & James, S. (1997). *Thompson's pediatric nursing: An introductory text* (7th ed.). Philadelphia: W. B. Saunders. p. 209.

BIBLIOGRAPHY

Ashwill, J., & Droske, S. (1977). *Nursing care of children: Principles and practice*. Philadelphia: W.B. Saunders.

Leifer, G. (1999). *Thompson's introduction to maternity and pediatric nursing* (3rd ed.). Philadelphia: W. B. Saunders.

Luckmann, J. (1997). *Saunders manual of nursing care*. Philadelphia: W. B. Saunders.

Schulte, E., Price, D., & James, S. (1997). *Thompson's pediatric nursing: An introductory text* (7th ed.). Philadelphia: W. B. Saunders.

CHAPTER 28

Neurological, Cognitive, and Psychosocial Disorders

· ·

I. Head Injury

A. Description
  1. The pathological result of any mechanical force to the skull, scalp, meninges, or brain
  2. Multiple trauma is the leading cause of death in children beyond infancy
  3. Manifestations depend on the type of injury and the subsequent amount of increased intracranial pressure (ICP)
◆ B. Data collection
  1. Increased ICP in infants
    a. Poor feeding or vomiting
    b. Irritability or restlessness
    c. Lethargy
    d. Increased head circumference, bulging fontanel, separation of cranial sutures
    e. Distended scalp veins
    f. Eyes deviated downward (sunset sign)
    g. Increased or decreased response to pain
  2. Increased ICP in children
    a. Headache
    b. Diplopia
    c. Mood swings
    d. Slurred speech
    e. Papilledema
    f. Altered level of consciousness (LOC)
    g. Nausea and vomiting
  3. Late signs of increased ICP
    a. Tachycardia leading to bradycardia
    b. Apnea
    c. Systolic hypertension and widening pulse pressure
    d. Decorticate/decerebrate posturing
◆ C. Implementation
  1. Monitor airway
  2. Monitor vital signs and neurological function
  3. Monitor for signs of decreased LOC
  4. Provide seizure precautions
  5. Check for injuries and immobilize the neck if a cervical injury is suspected
  6. Administer oxygen and monitor IV fluids as prescribed
  7. Monitor wound dressings and for nose or ear drainage, which could indicate leakage of cerebrospinal fluid (CSF)
  8. Monitor intake and output (I&O) and electrolyte status
  9. Avoid nasotracheal suction in a child with a basal or skull fracture

II. Hydrocephalus

A. Description
  1. An imbalance of CSF absorption or production, caused by malformations, tumors, hemorrhage, infections, or trauma
  2. Results in head enlargement and increased ICP
B. Types
  1. Communicating
    a. Occurs as a result of impaired absorption within the subarachnoid space
    b. No interference of CSF within the ventricular system occurs
  2. Noncommunicating: obstruction of CSF flow within the ventricular system occurs
C. Data collection
  1. Infant
    a. Increased head circumference; bones of head are thin and widely separated and scalp veins are dilated
    b. Anterior fontanel tense, bulging, and nonpulsating
    c. Frontal bossing and sunsetting eyes
  2. Child
    a. Behavior changes such as irritability and lethargy
    b. Headache upon awakening
    c. Nausea and vomiting
    d. Ataxia and nystagmus

e. High shrill cry and seizure activity are late signs

D. Surgical implementation
1. The goal of surgical treatment is to prevent further CSF accumulation by bypassing the blockage and draining the fluid from the ventricles, where it may be reabsorbed
2. Ventriculoperitoneal **shunt** (VP **shunt**): CSF drains into the peritoneal cavity from the lateral ventricle
3. Atrioventricular **shunt** (AV **shunt**): CSF drains into the right atrium of the heart from the lateral ventricle bypassing the obstruction

E. Postoperative implementation
1. Monitor vital signs
2. Monitor for signs of infection and check dressings for drainage
3. For the first 2 days, position on the nonoperated side as prescribed so that no weight is placed on the valve
4. The child is kept flat as prescribed to avoid rapid reduction of intracranial fluid
5. Observe for increased ICP; if increased ICP occurs, elevate the head of the bed 15 to 30 degrees to enhance gravity flow through the **shunt**
6. Measure head circumference
7. Monitor I&O
8. Provide comfort measures
9. Administer medications as prescribed, which may include diuretics, antibiotics, or anticonvulsants
10. Reinforce instructions to parents regarding how to recognize **shunt** infection or malfunction

III. Spina Bifida

A. Description
1. Central nervous system (CNS) defect that occurs as a result of neural tube failure to close during embryonic development
2. Associated deficits include sensory or motor disturbance, dislocated hips, club feet, and hydrocephalus
3. Defect closure usually done during infancy

B. Types
1. Spina bifida occulta
   a. Spinal cord remains intact and usually is not visible
   b. Meninges are not exposed on skin surface
   c. Neurological deficits are not usually present
2. Spina bifida cystica
   a. Protrusion of the spinal cord and/or its meninges
   b. Results in incomplete closure of the vertebral and neural tubes resulting in a saclike protrusion in the lumbar or sacral area, with varying degrees of nervous tissue involvement

c. Can include meningocele, myelomeningocele, lipomeningocele, and lipomeningomyelocele
3. Meningocele
   a. Protrusion involves meninges and a saclike cyst that contains CSF in the midline of the back, usually in the lumbosacral area
   b. No involvement of the spinal cord and neurological deficits are usually not present
4. Myelomeningocele
   a. Protrusion of meninges, CSF, nerve roots, and a portion of the spinal cord
   b. The sac is covered by a thin membrane that is prone to leakage or rupture
   c. Neurological deficits are evident
5. Data collection
   a. Depends on spinal cord involvement
   b. Visible spinal defect
   c. Flaccid paralysis of legs and hip and joint deformities
   d. Altered bladder and bowel function
6. Implementation
   a. Evaluate the sac and measure the lesion
   b. Monitor the neurological status and for signs of increased ICP
   c. Measure the head circumference and check the anterior fontanel for fullness
   d. Protect the sac and cover with a sterile saline dressing to maintain the moisture of the sac and contents as prescribed
   e. Place the child in a prone position to avoid stress or pressure on the sac
   f. Monitor the sac for redness or clear or purulent drainage; change the dressing whenever soiled using aseptic technique to prevent infection
   g. Assess for physical impairments
   h. Prepare the child and family for surgery
   i. Antibiotics may be prescribed to prevent infection, anticholinergics to improve urinary continence, antispasmodics to control bladder spasms, and laxatives to achieve bowel continence as prescribed

IV. Reye's Syndrome

A. Description
1. Acute encephalopathy characterized by a viral infection leading to hepatic, metabolic, and neurologic failure
2. The exact cause is not clear
3. It is recommended that aspirin not be administered to children with varicella or influenza because of its association with Reye's syndrome; acetaminophen (Tylenol) is considered the medication of choice for pediatric clients
4. The goal of treatment is to maintain effective cerebral perfusion and control increasing ICP

B. Data collection
1. History of systemic viral illness 4 to 7 days before the onset of symptoms

2. Malaise, nausea, and vomiting
3. Progressive neurological deterioration

C. Implementation
   1. Monitor neurological status and for signs of ICP
   2. Monitor cardiac and respiratory status
   3. Monitor hydration status and maintain fluid and electrolyte balance
   4. Monitor for signs of bleeding, which can occur with hepatic involvement

V. Meningitis

A. Description
   1. An infectious process of the CNS caused by bacteria and viruses that may be acquired as a primary disease or as a result of complications of neurosurgery, trauma, infection of the sinus or ears, or systemic infections
   2. Diagnosis is made by testing CSF obtained by lumbar puncture, which shows increased pressure, cloudy CSF, high protein, and low glucose
   3. Meningococcal meningitis is transmitted primarily by droplet infection
   4. Viral meningitis is associated with viruses such as mumps, paramyxovirus, herpes virus, and enterovirus

B. Data collection
   1. Signs and symptoms vary depending on the age of the child and the duration of the preceding illness; there is no one classic sign or symptom
   2. Fever
   3. Poor feeding, anorexia, and vomiting
   4. Diarrhea
   5. Headache
   6. Poor or high-pitched cry
   7. Altered level of consciousness such as lethargy or irritability
   8. Nuchal rigidity
   9. Bulging anterior fontanel in the infant
   10. Kernig's sign and Brudzinski's sign in children and adolescents
   11. Muscle or joint pain

C. Implementation
   1. Provide isolation and maintain for at least 24 hours after antibiotics are initiated
   2. Antibiotics are prescribed as necessary
   3. Monitor neurological status and for personality changes and irritability
   4. Monitor I&O and nutritional status
   5. Close contacts of the child are determined because they will need prophylactic treatment

VI. Seizures

A. Description
   1. Sudden, transient alterations in brain function resulting from excessive levels of electrical activity in the brain

2. Classified as either partial or generalized, depending on the area of the brain involved

B. Data collection
   1. Obtain information from the parents about the time of onset, precipitating events, and behavior before and after the seizure
   2. Determine the child's history related to seizures

C. Implementation
   1. Ensure patency of airway and monitor breathing during and after the seizure
   2. Stay with the child during the seizure
   3. Monitor skin color, respiratory rate, and for signs of respiratory distress
   4. Do not restrain the child or place anything in the child's mouth
   5. Place in a side-lying position with side rails up, protecting the child
   6. Loosen clothing around the child's neck
   7. Pad crib or bed and remove sharp objects from the bed
   8. Anticonvulsants are administered as prescribed
   9. Instruct parents in the administration and side effects of the prescribed anticonvulsants

VII. Cerebral Palsy

A. Description: A chronic disability characterized by a difficulty in controlling the muscles due to an abnormality in the extrapyramidal or pyramidal motor system

B. Data collection
   1. Irritability
   2. Feeding difficulties
   3. Delayed development and poor motor development
   4. Abnormal posturing
   5. Ataxic gait and poor muscle tone
   6. Persistence of infant reflexes

C. Implementation
   1. The goal to management is early recognition and intervention to maximize the child's abilities
   2. A multidisciplinary team approach is implemented to meet the many needs of the child
   3. Determine the child's developmental level and **intelligence**
   4. Encourage early intervention and participation in school programs
   5. Encourage communication and interaction with the child on a functional level not **chronological age** level
   6. Provide a safe environment by removing sharp objects, use of a protective helmet if the child falls frequently, and implementing seizure precautions if necessary
   7. Provide safe, appropriate toys for age and developmental level
   8. Position upright after meals

9. Reinforce speech therapy techniques, nonverbal methods to communicate, proper feeding techniques, and jaw control

VIII. Mental Retardation

A. Description
 1. Subaverage general intellectual functioning along with a deficit in adaptation in behavior
 2. Down's syndrome is a congenital condition that results in moderate to severe retardation and has been linked to an extra group G chromosome, chromosome 21 (trisomy 21)
B. Data collection
 1. Cognitive skills and level of adaptive functioning
 2. Delays in fine and gross motor skills; decreased spontaneous activity
 3. Speech delays
 4. Nonresponsiveness
 5. Irritability
 6. Poor eye contact during feeding
C. Implementation
 1. Medical strategies are focused at preventing and treating infections, correcting structural deformities, and treating associated behaviors
 2. Implement community and educational services using a multidisciplinary approach
 3. Promote care skills as much as possible; assist with communication and socialization skills
 4. Facilitate appropriate playtime
 5. Initiate safety precautions as necessary
 6. Assist the family with decisions regarding care and provide information regarding support services and community agencies

IX. Autism

A. Description
 1. A severe mental disorder beginning in infancy or toddlerhood; apparent to parents before the age of 3
 2. Characterized by impairment in reciprocal social interaction and in verbal and nonverbal communication
 3. The cause is unknown and the prognosis may be poor
 4. Diagnosis is established on the basis of symptoms and through the use of specialized autism assessment tools
 5. Also called infantile autism
B. Data collection
 1. Disturbance in the rate and appearance of physical, social, and language skills
 2. Abnormal responses of the body sensations
 3. Thinking capacity, but with absent or delayed speech and language
 4. Abnormal ways of relating to people, objects, and events
 5. Delusions and hallucinations are rare
 6. The child is self-absorbed and unable to relate to others

7. The child may play happily alone for hours, but have temper tantrums if interrupted
 8. Language disturbance often includes repetition of previously heard speech and reversal of the pronouns "I" and "you"
 9. If the child can talk, the child uses speech not for communication but to repeat words or phrases meaninglessly
 10. The child may develop an unusual attachment to a significant object and display frequent rocking, spinning, twirling, or other bizarre behaviors
C. Implementation
 1. Determine the child's routines, habits, and preferences and maintain consistency as much as possible
 2. Determine the specific ways in which the child communicates; facilitate communication through the use of picture boards
 3. Evaluate the child for safety and implement safety precautions as necessary for self-injurious behaviors such as head banging
 4. Monitor for stress and anxiety
 5. Avoid placing demands on the child
 6. Initiate referrals to special programs as required
 7. Provide support to parents

X. Attention Deficit Hyperactivity Disorder (ADHD)

A. Description
 1. A developmental disorder characterized by developmentally inappropriate degrees of inattention, overactivity, and impulsivity
 2. Childhood problems include lowered intellectual development, some minor physical abnormalities, sleeping disturbances, behavioral or emotional disorders, and difficulty in social relationships
 3. Diagnosis is established on the basis of self-reports, parent and teacher reports, and psychological assessments
B. Data collection
 1. Fidgets with the hands or feet or squirms in the seat
 2. Easily distracted with external or internal stimuli
 3. Difficulty with following through on instructions
 4. Poor attention span; shifts from one uncompleted activity to another
 5. Talks excessively
 6. Interrupts or intrudes on others
 7. Engages in physically dangerous activities without considering the possible consequences
C. Implementation
 1. Provide environmental and physical safety measures
 2. Enhance capabilities and self-esteem
 3. Encourage support groups for parents

4. Administer methylphenidate (Ritalin) as prescribed
5. Instruct the child and parents regarding medication administration
6. Inform the child and parents that positive effects of medication will be seen within 1 to 2 weeks if taken as prescribed

XI. Tourette's Disorder

A. Description: Appears between ages 2 and 15 and is characterized by recurrent involuntary and rapid movements affecting various parts of the body accompanied by vocal noises such as barks, grunts, or profanities
B. Implementation
   1. Establish a trusting one on one relationship
   2. Protect the client from harm by providing a helmet or protective padding
   3. Allow the child to have a favorite toy or other object
   4. Provide positive reinforcement for appropriate behaviors
   5. Maintain eye contact
   6. Assess suicide potential
   7. Remove dangerous objects from the environment
   8. Set limits on socially inappropriate or manipulative behaviors
   9. Encourage the client to confront tension and frustration before they emerge as inappropriate behaviors
   10. Provide noncompetitive group situations

XII. Child Abuse

A. Description: Involves emotional or physical **abuse** or neglect, as well as sexual exploitation or molestation by caretakers or other individuals
B. Data collection
   1. Physical **abuse**
      a. Unexplained bruises, burns, or fractures
      b. Bald spots on the scalp
      c. Apprehensive child
      d. Extreme aggressiveness or withdrawal
      e. Fear of parents
      f. Lack of crying when approached by a stranger
   2. Physical neglect
      a. Inadequate weight gain
      b. Poor hygiene
      c. Consistent hunger
      d. Inconsistent school attendance
      e. Constant fatigue
      f. Reports of lack of child supervision
      g. Delinquency
   3. Emotional **abuse**
      a. Speech disorders
      b. Habit disorders such as sucking, biting, or rocking
      c. Psychoneurotic reactions
      d. **Learning** disorders
      e. Suicide attempts

4. Sexual **abuse**
   a. Difficulty walking or sitting
   b. Torn, stained, or bloody underclothing
   c. Pain, swelling, or itching of the genitals
   d. Bruises, bleeding, or lacerations in the genital or anal area
   e. Unwillingness to change clothes or unwillingness to participate in gym activities
   f. Poor peer relations
   g. Delinquency
   h. Changes in sleep performance
   i. Self-disruptive behavior
C. Implementation
   1. Identify the parents' strengths and weaknesses, normal coping mechanisms, and presence or absence of support systems
   2. Support the child during a thorough physical assessment
   3. Check for injuries
   4. Report cases of suspected **abuse**
   5. Place the child in an environment that is safe, thereby preventing further injury
   6. Document in an objective manner information related to the suspected **abuse**
   7. Assist the family in identifying stressors, support systems, and resources
   8. Refer the family to appropriate support groups

PRACTICE QUESTIONS

1. The nurse is assisting in collecting data on a 6-month-old infant with a diagnosis of hydrocephalus. The nurse checks for the major symptom associated with hydrocephalus when the nurse
   1 Tests the urine for protein
   2 Takes the apical pulse
   3 Palpates the anterior fontanel
   4 Takes the blood pressure

2. A mother arrives at the emergency department with her 5-year-old child. The mother states that the child fell off a bunk bed. A head injury is suspected. The nurse checks the child for signs of increased ICP. Which of the following is a late sign of increased ICP?
   1 Bulging fontanel
   2 Altered level of consciousness
   3 Nausea
   4 Widening pulse pressure

3. The nurse is caring for a child with spina bifida who has a neurogenic bladder. As part of the nursing care plan, the nurse monitors for urinary tract infections. The nurse anticipates that the most likely medication to be prescribed prophylactically is
   1 Prednisone (Deltasone)
   2 Furosemide (Lasix)
   3 Sulfisoxazole (Gantrisin)
   4 Immune globulin IV

4. The nurse is caring for a child with Reye's syndrome. The nurse checks for the major symptom associated with Reye's syndrome when the nurse notes
   1 Persistent vomiting
   2 Protein in the urine
   3 A history of a staphylococcus infection
   4 Symptoms of hyperglycemia

5. The child is diagnosed with Reye's syndrome. The nurse assists in preparing a nursing care plan for this child and suggests to include
   1 Providing a quiet atmosphere with dimmed lights
   2 Checking for hearing loss
   3 Monitoring output
   4 Changing body position every 2 hours

6. The nurse reinforces home care instructions to the mother of a child with Reye's syndrome. Which of the following statements, if made by the mother, indicates a need for further instruction?
   1 "I need to decrease the stimuli at home to prevent intracranial pressure."
   2 "I need to give frequent, small, nutritious meals to decrease the amount of vomiting."
   3 "I need to have my child nap during the day to provide rest."
   4 "I need to check for jaundiced skin and eyes every day."

7. The nurse is assisting in collecting data on a child with seizures. The nurse is interviewing the child's parents to establish their adjustment to caring for a child with a chronic illness. Which of the following statements, if made by parents, indicates a need for further teaching?
   1 "Our child is involved in a swim program with neighbors and friends."
   2 "Our child sleeps in our bedroom at night."
   3 "Our baby-sitter just completed CPR training."
   4 "We worry about injuries when our child has a seizure."

8. Which of the following data if noted by the nurse indicates a potential complication associated with a seizure?
   1 Blood on the pillow
   2 Blanched toenails
   3 Migraine headaches
   4 High-pitched cry

9. The nurse plans for a safe environment when caring for an infant at risk for a grand mal seizure. In the plan of care, the seizure precautions most appropriately include placing which of the following items at the bedside?
   1 A suction apparatus and an airway
   2 Oxygen with a tracheotomy set
   3 Emergency cart
   4 Airway and a tracheotomy set

10. The nurse is reinforcing instructions with an adolescent with a history of grand mal seizures, who is on an anticonvulsant medication. Which of the following statements, if made by the adolescent, indicates an understanding of the teaching?
    1 "I will never be able to drive a car."
    2 "My anticonvulsant medication will clear up my skin."
    3 "I can't drink alcohol while I am taking my medication."
    4 "If I forget my morning medication, I can just take two pills at bedtime."

11. The nurse is collecting data on a child admitted with a diagnosis of grand mal seizures. The nurse checks for causes of the seizure activity when the nurse
    1 Tests the child's urine for specific gravity
    2 Obtains a family history of psychiatric illness
    3 Obtains a history of any factors that might precipitate seizure activity
    4 Asks the child what happens during a seizure

12. The nurse is caring for a child recently diagnosed with cerebral palsy. The parents of the child ask the nurse about the disorder. The nurse bases the response to the parents on the understanding that cerebral palsy is
    1 A chronic disability characterized by a difficulty in controlling the muscles.
    2 An infectious disease of the central nervous system.
    3 An inflammation of the brain as a result of a viral illness.
    4 A congenital condition that results in moderate to severe retardation.

13. The nurse is caring for a child with cerebral palsy. The primary goal to be included in the plan of care is to
    1 Eliminate the cause of the disease
    2 Prevent the occurrence of emotional disturbances
    3 Maximize the child's assets and minimize the limitations caused by the disease
    4 Improve muscle control and coordination

14. The nurse is caring for a child diagnosed with Down's syndrome. In describing the disorder to the parents, the nurse bases the explanation on the fact that Down's syndrome is a
    1 Condition characterized by above-average intellectual functioning with deficits in adaptive behavior
    2 Condition characterized by average intellectual functioning and the absence of deficits in adaptive behavior
    3 Congenital condition that results in moderate to severe retardation and has been linked to an extra group G chromosome

4 Condition characterized by subaverage intellectual functioning with the absence of deficits in adaptive behavior

15. The nurse is assigned to care for an 8-year-old child with a basilar skull fracture. Which of the following physician orders does the nurse question?
    1 Restrict fluid intake
    2 Keep an IV line patent
    3 Insert an indwelling urinary catheter
    4 Suction PRN

16. A lumbar puncture is performed on a child suspected of having bacterial meningitis. Cerebrospinal fluid (CSF) is obtained for analysis. The nurse understands that which of the following results will verify the diagnosis?
    1 Cloudy CSF with low protein and low glucose
    2 Cloudy CSF with high protein and low glucose
    3 Clear CSF with high protein and low glucose
    4 Decreased pressure and cloudy CSF with high protein

17. The nurse is caring for a child with meningococcal meningitis. Based on the mode of transmission of this infection, which of the following is included in the plan of care?
    1 No precautions are required as long as antibiotics have been started
    2 Maintain enteric precautions
    3 Maintain isolation precautions for at least 24 hours after the initiation of antibiotics
    4 Maintain neutropenic precautions

18. The nurse assists in developing a plan of care for the child with meningitis. Which of the following is the priority problem for this child?
    1 Altered cerebral tissue perfusion
    2 Parental knowledge deficit
    3 Altered family process
    4 Alteration in comfort

19. The nurse is observing a child diagnosed with autism. The nurse knows that the primary characteristic(s) of autism include which of the following?
    1 Consistent imitation of others' actions
    2 Normal social play
    3 Lack of social interaction and awareness
    4 Normal verbal but abnormal nonverbal communication

20. The emergency department nurse is collecting data on a child suspected of being sexually abused. Which of the following data most likely indicate this suspicion?
    1 Poor hygiene
    2 Bald spots on the scalp
    3 Fear of the parents
    4 Swelling of the genitals

ANSWERS

1. **3**

RATIONALE: An elevated or bulging anterior fontanel indicates an increase in cerebrospinal fluid collection in the cerebral ventricle. Proteinuria, apical pulse, and blood pressure changes are not specifically associated with increasing cerebrospinal fluid in the brain tissue.
TEST-TAKING STRATEGY: Use the principles associated with excessive fluid build-up in the cranial cavity and note the age of the infant. Additionally, correlate "hydrocephalus" in the question, with "anterior fontanel" in option 3, the correct option. If you had difficulty with this question, take time to review the symptoms associated with hydrocephalus.
LEVEL OF COGNITIVE ABILITY: Application
PHASE OF NURSING PROCESS: Data Collection
CLIENT NEEDS: Physiological Integrity
CONTENT AREA: Child Health
REFERENCE
Schulte, E., Price, D., & James, S. (1997). *Thompson's pediatric nursing: An introductory text* (7th ed.). Philadelphia: W. B. Saunders. p. 97.

2. **4**

RATIONALE: Late signs of increased ICP include tachycardia leading to bradycardia, apnea, systolic hypertension, widening pulse pressure, and posturing. A bulging fontanel is a sign of increased ICP in an infant. Nausea and altered level of consciousness are signs of increased ICP in a child. Options 1, 2, and 3 are not late signs.
TEST-TAKING STRATEGY: Note the age of the child and that the question asks for the "late" sign. Option 1 can be eliminated because the fontanels are closed in a child. Knowledge of the early and late signs will direct you to the correct option. Review these signs now if you had difficulty with this question.
LEVEL OF COGNITIVE ABILITY: Comprehension
PHASE OF NURSING PROCESS: Data Collection
CLIENT NEEDS: Physiological Integrity
CONTENT AREA: Child Health
REFERENCE
Schulte, E., Price, D., & James, S. (1997). *Thompson's pediatric nursing: An introductory text* (7th ed.). Philadelphia: W. B. Saunders. p. 230.

3. **3**

RATIONALE: The most likely medication to be prescribed to prevent urinary tract infection is an antibiotic. A common prescribed medication is sulfisoxazole (Gantrisin). The neurogenic bladder prevents the bladder from completely emptying due to the decrease in muscle tone. Prednisone relieves allergic reactions and inflammation rather than preventing infection. Lasix promotes diuresis and decreases edema caused by congestive heart failure. Immune globulin IV assists with antibody production with immune compromised clients. Option 3 is the correct answer.

TEST-TAKING STRATEGY: Knowledge of the actions and uses of these medications is required to answer this question. If you are unfamiliar with these medications, take time now to review their actions and purposes.
LEVEL OF COGNITIVE ABILITY: Comprehension
PHASE OF NURSING PROCESS: Planning
CLIENT NEEDS: Physiological Integrity
CONTENT AREA: Pharmacology
REFERENCE
Deglin, J., & Vallerand, A. (1999). *Davis's drug guide for nurses* (6th ed.). Philadelphia: F. A. Davis. pp. 414, 436, 939.

4. 1

RATIONALE: Persistent vomiting is a major symptom associated with intracranial pressure. Intracranial pressure and encephalopathy are major symptoms of Reye's syndrome. Options 2, 3, and 4 are incorrect. Protein is not present in the urine. Reye's syndrome is related to a history of viral infections, and hypoglycemia is a symptom of this disease.
TEST-TAKING STRATEGY: Knowledge related to the symptoms associated with Reye's syndrome is required to answer this question. Recalling that ICP is an associated characteristic will easily direct you to option 1. If you had difficulty with this question, take time now to review the symptoms of Reye's syndrome and the signs of intracranial pressure.
LEVEL OF COGNITIVE ABILITY: Comprehension
PHASE OF NURSING PROCESS: Data Collection
CLIENT NEEDS: Physiological Integrity
CONTENT AREA: Child Health
REFERENCE
O'Toole, M. (ed.). (1997). *Miller-Keane encyclopedia & dictionary of medicine, nursing, & allied health* (6th ed.). Philadelphia: W. B. Saunders. p. 1411.

5. 1

RATIONALE: The major elements of care are to maintain effective cerebral perfusion and control intracranial pressure. Decreasing stimuli in the environment decreases the stress on the cerebral tissue and neuron responses. Cerebral edema is a progressive part of this disease process. Hearing loss and output are not affected. Changing the body position every 2 hours does not affect the cerebral edema and intracranial pressure directly. The child should be in a head elevated position to decrease the progression of the cerebral edema and promote drainage of cerebrospinal fluid.
TEST-TAKING STRATEGY: Knowledge of the effect of environmental stimuli and the responses of the brain cells to stimuli are required to recognize how cerebral edema can result. If you had difficulty with this question, take time now to review the appropriate plan of nursing care for the child with Reye's syndrome.
LEVEL OF COGNITIVE ABILITY: Application
PHASE OF NURSING PROCESS: Planning
CLIENT NEEDS: Physiological Integrity
CONTENT AREA: Child Health
REFERENCE
Schulte, E., Price, D., & James, S. (1997). *Thompson's pediatric nursing: An introductory text* (7th ed.). Philadelphia: W. B. Saunders. pp. 230–231.

6. 2

RATIONALE: The vomiting that occurs in Reye's syndrome is caused by cerebral edema and is a symptom of

intracranial pressure. Small frequent meals will not affect the amount of vomiting. Options 1, 3, and 4 are all correct. Decreasing stimuli and providing rest decrease stress on the brain tissue. Checking for jaundice will assist in identifying the presence of liver complications, which are characteristic of Reye's syndrome.
TEST-TAKING STRATEGY: Knowledge regarding the causes of vomiting with Reye's syndrome will assist in answering this question. Note the key words "need for further education." Options 1, 3, and 4 are correct statements. If you had difficulty with this question, take time now to review the parent teaching points associated with the care of the child with Reye's syndrome.
LEVEL OF COGNITIVE ABILITY: Comprehension
PHASE OF NURSING PROCESS: Evaluation
CLIENT NEEDS: Health Promotion and Maintenance
CONTENT AREA: Child Health
REFERENCE
Schulte, E., Price, D., & James, S. (1997). *Thompson's pediatric nursing: An introductory text* (7th ed.). Philadelphia: W. B. Saunders. p. 241.

7. 2

RATIONALE: Parents are especially concerned about seizures that might go undetected at nighttime. The nurse should suggest a baby monitor. Reassurance by the nurse should ensure parental confidence and decrease overprotection. Options 1 and 3 demonstrate the parents' ability to choose respite care and activities appropriately. Option 4 is a common concern. The parents need to be reminded that, as the child grows, they cannot always observe their child, but that their knowledge of seizure activity and care are appropriate to minimize complications.
TEST-TAKING STRATEGY: Use the process of elimination and note the key words "need for further education." Option 2 identifies a need to provide the parents with an alternate manner to monitor for night seizures. Review parent teaching regarding seizures now, if you had difficulty with this question.
LEVEL OF COGNITIVE ABILITY: Comprehension
PHASE OF NURSING PROCESS: Evaluation
CLIENT NEEDS: Psychosocial Integrity
CONTENT AREA: Child Health
REFERENCE
Schulte, E., Price, D., & James, S. (1997). *Thompson's pediatric nursing: An introductory text* (7th ed.). Philadelphia: W. B. Saunders. p. 275.

8. 1

RATIONALE: The complications associated with seizures include airway compromise, extremity and teeth injuries, and tongue lacerations. Night seizures can cause the child to bite down on the tongue. Cyanosis can occur during the tonic-clonic part of the seizure activity, but blanching does not occur. Migraine headaches are not common in children with seizures. Seizures do not cause a high-pitched cry unless a tumor or intracranial pressure is the cause of the seizure diagnosis.
TEST-TAKING STRATEGY: Use knowledge of tonic-clonic activity and the involuntary tightening of all the body muscles that occurs during seizure activity when answering this question. Recall that the tongue can get easily caught by the child's teeth when the seizure activity occurs. This causes injury, swelling, and bleeding of the tongue tissue. Knowledge of the potential complications of seizures will assist in eliminating options 2, 3, and 4. If you had

difficulty with this question, take time now to review the complications associated with seizures.
LEVEL OF COGNITIVE ABILITY: Comprehension
PHASE OF NURSING PROCESS: Data Collection
CLIENT NEEDS: Physiological Integrity
CONTENT AREA: Child Health
REFERENCE
Schulte, E., Price, D., & James, S. (1997). *Thompson's pediatric nursing: An introductory text* (7th ed.). Philadelphia: W. B. Saunders. p. 275.

9. **1**

RATIONALE: Grand mal seizures cause tightening of all body muscles followed by tremors. Obstructive airway and increased oral secretions are the major complications during and following the seizure. Options 2 and 4 are incorrect because inserting a tracheostomy is not done. Suctioning is helpful to prevent choking and cyanosis. Option 3 is incorrect because this cart would not be left at the bedside, but would be available in the treatment room or on the nursing unit.
TEST-TAKING STRATEGY: Recall that grand mal seizures produce excessive oral secretions and airway obstruction. This will easily direct you to option 1. If you had difficulty with this question, take time now to review the plan of care associated with seizure precautions.
LEVEL OF COGNITIVE ABILITY: Application
PHASE OF NURSING PROCESS: Planning
CLIENT NEEDS: Safe, Effective Care Environment
CONTENT AREA: Child Health
REFERENCE
Schulte, E., Price, D., & James, S. (1997). *Thompson's pediatric nursing: An introductory text* (7th ed.). Philadelphia: W. B. Saunders. p. 275.

10. **3**

RATIONALE: Alcohol, marijuana, and street drugs will lower the seizure threshold. These substances need to be avoided. Adolescents can attain a driver's license, in most states, when they are seizure-free for one year. Anticonvulsants cause acne and oily skin; therefore, a dermatologist may need to be consulted. If an anticonvulsant medication is missed, the physician should be notified.
TEST-TAKING STRATEGY: Knowledge of medication administration, side effects, and the interactions of anticonvulsants with other medications and substances is needed. Laws of each state vary, but most consider 1 year of seizure-free activity as adequate to obtain a driver's license. Prescribed medications, if missed, require a physician or pharmacist's guidance. If you had difficulty with this question, take time now to review the client education points related to anticonvulsants.
LEVEL OF COGNITIVE ABILITY: Comprehension
PHASE OF NURSING PROCESS: Evaluation
CLIENT NEEDS: Health Promotion and Maintenance
CONTENT AREA: Pharmacology
REFERENCE
Ashwill, J., & Droske, S. (1997). *Nursing care of children: Principles and practice*. Philadelphia: W. B. Saunders. p. 1257.

11. **3**

RATIONALE: Fever and infections raise the body metabolism. This can cause seizure activity in children under the age of 5 years. Dehydration and electrolyte imbalance can also contribute to seizure occurrence. Falls can cause pres-

sure, which increases intracranial pressure or cerebral edema. Some medications could cause seizures. Specific gravity is not a reliable test as it varies depending on the existing condition. Psychiatric illness has no impact on seizure occurrence or cause. Children do not remember what happened during the seizure itself.
TEST-TAKING STRATEGY: Knowledge of the causes and precipitating factors associated with seizures is required to answer this question. Additionally, knowledge regarding the process of gathering appropriate data regarding the causes of a seizure will assist in eliminating the incorrect options. If you had difficulty with this question, take time now to review the precipitating factors associated with seizures.
LEVEL OF COGNITIVE ABILITY: Application
PHASE OF NURSING PROCESS: Data Collection
CLIENT NEEDS: Physiological Integrity
CONTENT AREA: Child Health
REFERENCE
Schulte, E., Price, D., & James, S. (1997). *Thompson's pediatric nursing: An introductory text* (7th ed.). Philadelphia: W. B. Saunders. p. 276.

12. **1**

RATIONALE: Cerebral palsy is a chronic disability characterized by difficulty in controlling the muscles due to an abnormality in the extrapyramidal or pyramidal motor system. Meningitis is an infectious process of the central nervous system. Encephalitis is an inflammation of the brain that occurs as a result of viral illness or CNS infection. Down's syndrome is an example of a congenital condition that results in moderate to severe retardation.
TEST-TAKING STRATEGY: Use the process of elimination. Eliminate options 2 and 3 first, noting that they are similar and basically stating a similar statement. Note the relationship between "palsy" in the question and "muscles" in option 1, the correct option. If you had difficulty with this question, take time now to review the characteristics associated with cerebral palsy.
LEVEL OF COGNITIVE ABILITY: Comprehension
PHASE OF NURSING PROCESS: Planning
CLIENT NEEDS: Physiological Integrity
CONTENT AREA: Child Health
REFERENCE
Schulte, E., Price, D., & James, S. (1997). *Thompson's pediatric nursing: An introductory text* (7th ed.). Philadelphia: W. B. Saunders. p. 227.

13. **3**

RATIONALE: The goal of managing the child with cerebral palsy is early recognition and intervention to maximize the child's abilities. The cause of the disease cannot be eliminated. The disease is caused by damage to the motor system that can occur during the prenatal, perinatal, and postnatal periods. It is best to minimize emotional disturbances if possible, but not to prevent them because it is healthy for the child to express emotions. Improvement of muscle control and coordination is a component of the plan, but the primary goal is to maximize the child's assets and minimize the limitations caused by the disease.
TEST-TAKING STRATEGY: Use knowledge regarding cerebral palsy and the process of elimination. Eliminate options 1 and 2 first because the cause of the disease cannot be eliminated nor can emotional disturbances be prevented. From the remaining two options, identify the option that is the most global, option 3.

LEVEL OF COGNITIVE ABILITY: Application
PHASE OF NURSING PROCESS: Planning
CLIENT NEEDS: Psychosocial Integrity
CONTENT AREA: Child Health
REFERENCE
Schulte, E., Price, D., & James, S. (1997). *Thompson's pediatric nursing: An introductory text* (7th ed.). Philadelphia: W. B. Saunders. p. 228.

14. **3**

RATIONALE: Down's syndrome is a form of mental retardation. It is a congenital condition that results in moderate to severe mental retardation. A high percentage of cases are linked to an extra group G chromosome, chromosome 21 (trisomy 21).
TEST-TAKING STRATEGY: Use the process of elimination. Eliminate options 1 and 2 first because average and above-average intelligence is not associated with this disorder. Eliminate option 4 because deficits in adaptive behavior do occur with Down's syndrome. Knowing that Down's syndrome is associated with an extra chromosome will assist in directing you to the correct option. If you had difficulty with this question, take time now to review the characteristics associated with Down's syndrome.
LEVEL OF COGNITIVE ABILITY: Comprehension
PHASE OF NURSING PROCESS: Implementation
CLIENT NEEDS: Physiological Integrity
CONTENT AREA: Child Health
REFERENCE
Schulte, E., Price, D., & James, S. (1997). *Thompson's pediatric nursing: An introductory text* (7th ed.). Philadelphia: W. B. Saunders. p. 114.

15. **4**

RATIONALE: Nasotracheal suctioning is contraindicated in a child with a basilar skull fracture. Because of the nature of the injury, the suction catheter may be introduced into the brain. The child may need a urinary catheter for accurate monitoring of I&O. Fluids are restricted to prevent fluid overload. An IV line is maintained to administer fluids or medications if necessary.
TEST-TAKING STRATEGY: Knowledge regarding care to a child with a basilar skull fracture is required to answer this question. Note that options 1, 2, and 3 are similar in that they all address the issue of fluid intake or output. If you had difficulty with this question, take time now to review the care of a child with this type of skull fracture.
LEVEL OF COGNITIVE ABILITY: Comprehension
PHASE OF NURSING PROCESS: Implementation
CLIENT NEEDS: Safe, Effective Care Environment
CONTENT AREA: Child Health
REFERENCE
Ashwill, J., & Droske, S. (1997). *Nursing care of children: Principles and practice.* Philadelphia: W. B. Saunders. p. 1261.

16. **2**

RATIONALE: A diagnosis of meningitis is made by testing CSF obtained by lumbar puncture. In the case of bacterial meningitis, findings usually include increased pressure, cloudy CSF, high protein, and low glucose.
TEST-TAKING STRATEGY: Use the process of elimination and knowledge regarding the diagnostic findings in meningitis. Eliminate options 3 and 4 first because clear CSF and decreased pressure are not likely to be found if an infectious process such as meningitis is suspected. From this point, knowledge that high protein indicates a possible diagnosis of meningitis is helpful. If you had difficulty with this question, take time now to review this diagnostic test.
LEVEL OF COGNITIVE ABILITY: Comprehension
PHASE OF NURSING PROCESS: Data Collection
CLIENT NEEDS: Physiological Integrity
CONTENT AREA: Child Health
REFERENCE
Schulte, E., Price, D., & James, S. (1997). *Thompson's pediatric nursing: An introductory text* (7th ed.). Philadelphia: W. B. Saunders. p. 177.

17. **3**

RATIONALE: Meningococcal meningitis is transmitted primarily by droplet infection; the risk increases as the number of contacts increase. Isolation is begun and maintained for at least 24 hours after antibiotics are given.
TEST-TAKING STRATEGY: Knowledge regarding the mode of transmission of meningococcal meningitis is required to answer this question. Use the process of elimination to eliminate options 2 and 4 first. Both enteric and neutropenic precautions are unrelated to the mode of transmission. Knowledge that it takes approximately 24 hours for antibiotics to reach a therapeutic blood level will assist in the selection of option 3 over option 2. If you had difficulty with this question, take time now to review the mode of transmission of meningococcal meningitis.
LEVEL OF COGNITIVE ABILITY: Application
PHASE OF NURSING PROCESS: Planning
CLIENT NEEDS: Safe, Effective Care Environment
CONTENT AREA: Child Health
REFERENCE
Schulte, E., Price, D., & James, S. (1997). *Thompson's pediatric nursing: An introductory text* (7th ed.). Philadelphia: W. B. Saunders. p. 177.

18. **1**

RATIONALE: Altered cerebral tissue perfusion is the priority nursing diagnosis for the child with meningitis. Pain related to meningeal irritation and altered family process related to a child with an acute illness may also be appropriate problems, but are not the priority. Parental knowledge deficit related to the seriousness of meningitis and the possible residual neurological deficits would be a secondary problem.
TEST-TAKING STRATEGY: Knowledge regarding the risk of intracranial pressure in the child with meningitis assists in answering the question. Use the ABCs, airway, breathing, and circulation, to assist in answering the question. Tissue perfusion relates to circulation.
LEVEL OF COGNITIVE ABILITY: Application
PHASE OF NURSING PROCESS: Planning
CLIENT NEEDS: Physiological Integrity
CONTENT AREA: Child Health
REFERENCE
Schulte, E., Price, D., & James, S. (1997). *Thompson's pediatric nursing: An introductory text* (7th ed.). Philadelphia: W. B. Saunders. p. 178.

19. **3**

RATIONALE: Autism is a severe developmental disorder that begins in infancy or toddlerhood. The primary characteristic is lack of social interaction and awareness. Social behaviors in autism include lack of or abnormal imitation of others' actions, and the lack of or abnormal social play. Additional characteristics include lack of or impaired verbal communication and markedly abnormal nonverbal communication.

TEST-TAKING STRATEGY: Use knowledge of the characteristics of autism and the process of elimination. Eliminate options 2 and 4 first because they address normal behaviors. Knowledge that the autistic child lacks social interaction and awareness will direct you to select option 3. If you had difficulty with this question, take time now to review the characteristics associated with autism.

LEVEL OF COGNITIVE ABILITY: Application
PHASE OF NURSING PROCESS: Data Collection
CLIENT NEEDS: Psychosocial Integrity
CONTENT AREA: Child Health
REFERENCE
Leifer, G. (1999). *Thompson's introduction to maternity and pediatric nursing* (3rd ed.). Philadelphia: W. B. Saunders. p. 838.

20. **4**

RATIONALE: The most likely findings in sexual abuse include difficulty walking or sitting; torn, stained, or bloody underclothing; pain, swelling, or itching of the genitals; and bruises, bleeding, or lacerations in the genital or anal area. Poor hygiene may be indicative of physical neglect. Bald spots on the scalp and fear of the parents are most likely associated with physical abuse.

TEST-TAKING STRATEGY: Note the key words "sexually abused." The only option that specifically addresses a finding related to sexual abuse is option 4. If you had difficulty with this question, take time now to review the findings in a child suspected of abuse.

LEVEL OF COGNITIVE ABILITY: Comprehension
PHASE OF NURSING PROCESS: Data Collection
CLIENT NEEDS: Physiological Integrity
CONTENT AREA: Child Health
REFERENCE
Leifer, G. (1999). *Thompson's introduction to maternity and pediatric nursing* (3rd ed.). Philadelphia: W. B. Saunders. p. 641.

BIBLIOGRAPHY

Ashwill, J., & Droske, S. (1997). *Nursing care of children: Principles and practice.* Philadelphia: W. B. Saunders.

Deglin, J., & Vallerand, A. (1999). *Davis's drug guide for nurses* (6th ed.). Philadelphia: F. A. Davis.

Leifer, G. (1999). *Thompson's introduction to maternity and pediatric nursing* (3rd ed.). Philadelphia: W. B. Saunders.

O'Toole, M. (ed.). (1997). *Miller-Keane encyclopedia & dictionary of medicine, nursing, & allied health* (6th ed.). Philadelphia: W. B. Saunders.

Schulte, E., Price, D., & James, S. (1997). *Thompson's pediatric nursing: An introductory text* (7th ed.). Philadelphia: W. B. Saunders.

CHAPTER 29

Eye, Ear, Throat, and Respiratory Disorders

I. Strabismus

A. Description
1. Called "squint" or "lazy eye"
2. A condition in which the eyes are not aligned because of lack of coordination of the extraocular muscles
3. Most often due to muscle imbalance or paralysis of extraocular muscles, but may also result from conditions such as a brain tumor, myasthenia gravis, or infection
4. Normal in the young infant but should not be present after about age 4 months

B. Data collection
1. Amblyopia or permanent loss of vision if not treated early
2. Loss of binocular vision
3. Impairment of depth perception
4. Frequent headaches
5. Squints or tilts the head to see

C. Implementation
1. Corrective lenses as indicated
2. Instruct the parents regarding eye-patching of the "good" eye to strengthen the weak eye
3. Prepare for surgery to realign the weak muscles if prescribed
4. Prepare the child for botulinum toxin (Botox) injection into the eye muscle, which produces temporary paralysis and allows muscles opposite the paralyzed muscle to straighten the eye
5. Inform the parents the injection of Botox wears off in about 2 months, and if successful, correction will occur
6. Instruct the parents in the need for follow-up visits

II. Conjunctivitis

A. Description
1. Also known as "pinkeye"
2. Inflammation of the conjunctiva
3. Usually caused by allergy, infection, or trauma
4. Bacterial and viral conjunctivitis is extremely contagious
5. Chlamydial conjunctivitis is rare in older children and if diagnosed in a nonsexually active child, the child should be assessed for possible sexual **abuse**

B. Data collection
1. Itching, burning, or scratchy eyelids
2. Redness, edema, discharge

C. Implementation
1. Instruct in infection control measures such as good handwashing and not sharing towels and washcloths
2. Administer antibiotic or antiviral eye drops or ointment as prescribed if infection is present
3. Administer antihistamines as prescribed if an allergy is present
4. Instruct the child and parents in the administration of the prescribed medications
5. Instruct the parents that the child should be kept home from school or day care until antibiotic eye drops have been administered for 24 hours
6. Instruct the child to avoid rubbing the eye to prevent injury
7. Instruct the child wearing contact lenses to discontinue wearing them and to obtain new lenses to eliminate the chance of reinfection
8. Instruct the adolescent that eye makeup should be discarded and replaced
9. Instruct in the use of cool compresses to lessen irritation, and in wearing dark glasses for photophobia

III. Otitis Media

A. Description
1. Infection of the middle ear occurring from a blocked eustachian tube, which prevents normal drainage

2. Otitis media is a common complication of an acute respiratory infection
3. Infants and children are more prone to otitis media because their eustachian tubes are shorter, wider, and straighter

B. Data collection
1. Fever, irritability, and restlessness
2. Earache or pain
3. Rolling of the head from side to side
4. Pulling or rubbing the ear
5. Loss of appetite
6. Hearing loss
7. Purulent drainage
8. Red, opaque, bulging, or retracting tympanic membrane

C. Implementation
1. Encourage fluids
2. Teach the parents to feed infants in an upright position
3. Instruct the child to avoid chewing during the acute period because chewing increases pain
4. Provide local heat and have the child lie with the affected ear down
5. Instruct the parents in the appropriate procedure to clean drainage from the ear with sterile cotton swabs
6. Instruct in the administration of analgesics or antipyretics such as acetaminophen (Tylenol) to decrease fever and pain
7. Instruct the parents in the administration of the prescribed antibiotics emphasizing that the 10- to 14-day period is necessary to eradicate positive organisms
8. Instruct the parents that screening for hearing loss may be necessary
9. If ear drops are prescribed, instruct the parents to pull the earlobe down and back in children younger than age 3, and to pull the pinna up and back for a child older than 3 years

D. Myringotomy
1. Description: insertion of tympanoplasty tubes into the middle ear to equalize pressure and keep the ear aerated
2. Implementation postoperatively
   a. Instruct the parents and child to keep the ears dry
   b. Ear plugs should be worn during bathing, shampooing, and swimming
   c. Diving and submerging in water is not allowed

IV. Tonsillectomy and Adenoidectomy

A. Description
1. Tonsillitis is a term commonly used to describe an inflammation and infection of the tonsils
2. Adenoiditis refers to infection and inflammation of the adenoids

B. Data collection
1. Persistent or recurrent sore throat
2. Enlarged bright red tonsils, which may be covered with white exudate

3. Difficulty swallowing
4. Mouth breathing and an unpleasant mouth odor
5. Fever
6. Cough
7. Enlarged adenoids may cause nasal quality of speech, mouth breathing, hearing difficulty, snoring, or obstructive sleep apnea

C. Implementation preoperatively
1. Monitor for signs of active infection
2. Monitor bleeding and clotting studies because the throat is very vascular
3. Prepare the child for a sore throat postoperatively and inform of the need to drink liquids
4. Check for any loose teeth to decrease the risk of aspiration during surgery

D. Implementation postoperatively
1. Position prone or side-lying to facilitate drainage
2. Have suction equipment available but do not suction unless there is an airway obstruction
3. Monitor for signs of hemorrhage; if hemorrhage occurs, turn the child to the side and notify the physician
4. Discourage coughing or clearing the throat
5. Provide clear, cool, noncitrus, and noncarbonated fluids
6. Avoid milk products initially as they will coat the throat
7. Avoid red liquids, which will indicate the appearance of blood if the child vomits
8. Do not give the child any straws, forks, or sharp objects that can be put in the mouth
9. Administer acetaminophen (Tylenol) for a sore throat as prescribed
10. Instruct the parents to notify physician if bleeding, persistent earache, or fever occurs
11. Instruct the parents to keep child away from crowds until healing has occurred

V. Epiglottitis

A. Description
1. A bacterial form of croup
2. An inflammation of the epiglottis most commonly caused by *Haemophilus influenzae* type B or *Streptococcus pneumoniae*
3. Occurs most frequently in age group 3 to 7 years
4. The onset is abrupt and occurs most often in the winter
5. Considered an emergency situation

B. Data collection
1. High fever
2. Red and inflamed sore throat
3. Difficulty swallowing, and drooling
4. Muffled voice
5. Inspiratory **stridor**
6. Absence of spontaneous cough
7. Tripod positioning; while supporting body with hands, the child thrusts the chin forward

and opens the mouth in an attempt to widen the airway

C. Implementation
1. Monitor airway status
2. Monitor respiratory status noting **nasal flaring,** the use of accessory muscles, and the presence of **stridor**
3. Monitor vital signs by taking the temperature by the axillary not the oral route
4. Do not leave the child unattended
5. Do not force the child to lie down
6. Do not restrain the child
7. NO attempts should be made to visualize posterior pharynx or to obtain throat culture to prevent spasm of epiglottis and airway occlusion
8. Maintain NPO status
9. Monitor hydration status and intake and output (I&O) status
10. Prepare the child for lateral neck films to confirm diagnosis
11. Antibiotics and IV fluids may be prescribed
12. Administer analgesics and antipyretics (acetaminophen [Tylenol]) to reduce fever and throat pain as prescribed
13. Provide cool-mist oxygen therapy as prescribed
14. Provide high humidification to cool the airway and decrease swelling
15. Have resuscitation equipment available
16. Prepare for endotracheal intubation or tracheotomy for severe respiratory distress
17. Question the physician regarding the need for immunization (*Haemophilus* type B) to prevent recurrence

VI. Laryngotrachcobronchitis (Croup)

A. Description
1. Inflammation of the larynx, trachea, and bronchi
2. May be viral or bacterial
3. Has a gradual onset and may be preceded by an upper respiratory infection
B. Data collection
1. Fever
2. Irritability, restlessness
3. Hoarse voice, seal bark, and brassy cough
4. Inspiratory **stridor** and labored respirations
5. Use of accessory muscles for breathing
6. Anorexia, nausea, and vomiting
7. Cyanosis
C. Implementation
1. Maintain patent airway
2. Assess respiratory status, monitoring for **nasal flaring,** sternal retraction, and inspiratory **stridor**
3. Monitor for cyanosis or pallor
4. Monitor vital signs
5. Elevate the head of the bed and provide bed rest

6. Provide humidified oxygen via cool-mist tent
7. Provide fluids and monitor IVs as prescribed to maintain hydration status
8. Administer acetaminophen (Tylenol) to reduce fever
9. Avoid cough syrups and cold medicines, which may dry and thicken secretions
10. Administer antibiotics as prescribed, noting that they are not indicated unless a bacterial infection is present
11. Administer bronchodilators if prescribed to relax smooth muscle and relieve **stridor**
12. Administer corticosteroids if prescribed for anti-inflammatory effect
13. Have resuscitation equipment available

VII. Bronchitis

A. Description: infection of the major bronchi
B. Data collection
1. Fever
2. Hacking and productive cough
3. Rhonchi and rales
C. Implementation
1. Monitor for respiratory distress
2. Monitor vital signs
3. Provide humidified air
4. Monitor for signs of dehydration such as sunken fontanels, poor skin turgor, and decreased and concentrated urinary output
5. Increase fluid intake
6. Monitor weight
7. Administer acetaminophen (Tylenol) for fever as prescribed
8. Administer respiratory treatments as prescribed

VIII. Bronchiolitis

A. Description
1. An inflammation of the bronchioles that causes a thick production of mucus that occludes the bronchiole tubes and small bronchi
2. Respiratory syncytial virus (RSV) is a common cause
3. RSV, although not airborne, is highly communicable and is usually transferred by the hands
B. Data collection
1. Upper respiratory infection (URI) symptoms
2. Fever
3. Nasal drainage
4. Tachypnea
5. Increased difficulty breathing
6. **Nasal flaring, retractions**
7. Expiratory wheeze and grunt
8. Harsh cough
C. Implementation
1. Maintain patent airway
2. Monitor vital signs
3. Position at a 30- to 40-degree angle with the

neck slightly extended to maintain an open airway and decrease pressure on the diaphragm
4. Provide cool, humidified oxygen
5. Monitor for signs of dehydration such as sunken fontanels, poor skin turgor, or decreased and concentrated urinary output

D. The child with RSV
1. Isolate in a single room or place in a room with another RSV child
2. Maintain good handwashing procedures
3. Nurses caring for these children do not care for other high-risk children
4. Wear gowns when soiling of clothing may occur
5. Ribavirin (Virazole), an antiviral respiratory medication, may be prescribed
6. The nurse wearing contact lenses should wear goggles when coming in contact with ribavirin because the mist may dissolve soft lenses

IX. Asthma (Fig. 29–1)

A. Description
1. Includes bronchospasm, edema, and inflammation of the bronchial airways
2. Is commonly caused by physical and chemical irritants such as foods, pollens, dust, smoke, animal dander, temperature changes, URI, activity, and stress

B. Data collection
1. Dyspnea, expiratory **wheezing**
2. Hacking, nonproductive cough
3. Hoarse, loud breath sounds
4. Tachycardia
5. Orthopnea
6. Apprehension and restlessness

C. Implementation
1. Acute episode
a. Monitor cardiac and respiratory status and pulse oximetry

b. Prepare the child for chest x-ray
c. Administer humidified oxygen by nasal prongs or face mask as prescribed
d. Bronchodilator via nebulizer and corticosteroids may be prescribed
e. Prepare the child for blood gases if prescribed
f. Prepare to administer subcutaneous epinephrine if the child does not respond to treatment
g. Be alert to decreased **wheezing** or a silent chest, which may signal the inability to move air
2. Long-term management
a. Eliminate or avoid allergens or environmental factors that can precipitate an attack
b. Avoid exposure to individuals with a viral respiratory infection
c. Instruct the child how to recognize early symptoms of an asthma attack, which may include an itchy chest or chin, cough, irritability or tired feeling, increased breathing rate, dry mouth, or unusual dark circles under the eyes
d. Instruct in the administration of bronchodilators and anti-inflammatory medications as prescribed
e. Encourage adequate rest, sleep, and a well-balanced diet
f. Instruct in the importance of adequate fluid intake to liquefy secretions
g. Assist in developing an exercise program
h. Instruct in the procedure for respiratory treatments and exercises as prescribed
i. Encourage the parents to keep immunizations up to date
j. Inform other health care providers of the asthma condition
k. Allow the child to take control of self-care measures based on age appropriateness

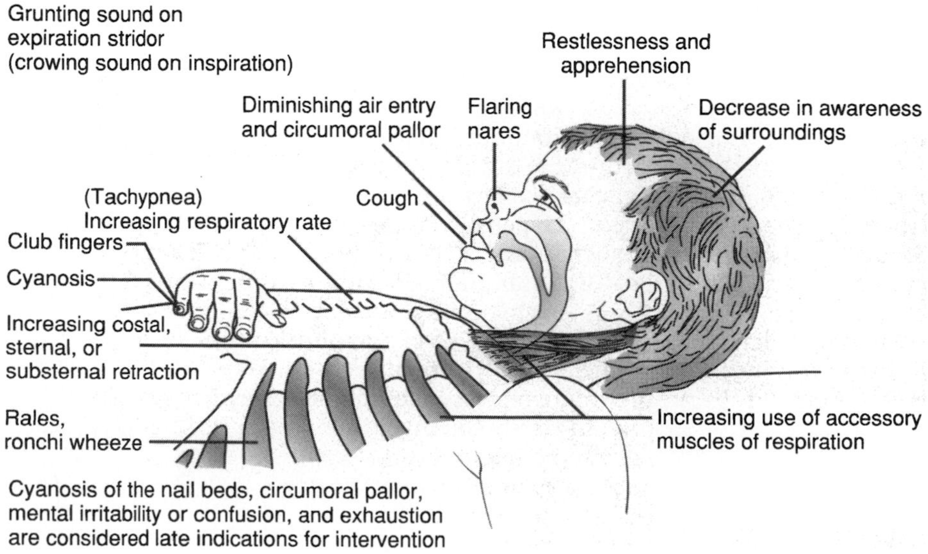

Grunting sound on expiration stridor (crowing sound on inspiration)

Restlessness and apprehension

Diminishing air entry and circumoral pallor

Flaring nares

Decrease in awareness of surroundings

(Tachypnea) Increasing respiratory rate

Cough

Club fingers

Cyanosis

Increasing costal, sternal, or substernal retraction

Rales, ronchi wheeze

Increasing use of accessory muscles of respiration

Cyanosis of the nail beds, circumoral pallor, mental irritability or confusion, and exhaustion are considered late indications for intervention

FIGURE 29–1. Signs of respiratory distress in infants and children. (From Leifer, G. [1999]. *Thompson's introduction to maternity and pediatric nursing* [3rd ed.]. Philadelphia: W. B. Saunders. p. 650.)

X. Pneumonia

A. Description: inflammation of the alveoli caused by bacteria, virus, organisms, and aspiration

B. Data collection
   1. Pneumococcal pneumonia
      a. Fever
      b. Increased pulse and respiratory rate
      c. **Retractions**
      d. Productive cough
   2. Viral pneumonia
      a. Follows URI
      b. Low-grade fever
      c. Nonproductive cough
      d. Increased respiratory rate
   3. Staphylococcal pneumonia
      a. Fever
      b. Cough
      c. Respiratory distress
      d. Cyanosis

C. Implementation
   1. Monitor breath sounds and respiratory rate
   2. Monitor vital signs
   3. Elevate the head of the bed
   4. Monitor cardiac and respiratory status and pulse oximetry
   5. Provide humidified oxygen as prescribed
   6. Monitor for restlessness
   7. Monitor I&O and weight
   8. Monitor for signs of dehydration
   9. Encourage fluid intake of warm liquids to loosen secretions
   10. Administer antipyretics (acetaminophen [Tylenol]) for fever
   11. Administer antibiotics as prescribed
   12. Assist with coughing and deep breathing
   13. Schedule chest physiotherapy before meals and bedtime
   14. Monitor for tension pneumothorax or empyema with staphylococcal pneumonia
   15. Maintain isolation with pneumococcal and staphylococcal pneumonia
   16. Avoid the use of infant seats because pressure may be placed on the diaphragm, decreasing lung expansion

XI. Cystic Fibrosis (CF) (Fig. 29–2)

A. Description
   1. A chronic multisystem disorder affecting exocrine gland function
   2. The mucus produced by the exocrine gland is abnormally thick, causing obstruction of the small passageways of these organs
   3. An autosomal recessive trait disorder

B. Data collection
   1. Respiratory system
      a. **Wheezing** and dry nonproductive cough
      b. Repeated episodes of bronchitis and pneumonia
      c. Purulent and copious sputum with infections
      d. Crackles and diminished breath sounds
      e. **Retractions,** accessory muscle use
      f. Hypoxia, cyanosis
      g. Barrel chest
      h. Clubbing of fingers (Fig. 29–3)
      i. Emphysema and atelectasis as the airways become increasingly obstructed
   2. Gastrointestinal system
      a. Steatorrhea
      b. Malnutrition and **growth** failure
      c. Protuberant abdomen
      d. Meconium ileus in the neonate
      e. Rectal prolapse and intussusception
      f. Biliary cirrhosis, portal hypertension, and esophageal varices as a result of obstruction of bile ducts
   3. Integumentary system
      a. Abnormally high concentrations of sodium and chloride in sweat
      b. Electrolyte imbalances especially during the hot weather
      c. Dry mouth
      d. Increased susceptibility to infection
   4. Reproductive system
      a. An average of 2 years' delay in development
      b. Difficulty becoming pregnant because of thick cervical mucus
      c. Increases incidence of fetal loss and preterm birth

C. Sweat test
   1. Sweating is stimulated on the child's forearm with pilocarpine, and the amount of sodium and chloride is measured
   2. A chloride level greater than 60 mEq/L is a positive test result
   3. A chloride level of 40 mEq/L is suggestive of CF and requires a repeat test

D. Implementation
   1. Monitor respiratory status
   2. Elevate the head of the bed or support the child in an upright position if he or she is having difficulty breathing
   3. Administer humidified low-flow oxygen
   4. Encourage coughing and deep breathing
   5. Teach the child forced expiratory technique to mobilize secretions
   6. Perform respiratory treatments as prescribed
   7. Administer CPT before meals
   8. Monitor weight; promote optimal nutrition and hydration
   9. Administer expectorants and bronchodilators as prescribed to facilitate thinning and mobilization of secretions
   10. Instruct the parents not to give cough suppressants because they will inhibit expectoration of secretions and promote infection
   11. Protect the child from exposure to infections

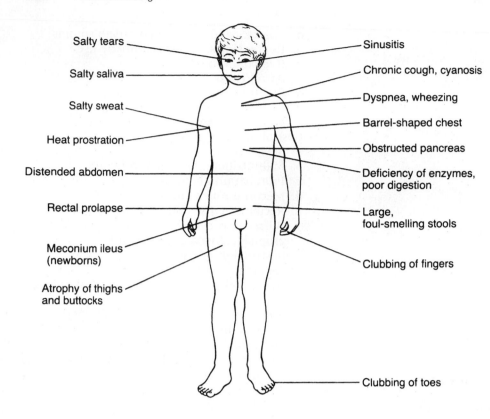

Salty tears

Salty saliva

Salty sweat

Heat prostration

Distended abdomen

Rectal prolapse

Meconium ileus
(newborns)

Atrophy of thighs
and buttocks

Sinusitis

Chronic cough, cyanosis

Dyspnea, wheezing

Barrel-shaped chest

Obstructed pancreas

Deficiency of enzymes,
poor digestion

Large,
foul-smelling stools

Clubbing of fingers

Clubbing of toes

FIGURE 29–2. Manifestations of cystic fibrosis. (From Leifer, G. [1999]. *Thompson's introduction to maternity and pediatric nursing* [3rd ed.]. Philadelphia: W. B. Saunders. p. 665.)

12. Instruct the parents to be sure immunizations are up to date
13. Administer pancreatic enzymes as prescribed within 30 minutes of eating meals and snacks
14. Do not mix pancreatic enzymes with hot or starchy foods but with a small amount of nonfat, nonprotein food
15. Enteric coated pancreatic enzymes should not be crushed or chewed
16. Pancreatic enzymes should not be given if the child is NPO
17. Administer multivitamins and iron supplements as prescribed
18. Supplement the child's diet with salt during extremely hot weather or if the child has a fever
19. Instruct in the administration of antibiotics if prescribed
20. Instruct in the use of mucolytics,

bronchodilators, hydrating agents, and corticosteroids as prescribed

XII. Sudden Infant Death Syndrome (SIDS)

A. Description
   1. Unexpected death of an apparently healthy infant under age 1 year for which a thorough autopsy fails to demonstrate an adequate cause of death
   2. The cause is not known
B. Characteristics
   1. Maternal risk factors
      a. Maternal smoking
      b. Younger mothers
      c. Any condition that places the mother at risk during pregnancy increases the risk of SIDS
   2. Birth factors
      a. Prematurity

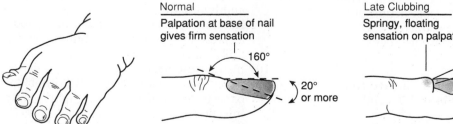
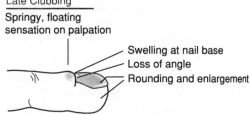

Normal

Palpation at base of nail
gives firm sensation

160°

20°
or more

Late Clubbing

Springy, floating
sensation on palpation

Swelling at nail base
Loss of angle
Rounding and enlargement

FIGURE 29–3. Clubbing of the fingers. (From Leifer, G. [1999]. *Thompson's introduction to maternity and pediatric nursing* [3rd ed.]. Philadelphia: W. B. Saunders. p. 666.)

b. Low-birthweight infants
c. Multiple births
d. Infants with central nervous system (CNS) problems
3. Time of year: most frequently during winter months
4. Time of death: usually occurs during sleep
5. Age: most frequently occurs during the first 2 to 4 months of life
6. Sex/race
a. Higher in males
b. Higher in Native Americans

C. Appearance when found
1. Apneic
2. Blue
3. Lifeless
4. Frothy blood-tinged fluid in nose and mouth
5. May be found in any position
6. May be clutching bedding

D. Prevention
1. Healthy infants should be placed for sleep on their sides or backs rather than prone
2. Soft bedding should be avoided because the infant may suffocate by rebreathing CO_2 expired air

XIII. Tuberculosis (TB) in Children

A. Description
1. A reportable contagious disease caused by *Mycobacterium tuberculosis*
2. The route of transmission is through inhalation of droplets from an individual with active TB
3. Most children are infected by a family member or by another individual with whom they have frequent contact, such as a baby-sitter

B. Data collection
1. Children ages 3 to 15 are usually asymptomatic, have normal chest x-ray results, and can be diagnosed only through a positive skin test
2. Some children develop malaise, fever, cough, weight loss, anorexia, and lymphadenopathy

C. Mantoux test
1. In most children, skin testing will produce a positive reaction 3 to 6 weeks after the initial infection and occasionally as long as 3 months after infection
2. An area of induration of 15 mm or greater is considered to be a positive sign in all children
3. Induration measuring 10 mm or greater is considered to be a positive result in children younger than 4 years of age and in those with chronic illness or high risk for exposure to TB
4. A reaction of 5 mm or greater is considered to be positive for the highest risk groups, such as in a child with AIDS

D. Sputum test: because children often swallow sputum rather than expectorate, gastric washings may be done to obtain swallowed sputum

E. Implementation
1. Bacille Calmette-Guérin vaccine (BCG), the vaccine used to prevent TB, is used mainly for children with negative chest x-ray and skin test results who have had repeated exposures to TB, and for asymptomatic human immunodeficiency virus (HIV)–infected children who are at increased risk for developing TB
2. Antituberculin medication for 9 months and for 12 months if the child has an HIV infection
3. Stress the importance of adequate rest and adequate diet
4. Instruct in measures to prevent transmission of TB to others

PRACTICE QUESTIONS

1. The day care nurse is observing a 2-year-old child. The nurse suspects that the child may have strabismus. Which of the following observations might be indicative of this condition?
   1 The child consistently tilts the head to see
   2 The child consistently turns the head to see
   3 The child does not respond when spoken to
   4 The child has difficulty hearing

2. The nurse prepares a teaching plan for a mother of a child diagnosed with bacterial conjunctivitis. Which of the following, if stated by the mother, indicates a need for further education?
   1 "I need to wash my hands frequently."
   2 "I need to clean the eye as prescribed."
   3 "I need to give the eye drops as prescribed."
   4 "It is OK to share towels and washcloths."

3. The nurse provides instructions to parents regarding the methods that will decrease the risk of recurrent otitis media in infants. Which of the following is included in the instructions?
   1 Feed the infant in an upright position
   2 Allow the infant to have a bottle during naptime
   3 Maintain bottle-feeding as long as possible
   4 Discontinue breast-feeding as soon as possible

4. The nurse is assigned to care for a child following myringotomy with insertion of tympanostomy tubes. The nurse notes a small amount of reddish drainage from the child's ear following the surgery. Which of the following is the most appropriate nursing action?
   1 Notify the registered nurse (RN) immediately
   2 Change the ear tubes so that they do not become blocked
   3 Document the findings
   4 Check the ear drainage for the presence of cerebrospinal fluid (CSF)

5. The nurse prepares a teaching plan regarding the administration of ear drops for the parents of a 6-year-old child. Which of the following is included in the plan?
   1. Pull the ear up and back
   2. Wear gloves when administering the medication
   3. Hold the child in a sitting position when administering the ear drops
   4. Pull the ear down, back, and out

6. The child is scheduled for a tonsillectomy. Which of the following presents the highest risk of aspiration during surgery?
   1. Difficulty swallowing
   2. The presence of loose teeth
   3. Bleeding during surgery
   4. Exudate in the throat area

7. The most appropriate child position following a tonsillectomy is which of the following?
   1. Supine
   2. Trendelenburg
   3. Side-lying
   4. High Fowler's

8. Following tonsillectomy, the child begins to vomit bright red blood. The most appropriate initial nursing action is to
   1. Administer the prescribed antiemetic
   2. Turn the child to the side
   3. Notify the registered nurse (RN)
   4. Maintain an NPO status

9. Following tonsillectomy, which of the following fluid or food items is appropriate to offer to the child?
   1. Cool cherry Kool-Aid
   2. Vanilla pudding
   3. Cold ginger ale
   4. Jell-O

10. The nurse is reinforcing instructions to the mother of an 8-year-old child who had a tonsillectomy. The mother tells the nurse that the child loves tacos and asks when the child can safely eat one. The most appropriate response is
    1. "In 1 week."
    2. "In 3 weeks."
    3. "Two days following surgery."
    4. "When the physician says it's OK."

11. The nurse reinforces instructions to the mother of a child with croup. The mother expresses concern regarding the occurrence of an acute spasmodic episode. Which of the following suggestions is not provided to the mother regarding management if an acute episode occurs?
    1. Place a steam vaporizer in the child's room
    2. Sit with the child in a closed bathroom and allow the child to inhale steam from the running water
    3. Place a cool-mist humidifier in the child's room
    4. Take the child out into the cool humid night air

12. The nurse reinforces instructions to the mother of a child hospitalized with croup. Which of the following statements, if made by the mother, indicates a need for further instruction?
    1. "I will give my child cough syrup if a cough develops."
    2. "I will be sure that my child drinks at least 2 to 4 glasses of fluids every day."
    3. "I will give Tylenol if my child develops a fever."
    4. "Sips of warm fluid will help if my child develops a croup attack."

13. The nurse working in the emergency department is caring for a child diagnosed with epiglottitis. Indications that the child may be experiencing airway obstruction include which of the following?
    1. The child is leaning backward supporting self with the hands and arms
    2. A low-grade fever and complaints of a sore throat
    3. The child is leaning forward with the chin thrust out
    4. Nasal flaring and bradycardia

14. The nurse is caring for an infant with bronchiolitis. Diagnostic tests have confirmed respiratory syncytial virus (RSV). Based on this finding, which of the following is the most appropriate nursing action?
    1. Plan to move the infant to another room with another RSV child
    2. Leave the infant in the present room because RSV is not contagious
    3. Wear a mask when caring for the child
    4. Initiate strict enteric precautions

15. A child is brought to the emergency department for treatment of an acute asthma attack. The nurse prepares to administer which of the following medications first?
    1. Subcutaneous epinephrine
    2. Subcutaneous terbutaline
    3. Oral corticosteroids
    4. A bronchodilator via nebulizer

16. The nursing student is asked to discuss sudden infant death syndrome (SIDS) at the clinical conference being held at the end of the clinical day. The student plans to include which of the following in the discussion during the conference?
    1. SIDS usually occurs during sleep and is more common in infants from lower socioeconomic groups
    2. SIDS usually occurs during sleep and is more common in girls

3 SIDS usually occurs during sleep and most frequently occurs between 8 and 10 months of age

4 SIDS usually occurs during sleep and is more common in high-birthweight infants

17. The home health nurse is instructing the mother of a child with cystic fibrosis (CF) about the appropriate dietary measures. Which of the following diets will be included in the instructions?
   1 Low-calorie, low-fat diet
   2 High-calorie, high-protein diet
   3 High-calorie, low-protein diet
   4 High-calorie, restricted fat

18. The nurse prepares to administer a pancreatic enzyme powder to the child with CF. Which of the following food items does the nurse plan to mix with the medication?
   1 Apple sauce
   2 Tapioca

3 Mashed potatoes
4 Hot oatmeal

19. The nurse reviews the results of a Mantoux test performed on a 3-year-old child. The results indicate an area of induration measuring 10 mm. The nurse interprets these results as
   1 Negative
   2 Positive
   3 Inconclusive
   4 Definitive, requiring a repeat test

20. Isoniazid (INH) is prescribed for a 2-year-old child with a positive Mantoux test. The mother of the child asks the nurse how long the child will need to take the medication. The most appropriate response is
   1 6 months
   2 9 months
   3 15 months
   4 18 months

ANSWERS

1. **1**

RATIONALE: The nurse may suspect strabismus in a child when the child complains of frequent headaches, squints, or tilts the head to see. Options 2, 3, and 4 are not indicative of this condition.
TEST-TAKING STRATEGY: Begin by eliminating option 3 and 4 because they are similar. Knowledge regarding the signs of this condition will assist in directing you to option 1. Review these signs now if you had difficulty with this question.
LEVEL OF COGNITIVE ABILITY: Comprehension
PHASE OF NURSING PROCESS: Data Collection
CLIENT NEEDS: Physiological Integrity
CONTENT AREA: Child Health
REFERENCE
Schulte, E., Price, D., & James, S. (1997). *Thompson's pediatric nursing: An introductory text* (7th ed.). Philadelphia: W. B. Saunders. p. 271.

2. **4**

RATIONALE: Bacterial conjunctivitis is highly contagious and infection control measures should be taught. These include good handwashing and not sharing towels and washcloths. Options 2 and 3 are correct treatment measures.
TEST-TAKING STRATEGY: Note the key words "indicates a need for further education." Knowledge that bacterial conjunctivitis is highly contagious will easily direct you to option 4. If you had difficulty with this question, take time now to review infection control measures for bacterial conjunctivitis.
LEVEL OF COGNITIVE ABILITY: Comprehension
PHASE OF NURSING PROCESS: Evaluation
CLIENT NEEDS: Health Promotion and Maintenance
CONTENT AREA: Child Health

REFERENCE
Leifer, G. (1999). *Thompson's introduction to maternity and pediatric nursing* (3rd ed.). Philadelphia: W. B. Saunders. p. 592.

3. **1**

RATIONALE: To decrease the risk of recurrent otitis media, parents should be encouraged to breast-feed during infancy, discontinue bottle-feeding as soon as possible, feed the infant in an upright position, and never give the infant a bottle in bed. Parents should be told not to smoke in the child's presence because passive smoking increases the incidence of otitis media.
TEST-TAKING STRATEGY: Knowledge of the physiology related to otitis media will assist in answering the question. Option 2 can be easily eliminated. Recalling that breast-feeding offers some protection by providing maternal antibodies will assist in eliminating options 3 and 4. Review measures that will assist in preventing otitis media if you had difficulty with this question.
LEVEL OF COGNITIVE ABILITY: Application
PHASE OF NURSING PROCESS: Implementation
CLIENT NEEDS: Health Promotion and Maintenance
CONTENT AREA: Child Health
REFERENCE
Leifer, G. (1999). *Thompson's introduction to maternity and pediatric nursing* (3rd ed.). Philadelphia: W. B. Saunders. p. 586.

4. **3**

RATIONALE: Following myringotomy with insertion of tympanostomy tubes, the child is monitored for ear drainage. A small amount of reddish drainage is normal for the first few days after surgery. Any heavy bleeding or bleeding that occurs after 3 days should be reported. The nurse should document the findings. Options 1, 2, and 4 are not necessary.
TEST-TAKING STRATEGY: Note the key words "small amount." Considering both the anatomical location of the surgery and these key words, you should easily be directed

to the correct option. Review postoperative findings following this type of surgery now if you had difficulty with this question.
LEVEL OF COGNITIVE ABILITY: Application
PHASE OF NURSING PROCESS: Implementation
CLIENT NEEDS: Physiological Integrity
CONTENT AREA: Child Health
REFERENCE
Schulte, E., Price, D., & James, S. (1997). *Thompson's pediatric nursing: An introductory text* (7th ed.). Philadelphia: W. B. Saunders. p. 155.

5. 4

RATIONALE: To administer ear drops in a child, the ear should be pulled down, back, and out. In adults, the ear is pulled up and back. Gloves do not need to be worn by the parents but handwashing before and after the procedure needs to be performed. The child needs to be in a side-lying position with the affected ear facing upward to facilitate the flow of medication down the ear canal by gravity.
TEST-TAKING STRATEGY: Options 2 and 3 can be eliminated first. From the remaining options, recalling the anatomy of the child's ear canal will direct you to option 4. Review this procedure now if you had difficulty with this question.
LEVEL OF COGNITIVE ABILITY: Application
PHASE OF NURSING PROCESS: Planning
CLIENT NEEDS: Health Promotion and Maintenance
CONTENT AREA: Child Health
REFERENCE
Schulte, E., Price, D., & James, S. (1997). *Thompson's pediatric nursing: An introductory text* (7th ed.). Philadelphia: W. B. Saunders. p. 155.

6. 2

RATIONALE: In the preoperative period, the child should be observed for the presence of loose teeth to decrease the risk of aspiration during surgery. Options 1 and 4 are incorrect. Bleeding during surgery will be controlled via packing and suction during the surgical procedure as needed.
TEST-TAKING STRATEGY: The issue of the question relates to aspiration. Note the key word "highest." Options 1 and 4 can be easily eliminated. Recalling that the tonsillar area is vascular, anticipation of bleeding during surgery is expected and would be controlled. Review preoperative assessment procedures related to tonsillectomy now if you had difficulty with this question.
LEVEL OF COGNITIVE ABILITY: Comprehension
PHASE OF NURSING PROCESS: Data Collection
CLIENT NEEDS: Physiological Integrity
CONTENT AREA: Child Health
REFERENCE
Ashwill, J., & Droske, S. (1997). *Nursing care of children: Principles and practice.* Philadelphia: W. B. Saunders. p. 830.

7. 3

RATIONALE: The child should be placed in a prone or side-lying position following tonsillectomy to facilitate drainage. Options 1, 2, and 4 will not achieve this goal.
TEST-TAKING STRATEGY: Visualize each of the positions described in the options. Keeping in mind that the goal is to facilitate drainage will easily direct you to option 3. Review positioning procedures following tonsillectomy now if you had difficulty with this question.
LEVEL OF COGNITIVE ABILITY: Application
PHASE OF NURSING PROCESS: Implementation

CLIENT NEEDS: Physiological Integrity
CONTENT AREA: Child Health
REFERENCE
Schulte, E., Price, D., & James, S. (1997). *Thompson's pediatric nursing: An introductory text* (7th ed.). Philadelphia: W. B. Saunders. p. 272.

8. 2

RATIONALE: Following tonsillectomy, if bleeding occurs, the child is turned to the side and the RN is notified, who will then contact the physician. An NPO status is maintained and an antiemetic may be prescribed; however, the initial nursing action is to turn the child to the side.
TEST-TAKING STRATEGY: Note the key word "initial." Although all of the options may be appropriate, to maintain physiological integrity, the initial action is to turn the child to the side.
LEVEL OF COGNITIVE ABILITY: Application
PHASE OF NURSING PROCESS: Implementation
CLIENT NEEDS: Physiological Integrity
CONTENT AREA: Child Health
REFERENCE
Schulte, E., Price, D., & James, S. (1997). *Thompson's pediatric nursing: An introductory text* (7th ed.). Philadelphia: W. B. Saunders. p. 272.

9. 4

RATIONALE: Following tonsillectomy, clear, cool liquids should be administered. Citrus, carbonated, and extremely hot or cold liquids need to be avoided because they may irritate the throat. Red liquids need to be avoided because they give the appearance of blood if the child vomits. Milk and milk products (pudding) are avoided because they coat the throat, cause the child to clear the throat, and increase the risk of bleeding.
TEST-TAKING STRATEGY: Knowledge regarding the foods and fluids that should be avoided following tonsillectomy is required to answer this question. Avoiding foods and fluids that may irritate or cause bleeding is the concern. This will assist in eliminating options 2 and 3. The word "cherry" in option 1 should be the clue that this is not an appropriate food item. Review dietary measures following tonsillectomy if you had difficulty with this question.
LEVEL OF COGNITIVE ABILITY: Application
PHASE OF NURSING PROCESS: Implementation
CLIENT NEEDS: Physiological Integrity
CONTENT AREA: Child Health
REFERENCE
Schulte, E., Price, D., & James, S. (1997). *Thompson's pediatric nursing: An introductory text* (7th ed.). Philadelphia: W. B. Saunders. p. 273.

10. 2

RATIONALE: Citrus juices, which irritate the throat, need to be avoided for 10 days. Red liquids are avoided because they will give the appearance of blood if the child vomits. The mother is instructed to add full liquids on the second day and soft foods as the child tolerates them. Rough or scratchy foods or spicy foods are to be avoided for 3 weeks.
TEST-TAKING STRATEGY: Knowledge regarding the specific instructions related to food and fluids following tonsillectomy is required to answer this question. Review the dietary instructions now if you had difficulty with this question.
LEVEL OF COGNITIVE ABILITY: Application
PHASE OF NURSING PROCESS: Implementation

CLIENT NEEDS: Health Promotion and Maintenance
CONTENT AREA: Child Health
REFERENCE
Schulte, E., Price, D., & James, S. (1997). *Thompson's pediatric nursing: An introductory text* (7th ed.). Philadelphia: W. B. Saunders. p. 273.

11. **1**

RATIONALE: Steam from running water in a closed bathroom and cool mist from a bedside humidifier are effective in reducing mucosal edema. Cool-mist humidifiers are recommended over steam vaporizers, which present a danger of scald burns. Taking the child out into the cool humid night air may also relieve mucosal swelling. Remember, however, that a cold mist may precipitate bronchospasm.
TEST-TAKING STRATEGY: The issue of the question is to reduce mucosal edema and to provide a safe environment. Note the key word "not." Option 1 is the option that would provide an unsafe environment for the child. Review management of acute spasmodic croup now if you had difficulty with this question.
LEVEL OF COGNITIVE ABILITY: Application
PHASE OF NURSING PROCESS: Implementation
CLIENT NEEDS: Safe, Effective Care Environment
CONTENT AREA: Child Health
REFERENCE
Schulte, E., Price, D., & James, S. (1997). *Thompson's pediatric nursing: An introductory text* (7th ed.). Philadelphia: W. B. Saunders. p. 224.

12. **1**

RATIONALE: Cough syrups and cold medicines are not to be given because they may dry and thicken secretions. Adequate hydration of 500 to 1000 mL of fluids daily is important in thinning secretions. Tylenol is used if a fever develops. Sips of warm fluids during a croup attack help relax the vocal cords and thin mucus.
TEST-TAKING STRATEGY: Note the key words "a need for further instruction." Options 2 and 3 can be easily eliminated. Recalling that warm fluids can relax membranes and thin secretions will assist in directing you to option 1. Review the effects of cough medicines now if you had difficulty with this question.
LEVEL OF COGNITIVE ABILITY: Comprehension
PHASE OF NURSING PROCESS: Evaluation
CLIENT NEEDS: Physiological Integrity
CONTENT AREA: Child Health
REFERENCE
Ashwill, J., & Droske, S. (1997). *Nursing care of children: Principles and practice.* Philadelphia: W. B. Saunders. p. 838.

13. **3**

RATIONALE: Clinical manifestations suggestive of airway obstruction include tripod positioning (leaning forward supported by arms, chin thrust out, mouth open), nasal flaring, tachycardia, a high fever, and sore throat.
TEST-TAKING STRATEGY: Eliminate option 4 first because tachycardia rather than bradycardia will occur in a child experiencing respiratory distress. Eliminate option 2 next, knowing that a high fever occurs with epiglottitis. From the remaining options, visualize the descriptions in each, and determine which position would best assist a child experiencing respiratory distress. Review the tripod position now if you had difficulty with this question.
LEVEL OF COGNITIVE ABILITY: Comprehension
PHASE OF NURSING PROCESS: Data Collection

CLIENT NEEDS: Physiological Integrity
CONTENT AREA: Child Health
REFERENCE
Schulte, E., Price, D., & James, S. (1997). *Thompson's pediatric nursing: An introductory text* (7th ed.). Philadelphia: W. B. Saunders. pp. 225–226.

14. **1**

RATIONALE: RSV is a highly communicable disorder. It is not transmitted via the airborne route. It is usually transferred by the hands, and meticulous handwashing is necessary to decrease the spread of organisms. The infant with RSV is isolated in a single room or placed in a room with another RSV child. Enteric precautions are not necessary; however, the nurse should wear a gown when soiling of clothing may occur.
TEST-TAKING STRATEGY: Knowledge regarding the transmission of RSV will easily direct you to option 1. Take time now to review the care of the child with RSV if you had difficulty with this question.
LEVEL OF COGNITIVE ABILITY: Application
PHASE OF NURSING PROCESS: Implementation
CLIENT NEEDS: Safe, Effective Care Environment
CONTENT AREA: Child Health
REFERENCE
Schulte, E., Price, D., & James, S. (1997). *Thompson's pediatric nursing: An introductory text* (7th ed.). Philadelphia: W. B. Saunders. p. 158.

15. **4**

RATIONALE: In treating an acute asthma attack, a bronchodilator (usually albuterol) is administered via a powdered nebulizer first. IV corticosteroids may also be administered following the broncodilator. Subcutaneous epinephrine or terbutaline may then be given if the child is not responding to treatment.
TEST-TAKING STRATEGY: Knowledge that asthma is a reversible obstructive airway disease should assist in directing you to option 4. It seems logical that the first action would be to dilate the bronchi. If you had difficulty with this question, take time now to review the treatment for an acute asthma episode.
LEVEL OF COGNITIVE ABILITY: Application
PHASE OF NURSING PROCESS: Planning
CLIENT NEEDS: Physiological Integrity
CONTENT AREA: Child Health
REFERENCE
Schulte, E., Price, D., & James, S. (1997). *Thompson's pediatric nursing: An introductory text* (7th ed.). Philadelphia: W. B. Saunders. p. 332.

16. **1**

RATIONALE: SIDS usually occurs during sleep. It most frequently occurs between the second and fourth months of life. It is more common in boys, low-birthweight infants, and infants from lower socioeconomic groups. It occurs more often in the winter. The highest incidence is in Native Americans followed by African-Americans.
TEST-TAKING STRATEGY: Knowledge regarding the characteristics related to the etiology and incidence of SIDS is required to answer this question. If you are unfamiliar with this information, take time now to review.
LEVEL OF COGNITIVE ABILITY: Comprehension
PHASE OF NURSING PROCESS: Planning
CLIENT NEEDS: Physiological Integrity
CONTENT AREA: Child Health

REFERENCE
Schulte, E., Price, D., & James, S. (1997). *Thompson's pediatric nursing: An introductory text* (7th ed.). Philadelphia: W. B. Saunders. p. 184.

17. **2**

RATIONALE: Children with CF are managed with a high-calorie, high-protein diet. Pancreatic enzyme replacement therapy and fat-soluble vitamin supplements are administered. If nutritional problems are severe, nighttime gastrostomy feedings or total parenteral nutrition (TPN) is administered. Fats are not restricted unless steatorrhea cannot be controlled by increased pancreatic enzymes.
TEST-TAKING STRATEGY: Knowledge regarding the appropriate diet in the child with CF is required to answer this question. If you are unfamiliar with this diet plan, take time now to review.
LEVEL OF COGNITIVE ABILITY: Application
PHASE OF NURSING PROCESS: Implementation
CLIENT NEEDS: Physiological Integrity
CONTENT AREA: Child Health
REFERENCE
Schulte, E., Price, D., & James, S. (1997). *Thompson's pediatric nursing: An introductory text* (7th ed.). Philadelphia: W. B. Saunders. p. 171.

18. **1**

RATIONALE: Pancreatic enzyme powders are not to be mixed with hot foods or foods containing tapioca or other starches. Enzyme powder should be mixed with nonfat, nonprotein foods such as apple sauce. Pancreatic enzymes are inactivated by heat and are partially degraded by gastric acids.
TEST-TAKING STRATEGY: Eliminate option 4 first because of the word "hot." Knowledge regarding the administration of pancreatic enzymes is helpful in making the correct selection. If you had difficulty with this question, be sure to review the procedures for administering pancreatic enzyme powder.
LEVEL OF COGNITIVE ABILITY: Application
PHASE OF NURSING PROCESS: Planning
CLIENT NEEDS: Physiological Integrity
CONTENT AREA: Child Health
REFERENCE
Schulte, E., Price, D., & James, S. (1997). *Thompson's pediatric nursing: An introductory text* (7th ed.). Philadelphia: W. B. Saunders. p. 170.

19. **2**

RATIONALE: Induration measuring 10 mm or greater is considered to be a positive result in children younger than 4 years of age and in those with chronic illness or high risk for environmental exposure to tuberculosis. A reaction of 5 mm or greater is considered to be a positive result for the highest risk groups, such as in the child with AIDS.
TEST-TAKING STRATEGY: Knowledge regarding a positive Mantoux test in children is required to answer this question. Option 4 can be easily eliminated first. Note the child's age in the question to determine the correct option from the remaining three. If you had difficulty with this question, take time now to review the analysis of a Mantoux test in children.
LEVEL OF COGNITIVE ABILITY: Comprehension
PHASE OF NURSING PROCESS: Data Collection
CLIENT NEEDS: Physiological Integrity
CONTENT AREA: Child Health
REFERENCE
Schulte, E., Price, D., & James, S. (1997). *Thompson's pediatric nursing: An introductory text* (7th ed.). Philadelphia: W. B. Saunders. p. 124.

20. **2**

RATIONALE: INH is given to prevent TB infection from progressing to active disease. A chest x-ray film is obtained prior to initiation of preventive therapy. In infants and children the recommended duration of INH therapy is 9 months. For children with HIV infection, a minimum of 12 months is recommended.
TEST-TAKING STRATEGY: Knowledge regarding treatment with INH in a 2-year-old child is required to answer this question. If you are unfamiliar with treatment plans for TB in children, take time now to review.
LEVEL OF COGNITIVE ABILITY: Application
PHASE OF NURSING PROCESS: Implementation
CLIENT NEEDS: Health Promotion and Maintenance
CONTENT AREA: Child Health
REFERENCE
Schulte, E., Price, D., & James, S. (1997). *Thompson's pediatric nursing: An introductory text* (7th ed.). Philadelphia: W. B. Saunders. p. 124.

BIBLIOGRAPHY

Ashwill, J., & Droske, S. (1997). *Nursing care of children: Principles and practice.* Philadelphia: W. B. Saunders.

Bowden, V., Dickey, S., & Greenberg, C. (1998). *Children and their families: The continuum of care.* Philadelphia: W. B. Saunders.

Leifer, G. (1999). *Thompson's introduction to maternity and pediatric nursing* (3rd ed.). Philadelphia: W. B. Saunders.

Luckmann, J. (1997). *Saunders manual of nursing care.* Philadelphia: W. B. Saunders.

Nichols, F., & Zwelling, E. (1997). *Maternal-newborn nursing: Theory and practice.* Philadelphia: W. B. Saunders.

O'Toole, M. (ed.). (1997). *Miller-Keane encyclopedia & dictionary of medicine, nursing, & allied health* (6th ed.). Philadelphia: W. B. Saunders.

Peckenpaugh, N. & Poleman, C. (1999). *Nutrition essentials and diet therapy* (8th ed.). Philadelphia: W. B. Saunders.

Schulte, E., Price, D., & James, S. (1997). *Thompson's pediatric nursing: An introductory text* (7th ed.). Philadelphia: W. B. Saunders.

CHAPTER 30

Cardiovascular Disorders

I. Congestive Heart Failure

A. Description
1. Inability of the heart to pump sufficiently to meet the metabolic needs of the body
2. In infants and children, inadequate cardiac output is most commonly caused by congenital heart defects that produce an excessive volume or pressure load on the myocardium
3. In children a combination of both left-sided and right-sided heart failure is usually present

B. Data collection of early symptoms
1. Tachypnea and diaphoresis during feeding
2. Poor feeding
3. Failure to thrive or grow as evidenced on growth chart

C. Implementation
1. Elevate the head of the bed
2. Administer oxygen as prescribed during stressful periods such as bouts of crying or invasive procedures
3. Feed in a relaxed environment
4. Provide small, frequent feedings, which will be less tiring
5. Monitor intake and output (I&O) and daily weight to monitor for fluid retention
6. Weigh diapers; a weight gain of more than 50 g/day may indicate fluid overload
7. Monitor for facial or peripheral edema
8. Monitor electrolyte levels
9. Administer digoxin (Lanoxin) and furosemide (Lasix) as prescribed
10. Administer vasodilators or angiotensin-converting enzyme (ACE) inhibitors as prescribed
11. Prostaglandin E_1 (PGE_1) may be administered in the neonatal period for ductal-dependent congenital heart defects with cardiovascular collapse to maintain patency of the ductus arteriosus before surgery
12. Reinforce instructions to the parents regarding description of diagnosis and administration of medications
13. Instruct the parents in cardiopulmonary resuscitation (CPR)

II. Intracardiac Shunt

A. Description: occurs when the blood flow is forced by a higher pressure to go through an opening that is not normally present

B. Left-to-right **shunts** (acyanotic heart defects)
1. Description (Box 30–1)
   a. Blood is shunted to the right side of the heart because the left side is normally functioning under a higher pressure than the right
   b. Oxygenated and unoxygenated blood mix
2. Data collection
   a. May be asymptomatic
   b. May show signs and symptoms of congestive heart failure (CHF)
   c. Poor feeding; may exhibit failure to thrive
   d. **Growth** retardation
   e. Diaphoresis
   f. Signs of fatigue
   g. Tachypnea, dyspnea, hypoxemia
3. Implementation
   a. Monitor respiratory status for the presence of **nasal flaring** and use of accessory muscles
   b. Monitor vital signs

BOX 30–1. Types of Left-to-Right Shunts

Atrial septal defect (ASD)
Ventricular septal defect (VSD)
Patent ductus arteriosus (PDA)
Atrioventricular canal defect (AVC)

> **BOX 30–2. Types of Right-to-Left Shunts**
>
> Tetralogy of Fallot
> Transposition of the great arteries
> Truncus arteriosus
> Pulmonary atresia
> Tricuspid atresia
> Hypoplastic left heart syndrome

   c. Monitor for signs of CHF such as fluid retention in the eyes, hands, feet, and chest
   d. Monitor urine output; weighing diapers is necessary
   e. Monitor calorie intake
   f. Plan interventions to allow maximal rest for the child
   g. Allow the parent or child if appropriate, to verbalize feelings and concerns regarding disorder
C. Right-to-left **shunts** (cyanotic heart defects)
   1. Description (Box 30–2)
      a. Occur when blood is shunted to the left side of the heart because one of the right heart chambers has a higher pressure
      b. Oxygenated blood mixes with unoxygenated blood; cyanosis occurs
      c. May be treated with PGE₁, which temporarily maintains patency of ductus arteriosus until surgery is performed
   2. Data collection
      a. Symptoms occur in the first week of life
      b. Dyspnea after feeding, crying, or other activities
      c. Hypercyanotic or "tet spells" characterized by increased respiratory rate and depth and increased hypoxemia with tetralogy of Fallot
      d. Squatting episodes with tetralogy of Fallot
      e. Signs of CHF
      f. Respiratory distress and tachycardia
      g. Clubbing of the digits
      h. Poor **growth**
   3. Implementation
      a. Monitor vital signs
      b. Monitor respiratory status and report findings if any changes occur
      c. Monitor for signs of CHF
      d. Keep the child as stress free as possible
      e. If respiratory effort is increased, place child in a reverse Trendelenburg (elevate the head and upper body) to decrease the work of breathing and report findings
      f. Monitor for hypercyanosis and place the child in a knee-chest position and report findings
      g. Administer humidified oxygen as prescribed
      h. Monitor body weight
      i. Monitor I&O and report findings if a decrease in urine output occurs

   j. Administer diuretics as prescribed
   k. Administer propranolol (Inderal) for hypercyanotic episodes as prescribed and monitor glucose levels during treatment; report findings if glucose level is less than 60 mg/dL
   l. Prepare for endotracheal tube insertion as prescribed (restrain the hands of an intubated child)

III. Stenotic Lesions (Box 30–3)

A. Description: narrowing or constriction of an opening in a valve or vessel that results in obstruction of blood flow through the area
B. Data collection
   1. Murmurs
   2. Signs of CHF
   3. Tachycardia
   4. Tachypnea, dyspnea, pallor
   5. Decreased peripheral pulses
   6. Cardiomegaly
C. Implementation
   1. Monitor vital signs
   2. Measure blood pressure in all four extremities
   3. Monitor peripheral pulses
   4. Administer oxygen as prescribed
   5. Monitor for signs of CHF
   6. Monitor I&O
   7. Maintain fluid restriction
   8. Obtain daily weight
   9. Administer cardiac medications and diuretics as prescribed

IV. Cardiac Surgery

A. Implementation postoperatively
   1. Monitor vital signs frequently
   2. Monitor temperature and report an elevation if it occurs
   3. Maintain aseptic technique
   4. Monitor for signs of sepsis such as fever, chills, diaphoresis, lethargy, and altered levels of consciousness
   5. Monitor lines, tubes, or catheters that are in place as prescribed and prepare to remove promptly as prescribed when no longer needed, to prevent infection
   6. Monitor for signs of discomfort such as irritability, changes in heart rate, respiratory rate and blood pressure, and inability to sleep
   7. Administer pain medications as prescribed, noting effectiveness

> **BOX 30–3. Types of Stenotic Lesions**
>
> Pulmonary stenosis
> Aortic stenosis
> Coarctation of the aorta

> ### BOX 30–4. Home Care Postoperative Cardiac Surgery
>
> Omit play outside for several weeks
> Avoid activities where the child could fall, such as bike riding, for several weeks
> Avoid crowds for 1 week after discharge
> Follow a no-added-salt diet if prescribed
> Do not add any new foods to an infant's eating schedule
> Review procedures for medication administration
> Do not place creams, lotions, or powders on the incision until completely healed
> The child may return to school the third week after discharge starting with half days
> No physical education for 2 months
> Instruct the parents to discipline the child normally
> Instruct the parents about the importance of the 2-week follow-up
> Avoid immunizations, invasive procedures, and dental visits for 2 months
> Advise the parents regarding the importance of a dental visit every 6 months after age 3 and to inform the dentist of the cardiac problem so that antibiotics can be prescribed if necessary
> Inform the parents to call the physician when coughing, tachypnea, cyanosis, vomiting, diarrhea, anorexia, pain, fever, or any swelling, redness, or drainage occurs at the site of the incision

8. Administer antibiotics and antipyretics as prescribed
9. Encourage rest periods
10. Facilitate parent-child contact as soon as possible

B. Postoperative home care (Box 30–4)

V. Rheumatic Fever

A. Description
1. An inflammatory autoimmune disease that affects the connective tissues of the heart, joints, subcutaneous tissues, and/or blood vessels of the central nervous system (CNS)
2. The most serious complication is rheumatic heart disease, which affects the cardiac valves
3. Presents 2 to 6 weeks following an untreated or partially treated group A beta-hemolytic streptococcal infection of the upper respiratory tract
4. Jones criteria are used in determining diagnosis

B. Data collection
1. Edema, inflammation of large joints
2. Joint pain
3. Fever
4. Erythema marginatum on the trunk and extremities
5. Chorea
6. Subcutaneous nodules in the joints, scalp, and spine
7. Arthritis

8. Aschoff's bodies, causing endocarditis
9. Fibrosis of mitral and aortic valves
10. Elevated antistreptolysin O titer
11. Elevated sedimentation rate
12. Elevated C-reactive protein

C. Implementation
1. Monitor vital signs
2. Monitor skin lesions and rash
3. Control joint pain and inflammation with massage and alternating hot and cold applications as prescribed
4. Provide bed rest during an acute febrile phase
5. Administer penicillin as prescribed to eradicate infection
6. Administer anti-inflammatory agents as prescribed, and if aspirin is prescribed it should not be given to a child who has chickenpox or other viral infections
7. Monitor for signs of carditis including shortness of breath, edema of the face, abdomen or ankles, and precordial pain
8. Limit physical exercise in a child with carditis
9. Initiate seizure precautions if the child is experiencing chorea
10. Advise the child to inform parents if anyone in school develops a strep throat

PRACTICE QUESTIONS

1. The nurse caring for an infant with congestive heart failure (CHF) is monitoring the infant closely for early signs of exacerbation. Which of the following alerts the nurse of the development of CHF?
   1 Bradycardia during feeding
   2 Diaphoresis during feeding
   3 Slow and shallow breathing
   4 Pallor

2. The physician has prescribed oxygen PRN for the child with CHF. In which of the following situations does the nurse administer the oxygen to the child?
   1 During sleep
   2 When the mother is holding the child
   3 When changing the child's diapers
   4 When drawing blood for electrolyte values

3. The infant with CHF is receiving diuretic therapy. Which of the following is the most appropriate method to assess urine output?
   1 Insert a Foley catheter
   2 Weigh the diapers
   3 Compare intake with output
   4 Measure the amount of water added to the formula

4. The nurse is monitoring the daily weight on an infant with CHF. Which of the following alerts the nurse to suspect fluid overload and the need to report the findings?
   1 A weight gain of more than 20 g in a 24-hour period
   2 A weight gain of more than 30 g in a 24-hour period
   3 A weight gain of more than 40 g in a 24-hour period
   4 A weight gain of more than 50 g in a 24-hour period

5. The nurse is reinforcing home care instructions to the parents of a child with CHF regarding the procedure for administration of digoxin (Lanoxin). Which of the following is not a component of the instructions?
   1 If the child vomits after medication administration, repeat the dose
   2 Take the child's pulse before administering the medication
   3 Do not mix the medication with food
   4 If more than one dose is missed, call the physician

6. The nurse reviews the chart of an infant admitted to the pediatric unit. The diagnosis is documented as a left-to-right cardiac shunt. The nurse understands that which of the following physiological alterations occurs in this condition?
   1 Blood is shunted to the left side of the heart
   2 The right side of the heart functions under greater pressure than the left side of the heart
   3 Oxygenated and unoxygenated blood mix
   4 Oxygenated and unoxygenated blood do not mix

7. The nurse is caring for a child with a diagnosis of a right-to-left shunt. The nurse collects data, knowing that the most common finding in this disorder is which of the following?
   1 Cyanosis
   2 Diaphoresis
   3 Growth retardation
   4 These children are asymptomatic

8. A child with transposition of the great arteries and patent ductus arteriosus (PDA) receives prostaglandin E_1 (PGE_1). The mother of the child asks the nurse why the child needs the medication. The nurse bases the response on which of the following actions of this medication?
   1 Maintains an adequate hormonal level
   2 Maintains the position of the great arteries
   3 Maintains patency of the ductus arteriosus
   4 Prevents cyanosis

9. The child with a right-to-left shunt is maintained on an NPO status. Propranolol (Inderal) is being administered to the child. Which of the following laboratory values is most important to monitor in this child?
   1 BUN

2 Creatinine
3 Glucose
4 Electrolytes

10. The nurse is caring for an infant with tetralogy of Fallot. The nurse recognizes that the infant is experiencing a hypercyanotic episode. The initial nursing action is to
    1 Ask the unit secretary to report the findings to the physician
    2 Place the infant in a knee-chest position
    3 Elevate the head of the bed
    4 Administer carbon dioxide whiffs

11. The nurse reviews the record of a child just seen by the physician. The physician has documented a diagnosis of suspected stenotic lesion. Which of the following symptoms documented in the record is most commonly found in this disorder?
    1 Subclavian bruit
    2 Cardiac murmur
    3 Pallor
    4 Gastric regurgitation

12. The nurse reinforces home care instructions to the mother of a child who is being discharged following heart surgery. The nurse describes the activity guidelines to the mother. Which of the following is not included in the instructions?
    1 Avoid large crowds of people for at least 1 month following surgery
    2 Resume regular nap and sleep schedules
    3 Omit play outside, allowing inside play as tolerated
    4 Avoid activities where the child could fall for 2 to 4 weeks

13. The nurse is assisting in collecting data from a child admitted to the nursing unit with a diagnosis of rheumatic fever (RF). The nurse plans to collect data regarding which of the following?
    1 History of sore throat or unexplained fever within the past 2 months
    2 History of unexplained nausea or vomiting
    3 History of unexplained headaches
    4 History of back pain

14. Acetylsalicylic acid (aspirin) is prescribed for the child with RF. The nurse questions this order if the child had which of the following?
    1 A viral infection
    2 Joint pain
    3 Facial edema
    4 Arthralgia

15. The nurse is reviewing the health record of a child with a suspected diagnosis of RF. Which of the following laboratory studies assists in confirming the diagnosis?
    1 White blood cell (WBC) count
    2 Red blood cell (RBC) count
    3 Immunoglobulin
    4 Antistreptolysin O titer

ANSWERS

1. **2**

RATIONALE: The early symptoms of CHF include tachypnea, poor feeding, and diaphoresis during feeding. Tachycardia rather than bradycardia occurs during feeding. Pallor may be noted in the infant with CHF, but it is not an early symptom.
TEST-TAKING STRATEGY: Think about the physiology and the effects on the heart when fluid overload occurs. These concepts will assist in directing you to option 2. If you had difficulty with this question, take time now to review the early signs of CHF in an infant.
LEVEL OF COGNITIVE ABILITY: Comprehension
PHASE OF NURSING PROCESS: Data Collection
CLIENT NEEDS: Physiological Integrity
CONTENT AREA: Child Health
REFERENCE
Schulte, E., Price, D., & James, S. (1997). *Thompson's pediatric nursing: An introductory text* (7th ed.). Philadelphia: W. B. Saunders. p. 107.

2. **4**

RATIONALE: Oxygen administration may be ordered for stressful periods especially during bouts of crying or invasive procedures. Drawing blood is an invasive procedure that would likely cause the child to cry.
TEST-TAKING STRATEGY: Recall the situations that would place stress and an increased workload on the heart. This concept should easily direct you to option 4. Review care to the child with CHF now if you had difficulty with this question.
LEVEL OF COGNITIVE ABILITY: Application
PHASE OF NURSING PROCESS: Implementation
CLIENT NEEDS: Physiological Integrity
CONTENT AREA: Child Health
REFERENCE
Schulte, E., Price, D., & James, S. (1997). *Thompson's pediatric nursing: An introductory text* (7th ed.). Philadelphia: W. B. Saunders. pp. 106–107.

3. **2**

RATIONALE: The most appropriate method to monitor urine output in an infant on diuretic therapy is to weigh the diapers. Comparing intake with output does not provide an accurate measure of urine output. Measuring the amount of water added to formula is unrelated to the amount of output. Although Foley catheter drainage is most accurate in determining output, it is not the most appropriate method in an infant.
TEST-TAKING STRATEGY: Eliminate options 3 and 4 first because they will not provide an indication of urine output. From the remaining two options, note the words "most appropriate." These words should direct you to option 2. Review methods of monitoring urine output now if you had difficulty with this question.
LEVEL OF COGNITIVE ABILITY: Comprehension
PHASE OF NURSING PROCESS: Implementation
CLIENT NEEDS: Physiological Integrity
CONTENT AREA: Child Health
REFERENCE
Ashwill, J., & Droske, S. (1997). *Nursing care of children: Principles and practice*. Philadelphia: W. B. Saunders. p. 950.

4. **4**

RATIONALE: A weight gain of more than 50 g/day may indicate fluid overload. The nurse should monitor urine output, monitor for evidence of facial or peripheral edema, and report significant findings.
TEST-TAKING STRATEGY: Knowledge regarding fluid overload and the abnormal parameters in an infant with CHF is required to answer this question. Take time now to review these parameters if you had difficulty with this question.
LEVEL OF COGNITIVE ABILITY: Comprehension
PHASE OF NURSING PROCESS: Data Collection
CLIENT NEEDS: Physiological Integrity
CONTENT AREA: Child Health
REFERENCE
Ashwill, J., & Droske, S. (1997). *Nursing care of children: Principles and practice*. Philadelphia: W. B. Saunders. p. 950.

5. **1**

RATIONALE: The parents need to be instructed that if the child vomits after the digoxin is administered, they are not to repeat the dose. Options 2, 3, and 4 are accurate instructions. The parents should be instructed that if a dose is missed and it is not identified until 4 or more hours later, the dose should not be administered. Additionally, vomiting may indicate medication toxicity.
TEST-TAKING STRATEGY: Note the key word "not" in the stem of the question. General knowledge regarding digoxin administration will assist in eliminating option 2. Principles related to administering medications to children will assist in eliminating option 3. From the remaining options, select option 1 over option 4 because if the child vomits it would be difficult to determine if the medication was also vomited or absorbed by the body. Review this medication now if you had difficulty with this question.
LEVEL OF COGNITIVE ABILITY: Application
PHASE OF NURSING PROCESS: Implementation
CLIENT NEEDS: Health Promotion and Maintenance
CONTENT AREA: Child Health
REFERENCE
Schulte, E., Price, D., & James, S. (1997). *Thompson's pediatric nursing: An introductory text* (7th ed.). Philadelphia: W. B. Saunders. p. 107.

6. **3**

RATIONALE: In a left-to-right cardiac shunt, blood is shunted to the right side of the heart because the left side is normally functioning under higher pressure than the right side. This shunting allows oxygenated and unoxygenated blood to mix.
TEST-TAKING STRATEGY: The key phrase is "left-to-right." Bearing this phrase in mind, eliminate options 1 and 2. Recall that unoxygenated blood returns to the right side of the heart from the body; therefore, it makes sense that oxygenated and unoxygenated blood would mix in this disorder. Review left-to-right cardiac disorders now if you had difficulty with this question.
LEVEL OF COGNITIVE ABILITY: Comprehension
PHASE OF NURSING PROCESS: Data Collection
CLIENT NEEDS: Physiological Integrity
CONTENT AREA: Child Health
REFERENCE
Ashwill, J., & Droske, S. (1997). *Nursing care of children: Principles and practice*. Philadelphia: W. B. Saunders. p. 842.

7. 1

RATIONALE: The child with a right-to-left shunt will be considerably sicker than a child with a left-to-right shunt. Many of these children will present with symptoms in the first week of life. The most common finding in these children is cyanosis. The child may also become dyspneic after feeding, crying, and other exertional activities. Many children with a left-to-right shunt may remain asymptomatic.
TEST-TAKING STRATEGY: Knowledge regarding the physiology associated with a right-to-left shunt will easily direct you to option 1. If you had difficulty with this question, take time now to review the manifestations associated with this disorder.
LEVEL OF COGNITIVE ABILITY: Comprehension
PHASE OF NURSING PROCESS: Data Collection
CLIENT NEEDS: Physiological Integrity
CONTENT AREA: Child Health
REFERENCE
Ashwill, J., & Droske, S. (1997). *Nursing care of children: Principles and practice.* Philadelphia: W. B. Saunders. p. 923.

8. 3

RATIONALE: A child with transposition of the great arteries and PDA may receive PGE₁ before surgery to maintain patency of the ductus arteriosus.
TEST-TAKING STRATEGY: Use knowledge regarding the purpose of this medication to answer the question. Understanding the physiology associated with the disorder will direct you to option 3. Review the purpose of this medication in this condition now if you had difficulty with this question.
LEVEL OF COGNITIVE ABILITY: Comprehension
PHASE OF NURSING PROCESS: Planning
CLIENT NEEDS: Physiological Integrity
CONTENT AREA: Child Health
REFERENCE
Ashwill, J., & Droske, S. (1997). *Nursing care of children: Principles and practice.* Philadelphia: W. B. Saunders. p. 926.

9. 3

RATIONALE: Propranolol, a beta blocker, is used in the palliative treatment of hypercyanotic episodes. It can cause hypoglycemia if administered in a child that is NPO or hypovolemic. The nurse should monitor glucose levels every 4 to 6 hours if the child is NPO or hypovolemic and receiving propranolol. The physician is notified if the glucose level is less than 60 mg/dL.
TEST-TAKING STRATEGY: Eliminate options 1 and 2 because they are similar and both relate to renal function studies. From the remaining two options, you may be tempted to select option 4, but familiarity with the medication will direct you to the correct option. Review this important medication now if you had difficulty answering.
LEVEL OF COGNITIVE ABILITY: Comprehension
PHASE OF NURSING PROCESS: Data Collection
CLIENT NEEDS: Physiological Integrity
CONTENT AREA: Child Health
REFERENCE
Ashwill, J., & Droske, S. (1997). *Nursing care of children: Principles and practice.* Philadelphia: W. B. Saunders. p. 928.

10. 2

RATIONALE: If a hypercyanotic episode occurs, place the infant in a knee-chest position and then notify the physician. This position is thought to increase pulmonary blood flow by increasing systemic vascular resistance. This position also improves systemic arterial oxygen saturation by decreasing venous return, so that smaller amounts of highly saturated blood reach the heart. Toddlers and children squat to obtain this position and relieve chronic hypoxia.
TEST-TAKING STRATEGY: Note the key word "initial." Eliminate option 4 first. Next, eliminate option 1 because a nursing intervention is required before notifying the physician. Remembering that a toddler or a child squats to achieve this position will assist in directing you to option 2.
LEVEL OF COGNITIVE ABILITY: Application
PHASE OF NURSING PROCESS: Implementation
CLIENT NEEDS: Physiological Integrity
CONTENT AREA: Child Health
REFERENCE
Schulte, E., Price, D., & James, S. (1997). *Thompson's pediatric nursing: An introductory text* (7th ed.). Philadelphia: W. B. Saunders. p. 105.

11. 2

RATIONALE: The child with a stenotic lesion will have varying symptoms, depending on the type and degree of the stenotic lesion. Most of them will have murmurs when first seen in the health care setting. Pallor may be noted, but is not specific to this type of disorder alone. Options 1 and 4 are not related to this disorder.
TEST-TAKING STRATEGY: Note the similarity of "stenotic lesion" in the question and "cardiac murmur" in the option. Review the manifestations associated with stenotic lesions now if you had difficulty with this question.
LEVEL OF COGNITIVE ABILITY: Comprehension
PHASE OF NURSING PROCESS: Data Collection
CLIENT NEEDS: Physiological Integrity
CONTENT AREA: Child Health
REFERENCE
Ashwill, J., & Droske, S. (1997). *Nursing care of children: Principles and practice.* Philadelphia: W. B. Saunders. p. 930.

12. 1

RATIONALE: The mother should be instructed that the child needs to avoid large crowds of people for 1 week following discharge. This includes day care centers and church. Options 2, 3, and 4 are accurate instructions regarding activity following heart surgery.
TEST-TAKING STRATEGY: Note the key word "not." Options 2 and 3 can easily be eliminated first. From the remaining two options, note the time frame in option 1. This seems rather lengthy. Review child activity guidelines following heart surgery now if you had difficulty with this question.
LEVEL OF COGNITIVE ABILITY: Application
PHASE OF NURSING PROCESS: Implementation
CLIENT NEEDS: Health Promotion and Maintenance
CONTENT AREA: Child Health
REFERENCE
Ashwill, J., & Droske, S. (1997). *Nursing care of children: Principles and practice.* Philadelphia: W. B. Saunders. p. 922.

13. 1

RATIONALE: RF characteristically presents 2 to 6 weeks following an untreated or partially treated group A beta-hemolytic streptococcal infection of the upper respiratory tract. Initially the nurse determines whether any family members have had a sore throat or unexplained fever within the past 2 months.

TEST-TAKING STRATEGY: Options 2, 3, and 4 are unrelated to RF. Note the similarity between rheumatic "fever" in the question and the word "fever" in the correct option. If you had difficulty with this question, take time now to review the etiology related to RF.
LEVEL OF COGNITIVE ABILITY: Application
PHASE OF NURSING PROCESS: Planning
CLIENT NEEDS: Physiological Integrity
CONTENT AREA: Child Health
REFERENCE
Ashwill, J., & Droske, S. (1997). *Nursing care of children: Principles and practice*. Philadelphia: W. B. Saunders. pp. 657, 659.

14. **1**

RATIONALE: Anti-inflammatory agents such as aspirin may be given to the child with RF. Aspirin should not be given to a child who has chickenpox or other viral infections. Options 2 and 4 are clinical manifestations of RF. Facial edema may be associated with the development of a cardiac complication.
TEST-TAKING STRATEGY: Options 2 and 4 can be eliminated because they are manifestations of RF. Knowledge that facial edema may indicate a cardiac complication will assist in eliminating this option. Review the contraindications related to the use of aspirin if you had difficulty with this question.

LEVEL OF COGNITIVE ABILITY: Application
PHASE OF NURSING PROCESS: Implementation
CLIENT NEEDS: Safe, Effective Care Environment
CONTENT AREA: Child Health
REFERENCE
Hodgson, B., & Kizior, R. (1999). *Saunders nursing drug handbook 1999*. Philadelphia: W. B. Saunders. p. 76.

15. **4**

RATIONALE: A diagnosis of RF is confirmed by the presence of two major manifestations or one major and two minor manifestations from the Jones criteria. Additionally, evidence of a recent streptococcal infection is confirmed by a positive antistreptolysin O titer, streptozyme or an anti-DNase B assay.
TEST-TAKING STRATEGY: Knowledge that RF is characteristically associated with streptococcal infection will easily direct you to option 4. If you had difficulty with this question take time now to review the Jones criteria.
LEVEL OF COGNITIVE ABILITY: Comprehension
PHASE OF NURSING PROCESS: Data Collection
CLIENT NEEDS: Physiological Integrity
CONTENT AREA: Child Health
REFERENCE
Ashwill, J., & Droske, S. (1997). *Nursing care of children: Principles and practice*. Philadelphia: W. B. Saunders. p. 658.

BIBLIOGRAPHY

Ashwill, J., & Droske, S. (1997). *Nursing care of children: Principles and practice*. Philadelphia: W. B. Saunders.
Burroughs, A. (1997). *Maternity nursing: An introductory text* (7th ed.). Philadelphia: W. B. Saunders.
Hodgson, B., & Kizior, R. (1999). *Saunders nursing drug handbook 1999*. Philadelphia: W. B. Saunders.

Leifer, G. (1999). *Thompson's introduction to maternity and pediatric nursing* (3rd ed.). Philadelphia: W. B. Saunders.
O'Toole, M. (ed.). (1997). *Miller-Keane encyclopedia & dictionary of medicine, nursing, & allied health* (6th ed.). Philadelphia: W. B. Saunders.
Shulte, E., Price, D., & James, S. (1997). *Thompson's pediatric nursing: An introductory text* (7th ed.). Philadelphia: W. B. Saunders.

CHAPTER 31

Metabolic, Endocrine, and Gastrointestinal Disorders

. . . .

I. Fever

A. Description
1. An abnormal body temperature elevation
2. A child's temperature can vary depending on activity, emotional stress, the type of clothing the child is wearing, and the temperature of the environment
3. Findings associated with the fever provide important indications of the seriousness of the fever

B. Data collection
1. Temperature elevation and increased heart rate
2. Flushed skin
3. Diaphoresis
4. Chills
5. Restlessness or lethargy

C. Implementation
1. Monitor vital signs
2. Administer a sponge bath with lukewarm water for 20 to 30 minutes
3. Administer antipyretics such as acetaminophen (Tylenol) as prescribed
4. Do not administer aspirin (acetylsalicylic acid, ASA) because of the risk of Reye's syndrome
5. Retake temperature 30 to 60 minutes after the antipyretic is administered
6. Provide adequate fluid intake as tolerated and as prescribed
7. Monitor for dehydration and fluid and electrolyte imbalance
8. Instruct the parents how to take the temperature, how to safely medicate their child, and when it is necessary to call the physician

II. Dehydration

A. Description
1. Dehydration is the most common fluid and electrolyte imbalance in children
2. Infants and children are more vulnerable to fluid-volume deficit because a greater amount of their body water is in the extracellular fluid compartment
3. In infants and children, the organs that conserve water are immature, placing them at risk for fluid-volume deficit
4. The causes can include decreased fluid intake, diaphoresis, vomiting, diarrhea, burns, or malnutrition

B. Data collection
1. Weight loss
2. Dry mucous membranes and decrease in skin turgor
3. Sunken eyeballs and depressed fontanels
4. Decreased urine output and increased urine-specific gravity
5. Absence of tears
6. Decreased blood pressure, tachycardia, and tachypnea
7. Excessive thirst
8. Prolonged capillary refill time and increased hemoglobin and hematocrit

C. Implementation
1. Monitor vital signs
2. Monitor skin turgor and for signs of dehydration
3. Monitor weight and monitor for changes including fluid gains and losses
4. Monitor I&O and urine for specific gravity
5. Intravenous (IV) fluids and electrolyte replacements may be prescribed if the child is unable to ingest sufficient fluids orally

6. Withhold a full diet until the child is well hydrated and the cause of the dehydration is under control
7. Provide clear liquids orally in small quantities such as 1 to 2 oz every hour

III. Vomiting

A. Description
1. The major concerns when a child is vomiting is the risk of dehydration, the loss of fluid and electrolytes, and the development of metabolic alkalosis
2. Additional concerns include aspiration, atelectasis, and the development of pneumonia
B. Data collection
1. Signs of aspiration
2. Character of vomitus
3. Abdominal cramping and pain
4. Dehydration and fluid and electrolyte imbalances
5. Metabolic alkalosis
6. Diarrhea
C. Implementation
1. Monitor vital signs
2. Monitor the character, amount, and frequency of vomiting
3. Monitor the force of the vomiting, as projectile vomiting is indicative of pyloric **stenosis** or increased intracranial pressure
4. Maintain a patent airway; position the child on the side to prevent aspiration
5. Monitor intake and output (I&O); monitor for signs of dehydration
6. Maintain NPO status and then provide adequate fluid intake as tolerated and as prescribed
7. Start feeding slowly with small amounts of fluid at frequent intervals
8. Advise parents to inform physician when signs of dehydration, blood in vomitus, forceful vomiting, or abdominal pain is present

IV. Diarrhea

A. Description: the major concerns when a child has diarrhea are dehydration, the loss of fluid and electrolytes, and metabolic acidosis
B. Data collection
1. Diarrhea
2. Abdominal cramping and pain
3. Dehydration and fluid and electrolyte imbalances
4. Metabolic acidosis
C. Implementation
1. Monitor vital signs
2. Monitor the character, amount, and frequency of diarrhea
3. Monitor skin integrity of perianal area
4. Monitor I&O and for dehydration
5. Monitor electrolyte levels

6. Maintain NPO status to place the bowel at rest and then provide adequate fluid intake as tolerated and as prescribed
7. Slowly refeed the child with fluids, and as diarrhea resolves begin easily digestible foods
8. Provide fluid and electrolyte replacement as prescribed
9. Provide isolation as required
10. Instruct the parents in good handwashing technique

V. Phenylketonuria (PKU)

A. Description
1. Genetic disorder that results in central nervous system (CNS) damage from toxic levels of phenylalanine in the blood
2. An autosomal recessive disorder
3. PKU is characterized by serum phenylalanine levels greater than 25 mg/dL (normal level is less than 2 mg/dL)
4. All 50 states require routine screening of all newborns for PKU
B. Data collection
1. In all children
a. Digestive problems and vomiting
b. Seizures
c. Musty odor of the urine
d. Mental retardation
2. In older children
a. Eczema
b. Hypopigmentation of the hair, skin, and irises
c. Hyperactive behavior
C. Implementation
1. Screening of newborns for PKU
2. If initial screening is positive, further diagnostic evaluation is required to verify the diagnosis
3. Rescreen infants by 14 days of age if initial screen was done before 24 to 48 hours of age
4. Restrict phenylalanine intake
5. Monitor physical, neurological, and intellectual development
6. Stress the importance of follow-up treatment
7. Encourage parents to express feelings about the diagnosis and the risk of PKU in future children

VI. Insulin-Dependent Diabetes Mellitus (Type 1 DM)

A. Description
1. Type 1 or juvenile-onset diabetes is caused by the partial or complete lack of the secretory capacity of the beta cells of the pancreas, resulting in insulin deficiency
2. Complete insulin deficiency requires the use of exogenous insulin to promote appropriate glucose use and to prevent complications related to elevated blood glucose levels such as hyperglycemia, diabetic ketoacidosis, and death

B. Data collection
 1. Polyuria, polydipsia, and polyphagia
 2. Hyperglycemia
 3. Weight loss
 4. Fruity odor to breath
 5. Dehydration
 6. Blurred vision
 7. Slow wound healing
 8. Weakness
 9. Changes in level of consciousness (LOC)
C. Long-term effects
 1. Failure to grow at a normal rate
 2. Delayed maturation
 3. Recurrent infections
 4. Neuropathy
 5. Cardiovascular disease
 6. Retinal microvascular disease
 7. Renal microvascular disease
D. Complications
 1. Hyperglycemia or hypoglycemia
 2. Diabetic ketoacidosis
 3. Coma
 4. Hypokalemia or hyperkalemia
 5. Microvascular changes
 6. Cardiovascular changes
E. Diet
 1. Total amount of calories are individualized based on the child's age and **growth** expectations
 2. As prescribed by the physician, the child may be instructed to follow the food exchange from the American Diabetic Association diet or the dietary guidelines for Americans (Food Guide Pyramid) issued by the U.S. Departments of Agriculture and Health Services
 3. Incorporate the diet into the individual child's needs, likes and dislikes, lifestyle, cultural, and socioeconomic patterns
 4. Allow the child to participate in making food choices to provide a sense of control
F. Exercise
 1. Instruct the child in dietary adjustments when exercising
 2. Extra food needs to be consumed for increased activity, usually 10 to 15 g of carbohydrate for every 30 to 45 minutes of activity
 3. Instruct the child to monitor blood glucose before exercising
 4. Plan with the child an appropriate exercise regimen incorporating the developmental stage
G. Insulin
 1. Diluted insulin may be required for some infants to provide small enough dosages to avoid hypoglycemia
 2. Diluted insulin should be clearly labeled to avoid dosage errors
 3. To prevent dosage errors, be certain that there is a match of the insulin concentration with the calibration of units on the insulin syringe

 4. Illness, infection, and stress increase the need for insulin, and insulin should not be withheld during illness, infection, or stress because hyperglycemia and ketoacidosis can result
 5. Instruct the parents and child to recognize symptoms of hypoglycemia and hyperglycemia
 6. Orange juice, sugar-sweetened beverages, or hard candy should be kept available and administered if a hypoglycemic reaction occurs
 7. Instruct the child and parents in the administration of the insulin
 8. Instruct the parents in administering glucagon by injection if the child has a hypoglycemic reaction and is unable to drink sugar-containing fluid
 9. Instruct the parents to always have a spare bottle of insulin available
 10. Advise the parents to obtain a Medic-Alert bracelet indicating the type and daily insulin dosage
H. Blood glucose monitoring
 1. Results provide the parents with information to maintain good glycemic control
 2. More accurate than urine testing
 3. Requires children to prick themselves several times a day as prescribed
 4. Instruct the parents and child in the proper procedure for obtaining blood glucose level
 5. Inform the parents and child that the procedure must be done precisely to obtain accurate results
 6. Stress the importance of handwashing before and after performing the procedure to prevent infection
 7. Stress the importance of following the manufacturer's instructions
 8. Instruct the parents and child to calibrate the monitor as instructed by the manufacturer
 9. Instruct the parents and child to check the expiration date on the test strips
 10. Instruct the parents and child that if blood glucose results do not seem reasonable, reread the instructions, reassess technique, check the expiration date of the test strips, and perform the procedure again to verify results
I. Urine testing
 1. Instruct the parents and child in the procedure for testing urine for ketones and glucose
 2. Teach the child that the second voided urine specimen is most accurate
 3. The presence of ketones may indicate impending ketoacidosis
 4. Urine glucose testing is not recommended as the only means of monitoring the child who is taking insulin, as it is a less reliable indicator as compared to blood glucose monitoring
J. Hypoglycemia

1. Description
    a. Described as a blood glucose level below 60 mg/dL
    b. Occurs as a result of too much insulin, not enough food, or excessive activity
2. Mild hypoglycemia
    a. Provide 15 g of carbohydrate and repeat the treatment in 10 to 15 minutes if symptoms do not subside
    b. Instruct the child to eat additional food or the next scheduled meal in 15 to 30 minutes
3. Moderate hypoglycemia
    a. Provide 15 to 30 g of carbohydrate and repeat the treatment in 10 to 15 minutes if symptoms do not subside
    b. Instruct the child to eat additional food such as low-fat milk or cheese after 15 to 30 minutes
4. Severe hypoglycemia
    a. Intramuscular (IM) or subcutaneous (SC) glucagon or dextrose IV may be prescribed
    b. Administer a second dose if the child remains unconscious
    c. Provide a small meal when the child wakes up and is no longer nauseated
    d. Instruct the parents on the administration of glucagon
K. Hyperglycemia
    1. Description: elevated blood glucose level over 200 mg/dL
    2. Implementation: instruct the parents to notify the physician when blood glucose results are greater than 200 mg/dL, when ketonuria is present, when unable to take food or fluids, and when illness persists
L. Diabetic ketoacidosis (DKA)
    1. Description
        a. A complication of diabetes mellitus that develops when a severe insulin deficiency occurs
        b. DKA is a life-threatening condition
        c. Hyperglycemia that progresses to metabolic acidosis occurs
        d. It develops over a period of several hours to days
        e. Serum glucose level is over 300 mg/dL and urine and serum ketones are positive
    2. Implementation
        a. Treatment is aimed at restoring circulating volume and protecting against cerebral, coronary, or renal hypoperfusion
        b. Hyperglycemia is treated with IV Regular Insulin
        c. Monitor vital signs, urine output, and mental status closely
        d. Dehydration is treated with IV infusions of 0.9% or 0.45% normal saline
        e. Administer oxygen as prescribed
        f. Monitor blood glucose closely
        g. Monitor child closely for signs of fluid overload

h. Monitor potassium closely because when the child receives insulin to lower the blood glucose level, the serum potassium will decrease as the acidosis improves, and potassium replacement may then be required
        i. Dextrose by IV may be prescribed when the blood glucose level reaches an appropriate level
M. Sick day rules for the diabetic (Box 31–1)

VII. Cleft Lip and Cleft Palate

A. Description
    1. A congenital anomaly that occurs due to failure of soft tissue or bony structure to fuse during embryonic development
    2. Involves abnormal openings in the lip or palate that may occur unilaterally or bilaterally and are readily apparent at birth
    3. Causes include genetic, **hereditary** and environmental factors; exposure to radiation or rubella virus; chromosome abnormalities; and teratogenic factors
    4. Surgical correction requires several stages
    5. Cleft lip repair is usually performed by age 4 weeks; in some cases, cleft lip repair is performed in the first 2 to 3 days of life, with cosmetic modifications performed at age 4 to 5 years
    6. Cleft palate repair is performed between the ages of 6 months to 2 years because early closure facilitates speech development
B. Data collection
    1. Cleft lip can range from a slight notch to a complete separation from the floor of the nose
    2. Cleft palate can include nasal distortion, midline, or bilateral cleft, with various extensions from the uvula and soft and hard palates
C. Implementation
    1. Check ability to suck, swallow, handle

BOX 31–1. Sick Day Rules for the Diabetic

Always give insulin even if the child does not have an appetite, or contact the physician for specific instructions
Test blood glucose levels at least every 4 hours
Test for urinary ketones with each voiding
Notify the physician if moderate or large amounts of urinary ketones are present
Follow the child's usual meal plan
Encourage calorie-free liquids to aid in clearing ketones
Encourage rest, especially if urinary ketones are present
Notify the physician if vomiting, fruity odor to the breath, deep rapid respirations, decreasing level of consciousness, or persistent hyperglycemia occurs

normal secretions, and breathe without distress
2. Encourage the parents to describe feelings related to deformity
3. Teach the parents special feeding or suctioning techniques
4. Modify feeding techniques to allow adequate **growth**
5. Plan to use specialized feeding techniques, obturators, and special nipples and feeders for the child unable to adequately suck on a standard nipple
6. Hold the child in upright position and direct the formula to the side and back of the mouth to prevent aspiration
7. Feed small amounts gradually; burp frequently
8. Encourage breast-feeding if appropriate
9. Reassure the parents that surgery usually is successful
10. Teach parents ESSR (enlarge, stimulate, swallow, rest) method of feeding (Box 31–2)

D. Implementation postoperatively
1. Position the infant on the side lateral to repair or on the back
2. Avoid the prone position to prevent rubbing of the surgical site on the mattress
3. Restrain with soft elbow or jacket restraints to keep the child from touching the repair site; remove restraints every 2 hours for skin care and range of motion exercises
4. Monitor the surgical site for redness, swelling, excessive bleeding, drainage, and monitor for fever
5. Provide analgesics for pain
6. Avoid contact with sharp objects near the surgical site; keep pacifiers, straws, spoons, forks, or fingers away from the mouth for 7 to 10 days
7. Avoid oral suction or placing objects in the mouth such as a tongue depressor or thermometer
8. Advance the diet as prescribed from clear liquids to a normal soft diet within 48 hours
9. For cleft palate repair, provide short nipples that don't rest on palatal sutures and give baby food or baby food mixed with water
10. Prevent sucking
11. If a palate repair was required, avoid

BOX 31–2. ESSR Method of Feeding

ENLARGE the nipple so that the food is delivered to the back of the throat without sucking
STIMULATE sucking by rubbing the nipple on the lower lip
SWALLOW
REST to allow the child to finish swallowing what has been placed in the mouth

---

inserting the spoon into the mouth, which may disrupt sutures
12. After feeding place the infant on his or her side lateral to the repair with the head elevated
13. Cleanse the lip suture line with sterile water after feeding and rinse the mouth with water after feedings to clean palate repair
14. Apply antibacterial ointment to surgical site as prescribed using a cotton-tipped applicator
15. Do not brush the child's teeth for 1 to 2 weeks
16. Encourage the parents to hold the child
17. Initiate appropriate referrals for speech impairment or language-based **learning** difficulties

VIII. Esophageal Atresia and Tracheoesophageal Fistula

A. Description
1. The esophagus terminates before it reaches the stomach and/or a fistula is present that forms an unnatural connection with the trachea
2. The condition causes oral intake to enter the lungs or a large amount of air to enter the stomach, and choking, coughing, and severe abdominal distention can occur
3. Aspiration pneumonia and severe respiratory distress will develop, and death will occur without surgical intervention
4. Surgical repair includes ligation of the fistula with anastomosis of the **atresia** to decrease the severity of stricture formation

B. Data collection
1. Cough and choking with feedings
2. Difficulty swallowing
3. Excessive oral secretions
4. **Regurgitation** and vomiting
5. **Nasal flaring** and **retractions**
6. Cyanosis
7. Abdominal distention
8. Failure to pass a suction catheter or nasogastric (NG) tube

C. Implementation preoperatively
1. Place in a supine or prone position with the head of the bed elevated
2. Keep the child warm and administer humidified oxygen to relieve respiratory distress as prescribed
3. Maintain NPO status
4. Assist with the placement of NG tube; aspiration of the NG tube may be prescribed to keep the proximal pouch clear of secretions
5. Maintain IV fluids as prescribed

D. Implementation postoperatively
1. Monitor respiratory status
2. Monitor I&O and daily weight
3. Monitor for dehydration and possible fluid overload

4. Note that a chest tube may be placed during surgery
5. Monitor for signs of pain
6. Monitor surgical site for redness, breakdown, or exudate
7. If cervical esophagostomy was performed, the area will be kept covered with gauze to absorb saliva, and skin care will be provided with half-strength hydrogen peroxide as prescribed
8. Assist with gastrostomy tube feedings when prescribed
9. The physician may prescribe elevation of the gastrostomy tube, which allows the gastric contents to pass to the small intestine and air to escape, thus decreasing the risk of leakage in the anastomosis
10. Do not offer the pacifier to the child until the child can tolerate oral secretions
11. Reinforce instructions to the parents in the techniques of gastrostomy tube feedings and skin site care

IX. Gastroesophageal Reflux (GER)

A. Description
 1. Backflow of gastric contents into the esophagus, as a result of relaxation or incompetence of the lower esophageal or cardiac sphincter
 2. Complications include esophagitis, esophageal strictures, aspiration of gastric contents, and aspiration pneumonia
 3. Treatment includes diet, positioning, medications, and surgery; however, surgery is considered as the last resort in treatment
B. Data collection
 1. Forceful chronic vomiting
 2. Aspiration
 3. Apnea with cyanosis
 4. Hematemesis and melena
 5. Weight loss and failure to thrive
 6. Recurrent respiratory infections
 7. Bitter taste as described in older children
C. Implementation
 1. Monitor amount and characteristics of emesis
 2. Monitor the relation of vomiting to the time of feedings and infant activity
 3. Burp the infant frequently when feeding
 4. Handle the child minimally after feedings
 5. Monitor for respiratory distress
 6. Suction equipment at bedside
 7. Monitor I&O and for signs and symptoms of dehydration
D. Positioning
 1. Place the infant in an upright angle 24 hours a day
 2. Position at a 60-degree upright angle when supine and a 30-degree upright angle when prone until asymptomatic
E. Diet
 1. Provide small, frequent feedings

2. For infants, thicken formula by adding 1 to 3 teaspoons of rice cereal per ounce of formula and cross-cut the nipple
3. For toddlers, feed solids first, followed by liquids
F. Medications
 1. Schedule medications around mealtimes
 2. Administer antacids as prescribed for symptom relief
 3. Administer H$_2$ receptor antagonists as prescribed to decrease acid secretions
 4. Administer prokinetic agents as prescribed to accelerate gastric emptying
G. Surgery
 1. If surgery is prescribed, it will require a procedure known as fundoplication, in which a wrap to the stomach fundus is made around the distal esophagus
 2. Instruct the parents that the child's ability to burp or vomit will eventually return
 3. Instruct the parents about the possibility of dumping syndrome, which begins 30 minutes after a feeding and may include diaphoresis, palpitations, weakness, syncope, abdominal fullness, nausea, or diarrhea

X. Pyloric Stenosis (Fig. 31–1)

A. Description: Hypertrophy of the circular muscles of the pylorus causes narrowing of the pyloric canal between the stomach and the duodenum
B. Data collection
 1. Vomiting that progresses from mild **regurgitation** to projectile and usually occurs after a feeding
 2. Vomitus contains gastric contents; may contain mucus, may be blood-tinged, and does not usually contain bile

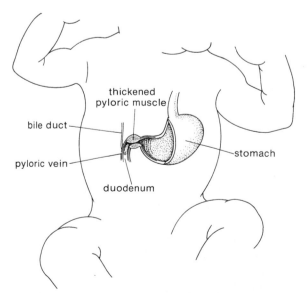

FIGURE 31–1. Pyloric stenosis. (From Betz, C., Hunsberger, M., & Wright, S. [1994]. *Family-centered nursing care of children* [2nd ed.]. Philadelphia: W. B. Saunders. p. 1446.)

3. Constant hunger
4. Fussiness and frequent crying
5. Decrease in size and number of stools
6. Failure to gain weight, dehydration, and malnutrition
7. Upper abdominal distention
8. Peristaltic waves visible from left to right across epigastrium during or immediately following a feeding
C. Implementation
   1. Monitor vital signs
   2. Monitor I&O and weight
   3. Monitor for signs of dehydration and electrolyte imbalances
   4. Monitor stools
   5. Administer antacids as prescribed to neutralize the acidity of refluxed contents and to prevent esophageal tissue damage
   6. Administer medications as prescribed to promote gastric emptying or pyloric sphincter relaxation
   7. Prepare the child and parents for pyloromyotomy if prescribed
D. Pyloromyotomy
   1. Description: an incision through the muscle fibers of the pylorus
   2. Implementation preoperatively
      a. Monitor frequency and amount of vomiting after feeding
      b. Prevent aspiration
      c. Monitor hydration status by daily weights, I&O, and urine for specific gravity
      d. Maintain IV fluids as prescribed
   3. Implementation postoperatively
      a. Maintain a patent airway
      b. Monitor vital signs
      c. Monitor for signs of shock
      d. Begin clear liquids 4 to 6 hours postoperatively as prescribed
      e. Advance diet to dilute then full-strength formula as prescribed
      f. Feed infant slowly, burping frequently
      g. Position in high Fowler's on the right side after feedings
      h. Handle infant minimally after feedings
      i. Monitor for abdominal distention
      j. Monitor surgical wound and for signs of infection
      k. Instruct parents about wound care, feeding, and positioning

XI. Lactose Intolerance

A. Description: inability to tolerate lactose as a result of an absence or deficiency of lactase, an enzyme found in the secretions of the small intestine that is required for the digestion of lactose
B. Data collection
   1. Diarrhea
   2. Abdominal distention
   3. Crampy abdominal pain
   4. Excessive flatus

C. Implementation
   1. Provide a lactose-free diet
   2. Encourage breast-feeding mother to limit dairy products
   3. Gradually add food containing small amounts of lactose such as yogurt, hard cheeses, and small amounts of milk to check the child's reaction
   4. Instruct the parents regarding alternative sources of calcium

XII. Celiac Disease

A. Description
   1. Intolerance to gluten, the protein component of wheat, barley, rye, and oats
   2. Symptoms of the disorder occur 3 to 6 months following the introduction of gluten-containing grains into the diet
   3. It results in the accumulation of the amino acid glutamine, which is toxic to intestinal mucosal cells
   4. Intestinal villi atrophy, which affects absorption of ingested nutrients
B. Data Collection
   1. Steatorrhea: frequent, bulky, greasy malodorous stools with a frothy appearance because of fat in the stool
   2. Abdominal distention
   3. Weight loss
   4. Signs of malnutrition
   5. **Growth** failure
   6. Irritability and apathy
   7. Anemia
C. Celiac crisis
   1. Precipitated by infection, fasting, and ingestion of gluten
   2. Can lead to electrolyte imbalance, rapid dehydration, and severe acidosis
   3. Causes profuse watery diarrhea and vomiting
D. Implementation
   1. Gluten-free diet and substituting corn and rice as a grain source
   2. Lifelong elimination of gluten sources such as wheat, rye, oats, and barley
   3. Mineral and vitamin supplements including fat-soluble supplements A, D, E, and K
   4. Teach the parents about a gluten-free diet (Box 31–3)
   5. Instruct in measures to prevent celiac crisis
   6. Instruct in the importance of preventing infection

XIII. Appendicitis

A. Description
   1. Inflammation of the appendix
   2. When the appendix becomes inflamed or infected, rupture may occur within a matter of hours leading to peritonitis and sepsis
B. Data collection

> **BOX 31-3. Basics of a Gluten-Free Diet**
>
> ### FOODS ALLOWED
>
> Meat such as beef, pork, and poultry, fish, eggs, milk and dairy products, vegetables, fruits, grains, rice, corn, gluten-free wheat flower, puffed rice, corn flakes, corn meal, precooked gluten-free cereals
>
> ### FOODS PROHIBITED
>
> Commercially prepared ice cream; malted milk; prepared puddings; grains, including anything made from wheat, rye, oats or barley such as breads, rolls, cookies, cakes, crackers, cereal, spaghetti, macaroni, beer, and ale

1. Pain in periumbilical area that descends to right lower quadrant
2. Abdominal pain that is most intense at McBurney's point
3. Rebound tenderness and abdominal rigidity
4. Elevated white blood cell (WBC) count
5. Side-lying position with abdominal guarding with legs flexed
6. Low-grade fever
7. Anorexia, nausea, and vomiting
8. Constipation or diarrhea

C. Ruptured appendix/peritonitis
  1. Description: inflammation of the peritoneum
  2. Data collection
    a. Increased fever
    b. Progressive abdominal distention and abdominal pain
    c. Right guarding of abdomen
    d. Tachycardia and tachypnea
    e. Pallor
    f. Chills
    g. Restlessness

D. Appendectomy
  1. Description: surgical removal of the appendix
  2. Implementation preoperatively
    a. Maintain NPO status
    b. Maintain IV fluids as prescribed to prevent dehydration
    c. Monitor for signs of ruptured appendix and peritonitis
    d. Antibiotics may be prescribed
    e. Monitor for changes in level of pain
    f. Monitor bowel sounds
    g. Position right side-lying or low to semi-Fowler's position to promote comfort
    h. Apply ice packs to abdomen for 20 minutes every hour as prescribed
    i. Avoid application of heat to abdomen
    j. Avoid laxatives or enemas
  3. Implementation postoperatively
    a. Monitor temperature for signs of infection
    b. Maintain NPO status until bowel function has returned
    c. Advance diet gradually as tolerated when bowel sounds return

    d. Monitor incision for signs of infection as redness, swelling, and pain
    e. If rupture of the appendix had occurred, a Penrose drain may be inserted or the incision may be left open to heal from the inside out
    f. Drainage from the Penrose may be profuse for the first 12 hours
    g. Position client in right side-lying or low to semi-Fowler's position with legs flexed to facilitate drainage
    h. Change the dressing as prescribed and record the type and amount of drainage
    i. Perform wound irrigations if prescribed
    j. Maintain NG suction and patency of NG tube as prescribed
    k. Administer antibiotics and analgesics as prescribed

XIV. Hirschsprung's Disease

A. Description
  1. A congenital anomaly also known as congenital aganglionosis or megacolon
  2. Occurs as the result of an absence of ganglion cells in the rectum and upward in the colon
  3. Results in mechanical obstruction from inadequate motility in an intestinal segment
  4. May be a familial congenital defect or may be associated with other anomalies such as Down's syndrome and genital urinary abnormalities
  5. Treatment for mild or moderate disease is based on relieving the chronic constipation with stool softeners and rectal irrigations
  6. Treatment for moderate to severe disease involves a two-step surgical procedure
  7. Initially, in the neonatal period, the obstruction is relieved by a temporary colostomy
  8. A complete surgical repair is performed when the child weighs 17.6 to 22 lb (8–10 kg) via a pull-through procedure to excise portions of the bowel; at this time, the colostomy is closed

B. Data collection
  1. In newborns, failure to pass meconium stool within 48 hours after birth
  2. In infants, failure to thrive
  3. In toddlers and older children, chronic constipation
  4. Ribbonlike and foul-smelling stools
  5. Abdominal distention
  6. Bowel obstruction
  7. Reluctance to ingest fluids
  8. Bile-stained vomitus
  9. Visible peristalsis
  10. Palpable fecal mass
  11. Signs of enterocolitis such as fever, severe prostration, or explosive watery diarrhea

C. Implementation
  1. Administer stool softeners as prescribed

2. Dietary management and cleansing enemas as prescribed until the child is able to tolerate surgery
D. Implementation preoperatively
   1. Monitor bowel function
   2. Administer bowel preparation as prescribed
   3. Maintain NPO status
   4. Maintain IV fluids as prescribed for hydration
   5. Administer antibiotics as prescribed to sterilize the bowel
   6. Monitor I&O and weight
   7. Monitor hydration and fluid and electrolyte status
   8. Measure abdominal girth
   9. Avoid rectal temperatures
   10. Monitor for respiratory distress associated with abdominal distention
E. Implementation postoperatively
   1. Monitor vital signs, avoiding rectal temperatures
   2. Measure abdominal circumference
   3. Monitor surgical site for redness, swelling, and drainage
   4. Monitor stoma for bleeding or skin breakdown
   5. Monitor anal area for the presence of stool, redness, or discharge
   6. Maintain NPO status as prescribed until bowel sounds return or flatus is passed
   7. Monitor for bowel sounds, which usually return within 48 to 72 hours
   8. Maintain NG to intermittent suction as prescribed until peristalsis returns
   9. Maintain IV as prescribed until child tolerates appropriate PO intake
   10. Begin diet with clear liquids, advancing to regular as tolerated and as prescribed
   11. Assess for dehydration and fluid overload
   12. Monitor I&O and weight

13. Assess pain and provide comfort measures as required
14. Provide the parents with instructions regarding colostomy care, skin care, and colostomy irrigations as required
15. Teach the parents about appropriate diet and adequate fluid intake

XV. Intussusception (Fig. 31–2)

A. Description
   1. Telescoping of one portion of the bowel into another portion
   2. Results in an obstruction to the passage of intestinal contents
B. Data collection
   1. Colicky, abdominal pain
   2. Pain causes the child to scream and draw knees to the abdomen
   3. Vomiting of gastric contents; bile-stained fecal emesis
   4. Currant jelly–like stools containing blood and mucus
   5. Hypoactive or hyperactive bowel sounds
   6. Tender distended abdomen, possibly with a palpable mass
   7. Lethargy
C. Implementation
   1. Monitor hydration status and for signs of dehydration
   2. Monitor I&O and weight
   3. Maintain NPO status and NG tube as prescribed if distention is present
   4. Maintain IV fluids as prescribed
   5. Monitor for signs of sepsis or peritonitis as evidenced by fever, increased heart rate, changes in level of consciousness (LOC) or blood pressure, and respiratory distress, and report immediately
   6. Prepare for hydrostatic reduction if prescribed

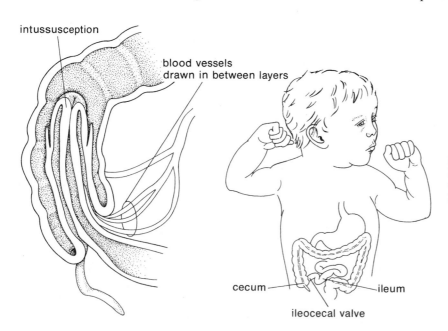

intussusception

blood vessels drawn in between layers

cecum — ileum

ileocecal valve

FIGURE 31–2. Intussusception. (From Betz, C., Hunsberger, M., & Wright, S. [1994]. *Family-centered nursing care of children* [2nd ed.]. Philadelphia: W. B. Saunders. p. 1462.).

7. Following hydrostatic reduction, administer clear fluids and advance the diet gradually as prescribed; monitor for the passage of barium and the characteristics of stool
8. If surgery is performed, maintain NPO status until bowel function returns, then begin clear liquids, advancing as tolerated as prescribed

XVI. Abdominal Wall Defects (Fig. 31–3)

A. Description
 1. Can include umbilical hernia, inguinal hernia, or hydrocele
 2. A hernia is a protrusion of the bowel through an abnormal opening in the abdominal wall
 3. In children, a hernia most commonly occurs at the umbilicus and through the inguinal canal
 4. A hydrocele is the presence of abdominal fluid in the scrotal sac
B. Data collection
 1. Umbilical hernia: soft swelling or protrusion around the umbilicus that is usually reducible with the finger
 2. Inguinal hernia
  a. Painless inguinal swelling that is reducible
  b. Swelling may disappear during periods of rest and is most noticeable when the infant cries or coughs
 3. Incarcerated hernia
  a. When the descended portion becomes tightly caught in the hernial sac, compromising blood supply
  b. A medical emergency requiring surgical repair
  c. Irritability
  d. Tenderness at site
  e. Anorexia
  f. Abdominal distention
  g. Difficulty defecating
  h. May lead to complete intestinal obstruction and gangrene

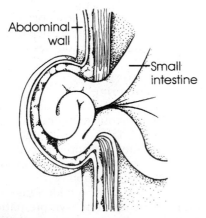

Abdominal wall

Small intestine

FIGURE 31–3. Diagram of an umbilical hernia. (From Milner, R., & Herber, S. [1984]. *Color atlas of the newborn.* Oradell, NJ: Medical Economics Books. p. 61.)

4. Noncommunicating hydrocele
  a. Occurs when residual peritoneal fluid is trapped with no communication to the peritoneal cavity
  b. Usually disappears by age 1 year
5. Communicating hydrocele
  a. Associated with a hernia that remains open from the scrotum to the abdominal cavity
  b. Data collection includes a bulge in the inguinal area or the scrotum that increases with crying or straining and decreases when the child is at rest
C. Implementation postoperatively (hernia)
 1. Monitor vital signs
 2. Assess for wound infection
 3. Monitor I&O and hydration status
 4. Advance the diet as tolerated
 5. Administer analgesics as prescribed
D. Implementation postoperatively (hydrocele)
 1. Provide ice bags and a scrotal support to relieve pain and swelling
 2. Instruct to avoid tub bathing until the incision heals
 3. Instruct to avoid strenuous physical activities

XVII. Constipation/Encopresis

A. Description
 1. Constipation is the infrequent and difficult passage of dry, hard stools
 2. Encopresis is fecal incontinence and children often complain that soiling is involuntary and occurs without warning
 3. If the child does not have a neurological or anatomical disorder, encopresis is usually the result of fecal impaction and an enlarged rectum caused by chronic constipation
B. Data collection
 1. Constipation
  a. Abdominal pain and cramping without distention
  b. Palpable movable fecal masses
  c. Normal or decreased bowel sounds
  d. Malaise and headache
  e. Anorexia, nausea, and vomiting
 2. Encopresis
  a. Evidence of soiling clothing
  b. Scratching or rubbing of the anal area
  c. Fecal odor
  d. Social withdrawal
C. Implementation
 1. Simple constipation may resolve using only dietary changes or methods to change the habit of retention
 2. Severe encopresis may require intervention to be continued over a period of 3 to 6 months
 3. Overcoming withholding
  a. Administer enemas as prescribed until impaction is cleared
  b. Monitor for hypernatremia or hyperphosphatemia when administering repeated enemas

    c. Administer stool softener or laxative as prescribed

    d. Administer mineral oil 30 to 75 mL BID as prescribed; administer mineral oil chilled or mixed with cold drinks to disguise the taste

  4. Dietary changes

    a. Increase water and fiber intake

    b. Decrease sugar and milk intake

    c. Administer fat-soluble vitamins during the use of mineral oil because the oil can interfere with vitamin absorption in the small intestine

  5. Changing the retention habit: have the child sit on the toilet for 5 to 10 minutes approximately 20 to 30 minutes after breakfast and dinner to assist with defecation

XVIII. Irritable Bowel Syndrome

A. Description

  1. Occurs as a result of increased motility that can lead to spasm and pain

  2. The diagnosis is based on the elimination of pathology

  3. It is a self-limiting, intermittent problem with no definitive treatment

  4. Stress and emotional factors may be contributed to its occurrence

B. Data collection

  1. Diffuse abdominal pain unrelated to meals or activity

  2. Alternating constipation and diarrhea with the presence of undigested food and mucus in the stool

  3. Normal **growth**

C. Implementation

  1. Reassure that the problem is self-limiting and intermittent and will resolve

  2. Encourage the maintenance of a healthy well-balanced, moderate-fiber diet

  3. Encourage health promotion activities such as exercise and school activities

  4. Inform the parents of psychosocial resources if required

XIX. Imperforate Anus

A. Description: incomplete development or absence of the anus in its normal position in the perineum

B. Data collection

  1. Failure to pass meconium stool

  2. Absence or **stenosis** of the anal rectal canal

  3. Anal membrane

  4. External fistula to the peritoneum

C. Implementation

  1. Determine patency of the anus

  2. Monitor for the presence of stool in the urine and vagina and report immediately

D. Implementation postoperatively

  1. Monitor the skin for signs of infection

  2. Position side-lying with legs flexed or a prone position to keep hips elevated to reduce edema and pressure on the surgical site

  3. Keep the anal surgical incision clean and dry and monitor for redness, swelling, or drainage

  4. Maintain NPO status and NG tube if in place as prescribed

  5. Maintain IV fluids as prescribed until GI motility returns

  6. Provide colostomy care if prescribed

  7. Colostomy site should be pink without drainage, swelling, or skin breakdown

  8. A fresh colostomy stoma will be red and edematous but this should decrease with time

  9. Reinforce instructions to the parents to perform anal dilatation if prescribed to achieve and maintain bowel patency

  10. Instruct the parents to use only dilators supplied by the physician, a water-soluble lubricant, and to insert the dilator no more than 1 to 2 cm into the anus to prevent damage to the mucosa

XX. Viral Hepatitis

A. Description

  1. An acute or chronic inflammation of the liver

  2. The most effective means of preventing hepatitis is immunization

  3. The most common mode of transmission of hepatitis A virus (HAV) is person-to-person by the fecal-oral route

  4. Hepatitis B virus (HBV) is primarily transmitted parenterally or by sexual contact

  5. Children who have had direct contact with a person infected with HAV should receive immune globulin as soon as possible after exposure

  6. Cases of hepatitis should be reported promptly to local public health officials

B. Data collection

  1. A history of exposure to jaundiced children, confirmed outbreaks in day care centers or schools, or exposure to blood or body fluids should raise the suspicion of hepatitis

  2. Right upper quadrant tenderness

  3. Hepatomegaly

  4. Pale clay-colored stools

  5. Dark and frothy urine

  6. Jaundice that is best assessed in the sclera, nailbeds, and mucous membranes

  7. Hepatitis A: in infants and preschool children, it is usually either asymptomatic or causes mild nonspecific symptoms such as anorexia, malaise, and easy fatigability

  8. Hepatitis B: may cause a wide range of symptoms ranging from asymptomatic infection to fatal acute fulminant hepatitis

C. Implementation

  1. Prevention of the spread of infection

2. Instruct on good handwashing
3. Instruct to thoroughly disinfect diaper-changing surfaces with a solution of 1/4 cup bleach to a gallon of water
4. Provide enteric precautions for at least 1 week after the onset of jaundice with HAV
5. Maintain comfort and provide adequate rest and sleep
6. Provide a low-fat, balanced diet
7. Instruct the parents that because hepatitis A is not infectious within 1 week after the onset of jaundice, the child may return to school at that time if feeling well enough
8. Instruct parents that jaundice may get worse before it resolves
9. Instruct parents in the signs indicating a worsening of the child's condition such as changes in the neurological status, bleeding, and fluid retention

XXI. Ingestion of Poisons

A. Lead poisoning
1. Description: excessive accumulation of lead in the blood
2. Causes
   a. Ingestion of lead through paint chips, soil contaminated with lead, canned food products, lead used in plumbing, vinyl miniblinds, and improperly glazed pottery
   b. A diet high in fat and low in iron and calcium increases lead absorption
3. Diagnostic test
   a. Erythrocyte protoporphyrin (EP) levels are used to screen children for lead levels and anemia
   b. An EP level greater than 9 μg/dL indicates the need for more frequent screening
   c. An EP level greater than 15 μg/dL indicates the need for nutritional and educational interventions and environmental investigation
   d. An EP level greater than 20 μg/dL requires pharmacological intervention
4. Data collection
   a. Anorexia, malaise, and headache
   b. Constipation or diarrhea
   c. Failure to thrive
   d. Abdominal pain
   e. Lead lines in gums around the teeth
   f. Tachycardia
   g. Hypertension or hypotension
   h. Lacrimation and nasal congestion
   i. Muscle pains
   j. Renal toxicity
5. Complications
   a. Cerebral edema
   b. Renal toxicity
   c. CNS toxicity
6. Implementation
   a. Remove the child from the lead source

   b. Administer chelating agents (EDTA with BAL) as prescribed
   c. Monitor kidney function for nephrotoxicity when medication is given
   d. Monitor calcium levels because medication enhances excretion of calcium
   e. Administer anticonvulsants as prescribed
   f. Administer oral or IM iron as prescribed
   g. Follow-up lead levels to monitor progress

B. Acetaminophen (Tylenol)
1. Description: seriousness of ingestion is determined by amount ingested and length of time before intervention
2. Data collection
   a. First 24 hours: malaise, nausea, vomiting, sweating, pallor, and weakness
   b. One to three days: elevated liver enzymes and bilirubin, right upper quadrant pain, prolonged prothrombin time (PT)
   c. One week: jaundice, liver necrosis, possible death from hepatic failure
3. Implementation
   a. Induce vomiting or gastric lavage depending on the amount ingested
   b. Administer activated charcoal or antidote acetylcysteine (Mucomyst)
   c. Administer acetylcysteine with juice or cola or via NG tube as prescribed
   d. Do not administer charcoal if a prescribed antidote is anticipated, because charcoal will make the antidote ineffective
   e. Monitor IV fluids as prescribed
   f. Provide sodium-restricted, high-calorie, high-protein diet as prescribed

C. Salicylates
1. Description
   a. Most common cause of drug poisoning in children
   b. Toxic dose: single dose exceeding 200 to 280 mg/kg
   c. Peak gastric absorption occurs within 2 hours of ingestion
2. Data collection
   a. GI effects: nausea, vomiting, and thirst
   b. CNS effects: hyperventilation, confusion, seizures, coma, respiratory failure, and circulatory collapse
   c. Renal effects: oliguria
   d. Hematopoietic effects: bleeding tendencies
   e. Metabolic effects: sweating, dehydration, fever, hyponatremia, hypokalemia, dehydration, and hypoglycemia
3. Implementation
   a. Induce vomiting as prescribed with syrup of ipecac or gastric lavage
   b. Administer activated charcoal to decrease absorption of salicylate as prescribed
   c. IVs, sodium bicarbonate, electrolytes, or volume expanders may be prescribed
   d. Administer vitamin K for bleeding tendencies as prescribed

e. Glucose may be prescribed for hypoglycemia

f. Prepare the child for dialysis as prescribed if the child is unresponsive to therapy

PRACTICE QUESTIONS

1. The nurse is caring for an 18-month-old child who has been vomiting. The most appropriate position for the child during sleep time is
   1 Side-lying position
   2 Prone with the face turned to the side
   3 Supine
   4 Prone with the head elevated

2. The nurse is monitoring for signs of dehydration in a 1-year-old child who has been hospitalized for diarrhea. The nurse prepares to take the child's temperature. Which of the following methods of measurement should be avoided?
   1 Tympanic
   2 Axillary
   3 Rectal
   4 Electronic

3. An infant returns to the nursing unit following a surgical repair of a cleft lip located on the right side of the lip. The best position to place this infant at this time is
   1 On the right side
   2 On the left side
   3 Prone
   4 Supine

4. The nurse reviews the record of an infant seen in the clinic. The nurse notes that a diagnosis of esophageal atresia with tracheoesophageal fistula (TEF) is suspected. The nurse understands that which of the following is not associated with this condition?
   1 Severe projectile vomiting
   2 Coughing
   3 Choking
   4 Cyanosis

5. The nurse is reviewing the record of a child with a diagnosis of pyloric stenosis. Which of the following data does the nurse expect to note documented in the child's record?
   1 Vomiting large amounts of bile
   2 Watery diarrhea
   3 Increased urine output
   4 Projectile vomiting

6. The nurse reinforces instructions to the mother about dietary measures for a 5-year-old child with lactose intolerance. The nurse tells the mother that which of the following supplements will be required due to the necessity of lactose avoidance in the diet?
   1 Zinc
   2 Protein

3 Calcium
4 Fats

7. The nurse reinforces home care instructions to the parents of a child with celiac disease. Which of the following food items does the nurse advise the parents to include in the child's diet?
   1 Rice
   2 Rye toast
   3 Oatmeal
   4 Wheat bread

8. The nurse is caring for a child who is scheduled for an appendectomy. When the nurse reviews the physician's preoperative orders, which of the following is questioned?
   1 Maintain IV fluids as prescribed
   2 Maintain NPO status
   3 Administer a Fleet enema
   4 Administer preoperative medication on call to the operating room

9. The clinic nurse reviews the record of a 3-week-old infant and notes that the physician has documented a diagnosis of suspected Hirschsprung's disease. The nurse understands that which of the following symptoms most likely led the mother to seek health care for the infant?
   1 Diarrhea
   2 Projectile vomiting
   3 Regurgitation of feedings
   4 Foul-smelling pellet-like stools

10. The nurse is caring for a child with a diagnosis of intussusception. Which of the following symptoms does the nurse expect to note in this child?
    1 Bright red blood and mucus in the stools
    2 Profuse projectile vomiting
    3 Watery diarrhea
    4 Ribbon-like stools

11. A child with a diagnosis of umbilical hernia has been scheduled for surgical repair in 2 weeks. The nurse reinforces instructions to the parents about the signs of possible hernial strangulation. The nurse tells the parents that which of the following signs requires physician notification by the parents?
    1 Fever
    2 Diarrhea
    3 Constipation
    4 Vomiting

12. The nurse reinforces home care instructions to the family of a child with hepatitis regarding care of the child and the prevention of transmission of the virus. Which of the following is not a component of the teaching?
    1 Handwashing techniques
    2 Cleaning household surfaces with bleach
    3 Providing a well-balanced, high-fat diet to the child
    4 The use of gloves

13. A child is hospitalized with a diagnosis of lead poisoning. The nurse assisting in caring for the child prepares to assist in administering which of the following medications?
    1 Activated charcoal
    2 Sodium bicarbonate
    3 Ipecac syrup
    4 EDTA in combination with BAL

14. The emergency department nurse is caring for a child brought to the emergency department following the ingestion of approximately one-half bottle of aspirin. The nurse anticipates that the most likely initial treatment will be
    1 The administration of syrup of ipecac
    2 The administration of sodium bicarbonate
    3 The administration of vitamin K
    4 Dialysis

15. The nurse is gathering supplies in preparation to administer a tepid bath to a child with a fever. Which of the following items is not necessary to obtain?
    1 Washcloths and towels
    2 A bottle of alcohol
    3 Toys
    4 Lightweight pajamas

16. A cooling blanket is prescribed for a child with a fever. Which of the following is not a component of the use of the cooling blanket?
    1 Place the cooling blanket on the bed and cover it with a sheet
    2 Check the skin condition of the child before, during, and after the use of the cooling blanket
    3 Keep the child uncovered to assist in reducing the fever
    4 Keep the child dry while on the cooling blanket to prevent the risk of frostbite

17. The nursing instructor asks a nursing student about phenylketonuria (PKU). Which of the following statements if made by the student indicates an understanding of this disorder?
    1 "PKU is an autosomal dominant disorder."
    2 "Treatment includes dietary restriction of tyramine."

3 "All 50 states require routine screening of all newborns for PKU."
    4 "PKU primarily affects the gastrointestinal (GI) system."

18. A school-aged child with insulin-dependent diabetes has soccer practice three afternoons a week. The nurse reinforces instructions regarding how to prevent hypoglycemia during practice. Which of the following is the most appropriate instruction?
    1 To take one half of the amount of prescribed insulin on practice days
    2 To eat twice the amount normally eaten at lunchtime
    3 To take the prescribed insulin at noontime rather than in the morning
    4 To eat six graham crackers or a cup of orange juice prior to soccer practice

19. The nurse is reinforcing instructions to an adolescent with insulin-dependent diabetes mellitus regarding insulin administration and rotation sites. Which of the following statements, if made by the adolescent, indicates effective teaching?
    1 "I need to use one major site for the morning injection and another site for the evening injection for 2 to 3 weeks before changing major sites."
    2 "I need to use a different site for each insulin injection."
    3 "I need to use the same site for 1 month before rotating to another site."
    4 "I should use my stomach and my thighs only for injections."

20. The mother of a 6-year-old insulin-dependent diabetic calls the clinic and tells the nurse that the child has been sick. The mother reports that she checked the child's urine and it showed positive ketones. Which of the following does the nurse instruct the mother to do?
    1 Come to the clinic immediately
    2 Hold the next dose of insulin
    3 Administer an additional dose of Regular Insulin
    4 Encourage the child to drink calorie-free liquids

ANSWERS

1. **1**

RATIONALE: The vomiting child should be placed in an upright or side-lying position to prevent aspiration. Options 2, 3, and 4 will place the child at risk for aspiration if vomiting occurs.

TEST-TAKING STRATEGY: Eliminate options 2 and 4 first because they are similar. Additionally, these positions would place the child at risk for aspiration if vomiting occurred. Visualize the remaining two positions. Option 3 is also inappropriate and would cause aspiration. Review appropriate positioning techniques now if you had difficulty with this question.
LEVEL OF COGNITIVE ABILITY: Application

PHASE OF NURSING PROCESS: Implementation
CLIENT NEEDS: Safe, Effective Care Environment
CONTENT AREA: Child Health
REFERENCE
Schulte, E., Price, D., & James, S. (1997). *Thompson's pediatric nursing: An introductory text* (7th ed.). Philadelphia: W. B. Saunders. p. 167.

2. **3**

RATIONALE: Rectal temperature measurements should be avoided if diarrhea is present. Use of a rectal thermometer can stimulate peristalsis and cause more diarrhea. Axillary and tympanic measurements of temperature would be acceptable. Most measurements are done via electronic devices.
TEST-TAKING STRATEGY: Eliminate option 4 first because most methods of temperature measurement are done through an electronic device. Note the diagnosis stated in the question. This should easily direct you toward option 3.
LEVEL OF COGNITIVE ABILITY: Comprehension
PHASE OF NURSING PROCESS: Implementation
CLIENT NEEDS: Physiological Integrity
CONTENT AREA: Child Health
REFERENCE
Ashwill, J., & Droske, S. (1997). *Nursing care of children: Principles and practice.* Philadelphia: W. B. Saunders. p. 687.

3. **2**

RATIONALE: Following cleft lip repair, the infant should be positioned supine or on the side lateral to the repair to prevent the contact of the suture lines with the bed linens. It is best to place the infant on the left side rather than supine immediately after surgery to prevent the risk of aspiration if the infant vomits.
TEST-TAKING STRATEGY: Consider the anatomical location of the surgical site and the key words "right side." You should easily be directed to the correct option using these concepts. Review postoperative positioning techniques now if you had difficulty with this question.
LEVEL OF COGNITIVE ABILITY: Application
PHASE OF NURSING PROCESS: Implementation
CLIENT NEEDS: Safe, Effective Care Environment
CONTENT AREA: Child Health
REFERENCE
Schulte, E., Price, D., & James, S. (1997). *Thompson's pediatric nursing: An introductory text* (7th ed.). Philadelphia: W. B. Saunders. p. 109.

4. **1**

RATIONALE: Any child who exhibits the "3 Cs" of coughing, choking with feedings, and cyanosis should be suspected of TEF. Failure to pass a suction catheter or nasogastric tube at birth, excessive oral secretions, vomiting, abdominal distention, and an airless, scaphoid abdomen (atresia without fistula) are also clinical manifestations.
TEST-TAKING STRATEGY: Recalling the "3 Cs" associated with this disorder will assist in directing you to the correct option. Review the clinical manifestations associated with this disorder now if you had difficulty with this question.
LEVEL OF COGNITIVE ABILITY: Comprehension
PHASE OF NURSING PROCESS: Data Collection
CLIENT NEEDS: Physiological Integrity
CONTENT AREA: Child Health
REFERENCE
Leifer, G. (1999). *Thompson's introduction to maternity and pediatric nursing* (3rd ed.). Philadelphia: W. B. Saunders. p. 723.

5. **4**

RATIONALE: Clinical manifestations of pyloric stenosis include projectile, nonbilious vomiting, irritability, hunger and crying, constipation, and signs of dehydration including a decrease in urine output.
TEST-TAKING STRATEGY: Considering the anatomical location of this disorder and its potential effects will assist in eliminating options 2 and 3. Recalling that a major clinical manifestation is projectile, nonbilious vomiting will assist in directing you to option 4. Review these clinical manifestations now if you had difficulty with this question.
LEVEL OF COGNITIVE ABILITY: Comprehension
PHASE OF NURSING PROCESS: Data Collection
CLIENT NEEDS: Physiological Integrity
CONTENT AREA: Child Health
REFERENCE
Leifer, G. (1999). *Thompson's introduction to maternity and pediatric nursing* (3rd ed.). Philadelphia: W. B. Saunders. p. 724.

6. **3**

RATIONALE: Lactose intolerance is the inability to tolerate lactose, the sugar found in dairy products. Removing milk from the diet can provide enough relief from symptoms. Additional dietary changes may be required to provide adequate sources of calcium and, if the child is an infant, protein and calories.
TEST-TAKING STRATEGY: Knowledge that lactose is the sugar found in dairy products will easily direct you to option 3 since dairy products contain high sources of calcium. Review the dietary management for lactose intolerance now if you had difficulty with this question.
LEVEL OF COGNITIVE ABILITY: Application
PHASE OF NURSING PROCESS: Implementation
CLIENT NEEDS: Health Promotion and Maintenance
CONTENT AREA: Child Health
REFERENCE
Peckenpaugh, N., & Poleman, C. (1999). *Nutrition essentials and diet therapy* (8th ed.). Philadelphia: W. B. Saunders. p. 257.

7. **1**

RATIONALE: Dietary management is the mainstay of treatment in celiac disease. All wheat, rye, barley, and oats should be eliminated from the diet and replaced with corn and rice. Vitamin supplements, especially fat-soluble vitamins and folate, may be needed in the early period of treatment to correct deficiencies. These restrictions are likely to be lifelong, although small amounts of grains may be tolerated after the ulcerations have healed.
TEST-TAKING STRATEGY: Knowledge regarding the dietary management in celiac disease is required to answer this question. Recalling that corn and rice are substitute food replacements in this disease will easily direct you to option 1. Review the dietary management in this disorder now if you had difficulty with this question.
LEVEL OF COGNITIVE ABILITY: Application
PHASE OF NURSING PROCESS: Implementation
CLIENT NEEDS: Health Promotion and Maintenance
CONTENT AREA: Child Health
REFERENCE
Ashwill, J., & Droske, S. (1997). *Nursing care of children: Principles and practice.* Philadelphia: W. B. Saunders. p. 733.

8. **3**

RATIONALE: In the preoperative period, enemas or laxatives should not be administered. No heat should be applied to the abdomen because this may increase the chance of

perforation secondary to vasodilation. IV fluids should be started and the child should be NPO. Prescribed preoperative medications most likely would be administered on call to the operating room.
TEST-TAKING STRATEGY: Consider the anatomical location and the concern of rupture in this disorder. Options 1, 2, and 4 are standard preoperative measures. Option 3 places the child at risk for a perforated appendix. Review preoperative care in the child with appendicitis now if you had difficulty with this question.
LEVEL OF COGNITIVE ABILITY: Comprehension
PHASE OF NURSING PROCESS: Implementation
CLIENT NEEDS: Safe, Effective Care Environment
CONTENT AREA: Child Health
REFERENCE
Schulte, E., Price, D., & James, S. (1997). *Thompson's pediatric nursing: An introductory text* (7th ed.). Philadelphia: W. B. Saunders. p. 346.

9. **4**
RATIONALE: Chronic constipation beginning in the first month of life resulting in pellet-like or ribbon stools that are foul-smelling is a clinical manifestation of this disorder. Delayed passage or absence of meconium stool in the neonatal period is the cardinal sign. Bowel obstruction, especially in the neonatal period, abdominal pain and distention, and failure to thrive are also clinical manifestations.
TEST-TAKING STRATEGY: Knowledge regarding the clinical manifestations associated with Hirschsprung's disease is required to answer this question. If you are unfamiliar with these symptoms, take time now to review.
LEVEL OF COGNITIVE ABILITY: Comprehension
PHASE OF NURSING PROCESS: Data Collection
CLIENT NEEDS: Physiological Integrity
CONTENT AREA: Child Health
REFERENCE
Leifer, G. (1999). *Thompson's introduction to maternity and pediatric nursing* (3rd ed.). Philadelphia: W. B. Saunders. p. 727.

10. **1**
RATIONALE: The child with intussusception classically presents with severe abdominal pain that is crampy and intermittent causing the child to draw in the knees to the chest. Vomiting may be present but it is not projectile. Bright red blood and mucus are passed through the rectum and is commonly described as currant jelly–like stools. Ribbon-like stools are not a manifestation of this disorder.
TEST-TAKING STRATEGY: Knowledge related to the clinical manifestations associated with intussusception is required to answer this question. Recalling that a classic manifestation is currant jelly–like stools will assist in directing you to option 1. Review this disorder now if you had difficulty with this question.
LEVEL OF COGNITIVE ABILITY: Comprehension
PHASE OF NURSING PROCESS: Data Collection
CLIENT NEEDS: Physiological Integrity
CONTENT AREA: Child Health
REFERENCE
Schulte, E., Price, D., & James, S. (1997). *Thompson's pediatric nursing: An introductory text* (7th ed.). Philadelphia: W. B. Saunders. p. 165.

11. **4**
RATIONALE: The parents of a child with an umbilical hernia need to be instructed in the signs of strangulation: vomiting, pain, and irreducible mass at the umbilicus. The parents should be instructed to contact the physician immediately if strangulation is suspected.

TEST-TAKING STRATEGY: Use the definition of the word "strangulation" to assist in answering this question. This will assist in eliminating options 1 and 2. From the remaining options, use knowledge regarding these signs to assist in answering the question. Review the signs of strangulation now if you had difficulty with this question.
LEVEL OF COGNITIVE ABILITY: Application
PHASE OF NURSING PROCESS: Implementation
CLIENT NEEDS: Health Promotion and Maintenance
CONTENT AREA: Child Health
REFERENCE
Schulte, E., Price, D., & James, S. (1997). *Thompson's pediatric nursing: An introductory text* (7th ed.). Philadelphia: W. B. Saunders. p. 163.

12. **3**
RATIONALE: The child with hepatitis should consume a well-balanced, low-fat diet in order to provide rest to the liver. Options 1, 2, and 4 are components of the home care instructions to the family of a child with hepatitis. Additionally, diapers should not be changed on or near surfaces used for preparing or serving food.
TEST-TAKING STRATEGY: Note the key word "not." Options 1, 2, and 4 can be easily eliminated by using the basic principles related to standard precautions. If you had difficulty with this question, take time now to review home care instructions to the family of a child with hepatitis.
LEVEL OF COGNITIVE ABILITY: Application
PHASE OF NURSING PROCESS: Implementation
CLIENT NEEDS: Health Promotion and Maintenance
CONTENT AREA: Child Health
REFERENCE
Schulte, E., Price, D., & James, S. (1997). *Thompson's pediatric nursing: An introductory text* (7th ed.). Philadelphia: W. B. Saunders. p. 295.

13. **4**
RATIONALE: n combination with BAL is a chelating agent that is administered IM for 5 days. It causes lead to be deposited in the bone and excreted in the kidneys. Sodium bicarbonate may be used in salicylate poisoning. Ipecac syrup is used in poisoning to induce vomiting. Activated charcoal is used to decrease absorption in certain poisoning situations.
TEST-TAKING STRATEGY: Knowledge regarding the treatment related to lead poisoning is required to answer this question. Review this treatment now if you are unfamiliar with it.
LEVEL OF COGNITIVE ABILITY: Application
PHASE OF NURSING PROCESS: Planning
CLIENT NEEDS: Physiological Integrity
CONTENT AREA: Child Health
REFERENCE
Schulte, E., Price, D., & James, S. (1997). *Thompson's pediatric nursing: An introductory text* (7th ed.). Philadelphia: W. B. Saunders. pp. 242–243.

14. **1**
RATIONALE: Initial treatment of salicylate overdose includes inducing vomiting with syrup of ipecac or gastric lavage. Activated charcoal may be administered to decrease absorption. IV fluids and sodium bicarbonate may be administered to enhance excretion but is not the initial treatment. Dialysis is used in extreme cases if the child is unresponsive to therapy. Vitamin K is the antidote for warfarin overdose.
TEST-TAKING STRATEGY: Knowledge regarding the treatment for aspirin overdose is required to answer this

question. Note the key word "initial" in the stem of the question. This key word will assist in directing you to option 1. Review the treatment for this common overdose now if you had difficulty with this question.
LEVEL OF COGNITIVE ABILITY: Comprehension
PHASE OF NURSING PROCESS: Planning
CLIENT NEEDS: Physiological Integrity
CONTENT AREA: Child Health
REFERENCE
Schulte, E., Price, D., & James, S. (1997). *Thompson's pediatric nursing: An introductory text* (7th ed.). Philadelphia: W. B. Saunders. p. 240.

15. 2

RATIONALE: Alcohol should never be used for bathing the child with a fever because it can cause rapid cooling, peripheral vasoconstriction, and chilling, thus elevating the temperature further. Washcloths can be used to squeeze water over the child's body. Towels are used to dry the child. Toys, especially water toys can be used to provide distraction during the bath. Lightweight clothing should be placed on the child after the child is dried.
TEST-TAKING STRATEGY: Note the key word "not." Options 1 and 4 can be easily eliminated. From the remaining options, select option 2 over option 3 because of the harmful effects of alcohol and the effect of potentially elevating the temperature. Review the procedure for administering a tepid bath now if you had difficulty with this question.
LEVEL OF COGNITIVE ABILITY: Application
PHASE OF NURSING PROCESS: Planning
CLIENT NEEDS: Safe, Effective Care Environment
CONTENT AREA: Child Health
REFERENCE
Schulte, E., Price, D., & James, S. (1997). *Thompson's pediatric nursing: An introductory text* (7th ed.). Philadelphia: W. B. Saunders. p. 428.

16. 3

RATIONALE: While on a cooling blanket, the child should be covered lightly to maintain privacy and reduce shivering. Options 1, 2, and 4 are important interventions to prevent shivering, frostbite, and skin breakdown.
TEST-TAKING STRATEGY: Note the key word "not." Knowledge regarding the physiological response associated with fever is helpful in answering this question. Review the procedure associated with the use of a cooling blanket now if you had difficulty with this question.
LEVEL OF COGNITIVE ABILITY: Application
PHASE OF NURSING PROCESS: Planning
CLIENT NEEDS: Safe, Effective Care Environment
CONTENT AREA: Child Health
REFERENCE
Ashwill, J., & Droske, S. (1997). *Nursing care of children: Principle and practice.* Philadelphia: W. B. Saunders. p. 459.

17. 3

RATIONALE: PKU is an autosomal recessive disorder. Treatment includes dietary restriction of phenylalanine intake. PKU is a genetic disorder that results in central nervous system (CNS) damage from toxic levels of phenylalanine in the blood. Option 3 is accurate.
TEST-TAKING STRATEGY: Knowledge regarding PKU is required to answer the question. Recalling that PKU is a recessive disorder will assist in eliminating option 1. Reading option 2 carefully will direct you to eliminate this option

because tyramine is restricted in clients on monoamine oxidase inhibitors (MAOIs) not in PKU. Recalling that PKU affects the CNS, not the GI system, will direct you in selecting option 3. Review the characteristics associated with this disorder now if you had difficulty with this question.
LEVEL OF COGNITIVE ABILITY: Comprehension
PHASE OF NURSING PROCESS: Evaluation
CLIENT NEEDS: Physiological Integrity
CONTENT AREA: Child Health
REFERENCE
Schulte, E., Price, D., & James, S. (1997). *Thompson's pediatric nursing: An introductory text* (7th ed.). Philadelphia: W. B. Saunders. p. 57.

18. 4

RATIONALE: An extra snack of 15 to 30 g of carbohydrate eaten before activities such as soccer practice will prevent hypoglycemia. Six graham crackers or a cup of orange juice will provide 15 to 30 g of carbohydrate. The child or parents should not be instructed to adjust the amount or time of insulin administration. Meal amounts should not be doubled.
TEST-TAKING STRATEGY: Options 1 and 3 can be eliminated first because insulin dosages and times should not be adjusted. From the remaining options, recalling the manifestations and treatment associated with hypoglycemia will direct you to option 4. Review treatment to prevent hypoglycemia now if you had difficulty with this question.
LEVEL OF COGNITIVE ABILITY: Application
PHASE OF NURSING PROCESS: Implementation
CLIENT NEEDS: Health Promotion and Maintenance
CONTENT AREA: Child Health
REFERENCE
Schulte, E., Price, D., & James, S. (1997). *Thompson's pediatric nursing: An introductory text* (7th ed.). Philadelphia: W. B. Saunders. p. 355.

19. 1

RATIONALE: To help decrease variations in absorption from day to day, the child should use one location within a major site for the morning injection. The child should then rotate to another site for the evening injection, and a third site for the bedtime injection. The child should follow this pattern for a period of 2 to 3 weeks before changing major sites.
TEST-TAKING STRATEGY: Eliminate option 4 first because of the word "only." From the remaining options, it is necessary to know the physiology associated with absorption of insulin. If you had difficulty with this question, take time now to review insulin administration.
LEVEL OF COGNITIVE ABILITY: Comprehension
PHASE OF NURSING PROCESS: Evaluation
CLIENT NEEDS: Physiological Integrity
CONTENT AREA: Child Health
REFERENCE
Schulte, E., Price, D., & James, S. (1997). *Thompson's pediatric nursing: An introductory text* (7th ed.). Philadelphia: W. B. Saunders. p. 354.

20. 4

RATIONALE: When the child is sick, the mother should test for urinary ketones with each voiding. If ketones are present, liquids are essential to aid in clearing. The child should be encouraged to drink calorie-free liquids. It is not necessary to take the child to the clinic immediately. Insulin doses should not be adjusted or changed.

TEST-TAKING STRATEGY: Eliminate options 2 and 3 first because insulin doses should not be adjusted or changed. From the remaining options, note the words "positive ketones." This finding does not require immediate physician referral. Review home care instructions for the sick diabetic child now if you had difficulty with this question.

LEVEL OF COGNITIVE ABILITY: Application
PHASE OF NURSING PROCESS: Implementation
CLIENT NEEDS: Health Promotion and Maintenance
CONTENT AREA: Child Health
REFERENCE
Ashwill, J., & Droske, S. (1997). *Nursing care of children: Principles and practice.* Philadelphia: W. B. Saunders. p. 1208.

BIBLIOGRAPHY

Ashwill, J., & Droske, S. (1997). *Nursing care of children: Principles and practice.* Philadelphia: W. B. Saunders.

Bowden, V., Dickey, S., & Greenberg, C. (1998). *Children and their families: The continuum of care.* Philadelphia: W. B. Saunders.

Leifer, G. (1999). *Thompson's introduction to maternity and pediatric nursing* (3rd ed.). Philadelphia: W. B. Saunders.

Luckmann, J. (1997). *Saunders manual of nursing care.* Philadelphia: W. B. Saunders.

Nichols, F., & Zwelling, E. (1997). *Maternal-newborn nursing: Theory and practice.* Philadelphia: W. B. Saunders.

O'Toole, M. (ed.). (1997). *Miller-Keane encyclopedia & dictionary of medicine, nursing, & allied health* (6th ed.). Philadelphia: W. B. Saunders.

Peckenpaugh, N., & Poleman, C. (1999). *Nutrition essentials and diet therapy* (8th ed.). Philadelphia: W. B. Saunders.

Schulte, E., Price, D., & James, S. (1997). *Thompson's pediatric nursing: An introductory text* (7th ed.). Philadelphia: W. B. Saunders.

CHAPTER 32

Renal and Urinary Disorders

I. Glomerulonephritis

A. Description
   1. A term that includes a variety of disorders, most of which are caused by an immunological reaction
   2. Destruction, inflammation, and sclerosis of the glomeruli of both kidneys occurs, and loss of kidney function develops
B. Causes
   1. Immunological or autoimmune diseases
   2. Streptococcal infection, group A beta hemolytic
   3. History of pharyngitis or tonsillitis 2 to 3 weeks prior to symptoms
C. Types
   1. Acute: occurs 2 to 3 weeks after a streptococcal infection
   2. Chronic: can occur after the acute phase or slowly over time
D. Data collection
   1. Pale and irritable
   2. Chills and fever
   3. Fatigue and weakness
   4. Vomiting
   5. Gross hematuria or dark, smoky, cola-colored, or red-brown urine
   6. Proteinuria that produces a persistent and excessive foam in the urine
   7. Oliguria or anuria
   8. Mid to high urine specific gravity, low urinary pH
   9. Increased BUN and creatinine
   10. Increased antistreptolysin O titer (used to diagnosis disorders caused by streptococcal infections)
   11. Edema in the face and periorbital area, feet, or generalized
   12. Hypertension
E. Implementation
   1. Monitor vital signs, especially temperature
   2. Monitor I&O and daily weight
   3. Provide a high-calorie, low-protein diet as prescribed
   4. Restrict fluid intake and sodium intake as prescribed
   5. Monitor for edema
   6. Provide bed rest and limited activity
   7. Administer diuretics, antihypertensives, and antibiotics as prescribed
   8. Reinforce to parents that the child needs to obtain treatment for infections, specifically a sore throat and upper respiratory infection

II. Nephrotic Syndrome

A. Description: Degenerative and noninflammatory disease of the kidneys, resulting in edema and large amounts of protein in the urine
B. Data collection
   1. Pale, irritable, and fatigued child
   2. Edema of the face and generalized edema over the entire body
   3. Abdominal ascites
   4. Respiratory distress
   5. Hypertension
   6. Anorexia
   7. Weight gain and decreased urine output
   8. Dark, frothy urine; hematuria may be present
   9. Proteinuria, and white blood cells (WBCs) in the urine
   10. Hyperlipidemia
C. Implementation
   1. Monitor vital signs, I&O, and daily weight
   2. Maintain bed rest if severe edema is present
   3. Provide a normal to low-protein, mild sodium restriction diet as prescribed
   4. Administer diuretics as prescribed to control edema, and steroids to control inflammation
   5. Prevent infections and provide meticulous skin care to prevent skin breakdown
   6. Teach the child and parents about home care,

medications, and measures to prevent infections

III. Cryptorchidism

A. Description: Occurs when one or both testes fail to descend through the inguinal canal into the scrotal sac
B. Data collection: Testes not palpable or easily guided into the scrotum
C. Implementation
   1. Monitored during the first 12 months of life to determine if spontaneous descent occurs
   2. After age 1, medical or surgical treatment may be instituted
   3. Human chorionic gonadotropin (hCG), a pituitary hormone that stimulates the production of testosterone, may be prescribed
   4. Surgical correction is done by orchiopexy
   5. Monitor for bleeding and infection if surgery is performed

IV. Hypospadias and Epispadias

A. Description: Congenital defects involving abnormal placement of the urethral orifice of the penis
B. Data collection
   1. Hypospadias: Urethral orifice located below the glans penis along the ventral surface
   2. Epispadias: Urethral orifice located on the dorsal surface of the penis
C. Surgical implementation
   1. Done before the age of toilet training
   2. Children with hypospadias should not be circumcised because the foreskin may be used in surgical reconstruction
D. Implementation postoperatively
   1. The child will have some type of urinary diversion to allow time for healing of the meatus
   2. Monitor vital signs
   3. Encourage high fluid intake
   4. Monitor urine for cloudiness or a foul smell
   5. Restrict activity for several days
   6. Parents need to be instructed in the care of the urinary diversion if present

V. Bladder Exstrophy

A. Description
   1. A congenital anomaly characterized by the extrusion of the urinary bladder to the outside of the body through a defect in the lower abdominal wall
   2. The cause is not known
   3. Treatment requires surgical management and occurs in a series of staged reconstructions
   4. The initial surgery for closure of the abdominal defect should occur within the first few days of life
   5. The goal of subsequent surgeries is to reconstruct the bladder and genitalia and enable the child to achieve urinary continence
B. Data collection
   1. Exposed bladder mucosa
   2. Displaced anal opening
   3. Defects of the external genitalia
C. Implementation
   1. Patency of the anus is determined
   2. Monitor adequacy of urine output
   3. Maintain integrity of the exposed bladder mucosa and protect from drying while allowing the drainage of urine
   4. Cover the bladder with a nonadhering plastic wrap
   5. Petroleum jelly gauze is avoided because this type of dressing can dry out, adhere to the mucosa, and damage the delicate tissues when the dressing is removed
   6. Administer antibiotics as prescribed
   7. Provide emotional support to the parents and encourage them to verbalize their fears and concerns

PRACTICE QUESTIONS

1. The nurse is reviewing the health record of a child recently diagnosed with glomerulonephritis. Which finding noted in the child's record is most often associated with the diagnosis of glomerulonephritis?
   1 Strep throat 2 weeks prior to diagnosis
   2 The child fell off a bike onto the handlebars
   3 Nausea and vomiting for the past 24 hours
   4 Urticaria and itching for 1 week prior to diagnosis

2. The nurse reviews the record of a child admitted for suspected glomerulonephritis. The nurse expects to note which of the following findings documented in the record?
   1 Elevated BUN
   2 Postural hypotension
   3 Low urinary-specific gravity
   4 Dark brown or rust-colored urine

3. The nurse is caring for a 7-year-old child diagnosed with acute glomerulonephritis. A priority nursing intervention that should be included in the nursing plan of care is
   1 Promote adequate bed rest while providing for quiet play
   2 Catheterize the child to monitor I&O strictly
   3 Force oral fluids to prevent hypovolemic shock
   4 Encourage classmates to visit and keep the child informed of school events

4. The nurse is caring for a 2-year-old child who has been diagnosed with nephrotic syndrome. The nurse plans to monitor the child for which

of the following most common characteristics associated with nephrotic syndrome?

1 Generalized edema
2 Frank blood in the urine
3 Increased urinary output
4 Hypotension

5. The nurse is preparing a 2-year-old child with suspected nephrotic syndrome for a renal biopsy to confirm the diagnosis. The mother asks the nurse, "Will my child ever look thin again?" The nurse most appropriately responds by saying

1 "Wearing loose-fitting clothing should help conceal the extra weight."
2 "In most cases, medication and diet will control fluid retention."
3 "Do you feel guilty because you didn't notice the weight gain?"
4 "When children are little, it's expected they'll look a little chubby."

6. The nurse is assisting in preparing a plan of care for a 4-year-old child hospitalized with nephrotic syndrome. The nurse suggests which intervention regarding diet therapy that is most appropriate for this child?

1 Provide a high-protein, high-salt diet
2 Discourage visitors at mealtimes
3 Encourage the child to eat in the playroom with others
4 Maintain a full liquid diet during the acute phase

7. The nurse is administering medications to a 6-year-old child with nephrotic syndrome. To reduce proteinuria, the nurse expects that which medication will be prescribed?

1 Prazosin hydrochloride (Minipress)
2 Furosemide (Lasix)
3 Prednisone (Deltasone)
4 Cyclophosphamide (Cytoxan)

8. A 7-year-old child is seen in the clinic, and the primary health care provider documents a diagnosis of primary nocturnal enuresis. The mother asks the nurse about the diagnosis. The nurse bases the response of the fact that primary nocturnal enuresis

1 Requires surgical intervention to improve the problem
2 Is caused by a psychiatric problem
3 Is common and most children will outgrow bed-wetting without therapeutic intervention
4 Does not respond to treatment

9. The nurse is caring for an 8-month-old infant. A urinalysis has been ordered and the nurse plans to collect the specimen. The nurse performs which of the following most appropriate methods to collect the specimen?

1 Catheterizing the infant, using a No. 5 French Foley
2 Obtaining the specimen from the diaper, using a syringe, after the infant voids
3 Attaching a urinary collection device to the infant's perineum
4 Monitoring the urinary patterns and prepare to collect the specimen into a cup when the infant voids

10. The nurse is assigned to care for an infant with cryptorchidism. The nurse anticipates that the most likely diagnostic studies to be prescribed are those that check

1 Kidney function
2 Babinski reflex
3 DNA synthesis
4 Chromosomal analysis

11. The child with cryptorchidism is being discharged following orchiopexy, which was performed on an outpatient basis. What care measure should take priority in the plan of care at home?

1 Administration of analgesics
2 Measurement of I&O
3 Application of cold to the surgical site
4 Prevention of infection at the surgical site

12. The nurse is assigned to care for a 2-year-old child who has been admitted to the hospital for surgical correction of cryptorchidism. The highest priority in the postoperative nursing care for this child is to

1 Force oral fluids
2 Prevent tension on the suture
3 Test urine for glucose
4 Encourage coughing

13. The nurse has reinforced discharge instructions for a 2-year-old child who has had an orchiopexy to correct cryptorchidism. Which of the following statements, if made by the mother of the child, indicates that further teaching is necessary?

1 "I'll check his temperature and report a fever."
2 "I'll let him decide when to return to his usual activities."
3 "I'll give him medication so he'll be comfortable."
4 "I'll check his voiding to be sure there are no problems."

14. The nurse collects a urine specimen preoperatively from a child with epispadias who is scheduled for surgical repair. The nurse reviews the child's record for the laboratory results of the urine and most likely expects to note which of the following?

1 Hematuria
2 Proteinuria
3 Bacteriuria
4 Glucosuria

15. A 1-year-old child with hypospadias is scheduled for surgery to correct this condition. The nurse is asked to assist in preparing a plan of care for this child and makes suggestions, knowing that this surgery is taking place at a time when
   1 Fears of separation and mutilation are great
   2 Sibling rivalry will cause regression to occur
   3 Embarrassment of voiding irregularities is common
   4 Concern over size and function of the penis is present

16. An 18-month-old child is being discharged following surgical repair of hypospadias. Which postoperative nursing care measure should the nurse stress to the parents as they prepare to take this child home?
   1 Encourage toilet training to ensure that flow of urine is normal
   2 Restrict fluid intake to reduce urinary output for the first few days
   3 Caution parents not to hold the child by straddling him on their hip
   4 Leave diapers off for the first 48 hours to allow the site to heal

17. The nurse is reviewing the treatment plan for a newborn infant with hypospadias. The infant is being discharged with the parents. Which statement by the parents indicates their understanding of the eventual outcome?
   1 Circumcision has been delayed to save tissue for surgical repair
   2 Catheterization will be necessary when the infant does not void
   3 Caution should be used when straddling the infant on a hip

   4 Vital signs should be taken daily to check for bladder infection

18. The parents of a newborn have been told that their child was born with bladder exstrophy. The parents ask the nurse about this condition. The nurse bases the response on knowledge that this condition is
   1 Caused by the use of medications taken by the mother during pregnancy
   2 A hereditary disorder that occurs in every other generation
   3 A condition in which the urinary bladder is abnormally located in the pelvic cavity
   4 An extrusion of the urinary bladder to the outside of the body through a defect in the lower abdominal wall

19. The nurse assists in preparing a plan of care for the infant with bladder exstrophy. The nurse knows that which problem will receive the highest priority?
   1 Altered elimination
   2 Impaired tissue integrity
   3 Parental knowledge deficit
   4 Potential for infection

20. The nurse is caring for an infant with a diagnosis of bladder exstrophy. The most appropriate intervention to protect the exposed bladder tissue from drying is to
   1 Cover the bladder with petroleum jelly gauze
   2 Keep the bladder tissue dry by covering it with dry sterile gauze
   3 Cover the bladder with a nonadhering plastic wrap
   4 Apply sterile distilled water dressings over the bladder mucosa

ANSWERS

1. **1**

RATIONALE: Group A beta-hemolytic streptococcal infection is a cause of glomerulonephritis. Often the child becomes ill with streptococcal infection of the upper respiratory tract and then develops symptoms of acute poststreptococcal glomerulonephritis after an interval of 1 to 2 weeks. The data in options 2, 3, and 4 are unrelated to a diagnosis of glomerulonephritis.
TEST-TAKING STRATEGY: Use knowledge regarding the causes of glomerulonephritis and the process of elimination to answer the question. Option 2 relates to a kidney injury. Options 3 and 4 are not related to the diagnosis of glomerulonephritis. If you had difficulty with this question, take time now to review the causes of glomerulonephritis.
LEVEL OF COGNITIVE ABILITY: Comprehension
PHASE OF NURSING PROCESS: Data Collection
CLIENT NEEDS: Physiological Integrity
CONTENT AREA: Child Health

REFERENCE
Luckmann, J. (1997). *Saunders manual of nursing care.* Philadelphia: W. B. Saunders. p. 1200.

2. **4**

RATIONALE: Gross hematuria resulting in dark brown or rust-colored urine is a classic symptom of glomerulonephritis. Hypertension is also common. BUN levels are elevated only when there is an 80% decrease in glomerular filtration rate. A mid to high urinary specific gravity is associated with glomerulonephritis.
TEST-TAKING STRATEGY: Eliminate options 2 and 3 first because hypertension and a high specific gravity is most likely to occur in this kidney disorder. Knowledge that BUN levels elevate only when there is an 80% decrease in glomerular filtration rate will assist in directing you to the correct option, option 4. If you had difficulty with this question, take time now to review the clinical manifestations associated with glomerulonephritis.
LEVEL OF COGNITIVE ABILITY: Comprehension

PHASE OF NURSING PROCESS: Data Collection
CLIENT NEEDS: Physiological Integrity
CONTENT AREA: Child Health
REFERENCE
Luckmann, J. (1997). *Saunders manual of nursing care.* Philadelphia: W. B. Saunders. p. 1201.

3. **1**

RATIONALE: Bed rest is required during the acute phase, and activity is gradually increased as the condition improves. Providing for quiet play according to the developmental stage of the child is important. Catheterization may cause a risk of infection. Fluids should not be forced. Visitors should be limited to allow for adequate rest.
TEST-TAKING STRATEGY: Use the process of elimination. Focusing on the child's diagnosis will assist in eliminating option 4. Eliminate option 3 because of the word "force." Eliminate option 2 because catheterization may cause a risk of infection. Review the appropriate nursing interventions for the child with glomerulonephritis if you had difficulty with this question.
LEVEL OF COGNITIVE ABILITY: Application
PHASE OF NURSING PROCESS: Planning
CLIENT NEEDS: Physiological Integrity
CONTENT AREA: Child Health
REFERENCE
Schulte, E., Price, D., & James, S. (1997). *Thompson's pediatric nursing: An introductory text* (7th ed.). Philadelphia: W. B. Saunders. p. 290.

4. **1**

RATIONALE: Massive edema resulting in dramatic weight gain is a characteristic finding in nephrotic syndrome. Urine is dark, foamy, and frothy, but only microscopic hematuria is present; frank bleeding does not occur. Urine output is decreased, and hypertension is likely to be present.
TEST-TAKING STRATEGY: Eliminate options 3 and 4 first because urine output is most likely to be decreased in a renal disorder, and hypertension is more likely to be present. Associate generalized edema with nephrotic syndrome to help you answer questions similar to this one. If you had difficulty with this question, take time now to review the characteristics of nephrotic syndrome.
LEVEL OF COGNITIVE ABILITY: Application
PHASE OF NURSING PROCESS: Data Collection
CLIENT NEEDS: Physiological Integrity
CONTENT AREA: Child Health
REFERENCE
Schulte, E., Price, D., & James, S. (1997). *Thompson's pediatric nursing: An introductory text* (7th ed.). Philadelphia: W. B. Saunders. p. 234.

5. **2**

RATIONALE: Most children experience remission with treatment and corticosteroids. It is important to give the parent information in a matter-of-fact manner and address the issue that is the parent's concern. Options 1, 3, and 4 do not address the parent's concern.
TEST-TAKING STRATEGY: The client of the question is the parent. Options 1 and 3 are nontherapeutic, adding to mother's guilt and putting down her concern. Option 4 doesn't acknowledge the concern and is a stereotypical answer. Use therapeutic communication techniques and always address the client's feelings and concerns.

LEVEL OF COGNITIVE ABILITY: Application
PHASE OF NURSING PROCESS: Implementation
CLIENT NEEDS: Psychosocial Integrity
CONTENT AREA: Child Health
REFERENCE
Schulte, E., Price, D., & James, S. (1997). *Thompson's pediatric nursing: An introductory text* (7th ed.). Philadelphia: W. B. Saunders. p. 235.

6. **3**

RATIONALE: Mealtimes should center on pleasurable socialization. Encourage the child to eat meals with other children on the unit. A diet that is normal in protein with a mild sodium restriction is normally prescribed.
TEST-TAKING STRATEGY: Use the process of elimination. Eliminate options 1 and 4 first. A diet that is normal in protein with a mild sodium restriction is normally prescribed. Option 2 diminishes the importance of socialization at mealtime. This leaves option 3 as the correct option. If you had difficulty with this question, take time now to review the diet normally prescribed for the child with nephrotic syndrome.
LEVEL OF COGNITIVE ABILITY: Application
PHASE OF NURSING PROCESS: Planning
CLIENT NEEDS: Physiological Integrity
CONTENT AREA: Child Health
REFERENCE
Schulte, E., Price, D., & James, S. (1997). *Thompson's pediatric nursing: An introductory text* (7th ed.). Philadelphia: W. B. Saunders. p. 236.

7. **2**

RATIONALE: The child is usually placed on diuretic therapy until protein loss is controlled. Corticosteroids, such as prednisone, may be prescribed to decrease inflammation. Corticosteroids also suppress the autoimmune response and stimulate vascular reabsorption of edema. Cyclophosphamide is an alkylating agent and may be used in maintaining remission. Prazosin hydrochloride is most commonly used to control hypertension.
TEST-TAKING STRATEGY: Use the process of elimination and knowledge regarding the actions of the medications to answer the question. Take time now to review the pharmacological treatments associated with nephrotic syndrome, if you had difficulty with this question. Additionally, review the actions and purposes of the medications listed in the options if you are unfamiliar with them.
LEVEL OF COGNITIVE ABILITY: Comprehension
PHASE OF NURSING PROCESS: Planning
CLIENT NEEDS: Physiological Integrity
CONTENT AREA: Child Health
REFERENCE
Ashwill, J., & Droske, S. (1997). *Nursing care of children: Principles and practice.* Philadelphia: W. B. Saunders. p. 790.

8. **3**

RATIONALE: Primary nocturnal enuresis is defined as a child who has never been dry at night for prolonged periods. It is common in children, and most children will eventually outgrow bedwetting without therapeutic intervention. Options 1, 3, and 4 are incorrect.
TEST-TAKING STRATEGY: Knowledge regarding the characteristics of enuresis is required to answer the question. Recalling that enuresis is common in children will

assist in directing you to the correct option. If you had difficulty with this question, take time now to review the characteristics associated with enuresis.
LEVEL OF COGNITIVE ABILITY: Comprehension
PHASE OF NURSING PROCESS: Planning
CLIENT NEEDS: Physiological Integrity
CONTENT AREA: Child Health
REFERENCE
Schulte, E., Price, D., & James, S. (1997). *Thompson's pediatric nursing: An introductory text* (7th ed.). Philadelphia: W. B. Saunders. p. 255.

9. **3**

RATIONALE: Although many methods have been used to collect urine from an infant, the most reliable method is the urine collection device. This device is a plastic bag that has an opening that is lined with adhesive so that it may be attached to the perineum. Urine for certain tests, such as specific gravity, may be obtained from a diaper. Urinary catheterization is not to be done unless specifically prescribed, because of the risk of infection. It is not reasonable to monitor urinary patterns and attempt to collect the specimen in a cup when the infant voids.
TEST-TAKING STRATEGY: Use the process of elimination and note the key words "most appropriate." Eliminate option 4, as this is unrealistic. Eliminate option 1, because catheterization is not prescribed and the risk of infection exists with this procedure. Eliminate option 2 because only certain tests can be obtained from the urine in a diaper. If you had difficulty with this question, take time now to review the procedure for collecting urine specimens from an infant.
LEVEL OF COGNITIVE ABILITY: Application
PHASE OF NURSING PROCESS: Implementation
CLIENT NEEDS: Safe, Effective Care Environment
CONTENT AREA: Child Health
REFERENCE
Schulte, E., Price, D., & James, S. (1997). *Thompson's pediatric nursing: An introductory text* (7th ed.). Philadelphia: W. B. Saunders. p. 429.

10. **1**

RATIONALE: Cryptorchidism may be the result of hormone deficiency, intrinsic abnormality of a testis, or a structural problem. Diagnostic tests assess kidney function because the kidneys and testes arise from the same germ tissue. Babinski reflex tests neurological function. DNA synthesis and a chromosomal analysis are unrelated to this diagnosis.
TEST-TAKING STRATEGY: Use the process of elimination and knowledge regarding the anatomical occurrence of cryptorchidism. Cryptorchidism, undescended or hidden testicles, relates to the genitourinary system. Option 2 relates to neurological function. Options 3 and 4 relate to the structure of cells. Option 1 is the only option that relates to the genitourinary system.
LEVEL OF COGNITIVE ABILITY: Comprehension
PHASE OF NURSING PROCESS: Data Collection
CLIENT NEEDS: Physiological Integrity
CONTENT AREA: Child Health
REFERENCE
Leifer, G. (1999). *Thompson's introduction to maternity and pediatric nursing* (3rd ed.). Philadelphia: W. B. Saunders. p. 764.

11. **4**

RATIONALE: The most common complications associated with orchiopexy is bleeding and infection. Parent instructions include demonstration of proper wound cleansing and dressing, and teaching parents to identify signs of infection such as redness, warmth, swelling, or discharge. Testicles will be held in a position to prevent movement, and great care should be taken to prevent contamination of the suture line.
TEST-TAKING STRATEGY: Note the word "priority." Use Maslow's Hierarchy of Needs theory. Of the options presented, the potential for infection is the physiological priority. Option 1 is important, but not the priority given the options listed. Use of cold, as suggested in option 3, is not necessary. Measurement of intake and output in option 2 is not required.
LEVEL OF COGNITIVE ABILITY: Comprehension
PHASE OF NURSING PROCESS: Planning
CLIENT NEEDS: Health Promotion and Maintenance
CONTENT AREA: Child Health
REFERENCE
Ashwill, J., & Droske, S. (1997). *Nursing care of children: Principles and practice*. Philadelphia: W. B. Saunders. p. 798.

12. **2**

RATIONALE: When a child returns from surgery, the testicle is held in position by an internal suture that passes through the testes and scrotum and is attached to the thigh. It is important not to dislodge this suture. Depending on the type of anesthesia used, option 4 may be appropriate, but is not the priority. Although it is important to maintain adequate hydration, it is not necessary to force fluids. Testing urine for glucose is not related to this type of surgery.
TEST-TAKING STRATEGY: Focus on the anatomical location of the surgery and the surgical procedure performed to direct you to option 2. If you had difficulty with this question, take time now to review the nursing care following the surgical correction of cryptorchidism.
LEVEL OF COGNITIVE ABILITY: Application
PHASE OF NURSING PROCESS: Implementation
CLIENT NEEDS: Physiological Integrity
CONTENT AREA: Child Health
REFERENCE
Leifer, G. (1999). *Thompson's introduction to maternity and pediatric nursing* (3rd ed.). Philadelphia: W. B. Saunders. p. 765.

13. **2**

RATIONALE: The child's activity should be restricted for 3 to 7 days after surgery to promote healing and prevent injury. This will prevent dislodging of the suture. Normally, 2-year-olds will want to be very active and it may be difficult to restrict activities. The parent should be taught to monitor the temperature, provide analgesics for pain as needed, and monitor the urine output.
TEST-TAKING STRATEGY: Note the key words "further teaching is necessary." Option 1 is an important action in order to recognize signs of infection. Option 3 is appropriate to keep pain to a minimum. Option 4 monitors the voiding pattern, which is also important following surgery. If you had difficulty with this question, take time now to review the discharge instructions following surgical correction of cryptorchidism.
LEVEL OF COGNITIVE ABILITY: Comprehension
PHASE OF NURSING PROCESS: Evaluation

CLIENT NEEDS: Health Promotion and Maintenance
CONTENT AREA: Child Health
REFERENCE
Leifer, G. (1999). *Thompson's introduction to maternity and pediatric nursing* (3rd ed.). Philadelphia: W. B. Saunders. p. 764.

14. **3**

RATIONALE: Epispadias is a congenital malformation with the absence of the upper wall of the urethra. The urethral opening is located anywhere on the dorsum of the penis. This anatomical characteristic leads to the easy access of bacterial entry into the urine. Options 1, 2, and 4 do not relate to the potential for infection, which is present in epispadias.
TEST-TAKING STRATEGY: Use knowledge regarding the anatomical characteristic of epispadias and the process of elimination to answer the question. If you had difficulty with this question, take time now to review the diagnostic findings associated with epispadias.
LEVEL OF COGNITIVE ABILITY: Comprehension
PHASE OF NURSING PROCESS: Data Collection
CLIENT NEEDS: Physiological Integrity
CONTENT AREA: Child Health
REFERENCE
O'Toole, M. (ed.). (1997). *Miller-Keane encyclopedia & dictionary of medicine, nursing, & allied health* (6th ed.). Philadelphia: W. B. Saunders. p. 547.

15. **1**

RATIONALE: At the age of 1, a child's fears of separation and mutilation are great, because the child is facing the developmental task of trusting others. As the child gets older, fears about virility and reproductive ability may surface. The question does not provide enough data to determine that siblings exist. Options 3 and 4 may be issues if the child were older.
TEST-TAKING STRATEGY: Focus on the age of the child and use knowledge regarding the stages of growth and development to answer the question. If you had difficulty with this question, take time now to review the stages of growth and development.
LEVEL OF COGNITIVE ABILITY: Application
PHASE OF NURSING PROCESS: Planning
CLIENT NEEDS: Psychosocial Integrity
CONTENT AREA: Child Health
REFERENCE
Leifer, G. (1999). *Thompson's introduction to maternity and pediatric nursing* (3rd ed.). Philadelphia: W. B. Saunders. p. 528.

16. **3**

RATIONALE: Parent teaching following hypospadias repair includes restricting the child from activities that put pressure on the surgical site. The parents should be instructed to use double diapers to hold the stent in place and should be instructed how to hold the child during the postoperative period. Leaving the diapers off can cause contamination of the surgical site. Fluids should be encouraged to maintain hydration. Toilet training should not be an issue during this stressful period.
TEST-TAKING STRATEGY: Focus on the anatomical location of the surgery and use the process of elimination. If you had difficulty with this question, take time now to review the postoperative care following surgical repair of hypospadias.

LEVEL OF COGNITIVE ABILITY: Application
PHASE OF NURSING PROCESS: Implementation
CLIENT NEEDS: Health Promotion and Maintenance
CONTENT AREA: Child Health
REFERENCE
Leifer, G. (1999). *Thompson's introduction to maternity and pediatric nursing* (3rd ed.). Philadelphia: W. B. Saunders. p. 755.

17. **1**

RATIONALE: The infant should not be circumcised because the dorsal foreskin tissue will be used for surgical repair of the hypospadias. This defect will most likely be corrected during the first year of life to limit the psychological effects on the child. Option 3 is important in the postoperative period, not before surgery. Vital signs do not need to be taken daily. Catheterization will only increase the risk of infection.
TEST-TAKING STRATEGY: Recalling that with this condition surgery will be planned during the first year of life will assist in directing you to the correct option. Take time now to review the surgical procedure related to the repair of the hypospadias if you had difficulty with this question.
LEVEL OF COGNITIVE ABILITY: Comprehension
PHASE OF NURSING PROCESS: Evaluation
CLIENT NEEDS: Physiological Integrity
CONTENT AREA: Child Health
REFERENCE
Ashwill, J., & Droske, S. (1997). *Nursing care of children: Principles and practice.* Philadelphia: W. B. Saunders. p. 799.

18. **4**

RATIONALE: Bladder exstrophy is a congenital anomaly characterized by the extrusion of the urinary bladder to the outside of the body through a defect in the lower abdominal wall. The cause is not known and a higher incidence occurs in the male. Options 1, 2, and 3 are incorrect.
TEST-TAKING STRATEGY: If you are unfamiliar with this condition, note the relationship of "ex"strophy to the word "ex"trusion in the correct option. This should provide you with the hint that this condition is located external to the body. If you had difficulty with this question, take time now to review the characteristics of bladder exstrophy.
LEVEL OF COGNITIVE ABILITY: Comprehension
PHASE OF NURSING PROCESS: Planning
CLIENT NEEDS: Physiological Integrity
CONTENT AREA: Child Health
REFERENCE
Leifer, G. (1999). *Thompson's introduction to maternity and pediatric nursing* (3rd ed.). Philadelphia: W. B. Saunders. p. 756.

19. **2**

RATIONALE: In bladder exstrophy, the bladder is exposed and external to the body. The highest priority is impaired tissue integrity related to the exposed bladder mucosa. Although the infant needs to be monitored for elimination patterns and kidney function, this is not the priority concern for this condition. Parental knowledge deficit will need to be addressed, but again is not the priority. Although infection related to the anatomically located defect is an appropriate problem, it is a potential problem and not an actual one.
TEST-TAKING STRATEGY: Use the process of elimination. Eliminate option 4 first because this addresses a poten-

tial problem rather than an actual one. Eliminate option 3 next because physiological needs take precedence over psychosocial needs. Knowledge that the bladder mucosa is exposed in this condition should direct you to the correct answer from the remaining two options. Review this condition now if you had difficulty with this question.
LEVEL OF COGNITIVE ABILITY: Comprehension
PHASE OF NURSING PROCESS: Planning
CLIENT NEEDS: Physiological Integrity
CONTENT AREA: Child Health
REFERENCE
Leifer, G. (1999). *Thompson's introduction to maternity and pediatric nursing* (3rd ed.). Philadelphia: W. B. Saunders. p. 756.

20. **3**

RATIONALE: Care should be taken to protect the exposed bladder tissue from drying while allowing the urine to drain. This is best accomplished by covering the bladder with a nonadhering plastic wrap. The use of petroleum jelly gauze should be avoided because this type of dressing can dry out, adhere to the mucosa, and damage the delicate tissue when removed. Dry sterile dressings and dressings soaked in solutions can also dry out and damage the mucosa when removed.
TEST-TAKING STRATEGY: Use the process of elimination. Note the similarities in options 1, 2, and 4. These types of dressings can dry out and cause damage to the bladder mucosa. Note the key word in the correct option, "nonadherent." If you had difficulty with this question, take time now to review care to the infant with bladder exstrophy.
LEVEL OF COGNITIVE ABILITY: Application
PHASE OF NURSING PROCESS: Implementation
CLIENT NEEDS: Physiological Integrity
CONTENT AREA: Child Health
REFERENCE
Leifer, G. (1999). *Thompson's introduction to maternity and pediatric nursing* (3rd ed.). Philadelphia: W. B. Saunders. p. 756.

BIBLIOGRAPHY

Ashwill, J., & Droske, S. (1997). *Nursing care of children: Principles and practice.* Philadelphia: W. B. Saunders.

Leifer, G. (1999). *Thompson's introduction to maternity and pediatric nursing* (3rd ed.). Philadelphia: W. B. Saunders.

Luckmann, J. (1997). *Saunders manual of nursing care.* Philadelphia: W. B. Saunders.

O'Toole, M. (ed.). (1997). *Miller-Keane encyclopedia & dictionary of medicine, nursing, & allied health* (6th ed.). Philadelphia: W. B. Saunders.

Schulte, E., Price, D., & James, S. (1997). *Thompson's pediatric nursing: An introductory text* (7th ed.). Philadelphia: W. B. Saunders.

CHAPTER 33

Integumentary Disorders

I. Eczema

A. Description
1. A superficial inflammatory process involving primarily the epidermis
2. A common allergic reaction in children; sometimes caused by an allergic sensitivity to foods such as milk, fish, or eggs
3. Childhood eczema often begins in infancy, and the rash appears on the face, neck, and folds of the elbows and knees; may persist for several years or return after the child is older
B. Data collection
1. Redness and itching
2. Minute papules and vesicles
3. Weeping, oozing, and crusting of lesions
C. Implementation
1. Cause needs to be identified
2. Alleviate itching by soothing baths or moisturizing creams
3. Administer topical steroids and oral antihistamines as prescribed

II. Impetigo

A. Description
1. Incubation period: 7 to 10 days
2. Infectious period: during the course of the infection
3. Transmission: contact
4. Season: summer
B. Data collection
1. Small, red macules that progress to vesicles and rupture and release serous fluid
2. Located around the mouth and nose and may be present on the extremities
C. Implementation
1. Contact isolation
2. Apply topical antibiotics and administer oral antibiotics as prescribed

III. Pediculosis Capitis (Lice)

A. Description
1. Incubation period: eggs incubate for about 1 week and lice reach sexual maturity in about 2 weeks
2. Infectious period: during infestation prior to treatment
3. Transmission: direct contact with infected person and indirect contact with infected person's belongings
4. Season: nonspecific; a common problem in schools
B. Data collection
1. Adult lice are difficult to see and appear as small gray specks that may crawl very fast
2. Nits are visible and are firmly attached to the hair shaft near the scalp; they are tiny silver or gray specks resembling dandruff
C. Implementation
1. antilice shampoo and medications

IV. Scabies

A. Description
1. Incubation period
a. Female mite burrows into epidermis, lays eggs, and dies in the burrow after 4 to 5 weeks
b. The eggs hatch in 3 to 5 days and larvae migrate to the skin to mature and complete their life cycle
2. Infectious period: during the course of the infestation
3. Transmission: by close personal contact with infected person
4. Season: any time of year
B. Data collection
1. Intense pruritus, especially at night
2. Burrows (fine grayish red lines that may be difficult to see) on the skin

C. Implementation
   1. Topical application of either lindane cream (Kwell, Scabene), crotamiton (Eurax), or permethrin 5% (Elimite)
   2. Lindane cream (Kwell, Scabene), should not be used in children younger than age 2 because of the risk of neurotoxicity
   3. Contacts of the infected individual need to be treated

V. Ringworm

A. Description
   1. Known as tinea capitis (scalp); tinea corporis (body); tinea pedis (feet)
   2. A fungal infection spread by direct contact
B. Data collection
   1. Papules and dry scales
   2. Itching
C. Implementation
   1. Provide meticulous skin care
   2. Apply antifungal ointments as prescribed
   3. Administer oral antifungal medications as prescribed

 ## VI. The Burned Child

A. Pediatric differences
   1. Very young children who have been severely burned have a higher mortality rate than older children and adults with comparable burns
   2. Lower burn temperatures and shorter exposure to heat can cause a more severe burn in a child than in an adult because a child's skin is thinner
   3. Severely burned children are at increased risk for fluid and heat loss, dehydration, and metabolic acidosis than are adults
   4. The higher proportion of body fluid to mass in children increases the risk of cardiovascular problems
   5. Burns involving greater than 10% total body surface area (TBSA) require some form of fluid resuscitation
   6. Infants and children are at increased risk for protein and calorie deficiency because they have smaller muscle mass and lower body fat than adults
   7. Scarring is more severe in a child
   8. An immature immune system presents an increased risk of infection for infants and young children
   9. A delay in **growth** may occur following a burn
B. Extent of burn injury (Fig. 33–1)
   1. The Rule of Nines gives an inaccurate estimate because of the differences in body proportion between children and adults

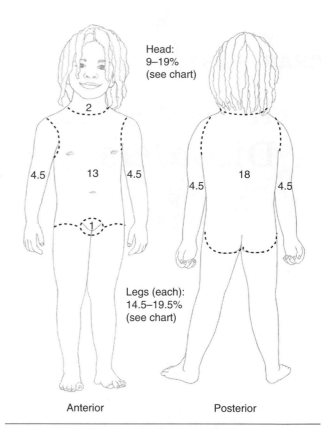

Anterior   Posterior

Child Burn Size Estimation Table
(percent total body surface area)

Burn area	Age (years)				
	1	1–4	5–9	10–14	15
Head	19	17	13	11	9
Neck	2	2	2	2	2
Anterior trunk	13	13	13	13	13
Posterior trunk	18	18	18	18	18
Genitalia	1	1	1	1	1
Upper extremity (each)	9	9	9	9	9
Lower extremity (each)	14.5	15.5	17.5	18.5	19.5

FIGURE 33–1. Calculating total body surface area (TBSA) burned in children. The standard Rule of Nines and standard body surface charts must be adapted because of the difference in body proportions between adults and children. (Child Burn Size Estimation Table reprinted from Lund, C. C., & Browder, N. C. [1944]. Estimation of burn size. Surg Gynecol Obstet 79: 352–358. By permission of Surgery, Gynecology, and Obstetrics, now known as the *Journal of the American College of Surgeons*.)

   2. The Lund and Browder method to estimate the extent of burn injury provides a body surface chart corrected for age

PRACTICE QUESTIONS

1. Corticream is prescribed by the physician for a child with atopic dermatitis (eczema). The nurse instructs the mother how to appropriately apply the cream. Which of the following instructions does the nurse provide to the mother?

1 Avoid cleansing the area before applying the cream

2 Apply the cream over the entire body

3 Apply a thin layer of cream and rub into the area thoroughly

4 Apply a thick layer of cream in affected areas only

2. The nurse assists in providing an instructional session to parents of the children attending the school regarding impetigo. Which of the following is not a component of the instructional session?

1 It is most common in humid weather

2 It begins in an area of broken skin, such as an insect bite

3 It is extremely contagious

4 Lesions are most often located on the arms and chest

3. The nurse provides instructions to the mother of a child with impetigo regarding the application of antibiotic ointment. The mother asks the nurse when the child can return to school. The most appropriate response is

1 24 hours after using antibiotic ointment

2 48 hours after using antibiotic ointment

3 1 week after using antibiotic ointment

4 10 days after using antibiotic ointment

4. The nurse prepares instructions regarding the use of permethrin 1% (Nix) for the parents of the children diagnosed with pediculosis (head lice). Which of the following is not included in the instructions?

1 The permethrin can be obtained over-the-counter in a local pharmacy

2 It is applied to the hair after shampooing and left on for 24 hours

3 It is applied to the hair after shampooing, left on for 10 minutes, and then rinsed out

4 The hair should not be shampooed for 24 hours following treatment

5. The nurse prepares a list of home care instructions for the parents of school children diagnosed with pediculosis. Which of the following is included in this list?

1 Use antilice sprays on all bedding and furniture

2 Take all bedding and linens to the cleaners to be dry cleaned

3 Boil combs and brushes in hot water for 1 hour

4 Vacuum floors, play areas, and furniture to remove any hairs that might carry live nits

6. The mother of a 3-year-old child tells the nurse that the child has been continuously scratching the skin and has developed a rash. The nurse inspects the child and suspects the presence of scabies. Which of the following most accurately describes the presence of this infestation?

1 Clusters of fluid-filled vesicles

2 Fine threadlike lines

3 Purple lesions

4 Thick, honey-colored crusts

7. Permethrin 5% (Elimite) is prescribed for a 4-year-old child with a diagnosis of the presence of scabies. The nurse instructs the mother regarding the use of this treatment. Which of the following instructions does the nurse provide to the mother?

1 The lotion should be applied from head to toe

2 Apply the lotion and leave on for 4 hours

3 Apply the lotion to cool dry skin at least ½ hour after bathing

4 Avoid clothing the child while the lotion is in place

8. A 2-year-old child is admitted to the burn unit with partial and full-thickness burns over 35% of the body. Following admission data collection, the nurse assisting in caring for the child plans care, understanding that the priority nursing intervention is

1 Sedating the child with morphine sulfate

2 Restricting IV fluids

3 Inserting a nasogastric tube

4 Inserting a Foley catheter

9. Griseofulvin (Fulvicin, Grisactin) is prescribed for a child with tinea capitis. The nurse provides instructions regarding administration of the medication. Which of the following is not a component of the instructions?

1 Administer 1 hour before meals

2 Shake the oral suspension before preparing the dose

3 Continue the therapy as long as prescribed

4 Avoid exposure to the sun

10. The nurse is providing home care instructions to an adolescent who has been diagnosed with tinea pedis. Which of the following statements if made by the adolescent indicates a need for further instruction?

1 "I need to dry my feet carefully, especially between the toes."

2 "I need to wear clean socks."

3 "I need to wear shoes that are well ventilated."

4 "I should wear plastic shoes as much as possible."

ANSWERS

1. 3

RATIONALE: Corticream is a topical corticosteroid. It should be applied sparingly and rubbed into the area thoroughly. The affected area should be cleansed gently before application. It should not be applied over extensive areas. Systemic absorption is more likely to occur with extensive application.

TEST-TAKING STRATEGY: Use the process of elimination. Eliminate option 1 because it does not make sense not to cleanse an affected area. Eliminate option 2 because cream should be applied only to areas that are affected. Eliminate option 4 because of the word "thick." Review the procedure for application of this cream now if you had difficulty with this question.

LEVEL OF COGNITIVE ABILITY: Application
PHASE OF NURSING PROCESS: Implementation
CLIENT NEEDS: Health Promotion and Maintenance
CONTENT AREA: Pharmacology
REFERENCE
Hodgson, B., & Kizior, R. (1999). *Saunders nursing drug handbook 1999*. Philadelphia: W. B. Saunders. pp.498–500.

2. 4

RATIONALE: Impetigo is most common during hot, humid summer months. It begins in an area of broken skin, such as an insect bite, scabies, or atopic dermatitis. It may be caused by *Staphylococcus aureus*, group A beta-hemolytic streptococci, or a combination of these bacteria. It is extremely contagious. Lesions are usually located around the mouth and nose, but may be present on the extremities.

TEST-TAKING STRATEGY: Knowledge regarding the etiology and manifestations is required to answer this question. Impetigo is the most common skin infection of childhood, and if you are unfamiliar with this disorder take time now to review.

LEVEL OF COGNITIVE ABILITY: Application
PHASE OF NURSING PROCESS: Implementation
CLIENT NEEDS: Health Promotion and Maintenance
CONTENT AREA: Child Health
REFERENCE
Leifer, G. (1999). *Thompson's introduction to maternity and pediatric nursing* (3rd ed.). Philadelphia: W. B. Saunders. p. 779.

3. 2

RATIONALE: The child should not attend school for 24 to 48 hours after the initiation of systemic antibiotics or 48 hours after using antibiotic ointment. The school should be notified of the diagnosis.

TEST-TAKING STRATEGY: Use knowledge related to the administration of antibiotics to answer the question. Eliminate options 3 and 4 first as the time frames are closely related and rather lengthy. Note the key word "ointment" in the stem of the question; this should assist in directing you to option 2.

LEVEL OF COGNITIVE ABILITY: Application
PHASE OF NURSING PROCESS: Implementation
CLIENT NEEDS: Safe, Effective Care Environment
CONTENT AREA: Child Health
REFERENCE
Ashwill, J., & Droske, S. (1997). *Nursing care of children: Principles and practice*. Philadelphia: W. B. Saunders. p. 1032.

4. 2

RATIONALE: Nix is an over-the-counter antilice product that kills both lice and eggs with one application and has residual activity for 10 days. It is applied to the hair after shampooing and left for 10 minutes before rinsing out. The hair should not be shampooed for 24 hours after the treatment.

TEST-TAKING STRATEGY: Note the key word "not" in the stem of the question. This should assist in directing you, by the process of elimination, to option 2. If you are unfamiliar with this treatment, take time now to review. Pediculosis is one of the largest and most exasperating problems in schools.

LEVEL OF COGNITIVE ABILITY: Application
PHASE OF NURSING PROCESS: Planning
CLIENT NEEDS: Health Promotion and Maintenance
CONTENT AREA: Child Health
REFERENCE
Ashwill, J., & Droske, S. (1997). *Nursing care of children: Principles and practice*. Philadelphia: W. B. Saunders. p. 1042.

5. 4

RATIONALE: Antilice sprays are unnecessary. Additionally, they should never be used on a child. Bedding and linens should be washed with hot water and dried on a hot setting. Items that cannot be washed should be dry cleaned or sealed in plastic bags in a warm place for 3 weeks. Combs and brushes should be boiled or soaked in antilice shampoo or hot water for 15 minutes. Thorough home cleaning is necessary to remove any remaining lice or nits.

TEST-TAKING STRATEGY: Eliminate option 1, knowing that antilice sprays should not be used. Knowing that bedding and linens can be washed will eliminate option 2. The time for boiling in option 3 is rather lengthy; therefore, eliminate this option. If you had difficulty with this question, take time now to review these important home care instructions.

LEVEL OF COGNITIVE ABILITY: Application
PHASE OF NURSING PROCESS: Planning
CLIENT NEEDS: Health Promotion and Maintenance
CONTENT AREA: Child Health
REFERENCE
Ashwill, J., & Droske, S. (1997). *Nursing care of children: Principles and practice*. Philadelphia: W. B. Saunders. p. 1042.

6. 2

RATIONALE: Scabies appears as burrows or fine, grayish threadlike lines. They may be difficult to see if they are obscured by excoriation and inflammation. Clusters of fluid-filled vesicles are seen in herpesvirus. Thick, honey-colored crusts are characteristic of impetigo. Purple lesions may be indicative of various disorders, including systemic conditions.

TEST-TAKING STRATEGY: Knowledge that scabies infestation produces burrows will assist in directing you to option 2. If you are unfamiliar with the clinical manifestations associated with scabies, take time now to review.

LEVEL OF COGNITIVE ABILITY: Comprehension
PHASE OF NURSING PROCESS: Data Collection
CLIENT NEEDS: Physiological Integrity
CONTENT AREA: Child Health
REFERENCE
Leifer, G. (1999). *Thompson's introduction to maternity and pediatric nursing* (3rd ed.). Philadelphia: W. B. Saunders. p. 781.

7. **3**

RATIONALE: Permethrin is applied from the neck downward, making sure the soles of the feet, behind the ears, and under the toenails and fingernails are covered. The lotion should be kept on for 8 to 14 hours, and then the child should be given a bath. The lotion should not be applied for at least 30 minutes after bathing and should be applied only to cool, dry skin. The child should be clothed during treatment.
TEST-TAKING STRATEGY: Options 1 and 4 can be easily eliminated. Knowledge regarding the treatment time will assist in directing you to option 3. Take time now to review this treatment if you had difficulty with this question.
LEVEL OF COGNITIVE ABILITY: Application
PHASE OF NURSING PROCESS: Implementation
CLIENT NEEDS: Health Promotion and Maintenance
CONTENT AREA: Child Health
REFERENCE
Leifer, G. (1999). *Thompson's introduction to maternity and pediatric nursing* (3rd ed.). Philadelphia: W. B. Saunders. p. 781.

8. **4**

RATIONALE: A Foley catheter is inserted into the child's bladder so that urine output can be accurately measured on an hourly basis. Although pain medication may be required, the child should not be sedated. IV fluids are not restricted and are administered at a rate sufficient to maintain adequate tissue perfusion. A nasogastric tube may or may not be required but is not the priority intervention.
TEST-TAKING STRATEGY: Option 1 can be eliminated first because the child should not be sedated. Eliminate option 2 next, knowing that fluid resuscitation is an important component of therapy to prevent burn shock. From the remaining options, knowledge that urine output reflects adequate tissue perfusion will direct you to option 4. Review the treatment of burns now if you had difficulty with this question.
LEVEL OF COGNITIVE ABILITY: Comprehension
PHASE OF NURSING PROCESS: Planning
CLIENT NEEDS: Physiological Integrity

CONTENT AREA: Child Health
REFERENCE
Leifer, G. (1999). *Thompson's introduction to maternity and pediatric nursing* (3rd ed.). Philadelphia: W. B. Saunders. p. 785.

9. **1**

RATIONALE: Griseofulvin is given with or after meals to avoid GI irritation and increase absorption. Suspensions should be shaken well. Parents are instructed to continue therapy as long as ordered and not to miss a dose. Exposure to the sun is avoided.
TEST-TAKING STRATEGY: Note the key word "not" in the stem of the question. Recalling that this medication causes GI irritation will easily direct you to option 1. Review this medication if you had difficulty with this question.
LEVEL OF COGNITIVE ABILITY: Application
PHASE OF NURSING PROCESS: Implementation
CLIENT NEEDS: Health Promotion and Maintenance
CONTENT AREA: Child Health
REFERENCE
Leifer, G. (1999). *Thompson's introduction to maternity and pediatric nursing* (3rd ed.). Philadelphia: W. B. Saunders. p. 780.

10. **4**

RATIONALE: Plastic shoes retain heat and should be avoided because the condition is aggravated by heat and moisture. Options 1, 2, and 3 are appropriate measures to treat this condition.
TEST-TAKING STRATEGY: Note the key words "a need for further instruction." Recalling that heat and moisture aggravate the condition will easily direct you to option 4. Review home care measures now if you had difficulty with this question.
LEVEL OF COGNITIVE ABILITY: Comprehension
PHASE OF NURSING PROCESS: Evaluation
CLIENT NEEDS: Health Promotion and Maintenance
CONTENT AREA: Child Health
REFERENCE
Leifer, G. (1999). *Thompson's introduction to maternity and pediatric nursing* (3rd ed.). Philadelphia: W. B. Saunders. p. 780.

BIBLIOGRAPHY

Ashwill, J., & Droske, S. (1997). *Nursing care of children: Principles and practice*. Philadelphia: W. B. Saunders.
Hodgson, B., & Kizior, R. (1999). *Saunders nursing drug handbook 1999*. Philadelphia: W. B. Saunders.
Leifer, G. (1999). *Thompson's introduction to maternity and pediatric nursing* (3rd ed.). Philadelphia: W. B. Saunders.
O'Toole, M. (ed.). (1997). *Miller-Keane encyclopedia & dictionary of medicine, nursing, & allied health* (6th ed.). Philadelphia: W. B. Saunders.

CHAPTER 34

Musculoskeletal Disorders

I. Dysplasia of the Hip

A. Description
1. A condition in which the head of the femur is improperly seated in the acetabulum or hip socket of the pelvis
2. Can range from very mild to severely dislocated
3. Can be congenital or develop after birth

B. Data collection (Fig. 34–1)
1. Neonates: laxity of the ligaments around the hip, which allows the femoral head to be displaced from the acetabulum upon manipulation
2. Infants beyond the newborn period
   a. Asymmetry of the gluteal skinfolds when placed prone and the legs are extended against the examining table
   b. Limited range of motion (ROM) in the affected hip
   c. Asymmetric abduction of the affected hip when placed supine with the knees and hips flexed
   d. Apparent short femur on the affected side (Galeazzi's sign)
3. The walking child: minimal to pronounced variations in gait with lurching toward the affected side
4. Positive Barlow's or Ortolani's maneuver

C. Implementation
1. In the neonatal period, splinting of the hips with Pavlik harness to maintain flexion and abduction and external rotation
2. Following the neonatal period, traction, and/or surgery to release muscles and tendons
3. Positioning and immobilization in a spica cast following surgery until healing is achieved
4. Osteotomy following traction in profoundly affected children

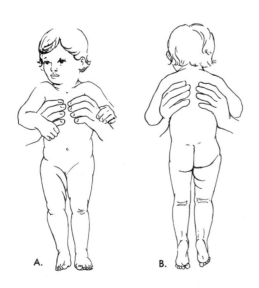
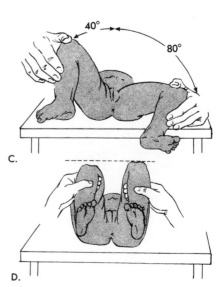

FIGURE 34–1. The three classic signs of congenital hip dysplasia. *A* and *B,* unequal skin folds; *C,* limitation of abduction; and *D,* unequal knee height. (From Tachdjian, M. [1990]. *Pediatric orthopedics* [2nd ed.]. Philadelphia: W. B. Saunders. p. 326.)

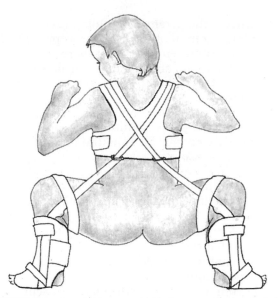

FIGURE 34–2. The child in a Pavlik harness. (From Tachdjian, M. O. [1990]. *Pediatric orthopedics* [2nd ed]. Philadelphia: W. B. Saunders, p. 336.)

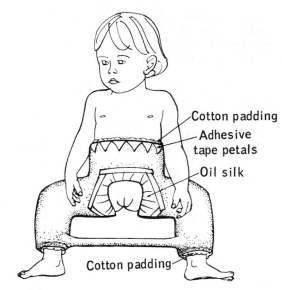

Cotton padding
Adhesive tape petals
Oil silk
Cotton padding

FIGURE 34–3. A body (spica) cast. (From Leifer, G. [1982]. *Principles and techniques in pediatrics nursing* [4th ed.]. Philadelphia: W. B. Saunders.)

5. Instruct parents regarding proper care of a Pavlik harness or spica cast (Fig. 34–2 and Fig. 34–3)

II. Congenital Clubfoot (Fig. 34–4)

A. Description
   1. A congenital malformation of the lower extremities
   2. The defect may be unilateral or bilateral
   3. Defects are rigid and cannot be manipulated into a neutral position
   4. Long-term interval follow-up is required until the child reaches skeletal maturity
B. Data collection: the foot is plantar flexed with an inverted heel and adducted forefoot
C. Implementation
   1. Treatment begins as soon after birth as possible
   2. Serial manipulation and casting are performed weekly, and if correction is not achieved in 3 to 6 months, surgery is indicated
   3. Monitor for pain
   4. Monitor neurovascular status of the toes
   5. Instruct parents in cast care and signs of

neurovascular impairment requiring physician notification

III. Scoliosis

A. Description
   1. A lateral curvature of the spine
   2. Surgical and nonsurgical interventions are employed and the type of treatment depends on the degree of curvature, the age of the child, and the amount of **growth** that is anticipated
   3. Long-term monitoring is essential to detect any progression of the curve
B. Data collection
   1. Visible curve fails to straighten when child bends forward and hangs arms down toward feet
   2. Hips, ribs, and shoulders are asymmetrical
   3. Apparent leg length discrepancy
C. Implementation
   1. Monitor progression of the curvature
   2. Prepare the child for the use of a brace if prescribed
   3. Prepare the child and parents for surgery

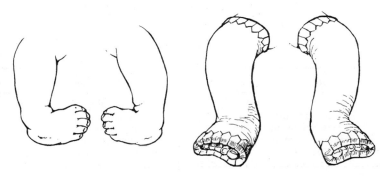

FIGURE 34–4. Clubfoot before and after application of plaster casts. (From Marlow, D. [1977]. *Textbook of pediatric nursing* [5th ed.]. Philadelphia: W. B. Saunders.)

(spinal fusion or internal instrumentation rods) if prescribed

D. Implementation postoperatively
  1. Maintain flat position
  2. Log roll the child when turning to maintain alignment
  3. Monitor extremities for neurovascular status
  4. Encourage coughing and deep breathing and use of incentive spirometry
  5. Monitor for pain and administer prescribed analgesics
  6. Monitor for incontinence
  7. Instruct in activity restrictions
  8. Instruct child to roll from a side-lying position to a sitting position and assist with ambulation

E. Braces
  1. Instruct the child to wear a brace as prescribed
  2. Inspect the skin for signs of redness or breakdown
  3. Keep the skin clean and dry, avoiding lotions and powders
  4. Advise the child to wear soft nonirritating clothing under the brace
  5. Instruct in prescribed exercises
  6. Encourage verbalization about body image

IV. Juvenile Rheumatoid Arthritis (JRA)

A. Description
  1. An autoimmune inflammatory disease affecting the joints
  2. The cause is unknown
  3. Juvenile onset is diagnosed before 16 years of age
  4. A leading cause of disability in children
  5. Treatment is supportive and directed toward preserving joint function, controlling inflammation, minimizing deformity, and reducing the impact that the disease may have on the development of the child
  6. Therapy includes medications, physical and occupational therapies, and family education
  7. Surgical intervention may be implemented when the child has problems with joint contractures and unequal growth of extremities

B. Data collection (Table 34–1)

C. Implementation
  1. Facilitate social, emotional, and development of **growth**

2. Instruct the parents and child in the administration of medications as prescribed, such as nonsteroidal anti-inflammatory drugs (NSAIDs) and antirheumatic medications
3. Assist the child with ROM and prescribed exercises
4. Instruct the parents and child in the use of hot or cold packs, splinting, and positioning the affected joint in a neutral position during painful episodes
5. Encourage and support prescribed physical and occupational therapy
6. Instruct in the importance of preventive eye care
7. Instruct in the importance of reporting visual disturbances
8. Determine the child's perception regarding the chronic illness
9. Encourage normal performance of activities of daily living (ADL)

V. Fractures (Fig. 34–5)

A. Description
  1. A break in the continuity of the bone caused by trauma, twisting, or bone decalcification
  2. Fractures in children usually result from increased mobility and inadequate or immature motor and cognitive skills
  3. Fractures in infancy are generally rare and warrant further investigation to rule out the possibility of child **abuse**
  4. The most frequently seen fracture in children is in the forearm

B. Data collection
  1. Pain or tenderness over the involved area
  2. Loss of function
  3. Obvious deformity
  4. Crepitation
  5. Erythema, ecchymosis, and edema
  6. Muscle spasm

C. Initial care of a fracture
  1. Immobilize affected extremity
  2. If compound fracture exists, splint the extremity and cover the wound with a sterile dressing

D. Implementation
  1. Reduction
    a. Restoring the bone to proper alignment
    b. Closed reduction: may require general

Table 34–1. **Characteristics of JRA**

Systemic JRA	Pauciarticular JRA	Polyarticular JRA
Fever	Mild joint pain and swelling	Morning joint stiffness
Salmon-pink rash	Affects large joints	Low-grade fever
Affects five or more joints	Affects no more than 4 joints	Affects weight-bearing joints
May also have anorexia, anemia, fatigue	Iridocyclitis and visual disturbances	Affects five or more joints

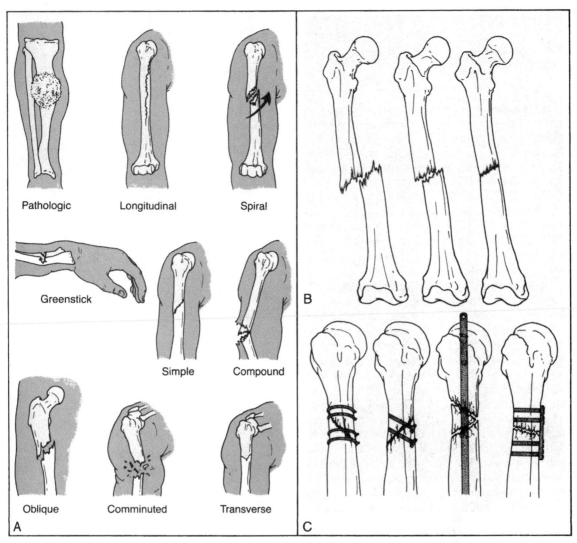

FIGURE 34–5. *A,* Types of Fractures. *B,* Reduction of a fractured bone. *C,* Various methods of internal fixation. (Redrawn from deWit, S.C. [1992]. *Keane's essentials of medical-surgical nursing* [3rd ed.]. Philadelphia: W. B. Saunders.)

anesthesia and is accomplished by manual alignment of the fragments followed by immobilization

    c. Open reduction: requires the surgical insertion of internal fixation devices such as rods, wires, or pins that help maintain alignment while healing occurs

  2. Retention: the application of traction or a cast to maintain alignment until healing occurs

E. Traction

  1. Cervical skin traction

    a. Relieves muscle spasms and compression in upper extremities and neck

    b. Uses a head halter and a chin pad to attach the traction

    c. Use powder to protect the ears from friction rub

    d. Position the child with the head of the bed elevated 20 to 30 degrees and attach the weights to a pulley system over the head of the bed

  2. Bryant's skin traction

    a. Used to stabilize a fractured femur

    b. Used to correct a congenital hip in children

    c. Position child flat with a 90-degree hip flexion

  3. Russell's skin traction

    a. Used to stabilize a fractured femur before surgery

    b. Similar to Buck's traction but provides a double pull with the use of a knee sling

    c. Traction pulls at the knee and foot

    d. Position the child with the foot of the bed slightly elevated

  4. Balanced suspension

    a. Used with skin or skeletal traction

    b. Used to approximate fractures of the femur, tibia, or fibula

    c. Produced by a counterforce other than the child

    d. Position the child in low-Fowler's position, either on the side or back

e. Maintain a 20-degree angle from the thigh to the bed

f. Protect the skin from breakdown

g. Provide pin care if pins are used with the skeletal traction

h. Clean pin site with normal saline and hydrogen peroxide or Betadine as prescribed

F. Casts

1. Description

a. Made of plaster or fiberglass to provide immobilization of bone and joints after a fracture or injury

b. Fractures of the hip and knee may require a body or spica cast

2. Implementation

a. Examine the cast for pressure areas

b. Monitor the extremity for circulatory impairment such as pain, swelling, discoloration, tingling, numbness, or coolness or diminished pulse

c. Notify the physician if circulatory compromise occurs

d. Prepare for bivalving or cutting the cast if circulatory impairment occurs

e. Instruct the child not to stick objects down the cast

f. Teach the child to keep cast clean and dry

g. Instruct the child on isometric exercises to prevent muscle atrophy

PRACTICE QUESTIONS

1. A 6-month-old infant is seen in the clinic and is diagnosed with unilateral hip dysplasia. The nurse reviews the health care record and understands which of the following assessment findings is not noted in this condition?
   1. An apparent short femur on the affected side
   2. Limited range of motion in the affected hip
   3. Asymmetric adduction of the affected hip when placed supine with the knees and hips flexed
   4. Asymmetry of the gluteal skinfolds when the infant is placed prone and the legs are extended against the examining table

2. The nurse is assisting a physician during the examination of an infant with hip dysplasia. The physician performs the Ortolani maneuver. The nurse determines that this maneuver is performed to
   1. Push the unstable femoral head out of the acetabulum
   2. Reduce the dislocated femoral head back into the acetabulum
   3. Determine the extent of range of motion
   4. Check for asymmetry on the affected side

3. The nurse reinforces instructions to the parents of an infant with hip dysplasia regarding care of the Pavlik harness. Which of the following does the nurse include in the instructions?

1. The harness should be worn 12 hours a day
2. The harness needs be removed for diaper changes and for feeding
3. The harness should be removed only to check the skin and for bathing
4. The infant should not be moved when out of the harness

4. The mother brings her 2-week-old infant to the clinic for treatment following a diagnosis of club-foot made at the time of birth. Which of the following statements, if made by the mother, indicates a need for further education regarding this disorder?
   1. "I need to bring my child back to the clinic in 1 month for a new cast."
   2. "Treatment needs to be started as soon as possible."
   3. "I need to come to the clinic every week with my child for the casting."
   4. "I realize my child will require follow-up care until full grown."

5. The nurse is assigned to care for a child following spinal fusion for the treatment of scoliosis. The child complains of abdominal discomfort and begins to have episodes of vomiting. On further data collection, the nurse notes abdominal distention. Which of the following nursing actions is most appropriate?
   1. Administer an antiemetic
   2. Place the child in a side-lying Sims' position
   3. Notify the registered nurse (RN)
   4. Increase the IV fluids

6. The nurse is providing instructions to the parents of a child with scoliosis regarding the use of a brace. Which of the following is not a component of the instructions?
   1. Apply lotion under the brace to prevent skin breakdown
   2. Avoid the use of powder because it will cake under the brace
   3. Have the child wear a soft fabric under the brace
   4. Encourage the child to perform prescribed exercises

7. A nursing student is asked to discuss juvenile rheumatoid arthritis (JRA) at a clinical conference scheduled at the end of the clinical day. Which of the following is not included in the discussion?
   1. It most often occurs before the age of 16
   2. It is twice as likely to occur in boys rather than girls
   3. Visual problems can occur in JRA
   4. Clinical manifestations include morning stiffness and painful, stiff, swollen joints

8. The mother of a child with juvenile rheumatoid arthritis (JRA) calls the nurse because the child

is experiencing a painful exacerbation of the disease. The mother asks the nurse if the child should perform the range of motion (ROM) exercises at this time. The most appropriate nursing response is

1 "The ROM exercises must be performed every day."
2 "Avoid all exercise during painful periods."
3 "Administer additional pain medication prior to performing ROM exercises."
4 "Have the child perform simple isometric exercises during this time."

9. A 2-year-old child is placed in Bryant's traction for treatment of a fractured femur. The nurse develops a plan of care for the child. Which of the following is not a component of the plan?

1 Restrain the child to maintain a supine position
2 Place the child supine with the legs flexed slightly less than 90 degrees
3 Ensure that the sacrum is resting on the mattress
4 Ensure the use of a footplate to keep the traction straps away from the child's ankles

10. A 4-year-old child sustains a fall at home and is brought to the emergency department by the mother. Following x-ray, it has been determined that the child has a fractured arm and a plaster cast is applied. The nurse provides instructions to the mother regarding cast care for the child. Which of the following statements, if made by the mother, indicates a need for further education?

1 "The cast may feel warm as the cast dries."
2 "If the cast becomes wet, a blow drier set on the cool setting may be used to dry the cast."
3 "A small amount of white shoe polish can touch up a soiled white cast."
4 "I can use lotion or powder around the cast edges to relieve itching."

11. The nurse is assigned to care for a child with a spica cast. The nurse avoids which of the following when caring for the child?

1 Checks neurovascular status of the extremities
2 Observes for nonverbal signs of pain
3 Places the child on a stretcher and brings the child to the playroom
4 Uses pillows to elevate the head and the shoulders

12. The student nurse is asked to discuss the topic of scoliosis at a clinical conference. Which of the following is not included in the discussion?

1 During adolescence, it is most common in boys
2 It refers to an S-shaped curvature of the spine
3 Many curvatures are not progressive and require only periodic evaluation

4 Untreated progressive scoliosis may lead to back pain, fatigue, disability, and heart and lung complications

13. The nurse is assigned to care for a child with a compound fracture of the arm that occurred as a result of a fall. The nurse understands that this type of fracture involves which of the following?

1 The bone is broken but the skin over the area of the break is not
2 The risk of infection is greater than in a simple fracture
3 One side of the bone is broken and the other side is bent
4 The entire bone is broken across its width

14. The child with a fractured femur is placed in Buck's skin traction. The nurse plans care, knowing that this type of traction

1 Requires frequent pin care
2 Places the child at risk for infection
3 Is a type of skin traction that pulls the hip and leg into extension
4 Uses skeletal traction and weights to provide a counterforce

15. The nurse is preparing to perform a neurovascular check for tissue perfusion in the child with an arm cast. Which of the following is the priority in performing this procedure?

1 Taking the blood pressure
2 Taking the temperature
3 Checking the apical heart rate
4 Checking the peripheral pulse in the affected arm

16. The nurse is checking the capillary refill in a child with a cast applied to the left arm. The nurse compresses the nailbed of a finger and it returns to its original color in 2 seconds. Based on this finding, the most appropriate action is to

1 Notify the registered nurse (RN)
2 Document the findings
3 Prepare the child for bivalving the cast
4 Elevate the extremity and recheck the capillary refill immediately

17. The nurse is performing a neurovascular check on a child with a cast applied to the lower leg. The child complains of tingling in the toes distal to the fracture site. The most appropriate nursing action is to

1 Ambulate the child with crutches
2 Elevate the extremity
3 Document the findings
4 Notify the registered nurse (RN)

18. The nurse is assigned to care for a child in skeletal traction. The nurse avoids which of the following when caring for the child?

1 Keeping the weights hanging freely
2 Placing the bed linen on the traction ropes
3 Ensuring that the ropes are on the pulleys

4 Ensuring that the weights are out of the child's reach

19. The nursing student is asked to discuss the topic of clubfoot at a clinical conference. The student plans to tell the group that clubfoot
    1 Is a rare deformity of the skeletal system
    2 Requires aggressive treatment for correction
    3 Affects girls more often than boys
    4 Is a congenital anomaly

20. The nurse is reinforcing information to the mother of a child about a synthetic cast that has been applied to the child for the treatment of a clubfoot. Which of the following information does the nurse provide to the mother?
    1 The cast takes 24 hours to dry
    2 The cast is heavier than a plaster cast
    3 It is stronger than a plaster cast
    4 It allows for greater mobility than a plaster cast

ANSWERS

1. **3**

RATIONALE: Asymmetric abduction of the affected hip, when placed supine with the knees and hips flexed, is a finding in hip dysplasia in infants beyond the newborn period. Options 1, 2, and 4 are accurate assessment findings in this disorder.
TEST-TAKING STRATEGY: Note the key word "not." Attempt to visualize each of the findings described in the options. This will assist in directing you to option 3. If you had difficulty with this question, take time now to review the assessment findings in hip dysplasia.
LEVEL OF COGNITIVE ABILITY: Comprehension
PHASE OF NURSING PROCESS: Data Collection
CLIENT NEEDS: Physiological Integrity
CONTENT AREA: Child Health
REFERENCE
Schulte, E., Price, D., & James, S. (1997). *Thompson's pediatric nursing: An introductory text* (7th ed.). Philadelphia: W. B. Saunders. p. 112.

2. **2**

RATIONALE: In Barlow's maneuver, the examiner pushes the unstable femoral head out of the acetabulum. In Ortolani's maneuver, the examiner reduces the dislocated femoral head back into the acetabulum. A positive finding in Ortolani's maneuver is a palpable clink upon entry or exit of the femoral head over the acetabular ring. Options 3 and 4 are data collection techniques for identification of the clinical manifestations of hip dysplasia but do not describe Ortolani's maneuver.
TEST-TAKING STRATEGY: Knowledge regarding findings in hip dysplasia and these maneuvers is required to answer this question. Review these maneuvers now if you had difficulty with this question. Remember that these maneuvers should only be performed by a physician or trained health care provider.
LEVEL OF COGNITIVE ABILITY: Comprehension
PHASE OF NURSING PROCESS: Data Collection
CLIENT NEEDS: Physiological Integrity
CONTENT AREA: Child Health
REFERENCE
Leifer, G. (1999). *Thompson's introduction to maternity and pediatric nursing* (3rd ed.). Philadelphia: W. B. Saunders. p. 357.

3. **3**

RATIONALE: The harness should be worn 23 hours a day and should be removed only to check the skin and for bathing. The hips and buttocks should be supported carefully when the infant is out of the harness. The harness does not need to be removed for diaper changes or feedings.

TEST-TAKING STRATEGY: Attempt to visualize this harness in answering the question. This will assist in eliminating options 2 and 4. Select option 3 over option 1 because the time frame in option 1 is rather low. Review home care instruction regarding this harness now if you had difficulty with this question.
LEVEL OF COGNITIVE ABILITY: Application
PHASE OF NURSING PROCESS: Implementation
CLIENT NEEDS: Health Promotion and Maintenance
CONTENT AREA: Child Health
REFERENCE
Schulte, E., Price, D., & James, S. (1997). *Thompson's pediatric nursing: An introductory text* (7th ed.). Philadelphia: W. B. Saunders. p. 112.

4. **1**

RATIONALE: Treatment for clubfoot is started as soon as possible after birth. Serial manipulation and casting are performed at least weekly. If sufficient correction is not achieved in 3 to 6 months, surgery is usually indicated. Because clubfoot can recur, all children with clubfoot require long-term interval follow-up until they reach skeletal maturity to ensure an optimal outcome.
TEST-TAKING STRATEGY: Knowledge regarding the treatment plan for clubfoot is required to answer the question. Note the key words "indicates a need for further education." This may assist in eliminating options 2 and 4. Recalling that serial manipulations and casting are required weekly will assist in directing you to option 1. Review these treatment procedures now if you had difficulty with this question.
LEVEL OF COGNITIVE ABILITY: Comprehension
PHASE OF NURSING PROCESS: Evaluation
CLIENT NEEDS: Physiological Integrity
CONTENT AREA: Child Health
REFERENCE
Schulte, E., Price, D., & James, S. (1997). *Thompson's pediatric nursing: An introductory text* (7th ed.). Philadelphia: W. B. Saunders. p. 110.

5. **3**

RATIONALE: A complication following surgical treatment of scoliosis is superior mesenteric artery syndrome. This disorder is caused by mechanical changes in the position of the child's abdominal contents, resulting from lengthening of the child's body. It causes vomiting and abdominal distention similar to that which occurs with intestinal obstruction or paralytic ileus. Postoperative vomiting in children with body casts or those who have undergone spinal fusion warrants attention because of the possibility of superior mesenteric artery syndrome.

TEST-TAKING STRATEGY: Eliminate option 4 first because it should not be implemented without a prescribed order. Eliminate option 2 next because this child requires log rolling, and the Sims' position may cause injury following surgery. From the remaining options, note the signs and symptoms in the question. These should alert you that the RN needs to be notified. Review superior mesenteric artery syndrome now if you had difficulty with this question.
LEVEL OF COGNITIVE ABILITY: Analysis
PHASE OF NURSING PROCESS: Implementation
CLIENT NEEDS: Physiological Integrity
CONTENT AREA: Child Health
REFERENCE
Ashwill, J., & Droske, S. (1997). *Nursing care of children: Principles and practice.* Philadelphia: W. B. Saunders. p. 1142.

6. **1**

RATIONALE: The use of lotions or powders should be avoided because they can become sticky or cake under the brace, causing irritation. Options 2, 3, and 4 are appropriate instructions to the parents of a child with a brace.
TEST-TAKING STRATEGY: Note the key word "not." Careful reading of the options will assist in directing you to option 1. Review home care instructions regarding the care of a child in a brace now if you had difficulty with this question.
LEVEL OF COGNITIVE ABILITY: Application
PHASE OF NURSING PROCESS: Implementation
CLIENT NEEDS: Health Promotion and Maintenance
CONTENT AREA: Child Health
REFERENCE
Schulte, E., Price, D., & James, S. (1997). *Thompson's pediatric nursing: An introductory text* (7th ed.). Philadelphia: W. B. Saunders. p. 392.

7. **2**

RATIONALE: JRA is twice as likely to occur in girls than boys. Options 1, 3, and 4 are accurate regarding this disorder.
TEST-TAKING STRATEGY: Note the key word "not." Knowledge regarding the etiology and clinical manifestations associated with JRA is required to answer this question. This knowledge will easily direct you to option 2. Review this disorder now if you are unfamiliar with JRA.
LEVEL OF COGNITIVE ABILITY: Comprehension
PHASE OF NURSING PROCESS: Planning
CLIENT NEEDS: Physiological Integrity
CONTENT AREA: Child Health
REFERENCE
Schulte, E., Price, D., & James, S. (1997). *Thompson's pediatric nursing: An introductory text* (7th ed.). Philadelphia: W. B. Saunders. p. 343.

8. **4**

RATIONALE: During painful episodes, hot or cold packs, and splinting and positioning the affected joint in a neutral position help reduce the pain. Although resting the extremity is appropriate, it is important to begin simple isometric or tensing exercises as soon as the child is able. These exercises do not involve joint movement.
TEST-TAKING STRATEGY: Eliminate options 1, 2, and 3 because of the words "must," "all," and "additional" in each of these options. Review pain management and care during exacerbations now if you had difficulty with this question.
LEVEL OF COGNITIVE ABILITY: Application
PHASE OF NURSING PROCESS: Implementation

CLIENT NEEDS: Physiological Integrity
CONTENT AREA: Child Health
REFERENCE
Schulte, E., Price, D., & James, S. (1997). *Thompson's pediatric nursing: An introductory text* (7th ed.). Philadelphia: W. B. Saunders. p. 345.

9. **3**

RATIONALE: In Bryant's traction, the sacrum should be off the mattress. Options 1, 2, and 4 are accurate interventions in the use of this traction.
TEST-TAKING STRATEGY: Note the key word "not." Attempt to visualize this type of traction in selecting the correct option. Review this type of traction and the associated nursing interventions now if you had difficulty with this question.
LEVEL OF COGNITIVE ABILITY: Application
PHASE OF NURSING PROCESS: Planning
CLIENT NEEDS: Physiological Integrity
CONTENT AREA: Child Health
REFERENCE
Schulte, E., Price, D., & James, S. (1997). *Thompson's pediatric nursing: An introductory text* (7th ed.). Philadelphia: W. B. Saunders. p. 277.

10. **4**

RATIONALE: The mother needs to be instructed not to use lotion or powders on the skin around the cast edges or inside the cast. Lotions or powders can become sticky or caked and cause skin irritation. Options 1, 2, and 3 are appropriate instructions.
TEST-TAKING STRATEGY: Note the key phrase "indicates a need for further education." Knowledge regarding routine cast care should easily direct you to option 4. Review home care instructions regarding cast care now if you had difficulty with this question.
LEVEL OF COGNITIVE ABILITY: Comprehension
PHASE OF NURSING PROCESS: Evaluation
CLIENT NEEDS: Health Promotion and Maintenance
CONTENT AREA: Child Health
REFERENCE
Schulte, E., Price, D., & James, S. (1997). *Thompson's pediatric nursing: An introductory text* (7th ed.). Philadelphia: W. B. Saunders. p. 111.

11. **4**

RATIONALE: Pillows should not be used to elevate the head or shoulders of a child in a body cast because the pillows will thrust the child's chest against the cast and cause discomfort and respiratory difficulty. Neurovascular checks are a critical component of care to ensure that the cast is not causing circulatory compromise. The nurse should observe for nonverbal signs of pain and should ask the older child if pain is experienced. A ride on a stretcher to the playroom or around the hospital provides changes of position and scenery.
TEST-TAKING STRATEGY: Note the key word "avoids." Visualize this type of cast and use the process of elimination to direct you to option 4. If you had difficulty with this question, take time now to review care to the child in a spica cast.
LEVEL OF COGNITIVE ABILITY: Application
PHASE OF NURSING PROCESS: Implementation
CLIENT NEEDS: Physiological Integrity
CONTENT AREA: Child Health

REFERENCE
Leifer, G. (1999). *Thompson's introduction to maternity and pediatric nursing* (3rd ed.). Philadelphia: W. B. Saunders. pp. 358–359, 361.

12. 1

RATIONALE: During adolescence, scoliosis is more common in girls. Options 2, 3, and 4 are accurate regarding scoliosis.
TEST-TAKING STRATEGY: Note the key word "not." Use knowledge regarding scoliosis and the process of elimination. If you are unfamiliar with this skeletal disorder, take time now to review.
LEVEL OF COGNITIVE ABILITY: Comprehension
PHASE OF NURSING PROCESS: Planning
CLIENT NEEDS: Physiological Integrity
CONTENT AREA: Child Health
REFERENCE
Leifer, G. (1999). *Thompson's introduction to maternity and pediatric nursing* (3rd ed.). Philadelphia: W. B. Saunders. p. 635.

13. 2

RATIONALE: In a compound fracture, a wound in the skin leads to the broken bone, and there is an added danger of infection. Option 1 describes a simple fracture. Option 3 describes a greenstick fracture. Option 4 describes a complete fracture.
TEST-TAKING STRATEGY: Use the process of elimination and knowledge regarding the various types of bone fractures to assist in answering the question. Take time now to review the various types of fractures if you had difficulty with this question.
LEVEL OF COGNITIVE ABILITY: Knowledge
PHASE OF NURSING PROCESS: Data Collection
CLIENT NEEDS: Physiological Integrity
CONTENT AREA: Child Health
REFERENCE
Leifer, G. (1999). *Thompson's introduction to maternity and pediatric nursing* (3rd ed.). Philadelphia: W. B. Saunders. p. 622.

14. 3

RATIONALE: Buck's skin traction (Buck's extension) is a type of skin traction used in fractures of the femur and in hip and knee contractures. It pulls the hip and leg into extension. Countertraction is supplied by the child's body. Options 1, 2, and 4 describe skeletal traction.
TEST-TAKING STRATEGY: Note the key word "skin" in the question. This will assist in directing you to option 3. If you had difficulty with this question, take time now to review Buck's skin traction.
LEVEL OF COGNITIVE ABILITY: Comprehension
PHASE OF NURSING PROCESS: Planning
CLIENT NEEDS: Physiological Integrity
CONTENT AREA: Child Health
REFERENCE
Leifer, G. (1999). *Thompson's introduction to maternity and pediatric nursing* (3rd ed.). Philadelphia: W. B. Saunders. p. 625.

15. 4

RATIONALE: The neurovascular check for tissue perfusion is performed on the toes or fingers distal to an injury or cast and includes peripheral pulse, color, capillary refill time, warmth, and motion and sensation. Options 1, 2, and 3 may be components of care but are not the priority in this situation.
TEST-TAKING STRATEGY: Note the key word "priority" and focus on the issue of the question. Option 4 is the only option that addresses a neurovascular check. Review the components of a neurovascular check now if you had difficulty with this question.
LEVEL OF COGNITIVE ABILITY: Application
PHASE OF NURSING PROCESS: Implementation
CLIENT NEEDS: Physiological Integrity
CONTENT AREA: Child Health
REFERENCE
Leifer, G. (1999). *Thompson's introduction to maternity and pediatric nursing* (3rd ed.). Philadelphia: W. B. Saunders. p. 627.

16. 2

RATIONALE: When checking capillary refill, the nurse expects to note that a compressed nailbed returns to its original color in less than 3 seconds. Options 1, 3, and 4 are unnecessary actions.
TEST-TAKING STRATEGY: Knowledge regarding a normal finding when checking the capillary refill is required to answer this question. If you are unfamiliar with this data collection technique, take time now to review.
LEVEL OF COGNITIVE ABILITY: Application
PHASE OF NURSING PROCESS: Implementation
CLIENT NEEDS: Physiological Integrity
CONTENT AREA: Child Health
REFERENCE
Leifer, G. (1999). *Thompson's introduction to maternity and pediatric nursing* (3rd ed.). Philadelphia: W. B. Saunders. p. 625.

17. 4

RATIONALE: Reduced sensation to touch, or if the child complains of numbness or tingling at a site distal to a fracture, may indicate poor tissue perfusion. This finding should be reported to the RN. Options 1, 2, and 3 are inappropriate and would delay the required and immediate interventions.
TEST-TAKING STRATEGY: Knowledge regarding the signs of circulatory compromise is required to answer this question. Note the child's complaint to assist in directing you to option 4. If you had difficulty with this question, take time now to review the signs of circulatory compromise.
LEVEL OF COGNITIVE ABILITY: Application
PHASE OF NURSING PROCESS: Implementation
CLIENT NEEDS: Physiological Integrity
CONTENT AREA: Child Health
REFERENCE
Leifer, G. (1999). *Thompson's introduction to maternity and pediatric nursing* (3rd ed.). Philadelphia: W. B. Saunders. p. 625.

18. 2

RATIONALE: Bed linens should not be placed on the traction ropes because of the risk of disrupting the traction apparatus. Options 1, 3, and 4 are appropriate measures when caring for a child in skeletal traction.
TEST-TAKING STRATEGY: Note the key word "avoids." Use the process of elimination and knowledge regarding the care to the child in traction to assist in directing you to option 2. Review these nursing measures now if you had difficulty with this question.
LEVEL OF COGNITIVE ABILITY: Application
PHASE OF NURSING PROCESS: Implementation
CLIENT NEEDS: Physiological Integrity
CONTENT AREA: Child Health
REFERENCE
Leifer, G. (1999). *Thompson's introduction to maternity and pediatric nursing* (3rd ed.). Philadelphia: W. B. Saunders. p. 625.

19. **4**

RATIONALE: Clubfoot, one of the most common deformities of the skeletal system, is a congenital anomaly characterized by a foot that has been twisted inward or outward. The condition generally affects both feet, and boys are affected twice as often as girls. Many mild forms resolve with little or no treatment if the extremity is allowed unrestricted activity.
TEST-TAKING STRATEGY: Knowledge regarding the characteristics associated with clubfoot is required to answer this question. If you are unfamiliar with this disorder, take time now to review.
LEVEL OF COGNITIVE ABILITY: Comprehension
PHASE OF NURSING PROCESS: Planning
CLIENT NEEDS: Physiological Integrity
CONTENT AREA: Child Health
REFERENCE
Schulte, E., Price, D., & James, S. (1997). *Thompson's pediatric nursing: An introductory text* (7th ed.). Philadelphia: W. B. Saunders. p. 110.

20. **4**

RATIONALE: Synthetic casts dry quickly (in less than 30 minutes) and are lighter than plaster casts. Synthetic casts allow for greater mobility than a plaster cast. However, synthetic casts are not as strong as plaster casts and are more expensive.
TEST-TAKING STRATEGY: Note the key word "synthetic." Use knowledge regarding the differences between a plaster and a synthetic cast to assist in directing you to option 4. If you had difficulty with this question, take time now to review these differences.
LEVEL OF COGNITIVE ABILITY: Application
PHASE OF NURSING PROCESS: Implementation
CLIENT NEEDS: Health Promotion and Maintenance
CONTENT AREA: Child Health
REFERENCE
Schulte, E., Price, D., & James, S. (1997). *Thompson's pediatric nursing: An introductory text* (7th ed.). Philadelphia: W. B. Saunders. pp. 110–111.

BIBLIOGRAPHY

Ashwill, J., & Droske, S. (1997). *Nursing care of children: Principles and practice.* Philadelphia: W. B. Saunders.

Bowden, V., Dickey, S., & Greenberg, C. (1998). *Children and their families: The continuum of care.* Philadelphia: W. B. Saunders.

Leifer, G. (1999). *Thompson's introduction to maternity and pediatric nursing* (3rd ed.). Philadelphia: W. B. Saunders.

Nichols, F., & Zwelling, E. (1997). *Maternal-newborn nursing: Theory and practice.* Philadelphia: W. B. Saunders.

O'Toole, M. (ed.). (1997). *Miller-Keane encyclopedia & dictionary of medicine, nursing, & allied health* (6th ed.). Philadelphia: W. B. Saunders.

Schulte, E., Price, D., & James, S. (1997). *Thompson's pediatric nursing: An introductory text* (7th ed.). Philadelphia: W. B. Saunders.

CHAPTER 35

Hematological and Oncological Disorders

I. Sickle Cell Anemia

A. Description
1. Caused by the inheritance of a gene for a structurally abnormal portion of the hemoglobin (Hgb) chain
2. The sickle hemoglobin is hemoglobin S (HbS)
3. HbS is sensitive to changes in the oxygen content of the red blood cell
4. Insufficient oxygen causes the cells to assume a sickle shape; the cells become rigid and clumped together, obstructing capillary blood flow
5. Situations that precipitate sickling include hypoxia, low environmental or body temperature, acidosis, strenuous exercise, dehydration, infections, or anesthesia
6. Risk factors include having parents heterozygous for HbS or being African-American
7. The process is reversible, but after repeated sickling the cell becomes permanently sickled
8. Treatment focuses on the prevention and treatment of crisis

B. Data collection
1. The clinical hallmark of sickle cell disease is the acute pain crisis, which occurs secondary to vaso-occlusion
2. Other significant crisis events are infections, acute splenic sequestration (blood is sequestered in the spleen), and bone marrow aplasia
3. Pain crisis causes pain in the back, ribs, joints, and extremities
4. Sequestration crisis causes splenomegaly, abdominal pain, hypotension, and shock
5. Acute chest syndrome caused by occlusion of the pulmonary vessels results in chest pain, pneumonia, leukocytosis, and hypoxia leading to congestive heart failure and myocardial infarction
6. Peripheral blood smear showing classic distorted sickled erythrocytes
7. Positive HbS screening test
8. Anemia
9. Renal ischemia causing decreased urine concentration

C. Implementation
1. Instruct the child and parents about the importance of avoiding activities that lead to hypoxia
2. Instruct the child and parents to recognize the early signs and symptoms of crisis
3. Inform the parents of the **hereditary** aspects of the disorder

D. Sickle cell crisis
1. Administer oxygen as prescribed
2. Administer pain medication as prescribed
3. Maintain adequate hydration and maintenance of blood flow with oral fluids and IV normal saline as prescribed
4. Remove any constrictive clothing
5. Maintain a position so that the child keeps extremities extended to promote venous return
6. Elevate the head of the bed no more than 30 degrees; do not raise the knee gatch of the bed
7. Maintain room temperature at or above 72°F
8. Monitor peripheral pulses, color, sensation, motion, and capillary refill of extremities
9. Monitor pulse oximetry in fingers and toes

II. Iron Deficiency Anemia

A. Description
1. Iron stores are depleted followed by a reduction in hemoglobin resulting in small red blood cells (RBCs)
2. Results in a decreased supply of iron for the manufacture of hemoglobin in RBCs
3. Commonly results from blood loss, increased

BOX 35–1. Iron-Rich Foods
Liver, especially pork and lamb
Red and organ meats
Kidney beans
Whole-wheat breads and cereals
Green, leafy vegetables
Carrots
Egg yolks
Raisins

metabolic demands, syndromes of gastrointestinal (GI) malabsorption, and dietary inadequacy

B. Data collection
   1. Manifestations of anemia
   2. Weakness
   3. Pallor
C. Implementation
   1. Increase the oral intake of iron and instruct parents and child in food choices that are high in iron (Box 35–1)
   2. Administer iron supplements as prescribed
   3. Instruct in measures to prevent staining of the teeth if liquid iron is prescribed
   4. Instruct in measures to prevent constipation when iron supplements are prescribed

III. Aplastic Anemia

A. Description
   1. A deficiency of circulating blood cells resulting from arrested development of cells within the bone marrow
   2. The cause is associated with chronic exposure to myelotoxic agents
B. Data collection: pancytopenia (a deficiency of erythrocytes, leukocytes, and thrombocytes)
C. Implementation
   1. Blood transfusions will be prescribed; note that transfusions are discontinued as soon as the bone marrow begins to produce RBCs
   2. Immunosuppressive therapy may be prescribed to prevent the destruction of normal RBCs
   3. Prepare the child for splenectomy, which may be prescribed for the child with an enlarged spleen that is destroying normal RBCs or suppressing their development

IV. Hemophilia

A. Description
   1. An X-linked recessive trait
   2. Hemophilia A (classic hemophilia) results from a deficiency of factor VIII
   3. Hemophilia B (Christmas disease) is a deficiency of factor IX
   4. Males inherit hemophilia from their mothers, and females inherit the carrier status from their fathers

   5. Some females who are carriers have an increased tendency to bleed, and, although it is rare, females can have hemophilia if their fathers have the disorder and their mothers are carriers of the genetic disorder
B. Data collection
   1. Abnormal bleeding in response to trauma, dental procedures, or surgery
   2. Joint and muscle hemorrhage
   3. Tendency to bruise easily
   4. Prolonged prothrombin time and a normal bleeding time
C. Implementation
   1. Intravenous factor VIII cryoprecipitate may be prescribed
   2. Monitor for bleeding and maintain bleeding precautions
   3. Monitor for joint pain; immobilize the affected extremity if joint pain occurs
   4. Instruct the parents and child regarding iron-rich foods
   5. Instruct the parents to obtain a Medic-Alert bracelet for the child
   6. Instruct the parents regarding activities for the child, emphasizing the avoidance of contact sports

V. Beta-Thalassemia Major

A. Description
   1. An autosomal recessive disorder
   2. Also called Cooley's anemia and includes a group of disorders characterized by reduced production of one of the globin chains in the synthesis of hemoglobin
   3. The incidence is highest in individuals of Mediterranean descent
B. Data collection
   1. Small size for age
   2. Severe anemia and hypoxia
   3. Fever
   4. Pallor and jaundice
   5. Bone pain
   6. Microcytic, hypochromic RBCs on blood cell analysis
C. Implementation
   1. Instruct in the administration of folic acid (vitamin B_9) as prescribed, which stimulates the production of blood cells
   2. Blood transfusion therapy may be prescribed
   3. Chelation therapy with deferoxamine (Desferal) may be prescribed to prevent organ damage from the elevated levels of iron caused by multiple blood transfusions
   4. Provide genetic counseling

VI. Leukemia (Table 35–1)

A. Description
   1. Malignant exacerbation in the number of leukocytes, usually at an immature stage, in the bone marrow

Table 35–1. Classification of Leukemia

Acute Lymphocytic Leukemia (ALL)	Acute Myelogenous Leukemia (AML)
Mostly lymphoblasts present in bone marrow	Mostly myeloblasts present in bone marrow
Age of onset is less than 15 years	Age of onset is between 15 and 39 years

2. Affects the bone marrow, causing anemia, leukopenia, the production of immature cells, thrombocytopenia, and a decline in immunity
3. The cause is unknown and appears to involve gene damage of cells, leading to the transformation of cells from a normal state to a malignant state
4. Risk factors include genetic, viral, immunological and environmental factors, and exposure to radiation, chemicals, and medications
5. Risk factors in children include those with Down's syndrome or a twin of a child who has had leukemia
6. Peak incidence is age 3 to 5 for acute lymphocytic leukemia (ALL)
7. Is more common in boys than girls after age 1 year

B. Data collection
   1. Anorexia, fatigue, weakness, and weight loss
   2. Pallor and anemia
   3. Bruising and bleeding from the nose or gums, rectal bleeding, and hematuria
   4. Prolonged bleeding after minor abrasions or lacerations
   5. Petechiae
   6. Elevated temperature
   7. Lymphadenopathy and splenomegaly
   8. Headache, bone pain, and joint swelling
   9. Normal, elevated, or a decline in white blood cell (WBC) count
   10. Decreased hemoglobin and hematocrit level and platelet count
   11. Positive bone marrow biopsy identifying leukemic blast phase cells

C. Infection (Box 35–2)
   1. A major cause of death in the immunosuppressed child
   2. Can occur through autocontamination or cross-contamination
   3. Most common sites of infection are the skin, respiratory tract, and GI tract

D. Bleeding (Box 35–3)
   1. During the period of greatest bone marrow suppression (the nadir), the platelet count may be extremely low
   2. Children with platelet counts below 20,000/mm³ may need a platelet transfusion
   3. For children with severe blood loss, packed red blood cells may be prescribed

E. Fatigue and nutrition

1. Assist the child in selecting a well-balanced diet
2. Provide small meals that require little chewing
3. Assist the child in self-care and mobility activities
4. Allow adequate rest periods during care
5. Do not perform activities unless they are essential

F. Chemotherapy
   1. Monitor for infection and bleeding
   2. Protect the child from life-threatening infections for at least 2 to 3 weeks following chemotherapy

---

BOX 35–2. Protecting the Child from Infection

Initiate protective isolation procedures

Maintain the child in a private room and a room with high efficiency particulate air (HEPA) filtration or laminar airflow system if possible

Frequent and thorough handwashing

Strict aseptic technique for all nursing procedures

Keeps supplies for child separate from supplies for other children

Limit the number of caregivers entering the child's room and ensure that anyone entering the child's room is wearing a mask

Reduce exposure to environmental organisms by eliminating raw fruits and vegetables and fresh flowers and by not leaving standing water in the child's room

Be sure that the child's room is cleaned daily

Assist the child with daily bathing using an antimicrobial soap

Assist the child to perform oral hygiene frequently

Initiate a bowel program to prevent constipation and rectal trauma

Avoid invasive procedures as injections, rectal temperatures, and urinary catheterization

Monitor for signs and symptoms of infection

Change wound dressings daily and inspect wounds for redness, swelling, or drainage

Assess urine for color and cloudiness

Assess skin and oral mucous membranes for signs of infection

Encourage the child to cough and deep breathe

Notify the physician if signs of infection are present and prepare to obtain specimens for culture of open lesions, urine, and sputum

Administer prescribed antibiotic, antifungal, and antiviral medication

Instruct the parents to keep the child away from crowds and those with infections

Instruct the parents that the child should not receive immunization with a live virus

Instruct the parents that siblings should receive inactivated polio vaccine (IPV) but may receive the measles-mumps-rubella (MMR) vaccine

Keep any child with chickenpox or any child who has been exposed to the virus away from the child who is immunocompromised

Instruct the parents to inform the teacher that they should be notified immediately if a case of chickenpox occurs in another child at school

---

BOX 35–3. Protecting the Child from Bleeding

Examine the child for signs and symptoms of bleeding

Handle the child gently

Instruct the child to use a soft toothbrush and to avoid dental floss

Provide soft foods that are cool to warm

Avoid injections if possible to prevent trauma to the skin and bleeding

Apply firm and gentle pressure to a needlestick site for at least 10 minutes

Pad side rails and sharp corners of the bed and furniture

Discourage the child from engaging in activities involving the use of sharp objects

Instruct the child to avoid constrictive or tight clothing

Use caution when taking blood pressures to prevent skin injury

Instruct the child to avoid blowing the nose

Avoid rectal suppositories, enemas, and thermometers

Examine all body fluids and excrement for the presence of blood

Count the number of pads or tampons used if the female adolescent is menstruating

Instruct the child in the signs and symptoms of bleeding

Instruct the parents to avoid administering nonsteroidal anti-inflammatory drugs (NSAIDs) and products that contain aspirin to the child

---

3. Monitor for nausea, vomiting, and diarrhea
4. Check the oral mucous membranes for stomatitis
5. Instruct the parents in signs and symptoms to monitor following chemotherapy and when to notify the physician
6. Inform the parents that hair loss may occur from chemotherapy
7. Reinforce information about the care of central venous access devices as necessary
8. Listen and encourage the child and family to verbalize their feelings and express their concerns
9. Introduce the family to other families of children with cancer
10. Consult social services and chaplains as necessary

VII. Hodgkin's Disease

A. Description
1. A malignancy of the lymph nodes that originates in a single lymph node or a single chain of nodes
2. Usually involves lymph nodes, tonsils, spleen, and bone marrow
3. Metastasis occurs to other adjacent lymph structures and eventually invades nonlymphoid tissue

4. Characterized by the presence of Reed-Sternberg cells in the lymph nodes
5. Possible causes include viral infections and previous exposure to chemical agents
6. Prognosis is dependent on the stage of disease
7. Occurs more often in boys in children under age 15
8. Diagnosis is usually made in the teenage to adult years

B. Data collection
1. Persistent fever and night sweats
2. Loss of appetite, fatigue, weakness, and significant weight loss
3. Anemia and thrombocytopenia
4. Enlarged lymph nodes, spleen, and liver
5. Positive biopsy of lymph nodes with cervical nodes most often affected first
6. Presence of Reed-Sternberg cells
7. Positive computed tomography (CT) scan of liver and spleen

C. Implementation
1. In the early stages without mediastinal node involvement, the treatment of choice is extensive external radiation of the involved lymph node regions; with more extensive disease, radiation along with chemotherapy is used
2. Monitor for side effects related to chemotherapy or radiation
3. Monitor for medication-induced blood disorders, which increases the risk for infection, bleeding, and anemia
4. Protect the child from infection
5. Provide a safe, hazard-free environment

VIII. Nephroblastoma (Wilms' Tumor)

A. Description
1. A tumor of the kidney that may present unilaterally and localized or bilaterally, sometimes with metastasis to other organs
2. Average age of occurrence is between 2 and 6 years
3. This tumor grows very rapidly and prognosis depends on the stage of the disease at the time of diagnosis
4. Treatment may include chemotherapy alone or in combination with radiation and nephrectomy

B. Data collection
1. Mobile abdominal mass
2. Abdominal pain
3. Urinary retention and/or hematuria
4. Hypertension
5. Fever
6. Malaise
7. Anemia

C. Implementation preoperatively
1. Monitor vital signs
2. Measure abdominal girth

3. Avoid palpation of the abdomen
4. Place a sign at bedside: "Do Not Palpate Abdomen"

D. Implementation postoperatively
 1. Monitor vital signs
 2. Monitor for changes in blood pressure
 3. Monitor for signs of hemorrhage and infection
 4. Maintain strict I&O measurements
 5. Monitor urine output closely
 6. Monitor for abdominal distention and for bowel sounds

IX. Neuroblastoma

A. Description
 1. An embryonal tumor found in children that arises from the neural crest
 2. Typically, the tumor infringes on adjacent normal tissue and organs
 3. Most commonly seen in the chest and neck, abdomen, and adrenal gland
 4. A 24-hour urine will be collected to assess for elevated catecholamines

B. Data collection
 1. Profuse diarrhea
 2. Anorexia, weight loss
 3. Fatigue and malaise, irritability
 4. Palpable mass
 5. Symptoms related to a neck and chest mass such as cough, respiratory dysfunction, and neck and facial edema
 6. Symptoms related to bone marrow involvement such as anemia, bleeding, and infection
 7. Symptoms related to cervical and thoracic masses
 8. Neurological symptoms and paralysis related to pressure of the mass on the spinal column

C. Implementation
 1. Treatment depends on the presence and extent of metastasis
 2. Early stage disease without metastasis may only require surgical excision of the tumor and follow-up evaluations
 3. Children with later-stage disease may receive radiation to tumor sites and chemotherapy for several months

D. Implementation preoperatively
 1. Monitor for signs and symptoms related to the location of the tumor
 2. Monitor vital signs
 3. Monitor neurological status and for signs of increased intracranial pressure (ICP)
 4. Obtain abdominal and cranial measurements
 5. Monitor for signs of infection
 6. Provide emotional support to the child and parents

E. Implementation postoperatively
 1. Monitor vital signs and neurological status
 2. Monitor abdominal girth and cranial measurements

3. Monitor I&O and for signs of fluid overload
4. Elevate the head of the bed to the semi-Fowler's position
5. Monitor for signs of infection
6. Provide pain relief measures
7. Instruct the parents about long-term management
8. Refer the parents to appropriate community services

X. Osteogenic Sarcoma

A. Description
 1. An aggressive tumor and the most common bone malignancy in children
 2. Usually found in the metaphysis of long bones, especially in the lower extremities
 3. Symptoms in its earliest stage are almost always attributed to extremity injury or normal growing pains
 4. Peak age of incidence is in the teenage years

B. Data collection
 1. Progressive intermittent pain
 2. Palpable mass
 3. Limping if weight-bearing limb is affected
 4. Progressive limited range of motion
 5. Pathological fractures at tumor site

C. Implementation
 1. Prepare the child and family for prescribed treatment modalities, which may include surgical resection by limb salvage to remove affected tissue, amputation, and chemotherapy
 2. Provide honesty and support for the child and family
 3. Prepare for prosthetic fitting as necessary
 4. Assist the child in dealing with problems of self-image

XI. Ewing's Sarcoma

A. Description
 1. A tumor that invades the soft tissue around the bone, especially the femur, vertebrae, ribs, and pelvic bones
 2. Peak incidence is age 7 to 12 years

B. Data collection
 1. Pain
 2. Soft tissue swelling around the affected bone
 3. Neurological symptoms if a vertebral tumor is present
 4. Respiratory symptoms if a rib tumor is present
 5. Anorexia, fever, malaise, fatigue, and weight loss if metastatic disease is present

C. Implementation: prepare the child and family for treatments that may include chemotherapy, radiation, or excision of the tumor

XII. Brain Tumors

A. Description
 1. The most common solid tumor and the

second most common type of cancer in children after leukemia

2. The cause is unknown, but heredity and environmental factors are both associated

3. Treatment can be devastating to the child's cognition and overall developmental progress

B. Data collection
1. Vomiting on arising, which becomes progressively more projectile
2. Headaches that worsen on arising and improve during the day
3. Lethargy
4. Behavioral changes
5. Ataxia, visual changes, papilledema
6. Seizures
7. Positive Babinski's sign
8. Cranial enlargement and bulging fontanel in infants
9. Nuccal rigidity

C. Implementation
1. Initial intervention is "debulking" or removal of as much of the tumor as possible while minimally disturbing surrounding brain tissue
2. A ventriculoperitoneal **shunt** may be inserted to relieve symptoms of hydrocephalus
3. Dexamethasone (Decadron) may be administered to reduce brain tissue swelling that occurs during surgery
4. Radiation and chemotherapy may be instituted

D. Implementation preoperatively
1. Monitor vital signs and neurological status
2. Institute safety measures and seizure precautions
3. Prepare the child as much as possible
4. The child's head will be shaved; provide a favorite cap or hat for the child
5. Prepare the child to wake up with a large head dressing

E. Implementation postoperatively
1. Monitor vital signs and neurological status frequently
2. Monitor for signs of increased ICP or hemorrhage
3. Monitor temperature, which may be elevated because of hypothalamus or brain stem involvement during surgery
4. Maintain a cooling blanket by the bedside
5. Monitor the back of the head dressing for posterior pooling of blood
6. Monitor for colorless drainage, which may indicate cerebrospinal fluid (CSF) and should be reported immediately
7. Check the physician's order for positioning, as the head of the bed is elevated to promote drainage; if a tumor was removed, the child may lie flat
8. Never place the child in the Trendelenburg position
9. Provide a quiet environment and administer pain medication as prescribed
10. Monitor for functional deficits

PRACTICE QUESTIONS

1. The pediatric nursing instructor asks the nursing student to describe the cause of the clinical manifestations that occur in sickle cell disease (SCD). Which of the following is the appropriate response by the nursing student?
   1 "Sickled cells increase the blood flow through the body and cause a great deal of pain."
   2 "The sickled cells mix with the unsickled cells and cause the immune system to become depressed."
   3 "Bone marrow depression occurs because of the development of sickled cells."
   4 "Sickled cells are unable to flow easily through the microvasculature and their clumping obstructs blood flow."

2. A child with sickle cell disease (SCD) is admitted to the hospital for treatment of vaso-occlusive pain crisis. The oxygen saturation level is 92%. The nurse prepares to administer care for the child. Which of the following is not a component of the plan of care?
   1 Monitoring IV fluids for rehydration
   2 Administering meperidine (Demerol) for pain management
   3 Administering oxygen
   4 Increasing fluid intake

3. The nurse instructs the mother of a child with sickle cell disease (SCD) regarding the precipitating factors related to pain crisis. The nurse provides instructions, knowing that which of the following is not a precipitating factor?
   1 Infection
   2 Trauma
   3 Fluid overload
   4 Stress

4. Oral iron supplements are prescribed for the 6-year-old child with iron deficiency anemia (IDA). The nurse instructs the mother to administer the iron with which of the following food items?
   1 Water
   2 Milk
   3 Apple juice
   4 Orange juice

5. The nurse caring for a child with aplastic anemia reviews the laboratory results and notes a WBC count of 6000/μl and a platelet count of 27,000/mm^3. Which of the following nursing interventions does the nurse suggest to incorporate into the plan of care?
   1 Maintain strict isolation precautions
   2 Encourage naps
   3 Encourage a diet high in iron
   4 Encourage quiet play activities

6. The nursing instructor asks a nursing student about the etiology of hemophilia. The student responds by telling the instructor that

1 Hemophilia is a Y-linked hereditary disorder
2 Males inherit hemophilia from their fathers
3 Females inherit hemophilia from their mothers
4 Hemophilia A results from deficiency of factor VIII

7. The nurse reinforces instructions regarding home care to the parents of a 3-year-old child hospitalized with hemophilia. Which of the following is not a component of the instructions?
   1 Supervise the child closely
   2 Pad corners of the furniture
   3 Remove household items that can easily fall over
   4 Avoid immunizations and dental hygiene

8. The nurse is reinforcing home care instructions to the mother of a 10-year-old child with hemophilia. Which of the following activities does the nurse suggest that the child could safely participate with peers?
   1 Basketball
   2 Swimming
   3 Soccer
   4 Field hockey

9. A nursing student is presenting a clinical conference and discusses the etiology related to beta thalassemia. The nursing student informs the group that the child at greatest risk of developing this disorder is
   1 A child whose intake of iron is extremely poor
   2 A breast-fed child by a mother with chronic anemia
   3 A child of Mediterranean descent
   4 A child of Mexican descent

10. A 4-year-old child is admitted to the hospital for abdominal pain. The mother reports that the child has been pale, excessively tired, and is bruising very easily. On physical examination, lymphadenopathy and hepatosplenomegaly are noted. Diagnostic studies are being performed on the child because acute lymphocytic leukemia (ALL) is suspected. The nurse understands that which of the following laboratory studies will confirm this diagnosis?
    1 White blood cell count
    2 A lumbar puncture
    3 Bone marrow biopsy
    4 A platelet count

11. The nurse reinforces instructions to the parents of a child with leukemia regarding measures related to monitoring for infection. Which of the following is not a component in the instructions?
    1 Proper handwashing techniques
    2 Taking a rectal temperature daily
    3 Inspecting the skin daily for redness
    4 Inspecting the mouth daily for lesions

12. A 6-year-old child with leukemia is hospitalized and is receiving chemotherapy. Laboratory results indicate that the child is neutropenic, and protective isolation procedures are initiated. The grandmother of the child visits and brings a fresh bouquet of flowers picked from her garden and asks the nurse for a vase for the flowers. Which of the following is the most appropriate response to the grandmother?
    1 "I have a vase in the utility room and I will get it for you."
    2 "The flowers from your garden are beautiful, but should not be placed in the child's room at this time."
    3 "I will get the vase and wash it well before you put the flowers in it."
    4 "When you bring the flowers into the room, place them on the bedside stand as far away from the child as possible."

13. A child with leukemia is complaining of nausea. The nurse suspects that the nausea is related to the medication therapy. The nurse, concerned about the child's nutritional status, most appropriately offers which of the following during this episode of nausea?
    1 The child's favorite foods
    2 Cool, clear liquids
    3 Low-protein foods
    4 Low-calorie foods

14. The nurse is reviewing the health record of a 10-year-old child suspected of having Hodgkin's disease. Which of the following does the nurse expect to note documented in the record that is most characteristic of this disease?
    1 Painful, enlarged inguinal lymph nodes
    2 Fever and malaise
    3 Painless, firm, and movable adenopathy in the cervical area
    4 Anorexia and weight loss

15. A 4-year-old child is hospitalized with a suspected diagnosis of Wilms' tumor. The nurse assists in developing a plan of care and suggests to include avoiding which of the following?
    1 Palpating the abdomen for a mass
    2 Checking the urine for the presence of hematuria
    3 Monitoring the temperature for the presence of fever
    4 Monitoring the blood pressure for the presence of hypertension

16. A diagnostic work-up is performed on a 1-year-old child suspected of a diagnosis of neuroblastoma. Which of the following findings most specifically associated with this type of tumor does the nurse expect to note documented in the child's record?
    1 Elevated VMA levels in the urine
    2 The presence of blast cells in the bone marrow

3 Projectile vomiting occurring most often in the morning

4 Positive Babinski's sign

17. The student nurse is conducting a clinical conference and is discussing osteogenic sarcoma. Which of the following is not a component of the information provided by the student during this conference?

   1 The symptoms of the disease in the early stage are almost always attributed to normal growing pains

   2 The femur is the most common site of this sarcoma

   3 Limping, if a weight-bearing limb is affected, is a clinical manifestation

   4 The child does not experience pain at the primary tumor site

18. A 13-year-old child is diagnosed with a Ewing's sarcoma of the femur. Following a course of chemotherapy, it has been decided that leg amputation is necessary. Following the amputation, the child becomes very frightened because of aching and cramping felt in the missing limb. Which of the following is the most appropriate nursing statement to assist in alleviating the child's fear?

   1 "This aching and cramping are normal and temporary and will subside."

   2 "This normally occurs after the surgery and we will teach you ways to deal with it."

   3 "The pain medication that I give you will take these feelings away."

   4 "This pain is not real pain and relaxation exercises will help it go away."

19. A child with a brain tumor is admitted to the hospital for "debulking" of the tumor. To ensure a safe environment for this child, the nurse suggests to include which of the following in the plan of care?

   1 Assisting the child with ambulation at all times

   2 Avoiding contact with other children on the nursing unit

   3 Initiating seizure precautions

   4 Using a wheelchair for out-of-bed activities

20. The nurse is monitoring for bleeding in a child following surgery for removal of a brain tumor. The nurse checks the head dressing for the presence of blood and notes a colorless drainage on the back of the dressing. Which of the following is the most appropriate nursing intervention?

   1 Circle the area of drainage and continue to monitor

   2 Reinforce the dressing

   3 Notify the registered nurse (RN)

   4 Document the findings and continue to monitor

ANSWERS

1. **4**

RATIONALE: All of the clinical manifestations of SCD are a result of the sickled cells being unable to flow easily through the microvasculature, and their clumping obstructs blood flow. With reoxygenation, most of the sickled RBCs resume their normal shape. Options 1, 2, and 3 are inaccurate.

TEST-TAKING STRATEGY: Recalling that sickled cells clump will assist in directing you to the correction option. Review the pathophysiology associated with SCD now if you had difficulty with this question.

LEVEL OF COGNITIVE ABILITY: Comprehension

PHASE OF NURSING PROCESS: Evaluation

CLIENT NEEDS: Physiological Integrity

CONTENT AREA: Child Health

REFERENCE

Schulte, E., Price, D., & James, S. (1997). *Thompson's pediatric nursing: An introductory text* (7th ed.). Philadelphia: W. B. Saunders. p. 160.

2. **2**

RATIONALE: Management of severe pain that occurs with vaso-occlusive crisis includes the use of strong narcotic analgesics such as morphine sulfate and hydromorphone hydrochloride. Demerol is contraindicated because of its side effects and increased risk of seizures. Oxygen is adminis-

tered when hypoxia is present and the oxygen saturation level is less than 95%. Increased fluid intake both orally and by IV are important components of care.

TEST-TAKING STRATEGY: Note the key word "not" in the stem of the question. Noting that the oxygen saturation level is 92% will assist in eliminating option 3. Eliminate options 1 and 4, knowing that hydration is necessary, and because these options are similar. Review care to the client with SCD now if you had difficulty with this question.

LEVEL OF COGNITIVE ABILITY: Application

PHASE OF NURSING PROCESS: Planning

CLIENT NEEDS: Physiological Integrity

CONTENT AREA: Child Health

REFERENCE

Bowden, V., Dickey, S., & Greenberg, C. (1998). *Children and their families: The continuum of care.* Philadelphia: W. B. Saunders. p. 1578.

3. **3**

RATIONALE: Pain crisis may be precipitated by infection, dehydration, hypoxia, trauma, or general stress. The mother of a child with SCD should encourage fluid intake of 1.5 to 2 times the daily requirement to prevent dehydration.

TEST-TAKING STRATEGY: Note the key word "not." Recalling that fluids are a main component of treatment in SCD to prevent dehydration and pain crisis will direct you to option 3. Review precipitating factors of pain crisis now if you had difficulty with this question.

LEVEL OF COGNITIVE ABILITY: Comprehension
PHASE OF NURSING PROCESS: Implementation
CLIENT NEEDS: Health Promotion and Maintenance
CONTENT AREA: Child Health
REFERENCE

Schulte, E., Price, D., & James, S. (1997). *Thompson's pediatric nursing: An introductory text* (7th ed.). Philadelphia: W. B. Saunders. p. 160.

4. **4**

RATIONALE: Vitamin C increases the absorption of iron by the body. The mother should be instructed to administer the medication with a citrus fruit or juice high in vitamin C.
TEST-TAKING STRATEGY: Recalling that vitamin C increases the absorption of iron will assist in eliminating options 1 and 2. From the remaining options, select option 4 because this food item contains the highest amount of vitamin C.
LEVEL OF COGNITIVE ABILITY: Application
PHASE OF NURSING PROCESS: Implementation
CLIENT NEEDS: Health Promotion and Maintenance
CONTENT AREA: Pharmacology
REFERENCE

Ashwill, J., & Droske, S. (1997). *Nursing care of children: Principles and practice*. Philadelphia: W. B. Saunders. p. 967.

5. **4**

RATIONALE: Precautionary measures to prevent bleeding should be taken when a child has a low platelet count. These include no injections, no rectal temperatures, use of a soft toothbrush, and abstinence from contact sports or activities that could cause an injury. Strict isolation is required if the WBC count is low. Options 2 and 3 are unrelated to the risk of bleeding.
TEST-TAKING STRATEGY: Note that the WBC count is normal and that the platelet count is low. Recall that a low platelet count places the client at risk for bleeding. This will assist in eliminating options 1, 2, and 3. Review normal WBC and platelet counts now if you had difficulty with this question.
LEVEL OF COGNITIVE ABILITY: Comprehension
PHASE OF NURSING PROCESS: Planning
CLIENT NEEDS: Physiological Integrity
CONTENT AREA: Child Health
REFERENCE

Chernecky, C., & Berger, B. (1997). *Laboratory tests and diagnostic procedures* (2nd ed.). Philadelphia: W. B. Saunders. p. 815.

6. **4**

RATIONALE: Males inherit hemophilia from their mothers and females inherit the carrier status from their fathers. Some females who are carriers have an increased tendency to bleed, and, although it is rare, females can have hemophilia if their fathers have the disorder and their mothers are carriers of the genetic disorder. Hemophilia is inherited in a recessive manner via a genetic defect on the X chromosome. Hemophilia A results from a deficiency of factor VIII. Hemophilia B (Christmas disease) is a deficiency of factor IX.
TEST-TAKING STRATEGY: Knowledge regarding hemophilia and related etiology is required to answer the question. Take time now to review this important disorder now if you had difficulty with this question.
LEVEL OF COGNITIVE ABILITY: Comprehension
PHASE OF NURSING PROCESS: Implementation

CLIENT NEEDS: Physiological Integrity
CONTENT AREA: Child Health
REFERENCE

Schulte, E., Price, D., & James, S. (1997). *Thompson's pediatric nursing: An introductory text* (7th ed.). Philadelphia: W. B. Saunders. p. 287.

7. **4**

RATIONALE: The nurse needs to stress the importance of immunizations, dental hygiene, and routine well-child care. Options 1, 2, and 3 are appropriate. The parents are also instructed in the event of blunt trauma, especially trauma involving the joints, and to apply prolonged pressure to superficial wounds until the bleeding has stopped.
TEST-TAKING STRATEGY: Note the key word "not." Knowledge that bleeding is a concern in this disorder will assist in eliminating options 1, 2, and 3 that include measures of protection and safety for the child. If you had difficulty with this question, take time now to review care to the child with hemophilia.
LEVEL OF COGNITIVE ABILITY: Application
PHASE OF NURSING PROCESS: Implementation
CLIENT NEEDS: Health Promotion and Maintenance
CONTENT AREA: Child Health
REFERENCE

Schulte, E., Price, D., & James, S. (1997). *Thompson's pediatric nursing: An introductory text* (7th ed.). Philadelphia: W. B. Saunders. p. 288.

8. **2**

RATIONALE: Children with hemophilia need to avoid contact sports and to take precautions such as wearing elbow and knee pads and helmets with other sports. The safest activity that will prevent injury is swimming.
TEST-TAKING STRATEGY: Note the key word "safely." Recalling that bleeding is a major concern in this condition will assist in directing you to option 2. Eliminate options 1, 3, and 4 because these activities present the potential for injury.
LEVEL OF COGNITIVE ABILITY: Comprehension
PHASE OF NURSING PROCESS: Implementation
CLIENT NEEDS: Health Promotion and Maintenance
CONTENT AREA: Child Health
REFERENCE

Schulte, E., Price, D., & James, S. (1997). *Thompson's pediatric nursing: An introductory text* (7th ed.). Philadelphia: W. B. Saunders. p. 288.

9. **3**

RATIONALE: Beta-thalassemia is inherited by an autosomal recessive pattern. This disorder is found primarily in individuals of Mediterranean descent. The disease has also been reported in Asian and African populations as well.
TEST-TAKING STRATEGY: Knowledge regarding the etiology associated with this disorder is required to answer this question. If you are unfamiliar with this disorder, take time now to review the information associated with its incidence and etiology.
LEVEL OF COGNITIVE ABILITY: Comprehension
PHASE OF NURSING PROCESS: Implementation
CLIENT NEEDS: Physiological Integrity
CONTENT AREA: Child Health
REFERENCE

Ashwill, J., & Droske, S. (1997). *Nursing care of children: Principles and practice*. Philadelphia: W. B. Saunders. p. 975.

10. **3**

RATIONALE: The confirmatory test for leukemia is microscopic examination of bone marrow obtained by bone marrow aspirate and biopsy. A lumbar puncture may be done to look for blast cells in the spinal fluid that are indicative of central nervous system (CNS) disease. The WBC count may be high or low in leukemia. An altered platelet count occurs as a result of chemotherapy.
TEST-TAKING STRATEGY: Note the key word "confirm." Use this key word and knowledge that the bone marrow is affected in leukemia. If you had difficulty with this question, review the significance of the bone marrow biopsy now.
LEVEL OF COGNITIVE ABILITY: Comprehension
PHASE OF NURSING PROCESS: Data Collection
CLIENT NEEDS: Physiological Integrity
CONTENT AREA: Child Health
REFERENCE

Schulte, E., Price, D., & James, S. (1997). *Thompson's pediatric nursing: An introductory text* (7th ed.). Philadelphia: W. B. Saunders. p. 284.

11. **2**

RATIONALE: The risk of injury to fragile mucous membranes is so great in the child with leukemia that only oral, axillary, or tympanic temperatures should be taken. Rectal abscesses can easily occur to damaged rectal tissue. No rectal temperatures should be taken. Additionally oral temperatures should be avoided if the child has oral ulcers. Options 1, 3, and 4 are appropriate teaching measures.
TEST-TAKING STRATEGY: Note the key word "not." Options 1 and 3 can be easily eliminated first. From the remaining options, note the word "rectal" in option 2. Recalling that rectal temperatures should be avoided will direct you to this option. Review home care instructions related to infection in the leukemic child now if you had difficulty with this question.
LEVEL OF COGNITIVE ABILITY: Application
PHASE OF NURSING PROCESS: Planning
CLIENT NEEDS: Health Promotion and Maintenance
CONTENT AREA: Child Health
REFERENCE

Schulte, E., Price, D., & James, S. (1997). *Thompson's pediatric nursing: An introductory text* (7th ed.). Philadelphia: W. B. Saunders. p. 286.

12. **2**

RATIONALE: For the hospitalized neutropenic child, flowers or plants should not be kept in the room because standing water and damp soil harbor *Aspergillus* and *Pseudomonas*, to which these children are very susceptible. Additionally unpeeled fruits and vegetables harbor molds and should be avoided until the WBC count rises.
TEST-TAKING STRATEGY: Knowledge regarding protective isolation procedures required in a neutropenic child will assist in answering this question. Note that options 1 and 3 are similar and should be eliminated first. From the remaining two options, select option 2 over option 4 because this nursing response maintains the procedure required. Review protective isolation procedures for the neutropenic child now if you had difficulty with this question.
LEVEL OF COGNITIVE ABILITY: Application
PHASE OF NURSING PROCESS: Implementation
CLIENT NEEDS: Safe, Effective Care Environment
CONTENT AREA: Child Health

REFERENCE

Schulte, E., Price, D., & James, S. (1997). *Thompson's pediatric nursing: An introductory text* (7th ed.). Philadelphia: W. B. Saunders. p. 285.

13. **2**

RATIONALE: When the child is nauseated, it is best to offer cool clear liquids because they are soothing and better tolerated. It is best not to offer favorite foods when the child is nauseated because foods eaten then will be associated with being sick. It is best to offer small frequent meals of high-protein, high-calorie content.
TEST-TAKING STRATEGY: The issue of the question relates to nutritional status in a child with nausea. You should easily be able to eliminate options 3 and 4. From the remaining two options, you may be tempted to select option 1. Recalling the issue related to nausea will assist in directing you to option 2. Review interventions related to these issues now if you had difficulty with this question.
LEVEL OF COGNITIVE ABILITY: Comprehension
PHASE OF NURSING PROCESS: Implementation
CLIENT NEEDS: Physiological Integrity
CONTENT AREA: Child Health
REFERENCE

Ashwill, J., & Droske, S. (1997). *Nursing care of children: Principles and practice*. Philadelphia: W. B. Saunders. p. 1005.

14. **3**

RATIONALE: Clinical manifestations specifically associated with Hodgkin's disease include painless, firm, and movable adenopathy in the cervical and supraclavicular area. Hepatosplenomegaly is also noted. Although anorexia, weight loss, fever, and malaise are associated with Hodgkin's disease, these manifestations are seen in many disorders.
TEST-TAKING STRATEGY: Note the key word "most." Eliminate options 2 and 4 first because these symptoms are general and vague. Recalling that painless adenopathy is associated with Hodgkin's disease will direct you to option 3. Review the clinical manifestations related to Hodgkin's disease now if you had difficulty with this question.
LEVEL OF COGNITIVE ABILITY: Comprehension
PHASE OF NURSING PROCESS: Data Collection
CLIENT NEEDS: Physiological Integrity
CONTENT AREA: Child Health
REFERENCE

Schulte, E., Price, D., & James, S. (1997). *Thompson's pediatric nursing: An introductory text* (7th ed.). Philadelphia: W. B. Saunders. p. 412.

15. **1**

RATIONALE: If Wilms' tumor is suspected, the tumor mass should not be palpated. Excessive manipulation can cause seeding of the tumor and cause spread of the cancerous cells. Fever, hematuria, and hypertension are clinical manifestations associated with Wilms' tumor.
TEST-TAKING STRATEGY: Note the key word "avoid." Knowledge that this tumor is located in the kidney will assist in eliminating options 2, 3, and 4 because of the relationship of these options to renal function. If you are unfamiliar with the care of the child with Wilms' tumor, take time now to review.
LEVEL OF COGNITIVE ABILITY: Analysis
PHASE OF NURSING PROCESS: Planning
CLIENT NEEDS: Physiological Integrity
CONTENT AREA: Child Health

REFERENCE
Schulte, E., Price, D., & James, S. (1997). *Thompson's pediatric nursing: An introductory text* (7th ed.). Philadelphia: W. B. Saunders. pp. 238–239.

16. **1**

RATIONALE: Neuroblastoma is a solid tumor found only in children. It arises from neural crest cells, which develop into the sympathetic nervous system and the adrenal medulla. Typically the tumor infringes on adjacent normal tissue and organs. Neuroblastoma cells may excrete catecholamines and their metabolites. Urine samples will indicate elevated VMA levels. The presence of blast cells in the bone marrow occurs in leukemia. Projectile vomiting occurring most often in the morning and a positive Babinski's sign are clinical manifestations of a brain tumor.
TEST-TAKING STRATEGY: Use the process of elimination. If you are unfamiliar with this type of tumor, recall that blast cells are noted in leukemia, and eliminate option 2. Next eliminate options 3 and 4, noting that these manifestations are found in the child with a brain tumor. Review the manifestations associated with neuroblastoma now if you had difficulty with this question.
LEVEL OF COGNITIVE ABILITY: Comprehension
PHASE OF NURSING PROCESS: Data Collection
CLIENT NEEDS: Physiological Integrity
CONTENT AREA: Child Health
REFERENCE
Ashwill, J., & Droske, S. (1997). *Nursing care of children: Principles and practice*. Philadelphia: W. B. Saunders. p. 1018.

17. **4**

RATIONALE: A clinical manifestation of osteogenic sarcoma is progressive, insidious, intermittent pain at the tumor site. By the time these children receive medical attention, they may be in considerable pain from the tumor. Options 1, 2, and 3 are accurate regarding osteogenic sarcoma.
TEST-TAKING STRATEGY: Note the key word "not." Knowledge that osteogenic sarcoma is a malignant tumor of the bone will easily direct you to option 4. Review the clinical manifestations associated with osteogenic sarcoma now if you had difficulty with this question.
LEVEL OF COGNITIVE ABILITY: Comprehension
PHASE OF NURSING PROCESS: Implementation
CLIENT NEEDS: Physiological Integrity
CONTENT AREA: Child Health
REFERENCE
Leifer, G. (1999). *Thompson's introduction to maternity and pediatric nursing* (3rd ed.). Philadelphia: W. B. Saunders. p. 663.

18. **1**

RATIONALE: Following amputation, phantom limb pain is a temporary condition that some children may experience. This sensation of burning, aching, or cramping in the missing limb is most distressing to the child. The child needs to be reassured that the condition is normal and only temporary.
TEST-TAKING STRATEGY: Use therapeutic communication techniques to answer this question. Note that the issue of the question relates to alleviating the child's fear. Option 1 is the only option that will alleviate fear. Options 2, 3, and 4 infer that this pain may be permanent.
LEVEL OF COGNITIVE ABILITY: Application
PHASE OF NURSING PROCESS: Implementation
CLIENT NEEDS: Psychosocial Integrity
CONTENT AREA: Child Health
REFERENCE
Ashwill, J., & Droske, S. (1997). *Nursing care of children: Principles and practice*. Philadelphia: W. B. Saunders. p. 1020.

19. **3**

RATIONALE: Seizure precautions should be considered for any child with a brain tumor, both preoperatively and postoperatively. A thorough neurological assessment should be performed on the child, and the child's safety should be assessed prior to allowing the child to get out of bed without help. Options 1 and 4 are not required unless functional deficits exist. Option 2 is not necessary.
TEST-TAKING STRATEGY: Note the key words "safe environment." Eliminate options 1 and 4 first because they are similar. Additionally, note the words "all times" in option 1. Eliminate option 2 because it is unnecessary. If you had difficulty with this question, review nursing interventions related to the child with a brain tumor.
LEVEL OF COGNITIVE ABILITY: Application
PHASE OF NURSING PROCESS: Planning
CLIENT NEEDS: Safe, Effective Care Environment
CONTENT AREA: Child Health
REFERENCE
Leifer, G. (1999). *Thompson's introduction to maternity and pediatric nursing* (3rd ed.). Philadelphia: W. B. Saunders. p. 600.

20. **3**

RATIONALE: Colorless drainage on the dressing indicates the presence of cerebrospinal fluid and should be reported to the RN immediately. The RN should then contact the physician. Options 1, 2, and 4 delay required immediate interventions.
TEST-TAKING STRATEGY: Note the key words "colorless drainage." This should quickly alert you to the possibility of the presence of cerebrospinal fluid. You should easily be able to eliminate options 1, 2, and 4. If you had difficulty with this question, review the significance of the presence of colorless drainage following cranial surgery.
LEVEL OF COGNITIVE ABILITY: Application
PHASE OF NURSING PROCESS: Implementation
CLIENT NEEDS: Physiological Integrity
CONTENT AREA: Child Health
REFERENCE
Ashwill, J., & Droske, S. (1997). *Nursing care of children: Principles and practice*. Philadelphia: W. B. Saunders. p. 1017.

BIBLIOGRAPHY

Ashwill, J., & Droske, S. (1997). *Nursing care of children: Principles and practice*. Philadelphia: W. B. Saunders.
Bowden, V., Dickey, S., & Greenberg, C. (1998). *Children and their families: The continuum of care*. Philadelphia: W. B. Saunders.
Chernecky, C., & Berger, B. (1997). *Laboratory tests and diagnostic procedures* (2nd ed.). Philadelphia: W. B. Saunders.

Leifer, G. (1999). *Thompson's introduction to maternity and pediatric nursing* (3rd ed.). Philadelphia: W. B. Saunders.
O'Toole, M. (ed.). (1997). *Miller-Keane encyclopedia & dictionary of medicine, nursing, & allied health* (6th ed.). Philadelphia: W. B. Saunders.
Schulte, E., Price, D., & James, S. (1997). *Thompson's pediatric nursing: An introductory text* (7th ed.). Philadelphia: W. B. Saunders.

CHAPTER 36

Communicable Diseases and Acquired Immunodeficiency Syndrome

. . . .

I. Rubeola (Measles)

A. Description
   1. Incubation period: 7 to 14 days
   2. Infectious period: 1 to 2 days before onset of symptoms to 4 days after the rash appears
   3. Transmission: airborne or direct contact with infectious droplets
   4. Seasons: winter and spring
B. Data collection
   1. Koplik's spots—small, bright red spots with a bluish white speck in the center of each; they are located on the mucosa and last 3 days
   2. Rash is red and maculopapular, blanches easily with pressure, gradually turns a brownish color, and lasts 6 to 7 days
   3. Rash begins behind the ears and spreads downward to the feet
C. Implementation
   1. Respiratory isolation if hospitalized
   2. Restrict to quiet activities and bed rest
   3. Keep skin clean

II. Roseola (Exanthem Subitum)

A. Description
   1. Incubation period: 5 to 15 days
   2. Infectious period: unknown, but thought to extend from the febrile stage to the time the rash first appears
   3. Transmission: saliva
   4. Seasons: spring and fall
B. Data collection
   1. Fever for 3 to 5 days, followed by a rash composed of rose-pink maculas that blanches with pressure
   2. Rash is found on the neck and trunk and is surrounded by a whitish ring
   3. Rash lasts 24 to 48 hours before fading
C. Implementation: supportive

III. Rubella (German Measles)

A. Description
   1. Incubation period: 14 to 21 days
   2. Infectious period: 10 days before the onset of symptoms to 15 days after the rash appears
   3. Transmission
      a. Airborne or direct contact with infectious droplets
      b. Transplacental
   4. Seasons: winter and spring
B. Data collection
   1. Pinkish rose maculopapular rash that begins on the face and spreads to the entire body
   2. Petechial spots may occur on the soft palate
C. Implementation
   1. Contact isolation
   2. Supportive treatment
   3. Isolate from pregnant women

IV. Mumps (Parotitis)

A. Description
   1. Incubation period: 16 to 18 days but may extend to 25 days
   2. Infectious period: usually 1 to 2 days (7 days prior to swelling to 9 days after onset)
   3. Transmission
      a. Airborne droplets
      b. Saliva and possibly urine
   4. Seasons: late winter and spring
B. Data collection: fever, muscular pain, headache, and malaise, followed by parotid glandular swelling
C. Implementation
   1. Respiratory isolation is indicated until 9 days after the onset of parotid swelling
   2. Analgesics for pain
   3. Provide soft foods

V. Chickenpox (Varicella)

A. Description
   1. Incubation period: 10 to 21 days
   2. Infectious period: 1 to 2 days before the onset of rash to 5 days after the onset of lesions and crusting of lesions
   3. Transmission: direct contact with infectious droplets and airborne particles
   4. Seasons: late winter through early spring
B. Data collection
   1. Elevated temperature, malaise, and anorexia, followed by a macular rash that first appears on the trunk and scalp and moves to the extremities
   2. The lesions become pustules, begin to dry, and develop a crust
   3. They appear on the mucous membranes of the mouth, genital area, and rectum
C. Implementation
   1. In the hospital setting, strict isolation
   2. In the home setting, the child is isolated from all individuals susceptible to infection

VI. Pertussis (Whooping Cough)

A. Description
   1. Incubation period: 6 to 20 days
   2. Infectious period: catarrhal stage (1 to 2 weeks) until the fourth week
   3. Transmission: direct contact or respiratory droplets from coughing
   4. Season: can occur during any season
B. Data collection: Symptoms of respiratory infection followed by increased severity of cough
C. Implementation
   1. Hospitalized child is placed in respiratory isolation
   2. Supportive therapy
   3. Antibiotics

VII. Diphtheria

A. Description
   1. Incubation period: 2 to 5 days
   2. Infectious period: ranges from 2 weeks or less up to several months in an untreated individual
   3. Transmission: contact with carrier or disease droplets
   4. Seasons: fall and winter
B. Data collection
   1. Foul-smelling mucopurulent nasal discharge
   2. Gray membrane on tonsils and pharynx
   3. Neck edema
C. Implementation
   1. Respiratory isolation
   2. Supportive therapy
   3. Antibiotics

VIII. Polio (Infantile Paralysis; Poliomyelitis)

A. Description
   1. Incubation period

a. 3 to 6 days for abortive
b. 7 to 21 days for paralytic
   2. Infectious period
      a. Shortly before the onset of illness
      b. The virus is shed in the pharynx for 1 week after onset, and in the feces for several weeks to months
   3. Transmission: fecal-oral, oral-oral
   4. Seasons: summer and fall
B. Data collection
   1. Fever, malaise, anorexia, nausea, headache, and sore throat
   2. Abdominal pain, followed by soreness and stiffness of the trunk, neck, and limbs, which progresses to flaccid paralysis
C. Implementation
   1. Enteric precautions
   2. Supportive treatment
   3. Monitor for respiratory paralysis

IX. Scarlet Fever

A. Description
   1. Incubation period: 1 to 7 days
   2. Infectious period: acute stage until 36 hours after antibiotic therapy is started
   3. Transmission: airborne and direct contact
   4. Seasons: late fall, winter, and spring
B. Data collection
   1. A fine, red, papular rash in the axilla, groin, and neck, which spreads to cover the entire body
   2. The rash blanches with pressure except in areas of deep creases (Pastia's sign)
   3. The tongue has a white furry coating, which progresses to a red, swollen tongue (white strawberry tongue, strawberry tongue)
   4. Tonsils are edematous and covered with a gray-white exudate
   5. Petechial hemorrhage covers the soft palate
C. Implementation
   1. Antibiotics
   2. Supportive therapy

X. Infectious Mononucleosis (Epstein-Barr Virus)

A. Description
   1. Incubation period: 4 to 7 weeks
   2. Infectious period: unknown; virus is shed before onset of disease until 6 months or longer after recovery
   3. Transmission: saliva; close intimate contact, blood
   4. Season: can occur during any season
B. Data collection
   1. Fever, pharyngitis, malaise, headache, fatigue, nausea, and abdominal pain
   2. Lymphadenopathy and hepatosplenomegaly
C. Implementation
   1. Supportive
   2. Monitor for signs of splenic rupture, which

includes abdominal pain, left upper quadrant pain, or left shoulder pain

XI. Rocky Mountain Spotted Fever (RMSF)

A. Description
   1. Incubation period: 2 to 14 days
   2. Transmission: bite of an infected tick
   3. Season: April through September
B. Data collection
   1. Headache, fever, anorexia, restlessness, maculopapular or petechial rash that begins on the palms and soles and spreads to the rest of the body
   2. Hemorrhagic and necrotic lesions can occur
   3. Periorbital edema progressing to generalized edema
C. Implementation
   1. Antibiotic therapy
   2. Preventive teaching regarding the risk of exposure to ticks
   3. Antibiotics and supportive care for presenting symptoms

XII. Enterobius (Pinworm)

A. Transmission
   1. Ingestion or inhalation of eggs
   2. Hands to mouth
   3. Fecal-oral
B. Data collection: nocturnal anal itching and sleeplessness
C. Implementation
   1. Cellophane tape test to identify
   2. Enteric precautions
   3. Anthelmintic medications

XIII. Immunizations

A. Immunization schedule (Box 36–1)
B. Contraindications to immunizations

BOX 36–1. Recommended Immunization Schedule for Healthy Infants and Children

Birth	Hepatitis B
1 month	Hepatitis B
2 months	OPV, DTP, HIB
4 months	OPV, DTP, HIB
6 months	DTP, HIB, hepatitis B
12 months	HIB, OPV
15 months	MMR
18 months	DTP
12–18 months	Varicella vaccine
4–6 years	DTP, OPV, MMR
11–12 years	MMR (if not administered at 4–6 years)
11–16 years	TD booster

DTP, diphtheria, tetanus toxoids, and pertussis; HIB, *Haemophilus influenzae* type B; MMR, measles-mumps-rubella; OPV, oral poliovirus vaccine; TD, tetanus-diphtheria.

---

1. Severe febrile illness
2. Suppressed immune system (NO LIVE VACCINES)
3. Siblings and household contacts of immunosuppressed children should not recieve the oral polio vaccine (OPV) but may be given the inactivated poliovirus vaccine (IPV)
4. Received gamma globulin within past 6 weeks
5. Allergic to contents of immunization (prior to the administration of measles-mumps-rubella [MMR] vaccine, assess for known history of allergy to eggs, neomycin, or related antibiotics)
6. Recent chemotherapy

XIV. Acquired Immunodeficiency Syndrome (AIDS)

A. Description
   1. A disorder caused by the human immunodeficiency virus (HIV) and is characterized by a generalized dysfunction of the immune system
   2. Immunity is compromised
   3. Treatment includes a modified immunization schedule to prevent disease and to provide prophylaxis against opportunistic infections especially *Pneumocystis carinii* pneumonia (PCP)
   4. Medical therapy includes the administration of antiretroviral medications to inhibit viral reproduction and the aggressive use of medications to treat infections
B. Data collection
   1. During neonatal period
      a. Lymphadenopathy
      b. Hepatosplenomegaly
      c. Opportunistic infections
      d. Progressive encephalopathy
      e. Microcephaly
   2. Infants
      a. Failure to thrive
      b. Developmental delays
      c. Oral candidiasis
      d. Diarrhea
      e. Hepatosplenomegaly
      f. Chronic pneumonia and cough
      g. Chronic otitis media
   3. Children/adolescents
      a. Malaise and fatigue
      b. Night sweats
      c. Weight loss
      d. Diarrhea
      e. Fever
      f. **Regression** of developmental milestones
      g. Generalized lymphadenopathy
      h. Nephropathy
      i. Interstitial pneumonitis and *Pneumocystis carinii* pneumonia
      j. Encephalopathy

C. Diagnostic tests
1. ELISA
   a. Enzyme-linked immunosorbent assay (ELISA) determines response of antibodies to HIV virus
   b. Used in children older than 18 months
2. Western blot
   a. Confirms the presence of HIV antibodies
   b. Useful in children older than 18 months of age
   c. A positive HIV antibody test in children younger than 18 months of age indicates only that the mother is infected
3. p24 Antigen
   a. Used to detect HIV antigen in children younger than 18 months
   b. Test can be useful at any age
   c. Only a positive result is significant
   d. Two or more positive results are diagnostic for HIV infection
4. CD4+: Used to assess a child's immune status, risk for disease progression, and the need for PCP prophylaxis after 1 year of age

XV. Care of the Child with AIDS

A. Prophylaxis
1. Prophylaxis may be prescribed against PCP at 4 to 6 weeks of age if exposed perinatally to HIV
2. Continued prophylaxis is provided through 12 months of age for children diagnosed with HIV
3. For HIV-infected children older than 12 months, continued prophylaxis is based on CD4+ counts and whether PCP has previously occurred

B. Parent instructions
1. Frequent handwashing
2. Monitor for fever, malaise, fatigue, weight loss, vomiting and diarrhea, altered activity level, and oral lesions and notify the physician if these occur
3. The signs and symptoms of opportunistic infections
4. The administration of antiretroviral medications as prescribed, side effects, and medication interactions
5. The child should avoid exposure to other illnesses
6. Keep immunizations up to date
7. Keep the child home when sick
8. Do not kiss infant/child on the mouth
9. Monitor weight
10. Provide high-calorie, high-protein diet
11. Do not share eating utensils
12. Wash eating utensils in the dishwasher
13. Cover unused food and formula and refrigerate
14. Discard unused refrigerated formula after 24 hours
15. Wear gloves for care, especially when in contact with body fluids and changing diapers
16. Change diapers frequently away from food areas
17. Fold soiled disposable diapers inward and tab and dispose in a tightly covered plastic-lined container
18. Dispose of trash daily
19. Cover sandboxes when not in use to create a barrier to germs
20. Avoid contact with bird cages and animal litter
21. Clean up body fluid/excretion spills with bleach solution (10:1 ratio of water to bleach)
22. Available support systems

C. Immunizations: Inactivated poliovirus (IPV) is substituted for oral poliovirus (OPV) in the regular immunization schedule

PRACTICE QUESTIONS

1. A child with measles (rubeola) is being admitted to the hospital. In preparing for the admission of the child, which of the following does the nurse suggest to include in the plan of care?
   1 Contact precautions
   2 Enteric precautions
   3 Respiratory isolation
   4 Protective isolation

2. The mother of a 15-month-old child brings the child to the clinic and reports that the child has a fever and has developed a rash on the neck and trunk of the body. Roseola is diagnosed. The mother is concerned that her other children will contract the disease. Which of the following instructions does the nurse provide to the mother regarding the prevention of transmission of the disease?
   1 The disease is transmitted through the urine and feces, so the other children should use a separate bathroom
   2 The disease is transmitted through saliva, so the other children should not share eating utensils
   3 The disease is transmitted through the respiratory tract, so the child should be isolated from the other children as much as possible
   4 The disease is transmitted by contact with body fluids, so any items contaminated with body fluids need to discarded in a separate receptacle

3. The nurse is assigned to care for a child with rubella (German measles). Which of the following protective measures is not necessary when providing direct care to the child?
   1 Mask
   2 Gloves
   3 Gown
   4 Goggles

4. The nurse reinforces instructions to the mother of a child with mumps regarding respiratory isolation procedures. The mother asks the nurse about the length of time required for the respiratory isolation. The most appropriate nursing response is
   1 "Respiratory isolation is not necessary."
   2 "Mumps is not transmitted by the respiratory system."
   3 "Respiratory isolation is indicated for 9 days following the onset of parotid swelling."
   4 "Respiratory isolation is indicated for 18 days following the onset of parotid swelling."

5. The parents of a child with mumps express concern that their child will develop orchitis as a result of having mumps. The parents ask the nurse about the complication and about the signs that may indicate this complication. Which of the following is not a part of the nurse's response to the parents?
   1 Abrupt onset of pain
   2 Heacache and vomiting
   3 Fever and chills
   4 Difficulty urinating

6. The nurse reinforces home care instructions to the parents of a child hospitalized with pertussis. The child is in the convalescent stage and is being prepared for discharge. Which of the following is not a component of the instruction?
   1 Maintain respiratory isolation and a quiet environment for at least 2 weeks
   2 Coughing spells may be triggered by noises or episodes of fright
   3 Encourage fluid intake
   4 Good handwashing techniques must be instituted to prevent spreading the disease to others

7. A nursing instructor asks a nursing student about the contraindications associated with the administration of oral poliovirus vaccine (OPV). The student is asked information about the administration of OPV to siblings of an immunocompromised child. The most appropriate response by the nursing student is
   1 "The viruses in OPV multiply in the vaccinee's respiratory tract and can then be transmitted with breathing and coughing."
   2 "OPV is not contraindicated in siblings of an immunocompromised child."
   3 "The viruses in OPV multiply in the vaccinee's GI tract and can then be transmitted in saliva and feces."
   4 "OPV is not contraindicated as long as the siblings and immunocompromised child do not share food or utensils."

8. A child is diagnosed with scarlet fever. The nurse reviews the child's health record for documentation of the clinical manifestations associated with this disorder. Which of the following is not a clinical manifestation associated with this disease?
   1 Pastia's sign
   2 White strawberry tongue
   3 Petechial hemorrhages on the soft palate
   4 Koplik's spots

9. The nurse reinforces home care instructions to the parents of a child with Epstein-Barr virus (mononucleosis). Which of the following does the nurse include in the instructions?
   1 Maintain bed rest for 2 weeks
   2 Maintain respiratory isolation precautions for 1 week
   3 Notify the physician if the child develops a fever
   4 Notify the physician if abdominal pain or left shoulder pain occurs

10. The mother of a preschooler who attends day care calls the nurse at the clinic and tells the nurse that the child is constantly itching the perianal area and that the area is irritated. The nurse suspects the possibility of pinworm (enterobius) infection. The nurse instructs the mother to obtain a cellophane tape rectal specimen. Which of the following is the appropriate instruction regarding obtaining this specimen?
    1 Obtain the specimen when you put the child to bed
    2 Obtain the specimen after toileting
    3 Obtain the specimen after bathing
    4 Obtain the specimen in the morning when the child awakens

11. The nurse employed in a well-baby clinic prepares to administer immunizations. Which of the following conditions, if present in a child, is a contraindication for receiving an immunization?
    1 Cold
    2 Otitis media
    3 Diarrhea
    4 Fever

12. A child with an HIV-infected mother is seen in the clinic on a monthly basis and is being monitored for symptoms indicative of AIDS. The nurse understands that the most common disease indicative of AIDS in children is
    1 Gastorenteritis
    2 Meningitis
    3 *Pneumocystis carinii* pneumonia (PCP)
    4 Lymphoid interstitial pneumonia (LIP)

13. The clinic nurse is reinforcing instructions to the mother of a child with HIV regarding immunizations. Which of the following does the nurse include in the instructions?
    1 Household members need to avoid receiving the influenza vaccine

2 Siblings need to receive inactivated poliovaccine (IPV)

3 The hepatitis B vaccine is not to be given to the child

4 A Western blot needs to be evaluated prior to immunizations

14. The nurse is caring for a 4-year-old child with a diagnosis of HIV infection. In planning care to address the psychosocial issues, the nurse expects that this child
    1 Is unable to grasp the concept of illness and death
    2 Begins to understand that something is wrong

3 Begins to conceptualize the death process as involving physical harm

4 Will express fear, withdrawal, and denial

15. The home care nurse reinforces instructions regarding basic infection control to the parents of a child with HIV infection. Which of the following is not a component of these instructions?
    1 Carefully wash all fresh fruits and vegetables
    2 Wash baby bottles, nipples, and pacifiers in the dishwasher
    3 Discard any unused food and formula immediately
    4 Rub the inside of the nipple with salt and rinse well if it becomes slimy

ANSWERS

1. **3**

RATIONALE: Rubeola is transmitted via airborne particles or direct contact with infectious droplets. Respiratory isolation is required and a mask should be worn by those in contact with the child. Gowns and gloves are not indicated. Articles that are contaminated should be bagged and labeled. Options 1, 2 and 4 are not indicated in rubeola.
TEST-TAKING STRATEGY: Knowledge regarding the route of transmission is required to answer this question. This knowledge will easily direct you to option 3. Review the route of transmission and therapeutic management now if you had difficulty with this question.
LEVEL OF COGNITIVE ABILITY: Application
PHASE OF NURSING PROCESS: Planning
CLIENT NEEDS: Safe, Effective Care Environment
CONTENT AREA: Child Health
REFERENCE
Schulte, E., Price, D., & James, S. (1997). *Thompson's pediatric nursing: An introductory text* (7th ed.). Philadelphia: W. B. Saunders. p. 296.

2. **2**

RATIONALE: Roseola is transmitted via saliva; therefore, others should not share eating utensils. Options 1, 3, and 4 are not accurate transmission routes of roseola.
TEST-TAKING STRATEGY: Eliminate options 1 and 4 first because they are similar. From the remaining two options, recalling that roseola is transmitted via saliva will assist in directing you to option 2. Review the route of transmission of roseola now if you had difficulty with this question.
LEVEL OF COGNITIVE ABILITY: Application
PHASE OF NURSING PROCESS: Implementation
CLIENT NEEDS: Health Promotion and Maintenance
CONTENT AREA: Child Health
REFERENCE
Schulte, E., Price, D., & James, S. (1997). *Thompson's pediatric nursing: An introductory text* (7th ed.). Philadelphia: W. B. Saunders. p. 296.

3. **4**

RATIONALE: Care of the child with rubella involves contact isolation. Contact isolation requires masks, gowns, and gloves for contact with any infectious material. Contaminated articles must be bagged and labeled per agency protocol.
TEST-TAKING STRATEGY: Note the key words "not" and "direct" in the stem of the question. Recalling that rubella is transmitted via airborne particles or direct contact with infectious droplets will assist in directing you to option 4 as the item not required when providing direct care to this child. If you had difficulty with this question, take time now to review the modes of transmission for rubella.
LEVEL OF COGNITIVE ABILITY: Application
PHASE OF NURSING PROCESS: Implementation
CLIENT NEEDS: Safe, Effective Care Environment
CONTENT AREA: Child Health
REFERENCE
Schulte, E., Price, D., & James, S. (1997). *Thompson's pediatric nursing: An introductory text* (7th ed.). Philadelphia: W. B. Saunders. p. 296.

4. **3**

RATIONALE: Mumps is transmitted via airborne droplets, salivary secretions, and possibly by contact with urine. Uncomplicated mumps may require only symptomatic care. Respiratory isolation is indicated for 9 days following the onset of parotid swelling.
TEST-TAKING STRATEGY: Knowledge regarding the infectious period for mumps is required to answer this question. Options 1 and 2 can be eliminated first because they are similar. From the remaining two options, select option 3 because the time frame indicated in option 4 seems rather lengthy. Review the infectious period related to mumps now if you had difficulty with this question.
LEVEL OF COGNITIVE ABILITY: Comprehension
PHASE OF NURSING PROCESS: Implementation
CLIENT NEEDS: Safe, Effective Care Environment
CONTENT AREA: Child Health
REFERENCE
Schulte, E., Price, D., & James, S. (1997). *Thompson's pediatric nursing: An introductory text* (7th ed.). Philadelphia: W. B. Saunders. p. 296.

5. **4**

RATIONALE: Unilateral orchitis occurs more frequently than bilateral orchitis. About 1 week after the appearance of parotitis, there is an abrupt onset of pain, tenderness, fever, chills, headache, and vomiting. The affected testicle

becomes red, swollen, and tender. Atrophy resulting in sterility occurs only in a small number of cases. Difficulty urinating is not a sign of this complication.
TEST-TAKING STRATEGY: Note the key word "not." Knowledge regarding the signs associated with orchitis is required to answer this question. If you had difficulty identifying these signs, take time now to review orchitis.
LEVEL OF COGNITIVE ABILITY: Application
PHASE OF NURSING PROCESS: Implementation
CLIENT NEEDS: Health Promotion and Maintenance
CONTENT AREA: Child Health
REFERENCE
Schulte, E., Price, D., & James, S. (1997). *Thompson's pediatric nursing: An introductory text* (7th ed.). Philadelphia: W. B. Saunders. p. 296.

6. **1**

RATIONALE: Pertussis is transmitted by direct contact or respiratory droplets from coughing. The infectious period occurs during the catarrhal stage (1–2 weeks) until the fourth week. Respiratory isolation is not required during the convalescent phase. Options 2, 3, and 4 are components of home care instruction. Additionally, a quiet environment is encouraged.
TEST-TAKING STRATEGY: Note the key word "not." Options 3 and 4 can be easily eliminated because they are general interventions associated with convalescence. Knowing that coughing spells are associated with pertussis will assist in directing you to option 1. Additionally, 2 weeks of respiratory isolation is not required. If you had difficulty with this question, review home care instructions for the child with pertussis.
LEVEL OF COGNITIVE ABILITY: Application
PHASE OF NURSING PROCESS: Implementation
CLIENT NEEDS: Health Promotion and Maintenance
CONTENT AREA: Child Health
REFERENCE
Schulte, E., Price, D., & James, S. (1997). *Thompson's pediatric nursing: An introductory text* (7th ed.). Philadelphia: W. B. Saunders. p. 296.

7. **3**

RATIONALE: Immunocompetent persons receiving OPV represent a risk for persons who are immunocompromised. The viruses in OPV multiply in the vaccinee's GI tract and can then be transmitted in saliva and feces. The risk of transmission can be reduced by avoiding contact with saliva and by practicing rigorous hygiene, especially handwashing.
TEST-TAKING STRATEGY: Options 2 and 4 can be eliminated first, knowing that OPV is contraindicated in siblings of an immunocompromised child. From the remaining two options, knowledge that the virus in OPV can be transmitted in saliva and feces will easily direct you to option 3. Review the contraindications associated with the administration of OPV vaccine now if you had difficulty with this question.
LEVEL OF COGNITIVE ABILITY: Comprehension
PHASE OF NURSING PROCESS: Implementation
CLIENT NEEDS: Physiological Integrity
CONTENT AREA: Child Health
REFERENCE
Lehne, R. (1998). *Pharmacology for nursing care* (3rd ed.). Philadelphia: W. B. Saunders. p. 743.

8. **4**

RATIONALE: Pastia's sign describes a rash that will blanch with pressure except in areas of deep creases. The tongue initially has a white furry covering with red projecting papillae (white strawberry tongue). By the fourth day, the white strawberry tongue sloughs off, leaving a red swollen tongue (strawberry tongue). The tonsils are edematous and petechial hemorrhages cover the soft palate. Koplik's spots are associated with rubeola.
TEST-TAKING STRATEGY: Note the key word "not." Knowledge that Koplik's spots are associated with rubeola will assist in answering this question. If you are unfamiliar with the clinical manifestations associated with scarlet fever, take time now to review.
LEVEL OF COGNITIVE ABILITY: Comprehension
PHASE OF NURSING PROCESS: Data Collection
CLIENT NEEDS: Physiological Integrity
CONTENT AREA: Child Health
REFERENCE
Ashwill, J., & Droske, S. (1997). *Nursing care of children: Principles and practice.* Philadelphia: W. B. Saunders. pp. 597, 614, 615.

9. **4**

RATIONALE: The parents need to be instructed to notify the physician if abdominal pain, especially in the left upper quadrant, or left shoulder pain occurs, because this may indicate splenic rupture. Children with enlarged spleens are also instructed to avoid contact sports until splenomegaly resolves. Bed rest is not necessary and children usually self-limit their activity. No isolation precautions are required, although transmission can occur via saliva, close intimate contact, or contact with infected blood. Fever is treated with acetaminophen (Tylenol).
TEST-TAKING STRATEGY: Knowledge regarding the organs affected in mononucleosis will assist in answering this question. Options 1 and 2 can be eliminated first because they are unnecessary interventions in this disease. From the remaining two options, knowledge that splenic rupture is a concern will direct you to option 4.
LEVEL OF COGNITIVE ABILITY: Application
PHASE OF NURSING PROCESS: Implementation
CLIENT NEEDS: Health Promotion and Maintenance
CONTENT AREA: Child Health
REFERENCE
Schulte, E., Price, D., & James, S. (1997). *Thompson's pediatric nursing: An introductory text* (7th ed.). Philadelphia: W. B. Saunders. p. 298.

10. **4**

RATIONALE: Diagnosis is confirmed by direct visualization of the worms. Parents can view the sleeping child's anus with a flashlight. The worm is white, thin, about 1/2 inch long, and moves. A simple technique, the cellophane tape slide method, is used to capture worms and eggs. Transparent adhesive tape is lightly touched to the anus and then applied to a slide for examination. The best specimens are obtained as the child awakens, before toileting, or before bathing.
TEST-TAKING STRATEGY: Knowledge regarding the procedure related to the cellophane tape slide for the diagnosis of pinworm is required to answer this question. If you are unfamiliar with this procedure, take time now to review.

LEVEL OF COGNITIVE ABILITY: Application
PHASE OF NURSING PROCESS: Implementation
CLIENT NEEDS: Health Promotion and Maintenance
CONTENT AREA: Child Health
REFERENCE
Schulte, E., Price, D., & James, S. (1997). *Thompson's pediatric nursing: An introductory text* (7th ed.). Philadelphia: W. B. Saunders. p. 234.

11. **4**

RATIONALE: High fevers and severe illness are reasons to delay immunization, but only until the child has recovered from the acute stage of the illness. Minor illnesses such as a cold, otitis media, or mild diarrhea without fever are not contraindications to immunization.
TEST-TAKING STRATEGY: Use the process of elimination to answer this question. Recalling that high fevers and severe illnesses are contraindications to receiving immunizations will easily direct you to option 4. If you had difficulty with this question, take time now to review the contraindications associated with immunizations.
LEVEL OF COGNITIVE ABILITY: Comprehension
PHASE OF NURSING PROCESS: Data Collection
CLIENT NEEDS: Physiological Integrity
CONTENT AREA: Child Health
REFERENCE
Schulte, E., Price, D., & James, S. (1997). *Thompson's pediatric nursing: An introductory text* (7th ed.). Philadelphia: W. B. Saunders. p. 143.

12. **3**

RATIONALE: PCP is one of the most common diseases indicative of AIDS in children. Along with PCP, children may experience at least two serious bacterial infections in 2 years. These infections are sepsis, otitis media, chronic sinusitis, meningitis, gastroenteritis, and pneumonia. LIP is a form of chronic pneumonitis. Children with LIP usually have acquired HIV infection perinatally. LIP can progress to severe respiratory compromise.
TEST-TAKING STRATEGY: Knowledge regarding the most common indications related to AIDS is required to answer this question. Take time now to review the common manifestations associated with AIDS if you had difficulty with this question.
LEVEL OF COGNITIVE ABILITY: Comprehension
PHASE OF NURSING PROCESS: Data Collection
CLIENT NEEDS: Physiological Integrity
CONTENT AREA: Child Health
REFERENCE
Schulte, E., Price, D., & James, S. (1997). *Thompson's pediatric nursing: An introductory text* (7th ed.). Philadelphia: W. B. Saunders. p. 121.

13. **2**

RATIONALE: A child with HIV will receive the same immunizations as other children except for the polio vaccine. The child with HIV and the siblings receive IPV. All household members receive the influenza vaccine. Option 4 is not necessary and is inaccurate.
TEST-TAKING STRATEGY: Option 4 can be easily eliminated. From the remaining options, recalling that IPV needs to be administered to the child with HIV and siblings will assist in directing you to option 2. Review immunizations in the immunocompromised child now if you had difficulty with this question.
LEVEL OF COGNITIVE ABILITY: Application
PHASE OF NURSING PROCESS: Implementation
CLIENT NEEDS: Health Promotion and Maintenance
CONTENT AREA: Child Health
REFERENCE
Schulte, E., Price, D., & James, S. (1997). *Thompson's pediatric nursing: An introductory text* (7th ed.). Philadelphia: W. B. Saunders. p. 143.

14. **3**

RATIONALE: The preschool child will begin to conceptualize the death process as involving physical harm. A child from birth to 2 years of age will be unable to grasp the concept of illness and death. A school-aged child will begin to understand something is wrong. An adolescent will express fear, withdrawal, and denial.
TEST-TAKING STRATEGY: Noting the age of the child will assist in directing you to the correct option. Use concepts of growth and development and the related psychosocial issues to answer the question. Review these concepts now if you had difficulty with this question.
LEVEL OF COGNITIVE ABILITY: Comprehension
PHASE OF NURSING PROCESS: Data Collection
CLIENT NEEDS: Psychosocial Integrity
CONTENT AREA: Child Health
REFERENCE
Schulte, E., Price, D., & James, S. (1997). *Thompson's pediatric nursing: An introductory text* (7th ed.). Philadelphia: W. B. Saunders. p. 247.

15. **3**

RATIONALE: The parents should be instructed to cover unused food and formula and refrigerate. They should also be informed to discard unused refrigerated food or formula after 24 hours. Options 1, 2, and 4 are accurate instructions related to basic infection control.
TEST-TAKING STRATEGY: Knowledge regarding basic infection control measures is required to answer this question. Note the key word "not." This may assist in directing you to option 3. Review these important infection control measures now if you had difficulty with this question.
LEVEL OF COGNITIVE ABILITY: Application
PHASE OF NURSING PROCESS: Implementation
CLIENT NEEDS: Health Promotion and Maintenance
CONTENT AREA: Child Health
REFERENCE
Schulte, E., Price, D., & James, S. (1997). *Thompson's pediatric nursing: An introductory text* (7th ed.). Philadelphia: W. B. Saunders. p. 123.

BIBLIOGRAPHY

Ashwill, J., & Droske, S. (1997). *Nursing care of children: Principles and practice.* Philadelphia: W. B. Saunders.

Bowden, V., Dickey, S., & Greenberg, C. (1998). *Children and their families: The continuum of care.* Philadelphia: W. B. Saunders.

Lehne, R. (1998). *Pharmacology for nursing care* (3rd ed.). Philadelphia: W. B. Saunders.

Luckmann, J. (1997). *Saunders manual of nursing care.* Philadelphia: W. B. Saunders.

O'Toole, M. (ed.). (1997). *Miller-Keane encyclopedia & dictionary of medicine, nursing, & allied health* (6th ed.). Philadelphia: W. B. Saunders.

Schulte, E., Price, D., & James, S. (1997). *Thompson's pediatric nursing: An introductory text* (7th ed.). Philadelphia: W. B. Saunders.

CHAPTER 37

Pediatric Medication Administration

I. Medications and the Pediatric Client
(Fig. 37–1)

A. Pediatric clients are smaller than an adult and their medications have to be adapted to their size and age

B. Neonates and premature infants have immature body systems

C. The absorption, distribution, metabolism, and excretion of medications differ substantially, and the pediatric client will react more quickly to medication than an adult

D. Medication reactions are not as predictable in a pediatric client as they are in an adult

II. Administering Oral Medication

A. Most oral pediatric medications are in liquid or suspension form because children usually are not able to swallow a tablet

B. Solutions may be measured using an oral syringe; if an oral syringe is not available, hypodermic syringes without the needle can be used for dosage measurement

C. When volumes are extremely small, oral liquids are measured using a calibrated medication dropper

D. Be alert to liquid medications prepared as suspensions because a medication in suspension settles to the bottom of the bottle between uses, and thorough mixing is required prior to pouring the medication

E. Suspensions must be administered immediately after measurement to prevent settling and administering an incomplete dosage

F. Administer oral medications with the child sitting upright with the head elevated, to prevent aspiration if the child cries or resists

G. Never pinch the child's nostrils when administering medication

H. Do not place medication in a bottle

I. Draw the required dose of an unpleasant medication into a small syringe and place the syringe into the side and toward the back of the infant's mouth; administer the medication slowly, allowing the infant to swallow

J. Place the small child sideways on the lap; the child's closest arm should be placed under the adult's arm and behind the adult's back; cradle the child's head and hold the child's hand and administer the medication slowly with a plastic spoon or small plastic cup

K. Mix liquid medications with less than an ounce of fluid to disguise the taste if necessary

L. Check the child's mouth if a tablet or capsule has been administered to ensure that it has been swallowed; if swallowing is a problem, some tablets can be crushed and given in small amounts of food

M. Crush tablets if necessary and mix with 1 teaspoon of pureed fruit or flavored syrup; enteric-coated and time-released tablets or capsules cannot be crushed

III. Administering Parenteral Medications
(Fig. 37–2)

A. Subcutaneous (SC) and intramuscular (IM) medications
   1. Medications most often given via the subcutaneous route are insulin and most immunizations
   2. Any site with sufficient subcutaneous tissue may be used; the upper arm is the site of choice for most immunizations
   3. The recommended injection site for children under 3 years of age is the vastus lateralis; it is the largest muscle mass in infants and small children and has few major nerves and blood vessels
   4. After age 3 years, the ventrogluteal site may be used for intramuscular injections
   5. The dorsogluteal site should not be used in any child who has not been walking for at least 2 years, and it is generally avoided in children under 6 years of age

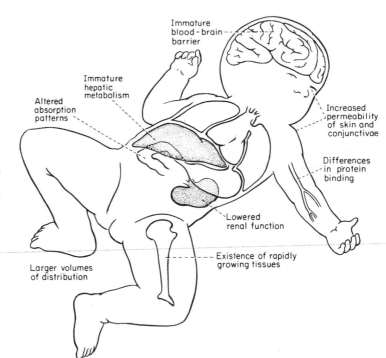

FIGURE 37–1. Some of the multiple factors that modify the drug disposition in the newborn infant. (Adapted from Hirata, T., in Smith D. [ed.]. [1977]. *Introduction to clinical pediatrics* [2nd ed.]. Philadelphia: W. B. Saunders.)

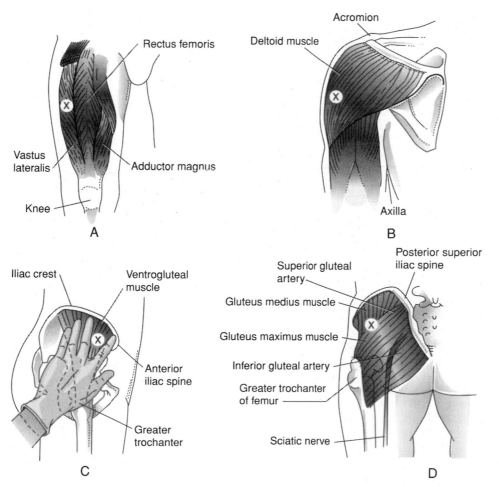

FIGURE 37–2. Injection sites. *A,* Vastus lateralis site; *B,* deltoid site; *C,* ventrogluteal site; *D,* dorsogluteal site. (From Betz C., Hunsberger, M., & Wright, S. [1994]. *Family-centered nursing care of children* [2nd ed.]. Philadelphia: W. B. Saunders. p. 876.)

6. The deltoid is also avoided in children under 6 years, and it should be used only for very small amounts of medication
7. Usually not more than 1 mL is injected per IM or SC sites, and sites are rotated regularly
8. Pediatric dosages for SC and IM administration are calculated to the nearest hundredth and measured using a tuberculin (TB) syringe
9. Usually a ⅝-inch needle is used to administer SC and IM injections to small infants
10. One-inch needles are appropriate for most IM injections in children
11. Place an adhesive bandage or decorated bandage over the puncture site, particularly for toddlers and preschoolers

B. Monitoring intravenous (IV) medications
1. When a child is receiving an IV medication, the IV site needs to be monitored for signs of infiltration and inflammation
2. Signs of inflammation include redness, heat, swelling, and tenderness
3. Signs of infiltration include swelling, coldness, pain, and lack of blood return
4. Signs of infiltration or inflammation need to be reported

IV. Calculation of Medication Dosage by Body Weight

A. Conversion of body weight
1. Pounds (lb) to kilograms (kg)
   a. 1 kg = 2.2 lb
   b. To convert from lb to kg, divide by 2.2
   c. The answer, in kg, will be smaller than the lb you are converting since you are dividing
   d. Answers are expressed to the nearest tenth
2. Kilograms (kg) to pounds (lb)
   a. 1 kg = 2.2 lb
   b. To convert from kg to lb, multiply by 2.2
   c. The answer, in lb, will be larger than the kg you are converting since you are multiplying
   d. Express weight to the nearest tenth

B. Calculating daily dosages
1. Dosages are expressed in terms of mg/kg/day, or mg/lb/day
2. The total daily dosage is usually administered in divided (more than one) doses per day
3. Express the child's body weight in kg or lb to correlate with the dosage specifications
4. Calculate the total daily dosage
5. Divide the total daily dosage by the number of doses to be administered in 1 day

V. Calculation of Body Surface Area (BSA)
(Fig. 37–3)

A. The body surface area is determined by comparing body weight and height with averages or norms on a graph called a nomogram

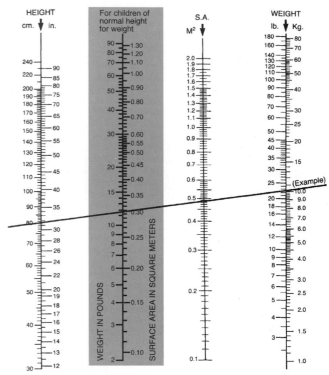

FIGURE 37–3. Nomogram for estimating body surface area. (Modified from data of E. Boyd by C. West. From Behrman R., & Kleigman R. [1992]. *Nelson textbook of pediatrics* [14th ed.]. Philadelphia: W. B. Saunders.)

B. Not all children are the same size at the same age; therefore, the nomogram chart is used to determine the BSA of a child
C. Look at the nomogram chart (see Fig. 37–3) and note that the height is on the left-hand side of the chart and the weight is on the right-hand side
D. Place a ruler on the chart
E. Line up the left side of the ruler on the height and the right side of the ruler on the weight; read the BSA where the point of the straight edge of the ruler intersects with the surface area (SA) column; this gives the estimated surface area in square meters (m²)

EXAMPLE:

Use the nomogram and calculate the BSA for a child whose height is 58 inches and weight is 12 kg.

ANSWER:

0.66 m²

VI. Calculation Based on Body Surface Area (BSA)

A. When dosage recommendations for children specify milligrams or units per square meter (m²), calculating the dosage is simple multiplication

EXAMPLE:

The dosage recommendation is 4 mg per m². The child has a BSA of 1.1 m². What is the dosage to be administered?

ANSWER:

$$1.1 \times 4 \text{ mg} = 4.4 \text{ mg}$$

B. When dosages are specified only for adults, a formula is used to calculate a child's dosage from the adult dosage

C. The average adult body surface area is approximately 1.7 square meters

EXAMPLE:

The physician has prescribed an antibiotic for a child. The average adult dose is 250 mg. The child has a BSA of 0.41 square meter (m²). What is the dose for the child?

ANSWER:

Formula:

$$\frac{\text{BSA of child}}{1.7 \text{ m}^2} \times \text{adult dose} = \text{child's dose}$$

$$\frac{0.41}{1.7} \times 250 \text{ mg} = 60.29 \text{ or } 60.3 \text{ mg}$$

PRACTICE QUESTIONS

1. Penicillin V (Veetids), 250 mg PO every 8 hours, is prescribed for a child with a respiratory infection. The child's weight is 45 lb. The safe pediatric dose is 25 to 50 mg/kg/day. The nurse determines that
   1 The dose is too low
   2 The dose is too high
   3 The dose is within the safe range
   4 There is not enough information to determine the safe dose

2. The physician has prescribed phenobarbital sodium (Luminal) 25 mg PO BID for a child with febrile seizures. The medication label reads: Luminal, 20 mg per 5 mL. The nurse has determined that the dosage prescribed is a safe dose for the child. How many milliliters does the nurse administer to the child per dose?
   1 2 mL
   2 4.5 mL
   3 6.25 mL
   4 7.0 mL

3. Cloxacillin (Tegopen), 100 mg PO q6h, is prescribed for a child with an elevated temperature suspected of having a respiratory tract infection. The child weighs 17 lb. The safe pediatric dose is 50 mg/kg/day. The nurse determines that
   1 The dose is too low
   2 The dose is too high
   3 The dose is within the safe range
   4 There is not enough information to determine the safe dose

4. Cloxacillin (Tegopen), 100 mg PO q6h, is prescribed for a child with an infection. The medication label reads: 125 mg per 5 mL. The nurse has determined that the dosage prescribed is a safe dose for the child. How many milliliters does the nurse administer to the child per dose?
   1 2 mL
   2 4 mL

   3 6 mL
   4 7 mL

5. Sulfisoxazole (Gantrisin) 1.0 g PO QID, is prescribed for an adolescent with a urinary tract infection. The medication label reads: 500-mg tablets. The nurse has determined that the dosage prescribed is safe. How many tablets does the nurse administer to the child per dose?
   1 0.5 tablet
   2 1 tablet
   3 2 tablets
   4 3 tablets

6. Promethazine hydrochloride (Phenergan), 20 mg IM every 8 hours PRN, is prescribed for the child with nausea. The medication label reads: 25 mg per mL. The nurse has determined that the dosage prescribed is safe. How many milliliters does the nurse administer to the child per dose?
   1 0.4 mL
   2 0.8 mL
   3 1 mL
   4 1.2 mL

7. Atropine sulfate, 0.2 mg IM, is prescribed for the child preoperatively. The medication label reads: 0.4 mg per mL. The nurse has determined that the dosage prescribed is safe. How many milliliters does the nurse administer to the child?
   1 0.5 mL
   2 0.8 mL
   3 1 mL
   4 1.2 mL

8. Penicillin G benzathine (Bicillin) 1,000,000 U IM, is prescribed for the child with an infection. The medication label reads: 600,000 Units per 1 mL. The nurse has determined that the dosage prescribed is safe. How many milliliters does the nurse administer to the child per dose?
   1 0.8 mL
   2 1.2 mL
   3 1.44 mL
   4 1.66 mL

9. The physician's order reads: acetaminophen (Tylenol) liquid, 450 mg PO every 4 hours PRN for pain. The medication label reads: 160 mg/5 mL. How many milliliters does the nurse give to administer one dose?
   1 0.1 mL
   2 5 mL
   3 10 mL
   4 14 mL

10. An adolescent is placed on a maintenance dosage of digoxin (Lanoxin) of 0.125 mg daily. The medication bottle reads 0.25 mg/mL. How much digoxin should the adolescent receive?
    1 0.25 mL
    2 0.37 mL
    3 0.50 mL
    4 2.50 mL

ANSWERS

1. **3**

RATIONALE:

Pounds to kilograms: 45 lb divided by 2.2 lb/kg
= 20.45 kg

Dosage parameters: 25 mg/kg × 20.45 kg
= 511.25 mg/day

50 mg/kg × 20.45 kg
= 1022.50 mg/day

Dosage frequency: 250 mg × 3 doses = 750 mg/day
Dosage is safe.

TEST-TAKING STRATEGY: Identify the key components of the question and what the question is asking. In this case, the question asks for the safe dosage range of the medication. Follow the formula steps. Change pounds to kilograms. Calculate the dosage parameters using the safe dose range identified in the question and the child's weight in kg. Remember to determine the total daily dosage prior to selecting an option.
LEVEL OF COGNITIVE ABILITY: Comprehension
PHASE OF NURSING PROCESS: Planning
CLIENT NEEDS: Safe, Effective Care Environment
CONTENT AREA: Child Health
REFERENCE
Schulte, E., Price, D., & James, S. (1997). *Thompson's pediatric nursing: An introductory text* (7th ed.). Philadelphia: W. B. Saunders. p. 435.

2. **3**

RATIONALE: Formula:

$$\frac{\text{desired}}{\text{available}} \times \text{volume} = \frac{25 \text{ mg}}{20 \text{ mg}} \times 5 \text{ mL} = 6.25 \text{ mL per dose}$$

TEST-TAKING STRATEGY: Identify the key components of the question and what the question is asking. In this case, the question asks for the milliliters per dose. Use the formula to determine the correct dosage. Label the answer before selecting an option.
LEVEL OF COGNITIVE ABILITY: Application
PHASE OF NURSING PROCESS: Implementation
CLIENT NEEDS: Safe, Effective Care Environment
CONTENT AREA: Child Health
REFERENCE:
Leahy, J., & Kizilay, P. (1998). *Foundations of nursing practice: A nursing process approach.* Philadelphia: W. B. Saunders. p. 453.

3. **3**

RATIONALE: Pounds to kilograms: 17 lb divided by 2.2 lb/kg = 7.72 kg
Dosage parameters: 50 mg/kg × 7.72 kg = 386 mg/day
Dosage frequency: 100 mg × 4 doses = 400 mg/day
Dosage is safe.
TEST-TAKING STRATEGY: Identify the key components of the question and what the question is asking. In this case, the question asks for the safe dosage range of the medication. Follow the formula steps. Change pounds to kilograms. Calculate the dosage parameters using the safe dose range identified in the question and the child's weight in kilograms. Remember to determine the total daily dosage prior to selecting an option.
LEVEL OF COGNITIVE ABILITY: Comprehension
PHASE OF NURSING PROCESS: Planning
CLIENT NEEDS: Safe, Effective Care Environment
CONTENT AREA: Child Health
REFERENCE
Leifer, G. (1999). *Thompson's introduction to maternity and pediatric nursing* (3rd ed.). Philadelphia: W. B. Saunders. p. 556.

4. **2**

RATIONALE: Formula:

$$\frac{\text{desired}}{\text{available}} \times \text{volume} = \frac{100 \text{ mg}}{125 \text{ mg}} \times 5 \text{ mL} = 4 \text{ mL per dose}$$

TEST-TAKING STRATEGY: Identify the key components of the question and what the question is asking. In this case, the question asks for the milliliters per dose. Use the formula to determine the correct dosage. Label the answer before selecting an option.
LEVEL OF COGNITIVE ABILITY: Application
PHASE OF NURSING PROCESS: Implementation
CLIENT NEEDS: Safe, Effective Care Environment
CONTENT AREA: Child Health
REFERENCE:
Leahy, J., & Kizilay, P. (1998). *Foundations of nursing practice: A nursing process approach.* Philadelphia: W. B. Saunders. p. 453.

5. **3**

RATIONALE: Change 1 g to mg
1000 mg = 1 g
When converting from g to mg, larger to smaller, move the decimal point 3 places to the right.
1 g = 1000 mg
Formula:

$$\frac{\text{desired}}{\text{available}} \times \text{tablet} = \frac{1000 \text{ mg}}{500 \text{ mg}} \times 1 \text{ tablet} = 2 \text{ tablets}$$

TEST-TAKING STRATEGY: Identify the key components of the question and what the question is asking. In this case, the question asks for tablets per dose. Change grams to milligrams first. Then use the formula to determine the correct dosage. Label the answer before selecting an option.
LEVEL OF COGNITIVE ABILITY: Application
PHASE OF NURSING PROCESS: Implementation
CLIENT NEEDS: Safe, Effective Care Environment
CONTENT AREA: Child Health
REFERENCE
Leifer, G. (1999). *Thompson's introduction to maternity and pediatric nursing* (3rd ed.). Philadelphia: W. B. Saunders. p. 556.

6. **2**

RATIONALE: Formula:

$$\frac{\text{desired}}{\text{available}} \times \text{volume} = \frac{20 \text{ mg}}{25 \text{ mg}} \times 1 \text{ mL} = 0.8 \text{ mL per dose}$$

TEST-TAKING STRATEGY: Identify the key components of the question and what the question is asking. In this case, the question asks for the milliliters per dose. Use the formula to determine the correct dosage. Label the answer before selecting an option!
LEVEL OF COGNITIVE ABILITY: Application
PHASE OF NURSING PROCESS: Implementation
CLIENT NEEDS: Safe, Effective Care Environment
CONTENT AREA: Child Health
REFERENCE
Leahy, J., & Kizilay, P. (1998). *Foundations of nursing practice: A nursing process approach.* Philadelphia: W. B. Saunders. p. 453.

7. 1

RATIONALE: Formula:

$$\frac{desired}{available} \times volume = \frac{0.2\ mg}{0.4\ mg} \times 1\ mL = 0.5\ mL\ per\ dose$$

TEST-TAKING STRATEGY: Identify the key components of the question and what the question is asking. In this case, the question asks for the milliliters per dose. Use the formula to determine the correct dosage. Label the answer before selecting an option.
LEVEL OF COGNITIVE ABILITY: Application
PHASE OF NURSING PROCESS: Implementation
CLIENT NEEDS: Safe, Effective Care Environment
CONTENT AREA: Child Health
REFERENCE
Leahy, J., & Kizilay, P. (1998). *Foundations of nursing practice: A nursing process approach*. Philadelphia: W. B. Saunders. p. 453.

8. 4

RATIONALE: Formula:

$$\frac{desired}{available} \times volume = \frac{1,000,000}{600,000} \times 1\ mL = 1.66\ mL\ per\ dose$$

TEST-TAKING STRATEGY: Identify the key components of the question and what the question is asking. In this case, the question asks for the milliliters per dose. Use the formula to determine the correct dosage. Label the answer before selecting an option.
LEVEL OF COGNITIVE ABILITY: Application
PHASE OF NURSING PROCESS: Implementation
CLIENT NEEDS: Safe, Effective Care Environment
CONTENT AREA: Child Health
REFERENCE
Leahy, J., & Kizilay, P. (1998). *Foundations of nursing practice: A nursing process approach*. Philadelphia: W. B. Saunders. p. 453.

9. 4

RATIONALE: Formula:

$$\frac{desired}{available} \times volume = \frac{450\ mg}{160\ mg} \times 5\ mL = 14\ mL\ per\ dose$$

TEST-TAKING STRATEGY: Set up the formula knowing that desired is 450 mg, available is 160 mg per 5 mL.
LEVEL OF COGNITIVE ABILITY: Application
PHASE OF NURSING PROCESS: Implementation
CLIENT NEEDS: Safe, Effective Care Environment
CONTENT AREA: Child Health
REFERENCE
Leahy, J., & Kizilay, P. (1998). *Foundations of nursing practice: A nursing process approach*. Philadelphia: W. B. Saunders, p. 453.

10. 3

RATIONALE: Formula:

$$\frac{desired}{available} \times volume = \frac{0.125\ mg}{0.25\ mg} \times 1\ mL = 0.5\ mL\ per\ dose$$

TEST-TAKING STRATEGY: Identify the key components of the question and what the question is asking. In this case, the question asks for milliliters per dose. Use the formula to determine the correct dosage. Label the answer before selecting an option.
LEVEL OF COGNITIVE ABILITY: Application
PHASE OF NURSING PROCESS: Implementation
CLIENT NEEDS: Safe, Effective, Care Environment
CONTENT AREA: Child Health
REFERENCE
Leifer, G. (1999). *Thompson's introduction to maternity and pediatric nursing* (3rd ed.). Philadelphia: W. B. Saunders. p. 556.

BIBLIOGRAPHY

Ashwill, J., & Droske, S. (1997). *Nursing care of children: Principles and practice*. Philadelphia: W. B. Saunders.

Hodgson, B., & Hizior, R. (2000). *Saunders nursing drug handbook 2000*. Philadelphia: W. B. Saunders.

Leahy, J., & Kizilay, P. (1998). *Foundations of nursing practice: A nursing process approach*. Philadelphia: W. B. Saunders.

Lehne, R. (1998). *Pharmacology for nursing care* (3rd ed.). Philadelphia: W. B. Saunders.

Leifer, G. (1999). *Thompson's introduction to maternity and pediatric nursing* (3rd ed.). Philadelphia: W. B. Saunders.

Luckmann, J. (1997). *Saunders manual of nursing care*. Philadelphia: W. B. Saunders.

O'Toole, M. (1997). *Miller-Keane encyclopedia & dictionary of medicine, nursing, & allied health* (6th ed.). Philadelphia: W. B. Saunders.

Schulte, E., Price, D., & James, S. (1997). *Thompson's pediatric nursing: An introductory text* (7th ed.). Philadelphia: W. B. Saunders.

UNIT VIII

....

The Adult Client with an Integumentary Disorder

PYRAMID TERMS

Burns—Cell destruction of the layers of the skin and the resultant depletion of fluid and electrolytes.

Chemical Burns—Caused by tissue contact with strong acids, alkalis, or organic compounds. Systemic toxicity from cutaneous absorption can occur.

Electrical Burns—Caused by heat generated by an electrical energy as it passes through the body. Results in internal tissue damage.

Fourth-Degree Burn—Involves injury to the muscle and bone. Injured area appears black. Edema is absent.

Full-Thickness (Third-Degree Burn)—Deep red, black, white, or brown area. Injured surface appears dry. Tissue disruption is noted, with fat exposed. Skin is edematous.

Partial-Thickness (Second-Degree Burn)—Mottled red base and broken epidermis with a wet, shiny, and weeping surface. Large blisters cover an extensive area. Skin is edematous and painful.

Smoke Inhalation Injury—Results when the victim is trapped in an enclosed, smoke-filled space.

Superficial (First-Degree Burn)—Mild to severe erythema, and the skin blanches with pressure.

Decubitus—Localized area of skin breakdown that occurs as a result of poor circulation to the area; also called pressure ulcer.

Kaposi's Sarcoma—Skin lesions that occur in individuals with a compromised immune system.

Lyme Disease—An infection acquired from a tick bite. Ticks live in wooded areas and survive by attaching to a host.

Skin Cancer—A malignant lesion of the skin that may or may not metastasize. Causes include chronic friction and irritation to a skin area and exposure to ultraviolet rays. Diagnosis is confirmed by a skin biopsy that is positive for cancer cells.

◆ PYRAMID TO SUCCESS

The Pyramid to Success focuses on the concept that the integumentary system provides the first line of defense against infections. Focus on the protective measures necessary to prevent infection. Pyramid points address the risk factors related to the development of integumentary disorders, the preventive measures related to skin cancer, and the content related to Kaposi's sarcoma and Lyme disease. Focus on the emergency measures related to a client with a burn, fluid resuscitation, monitoring for complications, and skin grafting. Psychosocial issues relate to the body image disturbances that can occur as a result of the integumentary disorder.

NURSING PROCESS

DATA COLLECTION

Change in skin color, texture, temperature, sensation, and turgor
Itching
Fever
Hair loss
Cleanliness
Changes of the hair and nails
Skin integrity and lesions

PLANNING	IMPLEMENTATION	EVALUATION
Skin integrity will remain intact.	Monitor client for risk for the development of alteration in skin integrity. Monitor skin condition. Monitor skin for breakdown or lesions. Initiate skin protective measures to prevent breakdown.	Client's skin remains intact and shows no signs of infection or drainage.
The client will not develop an infection.	Monitor temperature and for signs of infection. Monitor any lesions for drainage. Initiate body and fluid precautions as required.	Temperature remains within normal limits.
The client will maintain an adequate nutritional intake.	Encourage a well-balanced diet. Encourage adequate fluid intake. Monitor intake and output (I&O). Obtain weights.	Hydration and nutritional status of client is adequate.
Client will verbalize a need for pain medication.	Administer pain medication as prescribed. Monitor and document effectiveness of pain medication.	Client verbalizes reasonable comfort from pain medication.
Client reports sensation in extremities.	Monitor neurovascular status. Monitor color, motion, and sensation of affected area. Monitor peripheral pulses.	Neurovascular status remains intact.
The client acknowledges the actual change in body appearance. Client verbalizes the impact of the situation on existing personal relationships and lifestyle.	Encourage client to verbalize concerns regarding the skin disorder. Provide care in a nonjudgmental manner, maintaining the client's privacy and dignity.	Client verbalizes concerns related to skin disorder. Client verbalizes personal strengths. Client verbalizes available community resources.
The client will verbalize appropriate care to the skin.	Instruct client regarding the prescribed treatment plan. Allow client to demonstrate procedures related to the treatment plan.	Client demonstrates appropriate procedures for caring for skin disorder.

◢ CLIENT NEEDS

SAFE, EFFECTIVE CARE ENVIRONMENT

Informed consent for treatments and procedures
Confidentiality related to disorder
Asepsis
Handling infectious materials
Standard (universal) precautions

HEALTH PROMOTION AND MAINTENANCE

Disease prevention measures
Health promotion programs
Reinforcing instructions to the client regarding care to
  integumentary disorder

PSYCHOSOCIAL INTEGRITY

Body image changes
Utilizing coping mechanisms
Adapting to role changes
Use of support systems

PHYSIOLOGICAL INTEGRITY

Basic care and comfort
Adequate nutrition for healing
Comfort interventions
Monitoring laboratory values
Fluid and electrolyte imbalances
Monitoring for complications
Providing emergency care

BIBLIOGRAPHY

deWit, S. (1998). *Essentials of medical-surgical nursing* (4th ed.). Philadelphia: W. B. Saunders.

Hill, S., & Howlett, H. (1997). *Success in practical nursing: Personal and vocational issues* (3rd ed.). Philadelphia: W. B. Saunders.

Leahy, J., & Kizilay, P. (1998). *Foundations of nursing practice: A nursing process approach*. Philadelphia: W. B. Saunders.

Luckmann, J. (1997). *Saunders manual of nursing care*. Philadelphia: W. B. Saunders.

National Council of State Boards of Nursing (1998). *National Council detailed test plan for the NCLEX-PN examination*. Chicago: Author.

O'Toole, M. (1997). *Miller-Keane encyclopedia & dictionary of medicine, nursing, & allied health* (6th ed.). Philadelphia: W. B. Saunders.

CHAPTER 38

Integumentary System

. . . .

I. Anatomy and Physiology

A. The skin is the largest sensory organ of the body
B. Functions
   1. First line of defense against infections
   2. Protects underlying tissues and organs
   3. Receives stimuli from the external environment
   4. Maintains normal body temperature
   5. Excretes salts, water, and organic wastes
   6. Protects the body from dehydration
   7. Synthesizes vitamin D_3, that converts to calcitriol, for normal calcium metabolism
   8. Stores nutrients
   9. Protects the internal organs from injury
   10. Detects touch, pressure, pain, and temperature and relays that information to the nervous system
C. Layers
   1. Epidermis
   2. Dermis
   3. Subcutaneous fat
D. Accessory structures
   1. Nails
   2. Hair
   3. Glands
     a. Sebaceous
     b. Sweat
E. Normal bacterial flora
   1. A pH of 4.2 to 5.6 halts the growth of bacteria
   2. Organisms are shed with normal exfoliation
   3. Normal bacterial flora
     a. Gram-positive and gram-negative staphylococcus
     b. *Pseudomonas*
     c. *Streptococcus*

II. Risk Factors

A. Exposure to chemical and environmental pollutants
B. Exposure to radiation
C. Exposure to the sun
D. Lack of personal hygiene habits
E. Use of cosmetics and harsh soaps
F. Medications, such as long-term steroid and/or anticoagulant therapy
G. Nutritional deficiencies
H. Moderate to severe emotional stress
I. Injured areas with potential entry points for infection
J. Changes associated with developmental stages and aging

III. Psychosocial Impact

A. Change in body image
B. Fear of rejection
C. Social isolation (from embarrassment about changes in skin appearance)
D. Decreased self-esteem
E. Restrictions in physical activity
F. Pain
G. Disruption or loss of employment
H. Cost of medications, if prescribed
I. Cost of hospitalizations and follow-up care, including dressing supplies

IV. Diagnostic Tests

A. Skin biopsy
   1. Description: obtaining a small piece of skin tissue for histopathologic study
   2. Implementation preprocedure
     a. Obtain informed consent
     b. Cleanse the site as prescribed
   3. Implementation postprocedure
     a. Place the specimen when obtained by the physician in the appropriate container as directed and send to the pathology laboratory for analysis
     b. Use aseptic technique for biopsy site dressings
     c. Check the biopsy site for bleeding and infection
B. Skin cultures
   1. Description

a. Noninvasive procedure
b. A small skin culture sample is obtained, using a sterile applicator
c. A sample is sent to the laboratory to identify an existing organism

2. Implementation: ensure that skin culture samples are obtained prior to beginning antibiotic therapy
3. Implementation postprocedure: send a skin culture sample to the laboratory

C. Wood's light examination
1. Description: the skin is viewed under ultraviolet light through a special glass (Wood's glass) to identify superficial infections of the skin
2. Implementation preprocedure: darken the room prior to the examination
3. Implementation postprocedure: assist the client while adjustment from a darkened room occurs

D. Skin testing
1. Description
a. The administration of an allergen to the skin's surface or into the dermis
b. Administered by patch, scratch, or intradermal techniques
2. Implementation preprocedure
a. The client is instructed to discontinue systemic corticosteroids or antihistamine therapy for 48 hours prior to the test
b. Obtain informed consent
c. Resuscitation equipment needs to be available if a scratch test is performed, because it may induce an anaphylactic reaction
3. Implementation postprocedure
a. Instruct the client to keep the skin-testing patch area dry
b. Instruct the client to avoid activities that may produce sweating if a patch test was performed
c. Record the site, date, and time of the test and the date and the time for follow-up site reading
d. Inspect the site for erythema, papules, vesicles, edema, and induration
e. Provide the client with a list of potential allergens, if identified

V. Skin Disorders

A. Contact dermatitis
1. Description: an inflammatory response of the skin that produces skin changes after contact with a specific antigen
2. Data collection
a. Pruritus and burning
b. Edema
c. Erythema at the point of contact
d. Vesicles with drainage
3. Implementation

a. Elevation of the extremity to reduce edema
b. Application of cool, wet dressings and tepid baths as prescribed
c. Maintain a cool environment
d. Prevent scratching and rubbing of the affected area
e. Assist with skin testing as prescribed to determine allergen(s)
f. Instruct the client to avoid contact with the allergen when determined
g. Instruct the client to avoid harsh soaps
h. Instruct the client to avoid using heating pads or blankets
i. Prescribed medications may include antibiotics for infection, antipruritics or antihistamines for itching, or corticosteroids for inflammation

B. Poison ivy, poison oak, and poison sumac
1. Description: a dermatitis that develops from contact with urushiol from poison ivy, oak, or sumac plants
2. Data collection
a. Papulovesicular lesions
b. Severe itching
3. Implementation
a. Cleanse the skin of plant oils
b. Application of cool, wet dressings with Burrow's solution, as prescribed, to relieve the itching
c. Prescribed treatments may include the application of lotions or topical steroids, and/or oral corticosteroids

C. **Lyme disease**
1. Description
a. An infection caused by *Borrelia burgdorferi*, acquired from a tick bite
b. Ticks live in wooded areas and survive by attaching to a host
2. Data collection (Table 38–1)
3. Implementation
a. Gently remove the tick with tweezers or fingers, wash the skin with an antiseptic, and dispose of the tick by flushing it down the toilet
b. Obtain a blood test 4 to 6 weeks after a bite to detect the presence of the disease (testing before this time is not reliable)
c. Instruct the client in the administration of antibiotics, as prescribed, if the disease is confirmed
d. Instruct the client to avoid areas that contain ticks, such as wooded grassy areas, especially in the summer
e. Instruct the client to wear tight-fitting clothing while outside and to spray the body with tick repellent before going outside
f. Instruct the client to examine the body when returning inside
g. Lymerix, a vaccine for **Lyme disease**, is

Table 38–1. **Stages of Lyme Disease**

First Stage	Second Stage	Third Stage
Symptoms can occur several days to months following the bite A small red pimple develops that spreads into a ring-shaped rash Rash may be large or small or may not occur at all Flulike symptoms occur, such as headaches, stiff neck, muscle aches, and fatigue	Occurs several weeks following the tick bite Joint pain Neurological complications Symptoms of heart disease	Large joints become involved Arthritis progresses

available and may be recommended for high-risk individuals

D. Erysipelas and cellulitis
   1. Description
      a. Erysipelas is an acute, superficial rapidly spreading inflammation of the dermis and lymphatics caused by beta-hemolytic streptococcus group A that enters the tissue via an abrasion, bite, trauma, or wound
      b. Cellulitis is skin infection into the deeper dermis and subcutaneous fat, and the causative organism is usually *Streptococcus pyogenes*
   2. Data collection
      a. Pain and itching
      b. Swelling, redness, and warmth
      c. Presence of nodules
   3. Implementation
      a. Promote rest
      b. Apply warm compresses as prescribed to promote circulation and to decrease discomfort, erythema, and edema
      c. Antibiotics may be prescribed for infection (begin administration following a culture of the area)
E. Psoriasis
   1. Description
      a. A chronic, noninfectious skin inflammation involving keratin synthesis that results in psoriatic patches
      b. Possible causes of the disorder include stress, trauma, infection, and changes in climate
      c. The disorder may also be exacerbated by the use of certain medications
      d. Koebner's phenomenon is the development of psoriatic lesions at a site of injury, such as a scratched or sunburned area
   2. Data collection
      a. Pruritus
      b. Shedding, silvery white, scaling plaques; usually affects the scalp, knees, shins, elbows, and sacral regions
      c. A yellow discoloration, pitting, and a thickening of the nails
      d. Joint inflammation
   3. Implementation
      a. Administer and instruct the client

regarding daily soaks and tepid, wet compresses as prescribed to the affected areas
      b. Assist the client to remove the scales during the soak
      c. Apply corticosteroids and cover the areas with warm moist dressings or occlusive dressings as prescribed to decrease infection
      d. Use plastic wrap or plastic bags as the occlusive dressing, and apply rubber gloves on the client's hands
      e. Use a bed cradle to keep covers off the client's skin
      f. Instruct the client not to scratch the affected areas
      g. Monitor for and instruct the client to recognize the signs and symptoms of infection
      h. Administer antipsoriatics as prescribed, anticipating the use of anthralin (Anthra-Derm (coal tar), followed by exposure to ultraviolet light (tar preparations suppress miotic activity and produce an anti-inflammatory effect)
      i. Prepare the client for photochemotherapy (PUVA [psoralen and ultraviolet A] therapy) as prescribed anticipating the administration of methoxsalen (Oxsoralen) 2 hours prior to the ultraviolet light
      j. Prepare to administer keratolytics and antimicrobials as prescribed
      k. Instruct the client to wear light cotton clothing over affected areas
      l. Instruct clients to avoid over-the-counter medications
      m. Instruct clients regarding prescribed treatments and medications
      n. Assist the client to identify ways to reduce stress
F. **Skin cancer** (Box 38–1)
   1. Description
      a. A malignant lesion of the skin, which may or may not metastasize
      b. Causes include chronic friction and irritation to a skin area and exposure to ultraviolet rays
      c. Diagnosis is confirmed by a skin biopsy that is positive for cancer cells

---

BOX 38–1. Appearance of Skin Cancer Lesions

A waxy nodule
An irregular, circular, bordered lesion with hues of tan, black, or blue
A small, red, nodular lesion
An oozing, bleeding, crusting lesion

---

2. Types
   a. Basal cell: the most common form, arising from the basal cells contained in the epidermis
   b. Squamous cell: the second most common **skin cancer** in Caucasians; it is a tumor of the epidermal keratinocytes and can infiltrate surrounding structures, metastasize to lymph nodes, and be subsequently fatal
   c. Malignant melanoma: cancer of the melanocytes that can metastasize to the brain, lungs, bone, liver, and skin and is ultimately fatal
3. Data collection
   a. Change in color, size, or shape of preexisting lesion
   b. Pruritus
   c. Local soreness
4. Implementation
   a. Instruct clients regarding preventive measures
   b. Instruct clients to monitor for lesions that do not heal or that change characteristics
   c. Instruct the client to have moles or lesions removed that are subject to chronic irritation
   d. Instruct the client to avoid contact with chemical irritants
   e. Instruct clients to use sun-screening lotions and layered clothing when outdoors
   f. Assist with surgical excision of lesion as prescribed

G. **Kaposi's sarcoma**
   1. Description: skin lesions that occur primarily in individuals with a compromised immune system
   2. Data collection
      a. Purplish, reddish brown lesions on the skin
      b. Raised, oblong, tender, or nontender and slow-growing skin tumors
      c. Organ involvement includes the lymph nodes, airways or lungs, or any part of the gastrointestinal tract from the mouth to the anus
   3. Implementation
      a. Maintain body fluid precautions
      b. Provide protective isolation if the immune system is depressed
      c. Prepare the client for radiation as prescribed

   d. Prepare the client for chemotherapy as prescribed
   e. Immunotherapy may be prescribed to stabilize the immune system

H. Herpes zoster (shingles)
   1. Description
      a. An acute viral infection of the dorsal nerve root ganglion, caused by varicella-zoster virus
      b. Can be caused by the reactivation of the varicella-zoster virus or exposure to varicella-zoster or can occur during any immunocompromised state
      c. Diagnosis is determined by visual examination, skin cultures and skin stains that identify the organism, and by an antinuclear antibody (ANA) blood test that will produce a positive result
      d. A culture provides the definitive diagnosis
      e. Herpes zoster is contagious to individuals who have not had chickenpox
   2. Data collection
      a. Unilaterally clustered skin vesicles along peripheral sensory nerves on the trunk, thorax, or face
      b. Fever
      c. Burning and neuralgia
      d. Pruritus
      e. Paresthesia
   3. Implementation
      a. Isolate the client because exudate from lesions contain the virus
      b. Maintain strict wound and skin precautions
      c. Monitor vital signs
      d. Monitor for signs and symptoms of infection
      e. Keep blisters intact if formed
      f. Assist the client with acetic acid compresses and tepid baths as prescribed
      g. A nerve block using lidocaine (Xylocaine) may be performed
      h. Medications may include antiviral agents, analgesics, antianxiety agents, antipruritics, and corticosteroids
      i. Use an air mattress and a bed cradle on the client's bed
      j. Prevent the client from scratching and rubbing the affected area
      k. Instruct the client to wear lightweight, loose cotton clothing and to avoid wool and synthetic clothing

I. Paronychia
   1. Description
      a. An infection of the tissue around the nailbed
      b. The disorder most commonly occurs in middle-aged women and in diabetics
   2. Data collection
      a. Redness and swelling around the nailbed
      b. Soreness at the nailbed

3. Implementation
   a. Monitor temperature
   b. Monitor for infection around nails
   c. Assist the client with warm soaks as prescribed
   d. Prepare to assist with incision and drainage of the infected area if prescribed
   e. Antibiotic or fungicidal ointments may be prescribed

J. Impetigo
1. Description: a bacterial infection of the skin caused by *Streptococcus* or *Staphylococcus* or both
2. Data collection
   a. Skin lesions that appear as vesicles
   b. Lesions progress to crusted pustules
3. Implementation
   a. Allow lesions to dry by air exposure
   b. Assist the client with cleansing with hexachlorophene soap as prescribed
   c. Assist with compresses as prescribed to remove crusts and to allow for healing
   d. Apply and instruct the client in the use of antibiotic ointments as prescribed
   e. Apply and instruct the client in the use of emollients as prescribed to prevent the skin from cracking
   f. Instruct the client in methods to prevent the spread of the disease
   g. Instruct the client in the use of separate towels, linens, and dishes

K. Boils
1. Description
   a. A deep bacterial inflammation of a hair follicle caused by staphylococcus
   b. Commonly occur on the face, neck, arms, legs, and groin
2. Data collection
   a. Redness on skin
   b. Tender and painful furuncle
   c. Skin swelling at the site
   d. A yellow or white center at the furuncle
3. Implementation
   a. Instruct the client in good handwashing technique to prevent the spread of infection
   b. Apply hot, moist compresses until drainage occurs
   c. Assist the physician in incision and drainage, which relieves the pain and allows the escape of purulent drainage
   d. Instruct the client in the use of separate bath linens
   e. Instruct the client in daily cleanliness
   f. Instruct the client in the administration of antibiotics if prescribed

L. Frostbite
1. Description
   a. Damage to tissues and blood vessels as a result of prolonged exposure to cold
   b. Fingers, toes, nose, and ears are often affected

2. Data collection
   a. Numbness
   b. Paresthesia
   c. Pallor
   d. Severe pain, swelling, erythema, and blistering occur once the client is in a warm environment
   e. Necrosis and gangrene may develop in severe cases
3. Implementation
   a. Handle the tissues gently
   b. Rewarm the affected part with tepid water about 105°F as prescribed
   c. Do not massage the area because this may result in further tissue damage
   d. Do not open blisters
   e. Apply bulky dressings as prescribed to permit drainage and provide protection

M. Scabies
1. Description
   a. A parasitic skin disorder caused by an infestation of the *Sarcoptes scabiei* (itch mite)
   b. Is endemic among schoolchildren and institutionalized populations because of the contact
   c. Risk factors include contact with an infected person or contaminated article
   d. There is a 1-month delay between the initial infestation and the onset of pruritus in the host
   e. Common sites are the hands, feet, finger webs, nipples, umbilicus, penis, soles, and palms
2. Data collection
   a. Threadlike, brownish, linear burrows up to 1 cm long
   b. Secondary lesions consist of vesicles, crusts, reddish brown nodules, and excoriations
   c. Intense pruritus that worsens at night
3. Implementation
   a. Administer antihistamines or topical steroids to relieve itching as prescribed
   b. Apply topical antiscabies creams or lotions such as Kwell cream or Eurax, as prescribed, to kill the mites
   c. Instruct the client to apply antiscabies preparations to the entire body from the neck down and to leave on for 6 to 24 hours as prescribed
   d. Instruct clients to apply antiscabies creams to dry skin because moist skin increases absorption and the potential for side effects
   e. Following treatment with antiscabies preparations, instruct the client to remove the medication by washing with soap and water

N. Acne vulgaris
1. Description

a. A common, self-limiting, multifactorial disorder
b. Requires active treatment for control until it spontaneously resolves
c. The types of lesions are comedones (open and closed) pustules, papules, and nodules
d. The exact cause is unknown
e. There is no evidence that consumption of foods such as chocolate, nuts, or fatty foods affects acne
f. Exacerbations coincide with the menstrual cycle from hormonal activity
g. Heat, humidity, and excessive perspiration have a role in increased acne

2. Data collection
a. Closed comedone: whiteheads and noninflamed lesions that develop as a follicle and enlarge with retention of horny cells
b. Open comedones: blackheads that result from continuing accumulation of horny cells and sebum that dilate the follicles
c. Pustules and papules result as the inflammatory process progresses
d. Nodules result from total disintegration of a comedome and subsequent collapse of the follicle; deep scarring can result from nodules

3. Implementation
a. Instruct the client in the administration of topical antibiotics, such as clindamycin (Cleocin) and erythromycin (E.E.S.) or tretinoin (Retin-A), as prescribed
b. Provide the client with written instructions regarding the use of the medications
c. Instruct clients that improvement may not be apparent for 4 to 6 weeks
d. Instruct clients in the use of isotretinoin (Accutane) if prescribed, to inhibit inflammation
e. Instruct the client about the adverse effects of isotretinoin (Accutane), which include elevated triglycerides, skin dryness, cheilitis (lip inflammation), and eye discomfort
f. Instruct the client to stop taking vitamin A supplements during treatment with isotretinoin (Accutane)
g. Instruct clients in appropriate skin-cleansing methods, with emphasis on not scrubbing the face and using only the agreed-upon topicals
h. Instruct clients not to squeeze, prick, or pick at lesions
i. Instruct the client to use products labeled noncomedogenic, cosmetics that are water based, and to avoid contact with excessively oil-based products
j. Instruct the client on the importance of follow-up treatment

O. **Decubiti**
1. Description
a. An impairment of skin integrity
b. Localized areas of necrosis of the skin and subcutaneous tissue due to pressure
c. Prevention of skin breakdown is a major role of the nurse, particularly in caring for the bedridden or immobile client

2. Risk factors
a. Malnutrition
b. Incontinence
c. Immobility
d. Decreased sensory perception
e. Skin shearing

3. Data collection (Table 38–2)

4. Implementation
a. Institute measures to prevent **decubiti**
b. Monitor the nutritional status of the client
c. Provide adequate nutritional intake to promote tissue integrity
d. Monitor for an alteration in skin integrity
e. Relieve or remove pressure on the skin
f. Turn and reposition the immobile client every 2 hours, or more frequently if necessary
g. Ambulate the client
h. Provide active and passive exercises every 8 hours
i. Keep the skin clean and dry and the sheets wrinkle-free
j. Apply moisture barrier as prescribed to protect the skin
k. Use assistive devices to prevent pressure,

Table 38–2. **Stages of Decubitus**

Stage 1	Stage 2	Stage 3	Stage 4
A reddened area that returns to normal skin color after 15–20 minutes of pressure relief, such as turning the client to another position The skin is intact Area is red and does not blanch with external pressure	Area in which the top layer of skin is missing The ulcer usually is shallow with a pink to red base; a white or yellow eschar may be present	Deep ulcers that extend into the dermis and subcutaneous tissues White, gray, or yellow eschar usually is present at the bottom of the ulcer, and the ulcer crater may have a lip or edge Purulent drainage is common	Deep ulcers that extend into muscle and bone Foul-smelling Brown or black eschar Purulent drainage is common

such as an alternating air pressure mattress or sheepskin padding

l. Apply medications or dressings to the wound as prescribed

VI. Burn Injuries

A. Description: cell destruction of the layers of the skin and the resultant depletion of fluid and electrolytes

B. **Burn** size
1. Small **burns**: the body's response to injury is localized to the injured area
2. Large or extensive **burns**
   a. Consists of 25% or more of the total body surface area (TBSA)
   b. The body's response to the injury is systemic
   c. Affects all of the major systems of the body
C. Estimating the extent of injury (Table 38–3)
D. **Burn** depth
1. **Superficial—first degree**
   a. Mild to severe erythema
   b. Skin blanches with pressure
   c. Painful and tingling
   d. Pain is eased by cooling
   e. Discomfort lasts about 48 hours
   f. Healing occurs in about 3 to 7 days
   g. Skin grafts are not required
2. **Partial thickness—second degree**
   a. Large blisters covering an extensive area
   b. Edema
   c. Mottled red base and broken epidermis, with a wet, shiny, and weeping surface
   d. Painful; injured area is sensitive to cold air
   e. Superficial **partial thickness** heals in 14 to 21 days
   f. Deep **partial thickness** heals in 21 to 28 days
   g. Grafts may be used if the healing process is prolonged
3. **Full thickness—third degree**
   a. Deep red, black, white, or brown area
   b. Injured surface appears dry
   c. Edema
   d. Tissue disruption with fat exposed
   e. Little pain
   f. Spontaneous healing will not occur; healing takes weeks to months
   g. Requires removal of eschar and split- or full-thickness skin grafting

h. Scarring and wound contractures are likely to develop without preventive measures
4. **Fourth degree**
   a. Involves injury to the muscle and bone
   b. Injured area appears black
   c. Edema is absent
   d. Pain is absent
   e. No blisters
   f. Eschar is hard and inelastic
   g. Healing time takes weeks to months
   h. Grafts are required
E. **Burn** location
1. **Burns** of head, neck, and chest are associated with pulmonary complications
2. **Burns** of face are associated with corneal abrasion
3. **Burns** of ear are associated with auricular chondritis
4. Hands and joints require intensive therapy to prevent disability
5. The perineal area is prone to autocontamination by urine and feces
6. Circumferential **burns** of the extremities can produce a tourniquet-like effect and lead to vascular compromise
7. Circumferential thorax **burns** lead to inadequate chest wall expansion and pulmonary insufficiency

VII. Types of Burns

A. **Thermal burns**: caused by exposure to flames, hot liquids, steam, or hot objects
B. **Chemical burns**
1. Caused by tissue contact with strong acids, alkalis, or organic compounds
2. Systemic toxicity from cutaneous absorption can occur
C. **Electrical burns**
1. Caused by heat generated by an electrical energy as it passes through the body
2. Results in internal tissue damage
3. Cutaneous **burns** cause muscle and soft tissue damage that may be extensive, particularly in high-voltage electrical injuries
4. The voltage, type of current, contact site, and duration of contact are important to identify
5. Alternating current is more dangerous than direct current as it is associated with cardiopulmonary arrest, ventricular

Table 38–3. Methods to Estimate Extent of Burn Injury

Rule of Nines/Adult		*Lund and Browder Method*
Head and neck	9%	Modifies percentages for body segments according to age
Anterior trunk	18%	Provides a more accurate estimate of the burn size
Posterior trunk	18%	Uses a diagram of the body divided into sections, with the representative
Arms (9%)	18%	percentage of the TBSA for ages greater than 1 year
Legs (18%)	36%	Should be reevaluated after initial wound debridement
Perineum	1%	

fibrillation, tetanic muscle contractions, and long bone or vertebral fractures

D. **Radiation burns**: caused by exposure to a radioactive source

VIII. Inhalation Injuries

A. **Smoke inhalation injury**
1. Description: results when the victim is trapped in an enclosed, smoke-filled space
2. Data collection
   a. Facial **burns**
   b. Erythema
   c. Swelling of oropharynx and nasopharynx
   d. Singed nasal hairs
   e. Tachycardia
   f. Flaring nostrils, stridor, wheezing, and dyspnea
   g. Hoarse voice
   h. Sooty sputum and cough
B. Carbon monoxide poisoning
1. Carbon monoxide is a colorless, odorless, and tasteless gas that has an affinity for hemoglobin 200 times greater than that of oxygen
2. Oxygen molecules are displaced and carbon monoxide reversibly binds to hemoglobin to form carboxyhemoglobin
3. Tissue hypoxia occurs
C. Direct thermal heat injury
1. Description
   a. Can occur to the lower airways by the inhalation of steam or explosive gases or the aspiration of scalding liquids
   b. Can occur to the upper airways, which appear erythematous and edematous, with mucosal blisters and ulcerations
   c. Mucosal edema can lead to upper airway obstruction, especially during the first 24 to 48 hours
   d. All clients with head or neck **burns** should be monitored closely for the development of airway obstruction and are immediately considered for endotracheal intubation if obstruction occurs
2. Data collection
   a. Erythema and edema of upper airways
   b. Mucosal blisters and ulcerations

IX. Management of the Burn Injury

A. Emergent phase
1. Description
   a. Begins at the time of injury and ends with the restoration of capillary permeability, usually at 48 to 72 hours following the injury; includes resuscitative phase
   b. The primary goal is to prevent hypovolemic shock and preserve vital organ functioning

2. Prehospital care
   a. Begins at the scene of accident and ends when emergency care is obtained
   b. Remove the victim from the source of the **burn**
   c. Assess airway, breathing, and circulation
   d. Assess for associated trauma
   e. Conserve body heat
   f. Cover **burns** with sterile or clean cloths
   g. Remove constricting jewelry and clothing
   h. Transport
3. Emergency department care: continuation of care administered at the scene of the injury
4. Major **burns**
   a. A patent airway is established and 100% oxygen is administered as prescribed if the **burn** occurred in an enclosed area
   b. Prepare for the administration of IV fluids to maintain fluid balance
   c. Monitor vital signs closely
   d. Insert a Foley catheter as prescribed and maintain urine output at 50 mL/hour
   e. Maintain NPO status
   f. Prepare for insertion of a nasogastric tube as prescribed to prevent paralytic ileus, to prevent vomiting, and to reduce risk of aspiration
   g. Administer tetanus toxoid as prescribed
   h. Pain medication will be administered by IV route
   i. Prepare the client for an escharotomy or fasciotomy as prescribed
5. Minor **burns**
   a. Administer oral analgesics as prescribed
   b. Prepare to administer tetanus toxoid as prescribed if the client has not received tetanus within the past 5 years; clients not immunized should receive tetanus human immune globulin and the first series of active immunizations with tetanus toxoid
   c. Assist with wound care, which may include cleansing, debriding loose tissue, and removing any damaging agents, followed by application of topical antimicrobial cream and a sterile dressing
B. Resuscitative phase
1. Description
   a. Begins with the initiation of fluids and ends when capillary integrity returns to near-normal levels, and the large fluid shifts have decreased
   b. The amount of fluid administered is based on client's weight and extent of injury
   c. Most fluid replacement formulas are calculated from the time of injury and not from the time of arrival at the hospital
   d. The goal is to prevent shock by maintaining adequate circulating blood volume and maintaining vital organ perfusion
2. Fluid resuscitation
   a. Successful fluid resuscitation is evaluated

by stable vital signs, an adequate urine output, palpable peripheral pulses, and a clear sensorium
   b. Urinary output is the most common and most sensitive noninvasive assessment parameter for cardiac output and tissue perfusion
3. Implementation
   a. Monitor temperature and for signs of infection
   b. Monitor daily weights, expecting a weight gain of 15 to 20 lb in the first 72 hours
   c. Monitor gastric output and pH levels and for gastric discomfort and bleeding indicating a stress ulcer
   d. Administer antacids, H$_2$ receptor antagonists and mucosal barrier fortifier, sucralfate (Carafate), as prescribed
   e. Auscultate bowel sounds for ileus and monitor for abdominal distention and gastrointestinal (GI) dysfunction
   f. Monitor stools for occult blood
   g. Monitor pulses and capillary refill of the affected extremities and assess perfusion of the distal extremity with a circumferential **burn**
   h. Place client on an air-fluidized bed and use a bed cradle to keep sheets off the client's skin
4. Pain management
   a. Medicate the client prior to painful procedures
   b. Avoid IM or SC routes because absorption through the soft tissue is unreliable when hypovolemia and large fluid shifts are occurring
   c. Avoid oral route due to the possibility of GI dysfunction
5. Nutrition
   a. Essential to promote wound healing and prevent infection
   b. Maintain NPO status until the bowel sounds are heard, then advance to clear liquids as prescribed
   c. Nutrition may be provided via enteral tube feeding, peripheral parenteral nutrition, or total parenteral nutrition
6. Escharotomy
   a. A lengthwise incision is made through the **burn** eschar to relieve constriction and pressure and improve circulation

   b. Performed at the bedside without anesthesia because nerve endings have been destroyed by the **burn** injury
   c. Following the escharotomy, monitor pulses, color, movement, and sensation of affected extremity and control any bleeding with pressure
   d. Apply topical antimicrobial agents and dressings to the area as prescribed following the procedure
7. Fasciotomy
   a. An incision is made extending through the subcutaneous tissue and fascia
   b. The procedure is performed if adequate tissue perfusion does not return following an escharotomy
   c. Performed in the operating room with the client under general anesthesia
   d. Postprocedure care similar to escharotomy
C. Wound care
   1. Description: the cleansing, debridement, and dressing of the **burn** wounds
   2. Hydrotherapy
      a. Wounds are cleansed by immersion, showering, or spraying
      b. Hydrotherapy is generally not used for clients who are hemodynamically unstable or those with new skin grafts
   3. Debridement (Table 38–4)
      a. Removal of eschar to prevent bacterial proliferation under the eschar and to promote wound healing
      b. Debridement may be mechanical, enzymatic, or surgical
D. Wound closure (Table 38–5)
   1. Description
      a. Prevents infection and loss of fluid
      b. Promotes healing and prevents contractures
      c. Performed on the 5th to 21st day depending on the extent of the **burn**
   2. Temporary wound coverings (Boxes 38–2 and 38–3)
   3. Autografting
      a. Permanent wound coverage
      b. Surgical removal of a thin layer of the client's own unburned skin and application of the client's skin to the excised **burn** wound
      c. Performed in the operating room under anesthesia

Table 38–4. Debridement

Mechanical	Enzymatic	Surgical
Use of scissors and forceps to lift and trim away loose eschar	Application of prepared proteolytic and fibrinolytic topical enzymes that digest necrotic tissue and facilitate eschar removal	Excision of eschar and coverage of wound *Tangential:* Very thin layers of eschar are shaved until viable tissue is reached
Wet to dry or wet to wet dressing changes	Requires a moist environment to be effective and is applied directly to the burn wound	*Fascial:* Used for very deep burns and removes burn tissue and underlying fat down to the fascia
A painful procedure	Pain and bleeding are major problems	

Table 38–5. Open Method versus Closed Method of Wound Care

Method	Advantages	Disadvantages
Open		
Antimicrobial cream is applied, and wound is left open to the air without a dressing	Visualization of the wound	Increased chance of hypothermia from exposure
Application of antimicrobial cream is done every 12 hours	Easier mobility and joint range of motion	
	Simplicity in wound care	
Closed		
Gauze dressings are carefully wrapped from the distal to the proximal area of the extremity to ensure circulation is not compromised	Decreases evaporative fluid and heat loss	Mobility limitations
No two burn surfaces should be allowed to touch; touching promotes webbing of digits, contractures, and poor cosmetic outcome	Aids in debridement	Prevents effective range of motion exercises
Dressings are changed every 8–12 hours		Wound assessment is limited

    d. Monitor for bleeding following the graft because bleeding beneath an autograft can prevent adherence

    e. Autografts are immobilized following surgery for 3 to 7 days to allow time to adhere and attach to the wound bed

    f. Position for immobilization and elevation of the graft site to prevent movement and shearing of the graft

  4. Care to the graft site

    a. Elevate and immobilize the graft site

    b. Keep the site free from pressure

    c. Avoid weight bearing

    d. Monitor for foul-smelling drainage, increased temperature, increased WBC, hematoma, and fluid accumulation

  5. Care to the donor site

    a. The fine-mesh gauze dressing is allowed to dry

    b. Cover with nonadherent dressing and absorbent gauze as prescribed

    c. Nonadherent dressing will separate as healing occurs

    d. The gauze can be gently lifted and trimmed away as new epithelium forms below it

    e. Keep site dry, open to air, and free from pressure

    f. Prevent the client from scratching the donor site

    g. Apply lubricating lotions to soften the area and reduce itching after the donor site is healed

    h. Donor site can be reused once healing has occurred

E. Physical therapy

  1. An individualized program of splinting, positioning, exercises, ambulation, activities of

---

BOX 38–2. Types of Skin Grafts

SPLIT THICKNESS

Graft of half of the epidermis

FULL THICKNESS

Graft consisting of epidermis and dermis

PINCH GRAFT

Graft of a small piece of skin

SHEET GRAFT

Used to graft burns in visible areas; applied to the wound without alteration in its integrity

MESH GRAFT

Contains many little slits that allow for expansion of donor skin

Can cover large areas or irregularly shaped wounds

Allows for drainage from bleeding wounds

When healed, the mesh pattern of the skin graft remains visible

Used on hidden body areas

BOX 38–3. Temporary Wound Coverings

BIOLOGIC

Amnion

Amniotic membranes from human placenta

Dressing is changed every 48 hours with amnion

Allograft Homograft

Donated human cadaver skin is harvested within 24 hours after death

Rejection can occur within 24 hours

Monitor for wound exudate and signs of infection

Xenograft Heterograft

Porcine skin is harvested after slaughter and preserved for storage

Rejection can occur within 24 to 72 hours

Xenograft over granulation tissue is replaced every 2 to 5 days until the wound heals naturally or until closure with autograft is complete

BIOSYNTHETIC AND SYNTHETIC

Visual inspection of wound is possible because dressings are transparent or translucent

Monitor for wound exudate and signs of infection

BOX 38–4. Surgical Options for Contractures and Scarring

Split-thickness and full-thickness skin grafts
Skin flaps
Z-plasties
Tissue expansion

daily living, and physical therapy is implemented early in the acute phase of recovery to maximize functional and cosmetic outcomes

2. Apply splints as prescribed to maintain proper joint position and prevent contractures; do not apply pressure to skin areas with splints as it could lead to further tissue and nerve damage

3. Scarring is controlled by elastic wraps and bandages that apply continuous pressure to the healing skin during the period of time when the skin is vulnerable to shearing

4. Antiburn scar support garments are worn 23 hours a day until the **burn** scar tissue has matured, which takes 18 months to 2 years

F. Rehabilitative phase (Box 38–4)
   1. Description
      a. Final phase of **burn** care
      b. Overlaps the acute-care phase and goes well beyond hospitalization
      c. Goals of this phase are designed so that the client can gain independence and achieve maximal function
   2. Goals
      a. Promoting wound healing
      b. Minimizing deformities
      c. Increasing strength and function
      d. Providing emotional support

PRACTICE QUESTIONS

1. Which of the following individuals is at the greatest risk for development of an integumentary disorder?
   1 An elderly female
   2 An adolescent
   3 An outdoor construction worker
   4 A physical education teacher

2. The client scheduled for a skin biopsy asks the nurse how painful the procedure is. The most appropriate response by the nurse is
   1 "There is no pain associated with this procedure."
   2 "There is some pain, but the physician will prescribe an analgesic following the procedure."
   3 "The local anesthetic may cause a burning or stinging sensation."
   4 "A preoperative medication will be given so you will be sleeping and will not feel any pain."

3. The nurse is reinforcing the discharge instructions to a client who had a skin biopsy. Which of the following statements, if made by the client, indicates a need for further instruction?
   1 "I will call the physician if I see any drainage from the wound."
   2 "I will return in 7 days to have the sutures removed."
   3 "I will use the antibiotic ointment as prescribed."
   4 "I will remove the dressing when I get home and wash the site with tap water."

4. The nurse prepares to assist the physician to examine the client's skin with a Wood's light. Which of the following is included in the plan for this procedure?
   1 Obtain an informed consent
   2 Darken the room for the examination
   3 Shave the skin and scrub with Betadine solution
   4 Prepare a local anesthetic

5. The nurse is checking for the presence of cyanosis in a dark-skinned client. Which body area provides the best information?
   1 Back of the hands
   2 Earlobes
   3 Palms of the hands
   4 Sacrum

6. The nurse reinforces instructions to a client who is to return to the physician's office in 1 week for a patch test. The patch test will be done to identify the allergen causing the dermatitis. Which of the following instructions is most appropriate to provide to this client?
   1 Remain NPO prior to the test
   2 Shower using an antibacterial soap on the morning of the test
   3 Discontinue the prescribed antihistamine 2 days before the test
   4 Consume fluids only, on the day of the test

7. The nurse reinforces discharge instructions to a client following patch testing. Which of the following statements, if made by the client, indicates the need for further instruction?
   1 "I will return to the clinic in 2 days for the initial reading."
   2 "If the patch comes off I need to reapply it."
   3 "I need to avoid activities that will cause me to sweat."
   4 "I need to keep the test sites dry at all times."

8. The nurse reinforces instructions to the client who has complained of chronic dry skin and episodes of pruritus. Which of the following, if stated by the client, indicates a need for further teaching?
   1 "I should drink 8 to 10 glasses of water a day."

2 "I need to avoid using astringents on my skin."

3 "I should limit myself to one shower a day and apply emollient to my skin after the shower."

4 "I should use a dehumidifier, especially during the winter months."

9. The nurse prepares to assist in instructing a client about Lyme disease. Which of the following information does the nurse include in the instructions?
   1 Can be contagious by skin contact with an infected individual
   2 Can be caused by the inhalation of spores from bird droppings
   3 Is caused by contamination from cat feces
   4 Is caused by a tick carried by deer

10. The client is diagnosed with stage 1 of Lyme disease. The nurse reviews the client's health record, knowing that which of the following is characteristic of this stage?
    1 Signs of neurological disorders
    2 Enlarged and inflamed joints
    3 Arthralgias
    4 Flulike symptoms

11. Following diagnostic evaluation, it has been determined that the client has Lyme disease, stage 2. The nurse understands that which of the following is most indicative of this stage?
    1 Erythematous rash
    2 Neurological deficits
    3 Arthralgias
    4 Joint enlargements

12. The nurse reads the chart of a client who was seen by the physician and notes that the physician has documented that the client has Lyme disease stage 3. Which of the following clinical manifestations does the nurse expect to note in the client?
    1 A generalized skin rash
    2 A cardiac irregularity
    3 Enlarged and inflamed joints
    4 Paralysis in the extremity where the tick bite occurred

13. The client arrives at the health care clinic and tells the nurse that he or she was just bitten by a tick and would like to be tested for Lyme disease. The client tells the nurse that after removing the tick it was flushed down the toilet. Which of the following nursing actions is most appropriate?
    1 Tell the client that a blood test is needed immediately
    2 Inform the client that there is no test available for Lyme disease
    3 Inform the client that he or she will need to return in 4 to 6 weeks to be tested because testing before this time is not reliable

4 Tell the client that testing is not necessary unless arthralgia develops

14. Following diagnosis of Lyme disease stage 1, the nurse anticipates that which of the following will be part of the treatment plan for the client?
    1 No treatment unless symptoms develop
    2 A 3-week course of oral antibiotic therapy
    3 Treatment with intravenous (IV) penicillin G
    4 Daily oatmeal baths for 2 weeks

15. A nurse is reinforcing instructions regarding methods to prevent Lyme disease. Which of the following is not part of these instructions?
    1 Avoid the use of insect repellents because it will attract the ticks
    2 Wear long-sleeved tops and long pants in wooded areas
    3 Wear a hat in wooded areas
    4 Wear closed shoes and socks that can be pulled up over the pants when walking in the woods

16. A male client calls the emergency department and tells the nurse that he has been cleaning a wooded area in the backyard and came directly in contact with poison ivy shrubs. The client tells the nurse that there is no skin eruption. The client asks the nurse what to do. Which of the following is the most appropriate nursing response?
    1 "Come to the emergency department."
    2 "It is not necessary to do anything if you cannot see anything on your skin."
    3 "Take a shower immediately, lathering and rinsing several times."
    4 "Apply calamine lotion immediately to the exposed skin areas."

17. The client with acquired immunodeficiency syndrome (AIDS) is diagnosed with cutaneous Kaposi's sarcoma. Based on this diagnosis, the nurse understands that this has been determined by which of the following?
    1 Appearance of reddish blue lesions on the skin
    2 Swelling in the lower extremities
    3 Punch biopsy of the cutaneous lesions
    4 Swelling in the genital area

18. Which of the following individuals is least likely at risk for the development of Kaposi's sarcoma?
    1 A male with a history of same sex partners
    2 A renal transplant client
    3 A client receiving antineoplastic medications
    4 An individual working in an environment where exposure to asbestos exists

19. The nurse prepares to give a bath and change the bed linens on a client with cutaneous Kaposi's sarcoma lesions. The lesions are open and draining a scant amount of serous fluid. Which of

the following does the nurse most appropriately incorporate in the plan for bathing this client?
1 Wearing a gown, gloves, and a mask
2 Wearing a gown and gloves
3 Wearing gloves
4 Wearing a gown and gloves to change the bed linens and gloves only for the bath

20. The client is being admitted to the hospital for treatment of acute cellulitis of the lower left leg. The client asks the nurse to explain what cellulitis means. The nurse plans to base the response on the understanding that cellulitis is
1 A skin infection into the deep dermis and subcutaneous fat
2 An acute superficial infection
3 An inflammation of the epidermis
4 An epidermal infection caused by Staphylococcus

21. The nurse prepares to care for a client with acute cellulitis of the lower leg. Which of the following does the nurse anticipate to be prescribed for the client?
1 Warm compresses to the affected area
2 Cold compresses to the affected area
3 Intermittent heat lamp treatments four times daily
4 Alternating hot and cold compresses continuously

22. Which of the following individuals is least likely at risk for the development of psoriasis?
1 A 32-year-old African-American
2 A client with a systemic illness
3 An individual who has experienced a significant amount of emotional distress
4 A woman experiencing menopause

23. The nurse is caring for a client with a diagnosis of psoriasis. The nurse reviews the health record, knowing that which of the following characteristics is not associated with this skin disorder?
1 A discoloration and pitting of the nails
2 Silvery, white scaly patches on the scalp, elbows, knees, and sacral regions
3 Complaints of pruritus
4 Red-purple scaly lesions

24. Ultraviolet light (UVL) therapy is prescribed as a component of the treatment plan for a client with psoriasis. Which of the following is not a component of the plan of care related to this light treatment?
1 Eye goggles need to be worn to prevent exposure to UVL
2 The face needs to be shielded with a loosely applied covering
3 The client will stand in a light treatment chamber for 30 minutes
4 Only the area requiring treatment should be exposed to the UVL

25. The nurse notes that the physician has documented a diagnosis of herpes zoster in the client's chart. Based on an understanding of the cause of this disorder, the nurse determines that this definitive diagnosis was made following which diagnostic test?
1 Skin biopsy
2 Wood's light examination
3 Culture of the lesion
4 Patch test

26. The nurse is assigned to care for a client with herpes zoster. Which of the following characteristics does the nurse expect to note when assessing the lesions of this infection?
1 A generalized body rash
2 Small blue-white spots with a red base
3 A fiery red edematous rash on the cheeks
4 Clustered skin vesicles

27. The nurse employed in a long-term care facility is planning the clinical assignments for the day. Which of the following staff members is not assigned to the client with a diagnosis of herpes zoster?
1 A staff member who never had mumps
2 An experienced certified nursing assistant (CNA) who never had chickenpox
3 A staff member who never had roseola
4 A CNA who never had German measles

28. A client returns to the clinic for follow-up treatment following a skin biopsy of a suspicious lesion performed 1 week ago. The biopsy report indicates that the lesion is a melanoma. The nurse understands that which of the following describes a characteristic of this type of lesion?
1 Is highly metastatic
2 Metastasis is rare
3 Is characterized by local invasion
4 Is encapsulated

29. The nurse is reviewing the health care record of a client with a lesion diagnosed as malignant melanoma. The nurse most likely expects to note which of the following characteristics of this type of lesion documented in the client's record?
1 A small papule with a dry, rough scale
2 A firm nodular lesion topped with crust
3 A pearly papule with a central crater and a waxy border
4 An irregularly shaped lesion

30. The nurse reinforces discharge instructions following cryosurgery for treatment of a malignant skin lesion. Which of the following does the nurse plan to include in instructions?
1 To clean the site with hydrogen peroxide to prevent infection
2 To apply ice to the site for comfort
3 To apply alcohol-soaked dressings twice a day
4 To avoid showering for 7 to 10 days

31. The nurse reinforces instructions to a group of clients regarding measures that will assist in preventing skin cancer. Which of the following is not a part of the instructions?
    1 Use sunscreen when participating in outdoor activities
    2 Examine the body monthly for any lesions that may be suspicious
    3 Wear a hat, opaque clothing, and sunglasses when in the sun
    4 Avoid sun exposure before 11:00 a.m. and after 3:00 p.m.

32. The nurse reviews the client's chart and notes that the physician has documented a diagnosis of paronychia. Based on this diagnosis, which of the following does the nurse expect to note during the data collection?
    1 Swelling of the skin near the parotid gland
    2 Red, shiny skin around the nailbed
    3 White, silvery patches on the elbows
    4 White, taut skin in the popliteal area

33. The nurse reinforces instructions to a client diagnosed with impetigo. Which of the following is not a component of the instructions?
    1 Continue with antibiotics as prescribed
    2 Separate washing of dishes from other household members
    3 It is not necessary to separate laundry from other household members
    4 To wash hands thoroughly and frequently throughout the day

34. The client arrives at the emergency department and has experienced frostbite to the right hand. Which of the following does the nurse note on data collection of the client's hand?
    1 A fiery, red skin with edema in the nailbeds
    2 A pink, edematous hand
    3 Black fingertips surrounded by an erythematous rash
    4 A white color to the skin that is insensitive to touch

35. The nurse is assigned to assist in caring for a client with frostbite of the toes. Which of the following does the nurse anticipate to be prescribed for this condition?
    1 Rapid and continuous rewarming of the toes in a warm water bath until flushing of the skin occurs
    2 Rapid and continuous rewarming of the toes in hot water for 15 to 20 minutes
    3 Rapid and continuous rewarming of the toes when flushing occurs
    4 Rapid and continuous rewarming of the toes in cold water for 45 minutes

36. The evening nurse reviews the client's chart and notes that the day nurse has documented that the client has a stage 2 pressure ulcer (decubitus) in the sacral area. Which of the following does the nurse expect to note when checking the client's sacral area?
    1 Skin is intact
    2 Partial-thickness skin loss of the epidermis
    3 A deep crater-like appearance
    4 The presence of sinus tracts

37. Which of the following conditions would least likely be a risk factor for the development of skin breakdown?
    1 A client who is unable to move about and is confined to bed
    2 A client incontinent of urine and feces
    3 A client with chronic nutritional deficiencies
    4 A client with a lowered mental awareness status

38. The nurse inspects the oral cavity of a client with candidiasis (thrush). Which of the following does the nurse expect to note?
    1 The presence of numerous, small, red pinpoint lesions
    2 The presence of blisters
    3 The presence of white patches
    4 The presence of purple patches

39. The nurse plans to instruct a client with candidiasis (thrush) of the oral cavity on how to care for the disorder. Which of the following is not a component of the instructions?
    1 To rinse the mouth four times daily with a commercial mouthwash
    2 To avoid spicy foods
    3 To avoid citrus juices and hot liquids
    4 To eat foods that are liquid or pureed

40. The nurse is caring for a client with a diagnosis of pemphigus. The nurse understands that a hallmark sign characteristic of this condition is
    1 Homans' sign
    2 Chvostek's sign
    3 Trousseau's sign
    4 Nikolsky's sign

41. The client asks the nurse about the causes of acne. The nurse most appropriately responds by telling the client
    1 "It is caused by eating chocolate, nuts, and fatty foods."
    2 "It is caused by oily skin."
    3 "The exact cause is not known."
    4 "It is caused as a result of exposure to heat and humidity."

42. Isotretinoin (Accutane) is prescribed for a client with severe cystic acne. Which of the following, if stated by the client, indicates a need for further instruction regarding this medication?
    1 "I need to continue to take my vitamin A supplements."

2 "I need to use emollients and lip balms for my dry skin."

3 "The medication may cause dryness and burning in my eyes."

4 "I will need to return for a blood test to check my triglyceride level."

43. The nurse inspects the skin of a client suspected of having scabies. Which of the following findings does the nurse note if this disorder is present?
    1 The appearance of vesicles or pustules with a thick, honey-colored crust
    2 The presence of white patches scattered about the trunk
    3 Multiple straight or wavy threadlike lines beneath the skin
    4 Patchy hair loss and round red macules with scales

44. A nurse is told that an assigned client is suspected of having scabies. Which of the following precautions does the nurse institute during the care of the client?
    1 Wear a mask and gloves
    2 Wear gloves only
    3 Wear a gown and gloves
    4 Avoid touching the client's clothes

45. The adult client was burned as a result of an explosion. The burn initially affected the client's entire face (anterior half of the head) and upper half of the anterior torso, and caused circumferential burns to the lower half of both arms. The client's clothes caught on fire, and the client ran, causing subsequent burn injuries to the posterior surface of the head, and the upper half of the posterior torso. Using the rule of nines, the extent of the burn injury is which of the following?
    1 31.5%
    2 36%
    3 40.5%
    4 45%

46. The nurse is caring for a client who has just been admitted to the nursing unit following flame burns to the face and chest. The nurse notes a hoarse cough that produces sputum with black flecks. The client's eyelashes and eyebrows are singed. The eyelids are swollen. The client becomes restless and the color becomes dusky. The nurse interprets these data to indicate which of the following?
    1 The client is afraid and is having a panic attack due to the unfamiliar surroundings
    2 Pain is present from the burn injury
    3 The client is hypotensive
    4 The burn has probably caused laryngeal edema, which has occluded the airway

47. Which of the following is the anticipated therapeutic outcome of an escharotomy procedure performed for a third-degree circumferential arm burn?

1 Brisk bleeding from the site
2 Formation of granulation tissue
3 Decreasing edema formation
4 Return of distal pulses

48. The client is undergoing radiation therapy to treat lung cancer. Following the treatment, the nurse notes that the chest and neck are red, and the client is complaining of pain at the radiation site. The nurse interprets this as
    1 A superficial injury to tissue from the radiation
    2 An allergic reaction to the radiation
    3 A cutaneous reaction to products formed by the lysis of the neoplastic cells
    4 An ischemic injury, much like decubitus formation, due to pressure from the linear accelerator

49. The nurse is caring for a client with circumferential burns of both legs. Which of the following leg positions is most appropriate for this type of a burn?
    1 In a dependent position
    2 Flat without elevation
    3 Elevation above the level of the heart
    4 Elevation of the knee gatch on the bed

50. The nurse is caring for a burn client in protective isolation. Which of the following is not a component of protective isolation techniques?
    1 Using sterile sheets and linens
    2 Strict handwashing
    3 Wearing gloves and a gown when caring for the client
    4 Wearing protective garb including a mask, cap, shoe covers, and plastic apron

51. The nurse is caring for a client following an autograft and grafting to a burn wound on the right knee. Which of the following does the nurse anticipate to be prescribed for the client?
    1 Immobilization for 3 to 7 days
    2 Placing the affected leg flat
    3 Placing the affected leg in a dependent position
    4 Immobilization for 24 hours

52. The nurse reinforces discharge instructions regarding skin care to a client following grafting to burn injuries sustained to the left chest and left arm. Which of the following is not a component of the discharge instructions?
    1 Bathe, using a mild soap and rinsing thoroughly
    2 Avoid the use of lanolin products to the newly healed skin area
    3 Avoid direct sunlight to the newly healed skin area
    4 Never wear warm clothing over the newly healed skin area

ANSWERS

1. 3

RATIONALE: Prolonged exposure to the sun, unusual cold, or other conditions can damage the skin. An elderly client may be at a higher risk than a younger individual; immobility and lack of nutrition increase the elder person's risk. An adolescent may be prone to the development of acne, but this does not occur in all adolescents. The physical education teacher is at low or no risk of developing an integumentary problem.
TEST-TAKING STRATEGY: Note the key words "greatest risk." Eliminate option 4 first. Eliminate options 1 and 2 next because not all elderly or adolescents are at risk for the development of integumentary disorders. If you had difficulty with this question, take time now to review the risk factors associated with integumentary disorders.
LEVEL OF COGNITIVE ABILITY: Comprehension
PHASE OF NURSING PROCESS: Data Collection
CLIENT NEEDS: Health Promotion and Maintenance
CONTENT AREA: Adult Health/Integumentary
REFERENCE
deWit, S. (1998). *Essentials of medical-surgical nursing* (4th ed.). Philadelphia: W. B. Saunders. p. 910.

2. 3

RATIONALE: Depending on the size and location of the lesion, a biopsy is usually a quick and almost painless procedure. The most common source of pain is the initial local anesthetic, which can produce a burning or stinging sensation.
TEST-TAKING STRATEGY: Use the process of elimination. Eliminate option 1 first. Eliminate option 2 because this option addresses postprocedure, which is not the issue of the client's question to the nurse. Eliminate option 4 because a preoperative medication that puts the client to sleep is not a part of the procedure for a skin biopsy. If you had difficulty with this question, take time now to review the procedure related to a skin biopsy.
LEVEL OF COGNITIVE ABILITY: Application
PHASE OF NURSING PROCESS: Implementation
CLIENT NEEDS: Psychosocial Integrity
CONTENT AREA: Adult Health/Integumentary
REFERENCE
deWit, S. (1998). *Essentials of medical-surgical nursing* (4th ed.). Philadelphia: W. B. Saunders. p. 897.

3. 4

RATIONALE: Following a skin biopsy, the nurse instructs the client to keep the dressing dry and in place for a minimum of 8 hours. After the dressing is removed, the site is cleaned once a day with tap water or saline to remove any dry blood or crusts. The physician may prescribe an antibiotic ointment to minimize local bacterial colonization. The nurse instructs the client to report any redness or excessive drainage at the site. Sutures are usually removed 7 to 10 days after biopsy.
TEST-TAKING STRATEGY: Use the process of elimination. Eliminate option 3 first because the client verbalizes a physician's prescription. Eliminate options 1 and 2 next. A client needs to report signs of drainage and needs to return to the physician for follow-up and suture removal. Consider the alteration in skin integrity that occurs with a skin biopsy. This should assist in directing you to the correct option.

LEVEL OF COGNITIVE ABILITY: Comprehension
PHASE OF NURSING PROCESS: Evaluation
CLIENT NEEDS: Health Promotion and Maintenance
CONTENT AREA: Adult Health/Integumentary
REFERENCE
Monahan, F., & Neighbors, M. (1998). *Medical-surgical nursing. Foundations for clinical practice* (2nd ed.). Philadelphia: W. B Saunders. p. 1578.

4. 2

RATIONALE: Examination of the skin under a Wood's light is always carried out in a darkened room. This is a noninvasive examination; therefore, an informed consent is not required. A handheld long-wavelength ultraviolet light or Wood's light is used. The skin does not need to be shaved nor is a local anesthetic necessary. Areas of blue-green or red fluorescence are associated with certain skin infections. The procedure is painless.
TEST-TAKING STRATEGY: Use knowledge regarding the procedure for examining the skin with a Wood's light to answer the question. Knowing that this is a noninvasive procedure will assist in eliminating options 1, 3, and 4. Take time to review this procedure if you had difficulty answering this question.
LEVEL OF COGNITIVE ABILITY: Application
PHASE OF NURSING PROCESS: Planning
CLIENT NEEDS: Physiological Integrity
CONTENT AREA: Adult Health/Integumentary
REFERENCE
deWit, S. (1998). *Essentials of medical-surgical nursing* (4th ed.). Philadelphia: W. B. Saunders. p. 898.

5. 3

RATIONALE: In a dark-skinned client, the nurse examines the lips, tongue, nailbeds, conjunctivae, and palms and soles at regular intervals for subtle color changes. In a client with cyanosis, the lips and tongue are gray, and the palms, soles, conjunctivae, and nailbeds have a bluish tinge.
TEST-TAKING STRATEGY: Focus on the key words "dark-skinned" and use the process of elimination. Take time now to review this important assessment technique if you had difficulty with this question.
LEVEL OF COGNITIVE ABILITY: Application
PHASE OF NURSING PROCESS: Data Collection
CLIENT NEEDS: Physiological Integrity
CONTENT AREA: Adult Health/Integumentary
REFERENCE
deWit, S. (1998). *Essentials of medical-surgical nursing* (4th ed.). Philadelphia: W. B. Saunders. p. 477.

6. 3

RATIONALE: Client preparation for a patch test includes informing the client to discontinue the administration of systemic corticosteroids or antihistamines for at least 48 hours before the test. Topical steroid therapy may be continued as long as the agent is not applied on the area to be tested. To prevent suppression of the inflammatory response to an allergen, these medications must be discontinued. Options 1, 2, and 4 are unnecessary.
TEST-TAKING STRATEGY: Use the process of elimination. Eliminate option 1 and 4 first because they are similar and there is no need to restrict food or remain NPO prior to the procedure. A patch test does not require a body shower with an antibacterial soap. Note the relationship between "allergen" in the question and "antihistamine" in

the response. This should assist in directing you to the correct option.
LEVEL OF COGNITIVE ABILITY: Application
PHASE OF NURSING PROCESS: Implementation
CLIENT NEEDS: Health Promotion and Maintenance
CONTENT AREA: Adult Health/Integumentary
REFERENCE
deWit, S. (1998). *Essentials of medical-surgical nursing* (4th ed.). Philadelphia: W. B. Saunders. p. 898.

7. 2

RATIONALE: The nurse instructs the client to keep the test sites dry at all times. The nurse also discourages excessive physical activity that will result in sweating. Reapplying the patch can interfere with an accurate interpretation of the allergic reactions. The nurse reinforces the necessity of removing loose or nonadherent test patches for reapplication at a later date. The initial reading is performed 2 days after application and the final reading is performed 2 to 5 days later.
TEST-TAKING STRATEGY: Note the key words "need for further instruction." Use the process of elimination. Eliminate options 3 and 4 first because keeping the test site dry and avoiding sweating are similar. Knowledge that follow-up is important after any procedure should assist in directing you to option 2. If you had difficulty with this question, take time now to review the client teaching points following a patch test.
LEVEL OF COGNITIVE ABILITY: Comprehension
PHASE OF NURSING PROCESS: Evaluation
CLIENT NEEDS: Health Promotion and Maintenance
CONTENT AREA: Adult Health/Integumentary
REFERENCE
deWit, S. (1998). *Essentials of medical-surgical nursing* (4th ed.). Philadelphia: W. B. Saunders. p. 898.

8. 4

RATIONALE: Clients should avoid using a dehumidifier because this will further dry room air. Instead, they should use a room humidifier during the winter months or whenever the furnace is in use. Clients should be taught to maintain a daily fluid intake of 3000 mL unless contraindicated, and should avoid alcohol and caffeine ingestion. They should avoid applying rubbing alcohol, astringents, or other drying agents to the skin. One bath or one shower per day for 15 to 20 minutes with warm water and a mild soap should be immediately followed by the application of an emollient to prevent evaporation of water from the hydrated epidermis.
TEST-TAKING STRATEGY: Use the process of elimination and note the key words "need for further teaching." Knowledge that a dehumidifier is going to dry the air in the environment will assist in directing you to option 4. If you had difficulty with this question, take time now to review client teaching points related to dry skin and pruritus.
LEVEL OF COGNITIVE ABILITY: Comprehension
PHASE OF NURSING PROCESS: Evaluation
CLIENT NEEDS: Health Promotion and Maintenance
CONTENT AREA: Adult Health/Integumentary
REFERENCE
Monahan, F., & Neighbors, M. (1998). *Medical-surgical nursing: Foundations for clinical practice* (2nd ed.). Philadelphia: W. B. Saunders. p. 1570.

9. 4

RATIONALE: Lyme disease is a multisystem infection that results from a bite by a tick carried by several species of deer. People bitten by the *Ixodes* ticks are infected with the spirochete *Borrelia burgdorferi*. Histoplasmosis is caused by the inhalation of spores from bat or bird droppings. Toxoplasmosis is caused from the ingestion of cysts from contaminated cat feces. Lyme disease cannot be transmitted from one person to another.
TEST-TAKING STRATEGY: Knowledge regarding the cause of Lyme disease is required to answer this question. Knowing that this disease is caused by a bite will assist in eliminating the incorrect options. If you had difficulty with this question, take time now to review the cause of Lyme disease.
LEVEL OF COGNITIVE ABILITY: Application
PHASE OF NURSING PROCESS: Planning
CLIENT NEEDS: Health Promotion and Maintenance
CONTENT AREA: Adult Health/Integumentary
REFERENCE
Luckmann, J. (1997). *Saunders manual of nursing care*. Philadelphia: W. B. Saunders. p. 1654.

10. 4

RATIONALE: The hallmark of stage 1 is the development of a skin rash within 2 to 30 days of infection, generally at the site of the tick bite. The rash develops into a concentric ring, giving it a bull's-eye appearance. The lesion enlarges up to 50 to 60 cm, and smaller lesions develop farther away from the original tick bite. In stage 1, most infected people develop flulike symptoms that last 7 to 10 days, and these symptoms may reoccur later.
TEST-TAKING STRATEGY: Use the process of elimination and eliminate options 2 and 3 first because they are similar. Next, note that the question asks for the characteristic of stage 1. From the remaining two options, select the less serious since the issue of the question relates to stage 1. If you had difficulty with this question, take time now to review the stages of Lyme disease.
LEVEL OF COGNITIVE ABILITY: Comprehension
PHASE OF NURSING PROCESS: Data Collection
CLIENT NEEDS: Physiological Integrity
CONTENT AREA: Adult Health/Integumentary
REFERENCE
Luckmann, J. (1997). *Saunders manual of nursing care*. Philadelphia: W. B. Saunders. pp. 1654–1656.

11. 2

RATIONALE: Stage 2 of Lyme disease develops within 1 to 6 months in the majority of untreated individuals. The most serious problems include cardiac conduction defects and neurological disorders, such as Bell's palsy and paralysis. These problems are not usually permanent. Arthralgias and joint enlargements are noted in stage 3. A rash appears in stage 1.
TEST-TAKING STRATEGY: Knowledge regarding the clinical manifestations that occur in the stages of Lyme disease is helpful in answering the question. Eliminate options 3 and 4 first because they are similar. Knowledge that a rash appears following the tick bite will assist in eliminating option 1. If you had difficulty with this question, take time now to review the clinical manifestations associated with each stage of Lyme disease.

LEVEL OF COGNITIVE ABILITY: Comprehension
PHASE OF NURSING PROCESS: Data Collection
CLIENT NEEDS: Physiological Integrity
CONTENT AREA: Adult Health/Integumentary
REFERENCE
Luckmann, J. (1997). *Saunders manual of nursing care*. Philadelphia:
W. B. Saunders. p. 1656.

12. 3

RATIONALE: Stage 3 develops within a month to several months after initial infection. It is characterized by arthritic symptoms, such as arthralgias and enlarged or inflamed joints, which can persist for several years after the initial infection. Cardiac and neurological dysfunctions occur in stage 2. A rash occurs in stage 1. Paralysis of the extremity where the tick bite occurred is not a directly related characteristic of Lyme disease.
TEST-TAKING STRATEGY: Knowledge regarding the stages of Lyme disease is helpful in answering the question. Remember that a rash occurs in stage 1, cardiac and neurological disorders in stage 2, and joint involvement in stage 3. If you had difficulty with this question, take time now to review the clinical manifestations associated with Lyme disease.
LEVEL OF COGNITIVE ABILITY: Comprehension
PHASE OF NURSING PROCESS: Data Collection
CLIENT NEEDS: Physiological Integrity
CONTENT AREA: Adult Health/Integumentary
REFERENCE
Luckmann, J. (1997). *Saunders manual of nursing care*. Philadelphia:
W. B. Saunders. p. 1654.

13. 3

RATIONALE: There is a blood test available to detect Lyme disease; however, it is not a reliable test if performed prior to 4 to 6 weeks following the tick bite. Options 1, 2, and 4 are incorrect.
TEST-TAKING STRATEGY: Use the process of elimination. Eliminate option 1 first because of the word "immediately." A blood test is available; therefore, eliminate option 2. Eliminate option 4 because treatment should begin before the arthralgia develops. If you had difficulty with this question, take time now to review the method of diagnosing Lyme disease.
LEVEL OF COGNITIVE ABILITY: Application
PHASE OF NURSING PROCESS: Implementation
CLIENT NEEDS: Physiological Integrity
CONTENT AREA: Adult Health/Integumentary
REFERENCE
Monahan, F., & Neighbors, M. (1998). *Medical-surgical nursing: Foundations for clinical practice* (2nd ed.). Philadelphia: W. B Saunders.
p. 902.

14. 2

RATIONALE: Prevention, public education, and early diagnosis are vital to the control and treatment of Lyme disease. A 3-week course of oral antibiotic therapy is recommended during stage 1. Later stages of Lyme disease may require therapy with intravenous antibiotics, such as penicillin G. Oatmeal baths will not help a systemic disorder.
TEST-TAKING STRATEGY: Note the key words "stage 1." Eliminate option 3 because intravenous antibiotics will not be administered in this stage. Eliminate option 4 because, although oatmeal baths may be helpful for pruritus, they are not helpful to a systemic disorder. Waiting for symptoms to develop is an incorrect option. Take time to

review the treatment associated with Lyme disease now if you had difficulty with this question.
LEVEL OF COGNITIVE ABILITY: Comprehension
PHASE OF NURSING PROCESS: Planning
CLIENT NEEDS: Physiological Integrity
CONTENT AREA: Adult Health/Integumentary
REFERENCE
Luckmann, J. (1997) *Saunders manual of nursing care*. Philadelphia:
W. B. Saunders. p. 1656.

15. 1

RATIONALE: In the prevention of Lyme disease, individuals need to be instructed to use an insect repellent on the skin and clothes when in an area where ticks are likely to be found. Long-sleeved tops and long pants, closed shoes, and a hat or cap, should be worn. If possible, heavily wooded areas or areas with thick underbrush should be avoided. Socks can be pulled up and over pant legs to prevent ticks from entering under clothing.
TEST-TAKING STRATEGY: Note the key word "not." Use the process of elimination, noting that option 1 uses the word "avoid." If you had difficulty with this question, take time now to review measures to prevent contact with ticks.
LEVEL OF COGNITIVE ABILITY: Application
PHASE OF NURSING PROCESS: Planning
CLIENT NEEDS: Safe, Effective Care Environment
CONTENT AREA: Adult Health/Integumentary
REFERENCE
Monahan, F., & Neighbors, M. (1998). *Medical-surgical nursing: Foundations for clinical practice* (2nd ed.). Philadelphia: W. B. Saunders.
p. 902.

16. 3

RATIONALE: When an individual comes in contact with a poison ivy plant, the sap from the plant forms an invisible film on the human skin. The client should be instructed to immediately shower and to lather the skin several times, rinsing each time in running water. Calamine lotion is a treatment that is used if dermatitis develops. It is not necessary for the client to be seen in the emergency department at this time.
TEST-TAKING STRATEGY: Knowledge that dermatitis can develop from contact with an allergen will assist in selecting the correct option. Also, knowledge that contact with poison ivy results in an invisible film will assist in directing you to option 3. Take time now to review the immediate treatment for contact with poison ivy if you had difficulty with this question.
LEVEL OF COGNITIVE ABILITY: Application
PHASE OF NURSING PROCESS: Implementation
CLIENT NEEDS: Health Promotion and Maintenance
CONTENT AREA: Adult Health/Integumentary
REFERENCE
O'Toole, M. (1997). *Miller-Keane encyclopedia & dictionary of medicine, nursing, & allied health* (6th ed.). Philadelphia: W. B. Saunders.
pp. 1274–1275.

17. 3

RATIONALE: Kaposi's sarcoma lesions begin as red, dark blue, or purple macules on the lower legs that change into plaques. These large plaques ulcerate or open and drain. The lesions spread by metastasis through the upper body, then to the face and oral mucosa. They can move to the lymphatic system, lungs, and gastrointestinal (GI) tract. Late disease results in swelling and pain in the lower extremities, penis, scrotum, or face. Diagnosis is made by punch biopsy of cutaneous lesions and biopsy of pulmonary and GI lesions.

TEST-TAKING STRATEGY: Use the process of elimination, eliminating options 2 and 4 first. These symptoms occur late in the development of Kaposi's sarcoma. Note the key words "this has been determined." This should assist in directing you to the option that will confirm the diagnosis, which will be the biopsy of the lesions.
LEVEL OF COGNITIVE ABILITY: Comprehension
PHASE OF NURSING PROCESS: Data Collection
CLIENT NEEDS: Physiological Integrity
CONTENT AREA: Adult Health/Integumentary
REFERENCE

Luckmann, J. (1997). *Saunders manual of nursing care*. Philadelphia: W. B. Saunders. p. 1936.

18. **4**

RATIONALE: Kaposi's sarcoma is a vascular malignancy that presents as a skin disorder. It is a common AIDS indicator. Malignancy is seen most frequently in men with a history of same sex partners. Although the cause of Kaposi's sarcoma is not known, it is considered to be due to an alteration or failure in the immune system. The renal transplant client and the client receiving antineoplastic medications are at risk for immunosuppression. Exposure to asbestos is not related to the development of Kaposi's sarcoma.
TEST-TAKING STRATEGY: Note the key words "least likely." You can easily eliminate option 1. Note the similarity between options 2 and 3. These clients are at risk for immunosuppression. With this in mind, these options can be eliminated, leaving option 4 as the correct option. If you had difficulty with this question, take time now to review the risk factors associated with Kaposi's sarcoma.
LEVEL OF COGNITIVE ABILITY: Comprehension
PHASE OF NURSING PROCESS: Data Collection
CLIENT NEEDS: Physiological Integrity
CONTENT AREA: Adult Health/Integumentary
REFERENCE

Luckmann, J. (1997). *Saunders manual of nursing care*. Philadelphia: W. B. Saunders. p. 1936.

19. **2**

RATIONALE: Gowns and gloves are required if the nurse anticipates contact with soiled items such as wound drainage. Masks are not required unless droplet or airborne precautions are necessary.
TEST-TAKING STRATEGY: Think about the method of transmission when answering a question of this type. Read the question, noting the task that is presented; in this case, it is bathing and changing linens. Eliminate option 1 because the method of transmission is not respiratory in nature. Eliminate options 3 and 4 because neither provides adequate protection based on the method of transmission. If you had difficulty with this question, take time now to review standard precautions.
LEVEL OF COGNITIVE ABILITY: Application
PHASE OF NURSING PROCESS: Planning
CLIENT NEEDS: Safe, Effective Care Environment
CONTENT AREA: Adult Health/Integumentary
REFERENCE

Monahan, F., & Neighbors, M. (1998). *Medical-surgical nursing: Foundations for clinical practice* (2nd ed.). Philadelphia: W. B. Saunders. p. 1472.

20. **1**

RATIONALE: Cellulitis is a skin infection into deeper dermis and subcutaneous fat that results in deep red erythema without sharp borders that spreads widely through tissue spaces. The skin is erythematous, edematous, tender, and sometimes nodular. Erysipelas is an acute, superficial, rapidly spreading inflammation of the dermis and lymphatics.
TEST-TAKING STRATEGY: Knowledge regarding the characteristics of cellulitis is required to answer the question. If you had difficulty with this question, take time now to review the characteristics of cellulitis and erysipelas.
LEVEL OF COGNITIVE ABILITY: Comprehension
PHASE OF NURSING PROCESS: Planning
CLIENT NEEDS: Physiological Integrity
CONTENT AREA: Adult Health/Integumentary
REFERENCE

deWit, S. (1998). *Essentials of medical-surgical nursing* (4th ed.). Philadelphia: W. B. Saunders. p. 510.

21. **1**

RATIONALE: Warm compresses may be used to decrease the discomfort, erythema, and edema. After tissue and blood cultures are obtained, antibiotics will be initiated. Heat lamps can cause more disruption to already inflamed tissue. Cold and hot are not the best measures.
TEST-TAKING STRATEGY: Use the process of elimination, noting that option 1 is different from the others. Option 1 addresses "warm" compresses. If you had difficulty with this question, take time now to review the treatment associated with cellulitis.
LEVEL OF COGNITIVE ABILITY: Application
PHASE OF NURSING PROCESS: Planning
CLIENT NEEDS: Physiological Integrity
CONTENT AREA: Adult Health/Integumentary
REFERENCE

Luckmann, J. (1997). *Saunders manual of nursing care*. Philadelphia: W. B. Saunders. p. 1613.

22. **1**

RATIONALE: Psoriasis occurs equally among women and men, although the incidence is lower in darker-skinned races. The disorder may begin at any time throughout the life span, but most commonly affects people ages 10 to 40. Emotional distress, trauma, systemic illness, seasonal changes, and hormonal changes are linked to exacerbations.
TEST-TAKING STRATEGY: Use knowledge regarding what psoriasis is and the etiology associated with the disorder to answer the question. If you had difficulty with the question, take time now to review the causes of the disorder and the factors that affect exacerbations.
LEVEL OF COGNITIVE ABILITY: Comprehension
PHASE OF NURSING PROCESS: Data Collection
CLIENT NEEDS: Health Promotion and Maintenance
CONTENT AREA: Adult Health/Integumentary
REFERENCE

Luckmann, J. (1997). *Saunders manual of nursing care*. Philadelphia: W. B. Saunders. p. 1639.

23. **4**

RATIONALE: Psoriatic patches are covered with silvery white scales. Affected areas include the scalp, elbows, knees, shins, sacral area, and trunk. Thickening, pitting, and discoloration of the nails occurs. Pruritus may occur. The lesions in psoriasis are not red-purple scaly lesions.

TEST-TAKING STRATEGY: Knowledge regarding the clinical manifestations associated with psoriasis is required to answer the question. From this knowledge, you should be able to identify that option 4 is not associated with this condition. If you had difficulty with this question, take time now to review the manifestations associated with psoriasis.
LEVEL OF COGNITIVE ABILITY: Comprehension
PHASE OF NURSING PROCESS: Data Collection
CLIENT NEEDS: Physiological Integrity
CONTENT AREA: Adult Health/Integumentary
REFERENCE
Luckmann, J. (1997). *Saunders manual of nursing care*. Philadelphia: W. B. Saunders. p. 1639.

24. **3**

RATIONALE: Safety precautions are required during UVL therapy. Most UVL treatments require the client to stand in a light treatment chamber for up to 15 minutes. It is best to expose only those areas requiring treatment to the UVL. Protective wrap-around goggles prevent exposure of the eyes to UVL. The face should be shielded with a loosely applied covering if it is unaffected. Direct contact with the light bulbs of the treatment unit should be avoided to prevent burning the skin.
TEST-TAKING STRATEGY: Note the key word "not." Note that option 3 addresses a time frame of 30 minutes, which is an extensive period for exposure to UVL. If you had difficulty with this question, take time now to review client education for UVL treatments.
LEVEL OF COGNITIVE ABILITY: Application
PHASE OF NURSING PROCESS: Planning
CLIENT NEEDS: Safe, Effective Care Environment
CONTENT AREA: Adult Health/Integumentary
REFERENCE
Luckmann, J. (1997). *Saunders manual of nursing care*. Philadelphia: W. B. Saunders. p. 1640.

25. **3**

RATIONALE: Herpes zoster is caused by a reactivation of the varicella zoster virus, the cause of the virus for chickenpox. A viral culture of the lesion provides the definitive diagnosis. In a Wood's light examination, the skin is viewed under ultraviolet light to identify superficial infections of the skin. A patch test is a skin test that involves the administration of an allergen to the skin's surface to identify specific allergies. A biopsy determines tissue type.
TEST-TAKING STRATEGY: Knowledge that herpes zoster is caused by a virus will direct you toward the correct option. Eliminate options 2 and 4 first. From the remaining two options, remember that a biopsy determines tissue type, whereas a culture identifies an organism.
LEVEL OF COGNITIVE ABILITY: Comprehension
PHASE OF NURSING PROCESS: Data Collection
CLIENT NEEDS: Physiological Integrity
CONTENT AREA: Adult Health/Integumentary
REFERENCE
Luckmann, J. (1997). *Saunders manual of nursing care*. Philadelphia: W. B. Saunders. p. 1635.

26. **4**

RATIONALE: The primary lesion of herpes zoster is a vesicle. The classic presentation is grouped vesicles on a erythematous base along a dermatome. Because they follow nerve pathways, the lesions do not cross the body's midline. Options 1, 2, and 3 are incorrect descriptions.
TEST-TAKING STRATEGY: Knowledge regarding the characteristics of herpes zoster lesions is required to answer the question. Remembering that these lesions occur as grouped vesicles along a nerve pathway will assist in answering the question. If you had difficulty with this question, take time now to review the characteristics of herpes zoster lesions.
LEVEL OF COGNITIVE ABILITY: Comprehension
PHASE OF NURSING PROCESS: Data Collection
CLIENT NEEDS: Physiological Integrity
CONTENT AREA: Adult Health/Integumentary
REFERENCE
deWit, S. (1998). *Essentials of medical-surgical nursing* (4th ed.). Philadelphia: W. B. Saunders. p. 906.

27. **2**

RATIONALE: Herpes zoster is caused by a reactivation of the varicella zoster virus, the causative virus for chickenpox. Individuals who have not been exposed to the varicella zoster virus are susceptible to chickenpox. Options 1, 3, and 4 are not associated with the herpes zoster virus.
TEST-TAKING STRATEGY: Knowledge that herpes zoster is caused by a reactivation of the varicella zoster virus, the causative virus for chickenpox, will assist in answering the question. Review the relationship between herpes zoster and chickenpox now if you had difficulty with this question.
LEVEL OF COGNITIVE ABILITY: Application
PHASE OF NURSING PROCESS: Implementation
CLIENT NEEDS: Safe, Effective Care Environment
CONTENT AREA: Adult Health/Integumentary
REFERENCE
Luckmann, J. (1997). *Saunders manual of nursing care*. Philadelphia: W. B. Saunders. p. 1636.

28. **1**

RATIONALE: Melanomas are pigmented malignant lesions originating in the melanin-producing cells of the epidermis. This skin cancer is highly metastatic, and a person's survival depends on early diagnosis and treatment. Basal cell carcinomas arise in the basal cell layer of the epidermis. Early malignant basal cell lesions often go unnoticed and although metastasis is rare, underlying tissue destruction can progress to include vital structures. Squamous cell carcinomas are malignant neoplasms of the epidermis. They are characterized by local invasion and the potential for metastasis.
TEST-TAKING STRATEGY: Knowledge regarding the various types of skin cancers is required to answer this question. Knowing that melanomas are highly metastatic will assist in directing you to the correct option. If you had difficulty with this question, take time now to review the characteristics of skin cancers.
LEVEL OF COGNITIVE ABILITY: Comprehension
PHASE OF NURSING PROCESS: Data Collection
CLIENT NEEDS: Physiological Integrity
CONTENT AREA: Adult Health/Integumentary
REFERENCE
deWit, S. (1998). *Essentials of medical-surgical nursing* (4th ed.). Philadelphia: W. B. Saunders. p. 912.

29. 4

RATIONALE: A melanoma is an irregularly shaped red, white, or blue-toned pigmented papule or plaque. Basal cell carcinoma appears as a pearly papule with a central crater and rolled waxy border. Squamous cell carcinoma is a firm nodular lesion topped with a crust or a central area of ulceration. Actinic keratosis, a premalignant lesion, appears as a small macule or papule with dry, rough, adherent yellow or brown scales.
TEST-TAKING STRATEGY: Knowledge regarding the characteristics of melanoma is required to answer this question. Remembering that irregularly shaped lesions are a cause for concern will assist you in answering the question. If you had difficulty with this question, take time now to review the characteristics of malignant skin lesions.
LEVEL OF COGNITIVE ABILITY: Comprehension
PHASE OF NURSING PROCESS: Data Collection
CLIENT NEEDS: Physiological Integrity
CONTENT AREA: Adult Health/Integumentary
REFERENCE
deWit, S. (1998). *Essentials of medical-surgical nursing* (4th ed.). Philadelphia: W. B. Saunders. p. 912.

30. 1

RATIONALE: Cryosurgery involves the local application of liquid nitrogen to isolated lesions and causes cell death and tissue destruction. The nurse prepares the client for swelling and increased tenderness of the treated area when the skin thaws. Tissue freezing is followed in 1 to 2 days by hemorrhagic blister formation. The nurse instructs the client to clean the treatment site with hydrogen peroxide to prevent secondary infection. A topical antibiotic may also be prescribed. Application of a warm damp washcloth intermittently to the site will provide relief from any discomfort. Alcohol-soaked dressings will cause irritation. It is not necessary to avoid showering.
TEST-TAKING STRATEGY: Use the process of elimination. Eliminate option 4 first because there is no reason for the client to avoid showers. Eliminate option 3 (alcohol-soaked dressing) next. From the remaining two options, note that option 1 addresses the prevention of infection. If you had difficulty with this question, take time now to review client instructions following cryosurgery.
LEVEL OF COGNITIVE ABILITY: Application
PHASE OF NURSING PROCESS: Planning
CLIENT NEEDS: Health Promotion and Maintenance
CONTENT AREA: Adult Health/Integumentary
REFERENCE
Black, J. & Matassarin-Jacobs, E. (1997). *Medical surgical nursing: Clinical management for continuity of care* (5th ed.). Philadelphia: W. B. Saunders. p. 2225.

31. 4

RATIONALE: The client should be instructed to avoid sun exposure between the hours of 11:00 A.M. and 3:00 P.M. Sunscreen, a hat, opaque clothing, and sunglasses should be worn for outdoor activities. The client should be instructed to examine the body monthly for the appearance of any possible cancerous or any precancerous lesions.
TEST-TAKING STRATEGY: Note the key word "not." Careful reading of the question will easily direct you to option 4. Take time to review client teaching in the prevention of skin cancer now if you had difficulty with this question.
LEVEL OF COGNITIVE ABILITY: Application
PHASE OF NURSING PROCESS: Implementation

CLIENT NEEDS: Health Promotion and Maintenance
CONTENT AREA: Adult Health/Integumentary
REFERENCE
deWit, S. (1998). *Essentials of medical-surgical nursing* (4th ed.). Philadelphia: W. B. Saunders. pp. 910–912.

32. 2

RATIONALE: Paronychia or infection around the nail is characterized by red, shiny skin often associated with painful swelling. These infections frequently result from trauma, picking at the nail, or disorders such as dermatitis. Often these become secondarily infected with bacteria or fungus, which later involves the nail. Options 1, 3, and 4 are incorrect descriptions of this disorder.
TEST-TAKING STRATEGY: Knowledge regarding the characteristics of paronychia is required to answer the question. If you know that this disorder is related to an infection of the nail, you will easily be directed toward the correct option. If you had difficulty with this question, take time now to review the definition of this disorder.
LEVEL OF COGNITIVE ABILITY: Comprehension
PHASE OF NURSING PROCESS: Data Collection
CLIENT NEEDS: Physiological Integrity
CONTENT AREA: Adult Health/Integumentary
REFERENCE
deWit, S. (1998). *Essentials of medical-surgical nursing* (4th ed.). Philadelphia: W. B. Saunders. p. 911.

33. 3

RATIONALE: The nurse would not tell a client that it is not necessary to separate laundry from other household members. Thorough handwashing, separating laundry, and separating washing of the client's dishes is required, because the infection is contagious as long as skin lesions are present. Antibiotics are administered and should be continued as prescribed.
TEST-TAKING STRATEGY: Knowledge regarding the transmission of impetigo is required to answer the question. Note the key word "not." If you had difficulty with this question, take time now to review client instructions related to home care and the prevention of transmission.
LEVEL OF COGNITIVE ABILITY: Application
PHASE OF NURSING PROCESS: Implementation
CLIENT NEEDS: Health Promotion and Maintenance
CONTENT AREA: Adult Health/Integumentary
REFERENCE
Black, J., & Matassarin-Jacobs, E. (1997). *Medical-surgical nursing: Clinical management for continuity of care* (5th ed.). Philadelphia: W. B. Saunders. p. 2221.

34. 4

RATIONALE: Findings in frostbite include a white or blue color and the skin will be hard, cold, and insensitive to touch. As thawing occurs, flushing of the skin, the development of blisters or blebs, or tissue edema appears. Gangrene develops in 9 to 15 days.
TEST-TAKING STRATEGY: Knowledge regarding the characteristics of frostbite is required to answer the question. The words "insensitive to touch" should assist in directing you toward this option. If you had difficulty with this question, take time now to review the characteristics associated with frostbite.

LEVEL OF COGNITIVE ABILITY: Comprehension
PHASE OF NURSING PROCESS: Data Collection
CLIENT NEEDS: Physiological Integrity
CONTENT AREA: Adult Health/Integumentary
REFERENCE
Luckmann, J. (1997). *Saunders manual of nursing care*. Philadelphia: W. B. Saunders. p. 1736.

35. **1**

RATIONALE: Frostbite is ideally treated with rapid and continuous rewarming of the tissue in a water bath for 15 to 20 minutes or until flushing of the skin occurs. Hot or cold water is not used in the treatment of frosbite.
TEST-TAKING STRATEGY: Use the process of elimination. Eliminate options 2 and 4 first, because these options address "hot" and "cold." Eliminate option 3 because interventions should begin immediately. If you had difficulty with this question, take time now to review the interventions associated with frostbite.
LEVEL OF COGNITIVE ABILITY: Comprehension
PHASE OF NURSING PROCESS: Planning
CLIENT NEEDS: Physiological Integrity
CONTENT AREA: Adult Health/Integumentary
REFERENCE
Luckmann, J. (1997). *Saunders manual of nursing care*. Philadelphia: W. B. Saunders. p. 1736.

36. **2**

RATIONALE: In a stage 2 pressure ulcer, the skin is not intact. There is partial-thickness skin loss of the epidermis or dermis. The ulcer is superficial and may look like an abrasion, blister, or shallow crater. The skin is intact in stage 1. A deep crater-like appearance occurs in stage 3, and sinus tracts develop in stage 4.
TEST-TAKING STRATEGY: Use the process of elimination and knowledge of the characteristics associated with each stage of pressure ulcers. If you had difficulty with this question, take time now to review the characteristics associated with each stage of pressure ulcers.
LEVEL OF COGNITIVE ABILITY: Comprehension
PHASE OF NURSING PROCESS: Data Collection
CLIENT NEEDS: Physiological Integrity
CONTENT AREA: Adult Health/Integumentary
REFERENCE
de Wit, S. (1998). *Essentials of medical-surgical nursing* (4th ed.). Philadelphia: W. B. Saunders. p. 267.

37. **4**

RATIONALE: Bed or chair confinement, inability to move, loss of bowel or bladder control, poor nutrition, absent or inconsistent caregiving, and a lowered mental awareness can all contribute to the development of skin breakdown. The least likely risk as presented in the options, is the lowered mental awareness status. Options 1, 2, and 3 identify physiological conditions, which are the risk priorities.
TEST-TAKING STRATEGY: Note the key words "least likely." Use Maslow's hierarchy of needs theory. Remember that physiological needs are the priority. This will assist you in eliminating options 1, 2, and 3.
LEVEL OF COGNITIVE ABILITY: Comprehension
PHASE OF NURSING PROCESS: Data Collection
CLIENT NEEDS: Physiological Integrity
CONTENT AREA: Adult Health/Integumentary

REFERENCE
Luckmann, J. (1997). *Saunders manual of nursing care*. Philadelphia: W. B. Saunders. p. 194.

38. **3**

RATIONALE: Candidiasis (thrush) is noted as white patches on the tongue, palate, and buccal mucosa. The lesions adhere firmly to the tissues and are difficult to remove. The lesions are often referred to as milk curds because of their appearance. Clients often describe the lesions as dry and hot.
TEST-TAKING STRATEGY: Remembering that candidiasis presents as white patches will assist in answering the question. If you had difficulty with this question, take time now to review the characteristics associated with candidiasis.
LEVEL OF COGNITIVE ABILITY: Comprehension
PHASE OF NURSING PROCESS: Data Collection
CLIENT NEEDS: Physiological Integrity
CONTENT AREA: Adult Health/Integumentary
REFERENCE
de Wit, S. (1998). *Essentials of medical-surgical nursing* (4th ed.). Philadelphia: W. B. Saunders. p. 191.

39. **1**

RATIONALE: Clients cannot tolerate commercial mouthwashes because the high alcohol concentration in these products can cause pain and discomfort to the lesions. A solution of warm water, half-strength peroxide, or mouthwash formulas without alcohol are better tolerated and may promote healing. A change in diet to liquid or pureed food often eases the discomfort of eating. The client should avoid spicy foods, citrus juice, and hot liquids.
TEST-TAKING STRATEGY: Note the key word "not" and use the process of elimination. Take time now to review the client education teaching points related to candidiasis (thrush) if you had difficulty with this question.
LEVEL OF COGNITIVE ABILITY: Application
PHASE OF NURSING PROCESS: Planning
CLIENT NEEDS: Health Promotion and Maintenance
CONTENT AREA: Adult Health/Integumentary
REFERENCE
de Wit, S. (1998). *Essentials of medical-surgical nursing* (4th ed.). Philadelphia: W. B. Saunders. p. 190.

40. **4**

RATIONALE: A hallmark sign of pemphigus is Nikolsky's sign, which is when the epidermis can be rubbed off by slight friction or injury. Trousseau's is a sign for tetany in which carpal spasm can be elicited by compressing the upper arm and causing ischemia to the nerves distally. Chvostek's sign seen in tetany is a spasm of the facial muscles elicited by tapping the facial nerve in the region of the parotid gland. Homans' sign, a sign of thrombosis in the leg, is discomfort behind the knee on forced dorsiflexion of the foot.
TEST-TAKING STRATEGY: Use the process of elimination. If you knew that Homans' sign is related to thrombophlebitis and that Chvostek's sign and Trousseau's sign are related to tetany, then by the process of elimination, you would select option 4. If you had difficulty with this question, take time now to review these various signs.
LEVEL OF COGNITIVE ABILITY: Comprehension
PHASE OF NURSING PROCESS: Data Collection
CLIENT NEEDS: Physiological Integrity
CONTENT AREA: Adult Health/Integumentary

REFERENCE
O'Toole, M. (1997). *Miller-Keane encyclopedia & dictionary of medicine, nursing, & allied health* (6th ed.). Philadelphia: W. B. Saunders. pp. 328, 751, 1658.

41. 3

RATIONALE: The exact cause of acne is unknown. There is no scientific evidence that consumption of foods such as chocolate, nuts, or fatty foods affects acne. Exacerbations that coincide with the menstrual cycle result from hormonal activity. Heat, humidity, and excessive perspiration also play a role in increased acne.
TEST-TAKING STRATEGY: Use the process of elimination and knowledge regarding factors that exacerbate acne. Options 1, 2, and 4 relate specifically to factors that exacerbate acne. Take time now to review this disorder if you had difficulty with this question.
LEVEL OF COGNITIVE ABILITY: Application
PHASE OF NURSING PROCESS: Implementation
CLIENT NEEDS: Physiological Integrity
CONTENT AREA: Adult Health/Integumentary
REFERENCE
Schulte, E., Price, D., & James, S. (1997). *Thompson's pediatric nursing: An introductory text* (7th ed.). Philadelphia: W. B. Saunders. p. 413.

42. 1

RATIONALE: In severe cystic acne, isotretinoin (Accutane) is used to inhibit inflammation. Adverse effects include elevated triglycerides, skin dryness, eye discomfort such as dryness and burning, and cheilitis (lip inflammation). Close medical follow-up is required and dry skin and cheilitis can be decreased by the use of emollients and lip balms. Vitamin A supplements are stopped during this treatment.
TEST-TAKING STRATEGY: Note the key words "need for further instruction." Knowledge regarding the adverse effects related to this medication is required to answer this question. If you had difficulty with this question take time now to review the action, side effects, and adverse effects of isotretinoin.
LEVEL OF COGNITIVE ABILITY: Comprehension
PHASE OF NURSING PROCESS: Evaluation
CLIENT NEEDS: Health Promotion and Maintenance
CONTENT AREA: Adult Health/Integumentary
REFERENCE
Hodgson, B., & Kizior, R. (2000). *Saunders nursing drug handbook 2000*. Philadelphia: W. B. Saunders. p. 557.

43. 3

RATIONALE: Scabies can be identified by the multiple straight or wavy threadlike lines noted beneath the skin. The skin lesions are caused by the female, which burrows beneath the skin and lays its eggs. The eggs hatch in a few days and the baby mites find their way to the skin surface where they mate and complete the life cycle. Options 1, 2, and 4 are not characteristics of scabies.
TEST-TAKING STRATEGY: Knowledge that scabies mites burrow beneath the skin surface will assist in the process of elimination and provide direction toward selection of the correct option. If you had difficulty with this question, take time now to review the characteristics associated with scabies.
LEVEL OF COGNITIVE ABILITY: Comprehension
PHASE OF NURSING PROCESS: Data Collection

CLIENT NEEDS: Physiological Integrity
CONTENT AREA: Adult Health/Integumentary
REFERENCE
deWit, S. (1998). *Essentials of medical-surgical nursing* (4th ed.). Philadelphia: W. B. Saunders. p. 907.

44. 3

RATIONALE: The Centers for Disease Control and Prevention recommend wearing gowns and gloves for close contact with a person infested with scabies. Masks are not necessary. Transmission via clothing and other inanimate objects is uncommon. Scabies is usually transmitted from person to person by direct skin contact. All contacts that the client has had should be treated at the same time.
TEST-TAKING STRATEGY: Consider the mode of transmission of scabies and use the process of elimination. Since scabies is transmitted by direct skin contact, eliminate options 1, 2, and 4. If you had difficulty with this question, take time now to review standard precautions and the transmission mode of scabies.
LEVEL OF COGNITIVE ABILITY: Application
PHASE OF NURSING PROCESS: Implementation
CLIENT NEEDS: Safe, Effective Care Environment
CONTENT AREA: Adult Health/Integumentary
REFERENCE
O'Toole, M. (1997). *Miller-Keane encyclopedia & dictionary of medicine, nursing, & allied health* (6th ed.). Philadelphia: W. B. Saunders. p. 1444.

45. 2

RATIONALE: According to the rule of nines, with the initial burn, the anterior half of the head equals 4.5%, the upper half of the anterior torso equals 9%, and the lower half of both arms equals 9%. The subsequent burn included the posterior half of the head equaling 4.5% and the upper half of the posterior torso equaling 9%. This totals 36%.
TEST-TAKING STRATEGY: Knowledge regarding the rule of nines is required to answer this question. Remember: 9 (head), 18 (arms), 36 (thorax), 36 (legs), 1 (perineum), equaling 99. If you had difficulty with this question, take time now to review the rule of nines.
LEVEL OF COGNITIVE ABILITY: Comprehension
PHASE OF NURSING PROCESS: Data Collection
CLIENT NEEDS: Physiological Integrity
CONTENT AREA: Adult Health/Integumentary
REFERENCE
deWit, S. (1998). *Essentials of medical-surgical nursing* (4th ed.). Philadelphia: W. B. Saunders. p. 912.

46. 4

RATIONALE: The client exhibited several warning signs of an inhalation injury, namely, a history of flame burn to the face, hoarseness, cough, carbonaceous sputum, singed facial hair, facial edema, and then color change. Additionally, one of the cardinal signs of hypoxia is restlessness and anxiety.
TEST-TAKING STRATEGY: Use the ABCs (airway, breathing, and circulation) to answer the question. The only option that addresses airway is option 4. If you had difficulty with this question, take time now to review the clinical manifestations associated with burns to the face.
LEVEL OF COGNITIVE ABILITY: Comprehension
PHASE OF NURSING PROCESS: Data Collection
CLIENT NEEDS: Physiological Integrity
CONTENT AREA: Adult Health/integumentary

REFERENCE
deWit, S. (1998). *Essentials of medical-surgical nursing* (4th ed.). Philadelphia: W. B. Saunders. 915.

47. **4**

RATIONALE: Escharotomies are performed to alleviate the compartment syndrome, which can occur when edema forms under nondistensible eschar in a circumferential third-degree burn. Escharotomies are performed through avascular eschar to subcutaneous fat. Although bleeding may occur from the site, it is considered a complication rather than an anticipated therapeutic outcome. Formation of granulation tissue is not the intent of an escharotomy. An escharotomy will not affect the formation of edema.
TEST-TAKING STRATEGY: Use the ABCs, airway, breathing, and circulation, to answer the question. The only option that addresses circulation is option 4. If you had difficulty with this question, take time now to review the purpose of an escharotomy.
LEVEL OF COGNITIVE ABILITY: Comprehension
PHASE OF NURSING PROCESS: Evaluation
CLIENT NEEDS: Physiological Integrity
CONTENT AREA: Adult Health/Integumentary
REFERENCE
Monahan, F., & Neighbors, M. (1998). *Medical-surgical nursing: Foundations for clinical practice* (2nd ed.). Philadelphia: W. B. Saunders. p. 1664.

48. **1**

RATIONALE: Superficial injury from radiation causes erythema and pain, hyperpigmentation, dry desquamation, or moist desquamation. Options 2, 3, and 4 are not associated with the description presented in the question.
TEST-TAKING STRATEGY: Knowledge regarding the physiological manifestations that occur with radiation burns is helpful to answer this question. Focus on the description in the question and note the word "superficial" in the correct option. If you had difficulty with this question, take time now to review the effects of radiation burns.
LEVEL OF COGNITIVE ABILITY: Comprehension
PHASE OF NURSING PROCESS: Data Collection
CLIENT NEEDS: Physiological Integrity
CONTENT AREA: Adult Health/Integumentary
REFERENCE
Monahan, F., & Neighbors, M. (1998). *Medical-surgical nursing: Foundations for clinical practice* (2nd ed.). Philadelphia: W. B. Saunders. p. 1520.

49. **3**

RATIONALE: Circumferential burns of the extremities may compromise circulation. Elevating injured extremities above the level of the heart and active exercise help to reduce dependent edema formation. Options 1, 2, and 4 are incorrect.
TEST-TAKING STRATEGY: Use the process of elimination, remembering that when an injury such as a burn occurs, edema results. Option 3 addresses a position that will reduce edema. If you had difficulty with this question, take time now to review care to the client experiencing this type of burn injury.
LEVEL OF COGNITIVE ABILITY: Application
PHASE OF NURSING PROCESS: Implementation
CLIENT NEEDS: Physiological Integrity
CONTENT AREA: Adult Health/Integumentary

REFERENCE
Monahan, F., & Neighbors, M. (1998). *Medical-surgical nursing: Foundations for clinical practice* (2nd ed.). Philadelphia: W. B. Saunders. p. 1664.

50. **3**

RATIONALE: Thorough handwashing should be done before and after each contact with the burn-injured client. Sterile sheets and linens are used. Protective garb including gloves, cap, masks, shoe covers, scrub clothes, and plastic aprons need to be worn when caring for the client.
TEST-TAKING STRATEGY: Note the key word "not." Option 2 can easily be eliminated from the remaining options. Select option 3 because this is the least thorough technique to prevent infection. If you had difficulty with this question, take time now to review protective isolation techniques when caring for a burn client.
LEVEL OF COGNITIVE ABILITY: Application
PHASE OF NURSING PROCESS: Implementation
CLIENT NEEDS: Safe, Effective Care Environment
CONTENT AREA: Adult Health/Integumentary
REFERENCE
deWit, S. (1998). *Essentials of medical-surgical nursing* (4th ed.). Philadelphia: W. B. Saunders. p. 151.

51. **1**

RATIONALE: Autografts placed over joints or on the lower extremities are often elevated and immobilized following surgery for 3 to 7 days. This period of immobilization allows the autograft time to adhere and attach to the wound bed.
TEST-TAKING STRATEGY: Eliminate options 2 and 3 first because they are similar. Note that the autograft was placed over a joint. This should direct you toward selecting the option that identifies the longer period of immobilization. If you had difficulty with this question, take time now to review care to an autograft placed over a joint.
LEVEL OF COGNITIVE ABILITY: Comprehension
PHASE OF NURSING PROCESS: Planning
CLIENT NEEDS: Physiological Integrity
CONTENT AREA: Adult Health/Integumentary
REFERENCE
deWit, S. (1998). *Essentials of medical-surgical nursing* (4th ed.). Philadelphia: W. B. Saunders. p. 918.

52. **4**

RATIONALE: Newly healed skin is more sensitive to the cold and the client should be instructed to wear warm clothing. The client should wash using a mild soap, rinsing thoroughly, and patting the skin dry using a clean towel. Newly healed skin sunburns easily and direct sunlight needs to be avoided. Products that contain perfume, alcohol, or lanolin should be avoided because they tend to irritate newly healed skin.
TEST-TAKING STRATEGY: Read each option carefully noting that the correct option uses the absolute term "never." Absolute terms should be avoided. If you had difficulty with this question, take time now to review home care instructions regarding skin care.
LEVEL OF COGNITIVE ABILITY: Application
PHASE OF NURSING PROCESS: Planning
CLIENT NEEDS: Health Promotion and Maintenance
CONTENT AREA: Adult Health/Integumentary
REFERENCE
Monahan, F., & Neighbors, M. (1998). *Medical-surgical nursing: Foundations for clinical practice* (2nd ed.). Philadelphia: W. B. Saunders. p. 1683.

BIBLIOGRAPY

Black, J., & Matassarin-Jacobs, E. (1997). *Medical-surgical nursing: Clinical management for continuity of care* (5th ed.). Philadelphia: W. B. Saunders.

deWit, S. (1998). *Essentials of medical-surgical nursing* (4th ed.). Philadelphia: W. B. Saunders.

Hodgson, B., & Kizior, R. (2000). *Saunders nursing drug handbook 2000*. Philadelphia: W. B. Saunders.

Luckmann, J. (1997). *Saunders manual of nursing care*. Philadelphia: W. B. Saunders.

Monahan, F., & Neighbors, M. (1998). *Medical-surgical nursing: Foundations for clinical practice* (2nd ed.). Philadelphia: W. B. Saunders.

O'Toole, M. (1997). *Miller-Keane encyclopedia & dictionary of medicine, nursing, & allied health* (6th ed.). Philadelphia: W. B. Saunders.

Schulte, E., Price, D., & James, S. (1997). *Thompson's pediatric nursing: An introductory text* (7th ed.). Philadelphia: W. B. Saunders.

CHAPTER 39

Integumentary Medications

I. Emollients and Lotions

A. Emollients (Box 39–1)
1. Oily or fatty substances that soften and soothe irritated skin by allowing the skin to retain water
2. Available as creams or ointments
3. Used for dry, scaly, itchy inflammatory conditions

B. Lotions (Box 39–2)
1. Liquid suspensions that require shaking before application
2. Although lotions are predominantly water, they have a drying effect on the skin when the water evaporates
3. Used as a skin wash, as soaks, or as wet dressings on ulcers or **burns**
4. Used for inflammatory lesions after the severe exudate phase has ceased
5. Medicated lotions are often used as anti-inflammatory agents because they provide a drying, protective, and cooling effect

II. Rubs and Liniments (Box 39–3)

A. Used for the temporary relief of muscular aches, rheumatism, arthritis, sprains, and neuralgia

B. Over-the-counter (OTC) products contain combinations of antiseptics, local anesthetics, analgesics, and counterirritants

C. Some products contain salicylates and, if used over a large area of the skin, may cause salicylate side effects such as tinnitus, nausea, or vomiting

D. A heating pad is not used with these products

because irritation or burning of the skin may occur

III. Anti-infective Agents

A. Description
1. Includes antiseptics, antibacterial, antifungal, antiviral, and antiparasitic medications
2. Topical antibiotics are safe and effective in certain conditions; extensive use may encourage the emergence of resistant bacteria

B. Antiseptics
1. Sodium hypochlorite (Dakin solution)
   a. A chloride solution that loosens, dissolves, and deodorizes necrotic tissue and blood clots
   b. It kills most common bacteria, including spores, amebas, fungi, protozoa viruses, and yeast
   c. It is used for irrigating and cleaning necrotic or purulent wounds
   d. Loses its potency during storage, so fresh solution is prepared frequently
   e. It should not be in contact with healing or normal tissue
2. Chlorhexidine gluconate (Hibiclens)
   a. Effective for cleaning wounds caused by staphylococci and other gram-positive bacteria
   b. Used for irrigating and cleansing wounds, but not for packing wounds because it may cause contact dermatitis

---

BOX 39–1. Emollients

Glycerin	Cold cream
Petrolatum	Zinc ointment
Lanolin	

BOX 39–2. Lotions

Calamine lotion (Caladryl lotion)
Aluminum acetate solution (Burow solution)
Potassium permanganate solution
Zinc stearate

3. Acetic acid
   a. Effective for irrigating, cleansing, and packing wounds infected by *Pseudomonas aeruginosa*
   b. Healthy skin surrounding the wound must be protected with a petroleum barrier because it excoriates the skin
4. Hydrogen peroxide
   a. Used to irrigate and clean necrotic tissue and pus from open wounds
   b. Not used to pack wounds because it decomposes too rapidly
   c. When epithelial tissue begins to form, hydrogen peroxide is discontinued because it inhibits tissue formation
5. Hexachlorophene (pHisoHex, Septisol)
   a. A combination of hexachlorophene and alcohol
   b. Hexachlorophene is a bacterial static agent with activity against staphylococci and other gram-positive bacteria
   c. Hexachlorophene is heavily absorbed through broken skin and can cause neurotoxicity; it should not be used on wounds
   d. Alcohol dries and irritates tissue, is not a very effective germicide, and forms a film that can actually promote infection
   e. All hexachlorophene products need to be well rinsed from the skin after their use to prevent systemic absorption
C. Antibacterials (Box 39–4)
  1. Description
   a. Not effective for acute, superficial, or relatively localized infections
   b. Applied one to five times daily to the infected area and covered if needed
  2. Mupirocin (Bactroban)
   a. Topical antibacterial active against impetigo caused by *Staphylococcus* or *Streptococcus* species
   b. Apply three times daily
   c. If improvement is not observed within 3 to 5 days, it is discontinued
D. Antifungals

1. May cause erythema, stinging, blistering, peeling, pruritus, urticaria, and general skin irritation
2. Client is reevaluated if no results are obtained after 4 weeks of treatment
E. Antivirals
  1. Acyclovir (Zovirax) inhibits DNA replication in the virus
  2. Used for herpes simplex types 1 and 2, varicella-zoster, Epstein-Barr virus, and cytomegalovirus
  3. Can cause mild pain and transient burning and stinging
  4. Applied completely over the lesion every 3 hours six times daily for 1 week as prescribed
  5. Rubber gloves are used to apply the ointment to prevent the spread of infection
F. Antiparasitics
  1. Used to treat scabies (mites) and pediculosis (lice)
  2. May be harmful during pregnancy and in young children
  3. May irritate the skin, eyes, and mucous membranes
  4. May cause allergic reactions

IV. Antipruritics (Box 39–5)

A. Used to allay itching
B. Applied as wet dressings, pastes, lotions, creams, or ointments
C. People with dry skin should be instructed to bathe less frequently

V. Keratolytics (Box 39–6)

A. Description
  1. Preparations that dissolve keratin
  2. Soften scales and loosen the horny layer of skin, resulting in minimal peeling or extensive desquamation

3. Used to treat superficial fungal infections, dermatitis, psoriasis, and localized dermatitis

B. Salicylic acid
1. Used to treat seborrheic dermatitis, acne, and psoriasis, and to thin and remove calluses
2. Can be absorbed systematically and can cause salicylism, characterized by dizziness and tinnitus; it is not applied to large surface areas or open wounds

C. Podophyllum resin
1. Used for various types of **skin cancer**
2. Causes lesions to slough off, leaving a superficial ulcer and moderate dermatitis
3. After the therapy is discontinued, the lesions are dressed with a mild antiseptic ointment; healing usually occurs within a few days

D. Cantharidin (Cantharone)
1. Used in treating warts
2. Has an exfoliation effect only on the epidermal cells
3. May cause tingling, itching, and burning
4. Site may be very tender for 2 to 6 days

E. Masoprocol (Actinex)
1. Has antiproliferative activity and is used to treat keratosis
2. Occlusive dressings are not to be used
3. Transient burning may be experienced after administration

VI. Stimulants and Irritants (Box 39–7)

A. Description: produce a mild irritation to the surface of the skin, causing hyperemia and inflammation, which promote the healing process

B. Coal tar
1. Used in treating psoriasis, seborrheic dermatitis, and atopic dermatitis
2. Has an unpleasant odor and frequently stains the skin and hair
3. Can cause phototoxicity

C. Compound benzoin tincture
1. Protects the skin when the client has bed sores, ulcers, cracked nipples, and fissures of any orifice
2. Causes a mild irritation that produces increased blood flow and healing

VII. Protectives (Box 39–8)

A. Description
1. Preparations that form a film on the skin to protect it from irritations such as light, moisture, air, and dust
2. Promote natural healing without the usual

BOX 39–7. Stimulants and Irritants
Coal tar
Compound benzoin tincture

BOX 39–8. Protectives	
Tegaderm	Uniflex
DuoDerm	Mediskin and Silver
PolySkin	Zinc oxide paste
Ensure-It (Deseret)	(Unna's boot)
Op-Site	Vigilon
Tegasorb	

formation of dry crust over the wound; hydrate the wound surface
3. Allow exudate to collect beneath the dressing, forming an artificial blister
4. Uniflex, PolySkin, and Ensure-It may be used to cover IV sites
5. Op-Site, Tegasorb, Mediskin and Silver, and Vigilon may be used for skin **burns**

B. Sunscreens
1. Act by absorbing ultraviolet rays
2. The best sunscreens contain PABA (para-aminobenzoic acid)
3. Most effective when applied about 30 minutes to 1 hour before exposure to the sun; should be reapplied after swimming or sweating
4. Can cause contact dermatitis and photosensitivity reactions

VIII. Growth Factors

A. Description
1. Used to promote wound healing
2. Stimulate cells to divide and migrate, which results in wound healing, formation of granulation tissue, and new epidermis

B. Procuren solution
1. Promotes healing by actively stimulating growth and granulation tissue, capillaries, and epithelium
2. Applied to the wound and is covered with petrolatum-impregnated gauze
3. The material is left in place for 12 hours and then washed off with tapwater irrigation; during the remaining 12 hours of the day, the wound is covered with silver sulfadiazine (Silvadene)

IX. Enzymes

A. Description
1. Used to promote healing of wounds and to debride skin ulcers
2. Reduce inflammation resulting from trauma and infection
3. Dissolve fibrin clots, which helps to reduce the size of surface hematomas
4. To be effective, must be in contact with affected tissue in adequate concentrations for a sufficient length of time
5. Wound may need to be surgically debrided prior to application; if not administered to a

---

BOX 39–9. Enzymes That Promote Wound Healing

Papain (Panafil) (Panafil White)
Hyaluronidase (Wydase)

---

clean, debrided wound, healing may be delayed
B. Enzymes that promote wound healing (Box 39–9)
  1. Papain (Panafil) (Panafil White)
    a. Does not injure or affect healthy tissue or cells
    b. Enzyme must be in immediate contact with the purulent wound material
    c. Wounds are cleansed with prescribed irrigating solution between doses
    d. Hydrogen peroxide cannot be used to irrigate the wound because it inactivates the papain
    e. Light dressings and cellophane wrap may be used over the wound to prevent soiling of clothing
    f. Dressings are changed frequently to prevent contamination and to remove necrotic debris
  2. Hyaluronidase (Wydase)
    a. Facilitates the absorption of fluids given by subcutaneous hypodermoclysis
    b. It reduces the sloughing of tissue likely to occur secondarily to IV infiltration
C. Enzymes to remove exudates (Box 39–10)
  1. Description
    a. They alter the thick, purulent drainage to a thin, liquid material that can be easily wiped or irrigated off the wound
    b. Enzyme contact with the wound is necessary to promote wound healing
    c. The wound needs to be cleansed, and cross-hatching of eschar on **burns** is performed prior to application
  2. Sutilains (Travase)
    a. Used to remove nonviable or necrotic tissue and purulent enzymes from **second- or third-degree burns**, ulcers, traumatic injury, and peripheral vascular disease wounds
    b. Inactive on viable tissue
  3. Collagenase (Santyl)
    a. Used as a topical debriding agent
    b. Provides effective debridement of the collagen tissue at the wound edges where necrotic tissue is anchored

---

BOX 39–10. Enzymes to Remove Exudates

Sutilains (Travase)
Collagenase (Santyl)
Fibrinolysin and desoxyribonuclease (Elase)

---

    c. Encourages the formation of granulation tissue at the wound edges and quicker epithelialization of wounds
    d. Apply with tongue depressor directly into deep wounds
    e. Prior to application, cleanse wound of debris by gently rubbing with a gauze pad with sterile water or Dakin solution, followed by sterile saline
    f. Remove all excess ointment each time the dressing is changed
    g. Apply only to the injured area; causes erythema in healthy tissues
    h. Protect healthy tissue with zinc oxide paste
    i. Discontinued when necrotic tissue is gone
  4. Fibrinolysin and desoxyribonuclease (Elase)
    a. Used to debride wounds including **burns**, **decubitus** ulcers, and inflamed or infected lesions
    b. Clean the wound with sterile water, then pat dry
    c. Flush away necrotic debris with sterile saline
    d. Apply a thin layer and cover with petrolatum gauze
D. Dextranomer (Debrisan)
  1. Not a debriding agent but it is a cleansing agent
  2. Effective in wet wounds only
  3. Pack Debrisan into wounds tightly because maceration of surrounding tissue may occur

X. Corticosteroids

A. Have anti-inflammatory, antipruritic, and vasoconstrictive actions
B. Contraindications
  1. Clients demonstrating previous sensitivity to steroids
  2. Those with current systemic fungal, viral, or bacterial infections
  3. Those with current complications related to steroid therapy
C. Local adverse effects
  1. Hypopigmentation
  2. Acneiform eruptions
  3. Contact dermatitis
  4. Burning, dryness, irritation, itching
  5. Overgrowth of bacteria, fungi, and viruses
  6. Skin atrophy
D. Systemic adverse effects
  1. Occur rarely
  2. Adrenal suppression
  3. Cushing's syndrome
  4. Striae, skin atrophy
  5. Ocular effects (glaucoma and cataracts)
E. Topical steroids
  1. Apply products sparingly in a light film, rubbing gently
  2. Wash the area just prior to application to increase medication penetration

3. May apply to skin alone or with dry, occlusive dressing
4. Monitor for toxic reactions, liver dysfunction, or worsening of condition
5. Instruct the client to report burning, irritation, and infection to the physician

XI. Acne Products (Box 39–11)

A. Description
1. Mild acne can be treated with bar soaps, soap-free cakes, liquid cleansers, lotions, gels, and creams
2. For moderate acne, topical anti-inflammatory medication such as benzoyl peroxide, tretinoin (Retin-A), isotretinoin (Accutane), azelaic acid (Azelex), and adapalene (Differin) may be prescribed; antibiotics may also be prescribed
3. Side effects can include excessive redness, extreme dryness of the skin leading to blistering and crusting, temporary pigmentation changes, and peeling of the skin
4. All products are kept away from the eyes, inside the nose, mucous membranes, and hair
B. Benzoyl peroxide: a keratolytic agent that is bacteriostatic and may decrease the production of irritant free fatty acids in the follicle
C. Tretinoin and adapalene: acids of vitamin A that are used to treat acne vulgaris, **skin cancer**, and aging of the skin
D. Tretinoin (Retin-A)
1. Decreases cohesiveness of the epithelial cells, increasing cell mitosis and turnover; potentially irritating, particularly when used correctly
2. Within 48 hours of use the skin generally becomes red and begins to peel
3. Temporary hyperpigmentation and hypopigmentation can occur
4. The client should avoid sun exposure, because photosensitivity may occur
5. Applied liberally to the skin; the hands are washed thoroughly immediately after applying
6. Therapeutic results should be seen after 2 to 3 weeks but may not be optimal until after 6 weeks
7. Clients may use cosmetics, but the skin needs to be cleaned thoroughly before applying

BOX 39–11. Acne Products	
CLEANSERS	**DRYING AGENTS**
Acnomel	Acnomel
Brasivol	Dry and Clear
Clearasil Medicated Astringent	Ionax
	Listerex
Fostex	
pHisoDerm	
Stri-Dex	

BOX 39–12. Poison Ivy Treatment Products	
Calamine	Ivy-Rid
Calomox	Ivy-Chex
Rhuli cream/spray/gel	

E. Isotretinoin (Accutane)
1. A metabolite of vitamin A
2. Used to treat severe cystic acne, and its use is reserved for people who have not responded to other therapies, including systemic antibiotics
3. Can cause xerosis and facial desquamation, palmoplantar desquamation, pruritus, brittle nails, and hair loss
4. Is administered with meals two times daily for a 15- to 20-week course
5. If another course of therapy is needed, an 8-week lapse of time should occur
6. Photosensitivity may occur, so the client needs to be instructed to decrease sun exposure
7. Alcohol consumption should be eliminated during therapy because alcohol may potentiate the serum triglyceride elevation
F. Local antibiotics
1. Used to treat acne; include clindamycin phosphate (Cleocin T), erythromycin, tetracycline (Topicycline), and meclocycline sulfosalicylate (Meclan)
2. Therapeutic response generally requires 6 to 12 weeks of therapy
3. Side effects include acute contact dermatitis, transient stinging or burning, staining of the skin, erythema, and skin tenderness

XII. Poison Ivy Treatment (Box 39–12)

XIII. Burn Products

A. Nitrofurazone (Furacin)
1. Applied topically to the **burn** as a solution, ointment, or cream
2. Has a broad spectrum of antibacterial activity
3. Used in **second- or third-degree burns** when bacterial resistance to other agents is a problem
4. Topical: apply $1/16$-inch film directly to the burn
5. Side effects: contact dermatitis and rash
6. Less common side effects: pruritus, local edema
B. Mafenide acetate (Sulfamylon)
1. A water-soluble cream that is bacteriostatic for both gram-negative and gram-positive organisms
2. Is used to treat **second- and third-degree burns** to reduce the bacteria present in avascular tissues
3. Diffuses through the devascularized areas of the skin; may precipitate metabolic acidosis usually compensated by hyperventilation

4. Apply 1/16-inch film
5. Side effects can include local pain and rash
6. Systemic effects include bone marrow depression, hemolytic anemia, hyperventilation
7. Keep burn covered with mafenide acetate at all times
8. The physician is notified if hyperventilation occurs; if acidosis develops, mafenide acetate is washed off the skin

C. Silver sulfadiazine (Flint SSD, Silvadene)
1. Has a broad spectrum of activity against gram-negative and gram-positive bacteria, and yeast
2. Released slowly from the cream, which is selectively toxic to bacteria
3. Used primarily to prevent sepsis in clients with **second- and third-degree burns**
4. Rash and itching do occur from topical application
5. Apply 1/16-inch film (keep the burn covered at all times with silver sulfadiazine)
6. Side effects include rash and itching
7. Systemic effects include leukopenia and nephritis
8. The complete blood count (CBC), particularly the white blood cell count (WBC) is monitored frequently; if leukopenia develops, the medication is discontinued

D. Silver nitrate
1. An antiseptic solution active against gram-negative bacteria
2. Dressings are applied to the burn and kept moist with silver nitrate, which stains anything brown or black that it comes in contact with; this discoloration is not usually permanent
3. Used on extensive **burns** that may precipitate fluid and electrolyte imbalances
4. Apply to dressing; do not apply to wounds, cuts, or broken skin

PRACTICE QUESTIONS

1. The camp nurse asks the children preparing to swim in the lake if they have applied sunscreen. The nurse tells the children that sunscreen is most effective when applied
   1 1 hour before exposure to the sun
   2 Immediately before exposure to the sun
   3 15 minutes before exposure to the sun
   4 Immediately after swimming

2. DuoDerm is precribed for a client with a leg ulcer. The nurse is assisting in preparing a plan of care for the client and most appropriately includes which of the following in the plan?
   1 Change DuoDerm daily
   2 Apply DuoDerm over a dry, sterile dressing
   3 Change DuoDerm weekly
   4 Apply DuoDerm over a normal saline–soaked dressing

3. The nurse is assigned to care for a client with a burn injury to the lower legs. Nitrofurazone (Furacin) is precribed to be applied to the sites of injury. The nurse plans to
   1 Apply saline-soaked dressings over the medication
   2 Apply 1-inch film directly to the burn sites
   3 Apply 1/16-inch film directly to the burn sites
   4 Apply 1/2-inch film directly to the burn sites after cleansing the wounds

4. Mafenide acetate (Sulfamylon) is prescribed for the client with a burn injury. When applying the medication, the client complains of local discomfort and burning. The most appropriate nursing action is to
   1 Discontinue the medication
   2 Call the physician
   3 Apply a thinner film than prescribed to the burn site
   4 Inform the client that this is normal

5. The burn client is receiving treatments of topical mafenide acetate (Sulfamylon) to the site of injury. The nurse suspects that a systemic effect has occurred if which of the following is noted in the client?
   1 Local pain at the burn site
   2 Local rash at the burn site
   3 Hyperventilation
   4 Elevated blood pressure

6. A Vigilon burn dressing is prescribed for the client with a partial-thickness burn to the arm. The nurse assisting in developing a plan of care for the client understands that the dressing will need to be changed
   1 Daily
   2 Every 2 days
   3 Weekly
   4 Twice weekly

7. Sodium hypochlorite (Dakin) solution is prescribed for a client with a leg wound containing purulent drainage. The nurse is assisting in developing a plan of care for the client. Which of the following is not a component of the treatment plan with the use of this solution?
   1 Avoid contact with normal skin tissue
   2 Rinse off immediately following irrigation
   3 Soak a sterile dressing with solution and pack into the wound
   4 Prepare solution prior to use

8. Tretinoin (Retin-A) is prescribed for a client with acne. The client calls the physician's office and tells the nurse that the skin has become very red and is beginning to peel. The nurse most appropriately responds by telling the client
   1 To come to the clinic immediately
   2 To discontinue the medication

3 To notify the physician

4 That this is a normal occurrence with the use of this medication

9. The nurse provides instructions to a client regarding the use of tretinoin (Retin-A). Which of the following is not a component of the instructions regarding the use of this medication?

   1 Wash hands thoroughly after applying medication

   2 Optimal results will be seen after 6 weeks

   3 Apply a thin layer to the skin

   4 Cleanse the skin thoroughly before applying the medication

10. Isotretinoin (Accutane) is prescribed for a client to treat severe cystic acne. The nurse tells the client that the length of the usual prescribed course of treatment is:

   1 1 month

   2 8 weeks

   3 15 to 20 weeks

   4 1 year

11. Isotretinoin (Accutane) is prescribed for a client with severe acne. Prior to the administration of this medication, the nurse expects that which laboratory test will be prescribed?

   1 Complete blood count

   2 White blood cell count

   3 Triglyceride level

   4 Platelet count

12. A client with severe acne is seen at the physician's office. The physician prescribes isotretinoin (Accutane). The nurse reviews the client's health record and notifies the physician if the client is presently taking which of the following medications?

   1 Digoxin (Lanoxin)

   2 Phenytoin (Dilantin)

   3 Vitamin A

   4 Furosemide (Lasix)

13. Fibrinolysin and desoxyribonuclease (Elase) dry powder is prescribed to treat a skin ulcer. The nurse assists in developing a plan of care for the client. Which of the following nursing interventions is not a component of the plan regarding this treatment?

   1 Clean the wound with a sterile solution prior to applying Elase

   2 Prepare solution just prior to use

   3 Apply a thick layer of medication and cover with a dry, sterile dressing

   4 Apply a thin layer of medication and cover with a petrolatum gauze

14. The nurse is assigned to care for a client with a leg ulcer. Sutilains (Travase) treatments are prescribed. The nurse avoids which of the following when performing the treatment?

   1 Clean the wound with a sterile solution

   2 Cover the sutilains application with a dry, sterile dressing

   3 Moisten the wound with sterile normal saline and then apply the sutilains

   4 Place the sutilains in the refrigerator following use

15. Dextranomer (Debrisan) is prescribed for a client with a decubitus ulcer. The nurse prepares to perform the prescribed treatment, knowing that which of the following is inaccurate regarding this medication?

   1 It is effective in wet wounds only

   2 It should be packed lightly into the wound

   3 Maceration of tissue surrounding the wound can occur from the medication

   4 The wound bed must be thoroughly dried prior to applying the medication

16. Minoxidil solution (Rogaine) is prescribed for the client to treat hair loss. The nurse instructs the client regarding the medication, knowing that the usual dosage for this medication is

   1 0.5 mL applied two times a day

   2 1 mL applied at bedtime

   3 1 mL applied two times a day

   4 1 mL applied four times a day

17. The nurse employed in a physician's office is interviewing the client. The nurse notes that the client is taking azelaic acid (Azelex). Because of the medication prescription, the nurse suspects that the client is being treated for

   1 Herpes simplex

   2 Acne

   3 Eczema

   4 Hair loss

18. Collagenase (Santyl) is prescribed for a client with a severe burn to the hand. The nurse provides instructions to the client regarding the use of the medication. Which of the following statements if made by the client indicates an accurate understanding of the use of this medication?

   1 "I will apply the ointment once a day and leave it open to the air."

   2 "I will apply the ointment once a day and cover it with a sterile dressing."

   3 "I will apply the ointment twice a day and leave it open to the air."

   4 "I will apply the ointment at bedtime and in the morning and cover it with a sterile dressing."

19. Minoxidil (Rogaine) is prescribed for the client to treat hair loss. The client asks the nurse if the hair will continue to grow when the medication is stopped. The most appropriate nursing response is

1 "The hair will continue to grow."
2 "Newly gained hair is lost in 3 to 4 months."
3 "It depends on how long you have been taking the Rogaine."
4 "I'm not sure, you need to ask your physician."

20. Coal tar has been prescribed for a client with a diagnosis of psoriasis. The nurse is asked to describe the treatment to the client. Which of the following is not a component of the description of this treatment provided to the client?
1 The medication has an unpleasant odor
2 The medication can stain the skin and hair
3 The medication can cause systemic effects
4 The medication can cause phototoxicity

21. The client is diagnosed with herpes simplex type 1. The physician tells the nurse that a topical medication for treatment will be prescribed. The nurse expects that which of the following medications will be prescribed?
1 Triple antibiotic
2 Acyclovir (Zovirax)
3 Mupirocin (Bactroban)
4 Masoprocol (Actinex)

22. Salicylic acid is prescribed for a client with a diagnosis of psoriasis. The nurse suspects the presence of systemic toxicity from this medication if which of the following occurs in the client?
1 Decreased respirations
2 Diarrhea
3 Constipation
4 Tinnitus

23. The hospitalized client with severe seborrheic dermatitis is receiving treatments of topical glucocorticoid applications followed by the application of an occlusive dressing. The nurse monitors for which systemic effect that can occur from this treatment?
1 Adrenal suppression
2 Adrenal hyperactivity
3 Local infection
4 Thinning of the skin

24. The nurse is applying a topical glucocorticoid to a client with eczema. The nurse monitors for systemic absorption of the medication if the medication is being applied to which of the following body areas?
1 Back
2 Axilla
3 Palm of the hand
4 Sole of the foot

25. A topical glucocorticoid is prescribed for the client with dermatitis. The nurse provides instructions to the client regarding the use of the medication. Which of the following, if stated by the client, indicates a need for further instruction?

1 "I need to apply the medication in a thin film."
2 "I should gently rub the medication into the skin."
3 "I should place a bandage over the site after applying the medication."
4 "The medication will help to relieve the inflammation and itching."

26. Lindane (Kwell) is prescribed for the treatment of scabies. The nurse questions the order if the medication is prescribed for which of the following clients?
1 A 42-year-old female
2 An elderly client
3 A 6-year-old child
4 A 52-year-old male with hypertension

27. A client is seen in the clinic for complaints of skin itchiness that has been persistent over the past several weeks. Following an assessment, it has been determined that the client has scabies. Lindane (Kwell) is prescribed and the nurse is asked to provide instructions to the client regarding the use of the medication. The nurse tells the client to
1 Leave the cream on for 8 to 12 hours and then remove by washing
2 Apply a thick layer of cream to the entire body
3 Apply the cream as prescribed for 2 days in a row
4 Apply to the entire body and scalp, excluding the face

28. An outbreak of pediculosis capitus has occurred at the local school. The nurse is assisting in providing instructions to the mothers of the children attending the school regarding the application of permetrin (Nix, Elimite). The nurse tells the mothers to
1 Apply at bedtime and rinse off in the morning
2 Apply prior to washing the hair
3 Avoid saturating the hair and scalp when applying
4 Allow to remain on hair 10 minutes and then rinse with water

29. The physician has prescribed trolamine salicylate (Myoflex) topical cream for a client with a diagnosis of rheumatism who is complaining of muscular aches. The nurse provides which of the following instructions to the client regarding this medication?
1 Apply a heating pad to the area after applying the medication
2 The medication acts by decreasing muscle spasms
3 The medication is prescribed to cause the skin to peel
4 The medication will act as a local anesthetic

30. The female client tells the nurse that her skin is very dry and irritated. Which of the following products does the nurse suggest that the client apply to the dry skin?

1 A glycerin emollient
2 Aspercreme
3 Myoflex
4 Acetic acid solution

ANSWERS

1. **1**

RATIONALE: Sunscreens are most effective when applied about 30 minutes to 1 hour before exposure to the sun so that they can penetrate the skin. All sunscreens should be reapplied after swimming or sweating.
TEST-TAKING STRATEGY: Knowledge that sunscreens need to penetrate the skin will assist in eliminating options 2 and 3. Noting the key words "most effective" will direct you to option 1. Review protective skin measures now if you had difficulty with this question.
LEVEL OF COGNITIVE ABILITY: Application
PHASE OF NURSING PROCESS: Implementation
CLIENT NEEDS: Health Promotion and Maintenance
CONTENT AREA: Pharmacology
REFERENCE
Kuhn, M. (1998). *Pharmacotherapeutics: A nursing process approach* (4th ed.). Philadelphia: F. A. Davis. p. 993.

2. **3**

RATIONALE: DuoDerm contains hydroactive particles embedded in a polymer base, which are softened by wound moisture and act as a protective gel over healing tissue. It is applied directly to the wound and can be left in place up to 7 days.
TEST-TAKING STRATEGY: Knowledge regarding the use of DuoDerm is required to answer this question. If you are unfamiliar with this type of protective dressing, take time now to review.
LEVEL OF COGNITIVE ABILITY: Application
PHASE OF NURSING PROCESS: Planning
CLIENT NEEDS: Physiological Integrity
CONTENT AREA: Pharmacology
REFERENCE
Kuhn, M. (1998). *Pharmacotherapeutics: A nursing process approach* (4th ed.). Philadelphia: F. A. Davis. p. 993.

3. **3**

RATIONALE: Furacin is applied topically to the burn and has a broad spectrum of antibiotic activity. It is used in second- or third-degree burns where bacterial resistance to other agents is a real or potential problem. A film of $\frac{1}{16}$ inch is applied directly to the burn. Saline-soaked dressings are not used.
TEST-TAKING STRATEGY: Use the process of elimination. Option 1 can be eliminated because infection is a major concern with the burn client and a wet dressing can more easily harbor bacteria. Recalling that a very thin film is required will easily direct you to option 3. Review the use of this medication for burn therapy now if you had difficulty with this question.
LEVEL OF COGNITIVE ABILITY: Application
PHASE OF NURSING PROCESS: Implementation
CLIENT NEEDS: Physiological Integrity
CONTENT AREA: Pharmacology

REFERENCE
Kuhn, M. (1998). *Pharmacotherapeutics: A nursing process approach* (4th ed.). Philadelphia: F. A. Davis. p. 998.

4. **4**

RATIONALE: Mafenide acetate is bacteriostatic for both gram-negative and gram-positive organisms and is used to treat second- and third-degree burns to reduce bacteria present in avascular tissues. The client should be informed that the medication will cause local discomfort and burning.
TEST-TAKING STRATEGY: Eliminate options 1 and 3 because it is not within the scope of nursing practice to alter or discontinue a medication therapy. Knowledge that this is a normal expected occurrence will easily direct you to option 4. If you had difficulty with this question, take time now to review.
LEVEL OF COGNITIVE ABILITY: Application
PHASE OF NURSING PROCESS: Implementation
CLIENT NEEDS: Physiological Integrity
CONTENT AREA: Pharmacology
REFERENCE
Hodgson, B., & Kizior, R. (1999). *Saunders nursing drug handbook 1999*. Philadelphia: W. B. Saunders. p. 616.

5. **3**

RATIONALE: Mafenide acetate can suppress renal excretion of acid and cause acidosis evidenced by hyperventilation. Clients receiving this treatment should be monitored for acid-base status, and if the acidosis becomes severe the medication is discontinued for 1 to 2 days. Options 1 and 2 describe local rather than systemic effects. An elevated blood pressure may be expected in the client with pain.
TEST-TAKING STRATEGY: Note the key words "systemic effect." Options 1 and 2 can be eliminated because these are local rather than systemic effects. From the remaining options, recall that the client in pain likely has an elevated blood pressure. This should direct you to option 3. Review the systemic effects of this medication now if you had difficulty with this question.
LEVEL OF COGNITIVE ABILITY: Comprehension
PHASE OF NURSING PROCESS: Data Collection
CLIENT NEEDS: Physiological Integrity
CONTENT AREA: Pharmacology
REFERENCE
Hodgson, B., & Kizior, R. (1999). *Saunders nursing drug handbook 1999*. Philadelphia: W. B. Saunders. p. 616.

6. **1**

RATIONALE: A Vigilon dressing is used to clean small partial-thickness burns. It is a colloidal suspension on a polyethylene mesh support, is permeable to gases and water vapor, and provides a moist environment. It is changed daily.
TEST-TAKING STRATEGY: Eliminate options 2 and 4 first because they are similar time frames. Knowledge regarding the use of this type of burn covering will assist in

directing you to option 1. If you are unfamiliar with this type of burn covering, take time now to review.
LEVEL OF COGNITIVE ABILITY: Comprehension
PHASE OF NURSING PROCESS: Planning
CLIENT NEEDS: Physiological Integrity
CONTENT AREA: Pharmacology
REFERENCE
Kuhn, M. (1998). *Pharmacotherapeutics: A nursing process approach* (4th ed.). Philadelphia: F. A. Davis. p. 999.

7. **3**

RATIONALE: Dakin solution is a chloride solution that is used for irrigating and cleaning necrotic or purulent wounds. It can be used for packing necrotic wounds. It cannot be used to pack purulent wounds because the solution is inactivated by copious pus. It should not come in contact with healing or normal tissue, and it should be rinsed off immediately if used for irrigation. Solutions are unstable and must be prepared fresh for each use.
TEST-TAKING STRATEGY: Note the key word "not." Eliminate options 1 and 2 first because they are similar and indicate avoiding healthy tissue. It makes sense to prepare the solution prior to use; therefore, eliminate option 4. If you are unfamiliar with the use of this solution, take time now to review.
LEVEL OF COGNITIVE ABILITY: Application
PHASE OF NURSING PROCESS: Planning
CLIENT NEEDS: Physiological Integrity
CONTENT AREA: Pharmacology
REFERENCE
Kuhn, M. (1998). *Pharmacotherapeutics: A nursing process approach* (4th ed.). Philadelphia: F. A. Davis. p. 988.

8. **4**

RATIONALE: Tretinoin decreases cohesiveness of the epithelial cells, increasing cell mitosis and turnover. It is potentially irritating, particularly when used correctly. Within 48 hours of use, the skin generally becomes red and begins to peel.
TEST-TAKING STRATEGY: Options 1 and 3 can be eliminated first because they are similar. Eliminate option 2 next because it is not within the scope of nursing practice to advise a client to discontinue a medication. If you are unfamiliar with the use of this medication, take time now to review.
LEVEL OF COGNITIVE ABILITY: Application
PHASE OF NURSING PROCESS: Implementation
CLIENT NEEDS: Physiological Integrity
CONTENT AREA: Pharmacology
REFERENCE
Hodgson, B., & Kizior, R. (1999). *Saunders nursing drug handbook 1999*. Philadelphia: W. B. Saunders. p. 1018.

9. **3**

RATIONALE: Tretinoin is applied liberally to the skin. The hands are washed thoroughly immediately after applying. Therapeutic results should be seen after 2 to 3 weeks but may not be optimal until after 6 weeks. The skin needs to be cleansed thoroughly before applying the medication.
TEST-TAKING STRATEGY: Note the key word "not." Eliminate options 1 and 4 first, using the principles of asepsis. Knowledge regarding the use of the medication will assist in directing you to option 3. Review this medication now if you had difficulty with this question.
LEVEL OF COGNITIVE ABILITY: Application
PHASE OF NURSING PROCESS: Implementation

CLIENT NEEDS: Health Promotion and Maintenance
CONTENT AREA: Pharmacology
REFERENCE
Hodgson, B., & Kizior, R. (1999). *Saunders nursing drug handbook 1999*. Philadelphia: W. B. Saunders. pp. 1016–1018.

10. **3**

RATIONALE: Isotretinoin is administered two times daily for 15 to 20 weeks. If needed, a second course may be given, but not until 2 months have elapsed after completing the first course.
TEST-TAKING STRATEGY: Knowledge regarding the use of this medication is required to answer this question. If you are unfamiliar with this treatment, take time now to review.
LEVEL OF COGNITIVE ABILITY: Application
PHASE OF NURSING PROCESS: Implementation
CLIENT NEEDS: Health Promotion and Maintenance
CONTENT AREA: Pharmacology
REFERENCE
Lehne, R. (1998). *Pharmacology for nursing care* (3rd ed.). Philadelphia: W. B. Saunders. p. 1059.

11. **3**

RATIONALE: Isotretinoin can elevate triglyceride levels. Blood triglyceride content should be measured prior to treatment and periodically thereafter until effects of triglycerides have been evaluated.
TEST-TAKING STRATEGY: Eliminate options 1 and 2 first because a complete blood count will also measure the white blood cell count. From the remaining options, it is necessary to know that the medication can affect the triglyceride level in the client. Review this medication now if you had difficulty with this question.
LEVEL OF COGNITIVE ABILITY: Comprehension
PHASE OF NURSING PROCESS: Planning
CLIENT NEEDS: Physiological Integrity
CONTENT AREA: Pharmacology
REFERENCE
Lehne, R. (1998). *Pharmacology for nursing care* (3rd ed.). Philadelphia: W. B. Saunders. p. 1059.

12. **3**

RATIONALE: Vitamin A, being a relative of isotretinoin, can produce generalized intensification of isotretinoin toxicity. Because of the potential for increased toxicity, vitamin A supplements should be discontinued prior to isotretinoin therapy.
TEST-TAKING STRATEGY: Knowledge that isotretinoin is a derivative of vitamin A will easily direct you to the correct option. If you are unfamiliar with this medication, take time now to review the contraindications associated with its use.
LEVEL OF COGNITIVE ABILITY: Comprehension
PHASE OF NURSING PROCESS: Implementation
CLIENT NEEDS: Safe, Effective Care Environment
CONTENT AREA: Pharmacology
REFERENCE
Lehne, R. (1998). *Pharmacology for nursing care* (3rd ed.). Philadelphia: W. B. Saunders. p. 1059.

13. **3**

RATIONALE: The wound should be cleansed with a sterile solution and gently patted dry. A thin layer of Elase is applied and covered with a petrolatum gauze. If a dry powder is used, the solution should be prepared just prior to use.

TEST-TAKING STRATEGY: Note the word "not." Noting this key word should assist in directing you to option 3. Review the method of application of Elase now if you had difficulty with this question.
LEVEL OF COGNITIVE ABILITY: Application
PHASE OF NURSING PROCESS: Planning
CLIENT NEEDS: Physiological Integrity
CONTENT AREA: Pharmacology
REFERENCE
Kuhn, M. (1998). *Pharmacotherapeutics: A nursing process approach* (4th ed.). Philadelphia: F. A. Davis. p. 1010.

14. **2**

RATIONALE: The wound should be cleansed with a sterile solution prior to treatment. The nurse then should thoroughly moisten the wound with normal saline or sterile water and apply a loose, thin dressing after applying a thin film of sutilains extending ¼ to ½ inch beyond the area to be debrided. The ointment should be refrigerated.
TEST-TAKING STRATEGY: Note the word "avoids." Knowledge regarding the use of this medication is required to answer the question. Review the method of application of sutilains now if you had difficulty with this question.
LEVEL OF COGNITIVE ABILITY: Application
PHASE OF NURSING PROCESS: Implementation
CLIENT NEEDS: Physiological Integrity
CONTENT AREA: Pharmacology
REFERENCE
Kuhn, M. (1998). *Pharmacotherapeutics: A nursing process approach* (4th ed.). Philadelphia: F. A. Davis. p. 1010.

15. **4**

RATIONALE: Debrisan is a cleansing rather than a debriding agent. It is effective in wet wounds only. It should not be packed into wounds tightly because maceration of surrounding tissue may result.
TEST-TAKING STRATEGY: Note the key word "inaccurate." Knowledge regarding the use of this medication is required to answer this question. If you are unfamiliar with the use of Debrisan, take time now to review.
LEVEL OF COGNITIVE ABILITY: Comprehension
PHASE OF NURSING PROCESS: Planning
CLIENT NEEDS: Physiological Integrity
CONTENT AREA: Pharmacology
REFERENCE
Kuhn, M. (1998). *Pharmacotherapeutics: A nursing process approach* (4th ed.). Philadelphia: F. A. Davis. p. 1012.

16. **3**

RATIONALE: A 2% minoxidil solution is used for topical treatment of baldness. The usual dosage is 1 mL applied two times a day.
TEST-TAKING STRATEGY: Knowledge regarding the usual dosage for minoxidil solution is required to answer this question. If you are unfamiliar with this medication, take time now to review.
LEVEL OF COGNITIVE ABILITY: Comprehension
PHASE OF NURSING PROCESS: Implementation
CLIENT NEEDS: Physiological Integrity
CONTENT AREA: Pharmacology
REFERENCE
Lehne, R. (1998). *Pharmacology for nursing care* (3rd ed.). Philadelphia: W. B. Saunders. p. 1061.

17. **2**

RATIONALE: Azelex is a topical medication used to treat mild to moderate acne. It appears to work by suppressing growth of *Propionibacterium acnes* and by decreasing proliferation of keratinocytes.
TEST-TAKING STRATEGY: Knowledge regarding the use of Azelex is required to answer this question. It is a relatively new medication used to treat mild to moderate acne. If you are unfamiliar with this medication, take time now to review.
LEVEL OF COGNITIVE ABILITY: Comprehension
PHASE OF NURSING PROCESS: Data Collection
CLIENT NEEDS: Physiological Integrity
CONTENT AREA: Pharmacology
REFERENCE
Hodgson, B., & Kizior, R. (1999). *Saunders nursing drug handbook 1999*. Philadelphia: W. B. Saunders. p. 89.

18. **2**

RATIONALE: Collagenase is used to promote debridement of dermal lesions and severe burns. It is applied once daily and covered with a sterile dressing.
TEST-TAKING STRATEGY: Note the key word "accurate." Knowledge regarding the use of this medication is required to answer this question. If you are unfamiliar with this medication, take time now to review.
LEVEL OF COGNITIVE ABILITY: Comprehension
PHASE OF NURSING PROCESS: Evaluation
CLIENT NEEDS: Health Promotion and Maintenance
CONTENT AREA: Pharmacology
REFERENCE
Lehne, R. (1998). *Pharmacology for nursing care* (3rd ed.). Philadelphia: W. B. Saunders. p. 1061.

19. **2**

RATIONALE: Hair regrowth is most likely when baldness has developed recently and has been limited to a small area. Upon discontinuation of the medication, newly gained hair is lost in 3 to 4 months, and the natural progression of hair loss resumes.
TEST-TAKING STRATEGY: Option 4 can be easily eliminated because it places the client's question on hold. Knowledge regarding the clinical response and effects of this medication is required to select the correct answer from the remaining options. If you are unfamiliar with this medication, take time now to review.
LEVEL OF COGNITIVE ABILITY: Application
PHASE OF NURSING PROCESS: Implementation
CLIENT NEEDS: Physiological Integrity
CONTENT AREA: Pharmacology
REFERENCE
Lehne, R. (1998). *Pharmacology for nursing care* (3rd ed.). Philadelphia: W. B. Saunders. p. 1061.

20. **3**

RATIONALE: Coal tar is used to treat psoriasis and other chronic disorders of the skin. It suppresses DNA synthesis, mitotic activity, and cell proliferation. It has an unpleasant odor, can frequently stain the skin and hair, and can cause phototoxicity. Systemic toxicity does not occur.
TEST-TAKING STRATEGY: Note the key word "not." The name of the medication will assist in eliminating options 1 and 2. It is necessary to know that the medication does not cause systemic effects to answer this question correctly. If you had difficulty with this question, review this treatment now.

LEVEL OF COGNITIVE ABILITY: Application
PHASE OF NURSING PROCESS: Planning
CLIENT NEEDS: Physiological Integrity
CONTENT AREA: Pharmacology
REFERENCE
Lehne, R. (1998). *Pharmacology for nursing care* (3rd ed.). Philadelphia: W. B. Saunders. p. 1059.

21. **2**

RATIONALE: Acyclovir is a topical antiviral agent that inhibits DNA replication in the virus. It has activity against herpes simplex types 1 and 2, varicella-zoster, Epstein-Barr, and cytomegalovirus. Triple antibiotic would not be effective in treating herpes virus. Mupirocin is a topical antibacterial active against impetigo caused by staphylococcus or streptococcus. Masoprocol is a keratolytic.
TEST-TAKING STRATEGY: Knowledge that herpes simplex is a virus will direct you to the option that identifies an antiviral medication. If you are not familiar with these medications, take time now to review.
LEVEL OF COGNITIVE ABILITY: Comprehension
PHASE OF NURSING PROCESS: Planning
CLIENT NEEDS: Physiological Integrity
CONTENT AREA: Pharmacology
REFERENCE
Hodgson, B., & Kizior, R. (1999). *Saunders nursing drug handbook 1999*. Philadelphia: W. B. Saunders. pp. 12–15.

22. **4**

RATIONALE: Salicylic acid is readily absorbed through the skin and systemic toxicity (salicylism) can result. Symptoms include tinnitus, hyperpnea, dizziness, and psychologic disturbances. Constipation and diarrhea are not associated with salicylism.
TEST-TAKING STRATEGY: Noting the name of the medication will assist in directing you to the correct option if you can recall the toxic effects that occur with acetylsalicylic acid (aspirin). If you are unfamiliar with the toxic effects of salicylic acid, take time now to review.
LEVEL OF COGNITIVE ABILITY: Analysis
PHASE OF NURSING PROCESS: Data Collection
CLIENT NEEDS: Physiological Integrity
CONTENT AREA: Pharmacology
REFERENCE
Lehne, R. (1998). *Pharmacology for nursing care* (3rd ed.). Philadelphia: W. B. Saunders. p. 1056.

23. **1**

RATIONALE: Topical glucocorticoids can be absorbed in sufficient amounts to produce systemic toxicity. Principal concerns are growth retardation (in children), and adrenal suppression in all age groups. Options 3 and 4 identify local rather than systemic reactions.
TEST-TAKING STRATEGY: Use the process of elimination. Options 3 and 4 can be eliminated first because they are local reactions. From the remaining two options knowledge regarding the concerns related to systemic toxicity is required to answer the question. Review these systemic effects now if you had difficulty with this question.
LEVEL OF COGNITIVE ABILITY: Application
PHASE OF NURSING PROCESS: Implementation
CLIENT NEEDS: Physiological Integrity
CONTENT AREA: Pharmacology

REFERENCE
Lehne, R. (1998). *Pharmacology for nursing care* (3rd ed.). Philadelphia: W. B. Saunders. p. 1055.

24. **2**

RATIONALE: Topical glucocorticoids can be absorbed into the systemic circulation. Absorption is higher from regions where the skin is especially permeable (scalp, axilla, face, eyelids, neck, perineum, genitalia), and lower from regions where penetrability is poor (back, palms, soles).
TEST-TAKING STRATEGY: Focus on the issue of the question "systemic absorption." Eliminate options 3 and 4 because these body areas are similar in terms of skin substance. From the remaining options, think about permeability of the skin area. This will direct you to option 2.
LEVEL OF COGNITIVE ABILITY: Application
PHASE OF NURSING PROCESS: Implementation
CLIENT NEEDS: Physiological Integrity
CONTENT AREA: Pharmacology
REFERENCE
Lehne, R. (1998). *Pharmacology for nursing care* (3rd ed.). Philadelphia: W. B. Saunders. p. 1055.

25. **3**

RATIONALE: Clients should be advised not to use occlusive dressings (bandages or plastic wraps) to cover the affected site following the application of the topical glucocorticoid, unless the physician specifically prescribes wound coverage. Options 1, 2, and 4 are accurate statements related to the use of this medication.
TEST-TAKING STRATEGY: Note the key words "need for further instruction." Eliminate option 4, knowing that this is the action for glucocorticoids. The words "thin" in option 1 and "gently" in option 2 should assist you in eliminating these options. If you had difficulty with this question, take time now to review this medication.
LEVEL OF COGNITIVE ABILITY: Comprehension
PHASE OF NURSING PROCESS: Evaluation
CLIENT NEEDS: Health Promotion and Maintenance
CONTENT AREA: Pharmacology
REFERENCE
Lehne, R. (1998). *Pharmacology for nursing care* (3rd ed.). Philadelphia: W. B. Saunders. p. 1055.

26. **3**

RATIONALE: Lindane can penetrate the intact skin and can cause convulsions if absorbed in sufficient quantities. Clients at highest risk for convulsions are premature infants, children, and clients with preexisting seizure disorders. Lindane should not be used on pediatric clients unless safer medications have failed to control infection.
TEST-TAKING STRATEGY: Knowledge regarding the contraindications associated with the use of lindane is required to answer this question. If you are unfamiliar with these contraindications, learn them now.
LEVEL OF COGNITIVE ABILITY: Comprehension
PHASE OF NURSING PROCESS: Implementation
CLIENT NEEDS: Safe, Effective Care Environment
CONTENT AREA: Pharmacology
REFERENCE
Lehne, R. (1998). *Pharmacology for nursing care* (3rd ed.). Philadelphia: W. B. Saunders. p. 1003.

27. 1

RATIONALE: Lindane is applied in a thin layer to the entire body below the head. No more than 30 g (1 oz) should be used. The medication is removed by washing 8 to 12 hours later. As a rule, only one application is required.
TEST-TAKING STRATEGY: Knowledge regarding the use of lindane is required to answer this question. If you are unfamiliar with the use of this medication, take time now to review.
LEVEL OF COGNITIVE ABILITY: Application
PHASE OF NURSING PROCESS: Implementation
CLIENT NEEDS: Health Promotion and Maintenance
CONTENT AREA: Pharmacology
REFERENCE
Lehne, R. (1998). *Pharmacology for nursing care* (3rd ed.). Philadelphia: W. B. Saunders, p. 1003.

28. 4

RATIONALE: The instructions for the use of permetrin include wash, rinse, and towel-dry hair; apply a sufficient volume to saturate the hair and scalp; allow to remain on hair 10 minutes and then rinse with water. Options 1, 2, and 3 are incorrect instructions.
TEST-TAKING STRATEGY: Use the process of elimination. Note that both options 1 and 4 address a time frame for allowing the medication to remain on the hair. Recognizing this may provide you with the clue that one of these options is correct. If you are unfamiliar with the use of this treatment, review now.
LEVEL OF COGNITIVE ABILITY: Application
PHASE OF NURSING PROCESS: Implementation
CLIENT NEEDS: Health Promotion and Maintenance
CONTENT AREA: Pharmacology
REFERENCE
Kuhn, M. (1998). *Pharmacotherapeutics: A nursing process approach* (4th ed.). Philadelphia: F. A. Davis. p. 991.

29. 4

RATIONALE: Myoflex is used for the temporary relief of muscular aches, rheumatism, arthritis, sprains, and neural-

gia. It contains combinations of antiseptics, local anesthetics, analgesics, and counterirritants. They are not prescribed to cause the skin to peel and if this sort of reaction occurs, the physician should be notified. The medication does not act in a systemic manner. A heating pad should not be applied because irritation or burning of the skin may occur.
TEST-TAKING STRATEGY: Noting the key words "topical cream" may assist in eliminating option 2. Eliminate option 3, knowing that this is not an expected therapeutic effect. Recalling the principles related to heat application will assist in eliminating option 1. Review the action of this medication if you had difficulty with this question.
LEVEL OF COGNITIVE ABILITY: Application
PHASE OF NURSING PROCESS: Implementation
CLIENT NEEDS: Health Promotion and Maintenance
CONTENT AREA: Pharmacology
REFERENCE
Kuhn, M. (1998). *Pharmacotherapeutics: A nursing process approach* (4th ed.). Philadelphia: F. A. Davis. p. 988.

30. 1

RATIONALE: Glycerin is an emollient that is used for dry, cracked, and irritated skin. Aspercreme and Myoflex are used to treat muscular aches. Acetic acid solution is used for irrigating, cleansing, and packing wounds infected by *Pseudomonas aeruginosa*.
TEST-TAKING STRATEGY: Note the key words "skin is very dry and irritated." These key words and knowledge of the products indicated in the options will assist in directing you to option 1. Review these products now if you had difficulty with this question.
LEVEL OF COGNITIVE ABILITY: Application
PHASE OF NURSING PROCESS: Implementation
CLIENT NEEDS: Health Promotion and Maintenance
CONTENT AREA: Pharmacology
REFERENCE
Kuhn, M. (1998). *Pharmacotherapeutics: A nursing process approach* (4th ed.). Philadelphia: F. A. Davis. p. 988.

BIBLIOGRAPHY

Hodgson, B., & Kizior, R. (1999). *Saunders nursing drug handbook 1999*. Philadelphia: W. B. Saunders.
Kuhn, M. (1998). *Pharmacotherapeutics: A nursing process approach* (4th ed.). Philadelphia: F. A. Davis.
Lehne, R. (1998). *Pharmacology for nursing care* (3rd ed.). Philadelphia: W. B. Saunders.
Luckmann, J. (1997). *Saunders manual of nursing care*. Philadelphia: W. B. Saunders.
Monahan, F., & Neighbors, M. (1998). *Medical-surgical nursing: Foundations for clinical practice* (2nd ed.). Philadelphia: W. B. Saunders.
O'Toole, M. (1997). *Miller-Keane encyclopedia & dictionary of medicine, nursing, & allied health* (6th ed.). Philadelphia: W. B. Saunders.

UNIT IX

The Adult Client with an Oncological Disorder

PYRAMID TERMS

Benign—Usually refers to growths that are encapsulated, remain localized, and are slow growing.

Cancer—A neoplastic disorder that can involve all body organs. Cells lose their normal growth-controlling mechanism, and the growth of cells is uncontrolled.

Carcinogen—A physical, chemical, or biological stressor that causes neoplastic changes in normal cells.

Carcinoma in Situ—A lesion with all the histological characteristics of malignancies except invasion.

Carcinomas—Originate from epithelial cells, solid tumors, the skin, gastrointestinal (GI) tract, lungs, uterus, breast, and other organs.

Hospice—A concept of care for terminally ill clients that includes intensive caring rather than intensive care. The family and client are the focus of nursing care, and the goal is to relieve pain and facilitate the optimal quality of life.

Lymphomas—Originate from lymphoid tissue.

Leukemias or Myelomas—Originate from blood-forming organs.

Malignant—Refers to growths that are not encapsulated, metastasize, and grow; a cancerous lesion having the characteristics of disorderly, uncontrolled, and chaotic proliferation of cells.

Metastasis—The transfer of disease from one organ or part to another not directly connected with it. Secondary malignant lesions, orginating from the primary tumor, are located in anatomically distant places.

Nadir—The period when an antineoplastic medication has its most profound effects on the bone marrow.

Neoplasia—A new growth, which may be benign or malignant.

Sarcomas—Originate from muscle, bone, fat, or the lymph system or from connective tissues.

Staging—A method of classifying malignancies based on the presence and extent of the tumor within the body.

Tumor Markers—Specific bodily substances that seem to indicate tumor progression or regression.

Undifferentiated Cells—Cells that have lost the capacity for specialized functions.

◢ PYRAMID TO SUCCESS

Pyramid points focus on treatment modalities related to an oncological disorder, such as pain management, internal and external radiation, chemotherapy, and oncological disorders such as skin cancer, leukemia, breast cancer, and lung cancer. Specific focus relates to the nursing care related to these treatment modalities and disorders, and to client adaptation and the impact of the treatment or disorder. Specifically, focus on the complications related to chemotherapy and the nursing measures required in monitoring for these complications, and in preventing life-threatening conditions such as infection and bleeding. Specific laboratory values include the white blood cell count (WBC) and the platelet count.

NURSING PROCESS

DATA COLLECTION

- Risk factors
- Dietary factors
- Pain or discomfort
- Change in bowel or bladder habits
- Any sore that does not heal
- Recurrent infections
- Unusual bleeding or discharge
- Thickening or lump in breast or elsewhere in the body
- Anorexia, nausea, indigestion, or vomiting
- Unexplained weight loss
- Obvious change of wart or mole
- Nagging cough or hoarseness
- Expectorating or vomiting blood
- Blood in the urine or stools

PLANNING	IMPLEMENTATION	EVALUATION
The client consumes an adequate intake of food and fluids. The client remains free of nausea.	Monitor and document food intake. Monitor lab values. Develop a meal plan to include schedule of meals, and high-quality foods incorporating client's likes and dislikes.	The client maintains weight. The client consumes a balanced diet. The client is free of nausea and vomiting. The client tolerates the prescribed diet.
The client requests medication for discomfort. The client verbalizes relief of pain from comfort measures and medication.	Rate the client's pain on a scale of 0 to 10. Provide comfort measures and pain medications as required. Monitor and document the effects of pain control measures and pain medications. Describe pain management regimen to client and family.	The client verbalizes ability to cope with pain and measures for pain relief. The client obtains effective relief of pain.
The client acknowledges the need for care. The client is able to perform independent self-care activities.	Include the client in determining care routine. Encourage independence in the performance of self-care as much as possible. Instruct client and family in alternative methods for self-care.	The client participates in self-care to the optimum level.
The client verbalizes body image changes.	Encourage client to verbalize the effects of physical and emotional changes. Actively listen to client and family and acknowledge the reality of concerns about treatments, progress, and prognosis.	The client describes actual change in body function.
The client identifies behaviors that will reduce social isolation.	Identify with the client factors that might contribute to feelings of social isolation. Reinforce efforts by the client, family, and friends to maintain interactions and relationships.	The client identifies resources and support systems that will assist in decreasing social isolation.
The client identifies personal strengths that may promote effective coping.	Assist client to identify personal strengths. Encourage client to express concerns related to problem solving.	The client uses support systems. The client verbalizes a plan for accepting the personal health care situation.
The client verbalizes fears related to prognosis.	Encourage and assist client and family to express fears. Assist to mobilize support services such as hospice for client and family.	The client demonstrates behaviors that reduce fear.

CLIENT NEEDS

SAFE, EFFECTIVE CARE ENVIRONMENT

Advance directives
Advocacy related to client's decisions
Client rights
Confidentiality regarding diagnosis
Informed consent for treatments and procedures
Oncology-related consultations and referrals
Handling hazardous and infectious materials related to radiation and chemotherapy
Asepsis
Standard (universal) and protective precautions

HEALTH PROMOTION AND MAINTENANCE

Expected body image changes related to chemotherapy and treatments
Prevention of disease related to infection
Health screening measures for cancer
Health promotion programs regarding risks for cancer
Client lifestyle choices
Instructions regarding monthly self-breast or self-testicular exams

PSYCHOSOCIAL INTEGRITY

Ability to cope, adapt, and/or problem solve during illness or stressful events
Grief and loss related to death and the dying process
Religious, spiritual, and cultural preferences
Assisting the client and family to cope with alteration in body image

Assisting in mobilizing appropriate support and resource systems
Promoting a positive environment to maintain optimal quality of life

PHYSIOLOGICAL INTEGRITY

Providing basic care and comfort
Promoting nutrition
Managing pain
Diagnostic tests and laboratory values such as WBC and platelet counts
Monitoring for the expected and unexpected responses to radiation and chemotherapy
Protecting the client from the life-threatening side effects of treatments

BIBLIOGRAPHY

deWit, S. (1998). *Essentials of medical-surgical nursing* (4th ed.). Philadelphia: W. B. Saunders.

Hill, S., & Howlett, H. (1997). *Success in practical nursing: Personal and vocational issues* (3rd ed.). Philadelphia: W. B. Saunders.

Leahy, J., & Kizilay, P. (1998). *Foundations of nursing practice: A nursing process approach*. Philadelphia: W. B. Saunders.

Luckmann, J. (1997). *Saunders manual of nursing care*. Philadelphia: W. B. Saunders.

Monahan, F., & Neighbors, M. (1998). *Medical-surgical nursing: Foundations for clinical practice* (2nd ed.). Philadelphia: W. B. Saunders.

National Council of State Boards of Nursing (1998). *National Council detailed test plan for the NCLEX-PN examination*. Chicago: Author.

O'Toole, M. (1997). *Miller-Keane encyclopedia & dictionary of medicine, nursing, & allied health* (6th ed.). Philadelphia: W. B. Saunders.

CHAPTER 40

Oncological Disorders

. . . .

I. Cancer

A. Description
   1. A neoplastic disorder that can involve all body organs
   2. Cells lose their normal growth-controlling mechanism and the growth of cells is uncontrolled
B. **Metastasis:** can occur through the lymphatics, the bloodstream, seeding, or transfer and spread from one site to another
C. **Staging:** a method used to describe the tumor and includes the extent of the tumor, the extent to which malignancy has increased in size, the involvement of regional nodes, and metastatic development
D. Risk factors (Box 40–1)
E. Prevention
   1. Avoid obesity
   2. Decrease fat intake
   3. Increase total fiber in the diet
   4. Decrease alcohol consumption
   5. Avoid salt-cured/nitrate-cured foods
   6. Avoid exposure to **carcinogens**
   7. Obtain adequate rest and exercise to decrease stress
F. Early detection (Box 40–2)
   1. Mammography
   2. Papanicolaou (Pap) smear
   3. Stools for occult blood
   4. Sigmoidoscopy
   5. Breast self-examination
   6. Testicular self-examination
   7. Skin inspection

II. Breast Self-Examination (BSE)

A. Performing BSE
   1. Perform 7 to 10 days after menses
   2. Postmenopausal or clients who have had a hysterectomy should select a specific day of the month and perform BSE monthly on that day
B. Procedure
   1. Before a mirror

a. Inspect with arms at the side
b. Raise arms overhead to inspect for changes in size or contour, dimpling, or changes in the nipple
c. Inspect by resting the palms on the hips and pressing down firmly to flex chest muscles
   2. Lying down
a. Place a pillow under the right breast
b. Use the pads of the middle three fingers of the left hand, press firmly, and feel for lumps or changes using a rubbing, circular pattern to cover all breast tissue
c. Gently squeeze the nipple, looking for discharge
d. Perform BSE on the left breast using the same method
   3. In the shower
a. With fingers flat, move gently over every part of each breast
b. Check for lumps or thickening

III. Testicular Self-Examination (TSE)

A. Select a day of the month and perform the examination on the same day each month
B. Perform after a warm bath or shower
C. Hold the scrotum in one hand
D. Examine each testicle separately by gently rolling it between the thumb and fingers of the other hand
E. Check for hard lumps or knots

BOX 40–1. Risk Factors

Chemical carcinogens
Radiation carcinogens such as sunlight or x-rays
Viral factors
Genetic factors
Demographic/geographic factors
Dietary factors such as obesity, use of alcohol, and high-fat, low-fiber diets
Psychological factors such as stress

BOX 40–2. Warning Signs of Cancer

Change in bowel or bladder habits
Any sore that does not heal
Unusual bleeding or discharge
Thickening or lump in breast or elsewhere
Indigestion
Obvious change of wart or mole
Nagging cough or hoarseness

IV. Diagnostic Tests

A. Tomography
  1. Description
    a. X-ray films showing details of structures otherwise hidden by overlying radiopaque bone
    b. Allows views of tissues at various planes as if slices have been made through the tissue
  2. Implementation: no special preparation is required
B. Computed tomography (CT scan)
  1. Description
    a. X-ray technique that produces cross-sectional body images at progressive depths
    b. Can differentiate normal tissues from abnormal masses and accurately identify their size and location
    c. An oral or IV contrast agent may be administered to increase the sensitivity of the CT scan
  2. Implementation
    a. Obtain informed consent if a dye is injected
    b. Assess the client for allergies to the dye
    c. Clients should be told that they will lie on a table and the x-ray machine will move around them
    d. Clients should be told that the test is painless unless an IV contrast dye is used, which may cause a burning sensation on injection
    e. Inform the client that the dye may cause nausea, vomiting, flushing, itching, and a bitter taste in the mouth
    f. Clients should be told that the x-ray machine can be very noisy
C. Ultrasound
  1. Description
    a. Uses high-frequency sound waves to visualize organs and masses
    b. A noninvasive method of identifying and following the growth of neoplasms without radiation exposure
  2. Implementation
    a. Test preparation may include cleansing the bowel with enemas if the abdominal area is to be tested, and having the client drink 6 to 8 glasses of water without voiding before the test

b. Inform clients that they will not be allowed to void until after the test
    c. Inform the client that the test is painless and that only a slight pressure may be felt
    d. Inform the client that lubricant gel is applied to the area but is easily wiped off after the test
D. Magnetic resonance imaging (MRI) (refer to Chapter 54 for information regarding this diagnostic test)
E. Radioisotope scans
  1. Description
    a. Radioisotopes are used to locate tumors and lesions within the brain, kidneys, liver, lungs, pericardium, and bones
    b. When the radioisotope enters the client's body, the fate of the radioisotope can be followed or traced by the scanning machine
    c. Abnormal tissue appears different on the scan because the isotope is metabolized differently by this tissue
    d. A scan of the organ will reveal a high uptake of the radioisotope at the site of a tumor, and the area in which the concentration of the radioisotope is unusually high is called a hot spot
    e. The area of less concentration of a radioactive isotope is called a cold spot
  2. Implementation
    a. The client receives a tracer dose of the appropriate radioisotope, either orally or by injection
    b. Before the scanning procedure can be performed, the radioisotope must be assimilated by the organ under study; the length of time for organ assimilation of the radioisotope will vary
    c. During the procedure the client is asked to lie still and breathe normally while the scanner measures the radioactivity concentrated in the organ under study and records its findings
    d. Sedation before this procedure may be prescribed for the restless, agitated, or anxious client
F. Lymphangiogram
  1. Description
    a. Examines the lymphatic system, the primary site of **metastasis** for tumors with good lymphatic drainage
    b. The test is performed by injecting dye into the interdigital webs of the feet
    c. The dye is picked up by the lymphatic system; the dye may take several hours to infuse into the lymphatics of the abdomen
    d. X-ray studies are then obtained
  2. Implementation
    a. Obtain an informed consent
    b. Assess the client for allergies
    c. Note that the test cannot be performed for 48 hours after another contrast study

d. Inform the client that the test is fairly long and uncomfortable

e. Instruct the client to drink plenty of fluids after the test

f. Inform the client that the dye may continue to discolor the urine for several days

g. Inform client that he or she must return the following day for follow-up x-ray studies

G. Biopsy

1. Description

a. Surgical incision of a small piece of tissue for microscopic examination

b. Used to either rule out or confirm a diagnosis of malignancy

c. A total type of biopsy excises the entire tumor for examination

d. An excisional type of biopsy excises only a part of the tumor

e. Following excision, a frozen section or a permanent paraffin section is done in order to examine the specimen

f. The advantage of the frozen section is the speed with which the section can be prepared and the diagnosis made, because only minutes are required for this test

g. Permanent paraffin section takes about 24 hours; however, it provides clearer details than does the frozen section

2. Implementation

a. The procedure is usually performed in an outpatient surgical setting

b. Prepare the client for the surgery following the physician's instructions

c. Obtain an informed consent

H. Blood studies

1. Routine tests do not test for specific types of **cancer** but indicate the presence of any number of problems

2. Other blood tests, such as **tumor markers** and biochemical tests, identify the extent of a particular type of **cancer**

3. These specific tests are not used to make the diagnosis of **cancer** but only to check its progression

V. **Pain Control**

A. Causes of pain

1. Bone destruction
2. Obstruction of an organ
3. Compression of peripheral nerves
4. Infiltration/distention of tissue
5. Inflammation/necrosis
6. Psychological, such as fear or anxiety

B. Implementation

1. Collaborate with other members of the health care team to develop a pain management program

2. Administer oral preparations if possible and if they provide adequate relief of pain

3. Mild and moderate pain may be treated with salicylates, acetaminophen (Tylenol), and nonsteroidal anti-inflammatory drugs (NSAIDs)

4. Severe pain is treated with narcotics, such as codeine sulfate, meperidine (Demerol), morphine sulfate, and hydromorphone hydrochloride (Dilaudid)

5. Continuous IV and subcutaneous infusions of narcotics provide superior pain control

6. Monitor for side effects and effectiveness of medications

7. Provide nonpharmacological techniques of pain control such as relaxation, guided imagery, biofeedback, and diversion

8. Do not undermedicate the **cancer** client who is in pain

VI. **Surgery**

A. Description: used to diagnose, stage, and treat **cancer**

B. Curative surgery

1. For **cancer** that is localized to the organ of origin and regional lymph nodes

2. **Cancers** that recur locally can be excised, resulting in occasional cure or remission or both

3. Metastatic lesions that appear in the lungs, liver, or brain can be removed to attempt a surgical cure

4. Excision of a metastatic lesion is considered if no other evidence of disease exists and the metastatic lesion appeared after a relatively long disease-free period

C. Palliative surgery

1. Performed if the risk/benefit ratio is favorable and if it can benefit the client and improve quality of life

2. Reduces pain, relieves airway obstruction, relieves obstructions in the GI and urinary tracts

3. Performed to relieve pressure on the brain and spinal cord

4. Performed to prevent hemorrhage

5. Performed to remove infected and ulcerated tumors and drain abscesses

D. Reconstructive surgery: performed to improve the quality of life by restoring maximal function and appearance

E. Preventive surgery

1. Performed in clients with multiple high-risk factors

2. Performed in certain conditions that may increase the risk of **cancer,** such as polyps or ulcerative colitis

VII. **Chemotherapy** (refer to Chapter 41 for information regarding chemotherapy)

VIII. Radiation Therapy

A. Description
   1. Used as a primary, adjunctive, or palliative modality
   2. Involves therapeutic application of high-energy rays to tumors
   3. Damage to normal cells is the primary side effect and cause of toxicity

B. External radiation
   1. Description: radiation delivered from an external source
   2. Side effects
      a. Headache
      b. Nausea, vomiting, and diarrhea
      c. Skin irritation or injury
      d. Erythema and dryness of the skin
      e. Dry mouth, and change or loss of taste
      f. Esophagitis
      g. Cystitis
      h. Decreased white blood cell (WBC) count and platelets
   3. Implementation
      a. Monitor for signs of skin breakdown
      b. Monitor for signs of complications including cystitis, diarrhea, and nutritional alterations
      c. Increase fluids
      d. Provide a high-protein, high-carbohydrate, high-caloric diet, and provide dietary supplements as prescribed
      e. Instruct the client not to eat for several hours before a treatment if nausea occurs
      f. Administer antiemetics as prescribed and needed
      g. Do not wash off therapy markings
      h. Note that radiodermatitis occurs 3 to 6 weeks after treatments begin
      i. Avoid cream, lotion, or perfume on irradiated areas
      j. Wash irradiated area with lukewarm water and mild soap and pat dry
      k. Avoid exposure to sunlight or artificial heat
      l. Monitor for moist desquamation
   4. Moist desquamation
      a. Weeping of the skin due to the loss of the upper layer of the skin
      b. Cleanse the area with warm water and pat dry
      c. Apply antibiotic ointment or steroid cream as prescribed
      d. Expose the site to air

C. Internal radiation (Box 40–3)
   1. Description
      a. May be known as brachytherapy
      b. Intracavitary implants involve the temporary insertion of a sealed source into a body cavity
      c. Radioactive isotopes that are "sealed" are placed inside wires, needles, catheters, or seeds in interstitial implants to position the radioactive source directly into the tumor and surrounding tissue

---

BOX 40–3. Time, Distance, and Shielding Principles for Internal Radiation

Nursing assignments to a client with a radiation implant should be rotated

Limit time to 30 minutes per care provider per shift

Wear lead shields to reduce the transmission of radiation

A nurse should never care for more than one client with a radiation implant at one time

The nurse can spend more time with the client if he or she maintains a distance of 20 feet from the client, where exposure will be minimal

Communicate to the client from a distance

Stand as far away from the radiation source as possible

Provide nursing care by standing at the client's shoulder for cervical implants and the foot of the bed for head and neck implants

Identify the room with appropriate radiation signs

Wear a dosimeter badge to monitor the amount of radiation exposure

A cumulative radiation dose should not exceed 1250 rad every 3 months

Visitors should stand 6 feet away from the client

Pregnant women or individuals under 18 years of age should not go into the client's room

---

   2. Implementation
      a. Organize nursing tasks to minimize exposure to the client
      b. Maintain strict isolation and radiation precautions
      c. Place the client in a private room
      d. Maintain on bed rest, lying on the back, with head either flat or at less than 45 degrees to prevent dislodging of the radiation source (depending on the location of the radiation)
      e. Restrict visitors as necessary
      f. Nurses who are pregnant or attempting pregnancy should not be assigned to the client
      g. Avoid direct contact around the implant site; provide direct care from the head, foot, or side of the bed, depending on the source of the radiation
      h. Encourage increased fluids and maintain a patent Foley catheter
      i. Monitor for skin eruption, discharge, or abnormal vaginal bleeding
      j. Monitor for dehydration or paralytic ileus
      k. Place a sealed lead container with a long-handled forceps in the client's room
      l. Monitor for dislodging of the radiation source (Box 40–4)
      m. Note that body secretions are considered contaminated, and special techniques per agency policy are required for disposal with unsealed sources
      n. With sealed sources, the radioisotopes

cannot circulate through the body or contaminate body secretions
  o. Save dressings and linens until the radiation is removed, then dispose in the usual manner
3. Internal radiation removal
  a. The client is no longer radioactive
  b. Allow the client to be out of bed
  c. A normal diet may be resumed
  d. Sexual partners cannot "catch" **cancer**
  e. Provide a Betadine douche if prescribed if the implant was placed in the cervix
  f. Administer Fleet enema as prescribed
  g. Inform clients that they may resume sexual intercourse after 7 to 10 days if the implant was cervical or vaginal
  h. Advise the client to notify the physician if nausea, vomiting, diarrhea, frequent urination, excessive vaginal bleeding, rectal bleeding, hematuria, abdominal pain or distention, or an elevated temperature occurs

IX. Bone Marrow Transplantation

A. Description
  1. Used in the treatment of **leukemia** for clients who have closely matched donors and who are experiencing temporary remission with chemotherapy
  2. The goal of treatment is to rid the client of all leukemic or other **malignant** cells through treatment with high doses of chemotherapy and whole-body irradiation
  3. Since these treatments are lethal to bone marrow, without the replacement of bone marrow function through transplantation, the client would die of infection or hemorrhage
B. Transplantation: bone marrow is administered through the client's central IV line in a manner similar to a blood transfusion
C. Post-transplantation period
  1. The client remains without any natural immunity until the donor marrow begins to proliferate and engraftment (transfused bone marrow cells move to the marrow-forming sites of the recipient's bones) occurs
  2. Infection and severe thrombocytopenia are major concerns until engraftment occurs
  3. Major complications include failure to engraft and graft versus host disease (GVHD)

X. Skin Cancer (refer to Chapter 38 for information regarding skin cancer)

XI. Leukemia (Box 40–5)

A. Description
  1. **Malignant** exacerbation in the number of leukocytes, usually at an immature stage, in the bone marrow
  2. May be acute, with a sudden onset and short duration, or chronic, with a slow onset and persistent symptoms over a period of years
  3. Affects the bone marrow, causing anemia, leukopenia, the production of immature cells, thrombocytopenia, and a decline in immunity
  4. The cause is unknown and appears to involve gene damage of cells, leading to the transformation of cells from a normal state to a **malignant** state
  5. Risk factors include genetic, viral, immunological, and environmental factors and exposure to radiation, chemicals, and medications
B. Data collection
  1. Anorexia, fatigue, weakness, and weight loss
  2. Signs of bleeding
  3. Petechiae
  4. Prolonged bleeding after minor abrasions or lacerations
  5. Elevated temperature
  6. Lymphadenopathy and splenomegaly
  7. Normal, elevated, or reduced WBC count
  8. Decreased hemoglobin and hematocrit levels
  9. Decreased platelet count
  10. Positive bone marrow biopsy identifying leukemic blast phase cells
C. Infection
  1. A major cause of death in the immunosuppressed client

2. Can occur through autocontamination or cross-contamination
3. Common sites of infection are the skin, respiratory tract, and GI tract
4. Initiate protective isolation procedures
5. Perform frequent and thorough handwashing
6. Ensure that anyone entering the client's room is wearing a mask
7. Use strict aseptic technique for all procedures
8. Keep supplies for the client separate from supplies for other clients
9. Limit the number of caregivers entering the client's room
10. Maintain the client in a private room
11. Place the client in a room with high-efficiency particulate air (HEPA) filtration or a laminar airflow system if possible
12. Reduce exposure to environmental organisms by eliminating raw fruits and vegetables and fresh flowers and by not leaving standing water in the client's room
13. Be sure that the client's room is cleaned daily
14. Assist the client with daily bathing, using an antimicrobial soap
15. Assist the client to perform oral hygiene frequently
16. Initiate a bowel program for constipation and to prevent rectal trauma
17. Avoid invasive procedures such as injections, rectal temperature, and urinary catheterization
18. Monitor for signs and symptoms of infection
19. Change wound dressings daily, and inspect wounds for redness, swelling, or drainage
20. Monitor urine for color and cloudiness
21. Monitor skin and oral mucous membranes for signs of infection
22. Encourage the client to cough and deep breathe
23. Monitor temperature, pulse, and blood pressure
24. Monitor WBC and neutrophil count
25. The physician is notified if signs of infection are present, and prepare to obtain specimens for culture of open lesions, urine, and sputum
26. Antibiotic, antifungal, and antiviral medication may be prescribed
27. Instruct the client to avoid crowds and those with infections
28. Instruct the client that neither they nor their household contacts should receive immunization with a live virus

D. Bleeding
1. During the period of greatest bone marrow suppression (the **nadir**), the platelet count may be extremely low, less than 10,000/mm³
2. The client is at risk for bleeding when the platelet count falls below 50,000/mm³ and spontaneous bleeding frequently occurs when the platelet count is lower than 20,000/mm³
3. Clients with platelet counts below 20,000/mm³ may need a platelet transfusion

4. For clients with severe blood loss, packed red blood cells (RBCs) may be prescribed
5. Monitor laboratory values
6. Monitor the client for signs and symptoms of bleeding
7. Handle the client gently
8. Measure abdominal girth, which can indicate internal hemorrhage
9. Instruct the client to use a soft toothbrush and avoid dental floss
10. Instruct the client to use only an electric razor for shaving
11. Provide soft foods that are cool to warm
12. Avoid injection if possible to prevent trauma to the skin and bleeding
13. Apply firm and gentle pressure to a needlestick site for at least 10 minutes
14. Pad side rails and sharp corners of the bed and furniture
15. Discourage the client from engaging in activities involving sharp objects
16. Instruct the client to avoid constrictive or tight clothing
17. Use caution when taking blood pressures to prevent skin injury
18. Instruct the client to avoid blowing the nose
19. Avoid rectal suppositories, enemas, and thermometers
20. Examine all body fluids and excrement for the presence of blood
21. If the female client is menstruating, count the number of pads or tampons used
22. Instruct client to avoids NSAIDs and products that contain aspirin

E. Fatigue and nutrition
1. Assist the client in selecting a well-balanced diet
2. Provide small meals that require little chewing
3. Assist the client in self-care and mobility activities
4. Allow adequate rest periods during care
5. Do not perform activities unless they are essential

F. Chemotherapy (refer to Chapter 41 for information regarding chemotherapy and the client with leukemia)

XII. Hodgkin's Disease

A. Description
1. A malignancy of the lymph nodes that originates in a single lymph node or a single chain of nodes
2. **Metastasis** occurs to other adjacent lymph structures and eventually invades nonlymphoid tissue
3. Usually involves lymph nodes, tonsils, spleen, and bone marrow and is characterized by the presence of Reed-Sternberg cells in the lymph nodes
4. Possible causes include viral infections and

previous exposure to alkylating chemical agents

5. Prognosis is dependent on the stage of the disease

B. Data collection
1. Persistent fever
2. Night sweats
3. Loss of appetite and significant weight loss
4. Fatigue and weakness
5. Pruritus
6. Anemia and thrombocytopenia
7. Enlarged lymph nodes, spleen, and liver
8. Positive biopsy of lymph nodes with cervical nodes most often affected first
9. Presence of Reed-Sternberg cells
10. Positive CT scan of liver and spleen

C. Implementation
1. For the early stages without mediastinal node involvement, the treatment of choice is extensive external radiation of involved lymph node regions
2. With more extensive disease, radiation along with multiagent chemotherapy is used (Box 40–6)
3. Monitor for side effects related to chemotherapy or radiation
4. Discuss the possibility of sterility with the male client receiving radiation and inform the client of options related to sperm banks

XIII. Multiple Myeloma

A. Description
1. A **malignant** proliferation of plasma cells and tumors within the bone
2. Causes destruction to bone tissue, decreased production of immunoglobulin and antibodies, and increased levels of uric acid and calcium, which can lead to renal failure
3. The cause is unknown

B. Data collection
1. Bone (skeletal) pain, especially in the pelvis, spine, and ribs
2. Weakness and fatigue
3. Signs of respiratory infection
4. Anemia
5. Elevated temperature
6. Elevated calcium and uric acid levels
7. Decreased platelet count
8. Bone fractures
9. Spinal cord compression and paraplegia
10. Renal failure

BOX 40–6. MOPP Therapy for Hodgkin's Disease

Mechlorethamine (Mustargen)
Vincristine sulfate (Oncovin)
Procarbazine (Matulane)
Prednisone

C. Implementation
1. Force fluids up to 3 to 4 liters a day to maintain an adequate output
2. Monitor IV fluids and administer diuretics as prescribed to increase renal excretion of calcium
3. Encourage ambulation to prevent renal problems and to slow down bone resorption
4. Provide skeletal support during moving, turning, and ambulating to prevent pathological fractures
5. Provide a hazard-free environment
6. Monitor for signs of bleeding, infection, and skeletal fractures
7. Administer analgesics as prescribed to control pain and antibiotics as prescribed for infection
8. Chemotherapy will be prescribed

XIV. Testicular Cancer

A. Description
1. Arises from germinal epithelium from the sperm-producing germ cells or from nongerminal epithelium from other structure in the testicles
2. Most often occurs between ages of 20 and 40 years
3. **Metastasis** occurs to the lung, liver, bone, and adrenal glands

B. Prevention: routine testicular self-examination

C. Data collection
1. Painless testicular swelling
2. Dragging sensation in scrotum
3. Abdominal masses
4. Palpable lymphadenopathy
5. Gynecomastia
6. Infertility
7. Late signs include back or bone pain and respiratory symptoms

D. Implementation
1. Chemotherapy will be prescribed
2. Prepare the client for radiation therapy as prescribed
3. Prepare the client for unilateral orchiectomy if prescribed for diagnosis and primary surgical management
4. Prepare the client for radical retroperitoneal lymph node dissection if prescribed to stage the disease and reduce tumor volume so that chemotherapy and radiation therapy are more effective
5. Discuss reproduction, sexuality, and fertility information and options with the client
6. Identify with the client reproductive options such as sperm storage, donor insemination, and adoption

E. Postoperative implementation
1. Monitor vital signs
2. Monitor for signs of bleeding
3. Monitor for signs of wound infection
4. Monitor I&O
5. The physician is notified if chills, fever,

increasing pain or tenderness at the incision site, or drainage of the incision occurs

6. Instruct clients that they may resume normal activities except for lifting objects heavier than 20 pounds or stair climbing
7. Instruct the client to perform monthly testicular self-examination on the remaining testis

XV. Cervical Cancer

A. Description
  1. Preinvasive **cancer** is limited to the cervix
  2. Invasive **cancer** is in the cervix and other pelvic structures
  3. **Metastasis** is usually confined to the pelvis, but distant **metastasis** occurs through lymphatic spread
  4. Premalignant changes are described on a continuum from dysplasia, which is the earliest premalignancy change, to **carcinoma in situ** (CIS), the most advanced premalignant change (Box 40–7)
B. Precipitating factors
  1. Low socioeconomic groups
  2. Early first marriage
  3. Early and frequent intercourse
  4. Multiple sex partners
  5. High parity
  6. Poor hygiene
C. Data collection
  1. Painless vaginal bleeding postmenstrually and postcoitally
  2. Foul-smelling or serosanguineous vaginal discharge
  3. Pelvic, lower back, leg, or groin pain
  4. Anorexia and weight loss
  5. Leakage of urine and feces from the vagina
  6. Dysuria and hematuria
  7. Cytological changes on Papanicolaou test
D. Implementation (Box 40–8)
E. Laser therapy
  1. Used when all boundaries of the lesion are visible during colposcopic examination
  2. Energy from the beam is absorbed by fluid in the tissues, causing them to vaporize
  3. Minimal bleeding is associated with the procedure
  4. Slight vaginal discharge is expected following the procedure, and healing occurs in 6 to 12 weeks

---

BOX 40–7. Preinvasive Cancers

CERVICAL INTRAEPITHELIAL NEOPLASIA (CIN)

CIN I—mild dysplasia
CIN II—moderate dysplasia
CIN III—severe dysplasia to cancer in situ (CIS)

BOX 40–8. Treatment for Cervical Cancer

NONSURGICAL
External radiation
Internal radiation implants (intracavitary)
Chemotherapy
Laser therapy
Cryosurgery

SURGICAL
Conization
Hysterectomy
Pelvic exenteration

F. Cryosurgery
  1. Freezing of the tissues by a probe with subsequent necrosis
  2. No anesthesia is required, although cramping may occur during the procedure
  3. A heavy watery discharge will occur for several weeks following the procedure
  4. Instruct the client to avoid intercourse and the use of tampons while the discharge is present
G. Conization
  1. A cone-shaped area of cervix is removed
  2. Performed in women who desire future pregnancies
  3. Long-term follow-up care is needed as new lesions can develop
  4. The risks of the procedure include hemorrhage, uterine perforation, incompetent cervix, cervical stenosis, and preterm labor in future pregancies
H. Hysterectomy
  1. Description
    a. For microinvasive **cancer** if childbearing is not desired
    b. A vaginal approach is most commonly performed
    c. A radical hysterectomy and bilateral lymph node dissection may be performed for **cancer** that has spread beyond the cervix but not to the pelvic wall
  2. Postoperative implementation
    a. Monitor vital signs
    b. Assist with coughing and deep-breathing exercises
    c. Assist with ROM exercises and provide early ambulation
    d. Apply antiembolism stockings as prescribed
    e. Monitor I&O and hydration status
    f. Monitor bowel sounds
    g. Monitor vaginal bleeding; note that more than one saturated pad per hour may indicate excessive bleeding
    h. Assess incision site for signs of infection
    i. Monitor Foley catheter drainage
    j. Administer pain medication as prescribed

k. Instruct the client to limit stair climbing for 1 month and to avoid tub baths and sitting for long periods

l. Avoid strenuous activity or lifting anything weighing more than 20 pounds

m. Instruct the client to avoid sexual intercourse for 3 to 6 weeks

n. Instruct the client in the signs associated with complications

I. Pelvic exenteration (Box 40–9)

1. Description

   a. A radical surgical procedure performed for recurrent **cancer** if there is no evidence of tumor outside the pelvis and no lymph node involvement

   b. When the bladder is removed, an ileal conduit will be created and located on the right side of the abdomen to divert urine

   c. A colostomy may need to be created and will be located of the left side of the abdomen for the passage of feces

2. Postoperative implementation

   a. Nursing care measures are similar to postoperative care following hysterectomy

   b. Monitor the incision site for vaginal bleeding and infection

   c. Administer perineal irrigations with half-strength normal saline (NS) and hydrogen peroxide as prescribed

   d. Provide sitz baths as prescribed

   e. Instruct the client that the perineal opening, if present, may drain for several months

   f. Instruct the client in the care of the ileal conduit and colostomy

   g. Provide sexual counseling, as vaginal intercourse is not possible after anterior and total pelvic exenteration

XVI. Ovarian Cancer

A. Description

1. Grows rapidly, spreads fast, and is often bilateral

2. **Metastasis** occurs by direct spread to the organs in the pelvis, by distal spread through lymphatic drainage, or by peritoneal seeding

---

BOX 40–9. Types of Pelvic Exenteration

ANTERIOR

Removal of uterus, ovaries, fallopian tubes, vagina, bladder, urethra, and pelvic lymph nodes

POSTERIOR

Removal of uterus, ovaries, fallopian tubes, descending colon, rectum, and anal canal

TOTAL

Combination of anterior and posterior

---

3. Prognosis is usually poor because the tumor is usually detected late

4. An exploratory laparotomy is performed to diagnose and stage the tumor

B. Data collection

1. Abdominal discomfort or swelling

2. GI disturbances

3. Dysfunctional vaginal bleeding

4. Abdominal mass

C. Implementation

1. External radiation is used if the tumor has invaded other organs

2. Chemotherapy is used postoperatively for all stages of ovarian **cancer**

3. Intraperitoneal chemotherapy, which involves the instillation of chemotherapy into the abdominal cavity

4. Immunotherapy, which alters the immunological response of the ovary and promotes tumor resistance

5. Total abdominal hysterectomy and bilateral salpingo-oophorectomy

XVII. Endometrial Cancer

A. Description

1. A slow-growing tumor associated with menopausal years

2. **Metastasis** occurs through the lymphatic system to the ovaries and pelvis; via the blood to the lungs, liver, and bone; or intra-abdominally to the peritoneal cavity

B. Precipitating factors

1. History of uterine polyps

2. Nulliparity

3. Polycystic ovary disease

4. Estrogen stimulation

5. Late menopause

6. Family history

C. Data collection

1. Postmenopausal bleeding

2. Watery, serosanguineous discharge

3. Low back, pelvic, or abdominal pain

4. Enlarged uterus in advanced stages

D. Nonsurgical implementation

1. External radiation or internal radiation used alone or in combination with surgery, depending on the stage of **cancer**

2. Chemotherapy to treat advanced and recurrent disease

3. Progestational therapy with medroxyprogesterone (Depo-Provera) or megestrol acetate (Megace) for estrogen-dependent tumors

4. Tamoxifen (Nolvadex), an antiestrogen, may also be prescribed

E. Surgical implementation: total abdominal hysterectomy and bilateral salpingo-oophorectomy

XVIII. Breast Cancer

A. Description
  1. Classified as invasive when it penetrates the tissue surrounding the mammary duct and grows in an irregular pattern
  2. **Metastasis** occurs via lymph nodes
  3. Common sites of metastatic disease are the bone, lungs, brain, and liver
  4. Diagnosis is made by breast biopsy through a needle aspiration or by surgical removal of the tumor with microscopic examination made for **malignant** cells

B. Precipitating factors
  1. Family history
  2. Early menarche and late menopause
  3. Previous cancer of breast, uterus, or ovaries
  4. Nulliparity
  5. Obesity
  6. High-dose radiation exposure to the chest

C. Data collection
  1. Mass usually felt in the upper outer quadrant or beneath the nipple
  2. A fixed, irregular, nonencapsulated mass
  3. A painless mass except in the very late states
  4. Nipple retraction or elevation
  5. Asymmetry, with the affected breast being higher
  6. Bloody or clear nipple discharge
  7. Skin dimpling, retraction, or ulceration
  8. Skin edema or peau d'orange
  9. Axillary lymphadenopathy
  10. Lymphedema of affected arm
  11. Symptoms of bone or lung **metastasis**
  12. Presence of lesion on mammography

D. Prevention: monthly breast self-examination (BSE)

E. Nonsurgical implementation
  1. Chemotherapy
  2. Radiation therapy
  3. Hormonal manipulation via the use of estrogen in postmenopausal women or tamoxifen (Nolvadex) for estrogen receptor–positive tumors

F. Surgical implementation
  1. Surgical breast procedures (Box 40–10)
  2. Oophorectomy for estrogen receptor–positive tumors
  3. Ablative therapy with adrenalectomy or chemical ablation therapy

G. Postoperative implementation
  1. Monitor vital signs
  2. Position semi-Fowler's on the back or unaffected side with the affected arm above the level of the heart to promote drainage and prevent lymphedema
  3. Turn client only to the back and unaffected side
  4. Encourage coughing and deep breathing
  5. If a Hemovac or Jackson-Pratt drain is in place, maintain suction and record the amount of drainage and drainage characteristics
  6. Monitor operative site for swelling or the presence of fluid collection under the skin flaps
  7. Monitor for signs of infection
  8. Place a sign above the bed stating "No IVs, No IMs, No BPs, No Venipunctures"
  9. Provide the use of a pressure sleeve as prescribed if edema is severe
  10. Administer diuretics as prescribed for severe lymphedema
  11. Provide a low-salt diet as prescribed for severe lymphedema
  12. Monitor the site for restriction of dressing, impaired sensation, color changes of skin
  13. Assist with exercises as prescribed to decrease lymphedema and muscle weakness
  14. See Box 40–11 for client instructions following mastectomy

---

BOX 40–10. Surgical Breast Procedures

LUMPECTOMY

Excision and removal of the tumor
Lymph node dissection may also be performed

SIMPLE MASTECTOMY

Removal of the breast with no lymph node removal
The breast tissue is removed, but the anterior skin, axillary lymph nodes, and underlying muscles are left intact

PARTIAL MASTECTOMY

The tumor is removed along with a small amount of surrounding tissue

MODIFIED RADICAL MASTECTOMY

The breast tissue and nipple are totally removed, with partial excision of the skin, lymph nodes, and surrounding tissue

RADICAL MASTECTOMY

All breast tissue and nipple are removed along with partial removal of the overlying skin, chest muscles, axillary lymph tissue, and nearby adipose tissue

---

XIX. Gastric Cancer

A. Description
  1. An abnormal **malignant** growth in the stomach
  2. Risk factors include a diet high in complex carbohydrates, grains, and salt, and low in fresh, green leafy vegetables and fresh fruit; smoking; alcohol; foods containing nitrates; and a history of gastric ulcers
  3. Complications include hemorrhage, obstruction, and **metastasis**
  4. The goal of treatment is to remove the tumor and provide a nutritional program

BOX 40–11. Client Instruction following Mastectomy

Avoid overuse of the arm during the first few months

To prevent lymphedema, keep affected arm elevated

Perform incision care with lanolin to soften and prevent wound contracture

Encourage use of Reach for Recovery volunteers

Encourage the client to perform breast self-examination on the remaining breast

Protect affected hand and arm

Avoid strong sunlight to arm

Do not let arm hang dependent

Do not carry pocketbook or anything heavy over the affected arm

Avoid trauma, cuts, bruises, or burns to affected side

No constricting clothing or jewelry on affected side

Wear gloves when gardening

Use oven mitts when cooking

Use a thimble when sewing

Use cream cuticle remover

Call physician if signs of inflammation occur in affected arm

Wear Medic-Alert bracelet stating lymphedema arm

B. Data collection
   1. Fatigue
   2. Anorexia and weight loss
   3. Nausea and vomiting
   4. Indigestion and epigastric discomfort
   5. A sensation of pressure in the stomach
   6. Dysphagia
   7. Palpable mass
C. Implementation
   1. Monitor vital signs
   2. Monitor hemoglobin and hematocrit levels
   3. Monitor weight
   4. Monitor nutritional status
   5. Encourage small, bland, easily digestible meals with vitamin and mineral supplements
   6. Administer pain medication as prescribed
   7. Prepare the client for chemotherapy or radiation therapy as prescribed
   8. Prepare the client for surgical resection of the tumor as prescribed (Box 40–12)
D. Postoperative implementation (refer to Chapter 44 for information regarding postoperative care)

XX. Intestinal Tumors

A. Description
   1. **Malignant** lesions that develop in the cells lining the bowel wall or develop as polyps in the colon or rectum
   2. Complications include bowel perforation with peritonitis, abscess and/or fistula formation, frank hemorrhage, and complete intestinal obstruction
   3. Metastasis occurs via the circulatory or lymphatic system, or by direct extension to other areas in the colon or other organs

B. Data collection
   1. Blood in stools
   2. Anorexia, vomiting, and weight loss
   3. Malaise and anemia
   4. Abnormal stools
      a. Ascending colon tumor: diarrhea
      b. Descending colon tumor: constipation or some diarrhea, or flat, ribbonlike stool due to a partial obstruction
      c. Rectal tumor: alternating constipation and diarrhea
   5. Guarding or abdominal distention
   6. Abdominal mass (a late sign)
   7. Cachexia (a late sign)
C. Implementation
   1. Monitor for signs of complications, which include bowel perforation with peritonitis, abscess and/or fistula formation, frank hemorrhage, and complete intestinal obstruction
   2. Monitor for signs of intestinal perforation including low BP, rapid and weak pulse, distended abdomen, and elevated temperature
   3. Monitor for signs of intestinal obstruction, which may include vomiting (may be fecal contents), pain, constipation, and abdominal distention
   4. Note that an early sign of intestinal obstruction includes increased peristaltic

BOX 40–12. Surgical Implementation for Gastric Cancer

TOTAL GASTRECTOMY

Also called esophagojejunostomy

Removal of the stomach with attachment of the esophagus to the jejunum or duodenum

VAGOTOMY

Surgical division of the vagus nerve to eliminate the vagal impulses that stimulate hydrochloric acid secretion in the stomach

GASTRIC RESECTION

Also called antrectomy

Involves removal of the lower half of the stomach and usually includes a vagotomy

BILLROTH I

Also called gastroduodenostomy

Partial gastrectomy; remaining segment is anastomosed to duodenum

BILLROTH II

Also called gastrojejunostomy

Partial gastrectomy, with remaining segment anastomosed to the jejunum

PYLOROPLASTY

Enlarges the pylorus to prevent or decrease pyloric obstruction, thereby enhancing gastric emptying activity, which produces an increase in bowel sounds; as the obstruction progresses, hypoactive sounds are heard

5. Prepare for radiation preoperatively to facilitate surgical resection, and postoperatively to decrease the risk of recurrence or to reduce pain, hemorrhage, bowel obstruction, or **metastasis**
6. Chemotherapy is used postoperatively to assist in the control of symptoms and spread of the disease

D. Surgical implementation: bowel resection and creation of colostomy or ileostomy (refer to Chapter 44 for information regarding the preoperative and postoperative care related to surgery)

XXI. Lung Cancer

A. Description
   1. **Malignant** tumor of the lung that may be primary or metastatic
   2. The lungs are a common target for **metastasis** from other organs
   3. Bronchiogenic carcinoma spreads through direct extension and lymphatic dissemination
   4. The four major types of lung **cancer** include small cell (oat cell), epidermal (squamous cell), adenocarcinoma, and large cell anaplastic carcinoma
   5. Diagnosis is made by a chest x-ray, which will show a lesion or mass, and bronchoscopy and sputum studies, which will demonstrate a positive cytology for cancer cells
B. Causes
   1. Cigarette smoking
   2. Exposure to environmental pollutants
   3. Exposure to occupational pollutants
C. Data collection
   1. Cough and hemoptysis
   2. Dyspnea
   3. Hoarseness
   4. Chest pain
   5. Anorexia and weight loss
   6. Weakness
D. Implementation
   1. Monitor vital signs
   2. Monitor breathing patterns and for signs of respiratory impairment
   3. Administer analgesics as prescribed for pain management
   4. Position the client upright for ease in breathing
   5. Administer oxygen as prescribed and humidification to moisten and loosen secretions
   6. Monitor pulse oximetry
   7. Provide respiratory treatments as prescribed
   8. Administer bronchodilators and steroids as prescribed to decrease bronchospasm, inflammation, and edema
   9. Provide a high-protein, high-calorie diet
   10. Provide activity as tolerated, rest periods, and active and passive range of motion (ROM) exercises
   11. Monitor for bleeding, infection, and electrolyte imbalance
E. Nonsurgical implementation
   1. Radiation therapy for localized intrathoracic lung cancers
   2. Chemotherapy to promote tumor regression
   3. Immunotherapy directed at enhancing an effective response, which favorably affects the course of disease
   4. Nonspecific immune therapy with bacille Calmette-Guérin vaccine (BCG) as prescribed
F. Surgical implementation
   1. Laser therapy: to relieve endobronchial obstruction
   2. Thoracotomy with pneumonectomy: surgical removal of a lung for bronchiogenic carcinoma
   3. Thoracotomy with lobectomy: surgical removal of one lobe of the lung for tumors confined to a single lobe
   4. Thoracotomy with segmental resection: surgical removal of lobe segment for clients unable to tolerate lobectomy or pneumonectomy
G. Preoperative and postoperative implementation (refer to Chapter 46 for care to the client undergoing thoracic surgery)

XXII. Laryngeal Cancer

A. Description
   1. A **malignant** tumor of the larynx
   2. Laryngeal **cancer** presents as **malignant** ulcerations with underlying filtration
   3. **Metastasis** to the lung is common
   4. Diagnosis is made by laryngoscopy and biopsy showing a positive cytology for cancer cells
B. Causes
   1. Cigarette smoking
   2. Alcohol abuse
   3. Exposure to environmental pollutants
   4. Exposure to radiation
   5. Voice strain
C. Data collection
   1. Persistent hoarseness
   2. Persistent sore throat
   3. Painless neck mass
   4. A feeling of a lump in the throat
   5. Burning sensation in the throat
   6. Dysphagia
   7. Change in voice quality
   8. Dyspnea
   9. Hemoptysis
   10. Weakness and weight loss
   11. Foul breath
D. Implementation
   1. Position in Fowler's to promote optimal air exchange
   2. Monitor respiratory status

3. Monitor for signs of aspiration of food and fluid
4. Provide activity as tolerated
5. Provide a high-calorie, high-vitamin, high-protein diet
6. Provide nutritional support as prescribed
7. Administer oxygen as prescribed
8. Provide respiratory treatments as prescribed
9. Administer analgesic as prescribed

E. Nonsurgical implementation
1. Radiation therapy if the **cancer** is limited to a small area in one vocal cord
2. Chemotherapy, which may be done in combination with radiation and surgery

F. Surgical implementation
1. Small tumor excision or total laryngectomy: performed for infiltrate tumors that involve vocal cord paralysis and for tumors that do not respond to radiation therapy
2. Radical neck dissection: performed when lymph node involvement is present and involves a laryngectomy and tracheostomy

G. Preoperative and postoperative implementation (refer to Chapter 46 for care to the client undergoing surgery)

XXIII. Cancer of the Prostate

A. Description
1. A slow-growing **cancer** of the prostate gland, which is usually an androgen-dependent adenocarcinoma
2. The risk increases in the male with each decade after age 50
3. **Metastasis** occurs via direct invasion of surrounding tissues, spread through the bloodstream and lymphatics, and via **metastasis** to the bony pelvis and spine
4. Bone **metastasis** is a concern

B. Data collection
1. Asymptomatic in early stages
2. Hard pea-sized nodule palpated on rectal exam
3. Hematuria
4. Late symptoms include weight loss, urinary obstruction, and pain radiating from the lumbosacral area down the leg
5. Prostate-specific antigen (PSA) test does not necessarily indicate malignancy and is used routinely to monitor the client's response to therapy
6. Elevated serum acid phosphatase level indicates spread

C. Nonsurgical implementation
1. Prepare the client for hormone manipulation therapy as prescribed
2. Administer luteinizing hormone leuprolide acetate (Lupron), flutamide (Eulexin), or diethylstilbestrol (DES) as prescribed to slow the rate of growth of the tumor
3. Prepare the client for radiation (internal or external), which may be prescribed alone or in conjunction with surgery and may be prescribed pre- or postoperatively to reduce the lesion and limit **metastasis**
4. Prepare the client for the administration of chemotherapy in hormone-resistant tumors

D. Surgical implementation
1. Prepare the client for orchiectomy if prescribed, which will limit the production of testosterone
2. Prepare the client for transurethral resection (TUR) or prostatectomy if prescribed (refer to Chapter 50 for information regarding preoperative and postoperative care following TUR and prostatectomy)

XXIV. Bladder Cancer

A. Description
1. Papillomatous growths in the bladder urothelium that undergo **malignant** changes and may infiltrate the bladder wall
2. Predisposing factors include cigarette smoking, exposure to industrial chemicals, and exposure to radiation
3. Common sites of **metastasis** include the liver, bones, and lungs
4. As the tumor progresses, it can extend into the rectum, vagina, other pelvic soft tissues, and retroperitoneal structures

B. Data collection
1. Gross painless hematuria
2. Frequency, urgency, and dysuria
3. Clot-induced obstruction
4. Bladder biopsy confirms diagnosis

C. Radiation
1. Most bladder **cancers** are poorly radiosensitive and require high doses of radiation
2. Radiation therapy is more acceptable for advanced disease that cannot be eradicated by surgery
3. Palliative radiation may be used to relieve pain, bowel obstruction, and control potential hemorrhage and leg edema secondary to venous or lymphatic obstruction
4. Intracavitary radiation may be prescribed, which protects adjacent tissue
5. External radiation combined with chemotherapy or surgery may be prescribed because the external radiation alone may be ineffective
6. Complications of radiation
   a. Abacterial cystitis
   b. Proctitis
   c. Fistula formation
   d. Ileitis or colitis
   e. Bladder ulceration and hemorrhage

D. Chemotherapy
1. Intravesical instillation
   a. An alkylating chemotherapeutic agent is instilled in the bladder

b. Treat the urine as a biohazard and dispose of properly

c. For 6 hours following intravesical chemotherapy, disinfect the toilet with household bleach after voiding

2. Systemic chemotherapy: used to treat inoperable or late tumors

3. Complications of chemotherapy
   a. Bladder irritation
   b. Hemorrhagic cystitis

E. Surgical implementation

1. TURP: performed for very early tumors for cure or for inoperable tumors for palliation

2. Partial cystectomy
   a. The removal of up to half of the bladder
   b. Done in early tumors and for clients who cannot tolerate a radical cystectomy
   c. During the initial postoperative period, bladder capacity is markedly reduced to about 60 mL; however, as the bladder tissue expands, the capacity increases to 200 to 400 mL
   d. Maintenance of a continuous output of urine following surgery is critical to prevent bladder distention and stress on the suture line
   e. A urethral and suprapubic catheter may be in place, and the suprapubic catheter may be left in place for 2 weeks until healing occurs

3. Cystectomy and urinary diversion
   a. Removal of the bladder and urethra in women and the bladder, urethra, and usually prostate and seminal vesicles in men
   b. When the bladder and the urethra are removed, permanent urinary diversion is required
   c. The surgery may be performed in two stages if the tumor is extensive, with the creation of the urinary diversion first and the cystectomy several weeks later
   d. If a radical cystectomy is performed, lower extremity lymphedema may occur due to lymph node dissection, and impotence may occur in the male client

4. Ileal conduit
   a. Also called ureteroileostomy or Bricker procedure
   b. Ureters are implanted into a segment of the ileum with the formation of an abdominal stoma
   c. The urine flows into the conduit and is continually propelled out through the stoma by peristalsis
   d. The client is required to wear an appliance over the stoma to collect the urine
   e. Complications include obstruction, pyelonephritis, leakage at the anastomosis site, stenosis, hydronephrosis, calculi, skin irritation and ulceration, and stomal defects

5. Kock pouch or Indiana pouch
   a. Kock pouch: a continent internal ileal reservoir created from a segment of the ileum and ascending colon; the ureters are implanted into the side of the reservoir, and a special nipple valve is constructed to attach the reservoir to the skin
   b. Indiana pouch: a continent reservoir is created from the ascending colon and terminal ileum, making a pouch larger than the Kock pouch
   c. Postoperatively, the client will have a 24 to 26 Foley catheter in place to drain urine continuously until the pouch has healed
   d. The catheter is irrigated gently with normal saline to prevent obstruction from mucus or clots as prescribed
   e. Following removal of the catheter, the client is instructed how to self-catheterize and drain the reservoir at 4- to 6-hour intervals

6. Creation of a neobladder
   a. Similar to the creation of an internal reservoir with the difference being that instead of emptying through an abdominal stoma, it empties through a pelvic outlet into the urethra
   b. The client empties the neobladder by relaxing the external sphincter and creating abdominal pressure or by intermittent self-catheterization

7. Percutaneous nephrostomy or pyelostomy
   a. Used when the **cancer** is inoperable, to prevent obstruction
   b. Involves a percutaneous or surgical insertion of a nephrostomy tube into the kidney for drainage
   c. Nursing implementation involves stabilizing the tube to prevent dislodgment and monitoring output

8. Ureterostomy
   a. May be performed as a palliative procedure if the ureters are obstructed by the tumor
   b. The ureters are attached to the surface of the abdomen, where the urine flows directly into a drainage appliance without a conduit
   c. Potential problems include infection, skin irritation, and obstruction to urinary flow due to strictures at the opening

9. Vesicostomy
   a. The bladder is sutured to the abdomen, and a stoma is created in the bladder wall
   b. The bladder empties through the stoma

F. Preoperative implementation

1. Administer bowel preparation as prescribed, which may include clear liquid diet, laxatives and enemas, and antibiotics to lower the bacterial count in the bowel

2. Assist the surgeon and enterostomal nurse in selecting an appropriate skin site for creation of the abdominal stoma

BOX 40-13. Urinary Stoma Care

Instruct client to change appliance in the morning when urinary production is slowest

Collect equipment, remove collection bag, use water or commercial solvent to loosen adhesive

Hold a rolled gauze pad against stoma to collect and absorb urine during procedure

Cleanse skin around stoma and under drainage bag with mild nonresidue soap and water

Inspect skin for excoriation and instruct the client to prevent urine from coming in contact with the skin

After skin is dry, apply skin adhesive around stoma and to the appliance

Instruct client to cut stoma opening of the skin barrier just large enough to fit over the stoma (no more than 3 mm larger than the stoma)

Instruct client that the stoma will shrink, requiring a smaller stoma opening on the skin barrier

Apply skin barrier before attaching the pouch or faceplate

Place appliance over stoma and secure in place

Encourage self-care; teach client to use mirror

Instruct client that the pouch may be drained by a bedside bag or leg bag, especially at night

Instruct client to empty the urinary collection bag when it is one-third to one-half full to prevent pulling of the appliance and leakage

Instruct client to check the appliance seal if perspiring occurs

Instruct client to leave the urinary pouch in place as long as it is not leaking and change every 5 to 7 days

During appliance changes, leave the skin open to air as long as possible

Use a nonkaraya gum product as urine erodes karaya gum

To control odor, instruct the client to drink adequate fluids, to wash appliance thoroughly with soap and lukewarm water, to soak collection pouch in dilute white vinegar for 20 to 30 minutes, or to place a special deodorant tablet into the pouch while it is being worn

Instruct clients who take baths to keep the level of the water below the stoma and avoid oily soaps

If the client plans to shower, instruct client to direct flow of water away from the stoma

6. Monitor for prolapse or retraction of the stoma
7. Monitor for return of bowel function
8. Monitor for peristalsis, which will return in 3 to 4 days
9. Maintain NPO status as prescribed until bowel sounds return
10. Monitor urine flow, which is continuous (30 to 60 mL/hour) following surgery
11. The physician is notified if the urine output is less than 30 mL/hour or if there is no urine output for more than 15 minutes
12. Ureteral stents or catheters may be in place for 2 to 3 weeks or until healing occurs
13. Maintain stability with catheters to prevent dislodgment
14. Monitor for hematuria
15. Monitor for signs of peritonitis
16. Monitor for bladder distention following a partial cystectomy
17. Monitor for shock, hemorrhage, thrombophlebitis, and lower extremity lymphedema following a radical cystectomy
18. Monitor the urinary drainage pouch for leaks, and check skin integrity

BOX 40-14. Self-Irrigation and Catheterization of Stoma

IRRIGATION

Instruct client to wash hands and use clean technique

Instruct client to use a catheter and syringe to instill 60 mL of normal saline or water into the reservoir and to gently aspirate or allow to drain

Instruct client to irrigate until the drainage remains free of mucus but to be cautious not to overirrigate

CATHETERIZATION

Instruct client to wash hands and use a clean technique

Initially, the client is taught to insert a catheter every 2 to 3 hours to drain the reservoir; during each week thereafter, the interval is increased by 1 hour until the catheterization is done every 4 to 6 hours

Lubricate catheter well with water-soluble lubricant and instruct client never to force catheter into reservoir

If resistance is met, instruct client to pause, rotate catheter, and to apply gentle pressure to insert

Instruct client to notify physician if unable to insert catheter

When urine has stopped, instruct client to take several deep breaths and move the catheter in and out 2 to 3 inches to ensure that the pouch is empty

Instruct the client to withdraw the catheter slowly and to pinch the catheter when withdrawn so that it does not leak urine

Instruct clients to carry catheterization supplies with them

3. Encourage clients to talk about their feelings related to the stoma creation
G. Postoperative implementation
   1. Monitor vital signs
   2. Monitor incision site
   3. Assess stoma (should be red and moist) every hour for the first 24 hours (Box 40–13)
   4. Note edema in the stoma, which may be present in the immediate postoperative period
   5. If the stoma appears dark and dusky, the physician is notified immediately because this indicates necrosis

19. Monitor pH of the urine (do not place the dipstick in the stoma) because strongly alkali urine can cause skin irritation and facilitate crystal formation
20. Instruct the client regarding the potential for urinary tract infection (UTI) or the development of calculi
21. Instruct the client to assess skin for irritation, to monitor urinary drainage pouch for any leakage, and self-catheterization procedure (Box 40–14)
22. Encourage the client to express feelings about changes in body image, embarrassment, and sexual dysfunction

PRACTICE QUESTIONS

1. The nurse is instructing the client to perform a testicular self-examination (TSE). Which instruction does the nurse provide to the client?
   1 Examine the testicles while lying down
   2 The best time for the examination is after a shower
   3 Gently feel the testicle with one finger to feel for a growth
   4 Testicular exams should be done at least every 6 months

2. The nurse is assisting in conducting a health promotion program at a local school. Which of the following is not identified as a risk factor associated with cancer?
   1 Viral factors
   2 Stress
   3 Low-fat and high-fiber diets
   4 Exposure to radiation

3. The client with cancer is receiving chemotherapy and develops thrombocytopenia. Which goal should be given the highest priority in the nursing plan of care?
   1 Ambulation three times daily
   2 Monitoring temperature
   3 Monitoring for bleeding
   4 Monitoring for pathological fractures

4. The nurse inspects the oral cavity of a client with cancer and notes white patches on the mucous membranes. The nurse determines that this
   1 Is common
   2 Is characteristic of a thrush infection
   3 Is indicative that oral hygiene needs to be improved
   4 Suggests that the client is anemic

5. The nurse is monitoring the laboratory results of a client preparing to receive chemotherapy. The nurse determines that the white blood cell count (WBC) is normal if which of the following results is present?
   1 3000/mm^3
   2 7000/mm^3
   3 15,000/mm^3
   4 20,000/mm^3

6. The nurse is instructing a group of female clients about breast self-examination (BSE). The nurse instructs the clients to perform the examination
   1 At the onset of menstruation
   2 1 week after menstruation begins
   3 Every month during ovulation
   4 Weekly at the same time of day

7. The nurse is instructing the client in breast self-examination (BSE). The nurse tells the client to lie down and to examine the left breast. The nurse instructs the client that while examining the left breast she should place a pillow
   1 Under the right shoulder
   2 Under the left shoulder
   3 Under the small of the back
   4 Under the right scapula

8. The nurse is teaching breast self-examination (BSE) to a client who has had a hysterectomy. The most appropriate instruction regarding when the BSE should be performed is
   1 7 to 10 days after menses
   2 Just before menses begins
   3 At ovulation time
   4 At a specific day of the month and on that same day every month thereafter

9. A client suspected of having an abdominal tumor is scheduled for a computed tomography (CT scan) with dye injection. The nurse tells the client which of the following about the test?
   1 The test may be painful
   2 The dye injected may cause a warm, flushing sensation
   3 Fluids will be restricted following the test
   4 The test takes approximately 2 hours

10. The 32-year-old female client has a history of fibrocystic disorder of the breasts. The nurse gathering data from the client asks whether the breast lumps are more noticeable
    1 In the spring months
    2 In the autumn
    3 After menses
    4 Before menses

11. The client has undergone mastectomy. The nurse interprets that the client is making the best adjustment to the loss of the breast if which of the following behaviors is observed?
    1 Participating in the care of the surgical drain
    2 Reading the postoperative care booklet
    3 Refusing to look at the wound
    4 Asking for pain medication when needed

12. The client is preparing for discharge 10 days after radical vulvectomy. The nurse plans to tell this client that which of the following activities is

acceptable after discharge because it will not precipitate complications?
1 Sexual activity
2 Walking
3 Sitting for lengthy periods
4 Driving a car

13. The client has undergone vaginal hysterectomy. The nurse avoids which of the following in the care of this client?
1 Removal of antiembolism stockings twice daily
2 Assisting with range of motion leg exercises
3 Elevating the knee gatch on the bed
4 Checking placement of pneumatic compression boots

14. The client suspected of an ovarian tumor is scheduled for a pelvic ultrasound. The nurse plans to tell the client that preparation for the ultrasound includes which of the following?
1 NPO prior to the procedure
2 A light breakfast only
3 Drinking six to eight glasses of water without voiding prior to the test
4 Wearing comfortable clothing and shoes for the procedure

15. The client is diagnosed as having a bowel tumor. Several diagnostic tests are prescribed. The nurse understands that which of the following tests will confirm the diagnosis of malignancy?
1 Magnetic resonance imaging (MRI)
2 Computed tomography (CT) scan
3 Abdominal ultrasound
4 Biopsy of the tumor

16. A client is diagnosed with multiple myeloma. The client asks the nurse about the diagnosis. The nurse bases the response on which of the following characteristics of the disorder?
1 Malignant exacerbation in the number of leukocytes
2 Altered red blood cell production
3 Altered production of lymph nodes
4 Malignant proliferation of plasma cells and tumors within the bone

17. The nurse is reviewing the laboratory results of a client diagnosed with multiple myeloma. Which of the following does the nurse expect to specifically note with this diagnosis?
1 Decreased number of plasma cells in the bone marrow
2 Increased white blood cells
3 Increased calcium level
4 Decreased blood urea nitrogen (BUN)

18. The nurse is assisting in developing a plan of care for the client with multiple myeloma. A priority nursing intervention includes which of the following?

1 Coughing and deep breathing
2 Forcing fluids
3 Monitoring the red blood cell count
4 Providing frequent oral care

19. The nurse is assigned to assist in caring for a client with Hodgkin's disease. The nurse assists in planning care, knowing that which of the following is not a characteristic of this disease?
1 Presence of Reed-Sternberg cells
2 Involvement of lymph nodes, spleen, and liver
3 Occurs most often in older adults
4 Prognosis depends on the stage of the disease

20. The nurse is assisting in conducting a health promotion program regarding testicular cancer for community members. The nurse tells the members that which of the following is not a sign of testicular cancer?
1 Painless testicular swelling
2 Heavy sensation in the scrotum
3 Alopecia
4 Back pain

21. The nurse is reviewing the laboratory results of a client with leukemia who received a regimen of chemotherapy. Which of the following laboratory values does the nurse specifically note as a result of the massive cell destruction that occurred from the chemotherapy?
1 Anemia
2 Decreased platelets
3 Decreased leukocyte count
4 Increased uric acid level

22. The nurse is preparing a client with a bowel tumor for surgery. The physician has informed the client that the surgery is palliative in the treatment of the tumor. The nurse understands that this type of surgery is performed to
1 Restore maximal function and appearance
2 Eliminate high-risk factors
3 Reduce pain
4 Cure the client

23. The client is receiving external radiation to the neck for cancer of the larynx. The nurse plans care, knowing that the most likely side effect to be expected is
1 Constipation
2 Dyspnea
3 Sore throat
4 Diarrhea

24. The nurse inspects the skin of a client receiving external radiation therapy and documents a finding noted as moist desquamation. The nurse understands that the most appropriate description of moist desquamation is which of the following?

1. Reddened skin
2. A rash
3. Weeping of the skin
4. Dermatitis

25. The nurse is providing instructions to the client receiving external radiation therapy. Which of the following is not a component of the instructions?
    1. Avoid exposure to sunlight
    2. Wash the skin with a mild soap and pat dry
    3. Apply pressure on the irritated area to prevent bleeding
    4. Eat a high-protein diet

26. The nurse is caring for a client with an internal radiation implant. When caring for the client, the nurse should observe which of the following principles?
    1. Limit the time with the client to 1 hour per shift
    2. Do not allow pregnant women into the client's room
    3. Individuals under 16 years may be allowed to go into the room as long as they are 6 feet away from the client
    4. Remove dosimeter badge when entering the client's room

27. The client was hospitalized for a cervical radiation implant for the treatment of cervical cancer. The implant is removed and the client is to be discharged. The nurse plans to reinforce discharge instructions. Which of the following is not a component of the discharge instructions?
    1. Cream may be used to relieve dryness or itching
    2. Foul-smelling vaginal discharge is a sign of an infection
    3. Sexual intercourse may be resumed after 7 to 10 days
    4. Some vaginal bleeding is expected for 1 to 3 months

28. A cervical radiation implant is placed in the client for treatment of cervical cancer. What activity order is most appropriate for this client?
    1. Out of bed in a chair only
    2. Ambulate to the bathroom only
    3. Bed rest
    4. Out of bed ad lib

29. The nurse teaches skin care to the client receiving external radiation therapy. Which of the following statements, if made by the client, indicates the need for further instruction?
    1. "I will handle the area gently"
    2. "I will avoid the use of deodorants"
    3. "I will limit sun exposure to 1 hour daily"
    4. "I will wear loose-fitting clothing."

30. The client is hospitalized for insertion of an internal cervical radiation implant. While giving care, the nurse finds the radiation implant in the bed. The initial action by the nurse is to

1. Call the physician
2. Pick up the implant with gloved hands and flush it down the toilet
3. Reinsert the implant into the vagina immediately
4. Pick up the implant with long-handled forceps and place in a lead container

31. The nurse is assisting in developing a plan of care for a client experiencing hematological toxicity as a result of chemotherapy. Which of the following is included in the plan of care?
    1. Restricting all visitors
    2. Restricting fluid intake
    3. Inserting an indwelling urinary catheter to prevent skin breakdown
    4. Restricting fresh fruits and vegetables in the diet

32. The nurse is reviewing the laboratory results of a client receiving chemotherapy. The platelet count is 10,000/mm³. Based on this laboratory value, the priority nursing action is to monitor which of the following?
    1. Level of consciousness
    2. Temperature
    3. Bowel sounds
    4. Skin turgor

33. The nurse is assisting in conducting a teaching session for a group of community members regarding the risks of cervical cancer. Which of the following is not a risk factor associated with this type of cancer?
    1. Intercourse with circumcised males
    2. Early frequent intercourse
    3. Multiple sexual partners
    4. History of genital herpes

34. The nurse is caring for a client who is 4 days postoperative after a pelvic exenteration. The physician has changed the client's diet from NPO to clear liquids. The nurse checks which of the following before administering the clear liquids?
    1. Ability to ambulate
    2. Urine-specific gravity
    3. Incision appearance
    4. Bowel sounds

35. The client is admitted to the hospital with a diagnosis of suspected Hodgkin's disease. Which of the following assessment signs does the nurse most likely expect to note documented in the client's record?
    1. Weakness
    2. Fatigue
    3. Weight gain
    4. Enlarged lymph nodes

36. When reviewing the health care record of a client with ovarian cancer, the nurse recognizes which symptom as typical of the disease?

1 Hypermenorrhea
2 Abdominal distention
3 Diarrhea
4 Abnormal bleeding

37. The nurse is reviewing the complications of conization with a client who has microinvasive cervical cancer. Which of the following complications is not associated with this procedure?
1 Infection
2 Infertility
3 Ovarian perforation
4 Hemorrhage

38. The nurse is conducting a diet history with an elderly client who lives alone. The nurse finds that the client's typical 24-hour food intake consists of eggs and sausage for breakfast, a fast-food lunch of hamburger and french fries, take-out fried chicken for dinner, and ice cream in the evening. To decrease the risk of cancer, what information does the nurse provide to the client?
1 "You should not eat eggs"
2 "You should not eat sausage"
3 "Drinking a lot of alcohol increases the risk of liver cancer"
4 "A high-fat diet increases your risk for colon cancer"

39. The nurse is caring for a client dying of ovarian cancer. During care, the client states, "If I can just live long enough to attend my daughter's graduation, I'll be ready to die." Which phase of coping is this client experiencing?
1 Denial
2 Bargaining
3 Depression
4 Anger

40. The nurse is caring for a client following a modified radical mastectomy. Which of the following findings indicates that the client is experiencing a complication related to the surgery?
1 Sanguineous drainage in the drainage tube
2 Pain at the incisional site
3 Complaints of decreased sensation near the operative site
4 Arm edema on the operative side

41. The nurse is reviewing the health record of a client with laryngeal cancer. The nurse expects to note which of the following most common risk factors for this type of cancer in the record?
1 Use of chewing tobacco
2 Cigarette smoking
3 Urban living
4 Alcohol abuse

42. The female client who has been receiving radiation therapy for bladder cancer tells the nurse that it feels as if she is voiding through the vagina. The nurse interprets that the client may be experiencing

1 Extreme stress due to the diagnosis of cancer
2 Altered perineal sensation as a side effect of radiation therapy
3 The development of a vesicovaginal fistula
4 Rupture of the bladder

43. The client with leukemia is receiving busulfan (Myleran). Allopurinol (Zyloprim) is prescribed for the client. The nurse understands that the purpose of the allopurinol is to
1 Prevent gouty arthritis
2 Prevent hyperuricemia
3 Prevent stomatitis
4 Prevent diarrhea

44. The client receiving chemotherapy is experiencing stomatitis. The nurse advises the client to use which of the following as the best substance to rinse the mouth?
1 Hydrogen peroxide mixture
2 Weak salt and bicarbonate mouth rinse
3 Lemon-flavored mouthwash
4 Alcohol-based mouthwash

45. The nurse is assisting in conducting a health promotion program and the topic of the discussion relates to the risk factors of gastric cancer. Which of the following is not associated with the incidence of this type of cancer?
1 History of gastric polyps
2 History of pernicious anemia
3 A diet of smoked, highly salted, spiced food
4 High meat and carbohydrate consumption

46. The nurse is reviewing the preoperative orders of a client with a colon tumor who is scheduled for abdominal perineal resection. The nurse notes that the physician has prescribed neomycin sulfate (Mycifradin) for the client. The nurse determines that this medication has been prescribed:
1 Because the client has an infection
2 To prevent an infection
3 To decrease the bacteria in the bowel
4 Because the client is allergic to penicillin

47. The nurse is caring for a client following a radical neck dissection and creation of a tracheostomy performed for laryngeal cancer. The nurse is reinforcing discharge instructions to the client. Which of the following is not a component of the instructions regarding care to the stoma?
1 Apply a thin layer of petrolatum to the skin around the stoma to prevent cracking
2 Protect the stoma from water
3 Use an air conditioner to provide cool air to assist in breathing
4 Keep powders and sprays away from the stoma site

48. The nurse is caring for a client with cancer of the prostate following a prostatectomy. The nurse reinforces discharge instructions and plans to include which of the following?

1 Notify the physician if blood clots are noticed during urination
2 Driving in a car may be resumed in 1 week
3 Restrict fluid intake to prevent incontinence
4 Avoid lifting objects heavier than 20 pounds for at least 6 weeks

49. The nurse is assisting in providing a teaching session to a community group regarding the risks and causes of bladder cancer. Which of the following is not associated with this type of cancer?
1 It most often occurs in women
2 It is generally seen in clients older than age 40
3 Environmental health hazards have been attributed as a cause
4 Using cigarettes, artificial sweeteners, and coffee drinking can increase the risk

50. The nurse is reviewing the history of a client with bladder cancer. The nurse expects to note which common symptom of this type of cancer documented in the record?
1 Frequency of urination
2 Urgency on urination
3 Hematuria
4 Dysuria

51. The nurse is inspecting the stoma of a client following a ureterostomy. Which of the following does the nurse expect to note?
1 A pale stoma
2 A red, moist stoma
3 A dry stoma
4 A dark-colored stoma

52. The nurse is caring for a client following a radical mastectomy. Which of the following nursing interventions assists in preventing lymphedema of the affected arm?

1 Placing cool compresses on the affected arm
2 Elevating the affected arm on a pillow above heart level
3 Maintaining an IV site below the antecubital area on the affected side
4 Avoiding arm exercises in the immediate postoperative period

53. The nurse is preparing a client for a mammography. Which of the following instructions does the nurse provide to the client?
1 Mammography takes about 1 hour
2 Avoid the use of deodorants, powders, or creams on the day of the test
3 There is no discomfort associated with the procedure
4 Maintain an NPO status on the day of the test

54. A client is scheduled for a Papanicolaou smear at the next scheduled clinic visit. The nurse provides instructions to the client regarding preparation for this test. Which of the following does the nurse tell the client?
1 The test can be performed during menstruation
2 Fluids are restricted on the day of the test
3 The test is painless
4 Vaginal douching is required 2 hours before the test

55. The nurse is caring for a client with metastatic breast cancer. The client develops a new and sudden sharp pain in the back. The most appropriate nursing intervention is to
1 Reposition the client
2 Medicate the client for pain
3 Encourage ambulation
4 Notify the physician

ANSWERS

1. **2**

RATIONALE: The TSE is recommended monthly after a warm bath or shower when the scrotal skin is relaxed. The client should stand to examine the testicles. Using both hands, with fingers under the scrotum and thumbs on top, the client should gently roll the testicles, feeling for any lumps.
TEST-TAKING STRATEGY: Use the process of elimination. Eliminate option 4 first because of the words "6 months." Next, eliminate option 3 because of the word "one." From the remaining options, eliminate option 1 by trying to visualize the process of the self-examination. If you had difficulty with this question, take time now to review this important examination.
LEVEL OF COGNITIVE ABILITY: Application
PHASE OF NURSING PROCESS: Implementation
CLIENT NEEDS: Health Promotion and Maintenance
CONTENT AREA: Adult Health/Oncology

REFERENCE
Leahy, J., & Kizilay, P. (1998). *Foundations of nursing practice: A nursing process approach.* Philadelphia: W. B. Saunders. p. 334.

2. **3**

RATIONALE: Viruses may be one of the multiple agents acting to initiate carcinogenesis and have been associated with several types of cancer. Increased stress has been associated with causing the growth and proliferation of cancer cells. Two forms of radiation, ultraviolet and ionizing, can lead to cancer. High-fiber diets may reduce the risk of colon cancer. A diet high in fat may be a factor in the development of breast, colon, and prostate cancers.
TEST-TAKING STRATEGY: Note the key word "not." Read each option carefully, using the process of elimination. Familiarity with the risk factors related to cancer will easily direct you to option 3. Review these risk factors now if you had difficulty with this question.
LEVEL OF COGNITIVE ABILITY: Comprehension
PHASE OF NURSING PROCESS: Planning

CLIENT NEEDS: Health Promotion and Maintenance
CONTENT AREA: Adult Health/Oncology
REFERENCE
deWit, S. (1998). *Essentials of medical-surgical nursing* (4th ed.). Philadelphia: W. B. Saunders. p. 213.

3. 3

RATIONALE: Thrombocytopenia indicates a decrease in the number of platelets in the circulating blood. A major concern is monitoring for and preventing bleeding. Option 2 relates to monitoring for infection, particularly if leukopenia is present. Options 1 and 4, although important in the plan of care, are not directly related to thrombocytopenia.
TEST-TAKING STRATEGY: Note the key word "thrombocytopenia." Recalling that this condition places the client at risk of bleeding will assist in eliminating options 1, 2, and 4. If you are unfamiliar with the nursing interventions related to this disorder, review now.
LEVEL OF COGNITIVE ABILITY: Application
PHASE OF NURSING PROCESS: Planning
CLIENT NEEDS: Physiological Integrity
CONTENT AREA: Adult Health/Oncology
REFERENCE
O'Toole, M. (1997). *Miller-Keane encyclopedia & dictionary of medicine, nursing, & allied health* (6th ed.). Philadelphia: W. B. Saunders. p. 1610.

4. 2

RATIONALE: Candidiasis is a fungal infection caused by *Candida albicans*. In the mouth, it is called thrush, and appears as white plaques. Although it can occur in an immunocompromised client, it is not considered to be common. Options 3 and 4 are not accurate regarding this infection.
TEST-TAKING STRATEGY: Options 1 and 3 can be eliminated first. Recalling that the anemic client is more likely to exhibit pallor will direct you to option 2. If you are unfamiliar with the manifestations associated with thrush, take time now to review.
LEVEL OF COGNITIVE ABILITY: Comprehension
PHASE OF NURSING PROCESS: Data Collection
CLIENT NEEDS: Physiological Integrity
CONTENT AREA: Adult Health/Oncology
REFERENCE
deWit, S. (1998). *Essentials of medical-surgical nursing* (4th ed.). Philadelphia: W. B. Saunders. p. 191.

5. 2

RATIONALE: The normal WBC ranges from 4,500 to 11,000/mm³. Option 1 indicates a low value. Options 3 and 4 indicate elevated values.
TEST-TAKING STRATEGY: Knowledge regarding the normal WBC count is required to answer this question. If you are not familiar with this value, learn it now.
LEVEL OF COGNITIVE ABILITY: Comprehension
PHASE OF NURSING PROCESS: Data Collection
CLIENT NEEDS: Physiological Integrity
CONTENT AREA: Adult Health/Oncology
REFERENCE
deWit, S. (1998). *Essentials of medical-surgical nursing* (4th ed.). Philadelphia: W. B. Saunders. p, 467.

6. 2

RATIONALE: The BSE should be performed monthly 1 week after menstruation begins. It is not recommended to perform the examination weekly. At the onset of menstruation and during ovulation, hormonal changes occur that may alter breast tissue.
TEST-TAKING STRATEGY: Option 4 can be easily eliminated because of the word "weekly." Eliminate options 1 and 3 next because of the similarity that exists in regards to the hormonal changes that occur during these times. If you are unfamiliar with the procedure for performing BSE, review this important self-examination now.
LEVEL OF COGNITIVE ABILITY: Application
PHASE OF NURSING PROCESS: Implementation
CLIENT NEEDS: Health Promotion and Maintenance
CONTENT AREA: Adult Health/Oncology
REFERENCE
Leahy, J., & Kizilay, P. (1998). *Foundations of nursing practice: A nursing process approach*. Philadelphia: W. B. Saunders. pp. 332–333.

7. 2

RATIONALE: The nurse instructs the client to lie down and place a towel or pillow under the shoulder on the side of the breast to be examined. If the left breast is to be examined, the pillow is placed under the left shoulder. Options 3 and 4 are incorrect.
TEST-TAKING STRATEGY: Attempt to visualize this procedure to select the correct option. Remember to examine the left, the pillow is placed under the left; to examine the right, the pillow is placed under the right. If you are unfamiliar with the procedure for performing BSE, review this important self-examination now.
LEVEL OF COGNITIVE ABILITY: Application
PHASE OF NURSING PROCESS: Implementation
CLIENT NEEDS: Health Promotion and Maintenance
CONTENT AREA: Adult Health/Oncology
REFERENCE
Leahy, J., & Kizilay, P. (1998). *Foundations of nursing practice: A nursing process approach*. Philadelphia: W. B. Saunders. pp. 332–333.

8. 4

RATIONALE: If the client has had a hysterectomy or is no longer menstruating, the BSE should be performed on the same day every month. Options 1 and 2 are inappropriate because the client who has had a hysterectomy would not be menstruating. It is best not to perform the BSE at ovulation time because of the hormonal changes that occur.
TEST-TAKING STRATEGY: Note the key word "hysterectomy." Options 1 and 2 can be easily eliminated. Eliminate option 3 because of the hormonal changes that occur at this time. If you are unfamiliar with the procedure for performing BSE, review this important self-examination now.
LEVEL OF COGNITIVE ABILITY: Application
PHASE OF NURSING PROCESS: Implementation
CLIENT NEEDS: Health Promotion and Maintenance
CONTENT AREA: Adult Health/Oncology
REFERENCE
Leahy, J., & Kizilay, P. (1998). *Foundations of nursing practice: A nursing process approach*. Philadelphia: W. B. Saunders. pp. 332–333.

9. 2

RATIONALE: The CT scan causes no pain and can last for 15 to 60 minutes. The dye may cause a warm flushing sensation when injected. Fluids are encouraged following the procedure. If an iodine dye is used, the client should be asked about allergies to seafood or iodine.

TEST-TAKING STRATEGY: Note the key phrase "dye injection." This should provide you with the clue that the issue relates to the dye. If you are unfamiliar with this diagnostic test, review the important teaching points related to it now.

LEVEL OF COGNITIVE ABILITY: Comprehension
PHASE OF NURSING PROCESS: Implementation
CLIENT NEEDS: Physiological Integrity
CONTENT AREA: Adult Health/Oncology
REFERENCE

Leahy, J., & Kizilay, P. (1998). *Foundations of nursing practice: A nursing process approach.* Philedelphia: W. B. Saunders. pp. 755–756.

10. **4**

RATIONALE: The nurse asks the client with fibrocystic breast disorder about worsening of symptoms (breast lumps, painful breasts, and possible nipple discharge) before the onset of menses. This is associated with cyclical hormone changes. Options 1, 2, and 3 do not provide significant data regarding this disorder.

TEST-TAKING STRATEGY: The key words are "more noticeable." This implies that there is a predictable variation in symptoms. Use knowledge of the effects of various hormones in the body to analyze the options and choose correctly. Review fibrocystic disorder now if you had difficulty with this question.

LEVEL OF COGNITIVE ABILITY: Application
PHASE OF NURSING PROCESS: Data Collection
CLIENT NEEDS: Physiological Integrity
CONTENT AREA: Adult Health/Oncology
REFERENCE

Beare, P., & Myers, J. (1998). *Adult health nursing* (3rd ed.). St. Louis: Mosby–Year Book. p. 1685.

11. **1**

RATIONALE: The client demonstrates the best adaptation by participating in his or her care. This includes care of surgical drains that are in place for a short time after discharge. Asking for pain medication is also an action-oriented option, but it does not relate to acceptance of the loss of the breast. Reading the postoperative care booklet is useful, but is not the best of the options presented here. Refusing to look at the wound indicates no adaptation to the loss.

TEST-TAKING STRATEGY: Note the key word "best." This tells you that more than one or all of the responses may be partially or totally correct. Use prioritizing ability to determine the best option of those presented, keeping in mind the issue "best adjustment."

LEVEL OF COGNITIVE ABILITY: Comprehension
PHASE OF NURSING PROCESS: Data Collection
CLIENT NEEDS: Psychosocial Integrity
CONTENT AREA: Adult Health/Oncology
REFERENCE

Monahan, F., & Neighbors, M. (1998). *Medical-surgical nursing: Foundations for clinical practice* (2nd ed.). Philadelphia: W. B. Saunders. p. 1865.

12. **2**

RATIONALE: The client should resume activity slowly, but walking is a beneficial activity. The client should know to rest when fatigue occurs. Activities to be avoided include

driving, heavy housework, wearing tight clothing, crossing the legs, and prolonged standing or sitting. Sexual activity is prohibited for 4 to 6 weeks after surgery.

TEST-TAKING STRATEGY: Read the question carefully. Note the key words "not precipitate complications." With this in mind, evaluate each of the options in terms of the stress or harm it could cause to the perineal area. Review home care measures following vulvectomy now if you had difficulty with this question.

LEVEL OF COGNITIVE ABILITY: Application
PHASE OF NURSING PROCESS: Planning
CLIENT NEEDS: Physiological Integrity
CONTENT AREA: Adult Health/Oncology
REFERENCE

Monahan, F., & Neighbors, M. (1998). *Medical-surgical nursing: Foundations for clinical practice* (2nd ed.). Philadelphia: W. B. Saunders. p. 1829.

13. **3**

RATIONALE: The client is at risk of deep vein thrombosis or thrombophlebitis after this surgery, as for any other major surgery. For this reason, the nurse implements measures that will prevent this complication. Range of motion exercises, antiembolism stockings, and pneumatic compression boots are all helpful. The nurse should avoid using the knee gatch in the bed, which inhibits venous return, thus placing the client more at risk for deep vein thrombosis or thrombophlebitis.

TEST-TAKING STRATEGY: Note the key word "avoids." Use the process of elimination and basic nursing knowledge to choose correctly. Review postoperative nursing interventions now if you had difficulty with this question.

LEVEL OF COGNITIVE ABILITY: Application
PHASE OF NURSING PROCESS: Implementation
CLIENT NEEDS: Health Promotion and Maintenance
CONTENT AREA: Adult Health/Oncology
REFERENCE

Monahan, F., & Neighbors, M. (1998). *Medical-surgical nursing: Foundations for clinical practice* (2nd ed.). Philadelphia: W. B. Saunders. p. 1799.

14. **3**

RATIONALE: A pelvic ultrasound requires the ingestion of large volumes of water just prior to the procedure. A full bladder is necessary so that this organ will be visualized as such and not mistaken as a possible pelvic growth. An abdominal ultrasound may require that the client abstain from food or fluid for several hours before the procedure. Option 4 is unrelated to this specific procedure.

TEST-TAKING STRATEGY: Note the key word "pelvic." You should easily be able to eliminate option 4. From the remaining options, focusing on the key word will assist in directing you to option 3. Review preparation for a pelvic ultrasound now if you had difficulty with this question.

LEVEL OF COGNITIVE ABILITY: Application
PHASE OF NURSING PROCESS: Planning
CLIENT NEEDS: Physiological Integrity
CONTENT AREA: Adult Health/Oncology
REFERENCE

Leahy, J., & Kizilay, P. (1998). *Foundations of nursing practice: A nursing process approach.* Philadelphia: W. B. Saunders. p. 151.

15. **4**

RATIONALE: A biopsy is done to determine whether a tumor is malignant or benign. An MRI, CT scan, and ultra-

sound will visualize the presence of a mass but will not confirm a diagnosis of malignancy.
TEST-TAKING STRATEGY: Note the key word "confirm." This key word should easily direct you to option 4. If you are unfamiliar with the purpose of the tests identified in the options, review them now.
LEVEL OF COGNITIVE ABILITY: Comprehension
PHASE OF NURSING PROCESS: Data Collection
CLIENT NEEDS: Physiological Integrity
CONTENT AREA: Adult Health/Oncology
REFERENCE
O'Toole, M. (1997). *Miller-Keane encyclopedia & dictionary of medicine, nursing, & allied health* (6th ed.). Philadelphia: W. B. Saunders. p. 194.

16. **4**

RATIONALE: Multiple myeloma is a neoplastic condition characterized by abnormal malignant proliferation of plasma cells and the accumulation of mature plasma cells in the bone marrow. Option 1 describes the leukemic process. Options 2 and 3 are not characteristics of multiple myeloma.
TEST-TAKING STRATEGY: Knowledge regarding the pathophysiology associated with this disorder is required to answer the question. Review this information now if you are unfamiliar with this oncological disorder.
LEVEL OF COGNITIVE ABILITY: Comprehension
PHASE OF NURSING PROCESS: Planning
CLIENT NEEDS: Physiological Integrity
CONTENT AREA: Adult Health/Oncology
REFERENCE
deWit, S. (1998). *Essentials of medical-surgical nursing* (4th ed.). Philadelphia: W. B. Saunders. p. 492.

17. **3**

RATIONALE: Findings indicative of multiple myeloma are an increased number of plasma cells in the bone marrow, anemia, hypercalcemia due to the release of calcium from the deteriorating bone tissue, and an elevated BUN. An increased white blood cell count may be present but is not specifically related to multiple myeloma.
TEST-TAKING STRATEGY: This is a difficult question. Knowledge regarding the pathophysiology associated with this disorder and the effects it produces on the body are required to answer the question. Review this information now if you are unfamiliar with this oncological disorder.
LEVEL OF COGNITIVE ABILITY: Analysis
PHASE OF NURSING PROCESS: Data Collection
CLIENT NEEDS: Physiological Integrity
CONTENT AREA: Adult Health/Oncology
REFERENCE
O'Toole, M. (1997). *Miller-Keane encyclopedia & dictionary of medicine, nursing, & allied health* (6th ed.). Philadelphia: W. B. Saunders. p. 1024.

18. **2**

RATIONALE: Hypercalcemia secondary to bone destruction is a priority concern in the client with multiple myeloma. The nurse should administer fluids in adequate amounts to maintain an output of 1.5 to 2.0 L/day. Clients require about 3 liters of fluid per day. The fluid is needed not only to dilute the calcium overload but also to prevent protein from precipitating in the renal tubules. Options 1, 3, and 4 may be a component of the plan of care, but are not the priority in this client.

TEST-TAKING STRATEGY: Knowledge regarding the clinical manifestations that occur in multiple myeloma is required to answer the question. Recalling that forcing fluids is specific to the care of a client with this disorder will direct you to option 2. Review the specific manifestations of this disorder now if you had difficulty with this question.
LEVEL OF COGNITIVE ABILITY: Analysis
PHASE OF NURSING PROCESS: Planning
CLIENT NEEDS: Physiological Integrity
CONTENT AREA: Adult Health/Oncology
REFERENCE
deWit, S. (1998). *Essentials of medical-surgical nursing* (4th ed.). Philadelphia: W. B. Saunders. p. 492.

19. **3**

RATIONALE: Hodgkin's disease is a disorder of young adults and primarily occurs between the ages of 20 and 40. Options 1, 2, and 4 are characteristics of this disease.
TEST-TAKING STRATEGY: Note the key word "not." Recalling that Hodgkin's occurs in the young adult will easily direct you to option 3. Review the characteristics of this disorder now if you had difficulty with this question.
LEVEL OF COGNITIVE ABILITY: Analysis
PHASE OF NURSING PROCESS: Planning
CLIENT NEEDS: Physiological Integrity
CONTENT AREA: Adult Health/Oncology
REFERENCE
deWit, S. (1998). *Essentials of medical-surgical nursing* (4th ed.). Philadelphia: W. B. Saunders. p. 492.

20. **3**

RATIONALE: Alopecia is not a finding in testicular cancer. It may, however, occur as a result of radiation or chemotherapy. Options 1, 2, and 4 are findings in testicular cancer. Back pain may indicate metastasis to the retroperitoneal lymph nodes.
TEST-TAKING STRATEGY: Note the key word "not." Use the process of elimination, remembering that alopecia occurs as a result of chemotherapy rather than from the disease. Review the manifestations associated with testicular cancer now if you had difficulty with this question.
LEVEL OF COGNITIVE ABILITY: Application
PHASE OF NURSING PROCESS: Implementation
CLIENT NEEDS: Health Promotion and Maintenance
CONTENT AREA: Adult Health/Oncology
REFERENCE
deWit, S. (1998). *Essentials of medical-surgical nursing* (4th ed.). Philadelphia: W. B. Saunders. p. 867.

21. **4**

RATIONALE: Hyperuricemia is especially common following treatment for leukemias and lymphomas, since the therapy results in massive cell kill. Although options 1, 2, and 3 may also be noted, an increased uric acid level is specifically related to cell destruction.
TEST-TAKING STRATEGY: Note the key words "massive cell destruction" and "specifically note." Recalling the cell response to destruction will assist in directing you to option 4. Review this concept now if you had difficulty with this question.
LEVEL OF COGNITIVE ABILITY: Analysis
PHASE OF NURSING PROCESS: Data Collection
CLIENT NEEDS: Physiological Integrity
CONTENT AREA: Adult Health/Oncology

REFERENCE
Lehne, R. (1998). *Pharmacology for nursing care* (3rd ed.). Philadelphia: W. B. Saunders. p. 1017.

22. 3

RATIONALE: Use of surgery in palliative care is carefully considered and used only if the risk/benefit ratio is favorable. Palliative surgery that can benefit the client with cancer and improve quality of life includes procedures that reduce pain, relieve airway obstructions, relieve obstructions in the GI and urinary tracts, relieve pressure on the brain and spinal cord, and prevent hemorrhage. Options 1, 2, and 4 do not describe palliative surgery.
TEST-TAKING STRATEGY: Note the key word "palliative." Knowledge of the definition of this word will assist in directing you to option 3. Review the various types of surgery now if you had difficulty with this question.
LEVEL OF COGNITIVE ABILITY: Comprehension
PHASE OF NURSING PROCESS: Planning
CLIENT NEEDS: Physiological Integrity
CONTENT AREA: Adult Health/Oncology
REFERENCE
Black, J., & Matassarin-Jacobs, E. (1997). *Medical-surgical nursing: Clinical management for continuity of care* (5th ed.). Philadelphia: W. B. Saunders. p. 569.

23. 3

RATIONALE: In general, only the area in the treatment field is affected by the radiation. Skin reactions, fatigue, nausea, and anorexia may occur with radiation to any site, whereas other side effects occur only when specific areas are involved in treatment. A client receiving radiation to the larynx is most likely to experience a sore throat. Options 1 and 4 may occur with radiation to the GI tract. Dyspnea may occur with lung involvement.
TEST-TAKING STRATEGY: Eliminate options 1 and 4 first as they are similar and GI related. Consider the anatomical location of the radiation therapy to assist you in selecting option 3. Review the effects of radiation therapy now if you had difficulty with this question.
LEVEL OF COGNITIVE ABILITY: Comprehension
PHASE OF NURSING PROCESS: Planning
CLIENT NEEDS: Physiological Integrity
CONTENT AREA: Adult Health/Oncology
REFERENCE
Monahan, F. & Neighbors, M. (1998). *Medical-surgical nursing: Foundations for clinical practice* (2nd ed.). Philadelphia: W. B. Saunders. p. 1520.

24. 3

RATIONALE: Moist desquamation occurs when the basal cells of the skin are destroyed. The dermal level is exposed, which results in the leakage of serum. Reddened skin, a rash, and dermatitis may occur with external radiation but are not described as a moist desquamation.
TEST-TAKING STRATEGY: Noting the key word "moist" will easily direct you to option 3. Options 1, 2, and 4 are eliminated because they are similar and describe a dry rather than a moist skin alteration. Review the signs associated with a moist desquamation now if you had difficulty with this question.
LEVEL OF COGNITIVE ABILITY: Comprehension
PHASE OF NURSING PROCESS: Data Collection
CLIENT NEEDS: Physiological Integrity
CONTENT AREA: Adult Health/Oncology

REFERENCE
Monahan, F., & Neighbors, M. (1998). *Medical-surgical nursing: Foundations for clinical practice* (2nd ed.). Philadelphia: W. B. Saunders. p. 1520.

25. 3

RATIONALE: The client should avoid pressure on the irritated area and should wear loose-fitting clothing. Specific physician instructions are necessary if an alteration in skin integrity occurs as a result of the radiation therapy. Options 1, 2, and 4 are accurate instructions regarding radiation therapy.
TEST-TAKING STRATEGY: Note the key word "not." Use the process of elimination. The word "pressure" should be an indication that this is an inappropriate measure. Review client teaching points related to skin care and radiation therapy now if you had difficulty with this question.
LEVEL OF COGNITIVE ABILITY: Application
PHASE OF NURSING PROCESS: Implementation
CLIENT NEEDS: Health Promotion and Maintenance
CONTENT AREA: Adult Health/Oncology
REFERENCE
Monahan, F., & Neighbors, M. (1998). *Medical-surgical nursing: Foundations for clinical practice* (2nd ed.). Philadelphia: W. B. Saunders. p. 1523.

26. 2

RATIONALE: The time that the nurse spends in the room of a client with an internal radiation implant is 30 minutes per 8-hour shift. The dosimeter badge must be worn when in the client's room. Children younger than 16 years of age and pregnant women are not allowed in the client's room.
TEST-TAKING STRATEGY: Use the process of elimination. Option 4 can be eliminated first. Knowledge of the time frame related to exposure to the client will assist in eliminating option 1. From the remaining options, select option 2 because of the possible risks associated with exposure to the mother and fetus. Review these important principles now if you had difficulty with this question.
LEVEL OF COGNITIVE ABILITY: Application
PHASE OF NURSING PROCESS: Implementation
CLIENT NEEDS: Safe, Effective Care Environment
CONTENT AREA: Adult Health/Oncology
REFERENCE
Monahan, F., & Neighbors, M. (1998). *Medical-surgical nursing: Foundations for clinical practice* (2nd ed.). Philadelphia: W. B. Saunders. p. 1519.

27. 2

RATIONALE: Foul-smelling vaginal discharge is expected and will occur for some time following removal of a radiation implant from the cervix. Options 1, 3, and 4 are accurate discharge instructions.
TEST-TAKING STRATEGY: Note the key word "not." Knowledge regarding the client teaching points related to radiation implants is required to answer the question. Review these points now if you had difficulty with this question.
LEVEL OF COGNITIVE ABILITY: Application
PHASE OF NURSING PROCESS: Planning
CLIENT NEEDS: Health Promotion and Maintenance
CONTENT AREA: Adult Health/Oncology
REFERENCE
Monahan, F., & Neighbors, M. (1998). *Medical-surgical nursing: Foundations for clinical practice* (2nd ed.). Philadelphia: W. B. Saunders. p. 1835.

28. 3

RATIONALE: The client with a cervical radiation implant should be maintained on bed rest in the dorsal position to prevent movement of the radiation source. The head of the bed is elevated to a maximum of 10 to 15 degrees for comfort. Avoid turning the client on the side. If turning is absolutely necessary, place a pillow between the knees and, with the body in straight alignment, log roll the client.
TEST-TAKING STRATEGY: Consider the anatomical location of the implant and the risk of dislodgment to answer the question. Additionally, note that options 1, 2, and 4 are similar. If you had difficulty with this question, take time now to review care of the client with a radiation implant.
LEVEL OF COGNITIVE ABILITY: Application
PHASE OF NURSING PROCESS: Implementation
CLIENT NEEDS: Safe, Effective Care Environment
CONTENT AREA: Adult Health/Oncology
REFERENCE
Monahan, F., & Neighbors, M. (1998). *Medical-surgical nursing: Foundations for clinical practice* (2nd ed.). Philadelphia: W. B. Saunders. p. 1835.

29. 3

RATIONALE: The client needs to be instructed to avoid exposure to the sun. Options 1, 2, and 4 are accurate measures in the care of a client receiving external radiation therapy.
TEST-TAKING STRATEGY: Note the key words "need for further instruction." Eliminate option 1 because of the word "gently" and option 4 because of the word "loose." From the remaining options, recalling that sun exposure is to be avoided will assist in answering the question. Review skin care measures for the client receiving external radiation now if you had difficulty with this question.
LEVEL OF COGNITIVE ABILITY: Comprehension
PHASE OF NURSING PROCESS: Evaluation
CLIENT NEEDS: Health Promotion and Maintenance
CONTENT AREA: Adult Health/Oncology
REFERENCE
Monahan, F., & Neighbors, M. (1998). *Medical-surgical nursing: Foundations for clinical practice* (2nd ed.). Philadelphia: W. B. Saunders. p. 1523.

30. 4

RATIONALE: A lead container and long-handled forceps should be kept in the client's room at all times during internal radiation therapy. If the implant becomes dislodged, the nurse should pick up the implant with long-handled forceps and place it in the lead container. Options 1, 2, and 3 are inaccurate interventions.
TEST-TAKING STRATEGY: Note the key word "initial." Option 3 is not an appropriate action. Eliminate option 2 next because the implant would not be discarded. Although the physician should be notified, the initial action is option 4. Review the measures related to a dislodged implant now if you had difficulty with this question.
LEVEL OF COGNITIVE ABILITY: Application
PHASE OF NURSING PROCESS: Implementation
CLIENT NEEDS: Safe, Effective Care Environment
CONTENT AREA: Adult Health/Oncology
REFERENCE
Monahan, F., & Neighbors, M. (1998). *Medical-surgical nursing: Foundations for clinical practice* (2nd ed.). Philadelphia: W. B. Saunders. p. 1519.

31. 4

RATIONALE: In the immunocompromised client, a low-bacteria diet is implemented. This includes avoiding fresh fruits and vegetables and thorough cooking of all foods. Not all visitors are restricted, but the client is protected from people with known infections. Fluids should be encouraged. Invasive measures such as an indwelling urinary catheter should be avoided to prevent infections.
TEST-TAKING STRATEGY: Eliminate option 1 because of the word "all." Next, eliminate option 2 because it is not reasonable to eliminate fluids in a client receiving chemotherapy at risk for fluid and electrolyte imbalances. Eliminate option 3 because of the risk of infection that exists with this measure. Review interventions for the client with hematological toxicity now if you had difficulty with this question.
LEVEL OF COGNITIVE ABILITY: Application
PHASE OF NURSING PROCESS: Planning
CLIENT NEEDS: Safe, Effective Care Environment
CONTENT AREA: Adult Health/Oncology
REFERENCE
Monahan, F., & Neighbors, M. (1998). *Medical-surgical nursing: Foundations for clinical practice* (2nd ed.). Philadelphia: W. B. Saunders. pp. 1536–1537.

32. 1

RATIONALE: A high risk of hemorrhage exists when the platelet count is less than 20,000/mm³. Fatal central nervous system (CNS) hemorrhage or massive gastrointestinal (GI) hemorrhage can occur when the platelet count is less than 10,000/mm³. The client should be monitored for changes in level of consciousness, which may be an early indication of an intracranial hemorrhage. Option 2 is a priority when the WBC count is low and the client is at risk for an infection. Although options 3 and 4 are important, they are not the priority in this situation.
TEST-TAKING STRATEGY: Note the key word "priority." Recalling the normal platelet count and determining that a low count places the client at risk for bleeding will assist in eliminating options 2, 3, and 4. Review the normal platelet count and the nursing interventions for a client with a low count now if you had difficulty with this question.
LEVEL OF COGNITIVE ABILITY: Analysis
PHASE OF NURSING PROCESS: Implementation
CLIENT NEEDS: Physiological Integrity
CONTENT AREA: Adult Health/Oncology
REFERENCE
deWit, S. (1998). *Essentials of medical-surgical nursing* (4th ed.). Philadelphia: W. B. Saunders. p. 567.

33. 1

RATIONALE: Risk factors associated with cervical cancer include intercourse with uncircumcised males, early frequent intercourse with multiple sexual partners, multiparity, chronic cervicitis, history of genital herpes, or human papillomavirus infection. Cervical cancer is also higher in African-Americans.
TEST-TAKING STRATEGY: Note the key word "not." Read each option carefully. If you had difficulty with this question, review the risks of cervical cancer now.
LEVEL OF COGNITIVE ABILITY: Comprehension
PHASE OF NURSING PROCESS: Data Collection
CLIENT NEEDS: Health Promotion and Maintenance
CONTENT AREA: Adult Health/Oncology

REFERENCE
deWit, S. (1998). *Essentials of medical-surgical nursing* (4th ed.). Philadelphia: W. B. Saunders. p. 213.

34. **4**

RATIONALE: The client is kept NPO until peristalsis returns, usually in 4 to 6 days postoperatively. When signs of bowel function return, clear fluids are given to the client. If no distention occurs, the diet is advanced as tolerated. It is most important to monitor for bowel sounds prior to feeding the client. Options 1, 2, and 3 are unrelated to the issue of the question.
TEST-TAKING STRATEGY: Note the key words "NPO to clear liquids." Knowledge regarding general postoperative care measures will assist in selecting the correct option. Option 4 is the only option that relates to GI function, which is the issue of the question.
LEVEL OF COGNITIVE ABILITY: Comprehension
PHASE OF NURSING PROCESS: Data Collection
CLIENT NEEDS: Physiological Integrity
CONTENT AREA: Adult Health/Oncology
REFERENCE
Monahan, F., & Neighbors, M. (1998). *Medical-surgical nursing: Foundations for clinical practice* (2nd ed.). Philadelphia: W. B. Saunders. p. 1832.

35. **4**

RATIONALE: Hodgkin's disease is a chronic progressive neoplastic disorder of lymphoid tissue characterized by the painless enlargement of lymph nodes with progression to extralymphatic sites, such as the spleen and liver. Weight loss is most likely to be noted. Fatigue and weakness may occur, but are not significantly related to the disease.
TEST-TAKING STRATEGY: Knowledge that Hodgkin's affects the lymph nodes will easily direct you to option 4. Option 3 can be easily eliminated first because in such a disorder, weight loss is most likely to occur. Options 1 and 2 are similar and rather vague symptoms that can occur in many disorders. Review the manifestations associated with Hodgkin's disease now if you had difficulty with this question.
LEVEL OF COGNITIVE ABILITY: Comprehension
PHASE OF NURSING PROCESS: Data Collection
CLIENT NEEDS: Physiological Integrity
CONTENT AREA: Adult Health/Oncology
REFERENCE
deWit, S. (1998). *Essentials of medical-surgical nursing* (4th ed.). Philadelphia: W. B. Saunders. p. 492.

36. **2**

RATIONALE: Clinical manifestations of ovarian cancer include abdominal distention, urinary frequency and urgency, pleural effusion, malnutrition, pain from pressure caused by the growing tumor and the effects of urinary or bowel obstruction, constipation, ascites with dyspnea, and ultimately general severe pain. Abnormal bleeding, often resulting in hypermenorrhea, is associated with uterine cancer.
TEST-TAKING STRATEGY: Eliminate options 1 and 4 first because they are similar. From the remaining options, consider the anatomical location of the diagnosis. This will assist in directing you to option 2. Review the manifestations associated with ovarian cancer now if you had difficulty with this question.
LEVEL OF COGNITIVE ABILITY: Comprehension
PHASE OF NURSING PROCESS: Data Collection

CLIENT NEEDS: Physiological Integrity
CONTENT AREA: Adult Health/Oncology
REFERENCE
deWit, S. (1998). *Essentials of medical-surgical nursing* (4th ed.). Philadelphia: W. B. Saunders. p. 844.

37. **3**

RATIONALE: Conization is generally not performed on women who desire to bear children because it can lead to incompetence of the cervix or infertility. Complications of the procedure include hemorrhage, infection, and, less frequently, cervical stenosis.
TEST-TAKING STRATEGY: Note the key word "not" and the words "cervical cancer." Select option 3 because this option addresses an "ovarian" condition, not a cervical one. Review the complications associated with this procedure now if you had difficulty with this question.
LEVEL OF COGNITIVE ABILITY: Comprehension
PHASE OF NURSING PROCESS: Data Collection
CLIENT NEEDS: Physiological Integrity
CONTENT AREA: Adult Health/Oncology
REFERENCE
Monahan, F., & Neighbors, M. (1998). *Medical-surgical nursing: Foundations for clinical practice* (2nd ed.). Philadelphia: W. B. Saunders. p. 1784.

38. **4**

RATIONALE: A diet high in fat may be a factor in the development of breast, colon, and prostate cancers. High-fiber diets may reduce the risk of colon cancer. Excessive alcohol may increase the risk of cancer of the mouth, larynx, throat, esophagus, and liver.
TEST-TAKING STRATEGY: Eliminate option 3 first because the question does not address alcohol. Although the food items identified in options 1 and 2 are addressed in the question, option 4 is the global response and addresses both options 1 and 2.
LEVEL OF COGNITIVE ABILITY: Comprehension
PHASE OF NURSING PROCESS: Implementation
CLIENT NEEDS: Health Promotion and Maintenance
CONTENT AREA: Adult Health/Oncology
REFERENCE
Monahan, F., & Neighbors, M. (1998). *Medical-surgical nursing: Foundations for clinical practice* (2nd ed.). Philadelphia: W. B. Saunders. p. 1509.

39. **2**

RATIONALE: Denial, bargaining, anger, depression, and acceptance are recognized stages that a person facing a life-threatening illness experiences. Denial is expressed as shock and disbelief and may be the first response to hearing bad news. Depression may be manifested by hopelessness, weeping openly, or remaining quiet or withdrawn. Anger may also be a first response to upsetting news and the predominant theme is "why me?" or the blaming of others.
TEST-TAKING STRATEGY: Focus on the client's statement as identified in the question to assist in selecting the correct option. From this point, you should easily be able to eliminate options 1, 3, and 4. Review these stages now if you had difficulty with this question.
LEVEL OF COGNITIVE ABILITY: Analysis
PHASE OF NURSING PROCESS: Data Collection

CLIENT NEEDS: Psychosocial Integrity
CONTENT AREA: Adult Health/Oncology
REFERENCE
Leahy, J., & Kizilay, P. (1998). *Foundations of nursing practice: A nursing process approach*. Philadelphia: W. B. Saunders. pp. 1145-1149.

40. **4**

RATIONALE: Arm edema on the operative side (lymphedema) is a complication following mastectomy and can occur immediately postoperatively, or secondary edema may occur months or even years after surgery. Options 1, 2, and 3 are expected occurrences following mastectomy and are not indicative of a complication.
TEST-TAKING STRATEGY: Use the process of elimination considering the normal expected occurrences following a mastectomy. If you had difficulty with this question, take time now to review the complications following mastectomy.
LEVEL OF COGNITIVE ABILITY: Analysis
PHASE OF NURSING PROCESS: Data Collection
CLIENT NEEDS: Physiological Integrity
CONTENT AREA: Adult Health/Oncology
REFERENCE
Monahan, F., & Neighbors, M. (1998). *Medical-surgical nursing: Foundations for clinical practice* (2nd ed.). Philadelphia: W. B. Saunders. p. 1865.

41. **2**

RATIONALE: The most common risk factor associated with laryngeal cancer is cigarette smoking. Approximately three-quarters of those diagnosed with this form of cancer are either current or former smokers. Alcohol abuse seems to have a synergistic effect with cigarette smoking. Air pollution is also a contributing cause, as well as chronic laryngitis and voice abuse.
TEST-TAKING STRATEGY: Note the key words "most common." Begin to answer this question by eliminating options 3 and 4. Since cancer of the upper and lower airway is most often related to tobacco, these are the options that are most likely correct. To discriminate between the last two options, knowing that cigarettes are more harmful guides you to choose this option over chewing tobacco.
LEVEL OF COGNITIVE ABILITY: Comprehension
PHASE OF NURSING PROCESS: Data Collection
CLIENT NEEDS: Health Promotion and Maintenance
CONTENT AREA: Adult Health/Oncology
REFERENCE
Monahan, F., & Neighbors, M. (1998). *Medical-surgical nursing: Foundations for clinical practice* (2nd ed.). Philadelphia: W. B. Saunders. p. 616.

42. **3**

RATIONALE: A vesicovaginal fistula is a genital fistula that occurs between the bladder and the vagina. The fistula is an abnormal opening between these two body parts and if this occurs, the client may experience drainage of urine through the vagina. The client's complaint is not associated with options 1, 2, and 4.
TEST-TAKING STRATEGY: Noting the key words "voiding through the vagina" should easily direct you to option 3. Review the symptoms associated with vesicovaginal fistula now if you had difficulty with this question.
LEVEL OF COGNITIVE ABILITY: Analysis
PHASE OF NURSING PROCESS: Data Collection

CLIENT NEEDS: Physiological Integrity
CONTENT AREA: Adult Health/Oncology
REFERENCE
Monahan, F., & Neighbors, M. (1998). *Medical-surgical nursing: Foundations for clinical practice* (2nd ed.). Philadelphia: W. B. Saunders. p. 1821.

43. **2**

RATIONALE: Allopurinol decreases uric acid production and reduces uric acid concentrations in both serum and urine. In the client receiving chemotherapy, uric acid levels elevate as a result of the massive cell destruction that occurs from the chemotherapy. This medication prevents or treats hyperuricemia secondary to chemotherapy. Although the medication is used to treat gout, it is not the purpose in this client's situation. This medication is not used to prevent stomatitis or diarrhea.
TEST-TAKING STRATEGY: Knowledge regarding the action of this medication is required to answer this question. Recalling that hyperuricemia occurs as a result of chemotherapy will assist in directing you to option 2. If you had difficulty with this question or are unfamiliar with the action of this medication, take time now to review.
LEVEL OF COGNITIVE ABILITY: Analysis
PHASE OF NURSING PROCESS: Planning
CLIENT NEEDS: Physiological Integrity
CONTENT AREA: Adult Health/Oncology
REFERENCE
Hodgson, B., & Kizior, R. (1999). *Saunders nursing drug handbook 1999*. Philadelphia: W. B. Saunders. pp. 24–25.

44. **2**

RATIONALE: An acidic environment in the mouth is favorable for bacterial growth. Therefore, the client is advised to rinse the mouth at least before every meal and at bedtime with a weak salt and sodium bicarbonate solution. This lessens the growth of bacteria and limits plaque formation. The other substances are irritating to oral tissue, which is already at risk. If hydrogen peroxide must be used due to severe plaque, it should be a very weak solution, because it dries the mucous membranes.
TEST-TAKING STRATEGY: Specific knowledge regarding this complication of radiation and chemotherapy is needed to answer this question correctly. Options 3 and 4 can be eliminated first because of the irritating effects of these solutions. From the remaining options, note the word "weak" in the correct option. If needed, take a few moments now to review the treatment measures for stomatitis.
LEVEL OF COGNITIVE ABILITY: Application
PHASE OF NURSING PROCESS: Implementation
CLIENT NEEDS: Physiological Integrity
CONTENT AREA: Adult Health/Oncology
REFERENCE
Monahan, F., & Neighbors, M. (1998). *Medical-surgical nursing: Foundations for clinical practice* (2nd ed.). Philadelphia: W. B. Saunders. pp. 1529–1530.

45. **4**

RATIONALE: High meat and carbohydrate consumption plays a role in the development of cancer of the pancreas. Options 1, 2, and 3 are risk factors related to gastric cancer. Additionally, an increased risk exists in the male population in clients 50 years of age and older and in clients with a history of precancerous lesions and chronic gastritis.
TEST-TAKING STRATEGY: Note that the question asks about the risk factors associated with gastric cancer. Note

the key word "not." Eliminate options 1 and 2 because they are directly related to gastric disorders. Eliminate option 3, knowing that spicy foods cause gastric irritation. Review the risk factors associated with gastric cancer now if you had difficulty with this question.
LEVEL OF COGNITIVE ABILITY: Comprehension
PHASE OF NURSING PROCESS: Data Collection
CLIENT NEEDS: Health Promotion and Maintenance
CONTENT AREA: Adult Health/Oncology
REFERENCE

Monahan, F., & Neighbors, M. (1998). *Medical-surgical nursing: Foundations for clinical practice* (2nd ed.). Philadelphia: W. B. Saunders. pp. 1058, 1126.

46. **3**

RATIONALE: To reduce the risk of contamination at the time of surgery, the bowel is emptied and cleansed. Laxatives and enemas are given to empty the bowel. Intestinal anti-infectives such as neomycin or kanamycin are administered to decrease the bacteria in the bowel.
TEST-TAKING STRATEGY: Knowledge regarding the purpose of administering anti-infectives prior to bowel surgery is required to answer the question. Eliminate options 1 and 4 first because there is no reference made to this information in the question. Recalling the concepts related to the flora of the intestinal tract will assist in directing you to option 3 as the primary purpose of this medication. Review this important preoperative intervention now if you had difficulty with this question.
LEVEL OF COGNITIVE ABILITY: Analysis
PHASE OF NURSING PROCESS: Planning
CLIENT NEEDS: Physiological Integrity
CONTENT AREA: Adult Health/Oncology
REFERENCE

Monahan, F., & Neighbors, M. (1998). *Medical-surgical nursing: Foundations for clinical practice* (2nd ed.). Philadelphia: W. B. Saunders. p. 1101.

47. **3**

RATIONALE: Air conditioners need to be avoided to protect from excessive coldness. A humidifier in the home should be used if excessive dryness is a problem. Options 1, 2, and 4 are appropriate interventions regarding stoma care following radical neck dissection and creation of a tracheostomy.
TEST-TAKING STRATEGY: Note the key word "not." You should easily be able to eliminate options 2 and 4. From the remaining options, recalling that a humidifier rather than an air conditioner is recommended will assist you in selecting the correct option. If you had difficulty with this question, take time now to review discharge instructions following radical neck dissection.
LEVEL OF COGNITIVE ABILITY: Application
PHASE OF NURSING PROCESS: Implementation
CLIENT NEEDS: Health Promotion and Maintenance
CONTENT AREA: Adult Health/Oncology
REFERENCE

Monahan, F., & Neighbors, M. (1998). *Medical-surgical nursing: Foundations for clinical practice* (2nd ed.). Philadelphia: W. B. Saunders. p. 631.

48. **4**

RATIONALE: Small pieces of tissue or blood clots can be passed during urination for up to 2 weeks after surgery. Driving a car and sitting for long periods of time are restricted for at least 3 weeks. A daily fluid intake of 2.0 to 2.5 L/day should be maintained to limit clot formation and prevent infection. Option 4 is an accurate discharge instruction following prostatectomy.
TEST-TAKING STRATEGY: Option 3 can be easily eliminated first. Eliminate option 2 next, because 1 week is a rather short time. Recalling that blood clots are expected following this type of surgery will assist in directing you to option 4. Review client teaching points following prostatectomy now if you had difficulty with this question.
LEVEL OF COGNITIVE ABILITY: Application
PHASE OF NURSING PROCESS: Planning
CLIENT NEEDS: Health Promotion and Maintenance
CONTENT AREA: Adult Health/Oncology
REFERENCE

Monahan, F., & Neighbors, M. (1998). *Medical-surgical nursing: Foundations for clinical practice* (2nd ed.). Philadelphia: W. B. Saunders. p. 1720.

49. **1**

RATIONALE: The incidence of bladder cancer is three times greater in men than in women and affects the Caucasian population twice as often as African-Americans. Options 2, 3, and 4 are associated with the incidence of bladder cancer.
TEST-TAKING STRATEGY: Knowledge regarding the risk factors associated with bladder cancer is required to answer the question. Note the key word "not" in the question. If you had difficulty with this question, take time now to review these risks.
LEVEL OF COGNITIVE ABILITY: Comprehension
PHASE OF NURSING PROCESS: Data Collection
CLIENT NEEDS: Health Promotion and Maintenance
CONTENT AREA: Adult Health/Oncology
REFERENCE

Monahan, F., & Neighbors, M. (1998). *Medical-surgical nursing: Foundations for clinical practice* (2nd ed.). Philadelphia: W. B. Saunders. p. 1419.

50. **3**

RATIONALE: The most common symptom in clients with cancer of the bladder is hematuria. The client may also experience irritative voiding symptoms such as frequency, urgency, and dysuria, and these symptoms are often associated with cancer in situ.
TEST-TAKING STRATEGY: Note the key word "common." Options 1, 2, and 4 are symptoms that are also associated with bladder infection. If you need to make an educated guess, prioritize the options in a physiological manner and select option 3. Review the clinical manifestations associated with bladder cancer now if you had difficulty with this question.
LEVEL OF COGNITIVE ABILITY: Comprehension
PHASE OF NURSING PROCESS: Data Collection
CLIENT NEEDS: Physiological Integrity
CONTENT AREA: Adult Health/Oncology
REFERENCE

Monahan, F., & Neighbors, M. (1998). *Medical-surgical nursing: Foundations for clinical practice* (2nd ed.). Philadelphia: W. B. Saunders. p. 1419.

51. **2**

RATIONALE: Following ureterostomy, the stoma should be red and moist. A pale stoma may indicate an inadequate amount of vascular supply. A dry stoma may indicate body fluid deficit. Any sign of darkness or duskiness in the stoma

may mean loss of vascular supply and must be corrected immediately or necrosis can occur.
TEST-TAKING STRATEGY: You should easily be able to eliminate options 1 and 4. From the remaining options, note the key word "moist" in option 2. This should indicate that this is an expected and positive finding. If you had difficulty with this question, take time now to review expected and unexpected findings following ureterostomy.
LEVEL OF COGNITIVE ABILITY: Comprehension
PHASE OF NURSING PROCESS: Data Collection
CLIENT NEEDS: Physiological Integrity
CONTENT AREA: Adult Health/Oncology
REFERENCE
Monahan, F., & Neighbors, M. (1998). *Medical-surgical nursing: Foundations for clinical practice* (2nd ed.). Philadelphia: W. B. Saunders. p. 1421.

52. **2**

RATIONALE: Following mastectomy, the arm should be elevated above the level of the heart. Arm exercises should be encouraged. No BP readings, injections, IV lines, or blood draws should be performed on the affected arm. Cool compresses are not a suggested measure to prevent lymphedema from occurring.
TEST-TAKING STRATEGY: Note the key words "assists in preventing." Use the process of elimination and note the relationship between the words lymph "edema" in the question and "elevating" in the correct option. Review these important measures now if you had difficulty with this question.
LEVEL OF COGNITIVE ABILITY: Application
PHASE OF NURSING PROCESS: Implementation
CLIENT NEEDS: Physiological Integrity
CONTENT AREA: Adult Health/Oncology
REFERENCE
Monahan, F., & Neighbors, M. (1998). *Medical-surgical nursing: Foundations for clinical practice* (2nd ed.). Philadelphia: W. B. Saunders. p. 1864.

53. **2**

RATIONALE: Mammography takes about 15 to 30 minutes to complete. Some discomfort may be experienced because of the breast compression required to obtain a clear image. There is no reason to maintain an NPO status prior to the procedure. Option 2 is an accurate instruction.
TEST-TAKING STRATEGY: Use the process of elimination. Eliminate options 3 and 4 first. Attempt to visualize the procedure to assist in selecting the correct option. If you are unfamiliar with this important screening test, take time now to review.

LEVEL OF COGNITIVE ABILITY: Application
PHASE OF NURSING PROCESS: Implementation
CLIENT NEEDS: Physiological Integrity
CONTENT AREA: Adult Health/Oncology
REFERENCE
Monahan, F., & Neighbors, M. (1998). *Medical-surgical nursing: Foundations for clinical practice* (2nd ed.). Philadelphia: W. B. Saunders. p. 1848.

54. **3**

RATIONALE: A Pap smear is usually painless. The test cannot be performed during menstruation. The client needs to be instructed to avoid douching for at least 24 hours prior to the test. There is no reason to restrict fluids on the day of the test.
TEST-TAKING STRATEGY: Knowledge regarding the Pap test is required to answer the question. Eliminate option 2 first as an unlikely preparation measure. Eliminate options 1 and 4 next because both menstruation and douching will affect the results of the test. Review client preparation for a Pap test now if you had difficulty with this question.
LEVEL OF COGNITIVE ABILITY: Application
PHASE OF NURSING PROCESS: Implementation
CLIENT NEEDS: Physiological Integrity
CONTENT AREA: Adult Health/Oncology
REFERENCE
Monahan, F., & Neighbors, M. (1998). *Medical-surgical nursing: Foundations for clinical practice* (2nd ed.). Philadelphia: W. B. Saunders. p. 513.

55. **4**

RATIONALE: Spinal cord compression should be suspected in a client with metastatic disease particularly when a new and sudden onset of back pain occurs. Spinal cord compression causes back pain before neurological changes occur. Spinal cord compression is an oncological emergency and the physician should be notified.
TEST-TAKING STRATEGY: The key words "new and sudden" should easily direct you to option 4. If you had difficulty with this question or are unfamiliar with spinal cord compression, take time now to review this oncological emergency.
LEVEL OF COGNITIVE ABILITY: Application
PHASE OF NURSING PROCESS: Implementation
CLIENT NEEDS: Physiological Integrity
CONTENT AREA: Adult Health/Oncology
REFERENCE
Ignatavicius, D., Workman, M. & Mishler, M. (1999). *Medical surgical nursing: Across the health care continuum* (3rd ed.). Philadelphia: W. B. Saunders. p. 514.

BIBLIOGRAPHY

Beare, P., & Myers, J. (1998). *Adult health nursing* (3rd ed.). St. Louis: Mosby–Year Book. p. 1685.

Black, J., & Matassarin-Jacobs, E. (1997). *Medical-surgical nursing: Clinical management for continuity of care* (5th ed.). Philadelphia: W. B. Saunders.

Chernecky, C., & Berger, B. (1997). *Laboratory tests and diagnostic procedures* (2nd ed.). Philadelphia: W. B. Saunders.

deWit, S. (1998). *Essentials of medical-surgical nursing* (4th ed.). Philadelphia: W. B. Saunders.

Hodgson, B., & Kizior, R. (1999). *Saunders nursing drug handbook 1999*. Philadelphia: W. B. Saunders.

Ignatavicius, D., Workman, M., & Mishler, M. (1999). *Medical-surgical nursing: Across the health care continuum* (3rd ed.). Philadelphia: W. B. Saunders.

Leahy, J., & Kizilay, P. (1998). *Foundations of nursing practice: A nursing process approach*: Philadelphia: W. B. Saunders.

Lehne, R. (1998). *Pharmacology for nursing care* (3rd ed.). Philadelphia: W. B. Saunders.

Luckmann, J. (1997). *Saunders manual of nursing care*. Philadelphia: W. B. Saunders.

Monahan, F., & Neighbors, M. (1998). *Medical-surgical nursing: Foundations for clinical practice* (2nd ed.). Philadelphia: W. B. Saunders.

O'Toole, M. (1997). *Miller-Keane encyclopedia & dictionary of medicine, nursing, & allied health* (6th ed.). Philadelphia: W. B. Saunders.

CHAPTER 41

Antineoplastic Medications

I. Antineoplastic Medications

A. Description
1. Kill or inhibit the reproduction of neoplastic cells
2. The effect of antineoplastic medications may not be limited to neoplastic cells; normal cells are also affected by the medication
3. Cell cycle phase–specific medications affect cells only during a certain phase of the reproductive cycle of the cell
4. Cell cycle phase–nonspecific medications affect cells in any phase of the reproductive cycle of the cell
5. Usually several medications are used in combination to increase the therapeutic response and minimize toxicity
6. Antineoplastic therapy may be combined with other treatments, such as surgery and radiation
7. The routes of antineoplastic medication administration can vary
8. Side effects result from the effects of the antineoplastic medication on normal cells

B. Side effects
1. Mucositis/stomatitis
2. Alopecia
3. Anorexia, nausea, and vomiting
4. Diarrhea
5. Anemia
6. Low white blood cell (WBC) count (neutropenia)
7. Thrombocytopenia
8. Infertility

C. Implementation
1. Physiological Integrity
   a. The complete blood cell count (CBC), WBC, platelet count, and electrolytes are monitored closely
   b. Medications are held if the platelet count is less than 75,000 cells/µL or WBC count is less than 4000 cells/µL, and the physician is notified
   c. Bleeding precautions are initiated if thrombocytopenia occurs
   d. Monitor for petechiae, ecchymosis, bleeding of the gums, and nosebleeds because the decreased platelet count can precipitate bleeding tendencies
   e. Neutropenic precautions are initiated if the WBC count decreases
   f. Monitor for fever, sore throat, unusual bleeding, or signs and symptoms of infection
   g. Inform the client that loss of appetite may also be due to a bitter taste in the mouth from the medications
   h. Monitor for nausea and vomiting and provide a high-calorie diet with protein supplements
   i. Antiemetics are administered several hours before chemotherapy and for 12 to 48 hours after, as prescribed, because antineoplastic medications stimulate the vomiting center
   j. IV hydration is administered before and during therapy
   k. Promote a fluid intake of at least 2000 mL a day to maintain adequate renal function
   l. Allopurinol (Zyloprim) is administered as prescribed to lower the serum uric acid that occurs from the rapid destruction of body tissues by the antineoplastic medications
2. Safe, Effective Care Environment
   a. Monitor for phlebitis at the IV site because these medications irritate veins
   b. Monitor for extravasation, which causes tissue necrosis; if this occurs, an ice pack is applied and the physician is notified
   c. Antineoplastic medications are administered in short, high-dose,

intermittent courses as prescribed to maximize antineoplastic effects while allowing normal cells to recover
    d. Used intravenous (IV) equipment is discarded in designated containers
    e. Intramuscular (IM) injections and venipunctures are avoided to prevent bleeding
  3. Psychosocial Integrity
    a. Instruct the client of the potential for hair loss and that varying degrees of hair loss may occur after the first or second treatment
    b. Discuss the purchase of a wig before treatment starts
    c. Inform the client that new hair growth will occur several months after the final treatment
    d. Instruct the client about the need for contraception because these medications have teratogenic effects
    e. Discuss the potential effect of infertility, which may be irreversible
    f. Pretreatment counseling is encouraged
  4. Health Promotion and Maintenance
    a. Instruct the client that if diarrhea is a problem, avoid hot foods and high-fiber foods, which increase peristalsis
    b. Instruct the client to inspect oral mucosa for erythema and ulcers and to rinse the mouth after meals and provide good oral hygiene
    c. Instruct the client to use saline or sodium bicarbonate mouth rinses for mouth sores
    d. Instruct the client in the use of antifungal medications for mouth sores, if prescribed for the development of a superinfection
    e. Instruct the client to avoid crowds and persons with infections
    f. Instruct the client to report any fever, chills, or sore throat, or other signs of infection
    g. Instruct individuals with colds or infections to wear a mask or avoid visiting the client
    h. Instruct the client to use a soft toothbrush and an electric razor to minimize the risk of bleeding
    i. Instruct the client to avoid alcohol to minimize the risk of toxicity
    j. Instruct the client to avoid aspirin-containing products to minimize the risk of bleeding
    k. Instruct the client to consult a physician before receiving vaccinations

II. Alkylating Medications (Box 41–1)

A. Description
  1. Affects the synthesis of DNA to inhibit cell reproduction
  2. Cell cycle phase–nonspecific medications

BOX 41–1. Alkylating Medications

NITROGEN MUSTARDS
Chlorambucil (Leukeran)
Cyclophosphamide (Cytoxan)
Estramustine phosphate sodium (Emcyt)
Ifosfamide (Ifex)
Mechlorethamine HCl (Mustargen)
Melphalan (Alkeran)
Uracil mustard

NITROSOUREAS
Busulfan (Myleran)
Carmustine (BiCNU)
Lomustine (CeeNu)
Streptozocin (Zanosar)

ALKYLATING-LIKE MEDICATIONS
Altretamine (Hexalen)
Carboplatin (Paraplatin)
Cisplatin (Platinol)
Dacarbazine (DTIC)
Triethylenethiophosphoramide (thiotepa)

B. Side effects
  1. Anorexia, nausea, and vomiting
  2. Stomatitis
  3. Skin rash
  4. Pain during IV administration
  5. Busulfan (Myleran) may cause hyperuricemia
  6. Chlorambucil (Leukeran) may cause gonadal suppression and hyperuricemia
  7. Cisplatin (Platinol) may cause ototoxicity, tinnitus, hypokalemia, hypocalcemia, hypomagnesemia, and nephrotoxicity
  8. Cyclophosphamide (Cytoxan) may cause alopecia, gonadal suppression, hemorrhagic cystitis, and hematuria
  9. Mechlorethamine HCl (Mustargen) may cause gonadal suppression and hyperuricemia
C. Implementation
  1. CBC, WBC, platelet, uric acid, and electrolyte counts are monitored
  2. Pulmonary function tests, chest x-rays, and liver and renal function studies are monitored
  3. Monitor the IV site for irritation and phlebitis
  4. Monitor the client receiving cisplatin for dizziness, tinnitus, hearing loss, incoordination, and numbness or tingling of extremities
  5. Monitor clients receiving cyclophosphamide or ifosfamide (Ifex) therapy for signs of hemorrhagic cystitis such as hematuria or dysuria; encourage clients to drink increased fluids up to 2 to 3 liters per day
  6. Instruct the client taking cyclophosphamide orally to take the medication without food
  7. Instruct clients to follow a diet low in purines to alkalize urine and to avoid products containing citric acid

8. Instruct the client how to avoid infection and bleeding, and to report signs of either if they occur
9. Instruct the client to perform good oral hygiene with a soft toothbrush

III. Antitumor Antibiotic Medications (Box 41–2)

A. Description
   1. Interferes with DNA and ribonucleic acid synthesis
   2. Cell cycle phase–nonspecific medication
B. Side effects
   1. Nausea and vomiting
   2. Fever
   3. Bone marrow depression
   4. Skin rash
   5. Alopecia
   6. Stomatitis
   7. Gonadal suppression
   8. Hyperuricemia
   9. Vesication (blistering of tissue at IV site)
   10. Plicamycin (Mithracin) affects bleeding time
   11. Daunorubicin (Cerubidine) may cause congestive heart failure (CHF) and cardiac dysrhythmias
   12. Doxorubicin (Adriamycin) and idarubicin (Idamycin) may cause cardiotoxicity and cardiomyopathy; changes on the ECG will be noted
   13. Pulmonary toxicity can occur with bleomycin sulfate (Blenoxane)
C. Implementation
   1. CBC, WBC, platelet count, uric acid, bleeding time, and electrolyte counts are monitored
   2. Monitor for signs of CHF including dyspnea, peripheral edema, and weight gain
   3. Monitor IV site for irritation, phlebitis, and vesication
   4. Monitor for myocardial toxicity (dyspnea, dysrhythmias, hypotension, and weight gain) when the client is receiving doxorubicin or idarubicin
   5. Pulmonary status is monitored when the client is receiving bleomycin sulfate
   6. The use of aspirin, anticoagulants, and thrombolytic agents is avoided with plicamycin

---

BOX 41–2. Antitumor Antibiotic Medications

Bleomycin sulfate (Blenoxane)
Dactinomycin (actinomycin D, Cosmegen)
Daunorubicin (Cerubidine)
Doxorubicin (Adriamycin)
Idarubicin (Idamycin)
Mitomycin (Mutamycin)
Mitoxantrone (Novantrone)
Plicamycin (Mithracin)

BOX 41–3. Antimetabolite Medications

FOLIC ACID ANTAGONIST
Methotrexate (Folex)

PYRIMIDINE ANALOGS
Cytarabine HCl (ara-C; Cytosar-U)
Floxuridine (FUDR)
5-Fluorouracil (5-FU; Adrucil)
Procarbazine HCl (Matulane)

PURINE ANALOGS
6-Mercaptopurine (Purinethol)
Thioguanine

MISCELLANEOUS RIBONUCLEOTIDE REDUCTASE INHIBITORS
Hydroxyurea (Hydrea)
Trimetrexate glucuronate (NeuTrexin)

ANTIMICROTUBULE
Paclitaxel (Taxol)
Pentostatin (Nipent)

PODOPHYLLOTOXIN DERIVATIVE
Etoposide (VePesid, VP-16)
Teniposide (Vumon, VM-26)

OTHER ANTIMETABOLITE MEDICATIONS
Cladribine (Leustatin)
Fludarabine (Fludara)

IV. Antimetabolite Medications (Box 41–3)

A. Description
   1. Halts the synthesis of cell protein
   2. Cell cycle phase–specific
B. Side effects
   1. Anorexia, nausea, and vomiting
   2. Diarrhea
   3. Alopecia
   4. Stomatitis
   5. Depression of bone marrow
   6. Cytarabine HCl (ara-C; Cytosar-U,) may cause alopecia, stomatitis, hyperuricemia, and hepatotoxicity
   7. 5-Fluorouracil (5-FU; Adrucil) may cause alopecia, stomatitis, diarrhea, phototoxicity reactions, and cerebellar dysfunction
   8. 6-Mercaptopurine (Purinethol) may cause hyperuricemia and hepatotoxicity
   9. Methotrexate (Folex) may cause alopecia, stomatitis, hyperuricemia, photosensitivity, hepatotoxicity, and hematological, gastrointestinal (GI), and skin toxicity
C. Implementation
   1. CBC, WBC, platelet count, renal function studies, and uric acid are monitored
   2. When 5-fluorouracil is administered, monitor for signs of cerebellar dysfunction such as dizziness, weakness, and ataxia, and monitor for stomatitis and diarrhea, which may necessitate medication discontinuation

3. When methotrexate is administered in large doses, leucovorin (folinic acid or citrovorum factor) may be prescribed to prevent fatal medication toxicity (known as leucovorin rescue)

4. When 5-fluorouracil or methotrexate sodium is administered, the client is instructed to use sunscreen and wear protective clothing to prevent photosensitivity reactions

V. Vinca Alkaloids (Box 41–4)

A. Description
   1. Prevent mitosis, causing cell death
   2. Cell cycle phase–specific
B. Side effects
   1. Leukopenia
   2. Neurotoxicity with vincristine sulfate (Oncovin), manifested as numbness and tingling in the finger and toes
   3. Ptosis
   4. Hoarseness
   5. Motor instability
   6. Anorexia, nausea, vomiting
   7. Constipation
   8. Alopecia
   9. Stomatitis
   10. Hyperuricemia
   11. Phlebitis at IV site
C. Implementation
   1. WBC, CBC, uric acid, and platelet counts are monitored
   2. Monitor for hoarseness
   3. Monitor eyes for ptosis
   4. Monitor motor stability and initiate safety precautions as necessary
   5. Monitor for numbness and tingling in the fingers and toes

VI. Hormonal Medications and Enzymes
(Box 41–5)

A. Description
   1. Suppress the immune system and block normal hormones in hormone-sensitive tumors
   2. Change the hormonal balance and slow the growth rates of certain tumors
B. Side effects
   1. Anorexia, nausea, and vomiting
   2. Leukopenia
   3. Impaired pancreatic function with asparaginase (Elspar)
   4. Breast swelling

BOX 41–4. Vinca Alkaloids

Vinblastine sulfate (Velban)
Vincristine sulfate (Oncovin)
Vinorelbine (Navelbine)

BOX 41–5. Hormonal Medications and Enzymes

ANDROGENS
Progesterone (Gesterol 50)
Testolactone (Teslac)

HORMONAL ANTAGONISTS, ENZYMES
Aminoglutethimide (Cytadren)
Asparaginase (Elspar)
Diethylstilbestrol (DES; Stilphostrol)
Flutamide (Eulexin)
Goserelin acetate (Zoladex)
Leuprolide acetate (Lupron)
Megestrol acetate (Megace)
Mitotane (Lysodren)
Tamoxifen citrate (Nolvadex)

---

   5. Hot flashes
   6. Edema and weight gain
   7. Hypertension
   8. Thromboembolitic disorders
   9. Sex characteristic alterations
   10. Electrolyte imbalances
   11. Hemorrhagic cystitis, hypouricemia, and hypercholesterolemia can occur with mitotane (Lysodren)
   12. Tamoxifen citrate (Nolvadex) may cause edema and hypercalcemia
   13. Diethylstilbestrol (DES; Stilphostrol) may cause impotence and gynecomastia in males
   14. Tamoxifen citrate decreases the effects of estrogen
   15. Diethylstilbestrol may alter effects of insulin, oral anticoagulants, and oral hypoglycemic agents
C. Implementation
   1. Review medications that the client is currently taking
   2. Serum calcium levels are monitored when androgens are administered
   3. Monitor for signs of alterations in sexual characteristics
   4. Pancreatic function is monitored when asparaginase is administered
   5. Encourage 2 to 3 liters of fluids per day
   6. Uric acid and cholesterol levels are monitored
   7. Monitor for signs of hemorrhagic cystitis

PRACTICE QUESTIONS

1. The client with breast cancer is being treated with cyclophosphamide (Cytoxan). The nurse plans care knowing that this medication is
   1 Cell cycle phase–specific
   2 Cell cycle phase–nonspecific
   3 A hormonal medication
   4 An antimetabolite

2. The client with bladder cancer is receiving cisplatin (Platinol) and vincristine (Oncovin). The

nurse plans care knowing that the purpose of administering both of these medications is to
1 Prevent gastrointestinal side effects
2 Prevent alopecia
3 Decrease the destruction of cells
4 Decrease medication resistance and reduce drug toxicity

3. The nurse is instructed to initiate bleeding precautions on a client receiving an antineoplastic medication intravenously. The nurse reviews the laboratory results and expects to note which of the following?
1 A WBC of 3000 μL
2 A platelet count of 70,000 cells/μL
3 A clotting time of 10 minutes
4 An ammonia level of 20 μg/dL

4. The nurse is caring for a client who is receiving an IV infusion of an antineoplastic medication. During the infusion, the client complains of pain at the insertion site. On inspection of the site, the nurse notes redness and swelling, and that the infusion of the medication has slowed in rate. The most appropriate nursing action is to
1 Elevate the extremity of the IV site and slow the infusion
2 Apply ice and maintain the infusion rate as prescribed
3 Administer pain medication to reduce the discomfort
4 Notify the registered nurse

5. The client with leukemia is receiving busulfan (Myleran). Allopurinol (Zyloprim) is prescribed for the client. The nurse administers the allopurinol, knowing that its purpose is to
1 Prevent gouty arthritis
2 Prevent hyperuricemia
3 Prevent stomatitis
4 Prevent diarrhea

6. The nurse is reinforcing medication instructions to a client with breast cancer who will be taking cyclophosphamide (Cytoxan). Which of the following does the nurse plan to include in the instructions?
1 Take the medication with food
2 Increase fluid intake to 2000 to 3000 mL daily
3 Decrease sodium intake while taking the medication
4 Increase potassium intake while taking the medication

7. The nurse is assigned to care for a client with non-Hodgkin's lymphoma who is receiving daunorubicin (Cerubidine). Which of the following signs indicates to the nurse that the client is experiencing a toxic effect related to the medication?
1 Nausea and vomiting
2 Fever
3 Dyspnea
4 Diarrhea

8. The nurse is assigned to care for a client with testicular cancer who is receiving plicamycin (Mithracin). The nurse is preparing to administer the daily prescribed medications to the client. The nurse questions which of the following medications if noted on the client's medication record?
1 Warfarin (Coumadin)
2 Allopurinol (Zyloprim)
3 Acetaminophen (Tylenol)
4 Ondansetron (Zofran)

9. The client with squamous cell carcinoma of the larynx is receiving bleomycin sulfate (Blenoxane) by IV. The nurse assigned to the client receives a report and anticipates that which of the following diagnostic studies will be prescribed for this client?
1 Pulmonary function studies
2 Electrocardiogram
3 Cervical x-rays
4 Echocardiogram

10. Cytarabine HCl (Cytosar) is prescribed for the client with acute lymphocytic leukemia. The nurse plans care, knowing that this is a
1 Cell cycle–nonspecific medication
2 Hormone medication
3 Cell cycle–specific medication
4 A medication that affects cells in any phase of the reproductive cell cycle

11. The nurse is helping to prepare a teaching plan for the client receiving an antineoplastic medication. The nurse suggests including which of the following in the plan of care?
1 Take aspirin (acetylsalicylic acid, ASA) as needed for headache
2 Drink beverages containing alcohol in moderate amounts
3 Consult with the physician before receiving immunizations
4 Be sure to receive the flu and pneumonia vaccine

12. The client with lung cancer is receiving a high dose of methotrexate (Folex). Leucovorin (citrovorum factor, folic acid) is also prescribed. The nurse who is assisting in planning care for the client understands that the purpose of administering the leucovorin is to
1 Preserve normal cells
2 Promote DNA synthesis
3 Promote medication excretion
4 Promote the synthesis of nucleic acids

13. The client with ovarian cancer is being treated with vincristine (Oncovin). The nurse caring for the client monitors which side effect specific to this medication?

1 Diarrhea
2 Numbness and tingling in the fingers and toes
3 Chest pain
4 Hair loss

14. Asparaginase (Elspar), an antineoplastic agent, is prescribed for a client. The nurse assigned to care for the client collects data from the client. The nurse reports which of the following conditions contraindicated with the administration of asparaginase?
    1 Myocardial infarction
    2 Chronic obstructive pulmonary disease
    3 Diabetes mellitus
    4 Pancreatitis

15. Tamoxifen (Nolvadex) is prescribed for the client with metastatic breast carcinoma. The nurse assists in planning care, knowing that the primary action of this medication is to
    1 Increase DNA and RNA synthesis
    2 Compete with estradiol for binding to estrogen in tissues containing high concentrations of receptors
    3 Increase estrogen concentration and estrogen response
    4 Promote the biosynthesis of nucleic acids

16. The client with metastatic breast cancer is receiving tamoxifen (Nolvadex). The nurse assigned to care for the client monitors for signs of which of the following during therapy with this medication?
    1 Leukocytosis
    2 Weight loss
    3 Hypercalcemia
    4 Hypotension

17. Megestrol acetate (Megace), an antineoplastic medication, is prescribed for the client with metastatic endometrial carcinoma. The nurse assigned to care for the client collects data from the client. The nurse reports which of the following conditions that requires caution with the administration of megestrol acetate?
    1 Asthma
    2 Myocardial infarction
    3 Thrombophlebitis
    4 Gout

18. A female client with carcinoma of the breast is admitted to the hospital for treatment with intravenous vincristine (Oncovin). The client tells the nurse that she has been told by her friends that she is going to lose all of her hair. The most appropriate nursing response is which of the following?
    1 "You will not lose your hair."
    2 "Your friends are correct."
    3 "Hair loss may occur, but it will grow back just as it is now."
    4 "Hair loss may occur, and it will grow back, but it may have a different color or texture."

19. The nurse is assisting in preparing instructions for a client who developed stomatitis following the administration of a course of antineoplastic medications. Which of the following instructions does the nurse most appropriately suggest to include in the plan of care?
    1 To rinse the mouth with baking soda or saline
    2 To avoid foods and fluids for the next 24 hours
    3 To swab the mouth daily with lemon and glycerin pads
    4 To brush the teeth and use waxed dental floss three times a day

20. The client with acute myelocytic leukemia is being treated with busulfan (Myleran). The nurse monitors for signs of which of the following that specifically occurs from the administration of this medication?
    1 Hyperglycemia
    2 Renal failure
    3 Hyperkalemia
    4 Congestive heart failure

ANSWERS

1. **2**

RATIONALE: Cyclophosphamide is an antineoplastic medication of the alkylating classification. Medications in this classification are cell cycle phase–nonspecific and affect all phases of the reproductive cell cycle. Cell phase–specific medications affect cells only during a certain phase of the reproductive cycle.
TEST-TAKING STRATEGY: Knowledge regarding the classification of this medication and the specific action of alkylating agents is required to answer the question. If you had difficulty with this question, take time now to review the action of alkylating medications.
LEVEL OF COGNITIVE ABILITY: Comprehension

PHASE OF NURSING PROCESS: Planning
CLIENT NEEDS: Physiological Integrity
CONTENT AREA: Pharmacology
REFERENCE
Eckler, J., & Fair, J. (1996). *Pharmacology essentials*. Philadelphia: W. B. Saunders. p. 164.

2. **4**

RATIONALE: Cisplatin is an alkylating-like medication and vincristine is a vinca alkyloid. Alkylating medications are cell cycle phase–nonspecific. Vinca alkaloids are cell cycle phase–specific. Single-agent medication therapy is seldom used. Combinations of medications are used to enhance tumoricidal effects. Use of combination medications decreases medication resistance, increases destruction of cancer cells, and reduces medication toxicity.

TEST-TAKING STRATEGY: Knowledge regarding the rationale of combination medication therapy is required to answer the question. Use the process of elimination to answer the question. Eliminate option 3 first as the least likely option. Eliminate options 1 and 2 first. It may be possible, with some specific interventions, to reduce GI effects and alopecia, but it is unlikely that these occurrences can be prevented.
LEVEL OF COGNITIVE ABILITY: Comprehension
PHASE OF NURSING PROCESS: Planning
CLIENT NEEDS: Physiological Integrity
CONTENT AREA: Pharmacology
REFERENCE
Eckler, J., & Fair, J. (1996). *Pharmacology essentials*. Philadelphia: W. B. Saunders. p. 164.

3. **2**

RATIONALE: Bleeding precautions need to be initiated when the platelet count drops. Bleeding precautions include avoiding all trauma such as rectal temperatures or injections. The normal platelet count is 150,000 to 450,000 cells/μL. The normal WBC count is 5,000 to 10,000/μL. When the WBC count drops, neutropenic precautions need to be implemented. The normal clotting time is 8 to 15 minutes. The normal ammonia value is 15 to 45 μg/dL.
TEST-TAKING STRATEGY: Knowledge regarding normal laboratory values and the significance of the specific laboratory tests is required to answer the question. Options 3 and 4 identify normal laboratory values. To select between the last two options, correlate a low platelet count with the need for bleeding precautions, and a low WBC count with the need for neutropenic precaution.
LEVEL OF COGNITIVE ABILITY: Comprehension
PHASE OF NURSING PROCESS: Data Collection
CLIENT NEEDS: Safe, Effective Care Environment
CONTENT AREA: Pharmacology
REFERENCE
Kee, J., & Hayes, E. (1997). *Pharmacology: A nursing process approach* (2nd ed.). Philadelphia: W. B. Saunders. p. 413.

4. **4**

RATIONALE: When antineoplastic medications are administered by IV, great care must be taken to prevent the medication from escaping into the tissues surrounding the injection site, as pain, tissue damage, and necrosis can result. The nurse monitors for signs of extravasation such as redness or swelling at the insertion site and a decreased infusion rate. If extravasation occurs, the registered nurse needs to be notified who will then contact the physician.
TEST-TAKING STRATEGY: Use the process of elimination to answer the question. Eliminate options 1 and 2 first. The nurse would not slow the rate. Based on the information in the question, the nurse would not be able to maintain the prescribed rate. Administering pain medication to reduce discomfort at an IV site is not an appropriate action. Further investigation of the cause of the discomfort is required. This leaves option 4 as the correct nursing action.
LEVEL OF COGNITIVE ABILITY: Application
PHASE OF NURSING PROCESS: Implementation
CLIENT NEEDS: Physiological Integrity
CONTENT AREA: Pharmacology
REFERENCE
Eckler, J., & Fair, J. (1996). *Pharmacology essentials*. Philadelphia: W. B. Saunders. p. 163.

5. **2**

RATIONALE: Busulfan is an alkylating medication used in the treatment of acute myelocytic leukemia and in the palliative treatment of chronic myelogenous leukemia. Hyperuricemia can result from the use of this medication as it may produce uric acid nephropathy, renal stones, and acute renal failure. Allopurinol, an antigout medication, is used with chemotherapy to prevent or treat hyperuricemia secondary to blood dyscrasias caused by cancer chemotherapy. It may be used in mouthwash following fluorouracil therapy to prevent stomatitis. Allopurinol is not used to prevent diarrhea.
TEST-TAKING STRATEGY: Knowledge regarding the side effects associated with busulfan and the purpose of administering allopurinol during the administration of antineoplastic medication, is required to answer this question. Take time now to review both of these medications if you had difficulty with this question.
LEVEL OF COGNITIVE ABILITY: Comprehension
PHASE OF NURSING PROCESS: Implementation
CLIENT NEEDS: Physiological Integrity
CONTENT AREA: Pharmacology
REFERENCE
Hodgson, B., & Kizior, R. (1999). *Saunders nursing drug handbook 1999*. Philadelphia: W. B. Saunders. pp. 24, 134.

6. **2**

RATIONALE: Hemorrhagic cystitis is a toxic effect that can occur with the use of cyclophosphamide. The client needs to be instructed to drink copious amounts of fluid during the administration of this medication. Clients should also monitor urine output for hematuria. The medication should be taken on an empty stomach, unless GI upset occurs. Hyperkalemia can result from the use of the medication; therefore, the client should not be encouraged to increase potassium intake. The client is not instructed to alter sodium intake.
TEST-TAKING STRATEGY: Knowledge regarding the toxic effects of cyclophosphamide will assist to answer this question correctly. If you correlated cyclophosphamide with hemorrhagic cystitis, then, by the process of elimination, option 2 would be selected. If you had difficulty with this question, take time now to review the toxic effects associated with this medication.
LEVEL OF COGNITIVE ABILITY: Comprehension
PHASE OF NURSING PROCESS: Planning
CLIENT NEEDS: Health Promotion and Maintenance
CONTENT AREA: Pharmacology
REFERENCE
Hodgson, B., & Kizior, R. (1999). *Saunders nursing drug handbook 1999*. Philadelphia: W. B. Saunders. pp. 270–272.

7. **3**

RATIONALE: Cardiotoxicity and/or cardiomyopathy manifested as CHF is a toxic effect of daunorubicin. Bone marrow depression is also a toxic effect. Nausea and vomiting are frequent side effects associated with the medication that begin a few hours after administration, and last 24 to 48 hours. Fever is a frequent side effect, and diarrhea can occur occasionally.
TEST-TAKING STRATEGY: The ability to distinguish between side effects and toxic effects is required to answer the question. Use the process of elimination, keeping in mind that the question is asking for a toxic effect. This concept should direct you to the option addressing a sign

of CHF. Additionally, the correct option presents the most serious concern. If you had difficulty with this question, take time now to review the toxic effects associated with daunorubicin.

LEVEL OF COGNITIVE ABILITY: Analysis
PHASE OF NURSING PROCESS: Data Collection
CLIENT NEEDS: Physiological Integrity
CONTENT AREA: Pharmacology
REFERENCE
Hodgson, B., & Kizior, R. (1999). *Saunders nursing drug handbook 1999.* Philadelphia: W. B. Saunders. p. 288.

8. **1**

RATIONALE: Plicamycin is an antitumor antibiotic. Because plicamycin affects bleeding time, the use of aspirin, anticoagulants, and thrombolytic agents should be avoided. Warfarin is an anticoagulant, and the risk of hemorrhage is increased if administered during plicamycin therapy. Allopurinol, an antigout medication, may be used with chemotherapy to prevent or treat hyperuricemia secondary to blood dyscrasias caused by cancer chemotherapy. Acetaminophen may be used to treat mild discomfort. Ondansetron is an antiemetic used to prevent or treat nausea or vomiting during chemotherapy.

TEST-TAKING STRATEGY: Knowledge regarding the classifications of the medications identified in the options assists in answering the question. From this knowledge, use the process of elimination. If you are unfamiliar with these medications, take time now to review their classifications and use.

LEVEL OF COGNITIVE ABILITY: Comprehension
PHASE OF NURSING PROCESS: Implementation
CLIENT NEEDS: Safe, Effective Care Environment
CONTENT AREA: Pharmacology
REFERENCE
Hodgson, B., & Kizior, R. (1999). *Saunders nursing drug handbook 1999.* Philadelphia: W. B. Saunders. p. 838.

9. **1**

RATIONALE: Bleomycin sulfate is an antineoplastic medication that can cause interstitial pneumonitis, which can progress to pulmonary fibrosis. Pulmonary function studies along with hematologic, hepatic, and renal function tests need to be monitored. The nurse needs to monitor for dyspnea that may indicate pulmonary toxicity. The medication will be discontinued immediately if pulmonary toxicity occurs.

TEST-TAKING STRATEGY: Knowledge regarding the toxic effects of bleomycin sulfate is required to answer this question. Eliminate options 2 and 4 first because they are both cardiac related and therefore similar. From this point, prioritize and select option 1 as it relates to airway. If you had difficulty with this question, take time now to review the toxic effects of this medication.

LEVEL OF COGNITIVE ABILITY: Analysis
PHASE OF NURSING PROCESS: Planning
CLIENT NEEDS: Physiological Integrity
CONTENT AREA: Pharmacology
REFERENCE
Hodgson, B., & Kizior, R. (1999). *Saunders nursing drug handbook 1999.* Philadelphia: W. B. Saunders. pp. 120–122.

10. **3**

RATIONALE: Cytarabine is an antimetabolite. Antimetabolites are classified as cell cycle specific. Alkylating medica-

tions affect all phases of the cell reproductive cycle. Hormone medications suppress the immune system and block normal hormones in hormone-sensitive tumors.

TEST-TAKING STRATEGY: Eliminate options 1 and 4 first because they are similar. From this point, knowledge that this medication is an antimetabolite is required to answer the question. Take time now to review the action of this medication if you had difficulty with this question.

LEVEL OF COGNITIVE ABILITY: Comprehension
PHASE OF NURSING PROCESS: Planning
CLIENT NEEDS: Physiological Integrity
CONTENT AREA: Pharmacology
REFERENCE
Hodgson, B., & Kizior, R. (1999). *Saunders nursing drug handbook 1999.* Philadelphia: W. B. Saunders. p. 276.

11. **3**

RATIONALE: Since antineoplastic medications lower the body's resistance, clients must be informed not to receive immunizations or vaccines without a physician's approval. Clients also need to avoid contact with individuals who have recently taken oral polio vaccine. Aspirin and aspirin-containing products need to be avoided to minimize the risk of bleeding. Alcohol needs to be avoided to minimize the risk of toxicity.

TEST-TAKING STRATEGY: Knowledge regarding the contraindications and cautions associated with the administration of antineoplastic medications is required to answer this question. Use the process of elimination, remembering that antineoplastic medications lower the body's resistance. Take time now to review the client teaching points regarding these medications if you had difficulty with this question.

LEVEL OF COGNITIVE ABILITY: Application
PHASE OF NURSING PROCESS: Planning
CLIENT NEEDS: Health Promotion and Maintenance
CONTENT AREA: Pharmacology
REFERENCE
Hodgson, B., & Kizior, R. (1999). *Saunders nursing drug handbook 1999.* Philadelphia: W. B. Saunders. p. 430.

12. **1**

RATIONALE: High concentrations of methotrexate cause harm and damage to normal cells. To save normal cells, leucovorin is given. This is known as leucovorin rescue. Options 2, 3, and 4 do not identify the purpose for administering leucovorin.

TEST-TAKING STRATEGY: Knowledge regarding the action of leucovorin and the purpose of administering this medication with methotrexate is required to answer this question. Eliminate options 2 and 4 first because they are similar. Nucleic acids include RNA and DNA. Eliminate option 3 because increased fluids and diuretics are normally administered to promote medication excretion. If you had difficulty with this question, take time now to review leucovorin rescue.

LEVEL OF COGNITIVE ABILITY: Comprehension
PHASE OF NURSING PROCESS: Planning
CLIENT NEEDS: Physiological Integrity
CONTENT AREA: Pharmacology
REFERENCE
Lehne, R. (1998). *Pharmacology for nursing care* (3rd ed.). Philadelphia: W. B. Saunders. p. 1027.

13. **2**

RATIONALE: A side effect specific to vincristine is peripheral neuropathy, which occurs in nearly every client. This can be manifested as numbness and tingling in the fingers and toes. Constipation rather than diarrhea is most likely to occur with this medication, although diarrhea may occur occasionally. Hair loss occurs with nearly all of the antineoplastic medications. Chest pain is unrelated to this medication.

TEST-TAKING STRATEGY: Knowledge regarding the side effects associated with this medication is required to answer this question. Eliminate options 1 and 4 first because these side effects are associated with many of the antineoplastic agents. Note that the question asks for the side effect "specific" to this medication. Correlate peripheral neuropathy with vincristine.

LEVEL OF COGNITIVE ABILITY: Comprehension
PHASE OF NURSING PROCESS: Data Collection
CLIENT NEEDS: Physiological Integrity
CONTENT AREA: Pharmacology
REFERENCE

Hodgson, B., & Kizior, R. (1999). *Saunders nursing drug handbook 1999*. Philadelphia: W. B. Saunders. pp. 1053–1054.

14. **4**

RATIONALE: Asparaginase is contraindicated if hypersensitivity exists, in pancreatitis, or if the client has a history of pancreatitis. The medication impairs pancreatic function, and pancreatic function tests should be performed before therapy begins and when a week or more has elapsed between the administration of the doses. The client needs to be monitored for signs of pancreatitis, which include nausea, vomiting, and abdominal pain.

TEST-TAKING STRATEGY: Knowledge regarding the contraindications associated with asparaginase is required to answer this question. Take time now to review this medication if you had difficulty answering this question.

LEVEL OF COGNITIVE ABILITY: Application
PHASE OF NURSING PROCESS: Implementation
CLIENT NEEDS: Safe, Effective Care Environment
CONTENT AREA: Pharmacology
REFERENCE

Hodgson, B., & Kizior, R. (1999). *Saunders nursing drug handbook 1999*. Philadelphia: W. B. Saunders. pp. 72–74.

15. **2**

RATIONALE: Tamoxifen is an antineoplastic medication that competes with estradiol for binding to estrogen in tissues containing high concentrations of receptors. It is used in the treatment of metastatic breast carcinoma in women and men. It is also effective in delaying the recurrence of cancer following mastectomy. It reduces DNA synthesis and estrogen response.

TEST-TAKING STRATEGY: Eliminate options 1 and 4 first because they are similar. Nucleic acids include DNA and RNA. From this point, select option 2 because it is unlikely that treatment of metastatic breast carcinoma would focus toward increasing estrogen concentration and estrogen response. If you had difficulty with this question, take time now to review the action of this medication.

LEVEL OF COGNITIVE ABILITY: Comprehension
PHASE OF NURSING PROCESS: Planning
CLIENT NEEDS: Physiological Integrity
CONTENT AREA: Pharmacology
REFERENCE

Hodgson, B., & Kizior, R. (1999). *Saunders nursing drug handbook 1999*. Philadelphia: W. B. Saunders. p. 961.

16. **3**

RATIONALE: Tamoxifen may increase calcium, and cholesterol and triglyceride levels. The nurse should assess for hypercalcemia while the client is taking this medication. Signs of hypercalcemia include increased urine volume, excessive thirst, nausea, vomiting, constipation, hypotonicity of muscles, and deep bone or flank pain. Leukopenia, weight gain, and hypertension are most likely to occur.

TEST-TAKING STRATEGY: Knowledge regarding the side effects associated with this medication is required to answer this question. Take time now to review this important medication if you had difficulty answering this question.

LEVEL OF COGNITIVE ABILITY: Comprehension
PHASE OF NURSING PROCESS: Data Collection
CLIENT NEEDS: Physiological Integrity
CONTENT AREA: Pharmacology
REFERENCE

Hodgson, B., & Kizior, R. (1999). *Saunders nursing drug handbook 1999*. Philadelphia: W. B. Saunders. p. 962.

17. **3**

RATIONALE: Megestrol acetate suppresses the release of luteinizing hormone from the anterior pituitary by inhibiting pituitary function and regressing tumor size. It is used with caution if the client has a history of thrombophlebitis.

TEST-TAKING STRATEGY: Knowledge regarding the cautions associated with the administration of this medication is required to answer this question. Take time now to review this important medication if you had difficulty answering this question.

LEVEL OF COGNITIVE ABILITY: Application
PHASE OF NURSING PROCESS: Implementation
CLIENT NEEDS: Safe, Effective Care Environment
CONTENT AREA: Pharmacology
REFERENCE

Hodgson, B., & Kizior, R. (1999). *Saunders nursing drug handbook 1999*. Philadelphia: W. B. Saunders. p. 634.

18. **4**

RATIONALE: Alopecia can occur following the administration of many antineoplastic medications. Alopecia is reversible, but new hair growth may have a different color and texture.

TEST-TAKING STRATEGY: Use knowledge regarding the side effects of antineoplastic medications and therapeutic communication techniques to answer this question. Eliminate options 1 and 2 first. Option 1 is incorrect and option 2 is a nontherapeutic response. Recalling that new hair growth may have a different color and texture will assist in directing you to option 4. Take time now to review content related to hair loss and antineoplastic medications if you had difficulty with this question.

LEVEL OF COGNITIVE ABILITY: Application
PHASE OF NURSING PROCESS: Implementation
CLIENT NEEDS: Psychosocial Integrity
CONTENT AREA: Pharmacology
REFERENCE

Hodgson, B., & Kizior, R. (1999). *Saunders nursing drug handbook 1999*. Philadelphia: W. B. Saunders. p. 1054.

19. **1**

RATIONALE: Stomatitis (ulceration in the mouth) can occur as a result of the administration of antineoplastic medications. The client should be instructed to examine the mouth daily and to report any signs of ulceration. If stomatitis occurs, the client should be instructed to rinse the mouth with baking soda or saline. Food and fluid are important and should not be restricted. The client should avoid toothbrushing and flossing when stomatitis is severe. Lemon and glycerin swabs may cause pain and further irritation.

TEST-TAKING STRATEGY: Knowing that stomatitis involves ulcerations in the mucous membranes of the mouth will assist in the process of eliminating the incorrect options. Eliminate option 2 first because foods and fluids would not be restricted in a client that received antineoplastic medication. Eliminate option 3 because lemon can be irritating to ulcerated lesions. Eliminate option 4 because a toothbrush and floss will also irritate ulcerations and may cause bleeding. If you had difficulty with this question, take time now to review the client teaching points related to stomatitis.

LEVEL OF COGNITIVE ABILITY: Comprehension
PHASE OF NURSING PROCESS: Planning
CLIENT NEEDS: Physiological Integrity
CONTENT AREA: Pharmacology

REFERENCE
Eckler, J., & Fair, J. (1996). *Pharmacology essentials.* Philadelphia: W. B. Saunders. p. 163.

20. **2**

RATIONALE: Busulfan can cause an increase in the uric acid level. Hyperuricemia can produce uric acid nephropathy, renal stones, and acute renal failure. Options 1, 3, and 4 are unrelated to the administration of this medication.

TEST-TAKING STRATEGY: Knowledge regarding the adverse effects of this medication is required to answer this question. If you had difficulty with this question, take time now to review the effects of busulfan.

LEVEL OF COGNITIVE ABILITY: Comprehension
PHASE OF NURSING PROCESS: Data Collection
CLIENT NEEDS: Physiological Integrity
CONTENT AREA: Pharmacology
REFERENCE
Hodgson, B., & Kizior, R. (1999). *Saunders nursing drug handbook 1999.* Philadelphia: W. B. Saunders. pp. 133–134.

BIBLIOGRAPHY

Clark, J., Queener, S., & Karb V. (1997). *Pharmacologic basis of nursing practice* (5th ed.). St. Louis: Mosby–Year Book.

Eckler, J., & Fair, J. (1996). *Pharmacology essentials.* Philadelphia: W. B. Saunders.

Hodgson, B., & Kizior, R. (1999). *Saunders nursing drug handbook 1999.* Philadelphia: W. B. Saunders.

Kee, J., & Hayes, E. (1997). *Pharmacology: A nursing process approach* (2nd ed.). Philadelphia: W. B. Saunders.

Lehne, R. (1998). *Pharmacology for nursing care* (3rd ed.). Philadelphia: W. B. Saunders.

UNIT X

The Adult Client with an Endocrine Disorder

PYRAMID TERMS

Addisonian Crisis—A life-threatening disorder caused by adrenal hormone insufficiency. It is precipitated by infection, trauma, stress, or surgery. Death can occur from shock, vascular collapse, or hyperkalemia.

Addison's Disease—Hyposecretion of adrenal cortex hormones (glucocorticoids and mineralocorticoids) from the adrenal gland, resulting in deficiency of the steroid hormones. The condition is fatal if left untreated.

Adrenalectomy—The surgical removal of an adrenal gland. Lifelong steroid replacement is necessary with a bilateral adrenalectomy. Temporary steroid replacement, up to 2 years, is necessary for a unilateral adrenalectomy.

Chvostek's Sign—A spasm of the facial muscles elicited by tapping the facial nerve in the region of the parotid gland. It is noted in hypocalcemia.

Cushing's Syndrome—A condition resulting from the hypersecretion of glucocorticoids from the adrenal cortex.

Dawn Phenomenon—Results from a nocturnal release of growth hormone secretion that may cause blood glucose elevations at about 5 to 6 A.M. Treatment includes administering an evening dose of intermediate-acting insulin at 10 P.M.

Diabetic Ketoacidosis (DKA)—A complication of diabetes mellitus that develops when a severe insulin deficiency occurs. DKA is a life-threatening condition. Hyperglycemia that progresses to ketoacidosis occurs; Seen in clients with insulin-dependent diabetes mellitus (IDDM), undiagnosed diabetics, and persons who stop prescribed treatment for diabetes. It develops over a period of several hours to days.

Diabetes Insipidus—The hyposecretion of antidiuretic hormone (ADH) and a deficiency of vasopressin. Results in failure of tubular reabsorption of water in the kidneys.

Diabetes Mellitus—A chronic and potentially disabling disease characterized by elevated blood glucose levels. A chronic disorder of glucose intolerance and impaired carbohydrate, protein, and lipid metabolism because of a deficiency of insulin. A deficiency of insulin results in hyperglycemia.

Graves' Disease (Hyperthyroidism)—Known as thyrotoxicosis. A hyperthyroid state resulting from a hypersecretion of thyroid hormone.

Hyperglycemia—Elevated blood glucose level.

Hyperosmolar Hyperglycemia Nonketotic Syndrome (HHNS)—Extreme hyperglycemia without acidosis. Usually occurs in noninsulin-dependent diabetics when diabetes is uncontrolled or undiagnosed, or during stress or infection. The major difference between HHNS and DKA is the lack of ketone production with HHNS. Onset is usually slow, taking from hours to days.

Hypoglycemia (Insulin Reaction)—Described as a blood glucose level below 50 to 60 mg/dL. Occurs as a result of too much insulin, not enough food, or excessive activity.

Hypophysectomy—The removal of the pituitary gland.

Myxedema (Hypothyroidism)—A hypothyroid state resulting from a hyposecretion of thyroid hormone. The condition occurs in adulthood.

Myxedema Coma—A rare but serious disorder that results from a persistent low thyroid production. It can be precipitated by acute illness, rapid withdrawal of thyroid medication, anesthesia and surgery, hypothermia, and the use of sedatives and narcotics.

Somogyi's Phenomenon—A rebound phenomenon occurring in diabetes mellitus. Overtreatment with insulin induces hypoglycemia, which initiates the release of epinephrine, ACTH, glucagon, and growth hormone. It results in rebound hyperglycemia and ketosis. Occurs during the initial period of serum glucose control; develops at peak insulin times and during the night.

Thyroidectomy—Removal of the thyroid gland. Performed in conditions in which persistent hyperthryoidism exists.

Thyroid Storm—An acute and fatal thyroid condition that occurs from manipulation of the thyroid gland during surgery and the release of thyroid hormone into the bloodstream. It can also occur from severe infection and stress.

Trousseau's Sign—A sign found in hypocalcemia in which carpal spasm can be elicited by compressing the upper arm and causing ischemia to the nerves distally.

◢ PYRAMID TO SUCCESS

The endocrine system is made up of organs or glands that secrete hormones and release these hormones directly into the circulation. The endocrine system can be easily understood if you remember that basically one of two situations can occur: either hyposecretion or hypersecretion of hormones from the organ or gland. When an excess of the hormone occurs, treatment is aimed at blocking the hormone release through medication or surgery. When a deficit of the hormone exists, treatment is aimed at replacement therapy. Pyramid points focus on diabetes mellitus; the prevention and treatment of complications and insulin therapy, hypoglycemic and hyperglycemic reactions, and diabetic ketoacidosis; Addison's disease and addisonian crisis; Cushing's syndrome; thyroid disorders; thyroid storm; and care to the client following thyroidectomy or adrenalectomy.

NURSING PROCESS

DATA COLLECTION

Appetite changes
Growth imbalances
Weight gain or loss
Fluid and electrolyte
 imbalances
Gastrointestinal (GI)
 disturbances
Headache
Hypotension or
 hypertension
Hyperglycemia or
 hypoglycemia
Cardiac dysrhythmias
Abnormal skin pigmentation
Altered skin turgor
Signs of impaired healing
Fever and diaphoresis
Generalized weakness
Sensitivity to cold or heat
Exophthalmos
Visual disturbances
Hirsutism
Polyuria, polydipsia, and
 polyphagia
Mental status changes and
 emotional disturbances
Personality changes and
 mood swings
Menstrual changes
Impotence

PLANNING	IMPLEMENTATION	EVALUATION
The client will verbalize the prescribed diet plan. The client will maintain glucose levels to as near as normal as possible.	Instruct client in prescribed diet therapy. Instruct client and family how to shop and select items required to maintain prescribed dietary therapies.	The client maintains appropriate body weight. Blood glucose levels remain within the expected range.

PLANNING	IMPLEMENTATION	EVALUATION
The client will maintain normal fluid and electrolyte balance.	Monitor fluid and electrolyte balance closely. Administer replacement therapy as prescribed.	Maintenance of normal fluid balance is achieved as evidenced by balanced I&O, stable vital signs, stable weight, and normal laboratory values.

PLANNING	IMPLEMENTATION	EVALUATION
The client will identify factors that increase the risk for altered tissue perfusion.	Monitor neurological status. Monitor client for alterations in neurovascular and cardiovascular status.	Adequate tissue perfusion is maintained.
The client verbalizes the need for pain-relief measures.	Encourage client to verbalize measures that reduce pain.	The client remains comfortable.
The client remains free of infection.	Instruct client regarding measures to prevent infection. Instruct client in signs and symptoms of infection.	The client remains free of signs of infection.
The client will maintain intact skin.	Monitor skin integrity. Instruct client in measures to maintain skin integrity.	The client complies with treatment measures to prevent complications related to skin integrity.
The client will maintain an appropriate sensory and perceptual status.	Monitor vision and hearing abilities. Instruct client to obtain vision examinations every 6 to 12 months as prescribed.	Client remains free of sensory or perceptual disturbances.
The client will remain free of injury. The client verbalizes changes in feelings and mood.	Orient client to environment. Encourage client to discuss feelings related to personality changes. Discuss the causes of the changes that occur in personality. Promote a positive and calm environment.	The client is free of injury. The client is oriented to person, place, and time. The client describes altered feelings.
The client will experience an improvement in body image.	Encourage client to discuss feelings related to body image.	The client states that body image improves.
The client achieves a personal desired level of sexual functioning.	Identify problems that the client is experiencing related to sexual functioning. Encourage the client to express the effect that sexual dysfunction has had on the sexual partner.	The client participates in sexual activity as desired.
The client verbalizes the treatments prescribed. The client verbalizes the importance of the prescribed therapies. The client correctly demonstrates how to administer medications and injections.	Instruct client regarding the prescribed treatment plan. Instruct client on the disease process and the rationale for the prescribed plan. Instruct the client in measures to prevent complications. Instruct the client in the signs and symptoms of complications related to the disorder. Instruct client in preventive measures of complications. Instruct client and family regarding medications and the administration of injections.	The client complies with the prescribed treatment plan. The client obtains and carries or wears a Medic-Alert bracelet. The client notifies the physician when appropriate.

◢ **CLIENT NEEDS**

SAFE, EFFECTIVE CARE ENVIRONMENT

    Advocacy related to client's decisions
    Informed consent related to diagnostic tests and
       procedures
    Confidentiality related to client condition
    Accident prevention in the client with altered mental
       status

    Asepsis
    Handling hazardous and infectious materials

HEALTH PROMOTION AND MAINTENANCE

    Describing expected body image changes
    Disease prevention related to potential complications
    Health screening related to diabetes
    Addressing lifestyle choices
    Reinforcing instructions regarding the prescribed
       treatment plan

Reinforcing instructions regarding the effect of diet therapy, exercise, and the administration of insulin to the diabetic client

PSYCHOSOCIAL INTEGRITY

Coping mechanisms related to the endocrine disturbance
Sensory or perceptual alterations related to the disorder
Unexpected body image disturbances
Role changes and support systems

PHYSIOLOGICAL INTEGRITY

Basic carc and comfort measures
Expected effects of medication administration
Laboratory values of diagnostic tests
Identifying potential complications
Providing care in emergencies

BIBLIOGRAPHY

deWit, S. (1998). *Essentials of medical-surgical nursing* (4th ed.). Philadelphia: W. B. Saunders.

Hill, S., & Howlett, H. (1997). *Success in practical nursing: Personal and vocational issues* (3rd ed.). Philadelphia: W. B. Saunders.

Leahy, J., & Kizilay, P. (1998). *Foundations of nursing practice: A nursing process approach*. Philadelphia: W. B. Saunders.

Luckmann, J. (1997). *Saunders manual of nursing care*. Philadelphia: W. B. Saunders.

Monahan, F., & Neighbors, M. (1998). *Medical-surgical nursing: Foundations for clinical practice* (2nd ed.). Philadelphia: W. B. Saunders.

National Council of State Boards of Nursing (1998). *National Council detailed test plan for the NCLEX-PN examination*. Chicago: Author.

O'Toole, M. (1997). *Miller-Keane encyclopedia & dictionary of medicine, nursing, & allied health* (6th ed.). Philadelphia: W. B. Saunders.

CHAPTER 42

Endocrine System

I. Anatomy and Physiology of Endocrine Glands (Box 42–1)

A. Functions
   1. Maintenance and regulation of vital functions
   2. Response to stress and injury
   3. Growth and development
   4. Energy metabolism
   5. Reproduction
   6. Fluid, electrolyte, and acid-base balance

B. Pituitary gland (Box 42–2)
   1. The master gland
   2. Located at the base of the brain
   3. Influenced by the hypothalamus
   4. Directly affects the function of other endocrine glands
   5. Promotes growth of body tissue
   6. Influences water absorption by the kidney
   7. Controls sexual development and function

C. Adrenal gland
   1. Rests upon each kidney
   2. Regulates sodium and electrolyte balance
   3. Affects carbohydrate, fat, and protein metabolism
   4. Influences the development of sexual characteristics
   5. Sustains the "flight-or-fight" response
   6. Adrenal cortex
      a. The outer part of the adrenal gland
      b. Synthesizes glucocorticoids and mineralocorticoids and secretes small amounts of sex hormones (androgens, estrogens)
   7. Adrenal medulla
      a. The inner core of the adrenal gland
      b. Works as part of the sympathetic nervous system

   c. Produces epinephrine and norepinephrine

D. Thyroid gland
   1. Located in the anterior part of the neck
   2. Controls the rate of body metabolism and growth
   3. Produces thyroxine (T_4), triiodothyronine (T_3), and thyrocalcitonin

E. Parathyroid gland
   1. Located near the thyroid
   2. Controls calcium and phosphorus metabolism
   3. Produces parathyroid hormone (PTH)

F. Pancreas
   1. Located posterior to the liver
   2. Influences carbohydrate metabolism
   3. Indirectly influences fat and protein metabolism
   4. Produces insulin and glucagon

G. Ovaries and testes
   1. Ovaries
      a. Located in the pelvic cavity
      b. Produces estrogen and progesterone
   2. Testes
      a. Located in the scrotum
      b. Controls the development of the secondary sex characteristics
      c. Produces testosterone

BOX 42–1. Endocrine Glands

Pituitary	Parathyroid	Ovaries
Adrenal	Pancreas	Testes
Thyroid		

BOX 42–2. Pituitary Gland

ANTERIOR LOBE PRODUCTION

ACTH (adrenocorticotropic hormone)
TSH (thyroid-stimulating hormone)
STH (somatotropic growth-stimulating hormone)
FSH (follicle-stimulating hormone)
LH (luteinizing hormone)
PRL (prolactin)
GH (growth hormone)
MSH (melanocyte-stimulating hormone)

POSTERIOR LOBE PRODUCTION

ADH (vasopressin, antidiuretic hormone)
Oxytocin

II. Diagnostic Tests

A. Radioactive iodine (RAI) uptake
1. A thyroid function test that measures the absorption of the iodine isotope to determine how the thyroid gland is functioning
2. The amount of radioactivity is measured 2, 6, and 24 hours after ingestion of the capsule
3. Normal value is 5% to 35% in 24 hours
4. Elevated values are indicative of **hyperthyroidism,** thyrotoxicosis, decreased iodine intake, or increased iodine excretion
5. Decreased values indicate a low T_4, the use of antithyroid medications, thyroiditis, myxedema, or **hypothyroidism**

B. T_3 and T_4 resin uptake test
1. Blood tests for the diagnosis of thyroid disorders
2. T_3 and T_4 regulate thyroid-stimulating hormone
3. Normal values
   a. T_3: 25% to 35%
   b. T_4: 3.8% to 11.4%
4. The T_3 is elevated in **hyperthyroidism** and T_3 toxicosis, decreases with the aging process, and may be decreased in **hypothyroidism**
5. The T_4 is elevated in **hyperthyroidism** and decreased in **hypothyroidism**

C. Thyroid-stimulating hormone (TSH)
1. Blood test used to differentiate the diagnosis of primary **hypothyroidism**
2. Normal value is 0 to 6 µU/mL
3. Elevated values indicate primary **hypothyroidism**
4. Decreased values indicate **hyperthyroidism** or secondary **hypothyroidism**

D. Thyroid scan
1. Performed to identify nodules or growths in the thyroid gland
2. A radioisotope of iodine or technetium is administered prior to the scanning of the thyroid gland
3. Reassure the client that the level of radioactive medication is not dangerous to self and others
4. Determine whether the client has received radiographic contrast agents within the past 3 months, as these may invalidate the scan
5. Check with the physician regarding discontinuing medications containing iodine for 14 days prior to the test and the need to discontinue thyroid medication 4 to 6 weeks before the test
6. Instruct the client to maintain a NPO status after midnight on the day prior to the test; if iodine is used, the client will fast for an additional 45 minutes after ingestion of the oral isotope and the scan will be performed in 24 hours.
7. If technetium is used, it is administered IV 30 minutes before the scan

E. Needle aspiration of thyroid tissue
1. Aspiration of thyroid tissue for cytological examination
2. No special client preparation
3. Light pressure is applied to the aspiration site after the procedure

F. Glucose tolerance test (GTT)
1. Aids in the diagnosis of **diabetes mellitus**
2. If the glucose levels peak at higher than normal at 1 and 2 hours after injection or ingestion of glucose, and are slower than normal to return to fasting levels, then diabetes mellitus is confirmed
3. Instruct the client to eat a high-carbohydrate (200 to 300 g) diet for 3 days before the test
4. Instruct the client to avoid alcohol, coffee, and smoking for 36 hours before testing
5. Instruct the client to fast for 10 to 16 hours prior to the test
6. Instruct the client to avoid strenuous exercise for 8 hours before and after the test
7. Instruct diabetic clients to withhold morning insulin or oral hypoglycemic medication
8. Instruct clients that the test will take 3 to 5 hours, and requires IV or oral administration of glucose and multiple blood samples

G. Glycosylated hemoglobin (HbA_{1c})
1. HbA_{1c} is blood glucose bound to hemoglobin
2. HbA_{1c} is a reflection of how well blood glucose levels have been controlled in the prior 4 months
3. Hyperglycemia in diabetics is usually a cause of an increase in HbA_{1c}
4. Values are expressed as percentage of total hemoglobin
   a. Nondiabetic: 5.5% to 8.5%
   b. Diabetic with good control: 7.5% to 11.4%
   c. Diabetic with moderate control: 11.5% to 15%
   d. Diabetic with poor control: greater than 15%
5. Fasting is not required

III. Disorders of the Pituitary Gland (Box 42–3)

A. Acromegaly
1. Description
   a. The hypersecretion of growth hormone (GH) by the anterior pituitary gland

---

BOX 42–3. Pituitary Disorders

ANTERIOR PITUITARY
Acromegaly
Giantism
Dwarfism

POSTERIOR PITUITARY
Diabetes insipidus
SIADH (syndrome of inappropriate antidiuretic hormone)

b. Acromegaly occurs in middle age, after the closure of the epiphyses of the long bones

2. Data collection
   a. Large hands and feet
   b. Thickening and protrusion of the jaw
   c. Deepened voice
   d. Increased hair growth
   e. Headache and visual problems
   f. Joint pain
   g. Oily, rough skin
   h. Menstrual disturbances
   i. Impotence

3. Implementation
   a. Provide emotional support to client
   b. Encourage the client to express feelings related to altered body image
   c. Provide frequent skin care
   d. Provide pharmacologic and nonpharmacologic interventions for joint pain
   e. Prepare the client for radiation of the pituitary gland if prescribed
   f. Prepare the client for **hypophysectomy** if planned

B. Giantism
   1. Description
      a. The hypersecretion of growth hormone (GH) by the anterior pituitary gland
      b. Giantism occurs in childhood before the closure of the epiphyses of the long bones
   2. Data collection
      a. Overgrowth of long bones
      b. Increased height in early adulthood
      c. Deterioration of mental and physical status
   3. Implementation
      a. Provide emotional support to the client and family
      b. Encourage the client and family to express feelings related to altered body image
      c. Prepare the client for radiation of the pituitary gland if prescribed
      d. Prepare the client for **hypophysectomy** if planned

C. **Hypophysectomy**
   1. Description
      a. The removal of the pituitary gland
      b. Complications include increased intracranial pressure, bleeding, rhinorrhea, and meningitis
   2. Postoperative implementation
      a. Initiate postoperative care similar to craniotomy care
      b. Monitor vital signs
      c. Monitor level of consciousness and neurological status
      d. Monitor for increased ICP
      e. Monitor for bleeding
      f. Elevate the head of the bed
      g. Monitor for adrenal insufficiency
      h. Administer corticosteroids as prescribed on time
      i. Monitor fluids and electrolyte values

j. Monitor for temporary **diabetes insipidus** due to antidiuretic hormone (ADH) disturbances
k. Avoid water intoxication
l. Instruct the client to avoid sneezing, coughing, and blowing the nose
m. Instruct the client in the administration of prescribed medications

D. Dwarfism
   1. Description
      a. The hyposecretion of GH by the anterior pituitary gland
      b. Dwarfism occurs in childhood
   2. Data collection
      a. Retarded physical growth
      b. Premature aging
      c. Low intellectual development
      d. Dry skin
      e. Poor development of secondary sex characteristics
   3. Implementation
      a. Provide emotional support to the client and family
      b. Encourage the client and family to express feelings related to altered body image
      c. Prepare to administer hGH (human growth hormone)

E. **Diabetes Insipidus**
   1. Description
      a. The hyposecretion of ADH and a deficiency of vasopressin
      b. Results in failure of tubular reabsorption of water in the kidneys
   2. Data collection
      a. Polyuria of 4 to 24 L per day
      b. Polydipsia
      c. Dehydration
      d. Decreased skin turgor, dry mucous membranes
      e. Inability to concentrate urine; a low urinary-specific gravity of 1.006 or less
      f. Fatigue, muscle pain, and weakness
      g. Headache
      h. Postural hypotension
      i. Tachycardia
   3. Implementation
      a. Monitor vital signs and neurological and cardiovascular status
      b. Monitor electrolyte values
      c. Prepare to administer vasopressin tannate (Pitressin Tannate) or DDAVP (Desmopressin Acetate) as prescribed
      d. Monitor I&O, weights, specific gravity of urine
      e. Instruct the client to avoid foods or liquids with a diuretic-type action
      f. Maintain the intake of adequate fluids
      g. Instruct the client in the administration of medications as prescribed
      h. Instruct the client to wear a Medic-Alert bracelet

F. Syndrome of inappropriate antidiuretic hormone (SIADH) secretion
  1. Description
     a. A disorder of the posterior pituitary gland in which a continued release of the ADH occurs
     b. Results in water intoxication
  2. Data collection
     a. Changes in level of consciousness (LOC)
     b. Mental status changes
     c. Weight gain
     d. Hypertension
     e. Signs of fluid volume overload
     f. Tachycardia
     g. Anorexia, nausea, and vomiting
     h. Hyponatremia
  3. Implementation
     a. Monitor vital signs
     b. Monitor neurological and cardiac status
     c. Protect the client from injury
     d. Monitor I&O
     e. Obtain daily weights
     f. Restrict water intake as prescribed
     g. Monitor fluid and electrolyte balance
     h. Administer diuretics and monitor IV fluids as prescribed

IV. **Disorders of Adrenal Glands** (Box 42–4)

A. **Addison's disease**
  1. Description
     a. Hyposecretion of adrenal cortex hormones (glucocorticoids and mineralocorticoids)
     b. The condition is fatal if left untreated
  2. Data collection
     a. Weakness
     b. GI disturbances and weight loss
     c. Emotional disturbances
     d. Bronze pigmentation to the skin
     e. Electrolyte imbalances such as hyponatremia and hyperkalemia
     f. Hypotension
     g. **Hypoglycemia**
     h. Elevated blood urea nitrogen (BUN)
  3. Implementation
     a. Monitor vital signs
     b. Monitor weight and I&O
     c. Maintain fluid and electrolyte balance
     d. Monitor for infection

BOX 42–4. Disorders of Adrenal Glands

ADRENAL CORTEX
Addison's disease
Cushing's syndrome
Aldosteronism (Conn's syndrome)

ADRENAL MEDULLA
Pheochromocytoma

---

e. Instruct the client in a high-protein, high-carbohydrate diet
f. Instruct the client in the avoidance of stress
g. Instruct the client to avoid individuals with an infection
h. Instruct the client in the need for lifelong corticosteroids
i. Instruct clients to avoid over-the-counter medications
j. Instruct clients to avoid strenuous exercise
k. Instruct clients to wear a MedicAlert bracelet
l. Observe for **addisonian crisis** secondary to stress, infection, trauma, and surgery

B. **Addisonian crisis**
  1. Description
     a. A life-threatening disorder caused by acute adrenal insufficiency
     b. It is precipitated by infection, trauma, stress, or surgery
     c. Can cause hyponatremia, hyperkalemia, **hypoglycemia,** and shock
  2. Data collection
     a. Severe headache
     b. Severe abdominal, leg, and lower back pain
     c. Generalized weakness
     d. Irritability and confusion
     e. Severe hypotension
     f. Signs of shock
  3. Implementation
     a. Monitor vital signs
     b. Monitor neurological status, noting irritability and confusion
     c. Monitor I&O
     d. Monitor IV fluids as prescribed to restore electrolyte balance
     e. Administer adrenocorticosteroids as prescribed on time schedule
     f. Protect the client from infection
     g. Maintain bed rest and provide a quiet environment

C. **Cushing's syndrome**
  1. Description
     a. A condition resulting from the hypersecretion of glucocorticoids from the adrenal cortex
     b. Can result from the prolonged administration of corticosteroids
  2. Data collection
     a. Obesity with thin extremities
     b. Moonface
     c. Buffalo hump
     d. Fragile skin that easily bruises
     e. Hirsutism (masculine characteristics in female)
     f. Mood swings
     g. Muscular weakness
     h. Signs of infection
     i. Signs of osteoporosis

j. Hypertension
k. Hypokalemia
l. **Hyperglycemia** and glycosuria
m. Elevated white blood cells (WBC)
n. Sodium and water retention

3. Implementation
   a. Monitor I&O and weight
   b. Monitor for urinary glucose
   c. Provide good skin care
   d. Allow the client to discuss feelings related to body appearance
   e. High-protein, low-calorie diet with potassium supplements
   f. Prepare client for **adrenalectomy** if prescribed
   g. Prepare client for radiation if prescribed
   h. Administer hormone replacement therapy as prescribed
   i. Administer steroids as prescribed if **adrenalectomy** was performed
   j. Instruct clients in the administration of medications as prescribed
   k. Instruct clients to avoid infection, stress, and accidents
   l. Instruct the client in measures for adequate nutrition and rest

D. Aldosteronism (Conn's syndrome)
   1. Description
      a. A hypersecretion of aldosterone from the adrenal cortex of the adrenal gland
      b. Due to an adrenal lesion that is usually benign
   2. Data collection
      a. Generalized weakness
      b. Increased thirst, nocturia, and polyuria
      c. Weight gain and edema
      d. Headache
      e. Hypertension
      f. Positive **Chvostek's sign**
      g. Hypokalemia and hypernatremia
   3. Implementation
      a. Monitor vital signs
      b. Monitor I&O and weight
      c. Monitor muscular strength
      d. Monitor electrolytes
      e. Maintain sodium restriction as prescribed
      f. Administer antihypertensives and potassium supplements as prescribed
      g. Prepare the client for surgical removal of the tumor if prescribed

E. Pheochromocytoma
   1. Description
      a. A catecholamine-producing tumor, usually found in the adrenal gland but also may be found in the abdomen
      b. It causes hypersecretion of the hormones of the adrenal medulla and the secretion of excessive amounts of epinephrine and norepinephrine
      c. It is typically a benign tumor but can be malignant

      d. Surgical excision of the adrenal gland is the primary treatment
   2. Data collection
      a. Hypertension and headaches
      b. Hypermetabolism
      c. Diaphoresis, palpitations, and tachycardia
      d. Apprehension
      e. Emotional instability
      f. **Hyperglycemia** and glycosuria
      g. Pain in the chest or abdomen with nausea and vomiting
      h. Weight loss
   3. Implementation
      a. Monitor vital signs
      b. Monitor cardiovascular, neurological, and renal status
      c. Monitor for hypertensive attacks because hypertension can precipitate a CVA or sudden blindness
      d. Keep phentolamine (Regitine) at the bedside for hypertensive crisis
      e. Prepare to administer an alpha-adrenergic blocking agent, phenoxybenzamine (Dibenzyline) as prescribed to control blood pressure
      f. Be alert to stimuli that can precipitate a hypertensive crisis such as increased abdominal pressure, micturition, and vigorous abdominal palpation
      g. Avoid opiates preoperatively because they can precipitate a hypertensive crisis
      h. Monitor urine for glucose and acetone
      i. Promote rest and a nonstressful environment
      j. Provide a diet high in calories, vitamins, and minerals
      k. Prohibit caffeine-containing beverages and food

F. Adrenalectomy
   1. Description
      a. The surgical removal of an adrenal gland
      b. Lifelong steroid replacement is necessary with a bilateral **adrenalectomy**
      c. Temporary steroid replacement, up to 2 years, is necessary for a unilateral **adrenalectomy**
      d. Catecholamine levels drop as a result of surgery, which can result in cardiovascular collapse, hypotension, and shock; the client needs to be monitored closely
      e. Hemorrhage can also occur due to the high vascularity of the adrenal glands
   2. Implementation preoperative
      a. Prepare the client for surgical procedure
      b. Monitor electrolytes and correct electrolyte imbalances
      c. Monitor for cardiac irregularities
      d. Monitor for **hyperglycemia**
      e. Protect the client from infections
      f. Administer steroids as prescribed

3. Implementation postoperative
   a. Monitor vital signs
   b. Monitor I&O and if urinary output is less that 30 mL per hour notify the physician because this may be indicative of impending shock and renal failure
   c. Monitor daily weights
   d. Monitor electrolytes
   e. Monitor for signs of shock and hemorrhage particularly during first 24 to 48 hours
   f. Assess the dressing
   g. Monitor for paralytic ileus as manifested by abdominal distention and pain, nausea, vomiting, or diminished or absent bowel sounds because paralytic ileus can develop from internal bleeding
   h. Monitor IV fluids as prescribed to maintain blood volume
   i. Administer pain medication as prescribed, remembering that meperidine (Demerol) can cause hypotension
   j. Administer steroid replacement as prescribed
   k. Instruct the client in the importance of steroid therapy following surgery

V. Disorders of the Thyroid Gland (Box 42–5)

A. Cretinism
   1. Description: a severe thyroid hypofunction that results in hyposecretion of thyroid hormones in the fetus or soon after birth
   2. Data collection
      a. Severe physical and mental retardation
      b. Dry skin
      c. Coarse, dry, brittle hair
      d. Slow teething
      e. Large tongue
      f. Poor appetite
      g. Constipation
      h. Yellowish skin
      i. Potbelly with umbilical hernia
      j. Sensitivity to cold
   3. Implementation
      a. Provide emotional support
      b. Provide warmth and skin care
      c. Prevent injury
      d. Prevent constipation
      e. Encourage parents to discuss feelings regarding the disorder
      f. Administer hormone replacement of desiccated thyroid, thyroxine (Synthroid) or triiodothyronine (Cytomel) as prescribed

BOX 42–5. Disorders of the Thyroid Gland
Cretinism Myxedema Graves' disease (thyrotoxicosis, hyperthyroidism)

g. Instruct the parents regarding the administration of medication

B. **Myxedema (hypothyroidism)**
   1. Description
      a. A hypothyroid state resulting from a hyposecretion of thyroid hormone
      b. The condition occurs in adulthood
   2. Data collection
      a. Slowed rate of body metabolism
      b. Lethargy and fatigue
      c. Intolerance to cold
      d. Weight gain
      e. Dry skin and hair
      f. Loss of body hair
      g. Bradycardia
      h. Constipation
      i. Generalized puffiness and nonpitting edema
      j. Forgetfulness and loss of memory
      k. Menstrual disturbances
      l. Cardiac disorders
   3. Implementation
      a. Monitor vital signs
      b. Monitor for cardiac complications
      c. Administer and monitor thyroid replacement of desiccated thyroid, thyroxine (Synthroid) or triiodothyronine (Cytomel) as prescribed
      d. Instruct the client in low-calorie, low-cholesterol, low-saturated-fat diet
      e. Monitor the client for anorexia and constipation
      f. Provide roughage and fluids to prevent constipation
      g. Provide a warm environment for the client
      h. Avoid sedatives and narcotics due to intolerance
      i. Monitor for overdose of thyroid medications characterized by tachycardia, restlessness, nervousness, and insomnia

C. **Myxedema coma**
   1. Description
      a. A rare but serious disorder that results from a persistent low thyroid production
      b. It can be precipitated by acute illness, rapid withdrawal of thyroid medication, anesthesia and surgery, hypothermia, and the use of sedatives and narcotics
   2. Data collection
      a. Hypotension
      b. Hypothermia
      c. Bradycardia
      d. Mental depression
      e. Mood swings
      f. Hyponatremia
      g. **Hypoglycemia**
      h. Coma
   3. Implementation
      a. Maintain a patent airway
      b. Monitor vital signs and LOC
      c. Monitor the client's temperature frequently

d. Monitor IV fluids as prescribed
e. Monitor electrolytes and glucose level
f. Keep the client warm
g. Monitor for changes in mental status
h. Administer corticosteroids as prescribed
i. Avoid the use of sedatives and hypnotics

D. **Graves' disease (Hyperthyroidism)**
1. Description
   a. A hyperthyroid state resulting from a hypersecretion of thyroid hormone
   b. Also known as thyrotoxicosis
2. Data collection
   a. Increased rate of body metabolism
   b. Enlarged thyroid gland (goiter)
   c. Cardiac dysrhythmias such as tachycardia and palpitations
   d. Protruding eyeballs (exophthalmos)
   e. Hypertension
   f. Heat intolerance
   g. Diaphoresis
   h. Weight loss
   i. Smooth soft skin and hair
   j. Nervousness and fine hand tremors
   k. Personality changes
   l. Irritability and agitation
   m. Mood swings
3. Implementation
   a. Provide adequate rest
   b. Administer sedatives as prescribed
   c. Provide a cool and quiet environment
   d. Obtain daily weights
   e. Provide a high-calorie diet
   f. Avoid stimulants
   g. Provide psychosocial support
   h. Administer antithyroid medications, methimazole (Tapazole), or propylthiouracil, which blocks thyroid synthesis, as prescribed
   i. Administer iodine preparations, Lugol's solution, and saturated solution of potassium iodide (SSKI), which inhibits the release of thyroid hormone as prescribed
   j. Administer propranolol (Inderal) for tachycardia as prescribed
   k. Prepare the client for radioiodine therapy as prescribed to destroy thyroid cells
   l. Prepare the client for **thyroidectomy** if prescribed

E. **Thyroid storm**
1. Description
   a. An acute and fatal thyroid condition that occurs from manipulation of the thyroid gland during surgery and the release of thyroid hormone into the bloodstream
   b. It can also occur from severe infection and stress
2. Data collection
   a. Fever
   b. Diaphoresis
   c. Dehydration
   d. Tachycardia

e. Congestive heart failure and pulmonary edema
f. Nausea, vomiting, and diarrhea
g. Jaundice
h. Tremors
i. Irritability, agitation, and restlessness
j. Delirium and coma
3. Implementation
   a. Monitor vital signs
   b. Decrease temperature avoiding the use of salicylates as they increase free thyroid hormone levels
   c. Avoid palpating the thyroid gland
   d. Monitor I&O
   e. Monitor fluid and electrolyte balance
   f. Monitor for dehydration and overhydration
   g. Monitor pulmonary and cardiac status
   h. Administer iodine preparations, Lugol's solution, or a saturated solution of potassium iodide (SSKI), which inhibits the release of thyroid hormone as prescribed
   i. Administer propranolol (Inderal) for tachycardia and to reverse toxic manifestations of **thyroid storm** as prescribed
   j. Administer glucocorticoids as prescribed to allay stress effects
   k. Administer cardiac medications as prescribed to decrease heart activity

F. **Thyroidectomy**
1. Description
   a. Removal of the thyroid gland
   b. Performed in conditions where persistent hyperthyroidism exists
2. Implementation preoperative
   a. Obtain vital signs
   b. Obtain weight
   c. Monitor electrolyte levels
   d. Monitor for **hyperglycemia** and glycosuria
   e. Monitor level of consciousness
   f. Monitor for signs of **thyroid storm**
   g. Administer antithyroid medications as prescribed to deplete iodine and hormones
   h. Administer iodine as prescribed to decrease vascularity of the thyroid gland
3. Implementation postoperative
   a. Monitor for respiratory distress
   b. Have tracheotomy set, oxygen, and suction at the bedside
   c. Maintain a semi-Fowler's position
   d. Monitor for signs of bleeding
   e. Check the dressing anteriorly and at the back of the neck
   f. Limit talking and assess the level of hoarseness
   g. Monitor for laryngeal nerve damage as evidenced by respiratory obstruction, dysphonia, high-pitched voice, stridor, dysphagia, and restlessness

h. Monitor for signs of tetany, which can be due to trauma to the parathyroid gland
i. Prepare to administer calcium gluconate as prescribed for tetany (Box 42–6)

VI. Disorders of the Parathyroid Gland

A. Hypoparathyroidism
  1. Description
    a. A condition caused by hyposecretion of parathyroid hormone by the parathyroid gland
    b. The condition usually occurs following **thyroidectomy**
  2. Data collection
    a. Hypocalcemia and elevated phosphorus levels
    b. Numbness and tingling of extremeties
    c. Cramping
    d. Signs of tetany such as muscular spasms, irritability, seizures, positive **Trousseau's sign,** positive **Chvostek's sign,** laryngospasm, and cardiac dysrhythmias
    e. Signs of hypocalcemia such as weakness and tingling of the extremities, loss of hair, dry skin, dysrhythmias, personality changes, and renal stones
    f. Increased neuromuscular irritability
    g. Confusion
    h. Visual problems
    i. Depression
  3. Implementation
    a. Monitor vital signs
    b. Monitor cardiac status
    c. Monitor for tetany
    d. Initiate seizure precautions
    e. Place a tracheotomy set, oxygen, and suctioning at the bedside
    f. Provide a high-calcium, low-phosphorus diet
    g. Provide a quiet environment with no stimulants
    h. Administer aluminum hydroxide as prescribed to decrease phosphate levels
    i. Administer parathyroid hormone as prescribed
    j. Prepare for the administration of IV calcium gluconate for hypocalcemia
    k. Instruct the client in the administration of

calcium carbonate (Os-Cal) and vitamin D (Calciferol) as prescribed

B. Hyperparathyroidism
  1. Description: a condition caused by hypersecretion of parathyroid hormone by the parathyroid gland
  2. Data collection
    a. Bone deformities
    b. Fractures
    c. Calcium deposits in organs
    d. Gastric ulcers
    e. Nausea, vomiting, anorexia, and constipation
    f. Personality changes
    g. Polydypsia and polyuria
    h. Elevated calcium and low phosphorus levels
  3. Implementation
    a. Monitor cardiac function
    b. Monitor renal status
    c. Monitor I&O
    d. Provide hydration
    e. Monitor fluid and electrolyte balance
    f. Monitor calcium and phosphorus levels
    g. Administer furosemide (Lasix) as prescribed to lower calcium levels
    h. Monitor the administration of IV saline as prescribed to lower calcium levels
    i. The physician is notified immediately if a precipitous drop in the calcium level occurs
    j. Monitor the client for tingling and numbness in the muscles, which is caused by a sudden drop in calcium levels
    k. Administer phosphates as prescribed, which interfere with calcium absorption
    l. Prepare for the administration of calcitonin (Calcimar) as prescribed to decrease skeletal calcium release and increase renal clearance of calcium
    m. Prepare the client for parathyroidectomy as prescribed
C. Parathyroidectomy
  1. Description: removal of one or more of the parathyroid glands
  2. Implementation preoperative
    a. Monitor electrolytes, calcium, phosphate, and magnesium levels
    b. Ensure calcium levels are decreased to near normal
    c. Inform the client that talking may be painful for the first day or two postoperative
  3. Implementation postoperative
    a. Monitor for respiratory distress
    b. Place a tracheotomy set, oxygen, and suctioning at the bedside
    c. Monitor vital signs
    d. Position the client in semi-Fowler's
    e. Monitor the neck dressing for bleeding; 1 to 5 mL serosanguineous drainage is expected
    f. Monitor for hypocalcemic crisis as

BOX 42–6. Signs of Tetany

Positive Chvostek's sign
Positive Trousseau's sign
Numbness of extremities and spasm of glottis
Irritability
Wheezing and dyspnea
Visual disturbances
Muscle and abdominal cramps

evidenced by tingling and twitching in the extremities and face

    g. Monitor for positive **Trousseau's** and **Chvostek's sign,** which signals the potential of tetany

    h. Monitor for laryngeal nerve damage

    i. Monitor for changes in voice pattern and hoarseness

    j. Instruct the client in the administration of calcium and vitamin D as prescribed

VII. Disorders of the Pancreas

A. **Diabetes mellitus** (Table 42–1)

  1. Description

    a. A chronic disorder of impaired glucose intolerance and carbohydrate, protein, and lipid metabolism because of a deficiency of insulin

    b. A deficiency of insulin results in **hyperglycemia**

    c. Macrovascular complications include coronary disease, cardiomyopathy, hypertension, cerebrovascular disease, peripheral vascular disease, and infection

    d. Microvascular complications include retinopathy, nephropathy, and neuropathy

  2. Data collection

    a. Polyuria

    b. Polydipsia

    c. Polyphagia

    d. **Hyperglycemia**

    e. Weight loss

    f. Blurred vision

    g. Slow wound healing

    h. Weakness

    i. Paresthesias

    j. Signs of inadequate circulation to the feet

    k. Vaginal infections

  3. Diet

    a. Total amount of calories is individualized based on the client's current or desired weight

    b. Weight control centers around a diet high in complex carbohydrates and low in fat, behavior modification, and evaluation of eating habits

    c. As prescribed by the physician, the client

Table 42–1. Major Types of Diabetes

Type 1—Insulin-Dependent Diabetes Mellitus (IDDM)
Usually abrupt in onset
Clients require insulin injections
Occurs primarily in childhood or adolescence but can occur at any age

Type 2—Noninsulin-Dependent Diabetes Mellitus (NIDDM)
Generally slow in onset
Onset after the age of 30
Ability to produce some insulin with a favorable response to oral hypoglycemic agents

may be advised to follow the food exchange from the American Diabetic Association diet or the dietary guidelines for Americans (Food Guide Pyramid) issued by the U.S. Departments of Agriculture and Health Services

    d. Incorporate diet into individual client needs, lifestyle, cultural, and socioeconomic patterns

  4. Exercise

    a. Decreases cholesterol and triglyceride levels

    b. Decreases blood pressure

    c. Helps the body to burn excess sugar

    d. Improves circulation

    e. Encourages weight loss

    f. Decreases the body's need for oral hypoglycemic agents or insulin

    g. Instruct the client in dietary adjustments when exercising

    h. Instruct the client to monitor blood glucose prior to exercising

    i. If the exercise is of short duration and of low to moderate intensity, and if the blood glucose is less than 100 mg/dL, increase food intake by 10 to 15 g carbohydrate per hour (1 fruit or 1 starch/bread exchange)

    j. If the exercise is of moderate intensity, and if the blood glucose is less than 100 mg/dL, increase food intake by 25 to 50 g carbohydrate before exercise, then 10 to 15 g per hour of exercise (1 fruit or 1 starch/bread exchange)

    k. If the exercise is strenuous, and if the blood glucose is less than 100 mg/dL, increase food intake by 50 g carbohydrate (1 meat sandwich with a milk and fruit exchange) and monitor the blood glucose carefully

    l. If the exercise is strenuous, and if the blood glucose is between 100 and 180 mg/dL, increase food intake by 25 to 50 g carbohydrate (½ meat sandwich with a milk and fruit exchange) and monitor the blood glucose carefully

    m. If the blood glucose is 180 to 300 mg/dL or above, instruct the client not to exercise until the blood glucose is under better control

  5. Oral hypoglycemic medications

    a. Prescribed for clients with **diabetes mellitus** type 2

    b. Assess the client's knowledge of diabetes and the use of oral antidiabetic agents

    c. Monitor vital signs and blood glucose levels

    d. Assess the medications that the client is currently taking

    e. Aspirin, alcohol, sulfonamides, oral contraceptives, and MAO inhibitors increase the hypoglycemic effect

    f. Glucocorticoids, thiazide diuretics, and estrogen increase blood glucose levels

g. Instruct the client to recognize symptoms of **hypoglycemia** and **hyperglycemia**

h. Instruct the client to avoid over-the-counter medications unless prescribed by the physician

i. Instruct clients not to ingest alcohol with sulfonylureas

j. Inform the client that insulin may be needed during stress, surgery, or infection

k. Instruct the client in the necessity of compliance with prescribed medication

l. Advise the client to obtain a Medic-Alert bracelet

6. Insulin

a. Used in the treatment of insulin-dependent Type 1 diabetes mellitus and in noninsulin-dependent Type 2 diabetes mellitus when diet/weight control therapy has failed to maintain satisfactory blood glucose levels

b. Regular Insulin, the only type of insulin that can be administered by the IV route, is used in emergency treatment of ketoacidosis

c. Aspirin, alcohol, oral anticoagulants, oral hypoglycemics, beta blockers, tricyclic antidepressants, tetracycline, and MAO inhibitors increase the hypoglycemic effect when taking insulin

d. Glucocorticoids, thiazide diuretics, thyroid agents, oral contraceptives, and estrogen increase blood sugar levels

e. Illness, infection, and stress increase the need for insulin; insulin should not be withheld during illness, infection, or stress because **hyperglycemia** and ketoacidosis can result

f. Instruct the client to recognize symptoms of **hypoglycemia** and **hyperglycemia**

g. The peak action times of insulin is very important because of the possibility of hypoglycemic reactions occurring during that time

B. Complications of insulin therapy

1. **Dawn phenomenon**

a. Results from a nocturnal release of growth hormone secretion that may cause blood glucose elevations about 5:00 to 6:00 A.M.

b. Treatment includes administering an evening dose of intermediate acting insulin at 10:00 P.M.

2. **Somogyi's phenomenon**

a. A rebound phenomenon occurring in **diabetes mellitus**

b. Overtreatment with insulin induces **hypoglycemia,** which initiates the release of epinephrine, ACTH, glucagon, and growth hormone

c. Lipolysis, glyconeogenesis, and glycogenolysis result in rebound **hyperglycemia** and ketosis

d. Occurs during the initial period of serum glucose control; develops at peak insulin times and during the night

e. Treatment includes adjusting the insulin dose, the evening diet and bedtime snack and the exercise program to prevent **hypoglycemia**

C. Continuous subcutaneous infusion of insulin

1. Administered by an externally worn pump containing a syringe and reservoir with Regular Insulin connected to the client by an infusion set

2. Continuous infusion of a basal dose of insulin with meal-associated increases in insulin seems to be more effective than a multiple injection protocol in providing metabolic control

3. Buffered insulin is used to prevent the precipitation of insulin crystals within the catheter

4. Instruct the client to adjust the amount of insulin received by regulating the pump settings on the basis of blood glucose monitoring

5. To prevent infections, the needle insertion site is cleaned every 48 hours and the needle placement is changed every 3 days

6. The cessation of insulin administration quickly results in **hyperglycemia,** leading to ketoacidosis; the client is instructed to perform regular urine tests for the presence of ketones

D. Insulin pumps

1. Implanted in the peritoneal cavity where insulin can be absorbed in a more physiological manner

2. Buffered insulin is used

3. Mechanical problems are associated with the pump, the catheter, and insulin delivery

E. Blood glucose monitoring

1. Provides the client with current blood glucose levels

2. Results provide the client with information to maintain good glycemic control

3. More accurate than urine testing

4. Requires clients to prick themselves several times a day as prescribed

5. Must be used with caution with clients with diabetic retinopathy and neuropathy

6. Instruct clients in the proper procedure for obtaining blood glucose level

7. Inform the client that the procedure must be done precisely to obtain accurate results

8. Stress the importance of following the manufacturer's instructions

9. Stress the importance of handwashing before and after performing the procedure to prevent infection

10. Instruct the client to calibrate the monitor as instructed by the manufacturer

11. Instruct the client to check the expiration date on the test strips

12. Instruct the client that if blood glucose

results do not seem reasonable, reread the instructions, reassess technique, check the expiration date of the test strips, and perform the procedure again to verify results

F. Urine testing
1. Instruct clients in the procedure for testing the urine for ketones and glucose
2. Teach the client that the second voided urine specimen is most accurate
3. The presence of ketones may indicate impending ketoacidosis
4. Urine glucose testing is not recommended as a means of monitoring for clients taking insulin because it is a less reliable indicator compared with blood glucose monitoring

VIII. Acute Complications of Diabetes Mellitus

A. **Hypoglycemia (insulin reaction)**
1. Description
   a. Described as a blood glucose level below 50 mg/dL
   b. Occurs as a result of too much insulin, not enough food, or excessive activity
2. Data collection
   a. Cool, clammy skin
   b. Diaphoresis
   c. Irritable, nervous, and weepy
   d. Difficulty concentrating, speaking, focusing, and coordinating
   e. Shaky feeling, tremors, and dizziness
   f. Hunger
   g. Headache
   h. Shallow respirations
   i. Tachycardia
   j. Blood glucose below 50 mg/dL
   k. Negative ketones
   l. Late signs: hyperreflexia, dilated pupils, convulsions, shock, and coma
3. Implementation
   a. Monitor vital signs
   b. Monitor neurological status
   c. Monitor blood glucose
4. Mild **hypoglycemia** (Box 42–7)
   a. A capillary blood glucose level of 40 to 60 mg/dL
   b. Provide 10 to 15 g of carbohydrate and repeat the treatment in 10 to 15 minutes if symptoms do not subside; instruct the client to eat additional food or the next scheduled meal in 15 to 30 minutes

---

BOX 42–7. Food Items Providing 10 to 15 Grams of Carbohydrate

2–3 glucose tablets	6–10 hard candies
½ cup orange or grape juice	4 cubes sugar
½ cup regular soft drink	6 saltines
8 oz skim milk	3 graham crackers

---

5. Moderate **hypoglycemia**
   a. A capillary blood glucose level of 20 to 40 mg/dL
   b. Provide 15 to 30 g of carbohydrate and repeat the treatment in 10 to 15 minutes if symptoms do not subside
   c. Instruct the client to eat additional food such as low-fat milk or cheese after 15 to 30 minutes
6. Severe **hypoglycemia**
   a. The client who is unconscious or experiencing seizures
   b. Prepare for the administration of IM or SC glucagon or 50% dextrose IV as prescribed
   c. Administer a second dose if the client remains unconscious
   d. Provide a small meal when the client wakes up and is no longer nauseated
   e. Instruct the family on the administration of glucagon

B. **Hyperglycemia**
1. Description: described as an elevated blood glucose level
2. Data collection
   a. Gradual onset
   b. Lethargic, dulled sensorium, and confusion
   c. Thirst
   d. Weakness
   e. Nausea, vomiting, and abdominal pain
   f. Flushed
   g. Signs of dehydration
   h. Dry, crusty mucous membranes
   i. Deep rapid respirations and weak pulse
   j. Fruity, acetone breath
   k. Paresthesia and diminished reflexes
   l. Acidosis and coma
   m. Blood glucose as high as 250 mg/dL or more
   n. Ketones high
   o. Polyuria (early) to oliguria (late)
3. Implementation
   a. Instruct the client to monitor for signs of hyperglycemia
   b. Instruct clients to notify the physician when blood glucose results are greater than 250 mg/dL, when ketonuria is present for more than 24 hours, when unable to take food or fluids, and when illness persists for more than 2 days

C. **Diabetic ketoacidosis (DKA)**
1. Description
   a. A complication of **diabetes mellitus** that develops when a severe insulin deficiency occurs
   b. **DKA** is a life-threatening condition
   c. Hyperglycemia that progresses to metabolic acidosis occurs
   d. Seen in clients with IDDM, undiagnosed diabetics, and those who stop prescribed treatment for diabetes
   e. It develops over a period over several hours to days

2. Data collection
   a. Fatigue and weakness
   b. Headache
   c. Sunken eyeballs
   d. Dry mucous membranes
   e. Thirst
   f. Kussmaul's respirations
   g. Polyuria
   h. Fruity breath odor
   i. Warm, flushed skin
   j. Nausea, vomiting, and abdominal pain
   k. Tachycardia
   l. Drowsiness and stupor
   m. Urinary glucose and ketones
   n. Potassium imbalances
   o. Late signs include oliguria, anuria, and hypotension

3. Implementation
   a. Restoration of circulating volume to protect against cerebral, coronary, or renal hypoperfusion
   b. **Hyperglycemia** is corrected with IV Regular Insulin administration as prescribed
   c. Monitor vital signs, urine output, and mental status closely
   d. Correct dehydration with rapid IV infusions of 0.9% or 0.45% normal saline as prescribed
   e. Correct acidosis if pH is less than 7.10
   f. Correct electrolyte imbalance
   g. Administer oxygen as prescribed
   h. Monitor blood glucose closely
   i. Monitor client closely for signs of fluid overload
   j. Monitor potassium closely because when the client receives insulin to lower the blood glucose level, the serum potassium will decrease as the acidosis improves, and potassium replacement may be required
   k. Treat the cause of **hyperglycemia**
   l. Administer normal saline as prescribed until the blood pressure is normal; then the rate is decreased
   m. IV dextrose is added as prescribed when the blood glucose reaches 250 mg/dL
   n. Monitor potassium levels, glucose levels, urinary output, and for signs of increased intracranial pressure
   o. If blood glucose falls too far too fast before the brain has time to equilibrate, water is pulled from the blood to the CSF and the brain, causing cerebral edema and increased ICP
   p. The potassium level will fall rapidly within the first hour of treatment as fluids and insulin are replaced
   q. IV potassium is added to the IV as prescribed when the potassium reaches a normal level and urinary output is normal

D. **Hyperglycemia hyperosmolar nonketotic syndrome (HHNS)**
   1. Description
      a. Extreme **hyperglycemia** without acidosis
      b. Usually occurs in noninsulin-dependent diabetics when diabetes is uncontrolled, undiagnosed, or during stress or infection
      c. The major difference between **HHNS** and **DKA** is the lack of production of ketones with **HHNS**
      d. Onset is usually slow, taking from hours to days
   2. Data collection
      a. Polyuria, polydipsia, and polyphagia
      b. Glycosuria
      c. Dehydration
      d. Abdominal discomfort
      e. Hyperventilation
      f. Alterations in LOC
      g. Hypotension
      h. Blood glucose is extremely high from 800 up to 2400 mg/dL
      i. Absent ketones
      j. Shock and coma
   3. Implementation
      a. The most critical element is the choice and rate of fluid replacement
      b. The initial objective for fluid replacement is to raise the circulating blood volume
      c. Monitor vital signs, urine output, and mental status closely
      d. Monitor fluid and electrolyte levels closely
      e. Monitor potassium levels and glucose levels and for signs of increased intracranial pressure
      f. Hydration is corrected with IV fluids of 0.9% or 0.45% normal saline as prescribed
      g. Regular Insulin is administered IV to correct the **hyperglycemia** as prescribed
      h. Potassium is administered by IV as prescribed

IX. **Chronic Complications of Diabetes Mellitus**

A. Diabetic retinopathy
   1. Description
      a. A chronic and progressive noninflammatory impairment of the retinal circulation that eventually causes hemorrhage
      b. Permanent vision changes and blindness can occur
      c. The client has difficulty with carrying out the daily tasks of glucose testing and insulin injections
   2. Data collection
      a. A change in vision as a result of ruptured vessels
      b. Blurred vision due to macular edema
      c. Sudden loss of vision caused by retinal detachment
      d. Cataracts due to lens opacity

3. Implementation
   a. Maintain safety
   b. Early prevention by the control of hypertension and blood glucose levels
   c. Photocoagulation (laser therapy) to remove hemorrhagic tissue to decrease scarring
   d. Vitrectomy to remove vitreous hemorrhages and thus decrease tension on the retina, preventing detachment
   e. Cataract removal with lens implant

B. Diabetic nephropathy
   1. Description: a progressive decrease in kidney function as a result of the diabetes
   2. Data collection
      a. Microalbuminuria
      b. Thirst
      c. Fatigue
      d. Anemia
      e. Weight loss
      f. Signs of malnutrition
      g. Frequent urinary tract infections
      h. Signs of a neurogenic bladder
   3. Implementation
      a. Early prevention by the control of hypertension and blood glucose levels
      b. Monitor vital signs
      c. Monitor I&O
      d. Monitor BUN, creatinine, and for albuminuria
      e. Restrict dietary protein, sodium, and potassium as prescribed
      f. Avoid nephrotoxic medications
      g. Prepare the client for dialysis procedures as prescribed
      h. Prepare the client for kidney transplants as prescribed
      i. Prepare the client for pancreas transplants as prescribed

C. Diabetic neuropathy
   1. Description
      a. General deterioration of the nervous system as a result of the diabetes disease process
      b. Complications include foot injuries resulting from trauma and diabetic ulcers frequently requiring amputation
   2. Data collection
      a. Paresthesias
      b. Decreased or absent reflexes
      c. Decreased sensation to vibration or light touch
      d. Pain, aching, and burning in the lower extremities
      e. Poor peripheral pulses
      f. Skin breakdown and signs of infection
      g. Weakness or loss of sensation in cranial nerves III, IV, V, or VI
      h. Dizziness and postural hypotension
      i. Nausea and vomiting
      j. Diarrhea or constipation
      k. Incontinence
      l. Dyspareunia

BOX 42–8. Preventive Foot Care

Teach client meticulous skin care and proper foot care

Instruct client to inspect feet daily

Monitor feet for redness, swelling, or break in skin integrity; notify physician if any of these occurs

Instruct client to wash with lukewarm water and dry thoroughly

Do not soak feet

Do not treat corns, blisters, or ingrown toenails

Do not cross legs or wear tight garments that may constrict blood flow

Apply moisturizing lotion to the feet but not between the toes

Prevent moisture from accumulating between the toes

Wear loose socks and well-fitting shoes and instruct client not to go barefoot

Instruct client to avoid thermal injuries from hot water, heating pads, and baths

Change into clean cotton soaks daily

Wear socks to keep feet warm

Avoid tight-fitting garments and shoes

Do not wear the same pair of shoes 2 days in a row

Wear leather shoes

Do not wear open-toed shoes or shoes with a strap that goes between the toes

Check shoes for cracks or tears in the lining and for foreign objects before putting them on

Break in new shoes gradually

Cut toenails straight across and smooth them with an emery board

Do not smoke

---

      m. Impotence
      n. Hypoglycemic unawareness
   3. Implementation (Box 42–8)
      a. Early prevention by the control of hypertension and blood glucose levels
      b. Careful foot care to prevent trauma
      c. Apply topical capsaicin (Axsain, Zostrix) for temporary relief of neuralgia as prescribed
      d. Initiate bladder-training programs
      e. Instruct in the use of estrogen-containing lubricants for women with dyspareunia
      f. Prepare the male client with impotence for penile injections or implantable devices as prescribed
      g. Prepare for surgical decompression for compression lesions related to the cranial nerves as prescribed

X. Operative Care for the Diabetic Client

A. Preoperative care
   1. Discontinue sulfonyurea medications as prescribed 36 to 72 hours before surgery
   2. Monitor blood glucose
   3. Monitor IV fluids as prescribed
   4. Administer insulin as prescribed

5. In stable clients undergoing minor procedures, hold the prescribed morning dose of insulin or oral agent if the client is fasting; monitor blood glucose levels and notify the physician of results, because a supplemental short-acting insulin may be prescribed preoperatively

B. Postoperative care
  1. Monitor glucose and insulin infusions as prescribed until the client can tolerate oral feedings
  2. Administer supplemental short-acting insulin as prescribed based on blood glucose results
  3. Monitor blood glucose levels closely if the diabetic is receiving TPN
  4. When the client is tolerating food, ensure that the client receives an adequate amount of carbohydrates daily to prevent **hypoglycemia** and ketosis

C. Whole pancreas transplants
  1. The goal of pancreatic transplantation is to halt or reverse the complications of diabetes
  2. The pancreas is transplanted into the peritoneal cavity with drainage of exocrine secretions into the urinary bladder
  3. Monitor urinary amylase because a decrease indicates the need to treat the client for rejection
  4. **Hyperglycemia** is a late sign of rejection and indicates irreversible graft failure
  5. Immunosuppressive therapy is prescribed to prevent and treat rejection
  6. Inform the client that the potential for future insulin injections may be necessary to treat hyperglycemia caused by immunosuppressive medications

PRACTICE QUESTIONS

1. The nurse is caring for a client following hypophysectomy. The nurse notices clear nasal drainage from the client's nostril. The initial nursing action is to
   1 Continue to observe the drainage
   2 Test the drainage for glucose
   3 Lower the head of the bed
   4 Obtain a culture of the drainage

2. Following several diagnostic tests, a client is diagnosed with diabetes insipidus. The nurse understands that which of the following symptoms is indicative of this disorder?
   1 Diarrhea
   2 Polydipsia
   3 Weight gain
   4 Fatigue

3. The nurse caring for a client with Addison's disease expects to note which of the following?
   1 Obesity
   2 Edema
   3 Hypotension
   4 Hirsutism

4. The client with Cushing's syndrome verbalizes concern to the nurse regarding the appearance of the buffalo hump that has developed. Which of the following statements by the nurse is most appropriate?
   1 "This is permanent, but looks are deceiving and not that important."
   2 "Don't be concerned, this problem can be covered with clothing."
   3 "Try not to worry about it, there are other things to be concerned about."
   4 "Usually these physical changes slowly improve following treatment."

5. The nurse assists in developing a plan of care for a client with Graves' disease. Which of the following does the nurse include in the plan of care?
   1 Provide small meals
   2 Provide the client with extra blankets
   3 Provide a high-fiber diet
   4 Provide a restful environment

6. The nurse is caring for a client following thyroidectomy. The nurse notes that calcium gluconate is prescribed for the client. The nurse determines that this medication has been prescribed to
   1 Treat thyroid storm
   2 Prevent cardiac irritability
   3 Stimulate release of parathyroid hormone
   4 Treat hypocalcemic tetany

7. The nurse is collecting data on the client following a thyroidectomy. The nurse notes that the client has developed hoarseness and a weak voice. Which of the following nursing actions is appropriate?
   1 Notify the physician immediately
   2 Reassure the client that this is usually a temporary condition
   3 Check for signs of bleeding
   4 Administer calcium gluconate

8. A client is admitted to the emergency department and a diagnosis of myxedema coma is made. Which of the following nursing actions does the nurse prepare to carry out initially?
   1 Warming the client
   2 Replacing fluid
   3 Maintaining an airway
   4 Administrating thyroid hormone

9. The client is taking NPH Insulin daily every morning. The nurse instructs the client that the most likely time for a hypoglycemic reaction to occur is
   1 2 to 4 hours after administration
   2 6 to 12 hours after administration
   3 12 to 16 hours after administration
   4 18 to 24 hours after administration

10. The client with Type 1 diabetes is to begin an exercise program and the nurse is reinforcing instructions to the client regarding the program. Which of the following does the nurse include in the teaching plan?
    1 Exercise is best performed during peak times of insulin
    2 Administer insulin after exercising
    3 Take a blood glucose test before exercising
    4 Try to exercise prior to mealtime

11. The nurse is assisting in preparing a teaching plan for the diabetic client regarding proper foot care. Which of the following instructions should be included in the plan?
    1 Soak feet in hot water
    2 Apply a lanolin lotion to dry feet
    3 Always have a podiatrist cut your toenails, never cut them yourself
    4 Avoid using soap on the feet

12. The nurse provides dietary instructions to a diabetic client regarding the prescribed diabetic diet. Which statement, if made by the client, indicates a need for further teaching?
    1 "I need to drink diet soft drinks."
    2 "I'll follow a balanced meal plan."
    3 "I need to buy special dietetic foods."
    4 "I'll snack on fruit instead of cake."

13. An external insulin pump is prescribed for the client with diabetes. The client asks the nurse about the functioning of the pump. The nurse plans to base the response on the information that the pump
    1 Gives a small continuous does of regular insulin subcutaneously and the client can self-bolus with additional dosage from the pump prior to each meal
    2 Is timed to release programmed doses of Regular or NPH Insulin into the bloodstream at specific intervals
    3 Is surgically attached to the pancreas and infuses Regular Insulin into the pancreas, which in turn releases the insulin into the bloodstream
    4 Continuously infuses small amounts of NPH Insulin into the bloodstream while regularly monitoring blood glucose levels

14. The newly diagnosed client with diabetes mellitus has been stabilized with insulin injections daily. The nurse assists in preparing a discharge teaching plan regarding the insulin. The teaching plan reinforces which of the following concepts?
    1 Increase the amount of insulin prior to unusual exercise
    2 Acetone in the urine will signify a need for less insulin
    3 Always keep insulin vials refrigerated
    4 Systematically rotate insulin injection sites

15. The client received 20 units of NPH Insulin subcutaneously at 8:00 A.M. The nurse should monitor the client for a hypoglycemic reaction at
    1 10:00 A.M.
    2 11:00 A.M.
    3 5:00 P.M.
    4 11:00 P.M.

16. The nurse reinforces teaching with a diabetic client about differentiating between hypoglycemia and ketoacidosis. The client demonstrates an understanding of the teaching by stating that glucose will be taken if which of the following symptoms develops.
    1 Fruity breath odor
    2 Shakiness
    3 Blurred vision
    4 Polyuria

17. A diabetic client demonstrates acute anxiety when first admitted for the treatment of hyperglycemia. The most appropriate intervention to decrease the client's anxiety is to
    1 Administer a sedative
    2 Make sure the client knows all the correct medical terms to understand what is happening
    3 Ignore the signs and symptoms of anxiety so that they will soon disappear
    4 Convey empathy, trust, and respect toward the client

18. The nurse reinforces instructions to a newly diagnosed Type 1 diabetic client. The nurse evaluates accurate understanding of measures to prevent diabetic ketoacidosis (DKA) when the client says
    1 "I will stop taking my insulin if I'm too sick to eat."
    2 "I will decrease my insulin dose during times of illness."
    3 "I will notify my physician if my blood glucose level is greater than 250 mg/dL."
    4 "I will adjust my insulin dose according to the level of glucose in my urine."

19. The nurse assists in developing a plan of care for a client with hyperparathyroidism receiving calcitonin (Calcimar). Which of the following outcome criteria has the highest priority regarding this medication?
    1 Absence of side effects
    2 Achievement of normal serum calcium levels
    3 Relief of pain
    4 Verbalization of appropriate medication knowledge

20. The physician prescribes levothyroxine (Synthroid) 0.15 mg PO daily for the client with hypothyroidism. The nurse prepares to administer this medication
    1 Three times a day in equal doses of 0.5 mg each to ensure consistent serum drug levels
    2 In the morning to prevent sleeplessness

3 Only when the client complains of fatigue and cold intolerance

4 At various times of the day to prevent tolerance from occurring

21. The nurse is monitoring a client receiving chlorpropamide (Diabenese). The nurse understands that which of the following is not a therapeutic outcome for this client?
   1 A decrease in polyuria
   2 An FBS of 110
   3 A decrease in polyphagia
   4 A glycosylated hemoglobin of 10%

22. The nurse is monitoring a newly diagnosed diabetic client for signs of complications. Which of the following, if exhibited in the client, indicates hyperglycemia and warrants physician notification?
   1 Hypertension
   2 Diaphoresis
   3 Polyuria
   4 Increased pulse rate

23. The nurse is planning to reinforce instructions with a client with diabetes mellitus recovering from diabetic ketoacidosis (DKA) to develop a plan to prevent a recurrence. Which of the following is most important to include in the plan of care?
   1 Eat 6 small meals per day
   2 Receive appropriate follow-up health care
   3 Monitor blood glucose levels frequently
   4 Test urine for ketone levels

24. The nurse is collecting data from a client with Type 2 diabetes mellitus. Which statement by the client indicates an understanding of the medications?
   1 "I am taking oral insulin instead of shots."
   2 "The medications I'm taking help release the insulin I already make."
   3 "By taking these medications I am able to eat more."
   4 "When I become ill I need to increase the number of pills I take."

25. The client with IDDM is having trouble remembering the types, duration, and onset of action of insulin. The client's family members have not been supportive. The nurse's best response is
   1 "You can't always depend on your family to help."
   2 "Let me go over the types of insulin with you again."
   3 "It's not really necessary for you to remember this."
   4 "What is it you don't understand?"

26. A nurse is doing discharge teaching with a client who has Cushing's syndrome. Which of the following statements by the client indicates that instructions related to dietary management were understood?
   1 "I am fortunate that I do not need to follow any special diet."
   2 "I will need to limit the amount of protein in my diet."
   3 "I am fortunate that I can eat all the salty foods I enjoy."
   4 "I can eat foods that have a lot of potassium in them."

27. A client with Type 1 diabetes calls the nurse to report recurrent episodes of hypoglycemia. Which of the following statements by the client indicates an inadequate understanding of NPH Insulin and exercise?
   1 "The best time for me to exercise is every afternoon."
   2 "The best time for me to exercise is after lunch."
   3 "The best time for me to exercise is after dinner."
   4 "The best time for me to exercise is before bedtime."

28. The nurse is collecting data from an elderly client who is being admitted for a diagnostic workup for primary hyperparathyroidism. The nurse understands that which client complaint is characteristic of this disorder?
   1 Diarrhea
   2 Polyuria
   3 Polyphagia
   4 Weight gain

29. The nurse is caring for a postoperative parathyroidectomy client. Which client complaint indicates that a serious life-threatening complication may be developing requiring immediate notification of the physician?
   1 Difficulty voiding
   2 Abdominal cramps
   3 Laryngeal stridor
   4 Mild to moderate incisional pain

30. The nurse is preparing to discharge a client who has had parathyroidectomy. Part of your discharge instructions include medication administration for oral calcium supplements that the client will need daily. Which statement by the nurse is appropriate regarding oral calcium supplement therapy?
   1 Store the tablets in the refrigerator to maintain potency
   2 Check the pulse daily, if it is below 60 bpm, do not take the tablets
   3 Take the tablets with food or following a meal
   4 Avoid sunlight because it can cause skin color change

31. The nurse notes that the Type 1 diabetic has lipodystrophy on both upper thighs. The nurse appropriately inquires if the client
    1 Cleanses the skin with alcohol before each injection
    2 Rotates sites for injection
    3 Aspirates for blood prior to injection into the subcutaneous tissue
    4 Administers the insulin at a 45-degree angle

32. The nurse is caring for a Type 1 diabetic client. Which of the following client complaints alerts the nurse of a possible hypoglycemic reaction?
    1 Hot, dry skin
    2 Muscle cramps
    3 Anorexia
    4 Tremors

33. A young Type 1 male diabetic client tells the nurse that he might lose his job because he has been having frequent hypoglycemic reactions. His boss thinks that he is drunk during these episodes and that he has been drinking on the job. Which action by the nurse best assists this client to meet his needs?
    1 Contact the local employment office to help him find another job
    2 Ask the client if he indeed has been drinking at work
    3 Examine factors with the client that may be causing frequent hypoglycemic episodes
    4 Ask the client what he does to treat his hypoglycemia

34. The nurse needs to maintain food and fluid intake to minimize the risk of dehydration in a frail, elderly, diabetic client with gastroenteritis. An appropriate intervention for the nurse to perform is
    1 Offer water only, until the client is able to tolerate solid foods
    2 Withhold all fluids until vomiting has ceased for at least 4 hours
    3 Encourage the client to take 8 to 12 oz of fluid every hour while awake
    4 Maintain a clear liquid diet for at least 5 days before advancing to allow inflammation of the bowel to dissipate

35. A client who is currently taking levothyroxine (Synthroid) complains of cold intolerance, constipation, dry skin, weight gain, and puffy eyes. Based on these findings, the nurse anticipates which of the following prescriptions?
    1 Increase Synthroid dosage after checking T_4 level
    2 Decrease Synthroid dosage after checking T_4 level
    3 Discontinue Synthroid; the client is having an adverse reaction
    4 No change in medication, these are common side effects that will diminish with time

36. The nurse is caring for a client with diabetes insipidus receiving vasopressin (Pitressin). The nurse understands that which of the following is not a therapeutic effect of this medication?
    1 Increased gastrointestinal tract smooth muscle tone and contractions
    2 Decreased urine output
    3 Increases reabsorption of water by the renal tubules
    4 Vasodilation of vascular vessels

37. The client is diagnosed with pheochromocytoma. The nurse assists in preparing a nursing care plan for the client and understands that pheochromocytoma is a condition
    1 That causes profound hypotension
    2 That causes the release of excessive amounts of catecholamines
    3 That is not curable and is treated symptomatically
    4 That is manifested by severe hypoglycemia

38. The nurse is collecting data on a client admitted with a diagnosis of pheochromocytoma. The nurse observes for the major symptom associated with pheochromocytoma when:
    1 Testing the client's urine for glucose
    2 Taking the client's weight
    3 Palpating the skin for its temperature
    4 Taking the client's blood pressure

39. The nurse is caring for a client with pheochromocytoma. The client is scheduled for adrenalectomy. In the preoperative period, the priority nursing action is to monitor:
    1 Vital signs
    2 Urine for glucose and acetone
    3 Intake and output
    4 BUN (blood urea nitrogen) lab values

40. The nurse is caring for a client with pheochromocytoma. The client asks for a snack and something warm to drink. The most appropriate choice for this client to meet nutritional needs is which of the following?
    1 Graham crackers and warm milk
    2 Toast with peanut butter and cocoa
    3 Crackers with cheese and tea
    4 Vanilla wafers and coffee with cream and sugar

41. The nurse is caring for a client with pheochromocytoma. Which of the following data indicates a potential complication associated with pheochromocytoma?
    1 A urinary output of 50 mL per hour
    2 Rales heard on auscultation
    3 A BUN (blood urea nitrogen) of 20 mg/dL
    4 A coagulation time of 5 minutes

42. The client with pheochromocytoma is scheduled for surgery and says to the nurse, "I'm not sure

that surgery is the best thing to do." The most appropriate response by the nurse is which of the following?

1 "You have concerns about the surgical treatment for your condition."
2 "There is no reason to worry. Your doctor is a wonderful surgeon."
3 "You are very ill. Your physician has made the correct decision."
4. "I think you are making the right decision to have the surgery."

43. The nurse is caring for a client following thyroidectomy and is monitoring for signs of thyroid storm. The nurse understands that which of the following is a manifestation associated with this disorder?

1 Low-grade temperature
2 Bradycardia
3 Hypotension
4 Constipation

44. The nurse is providing instructions to the client with Addison's disease regarding diet therapy. The nurse understands that which of the following diets is most likely prescribed for this client?

1 Low sodium
2 High sodium
3 Low protein
4 Low carbohydrate

45. The nursing instructor asks the student to describe the pathophysiology that occurs in Cushing's disease. Which of the following statements by the student indicates an accurate understanding of this disorder?

1 "It is characterized by an oversecretion of glucocorticoid hormones."
2 "It is characterized by an undersecretion of glucocorticoid hormones."
3 "It is characterized by an oversecretion of insulin."
4 "It is characterized by an undersecretion of corticotropic hormones."

ANSWERS

1. **2**

RATIONALE: Following hypophysectomy, the client is monitored for rhinorrhea, which could indicate a CFS leak. If this occurs, the drainage should be collected and tested for the presence of CSF. The head of the bed should not be lowered, to prevent increased intracranial pressure. Clear nasal drainage does not indicate the need for a culture. Continuing to observe the drainage without taking action could result in a serious complication.

TEST-TAKING STRATEGY: Note the key word "initial." This indicates that an action is required. Option 3 can be easily eliminated. Option 4 can be easily eliminated because the drainage is clear. Because an action is required, eliminate option 1. Review the complications following hypophysectomy if you had difficulty with this question.

LEVEL OF COGNITIVE ABILITY: Application
PHASE OF NURSING PROCESS: Implementation
CLIENT NEEDS: Physiological Integrity
CONTENT AREA: Adult Health/Endocrine
REFERENCE
Black, J., & Matassarin-Jacobs, E. (1997). *Medical-surgical nursing: Clinical management for continuity of care* (5th ed.). Philadelphia: W. B. Saunders. p. 2064.

2. **2**

RATIONALE: Polydipsia and polyuria are classic symptoms of diabetes insipidus. The urine is pale in color and the specific gravity is low. Anorexia and weight loss occur.

TEST-TAKING STRATEGY: Eliminate option 4 first because this symptom is rather vague and occurs in many conditions. Knowledge of the manifestations of diabetes insipidus will assist in eliminating options 1 and 3. If you had difficulty with this question, review the clinical manifestations associated with diabetes insipidus.

LEVEL OF COGNITIVE ABILITY: Comprehension
PHASE OF NURSING PROCESS: Data Collection
CLIENT NEEDS: Physiological Integrity
CONTENT AREA: Adult Health/Endocrine
REFERENCE
Monahan, F., & Neighbors, M. (1998). *Medical-surgical nursing: Foundations for clinical practice* (2nd ed.). Philadelphia: W. B. Saunders. pp. 1274–1275.

3. **3**

RATIONALE: Common manifestations of Addison's disease include postural hypotension from fluid loss, syncope, muscle weakness, anorexia, nausea and vomiting, abdominal cramps, weight loss, depression, and irritability.

TEST-TAKING STRATEGY: Knowledge regarding the clinical manifestations associated with Addison's disease is required to answer this question. If you had difficulty with this question, be sure to review this very important endocrine disorder.

LEVEL OF COGNITIVE ABILITY: Comprehension
PHASE OF NURSING PROCESS: Data Collection
CLIENT NEEDS: Physiological Integrity
CONTENT AREA: Adult Health/Endocrine
REFERENCE
Monahan, F., & Neighbors, M. (1998). *Medical-surgical nursing: Foundations for clinical practice* (2nd ed.). Philadelphia: W. B. Saunders. p. 1278.

4. **4**

RATIONALE: The client with Cushing's syndrome should be reassured that most physical changes resolve with treatment. Options 1, 2, and 3 are not therapeutic responses.

TEST-TAKING STRATEGY: Use knowledge regarding the physical changes that occur in Cushing's syndrome to answer this question. If you are unfamiliar with this disorder, you can easily eliminate options 1, 2, and 3 because these statements are not therapeutic responses to a client.

LEVEL OF COGNITIVE ABILITY: Application
PHASE OF NURSING PROCESS: Implementation
CLIENT NEEDS: Psychosocial Integrity
CONTENT AREA: Adult Health/Endocrine
REFERENCE
Monahan, F., & Neighbors, M. (1998). *Medical-surgical nursing: Foundations for clinical practice* (2nd ed.). Philadelphia: W. B. Saunders. p. 1289.

5. 4

RATIONALE: Because of the hypermetabolic state, the client with Graves' disease needs to be provided with an environment that is restful both physically and mentally. Six full high-calorie, well-balanced meals a day are required because of the accelerated metabolic rate. Foods that increase peristalsis such as high-fiber foods need to be avoided. These clients suffer from heat intolerance and require a cool environment.
TEST-TAKING STRATEGY: The key concept to bear in mind when answering this question is that clients with Graves' disease experience an accelerated metabolic rate. This concept should assist you in eliminating options 1, 2, and 3.
LEVEL OF COGNITIVE ABILITY: Application
PHASE OF NURSING PROCESS: Planning
CLIENT NEEDS: Physiological Integrity
CONTENT AREA: Adult Health/Endocrine
REFERENCE
Monahan, F., & Neighbors, M. (1998). *Medical-surgical nursing: Foundations for clinical practice* (2nd ed.). Philadelphia: W. B. Saunders. p. 1307.

6. 4

RATIONALE: Hypocalcemia can develop after thyroidectomy if the parathyroid glands are accidentally removed during surgery. Manifestations develop 1 to 7 days after surgery. If the client develops numbness and tingling around the mouth, fingertips or toes; muscle spasms; or twitching, the physician is notified immediately. Calcium gluconate should be kept at the bedside.
TEST-TAKING STRATEGY: Noting the name of the medication (calcium gluconate) should easily direct you to option 4. Calcium is given if hypocalcemic tetany occurs.
LEVEL OF COGNITIVE ABILITY: Comprehension
PHASE OF NURSING PROCESS: Planning
CLIENT NEEDS: Physiological Integrity
CONTENT AREA: Pharmacology
REFERENCE
Monahan, F., & Neighbors, M. (1998). *Medical-surgical nursing: Foundations for clinical practice* (2nd ed.). Philadelphia: W. B. Saunders. p. 1314.

7. 2

RATIONALE: Weakness and hoarseness of the voice can occur due to trauma or damage of the laryngeal nerve. If this develops, the client should be reassured that the problem will subside in a few days. Unnecessary talking should be discouraged. It is not necessary to notify the physician. These signs do not indicate bleeding or the need to administer calcium gluconate.
TEST-TAKING STRATEGY: Knowledge regarding the complications following thyroidectomy will easily direct you to option 2. Options 3 and 4 can easily be eliminated because they are unrelated to the signs presented in the question. There are no data presented requiring physician notification.

LEVEL OF COGNITIVE ABILITY: Application
PHASE OF NURSING PROCESS: Implementation
CLIENT NEEDS: Physiological Integrity
CONTENT AREA: Adult Health/Endocrine
REFERENCE
Monahan, F., & Neighbors, M. (1998). *Medical-surgical nursing: Foundations for clinical practice* (2nd ed.). Philadelphia: W. B. Saunders. p. 1314.

8. 3

RATIONALE: The initial nursing action is to maintain a patent airway. Oxygen is administered followed by fluid replacement, keeping the client warm, monitoring vital signs, and administering thyroid hormones by IV.
TEST-TAKING STRATEGY: Note the key phrase "carry out initially." All of the options are appropriate interventions, but use the ABCs in selecting the correct option.
LEVEL OF COGNITIVE ABILITY: Application
PHASE OF NURSING PROCESS: Implementation
CLIENT NEEDS: Physiological Integrity
CONTENT AREA: Adult Health/Endocrine
REFERENCE
Monahan, F., & Neighbors, M. (1998). *Medical-surgical nursing: Foundations for clinical practice* (2nd ed.). Philadelphia: W. B. Saunders. p. 1298.

9. 2

RATIONALE: NPH is an intermediate-acting insulin. The onset of action is 1 to 2 hours, it peaks in 6 to 12 hours, and its duration of action is 18 to 24 hours. Hypoglycemic reactions most likely occur during peak time.
TEST-TAKING STRATEGY: Knowledge regarding the onset, peak, and duration of action for NPH Insulin is required to answer this question. Be sure to learn these characteristics of NPH Insulin.
LEVEL OF COGNITIVE ABILITY: Application
PHASE OF NURSING PROCESS: Implementation
CLIENT NEEDS: Health Promotion and Maintenance
CONTENT AREA: Pharmacology
REFERENCE
Lehne, R. (1998). *Pharmacology for nursing care* (3rd ed.). Philadelphia: W. B. Saunders. p. 580.

10. 3

RATIONALE: A blood glucose test performed before exercising lets the client know whether to eat a snack first. Exercising during the peak times of insulin or prior to mealtime places the client at risk for hypoglycemia. Insulin should be administered as prescribed.
TEST-TAKING STRATEGY: The issue of the question relates to the occurrence of a hypoglycemia reaction. Use the process of elimination, keeping in mind this issue and the action of insulin. You should easily be able to eliminate options 1, 2, and 4.
LEVEL OF COGNITIVE ABILITY: Application
PHASE OF NURSING PROCESS: Planning
CLIENT NEEDS: Health Promotion and Maintenance
CONTENT AREA: Adult Health/Endocrine
REFERENCE
Monahan, F., & Neighbors, M. (1998). *Medical-surgical nursing: Foundations for clinical practice* (2nd ed.). Philadelphia: W. B. Saunders. p. 1234.

11. 2

RATIONALE: The client should be instructed not to soak the feet and should avoid hot water to prevent burns. The client should cut toenails straight and even with the toe itself and consult a podiatrist if the toenails are thick, hard to cut, or vision is poor. The client should be instructed to wash the feet daily using a mild soap.

TEST-TAKING STRATEGY: Eliminate option 3 first because of the word "always." Options 1 and 4 can be easily eliminated, leaving option 2 as the correct choice. Review diabetic foot care instructions now if you had difficulty with this question.

LEVEL OF COGNITIVE ABILITY: Application
PHASE OF NURSING PROCESS: Planning
CLIENT NEEDS: Health Promotion and Maintenance
CONTENT AREA: Adult Health/Endocrine
REFERENCE
Monahan, F., & Neighbors, M. (1998). *Medical-surgical nursing: Foundations for clinical practice* (2nd ed.). Philadelphia: W. B. Saunders. p. 1252.

12. 3

RATIONALE: It is important to emphasize to the client and family that they are not eating a diabetic diet but rather following a balanced meal plan. Adherence to nutrition principles is an important component of diabetic management, and an individualized meal plan should be developed for the client.

TEST-TAKING STRATEGY: Careful reading of this question and the options will easily direct you to the correct answer. Note the key phrase "indicates a need for further teaching." By the process of elimination you will easily be directed to option 3.

LEVEL OF COGNITIVE ABILITY: Comprehension
PHASE OF NURSING PROCESS: Evaluation
CLIENT NEEDS: Health Promotion and Maintenance
CONTENT AREA: Adult Health/Endocrine
REFERENCE
Monahan, F., & Neighbors, M. (1998). *Medical-surgical nursing: Foundations for clinical practice* (2nd ed.). Philadelphia: W. B. Saunders. p. 1231.

13. 1

RATIONALE: An insulin pump provides a small continuous dose of Regular Insulin subcutaneously throughout the day and night and the client can self-bolus with additional dosage from the pump prior to each meal as needed. Regular Insulin is used in an insulin pump. An external pump is not surgically attached to the pancreas.

TEST-TAKING STRATEGY: Knowledge that Regular Insulin is used in an insulin pump will assist in eliminating options 2 and 4. Careful reading of the question and noting the word "external" will assist in eliminating option 3. Review the used of the insulin pump now if you are unfamiliar with it.

LEVEL OF COGNITIVE ABILITY: Comprehension
PHASE OF NURSING PROCESS: Planning
CLIENT NEEDS: Physiological Integrity
CONTENT AREA: Adult Health/Endocrine
REFERENCE
Monahan, F., & Neighbors, M. (1998). *Medical-surgical nursing: Foundations for clinical practice* (2nd ed.). Philadelphia: W. B. Saunders. pp. 1238–1239.

14. 4

RATIONALE: Insulin dosages should not be adjusted and should not be increased prior to unusual exercise. If acetone is found in the urine, it may possibly indicate the need for additional insulin. To minimize the discomfort associated with insulin injections, insulin should be administered at room temperature. Injection sites should be systematically rotated from one area to another. The client should be instructed to give injections in one area, about an inch apart, until the whole area has been used, then change to another site. This prevents dramatic changes in daily insulin absorption.

TEST-TAKING STRATEGY: Eliminate option 3 first because of the word "always." Knowledge regarding insulin administration and the significance of acetone in the urine will assist in eliminating options 1 and 2. If you had difficulty with this question, take time now to review insulin management.

LEVEL OF COGNITIVE ABILITY: Comprehension
PHASE OF NURSING PROCESS: Planning
CLIENT NEEDS: Health Promotion and Maintenance
CONTENT AREA: Pharmacology
REFERENCE
Monahan, F., & Neighbors, M. (1998). *Medical-surgical nursing: Foundations for clinical practice* (2nd ed.). Philadelphia: W. B. Saunders. p. 1224.

15. 3

RATIONALE: NPH is an intermediate-acting insulin. The onset of action is 1 to 2 hours, it peaks in 6 to 12 hours, and its duration of action is 18 to 24 hours. Hypoglycemic reactions most likely occur during peak time.

TEST-TAKING STRATEGY: Knowledge regarding the onset, peak, and duration of action for NPH Insulin is required to answer this question. Knowing that peak action is between 6 and 12 hours will easily direct you to option 3. Be sure to learn these characteristics of NPH Insulin

LEVEL OF COGNITIVE ABILITY: Application
PHASE OF NURSING PROCESS: Planning
CLIENT NEEDS: Physiological Integrity
CONTENT AREA: Pharmacology
REFERENCE
Lehne, R. (1998). *Pharmacology for nursing care* (3rd ed.). Philadelphia: W. B. Saunders. p. 580.

16. 2

RATIONALE: Shakiness is a sign of hypoglycemia and indicates the need for food, glucose, or glycogen. A fruity breath odor, blurred vision, and polyuria are signs of hyperglycemia.

TEST-TAKING STRATEGY: Knowledge regarding the signs and symptoms of hypoglycemia and hyperglycemia is required to answer this question. If you are unfamiliar with these signs, be sure to learn them.

LEVEL OF COGNITIVE ABILITY: Comprehension
PHASE OF NURSING PROCESS: Evaluation
CLIENT NEEDS: Health Promotion and Maintenance
CONTENT AREA: Adult Health/Endocrine
REFERENCE
Monahan, F., & Neighbors, M. (1998). *Medical-surgical nursing: Foundations for clinical practice* (2nd ed.). Philadelphia: W. B. Saunders. p. 1251.

17. 4

RATIONALE: The most appropriate intervention is to address the client's feelings related to the anxiety. Administering a sedative is not the most appropriate intervention. The nurse should not ignore the client's anxious feelings. A client will not relate to medical terms, particularly when anxious.

TEST-TAKING STRATEGY: Use therapeutic communica-

tion techniques to answer the question. Remember that the client's feelings come first. Keeping this in mind will easily direct you to option 4.
LEVEL OF COGNITIVE ABILITY: Application
PHASE OF NURSING PROCESS: Implementation
CLIENT NEEDS: Psychosocial Integrity
CONTENT AREA: Adult Health/Endocrine
REFERENCE
Leahy, J., & Kizilay, P. (1998). *Foundations of nursing practice: A nursing process approach.* Philadelphia: W. B. Saunders. p. 223.

18. **3**

RATIONALE: During illness, the client should monitor blood glucose levels and notify the physician if the level is over 250 mg/dL. Insulin should never be stopped; in fact, it may need to be increased. Doses should not be adjusted without the physician's advice.
TEST-TAKING STRATEGY: Note that options 1, 2, and 4 all relate to adjustment of insulin doses. Therefore, eliminate these options. Review diabetic management during illness now if you had difficulty with this question.
LEVEL OF COGNITIVE ABILITY: Comprehension
PHASE OF NURSING PROCESS: Evaluation
CLIENT NEEDS: Health Promotion and Maintenance
CONTENT AREA: Adult Health/Endocrine
REFERENCE
Monahan, F., & Neighbors, M. (1998). *Medical-surgical nursing: Foundations for clinical practice* (2nd ed.). Philadelphia: W. B. Saunders. pp. 1240–1241.

19. **2**

RATIONALE: Calcitonin can lower plasma calcium levels in clients with hypercalcemia secondary to hyperparathyroidism. The therapeutic effect in this client situation is a reduction in serum calcium levels. Calcitonin is a very safe medication. It is the medication of choice for rapid relief of pain associated with Paget's disease.
TEST-TAKING STRATEGY: Reading the question carefully and noting the client diagnosis will assist in directing you to option 2. Additionally, note the relationship between the name of the medication and the word "calcium" in option 2. If you are unfamiliar with this medication, take time now to review.
LEVEL OF COGNITIVE ABILITY: Analysis
PHASE OF NURSING PROCESS: Evaluation
CLIENT NEEDS: Physiological Integrity
CONTENT AREA: Adult Health/Endocrine
REFERENCE
Lehne, R. (1998). *Pharmacology for nursing care* (3rd ed.). Philadelphia: W. B. Saunders. pp. 820, 828.

20. **2**

RATIONALE: Synthroid is a synthetic thyroid hormone that increases cellular metabolism. It should be given in the morning in a single dose to prevent sleeplessness. It should be given at the same time each day to maintain drug level.
TEST-TAKING STRATEGY: Options 3 and 4 can be eliminated because it is not the nurse's decision to change or alter a physician's order. When choosing between options 1 and 2, option 2 has more validity based on common nursing sense, even if you do not know the action of Synthroid.
LEVEL OF COGNITIVE ABILITY: Application
PHASE OF NURSING PROCESS: Planning
CLIENT NEEDS: Physiological Integrity
CONTENT AREA: Adult Health/Endocrine

REFERENCE
Hodgson, B., & Kizior, R. (1999). *Saunders nursing drug handbook 1999.* Philadelphia: W. B. Saunders. pp. 589–590.

21. **4**

RATIONALE: Chlorpropamide is an oral hypoglycemic agent given to reduce serum glucose and the signs and symptoms of hyperglycemia. Therefore, a decrease in both polyuria and polyphagia and symptoms of hyperglycemia denote a beneficial response to chlorpropamide. Lab values are also used to assess the client's response to treatment. An FBS of 110 mg/dL is within normal limits. However, a glycosylated hemoglobin of 10% is at least 3% above normal, denoting poor glycemic control.
TEST-TAKING STRATEGY: Note the key word "not" in the stem of the question. Knowledge of chlorpropamide as an oral hypoglycemic agent tells you to look for an option that denotes hyperglycemia (lack of response to medication). Options 1 and 3 are similar, a clue that they are both either true or false and therefore could not be the correct option. Knowledge of the normal blood glucose level will easily direct you to option 4.
LEVEL OF COGNITIVE ABILITY: Comprehension
PHASE OF NURSING PROCESS: Evaluation
CLIENT NEEDS: Physiological Integrity
CONTENT AREA: Adult Health/Endocrine
REFERENCE
Lehne, R. (1998). *Pharmacology for nursing care* (3rd ed.). Philadelphia: W. B. Saunders. pp. 594–595.

22. **3**

RATIONALE: Regular monitoring may detect hyperglycemia early enough to prevent serious complications. Classic symptoms of hyperglycemia include polydipsia, polyuria, and polyphagia.
TEST-TAKING STRATEGY: Knowledge regarding the signs and symptoms of hyperglycemia is required to answer this question. Remember the 3 Ps, polyuria, polydipsia, and polyphagia. Learn the signs of hyperglycemia now if you had difficulty with this question.
LEVEL OF COGNITIVE ABILITY: Comprehension
PHASE OF NURSING PROCESS: Data Collection
CLIENT NEEDS: Physiological Integrity
CONTENT AREA: Adult Health/Endocrine
REFERENCE
Monahan, F., & Neighbors, M. (1998). *Medical-surgical nursing: Foundations for clinical practice* (2nd ed.). Philadelphia: W. B. Saunders. p. 1251.

23. **3**

RATIONALE: Client education following DKA should emphasize the need for home glucose monitoring two to four times per day. It is also important to instruct the client to notify the health care provider when illness occurs. The presence of urine ketones indicates that DKA has already occurred. The client should eat well-balanced meals with snacks as prescribed.
TEST-TAKING STRATEGY: Treatment of DKA focuses on maintenance of blood glucose levels; therefore, this knowledge is necessary to provide the client with correct instructions. Option 1 is not an accurate component of diabetic care. Option 2 will not prevent DKA, and option 4 does not prevent DKA but actually confirms the diagnosis.
LEVEL OF COGNITIVE ABILITY: Application
PHASE OF NURSING PROCESS: Planning
CLIENT NEEDS: Health Promotion and Maintenance

CONTENT AREA: Adult Health/Endocrine
REFERENCE
Monahan, F., & Neighbors, M. (1998). *Medical-surgical nursing: Foundations for clinical practice* (2nd ed.). Philadelphia: W. B. Saunders. pp. 1242–1243.

24. 2

RATIONALE: Clients with Type 2 diabetes have decreased or impaired insulin secretion. Oral hypoglycemic agents are given to these clients to facilitate glucose utilization. Insulin injections may be given during times of stress-induced hyperglycemia. Oral insulin is not available due to the breakdown of the insulin by digestion.
TEST-TAKING STRATEGY: Be careful and read the options completely to prevent any confusion. You must be able to determine specific treatment for Type 2 diabetes mellitus and analyze the client's response regarding medication. Option 1 is incorrect because there is no "oral insulin"; options 3 and 4 are not accepted treatments for diabetes.
LEVEL OF COGNITIVE ABILITY: Comprehension
PHASE OF NURSING PROCESS: Evaluation
CLIENT NEEDS: Health Promotion and Maintenance
CONTENT AREA: Adult Health/Endocrine
REFERENCE
Monahan, F., & Neighbors, M. (1998). *Medical-surgical nursing: Foundations for clinical practice* (2nd ed.). Philadelphia: W. B. Saunders. p. 1227.

25. 2

RATIONALE: Reinforcement of knowledge and behaviors is vital to the success of the client's self-care. Knowledge and understanding of insulin are essential in maintaining optimum health.
TEST-TAKING STRATEGY: Remember to be therapeutic in your interaction with the client. By analyzing the responses, you find option 1 may devalue a client's family, option 3 places the issue on hold, and option 4 requests an explanation by the client. Option 2 is the correct answer because it validates and clarifies previous information.
LEVEL OF COGNITIVE ABILITY: Application
PHASE OF NURSING PROCESS: Implementation
CLIENT NEEDS: Psychosocial Integrity
CONTENT AREA: Adult Health/Endocrine
REFERENCE
Leahy, J., & Kizilay, P. (1998). *Foundations of nursing practice: A nursing process approach*. Philadelphia: W. B. Saunders. pp. 222–225.

26. 4

RATIONALE: A diet low in calories, carbohydrates, and sodium but ample in protein and potassium is encouraged for a client with Cushing's syndrome. Such a diet promotes weight loss, reduction of edema and hypertension, control of hypokalemia, and rebuilding of wasted tissue. The client with Cushing's syndrome who also is experiencing diabetes mellitus or gastric ulcers needs further modifications in their diet.
TEST-TAKING STRATEGY: To measure whether teaching was understood, you must first recall the effect that Cushing's syndrome has on the body, particularly in relation to metabolic processes. Option 1 is the only option that says no change is necessary. Protein is usually only limited with renal disorders. Excess sodium is not healthy in general, so using the process of elimination, you should be directed to option 4.
LEVEL OF COGNITIVE ABILITY: Comprehension

PHASE OF NURSING PROCESS: Evaluation
CLIENT NEEDS: Health Promotion and Maintenance
CONTENT AREA: Adult Health/Endocrine
REFERENCE
Luckmann, J. (1997). *Saunders manual of nursing care*. Philadelphia: W. B. Saunders p. 1405.

27. 1

RATIONALE: Hypoglycemia reaction may occur in response to increased exercise. Clients should avoid exercise during the peak time of insulin. NPH Insulin peaks at 6 to 12 hours; therefore, afternoon exercise will occur during the peak of the medication. The client should be educated to adjust the exercise schedule.
TEST-TAKING STRATEGY: Knowledge that the client should not exercise within 1 hour of an insulin injection or at the peak time of insulin action is required to answer this question. Remember these important points and you will easily be able to answer questions similar to this one.
LEVEL OF COGNITIVE ABILITY: Comprehension
PHASE OF NURSING PROCESS: Evaluation
CLIENT NEEDS: Health Promotion and Maintenance
CONTENT AREA: Adult Health/Endocrine
REFERENCE
deWit, S. (1998). *Essentials of medical-surgical nursing* (4th ed.). Philadelphia: W. B. Saunders. p. 817.

28. 2

RATIONALE: Hypercalcemia is the hallmark of hyperparathyroidism. Elevated serum calcium levels produce osmotic diuresis, thus, option 2 would be the correct answer. This diuresis leads to dehydration; therefore, option 4 can be eliminated. Both options 1 and 3 are gastrointestinal (GI) symptoms but are not associated with the common GI symptoms typical of hyperparathyroidism (i.e., nausea, vomiting, anorexia, and constipation).
TEST-TAKING STRATEGY: Knowledge of the symptoms associated with hypercalcemia, the hallmark of hyperparathyroidism, is required to answer this question. If you were unsure of these symptoms, note that options 1, 3, and 4 are all GI symptoms, whereas option 2 is the only renal symptom.
LEVEL OF COGNITIVE ABILITY: Comprehension
PHASE OF NURSING PROCESS: Data Collection
CLIENT NEEDS: Physiological Integrity
CONTENT AREA: Adult Health/Endocrine
REFERENCE
deWit, S. (1998). *Essentials of medical-surgical nursing* (4th ed.). Philadelphia: W. B. Saunders. p. 781.

29. 3

RATIONALE: During the postoperative period, the nurse carefully observes the client for signs of hemorrhage that cause swelling and compression of adjacent tissue. Laryngeal stridor is a harsh, high-pitched sound heard on inspiration and expiration caused by compression of the trachea leading to respiratory distress. It is an acute emergency situation that requires immediate attention to avoid complete obstruction of the airway.
TEST-TAKING STRATEGY: Consider the anatomical location of the surgical procedure and use the ABCs to select the correct option. Options 1, 2, and 4 are usual postoperative problems that are not life-threatening. Option 3 addresses airway.
LEVEL OF COGNITIVE ABILITY: Comprehension
PHASE OF NURSING PROCESS: Data Collection

CLIENT NEEDS: Physiological Integrity
CONTENT AREA: Adult Health/Endocrine
REFERENCE
Black, J., & Matassarin-Jacobs, E. (1997). *Medical-surgical nursing: Clinical management for continuity of care* (5th ed.). Philadelphia: W. B. Saunders. p. 2035.

30. 3

RATIONALE: Oral calcium supplements need to be given with food in the stomach to enhance its absorption as well as decrease gastrointestinal irritation. All other options are inappropriate and unrelated to oral calcium therapy.
TEST-TAKING STRATEGY: Knowledge of the specifics about this medication is required to answer this question. Eliminate those choices that seem unusual. Checking for a pulse is usually done for cardiac medications. Avoidance of sunlight and refrigeration of tablets are required for some medications, but are not as common an intervention as option 3. Review this medication now if you had difficulty with this question.
LEVEL OF COGNITIVE ABILITY: Application
PHASE OF NURSING PROCESS: Implementation
CLIENT NEEDS: Health Promotion and Maintenance
CONTENT AREA: Adult Health/Endocrine
REFERENCE
Hodgson, B., & Kizior, R. (2000). *Saunders nursing drug handbook 2000.* Philadelphia: W. B. Saunders. p. 139.

31. 2

RATIONALE: Lipodystrophy (hypertrophy of subcutaneous tissue at the injection site) occurs in some diabetic clients when injection sites are used repeatedly. Thus, clients are instructed to adhere to a rotating injection site plan to avoid tissue changes. Cleansing with alcohol, aspiration, and angle of insulin administration do not produce tissue damage.
TEST-TAKING STRATEGY: Knowledge of the definition of lipodystrophy will easily direct you to the correct option. If you are unfamiliar with this complication, take time now to review this important component in diabetic teaching.
LEVEL OF COGNITIVE ABILITY: Comprehension
PHASE OF NURSING PROCESS: Data Collection
CLIENT NEEDS: Physiological Integrity
CONTENT AREA: Adult Health/Endocrine
REFERENCE
Monahan, F., & Neighbors, M. (1998). *Medical-surgical nursing: Foundations for clinical practice* (2nd ed.). Philadelphia: W. B. Saunders. p. 1237.

32. 4

RATIONALE: Decreased blood glucose levels produce automatic nervous system symptoms, which are classically manifested as nervousness, irritability, and tremors. Option 1 is more likely to occur with hyperglycemia. Options 2 and 3 are unrelated to the signs of hypoglycemia.
TEST-TAKING STRATEGY: Knowledge regarding the signs associated with a hypoglycemic reaction is required to answer the question. If you had difficulty with this question, take time now to review this important complication.
LEVEL OF COGNITIVE ABILITY: Comprehension
PHASE OF NURSING PROCESS: Data Collection
CLIENT NEEDS: Physiological Integrity
CONTENT AREA: Adult Health/Endocrine
REFERENCE
Monahan, F., & Neighbors, M. (1998). *Medical-surgical nursing: Foundations for clinical practice* (2nd ed.). Philadelphia: W. B. Saunders. p. 1251.

33. 3

RATIONALE: Hypoglycemic reactions present adrenergic symptoms of tremor, shakiness, and nervousness, which are similar to alcohol intoxication. The best strategy to deal with this client's psychosocial need is to decrease the episodes of hypoglycemia by first identifying and then eliminating those factors that precipitate this event. Frequent hypoglycemic reactions can affect the client's self-esteem as well as physiological integrity.
TEST-TAKING STRATEGY: This is a complex question because it involves a biophysical problem that is affecting the client's psychosocial functioning. Always remember that the nurse's role is to assist clients to adapt to their illness. Option 1 presumes that the problem is unavoidable and thus the client is at fault. Option 2 is absolutely nontherapeutic because it presumes that the client may be drinking, and option 4 is avoidance of the psychosocial aspects of the client's problem.
LEVEL OF COGNITIVE ABILITY: Application
PHASE OF NURSING PROCESS: Implementation
CLIENT NEEDS: Psychosocial Integrity
CONTENT AREA: Adult Health/Endocrine
REFERENCE
Monahan, F. & Neighbors, M. (1998). *Medical-surgical nursing: Foundations for clinical practice* (2nd ed.). Philadelphia: W.B. Saunders. p. 1251.

34. 3

RATIONALE: Offer liquids containing both glucose and electrolytes. Small amounts of fluid may be tolerated even when vomiting is present. Advance diet as tolerated including a minimum of 100 to 150 g carbohydrates daily.
TEST-TAKING STRATEGY: Eliminate options 1 and 2 because of the words "only" and "all." The time frame in option 4 seems unreasonable; therefore, select option 3. Review care to the diabetic client during illness now, if you had difficulty with this question.
LEVEL OF COGNITIVE ABILITY: Application
PHASE OF NURSING PROCESS: Implementation
CLIENT NEEDS: Physiological Integrity
CONTENT AREA: Adult Health/Endocrine
REFERENCE
Monahan, F., & Neighbors, M. (1998). *Medical-surgical nursing: Foundations for clinical practice* (2nd ed.). Philadelphia: W. B. Saunders. p. 1240.

35. 1

RATIONALE: Manifestations of hypothyroid syndrome include cold intolerance, constipation, loss of initiative, thick dry skin, a notably puffy appearance of the skin around the eyes, slowed intellectual function including retarded speech and apathy, and low metabolic rate. Synthroid is used to correct hypothyroid syndrome. This dosage appears to be subtherapeutic.
TEST-TAKING STRATEGY: Note the key phrase "currently taking Synthroid." Knowledge that the signs presented in the question relate to the manifestations associated with hypothyroidism will easily direct you to option 1. The dosage needs to be increased.
LEVEL OF COGNITIVE ABILITY: Comprehension
PHASE OF NURSING PROCESS: Planning
CLIENT NEEDS: Physiological Integrity
CONTENT AREA: Adult Health/Endocrine
REFERENCE
Hodgson, B., & Kizior, R. (2000). *Saunders nursing drug handbook 2000.* Philadelphia: W. B. Saunders. pp. 589–590.

36. **4**

RATIONALE: Vasopressin, an antidiuretic hormone, causes vasoconstriction with reduced blood flow in coronary, peripheral, cerebral, and pulmonary vessels. Options 1, 2, and 3 are therapeutic effects of the medication.
TEST-TAKING STRATEGY: Not the key word "not" in the stem of the question. Eliminate options 2 and 3 because they are similar. Knowledge regarding the therapeutic effects of this medication is required to answer this question. If you had difficulty with this question, take time now to review this important medication.
LEVEL OF COGNITIVE ABILITY: Comprehension
PHASE OF NURSING PROCESS: Evaluation
CLIENT NEEDS: Physiological Integrity
CONTENT AREA: Adult Health/Endocrine
REFERENCE
Hodgson, B., & Kizior, R. (2000). *Saunders nursing drug handbook 2000.* Philadelphia: W. B. Saunders. p. 1043.

37. **2**

RATIONALE: Pheochromocytoma is a catecholamine-producing tumor and causes secretion of excessive amounts of epinephrine and norepinephrine. Hypertension is the principal manifestation and the client has episodes of high blood pressure accompanied by pounding headaches. The release of excessive catecholamine also results in excessive conversion of glycogen into glucose in the liver. Consequently, hyperglycemia and glucosuria occur during attacks. Pheochromocytoma is curable. The primary treatment is surgical removal of one or both of the adrenal glands depending on whether the tumor is unilateral or bilateral.
TEST-TAKING STRATEGY: In both options 1 and 4, a similarity exists in the sense of hypotension and hypoglycemia. There is only one correct answer. If a similarity exists in the answers, then neither one is likely to be correct. The word "not" in 3 is an absolute term, and it is best to avoid selecting statements that include absolute terminology.
LEVEL OF COGNITIVE ABILITY: Comprehension
PHASE OF NURSING PROCESS: Planning
CLIENT NEEDS: Physiological Integrity
CONTENT AREA: Adult Health/Endocrine
REFERENCE
Monahan, F., & Neighbors, M. (1998). *Medical-surgical nursing: Foundations for clinical practice* (2nd ed.). Philadelphia: W. B. Saunders. p. 1292.

38. **4**

RATIONALE: Hypertension is the major symptom associated with pheochromocytoma. The blood pressure status is assessed by taking the client's blood pressure. Glycosuria, weight loss, and diaphoresis are also clinical manifestations of pheochromocytoma, yet hypertension is the major symptom.
TEST-TAKING STRATEGY: Use the principles associated with prioritizing when answering this question. Remember the ABCs, airway, breathing, and circulation. A method of assessing circulation is to take the blood pressure.
LEVEL OF COGNITIVE ABILITY: Application
PHASE OF NURSING PROCESS: Data Collection
CLIENT NEEDS: Physiological Integrity
CONTENT AREA: Adult Health/Endocrine
REFERENCE
Luckmann, J. (1997). *Saunders manual of nursing care.* Philadelphia: W. B. Saunders. p. 1411.

39. **1**

RATIONALE: Hypertension is the hallmark of pheochromocytoma. Severe hypertension can precipitate a cerebrovascular accident or sudden blindness. Although all of the responses are accurate nursing interventions for the client with pheochromocytoma, the priority nursing action is to monitor the vital signs, particularly the blood pressure.
TEST-TAKING STRATEGY: Use the principles associated with prioritizing when answering this question. Remember the ABCs, airway, breathing, and circulation. Monitoring vital signs is the nursing action that assesses airway, breathing, and circulation. You can use the strategy of selecting the response that is different. Options 2, 3, and 4 all refer to the assessment of the renal system, whereas option 1 does not. In this situation, it is more likely that the option that is different is the correct response.
LEVEL OF COGNITIVE ABILITY: Application
PHASE OF NURSING PROCESS: Data Collection
CLIENT NEEDS: Physiological integrity
CONTENT AREA: Adult Health/Endocrine
REFERENCE
Monahan, F., & Neighbors, M. (1998). *Medical-surgical nursing: Foundations for clinical practice* (2nd ed.). Philadelphia: W. B. Saunders. p. 1292.

40. **1**

RATIONALE: The client with pheochromocytoma needs to be provided with a diet high in vitamins, minerals, and calories. Of particular importance is that food or beverages that contain caffeine such as coffee, tea, or colas are prohibited.
TEST-TAKING STRATEGY: Be careful with the selection of your answer when it contains the word "and." Remember that the entire option needs to be correct. If you look at options 2, 3, and 4 you will find a similarity in that they all contain a drink that has caffeine. This strategy represents selection of the option that is different. Option 1 does not identify a caffeine-containing drink. Clients with pheochromocytoma are prohibited to eat or drink any caffeine containing products.
LEVEL OF COGNITIVE ABILITY: Application
PHASE OF NURSING PROCESS: Implementation
CLIENT NEEDS: Physiological Integrity
CONTENT AREA: Adult Health/Endocrine
REFERENCE
Luckmann, J. (1997). *Saunders manual of nursing care.* Philadelphia: W. B. Saunders. p. 1411.

41. **2**

RATIONALE: The complications associated with pheochromocytoma include hypertensive retinopathy and nephropathy, myocarditis, CHF, increased platelet aggregation, and CVA. Death can occur from shock, CVA, renal failure dysrhythmias, and dissecting aortic aneurysm. Rales heard on auscultation are indicative of CHF. A urinary output of 50 mL per hour is an appropriate output and the nurse becomes concerned if the output is below 30 mL per hour. A BUN (blood urea nitrogen) of 20 mg/dL is a normal finding. Normal BUN is 5 to 20 mg/dL. Normal coagulation time is 5–15 minutes.
TEST-TAKING STRATEGY: Use the principles associated with prioritizing when answering this question. Remember the ABCs, airway, breathing, and circulation. Rales heard on auscultation in the lungs are associated with airway. Additionally, if you knew the normal hourly expectations associated with urinary output and the normal laboratory

values for coagulation time and for /e BUN, by the process of elimination you can determine that option 2 is the correct answer.
LEVEL OF COGNITIVE ABILITY: Comprehension
PHASE OF NURSING PROCESS: Data Collection
CLIENT NEEDS: Physiological Integrity
CONTENT AREA: Adult Health/Endocrine
REFERENCE
Luckmann, J. (1997). *Saunders manual of nursing care.* Philadelphia: W. B. Saunders. p. 1412.

42. 1

RATIONALE: Paraphrasing is restating the client's messages in the nurse's own words. Option 1 addresses the therapeutic communication technique of paraphrasing. The client is reaching out for understanding. In the nurse's response in option 2, the nurse is offering a false reassurance, which will block communication. Option 3 also represents a communication block in that it reflects a lack of the client's right to an opinion. In option 4, the nurse is expressing approval, which can be harmful to a nurse-client relationship.
TEST-TAKING STRATEGY: Remember that therapeutic communication techniques enhance communication. Always select the answer that will enhance communication and always address the client's concerns and feelings.
LEVEL OF COGNITIVE ABILITY: Application
PHASE OF NURSING PROCESS: Implementation
CLIENT NEEDS: Psychosocial Integrity
CONTENT AREA: Adult Health/Endocrine
REFERENCE
Leahy, J., & Kizilay, P. (1998). *Foundations of nursing practice: A nursing process approach.* Philadelphia: W. B. Saunders. pp. 229-231.

43. 3

RATIONALE: Clinical manifestations associated with thyroid storm include a fever as high as 106°F, severe tachycardia, profuse diarrhea, extreme vasodilation, hypotension, atrial fibrillation, hyperreflexia, abdominal pain, diarrhea, and dehydration rapidly progressing to coma and cardiovascular collapse.
TEST-TAKING STRATEGY: Knowledge regarding the manifestations associated with thyroid storm is required to answer the question. This condition is a rare but potentially fatal hypermetabolic state. If you are unfamiliar with this disorder, take time now to review.
LEVEL OF COGNITIVE ABILITY: Comprehension

PHASE OF NURSING PROCESS: Data Collection
CLIENT NEEDS: Physiological Integrity
CONTENT AREA: Adult Health/Endocrine
REFERENCE
Monahan, F., & Neighbors, M. (1998). *Medical-surgical nursing: Foundations for clinical practice* (2nd ed.). Philadelphia: W. B. Saunders. p. 1308.

44. 2

RATIONALE: A high-sodium, high-complex carbohydrate, and high-protein diet is prescribed for the client with Addison's disease. To prevent excess fluid and sodium loss, the client is instructed to maintain adequate salt intake of up to 8 g sodium daily and to increase salt intake during hot weather, before strenuous exercise, and in response to fever, vomiting, or diarrhea.
TEST-TAKING STRATEGY: Knowledge regarding the pathophysiology associated with Addison's disease will assist in answering this question. If you were unfamiliar with this disorder, it is important to review now.
LEVEL OF COGNITIVE ABILITY: Comprehension
PHASE OF NURSING PROCESS: Planning
CLIENT NEEDS: Physiological Integrity
CONTENT AREA: Adult Health/Endocrine
REFERENCE
Monahan, F., & Neighbors, M. (1998). *Medical-surgical nursing: Foundations for clinical practice* (2nd ed.). Philadelphia: W. B. Saunders. p. 1284.

45. 1

RATIONALE: Cushing's syndrome is characterized by an oversecretion of glucocorticoid hormones. Addison's disease is characterized by the failure of the adrenal cortex to produce and secrete adrenalcortical hormones. Options 3 and 4 are inaccurate regarding Cushing's syndrome.
TEST-TAKING STRATEGY: Option 3 can be easily eliminated. Remembering that in C"u"shing's (up) syndrome, there is an oversecretion, and in A"dd"ison's (down), there is an undersecretion. This may assist in answering questions similar to this one.
LEVEL OF COGNITIVE ABILITY: Comprehension
PHASE OF NURSING PROCESS: Evaluation
CLIENT NEEDS: Physiological Integrity
CONTENT AREA: Adult Health/Endocrine
REFERENCE
Monahan, F., & Neighbors, M. (1998). *Medical-surgical nursing: Foundations for clinical practice* (2nd ed.). Philadelphia: W. B. Saunders. p. 1285.

BIBLIOGRAPHY

Black, J., & Matassarin-Jacobs, E. (1997). *Medical-surgical nursing: Clinical management for continuity of care* (5th ed.). Philadelphia: W. B. Saunders.
Burrell, L., Gerlach, M., & Pless, B. (1997). *Adult nursing: Acute & community care* (2nd ed.). Stamford, CT: Appleton & Lange.
Chernecky, C., & Berger, B. (1997). *Laboratory tests and diagnostic procedures* (2nd ed.). Philadelphia: W. B. Saunders.
Hodgson, B., & Kizior, R. (2000). *Saunders nursing drug handbook 2000.* Philadelphia: W. B. Saunders.
Ignatavicius, D., Workman, M., & Mishler, M. (1999). *Medical-surgical nursing across the health care continuum* (3rd ed.). Philadelphia: W. B. Saunders.
Lehne, R. (1998). *Pharmacology for nursing care* (3rd ed.). Philadelphia: W. B. Saunders.
Leahy, J., & Kizilay, P. (1998). *Foundations of nursing practice: A nursing process approach.* Philadelphia: W. B. Saunders.
Lewis, S., Collier, I., & Heitkemper, M. (1996). *Medical-surgical nursing: Assessment and management of clinical problems* (4th ed.). St. Louis: Mosby–Year Book.
Luckmann, J. (1997). *Saunders manual of nursing care.* Philadelphia: W. B. Saunders.
Lutz, C., & Przytulski, K. (1997). *Nutrition and diet therapy* (2nd ed.). Philadelphia: F. A. Davis.
Monahan, F., & Neighbors, M. (1998). *Medical-surgical nursing: Foundations for clinical practice* (2nd ed.). Philadelphia: W. B. Saunders.
O'Toole, M. (1997). *Miller-Keane encyclopedia & dictionary of medicine, nursing, & allied health* (6th ed.). Philadelphia: W. B. Saunders.
Potter, P., & Perry, A. (1997). *Fundamentals of nursing* (4th ed.). St. Louis: Mosby–Year Book.
Smeltzer, S., & Bare, B. (1996). *Brunner and Suddarth's textbook of medical-surgical nursing* (8th ed.). Philadelphia: Lippincott-Raven.

CHAPTER 43

Endocrine Medications

I. Pituitary Medications

A. Description
1. Anterior pituitary gland: secretes growth hormone (GH), thyroid-stimulating hormone (TSH), adrenocorticotropic hormone (ACTH), and gonadotropins (follicle-stimulating hormone, or FSH, and luteinizing hormone, or LH)
2. Posterior pituitary gland: secretes antidiuretic hormones (ADH, vasopressin) and oxytocin
B. Growth hormones (Box 43–1)
1. Description
   a. Secreted by the anterior pituitary gland
   b. Stimulate linear growth
   c. Used for pituitary dwarfism
2. Side effects
   a. Pain at injection site
   b. Glucose intolerance
   c. **Hypothyroidism**
   d. Giantism in children with excessive doses
3. Implementation
   a. Monitor the child's physical growth and compare growth with standards
   b. Recommend annual bone age determinations for children receiving growth hormones
   c. Teach the client and family about the importance of follow-up regarding blood and urine glucose testing

◆ II. Antidiuretic Hormones (Box 43–2)

A. Description
1. Enhance reabsorption of water in the kidneys, promoting an antidiuretic effect and regulating fluid balance
2. Used in **diabetes insipidus**

B. Side effects
1. Flushing and headache
2. Nausea and abdominal cramps
3. Water intoxication
4. Hypertension with water intoxication
5. Nasal congestion with nasal administration
C. Implementation
1. Monitor weight, I&O, and urine osmolality
2. Restrict intake as necessary to prevent water intoxication
3. Monitor for signs of water intoxication, such as drowsiness, listlessness, and headache
4. Instruct the client how to use the intranasal drug form
5. Instruct the client to report signs of water intoxication or symptoms of headache or shortness of breath

III. Thyroid Hormones (Box 43–3)

A. Description
1. Control the metabolic rate of tissues and accelerates heat production and oxygen consumption
2. Used to replace hormonal deficit in the treatment of **hypothyroidism, myxedema,** or cretinism
3. Enhance the action of oral anticoagulants and antidepressants, and decrease the action of insulin, oral hypoglycemics, and digitalis preparations
4. Phenytoin (Dilantin) and aspirin can enhance the action of thyroid hormone
B. Side effects
1. Nausea and vomiting

BOX 43-1. Growth Hormones

Somatrem (Protropin)
Somatropin (Humatrope)

BOX 43-2. Antidiuretic Hormones

Desmopressin acetate (DDAVP)
Desmopressin (Stimate)
Lypressin (Diapid)
Vasopressin (Pitressin)

BOX 43–3. Thyroid Hormones

Levothyroxine sodium (Synthroid)
Liothyronine sodium (Cytomel)
Liotrix (Euthroid, Thyrolar)
Thyroglobulin (Proloid)
Thyroid (Armour Thyroid, Thyrar)

---

2. Cramps and diarrhea
3. Weight loss
4. Nervousness and tremors
5. Headache
6. Hypertension
7. Tachycardia
8. Sweating and heat intolerance
9. Insomnia

C. Implementation
   1. Ask the client about a history regarding current medication therapy
   2. Monitor vital signs and weight
   3. Monitor triiodothyronine (T_3), thyroxine (T_4), and thyroid stimulating hormone (TSH) levels
   4. Instruct the client to take the medication at the same time each day, preferably in the morning without food
   5. Instruct the client to monitor the pulse rate
   6. Advise the client to report symptoms of **hyperthyroidism,** such as tachycardia, chest pain, palpitations, and excessive sweating
   7. Instruct the client to avoid foods that can inhibit thyroid secretion, such as strawberries, peaches, pears, cabbage, turnips, spinach, kale, Brussel sprouts, cauliflower, radishes, and peas
   8. Advise the client to avoid over-the-counter medications
   9. Instruct the client to wear a Medic-Alert bracelet

IV. Antithyroid Medications (Box 43–4)

A. Description
   1. Inhibit the synthesis of thyroid hormone
   2. Used for **hyperthyroidism** or **Graves' disease**
B. Side effects
   1. Nausea, vomiting, and diarrhea
   2. Hypersensitivity and rash
   3. Agranulocytosis
   4. **Hypothyroidism**
   5. Iodism characterized by vomiting, abdominal

BOX 43–4. Antithyroid Medications

Iodine solution (Lugol's solution, potassium iodide solution)
Methimazole (Tapazole)
Propylthiouracil (PTU)

---

pain, brassy taste, rash, and sore salivary glands
C. Implementation
   1. Monitor vital signs and weight
   2. Monitor T_3, T_4, and TSH levels
   3. Instruct the client to take medication with meals to avoid gastrointestinal (GI) upset
   4. Instruct the client how to take his or her pulse
   5. Advise the client to contact a physician if a fever or sore throat develops
   6. Instruct the client in the signs of **hypothyroidism**
   7. Instruct the client regarding the importance of compliance and that abruptly stopping the medication could cause thyroid crisis
   8. Monitor for signs and symptoms of thyroid crisis **(thyroid storm),** which include fever, flushed skin, confusion and behavioral changes, tachycardia, and heart failure
   9. Advise the client to consult a physician before eating iodized salt and iodine-rich foods
   10. Instruct the client to avoid aspirin and medications containing iodine

V. Parathyroid Medications (Table 43–1)

A. Description
   1. Parathyroid hormone regulates serum calcium levels
   2. Low serum levels of calcium stimulate parathyroid hormone release
   3. Hyperparathyroidism results in high serum calcium levels and bone demineralization, and medication is used to lower serum calcium levels
   4. Hypoparathyroidism results in low serum calcium levels, which increase neuromuscular excitability, and the treatment includes calcium and vitamin D supplements
   5. Calcium salts administered with digitalis increase the risk of digitalis toxicity
   6. Oral calcium salts reduce the absorption of tetracycline
B. Implementation
   1. Monitor electrolyte and calcium levels
   2. Monitor for symptoms of tetany in hypocalcemia, such as twitching of the

---

Table 43–1. Parathyroid Medications

For Hypoparathyroidism and Hypocalcemia

Calcifediol (Calderol)
Calcitriol (Rocaltrol)
Ergocalciferol (Drisdol)
Calcium carbonate (Os-Cal)
Calcium gluconate

For Hyperparathyroidism and Hypercalcemia

Calcitonin (human) (Cibacalcin)
Calcitonin (salmon) (Calcimar)
Etidronate (Didronel)

mouth, and tingling and numbness of the fingers

3. Monitor for signs and symptoms of hypercalcemia, such as bone pain, anorexia, nausea, vomiting, thirst, constipation, lethargy, bradycardia, and polyuria
4. Instruct the client in the signs and symptoms in hypercalcemia and hypocalcemia
5. Instruct the client to check over-the-counter medication labels for the possibility of calcium content
6. Instruct the client receiving oral calcium to maintain an adequate intake of vitamin D, as vitamin D enhances absorption of calcium

VI. Adrenocorticotropic Hormones (Box 43–5)

A. Description
1. Stimulate the adrenal cortex to secrete cortisol
2. Produce an anti-inflammatory effect
3. Used to treat acute multiple sclerosis
B. Side effects
1. Nausea and vomiting
2. Increased appetite
3. Mood swings
4. Petechiae
5. Water and sodium retention
6. Hypokalemia
7. Hypocalcemia
C. Implementation
1. Monitor vital signs
2. Monitor I&O, weight, and for edema
3. Monitor for signs of infection
4. Monitor electrolyte and calcium levels
5. Avoid administering to the client with adrenocortical hyperfunction
6. Instruct the client to decrease salt intake
7. Instruct the client to report muscle weakness, edema, petechiae, ecchymosis, decrease in growth, decreased wound healing, and menstrual irregularities
8. Monitor for adverse effects when the medication is discontinued
9. The dose should be tapered and not stopped abruptly, because adrenal hypofunction may result

VII. Corticosteroids

A. Description (Box 43–6)
1. Corticosteroids are normally secreted by the adrenal cortex
2. Alter the normal immune response and suppress inflammation

BOX 43–6. Use of Corticosteroids

Trauma
Surgery
Infections
Emotional upsets and anxiety
Autoimmune disorders
Inflammatory diseases
Allergic reactions
By organ transplant recipients to prevent rejection

3. Produce anti-inflammatory, antiallergic, and antistress effects
4. Promote sodium and water retention and potassium excretion
B. Contraindications and cautions
1. Contraindicated in hypersensitivity, psychosis, and fungal infections
2. Use with caution in **diabetes mellitus**
3. Dexamethasone decreases the effects of oral anticoagulants and oral hypoglycemic agents
4. Corticosteroids increase the potency of medications taken concurrently, such as aspirin, and nonsteroidal anti-inflammatory drugs (NSAIDs), thus increasing the risk of GI bleeding and ulceration
5. Use of potassium-wasting diuretics increases potassium loss, resulting in hypokalemia
6. Should be used with extreme caution in clients with infections because they mask the signs and symptoms of an infection
C. Glucocorticoids (Box 43–7)
1. Description: used as a replacement for adrenocortical insufficiency
2. Side effects
a. Hyperglycemia
b. Edema
c. Sodium and water retention
d. Hypokalemia
e. Cause muscle wasting, osteoporosis, growth retardation in children, peptic ulcer, increased serum glucose levels, hypertension, convulsions, mood swings, cataracts, glaucoma, fragile skin, hirsutism, altered fat distribution
f. Mask the signs and symptoms of infection

BOX 43–5. Adrenocorticotropic Hormones

Corticotropin (Acthar)
Corticotropin repository (Acthar gel)
Cosyntropin (Cortrosyn)

BOX 43–7. Glucocorticoids

Betamethasone (Celestone)
Cortisone acetate (Cortone Acetate)
Dexamethasone (Decadron)
Hydrocortisone (Cortef, Hydrocortone)
Methylprednisolone (Depo-Medrol, Medrol, Solu-Medrol)
Prednisolone (Delta-Cortef, Prelone)
Prednisone (Deltasone)
Triamcinolone (Aristocort, Kenalog, Kenacort)

3. Implementation
   a. Monitor vital signs
   b. Monitor serum electrolytes and blood glucose
   c. Monitor for hypokalemia and **hyperglycemia**
   d. Monitor weight
   e. Monitor for hypertension
   f. Monitor for edema
   g. Monitor urine output
   h. Check medical history for glaucoma, cataracts, peptic ulcer, mental health disorders, or diabetes
   i. Instruct the client that topical medication should be applied in a thin layer and to report any rashes, infections, or purpura
   j. Monitor the older client for signs and symptoms of increased osteoporosis
   k. Prepare a schedule for the client on short-term tapered doses
   l. Instruct the client to take at mealtime or with food
   m. Advise the client to eat foods high in potassium
   n. Advise clients to inform all health care providers that they are taking the medication
   o. Instruct clients to report signs and symptoms of a medication overdose or **Cushing's syndrome,** including a moon face, puffy eyelids, edema in the feet, increased bruising, dizziness, bleeding, and menstrual irregularities
   p. Note that the client may need additional doses during periods of stress, such as surgery
   q. Instruct clients not to stop the medication abruptly, as abrupt withdrawal can result in severe adrenal insufficiency
   r. Advise the client to consult with a physician before receiving vaccinations
   s. Advise the client to wear Medic-Alert bracelet

D. Mineralocorticoid (Box 43–8)
   1. Description
      a. Mineralocorticoid deficiency usually occurs with a glucocorticoid deficiency, frequently called corticosteroid deficiency
      b. Enhances reabsorption of sodium and chloride and promotes excretion of potassium thereby helping to maintain fluid and electrolyte balance
      c. Used for replacement therapy in primary and secondary adrenal insufficiency in **Addison's disease**

BOX 43–8. Mineralocorticoid

Fludrocortisone acetate (Florinef Acetate)

BOX 43–9. Androgens

Fluoxymesterone (Halotestin)
Methyltestosterone (Android, Oreton Methyl, Testred, Virilon)
Testosterone (Andronaq, Histerone)
Testosterone cypionate (Depotest, Depo-Testosterone)
Testosterone enanthate (Delatest)
Testosterone propionate (Testex)
Flutamide (Eulexin)
Leuprolide acetate (Lupron)

---

2. Side effects
   a. Sodium and water retention
   b. Hypokalemia
   c. Hypocalcemia
   d. Increased susceptibility to infection and delayed wound healing
   e. GI distress, such as abdominal distention, diarrhea, or constipation
   g. Increased appetite and weight gain
   f. Insomnia
   g. Mood swings
3. Implementation
   a. Monitor vital signs and weight
   b. Monitor electrolytes and calcium and glucose levels
   c. Instruct the client to take medication with food or milk
   d. Instruct clients to consume a high-potassium diet
   e. Instruct clients not to stop the medication abruptly
   f. Instruct the client to notify a physician if signs of infection, muscle aches, sudden weight gain, or headaches occur
   g. Instruct clients to avoid exposure to disease or trauma
   h. Instruct clients not to take aspirin or any other medication without consulting a physician
   i. Instruct the client to wear a Medic-Alert bracelet

VIII. Androgens (Box 43–9)

A. Description
   1. The androgens are steroids that stimulate the action of endogenous hormones
   2. Used to either replace deficient hormones or treat hormone-sensitive disorders
   3. Prescribed as a palliative treatment for androgen-sensitive breast cancer or fibrocystic breast disease, to treat endometriosis or advanced prostatic cancer
   4. Can cause bleeding if the client is taking oral anticoagulants
   5. Cause decreased serum glucose concentration, thereby reducing insulin requirements in the diabetic client

B. Side effects
1. Masculine secondary sexual characteristics, such as body hair growth, lowered voice, or muscle growth
2. Bladder irritation and urinary tract infections
3. Breast tenderness and impotence in men
4. Gynecomastia
5. Priapism
6. Menstrual irregularities
7. Sodium and water retention, edema, and weight gain
8. Mood swings
9. Hepatotoxicity

C. Implementation
1. Monitor vital signs
2. Monitor for edema, weight gain, and skin changes
3. Monitor mental status and neurological function
4. Monitor for signs of liver dysfunction, including right upper quadrant abdominal pain, malaise, fever, jaundice, pruritus
5. Monitor for the development of secondary sexual characteristics
6. Instruct client to take with meals or a snack
7. Instruct the client to notify physician if priapism develops
8. Instruct the client to notify the physician if fluid retention occurs
9. Instruct the diabetic client to monitor blood glucose levels
10. Instruct women to use a nonhormonal contraceptive while on therapy

IX. Estrogens and Progestins

A. Description
1. Used to stimulate the endogenous hormones to restore hormonal balance and treat hormone-sensitive tumors
2. Lactation suppressants decrease the serum prolactin level, thereby relieving postpartal breast engorgement
3. Fertility medications stimulate ovarian function by increasing levels of pituitary gonadotropins
4. Oxytoxic medications enhance uterine motility by directly stimulating uterine and smooth muscle contractions
5. Labor suppressants relax uterine muscles and decrease uterine contractions

B. Estrogens (Box 43–10)
1. Estrogen preparations suppress tumor growth

> **BOX 43–10. Estrogens**
>
> Diethylstilbestrol (DES, Stilphostrol)
> Ethinylestradiol (Estinyl)
> Chlorotrianisene (Tace)
> Conjugated estrogens (Premarin)

> **BOX 43–11. Progestins**
>
> Hydroxyprogesterone caproate (Duralutin)
> Medroxyprogesterone acetate (Depo-Provera)
> Megestrol acetate (Megace)

2. Estrogen therapy is a palliative treatment used in men to decrease the progression of prostatic cancer and in postmenopausal women to decrease the progression of breast cancer

C. Progestins: used for breast cancer, endometrial cancer, and renal cancer (Box 43–11)

D. Contraindications and cautions
1. Contraindicated in embolism, thrombophlebitis, undiagnosed breast neoplasms, and history of cerebral vascular accident (CVA)
2. Associated with an increased risk of endometrial cancer

E. Side effects
1. Nausea, vomiting, and diarrhea
2. Edema and fluid retention, weight gain
3. Rash
4. Headache
5. Insomnia
6. Hypertension
7. Thromboembolitic disorders

F. Implementation
1. Monitor vital signs
2. Monitor for hypertension
3. Monitor weight and for edema
4. Advise the client not to smoke
5. Advise the client to undergo routine breast and pelvic exams

X. Gonadotropin-Releasing Hormones
(Box 43–12)

A. Description
1. Stimulates synthesis and release of LH and FSH from the anterior pituitary
2. Used as palliative treatment for advanced prostatic cancer, to treat endometriosis, and to treat hypothalamic amenorrhea

B. Side effects
1. Headache
2. Nausea, vomiting, and abdominal discomfort
3. Light-headedness
4. Hot flashes

> **BOX 43–12. Gonadotropin-Releasing Hormones**
>
> Gonadorelin acetate (Lutrepulse)
> Gonadorelin hydrochloride (Factrel)
> Goserelin acetate (Zoladex)
> Leuprolide acetate (Lupron)
> Nafarelin acetate (Synarel)

5. Vaginitis
6. Decreased libido
C. Implementation
   1. Instruct the client to use contraceptive measures during therapy
   2. Monitor for side effects related to therapy
   3. Stress the importance of follow-up with the physician as scheduled

XI. Diabetic Medications

A. Insulin and oral hypoglycemic medications
   1. Description
      a. Insulin increases glucose transport into cells and promotes conversion of glucose to glycogen, decreasing serum glucose levels
      b. Oral hypoglycemic agents stimulate the pancreas to produce more insulin and increase the sensitivity of peripheral receptors to insulin, thereby decreasing serum glucose levels
      c. Used in **diabetes mellitus**
   2. Contraindications and concerns
      a. Insulin is contraindicated in clients with hypersensitivity
      b. Oral hypoglycemic agents are contraindicated in Type 1 insulin-dependent **diabetes mellitus** and in those individuals allergic to sulfonylureas
      c. Sulfonylureas can increase myocardial oxygen consumption and lead to cardiac dysrhythmias
      d. Use of antidiabetic medications with beta-adrenergic blocking agents mask signs and symptoms of **hypoglycemia**
      e. Use of antidiabetic medications with alcohol, steroids, salicylates, or MAO inhibitors may cause **hypoglycemia**
      f. Anticoagulants, chloramphenicol, and sulfonamides may cause **hypoglycemia**
      g. Use of insulin with corticosteroids, thiazide diuretics, thyroid preparations, oral contraceptives, and estrogen may cause **hyperglycemia**
   3. Implementation
      a. Monitor serum and urine glucose and ketone levels and for signs of **hypoglycemia** and **hyperglycemia**
      b. Note that stress, fever, trauma, and infection may increase insulin requirements or necessitate switching from an oral hypoglycemic agent to insulin
      c. Note that IV glucose or glucagon may be used to treat severe hypoglycemia
      d. Inform the client that antidiabetic agents control but do not cure diabetes and emphasize the need for lifelong therapy
      e. Instruct the client in the signs and symptoms of **hypoglycemia** and **hyperglycemia**
      f. Instruct clients about diet and the use of the exchange system when planning meals
      g. Instruct clients how to monitor serum and urine glucose levels
      h. Instruct the client in the importance of regular exercise
      i. Instruct the client about the importance of daily foot inspection
      j. Instruct the client regarding alcohol intake
      k. Instruct clients to notify the physician if unable to eat
      l. Instruct clients to carry sugar and to wear a Medic-Alert bracelet
B. Oral hypoglycemic medications
   1. Prescribed for clients with **diabetes mellitus** Type 2
   2. Sulfonylureas
      a. Classified as first- and second-generation sulfonylureas (Table 43–2)
      b. Stimulate the beta cells to produce more insulin
   3. Nonsulfonylureas

Table 43–2. First- and Second-Generation Sulfonylureas and Nonsulfonylureas

Medication	Implementation
First-Generation Sulfonylureas *Short-Acting*	
Tolbutamide (Orinase)	Administer 30 minutes before meals to provide the best reduction in postprandial hyperglycemia
Intermediate-Acting	
Acetohexamide (Dymelor)	Stress eating habits and patterns There is a high incidence of hypoglycemia in clients with renal impairment Monitor renal function
Tolazamide (Tolinase)	Administer with meals to avoid GI upset
Long-Acting	
Chlorpropamide (Diabenese)	Stress eating habits and patterns because the medication is associated with hypoglycemia
Second-Generation Sulfonylureas	
Glipizide (Glucotrol)	Administer 30 minutes before meals to provide the best reduction in postprandial hyperglycemia
Glyburide (DiaBeta, Micronase, Glynase)	Administer with meals to avoid GI upset Stress eating habits and patterns because the medication is associated with hypoglycemia
Glimepiride (Amaryl)	Administer with breakfast Contraindicated in clients with severe renal or hepatic impairment
Nonsulfonylureas	
Metformin (Glucophage)	Monitor renal function Should not be used in clients with renal impairment
Acarbose (Precose)	Intended for use in clients who do not achieve results with diet alone

a. Affect the hepatic and gastrointestinal production of glucose
b. May be used in combination with a sulfonylurea

4. Implementation
   a. Determine the client's knowledge of diabetes and the use of oral antidiabetic agents
   b. Monitor vital signs and blood glucose levels
   c. Identify the medications that the client is currently taking
   d. Instruct the client to recognize symptoms of **hypoglycemia** and **hyperglycemia**
   e. Instruct the client to avoid over-the-counter medications unless prescribed by the physician
   f. Instruct the client not to ingest alcohol with sulfonylureas
   g. Inform the client that insulin may be needed during stress, surgery, or infection
   h. Instruct the client in the necessity of compliance with prescribed medication
   i. Advise the client to obtain a Medic-Alert bracelet

C. Insulin (Table 43–3)
   1. Primarily acts in the liver, muscle, and adipose tissue by attaching to receptors on cellular membranes and facilitating the passage of glucose, potassium, and magnesium
   2. Prescribed for clients with **diabetes mellitus Type 1**
   3. Insulin injection sites
      a. Insulin injected into the abdomen may absorb more evenly and rapidly than other sites
      b. Insulin administered SC has a slower absorption rate than if administered IM
      c. Heat, massage, and exercise of the injected area can increase absorption rates
      d. Injection into scar tissue may delay absorption of insulin
      e. Insulin injection sites should be rotated to prevent hypertrophic lipodystrophy, a spongy swelling at or around the injection site, which can interfere with insulin absorption

f. Lipoatrophic lipodystrophy, a loss of fat at the injection site, is most often due to the use of animal insulins
g. Rotation within one anatomical site is preferred to rotation from one anatomical site to another
h. Administer the insulin in the same general area, rotating sites within that area, to predict absorption rate
i. Injections should be 1.5 inches apart at a site area each day

4. Storing insulin: vials of insulin not in use should be refrigerated
5. Administering insulin (Box 43–13)
   a. To prevent dosage errors, be certain that there is a match of the insulin concentration with the calibration of units on the insulin syringe
   b. Before use, roll, not shake, the insulin bottle to ensure that the insulin and ingredients are mixed well and to avoid bubbles, causing drawing an inaccurate dose
   c. When mixing insulin, inject an amount of air equal to the insulin dose into the longer-acting insulin first
   d. Always withdraw the shorter-acting insulin first
   e. Be careful not to inject any shorter-acting insulin into the NPH bottle
   f. Regular Insulin may be mixed with any other type of insulin
   g. Insulin zinc suspensions may be mixed only with each other and Regular Insulin, not with other types of insulin
   h. Administer a mixed dose of insulin within 5 minutes of preparation, because after this time the Regular Insulin binds with the NPH Insulin and its action is reduced
   i. Administer insulin at a 45° to 90° angle, and at a 45° to 60° angle in thin persons
   j. Regular Insulin is the only type of insulin that can be administered by IV

D. Glucagon
   1. A hormone secreted by the alpha cells of the islets of Langerhans in the pancreas

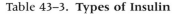

Table 43–3. Types of Insulin

Type	Onset	Peak	Duration
Short-Acting Insuln			
Humulin (Regular)	0.5–1 hour	2–4 hours	5–7 hours
Lispro (Humalog)	5 minutes	0.5–1 hour	2–4 hours
Intermediate-Acting Insulin			
Humulin N (NPH)	1–2 hours	6–12 hours	18–24 hours
Humulin L (Lente)	1–2 hours	6–12 hours	18–24 hours
Long-Acting Insulin			
Humulin U Ultralente	4–6 hours	16–18 hours	20–36 hours
Premixed Insulin			
70% NPH and 30% Regular	0.5 hour	2–12 hours	18–24 hours

BOX 43-13. Client Instructions for Insulin

Instruct client and family members in the administration of the insulin

Instruct client to keep insulin in use at room temperature and refrigerate any extra supplies of insulin

Instruct client to draw up Regular Insulin prior to NPH Insulin if a mix is prescribed

Illness, infection, and stress increase the need for insulin, and insulin should not be withheld at these times because hyperglycemia and ketoacidosis can result

Instruct the client to recognize symptoms of hypoglycemia and hyperglycemia

The peak action times of insulin is very important because of the possibility of hypoglycemic reactions occurring

Orange juice, sugar-sweetened beverages, or hard candy should be kept available and administered if a hypoglycemic reaction occurs

Instruct client that hypoglycemic reactions are likely to occur during peak times and that orange juice, sugar-containing drinks, and hard candy may be used when a hypoglycemic reaction occurs

Instruct family in administering glucagon by injection if the client has a hypoglycemic reaction and is unable to drink sugar-containing fluid

Instruct client to avoid over-the-counter medications unless prescribed by the physician

Instruct the client to always have a spare bottle of insulin available

Advise the client to obtain a Medic-Alert bracelet indicating the type and daily insulin dosage

---

2. Increases blood glucose by stimulating glycogenolysis in the liver
3. Can be administered SC, IM, or IV
4. Used to treat insulin-induced **hypoglycemia** when the client is semiconscious or unconscious and is unable to ingest liquids
5. The blood glucose level begins to increase within 5 to 20 minutes after administration

E. Diazoxide (Proglycem)
1. Increases blood glucose by inhibiting insulin release from the beta cells and stimulating the release of epinephrine from the adrenal medulla
2. Used to treat chronic **hypoglycemia** caused by hyperinsulinism due to islet cell cancer or hyperplasia
3. It is not used for **hypoglycemic** reactions from insulin

PRACTICE QUESTIONS

1. Somatren (Protropin) is administered to a client with pituitary dwarfism. The expected therapeutic effect of this medication is to
   1 Promote weight gain
   2 Stimulate linear growth
   3 Increase bone density
   4 Decrease the mobilization of fats

2. The nurse is monitoring a client receiving desmopressin (DDAVP). Which of the following if noted in the client indicates an adverse reaction to the medication?
   1 Increased urination
   2 Weight loss
   3 Drowsiness
   4 Insomnia

3. The nurse reinforces instructions to a client taking levothyroxine (Synthroid). The nurse determines that the teaching was effective if the client states to take the medication
   1 With food
   2 On an empty stomach
   3 At bedtime
   4 At lunch time

4. Thyroid replacement therapy is prescribed for the client diagnosed with hypothyroidism. The client asks the nurse when the medication will no longer be needed. The most appropriate nursing response is which of the following?
   1 "You will need to ask your physician."
   2 "Most clients require medication therapy for about 1 year."
   3 "It depends on the results of the laboratory values."
   4 "The medication will need to be continued for life."

5. The nurse reinforces medication instructions to a client taking levothyroxine (Synthroid). The nurse instructs the client to notify the physician if which of the following occurs?
   1 Cold intolerance
   2 Tremors
   3 Excessively dry skin
   4 Fatigue

6. The nurse reviews the health record of a client seen in the physician's office and notes that the client is taking propylthiouracil (PTU) daily. The nurse suspects that the client has a history of
   1 Cushing's syndrome
   2 Addison's disease
   3 Myxedema
   4 Graves' disease

7. The nurse is reinforcing instructions to a client regarding the administration of lypressin (Diapid). The nurse instructs the client that the medication will be taken by which of the following routes?
   1 Oral
   2 Subcutaneous
   3 Intranasal
   4 Intramuscular

8. A client is seen by the physician for complaints of fatigue, a lack of energy, constipation, and depression. Following diagnostic studies, hypothyroidism

is diagnosed. Levothyroxine (Synthroid) is prescribed. The nurse tells the client that the expected outcome of the medication is to
1 Increase energy levels
2 Achieve normal thyroid hormone levels
3 Increase blood glucose levels
4 Alleviate depression

9. Propylthiouracil (PTU) is prescribed for the client with hyperthyroidism. The nurse reinforces instructions to the client regarding the medication. The nurse informs the client to notify the physician if which of the following signs occur?
1 Drowsiness
2 Sore throat
3 Polyuria
4 Dry mouth

10. The client is scheduled for subtotal thyroidectomy. Iodine solution (Lugol's solution) is prescribed. The nurse understands that the therapeutic effect of this medication is to
1 Increase thyroid hormone production
2 Suppress thyroid hormone production
3 Replace thyroid hormone
4 Prevent the oxidation of iodide

11. The nurse reinforces instructions to the client taking fludrocortisone (Florinef). The nurse tells the client to notify the physician if which of the following occurs?
1 Weight loss
2 Nausea
3 Swelling of the feet
4 Fatigue

12. Calcium carbonate (Os-Cal) is prescribed for the client with hypocalcemia. The nurse most appropriately instructs the client to take the medication.
1 With meals
2 One hour after meals
3 Just before meals
4 Just before breakfast

13. Calcitriol (Rocaltrol) is prescribed for the client with hypocalcemia. The nurse provides dietary instructions to the client. Which of the following food items does the nurse instruct the client to avoid while taking this medication?
1 Dark green, leafy vegetables
2 Milk
3 Whole-grain cereals
4 Sardines

14. A daily dose of prednisone (Deltasone) is prescribed for the client. The nurse provides instructions to the client regarding administration of the medication. The nurse instructs the client that the best time to take this medication is
1 At bedtime
2 At noon

3 Early morning
4 Anytime, at the same time, each day

15. The hospitalized diabetic client received NPH Insulin in the morning. When would the nurse expect the peak action of the insulin dose to occur?
1 2 to 4 hours after administration
2 6 to 12 hours after administration
3 12 to 16 hours after administration
4 18 to 24 hours after administration

16. The nurse is teaching the client how to mix Regular Insulin and NPH Insulin in the same syringe. Which of the following actions, if performed by the client, indicates the need for further teaching?
1 Injects air into NPH Insulin vial first
2 Injects the amount of air equal to the desired dose of insulin into the vial
3 Withdraws the NPH Insulin first
4 Withdraws the Regular Insulin first

17. The nurse is reinforcing home care instructions to a client recently diagnosed with diabetes mellitus. The client is taking NPH Insulin daily. The client asks the nurse how to store the unopened vials of insulin. Which of the following instructions does the nurse provide to the client?
1 Freeze the insulin
2 Refrigerate the insulin
3 Keep the insulin at room temperature
4 In a dark dry place

18. A diabetic client is self-administering NPH Insulin from a vial that is kept at room temperature. The client asks the nurse about the length of time an unrefrigerated vial of insulin will maintain its potency. The most appropriate response is which of the following?
1 2 weeks
2 1 month
3 2 months
4 6 months

19. Lispro insulin (Humalog), a rapid-acting form of insulin, is prescribed for the client. The client is instructed to administer the insulin prior to meals. The nurse instructs the client to administer the insulin
1 Immediately before eating
2 30 minutes before eating
3 45 minutes before eating
4 60 minutes before eating

20. Tolbutamide (Orinase) is prescribed for the client with diabetes. The nurse instructs the client to avoid which of the following while taking this medication?
1 Carbonated beverages
2 Organ meats
3 Alcohol
4 Whole-grain cereals

ANSWERS

1. **2**

RATIONALE: Protropin is a growth stimulator used in the long-term treatment of growth failure due to growth hormone deficiency. It stimulates linear growth and increases the number and size of muscle cells and red cell mass. It affects carbohydrate metabolism by antagonizing the action of insulin, increasing mobilization of fats, and increasing cellular protein synthesis.

TEST-TAKING STRATEGY: Use the client diagnosis in the question to assist in the process of elimination in answering the question. Note the relationship between "dwarfism" in the question and "growth" in the correct option. Review the action of this medication now if you had difficulty with this question.

LEVEL OF COGNITIVE ABILITY: Comprehension
PHASE OF NURSING PROCESS: Evaluation
CLIENT NEEDS: Physiological Integrity
CONTENT AREA: Pharmacology
REFERENCE

Hodgson, B. & Kizior, R. (1999). *Saunders nursing drug handbook 1999.* Philadelphia: W. B. Saunders. p. 936.

2. **3**

RATIONALE: Water intoxication or hyponatremia is an adverse reaction to DDAVP. Early signs include drowsiness, listlessness, and headache. Decreased urination, rapid weight gain, confusion, seizures, and coma may also occur in overhydration.

TEST-TAKING STRATEGY: Knowledge that this medication is used in the treatment of diabetes insipidus will assist in eliminating options 1 and 2. Recalling the action of the medication will assist you in determining that water intoxication is an adverse reaction. This thought process will assist in directing you to option 3. Review the adverse reactions related to this important medication now if you had difficulty with this question.

LEVEL OF COGNITIVE ABILITY: Analysis
PHASE OF NURSING PROCESS: Data collection
CLIENT NEEDS: Physiological Integrity
CONTENT AREA: Pharmacology
REFERENCE

Hodgson, B., & Kizior, R. (1999). *Saunders nursing drug handbook 1999.* Philadelphia: W. B. Saunders. p. 295.

3. **2**

RATIONALE: Oral doses of levothyroxine should be taken on an empty stomach to enhance absorption. The medication should be taken in the morning before breakfast.

TEST-TAKING STRATEGY: Knowledge regarding the administration of levothyroxine is required to answer the question. If you are unfamiliar with this medication, review it now.

LEVEL OF COGNITIVE ABILITY: Comprehension
PHASE OF NURSING PROCESS: Evaluation
CLIENT NEEDS: Health Promotion and Maintenance
CONTENT AREA: Pharmacology
REFERENCE

Lehne, R. (1998). *Pharmacology for nursing care* (3rd ed.). Philadelphia: W. B. Saunders. p. 601.

4. **4**

RATIONALE: For most hypothyroid clients, replacement therapy must be continued for life. Treatment provides symptomatic relief but does not produce a cure. The client should be told that although therapy will cause symptoms to improve, these improvements do not constitute a reason to interrupt or discontinue the medication.

TEST-TAKING STRATEGY: Knowledge regarding the physiology associated with hypothyroidism is required to answer the question. If you are unfamiliar with this disorder and the medication therapy associated with it, take time now to review.

LEVEL OF COGNITIVE ABILITY: Application
PHASE OF NURSING PROCESS: Implementation
CLIENT NEEDS: Health Promotion and Maintenance
CONTENT AREA: Pharmacology
REFERENCE

Lehne, R. (1998). *Pharmacology for nursing care* (3rd ed.). Philadelphia: W. B. Saunders. p. 601.

5. **2**

RATIONALE: Excessive doses of levothyroxine can produce signs and symptoms of hyperthyroidism (thyrotoxicosis). These include tachycardia, angina, tremors, nervousness, insomnia, hyperthermia, heat intolerance, and sweating. The client should be instructed to notify the physician if these occur. Options 1, 3, and 4 are signs of hypothyroidism.

TEST-TAKING STRATEGY: Use the process of elimination recalling the symptoms associated with hypothyroidism, the purpose of administering levothyroxine and the effects of the medication. Options 1, 3, and 4 are symptoms related to hypothyroidism. Review the adverse effects of the medication now if you are unfamiliar with it.

LEVEL OF COGNITIVE ABILITY: Application
PHASE OF NURSING PROCESS: Implementation
CLIENT NEEDS: Health Promotion and Maintenance
CONTENT AREA: Pharmacology
REFERENCE

Lehne, R. (1998). *Pharmacology for nursing care* (3rd ed.). Philadelphia: W. B. Saunders. p. 601.

6. **4**

RATIONALE: PTU inhibits thyroid hormone synthesis and is used to treat hyperthyroidism or Graves' disease. Myxedema indicates hypothyroidism. Cushing's syndrome and Addison's disease are disorders related to adrenal function.

TEST-TAKING STRATEGY: Knowledge regarding the action of the medication and the treatment measures for Graves' disease is required to answer the question. If you are unfamiliar with either of these, review now.

LEVEL OF COGNITIVE ABILITY: Comprehension
PHASE OF NURSING PROCESS: Data Collection
CLIENT NEEDS: Physiological Integrity
CONTENT AREA: Pharmacology
REFERENCE

Lehne, R. (1998). *Pharmacology for nursing care* (3rd ed.). Philadelphia: W. B. Saunders. p. 601.

7. **3**

RATIONALE: Lypressin is administered by the intranasal route. It is used for diabetes insipidus. The usual adult dosage is 1 to 2 sprays into each nostril four times daily.

TEST-TAKING STRATEGY: Knowledge that lypressin is administered by the nasal route is required to answer the question. If you are unfamiliar with this medication, take time now to review.

LEVEL OF COGNITIVE ABILITY: Application
PHASE OF NURSING PROCESS: Implementation
CLIENT NEEDS: Health Promotion and Maintenance
CONTENT AREA: Pharmacology
REFERENCE
Lehne, R. (1998). *Pharmacology for nursing care* (3rd ed.). Philadelphia: W. B. Saunders. p. 613.

8. 2

RATIONALE: Laboratory determinations of serum TSH are an important means of evaluation of therapy with levothyroxine. Successful therapy will cause the elevated TSH levels to decrease. These levels will begin their decline within hours of the onset of therapy and will continue to drop as plasma levels of thyroid hormone build up. If an adequate dosage is established, TSH levels will remain suppressed for the duration of the therapy.
TEST-TAKING STRATEGY: Note the key words "expected outcome." Relate the diagnosis hypo"thyroidism" with "thyroid" hormone levels in the correct option. If you had difficulty with this question, take time now to review the therapeutic effect of levothyroxine.
LEVEL OF COGNITIVE ABILITY: Application
PHASE OF NURSING PROCESS: Implementation
CLIENT NEEDS: Physiological Integrity
CONTENT AREA: Pharmacology
REFERENCE
Lehne, R. (1998). *Pharmacology for nursing care* (3rd ed.). Philadelphia: W. B. Saunders. p. 601.

9. 2

RATIONALE: An adverse effect of PTU is agranulocytosis. The client needs to be informed of the early signs of this adverse effect, which includes fever or sore throat. Drowsiness is an occasional side effect of the medication. Polyuria and dry mouth are unrelated to this medication.
TEST-TAKING STRATEGY: Knowledge that agranulocytosis is an adverse effect of PTU is required to answer this question. If you are unfamiliar with this important medication, take time now to review.
LEVEL OF COGNITIVE ABILITY: Application
PHASE OF NURSING PROCESS: Implementation
CLIENT NEEDS: Health Promotion and Maintenance
CONTENT AREA: Pharmacology
REFERENCE
Lehne, R. (1998). *Pharmacology for nursing care* (3rd ed.). Philadelphia: W. B. Saunders. p. 606.

10. 2

RATIONALE: Lugol's solution is administered to hyperthyroid individuals in preparation for thyroidectomy to suppress thyroid function. Initial effects develop within 24 hours; peak effects develop in 10 to 15 days. Options 1, 3, and 4 are incorrect.
TEST-TAKING STRATEGY: Eliminate options 1 and 3 first because they are similar. From the remaining options, select option 2 because of its relationship to the issue of the question. If you had difficulty with this question, take time now to review the purpose of this medication.
LEVEL OF COGNITIVE ABILITY: Comprehension
PHASE OF NURSING PROCESS: Evaluation
CLIENT NEEDS: Physiological Integrity
CONTENT AREA: Pharmacology
REFERENCE
Lehne, R. (1998). *Pharmacology for nursing care* (3rd ed.). Philadelphia: W. B. Saunders. p. 604.

11. 3

RATIONALE: Excessive doses of fludrocortisone cause retention of sodium and water and excessive excretion of potassium resulting in expansion of blood volume, hypertension, cardiac enlargement, edema, and hypokalemia. The client needs to be informed about the signs of sodium and water retention, such as unusual weight gain, or swelling of the feet or lower legs. If these signs occur, the physician needs to be notified.
TEST-TAKING STRATEGY: Recalling that fludrocortisone can cause water retention will easily direct you to option 3. If you are unfamiliar with the adverse effects associated with this medication, review them now.
LEVEL OF COGNITIVE ABILITY: Application
PHASE OF NURSING PROCESS: Implementation
CLIENT NEEDS: Health Promotion and Maintenance
CONTENT AREA: Pharmacology
REFERENCE
Lehne, R. (1998). *Pharmacology for nursing care* (3rd ed.). Philadelphia: W. B. Saunders. p. 623.

12. 2

RATIONALE: The client should be instructed to take the medication exactly as prescribed and it is best administered 1 to 1.5 hours after meals. The client should take the medication with a full glass of water; however, it can be taken with milk.
TEST-TAKING STRATEGY: Knowledge regarding the administration of calcium carbonate is required to answer the question. If you are unfamiliar with the administration of this medication, take time now to review.
LEVEL OF COGNITIVE ABILITY: Application
PHASE OF NURSING PROCESS: Implementation
CLIENT NEEDS: Health Promotion and Maintenance
CONTENT AREA: Pharmacology
REFERENCE
Deglin, J., & Vallerand, A. (1999). *Davis's drug guide for nurses* (6th ed.). Philadelphia: F. A. Davis. p. 144.

13. 3

RATIONALE: The client taking an antihypocalcemic medication should be instructed to avoid eating too much spinach, rhubarb, bran, or whole-grain cereals because they decrease calcium absorption. Good dietary sources of calcium are milk products, dark green, leafy vegetables, clams, oysters, sardines, and orange juice fortified with calcium.
TEST-TAKING STRATEGY: Note that the diagnosis is "hypocalcemia." Note also the key word "avoid." Use the process of elimination and knowledge regarding food items high in calcium to assist in selecting the correct option. Review these foods now if you had difficulty with this question.
LEVEL OF COGNITIVE ABILITY: Application
PHASE OF NURSING PROCESS: Implementation
CLIENT NEEDS: Health Promotion and Maintenance
CONTENT AREA: Pharmacology
REFERENCE
Hodgson, B., & Kizior, R. (1999). *Saunders nursing drug handbook 1999*. Philadelphia: W. B. Saunders. p. 1058.

14. 3

RATIONALE: Glucocorticoids should be administered before 9 A.M. and the client should be instructed to do so. Administration at this time helps minimize adrenal insuffi-

ciency and mimics the burst of glucocorticoids released naturally by the adrenals each morning.
TEST-TAKING STRATEGY: Knowledge regarding the administration of glucocorticoids is required to answer this question. If you had difficulty with this question, take time now to review these concepts.
LEVEL OF COGNITIVE ABILITY: Application
PHASE OF NURSING PROCESS: Implementation
CLIENT NEEDS: Health Promotion and Maintenance
CONTENT AREA: Pharmacology
REFERENCE
Lehne, R. (1998). *Pharmacology for nursing care* (3rd ed.). Philadelphia: W. B. Saunders. p. 717.

15. **2**

RATIONALE: NPH Insulin is an intermediate-acting insulin. Its onset of action is 1 to 2 hours, it peaks in 6 to 12 hours, and its duration of action is 18 to 24 hours.
TEST-TAKING STRATEGY: Read the question carefully noting that the question is asking about NPH Insulin. Knowledge regarding the onset of action, peak, and duration of action is required to answer the question. Review these points regarding both NPH and Regular Insulin now if you are unfamiliar with them.
LEVEL OF COGNITIVE ABILITY: Comprehension
PHASE OF NURSING PROCESS: Planning
CLIENT NEEDS: Physiological Integrity
CONTENT AREA: Pharmacology
REFERENCE
Lehne, R. (1998). *Pharmacology for nursing care* (3rd ed.). Philadelphia: W. B. Saunders. p. 580.

16. **3**

RATIONALE: When preparing a mixture of Regular Insulin with another insulin preparation, the Regular Insulin should be drawn into the syringe first. This sequence will avoid contaminating the vial of Regular Insulin with insulin of another type.
TEST-TAKING STRATEGY: Knowledge regarding the appropriate method of preparing insulin for injection is required to answer the question. If you are unfamiliar with this procedure, review it now.
LEVEL OF COGNITIVE ABILITY: Comprehension
PHASE OF NURSING PROCESS: Evaluation
CLIENT NEEDS: Health Promotion and Maintenance
CONTENT AREA: Pharmacology
REFERENCE
Lehne, R. (1998). *Pharmacology for nursing care* (3rd ed.). Philadelphia: W. B. Saunders. p. 583.

17. **2**

RATIONALE: Insulin in unopened vials should be stored under refrigeration until needed. Vials should not be frozen. Open vials in use may be kept at room temperature and should be kept away from heat and direct light.
TEST-TAKING STRATEGY: Note the key word "store" in the question. Remembering that insulin should not be frozen will assist in eliminating option 1. Options 3 and 4 are similar and should be eliminated. Review client teaching points related to insulin now if you had difficulty with this question.
LEVEL OF COGNITIVE ABILITY: Application
PHASE OF NURSING PROCESS: Implementation

CLIENT NEEDS: Health Promotion and Maintenance
CONTENT AREA: Pharmacology
REFERENCE
Lehne, R. (1998). *Pharmacology for nursing care* (3rd ed.). Philadelphia: W. B. Saunders. p. 583.

18. **2**

RATIONALE: An insulin vial in current use can be kept at room temperature for up to 1 month without significant loss of activity. Direct sunlight and heat must be avoided.
TEST-TAKING STRATEGY: Note the key word "unrefrigerated." This word will assist in directing you to the correct option. However, if you are unfamiliar with the concepts related to insulin stability, review now.
LEVEL OF COGNITIVE ABILITY: Application
PHASE OF NURSING PROCESS: Implementation
CLIENT NEEDS: Health Promotion and Maintenance
CONTENT AREA: Pharmacology
REFERENCE
Lehne, R. (1998). *Pharmacology for nursing care* (3rd ed.). Philadelphia: W. B. Saunders. p. 583.

19. **1**

RATIONALE: The effect of Lispro insulin begins within 5 minutes of SC injection and persists for 2 to 4 hours. Lispro insulin acts more rapidly that Regular Insulin but has a shorter duration of action. Because of its rapid onset, it can be administered immediately before eating. In contrast, Regular Insulin is generally administered 30 to 60 minutes before meals.
TEST-TAKING STRATEGY: Note the key words "rapid acting." You should easily be able to eliminate options 3 and 4. From the remaining two options, remember that the question is asking about Lispro not Regular Insulin. Review this insulin now if you had difficulty with this question.
LEVEL OF COGNITIVE ABILITY: Application
PHASE OF NURSING PROCESS: Implementation
CLIENT NEEDS: Health Promotion and Maintenance
CONTENT AREA: Pharmacology
REFERENCE
Lehne, R. (1998). *Pharmacology for nursing care* (3rd ed.). Philadelphia: W. B. Saunders. p. 583.

20. **3**

RATIONALE: When alcohol is combined with tolbutamide, a disulfiram-like reaction may occur. This syndrome includes flushing, palpitations, and nausea. Alcohol can potentiate the hypoglycemic effects of tolbutamide. Clients must be warned about alcohol consumption while taking this medication.
TEST-TAKING STRATEGY: Use the process of elimination. Eliminate options 1, 2, and 4 because these food items are allowed in a diabetic diet. Remembering that alcohol can affect the action of many medications will assist in directing you to option 3. Review this medication now if you had difficulty with this question.
LEVEL OF COGNITIVE ABILITY: Application
PHASE OF NURSING PROCESS: Implementation
CLIENT NEEDS: Health Promotion and Maintenance
CONTENT AREA: Pharmacology
REFERENCE
Lehne, R. (1998). *Pharmacology for nursing care* (3rd ed.). Philadelphia: W. B. Saunders. p. 588.

BIBLIOGRAPHY

Deglin, J., & Vallerand, A. (1999). *Davis's drug guide for nurses* (6th ed.). Philadelphia: F. A. Davis.

Hodgson, B., & Kizior, R. (1999). *Saunders nursing drug handbook 1999*. Philadelphia: W. B. Saunders.

Leahy, J., & Kizilay, P. (1998). *Foundations of nursing practice: A nursing process approach*. Philadelphia: W. B. Saunders.

Lehne, R. (1998). *Pharmacology for nursing care* (3rd ed.). Philadelphia: W. B. Saunders.

Luckmann, J. (1997). *Saunders manual of nursing care*. Philadelphia: W. B. Saunders.

Monahan, F., & Neighbors, M. (1998). *Medical-surgical nursing: Foundations for clinical practice* (2nd ed.). Philadelphia: W. B. Saunders.

O'Toole, M. (1997). *Miller-Keane encyclopedia & dictionary of medicine, nursing, & allied health* (6th ed.). Philadelphia: W. B. Saunders.

UNIT XI

....

The Adult Client with a Gastrointestinal Disorder

PYRAMID TERMS

Ascites—The accumulation of fluid within the peritoneal cavity that results in venous congestion of the hepatic capillaries. This leads to plasma leaking directly from the liver surface and portal vein.

Asterixis—Also termed liver flap. A coarse tremor characterized by rapid, nonrhythmic extensions and flexions in the wrist and fingers.

Billroth I—Also called gastroduodenostomy; partial gastrectomy with the remaining segment anastomosed to the duodenum.

Billroth II—Also called gastrojejunostomy; partial gastrectomy with the remaining segment anastomosed to the jejunum.

Cholecystectomy—Removal of the gallbladder.

Cholecystitis—An inflammation of the gallbladder that may occur as an acute or chronic process. Acute inflammation is associated with gallstones (cholelithiasis). Chronic cholecystitis results when inefficient bile emptying and gallbladder muscle wall disease cause a fibrotic and contracted gallbladder.

Choledochotomy—Incision into the common bile duct to remove the stone.

Cirrhosis—A chronic, progressive disease of the liver characterized by diffuse damage to cells with fibrosis and nodular regeneration. Repeated destruction of hepatic cells causes the formation of scar tissue.

Crohn's Disease—An inflammatory disease that can occur anywhere in the gastrointestinal (GI) tract but most often affects the terminal ileum and leads to thickening and scarring, a narrowed lumen, fistulas, ulcerations, and abscesses. It is characterized by remissions and exacerbations.

Diverticulitis—Inflammation of one or more diverticuli. Results when diverticulum perforates, with local abscess formation. A perforated diverticulum can progress to intra-abdominal perforation with generalized peritonitis.

Diverticulosis—Outpouching or herniations of the intestinal mucosa. They can occur in any part of the intestine but are most common in the sigmoid colon.

Dumping Syndrome—Rapid emptying of the gastric contents into the small intestine. Occurs following gastric resection.

Esophageal Varices—Dilated and tortuous veins in the submucosa of the esophagus. They are caused by portal hypertension, are often associated with liver cirrhosis, and are at high risk for rupture if portal circulation pressure rises.

Fetor Hepaticus—The fruity musty breath odor associated with chronic liver disease.

Gastrectomy—Also called esophagojejunostomy; removal of the stomach with attachment of the esophagus to the jejunum or duodenum.

Gastric Resection—Also called antrectomy; involves removal of the lower half of the stomach and usually includes a vagotomy.

Hepatitis—An inflammation of the liver caused by a virus, bacteria, or exposure to medications or hepatotoxins.

Hiatus Hernia—Also known as esophageal or diaphragmatic hernia. A portion of the stomach herniates through the diaphragm and into the thorax. It results from weakening of the muscles of the diaphragm and is aggravated by factors that increase abdominal pressure such as pregnancy, ascites, obesity, tumors, and heavy lifting.

Pancreatitis—An acute or chronic inflammation of the pancreas, with associated escape of pancreatic enzymes into surrounding tissue. Acute pancreatitis occurs suddenly as one attack or can be recurrent, but resolves. Chronic pancreatitis is a continual inflammation and destruction of the pancreas, with scar tissue replacing pancreatic tissue.

Peristalsis—Wavelike rhythmic contractions that propel material through the GI tract.

Pyloroplasty—Enlarging the pylorus to prevent or decrease pyloric obstruction, thereby enhancing gastric emptying.

Ulcerative Colitis—Ulcerative and inflammatory disease of the bowel that results in poor absorption of nutrients. Acute ulcerative colitis results in vascular congestion, hemorrhage, edema, and ulceration of the bowel mucosa. Chronic ulcerative colitis causes muscular hypertrophy, fat deposits, and fibrous tissue with bowel thickening, shortening, and narrowing.

Vagotomy—Surgical division of the vagus nerve to eliminate the vagal impulses that stimulate hydrochloric acid secretion in the stomach.

◢ PYRAMID TO SUCCESS

Pyramid points focus on diagnostic tests, nursing care related to the various gastric or intestinal tubes, gastric surgery, cirrhosis, hepatitis, pancreatitis, and colostomy care. Focus on preprocedure and postprocedure care of the client undergoing a GI diagnostic test. Remember that an informed consent is required for any invasive procedure. Focus on diet restrictions before and following the diagnostic test, and remember that the gag reflex or bowel sounds must return before allowing a client to consume food or fluids. Pyramid points include instructions to the client and family regarding the prevention of GI disorders and the complications associated with the disorder. Focus on teaching the client and family about diet and nutrition specific to the disorder, tube and wound care, preventing the transmission of infection, and care to a colostomy or ileostomy. Remember that body image disturbances can occur in clients with a GI disorder. Specific focus relates to the client with a diversion, such as an ileostomy or colostomy, to the social isolation issues that can occur, and coping strategies.

NURSING PROCESS

DATA COLLECTION

Medical and family history
Socioeconomic status
Cultural and religious patterns
Vital signs, including respiratory pattern
Level of consciousness
Appearance as emaciated or obese
Dietary patterns
Nutritional and fluid intake
Weight changes

Nausea and vomiting
Condition of mouth, teeth, tongue, and gums
Swallowing ability and gag reflex
Skin color, turgor, and appearance
Pain
Edema and ascites
Bowel patterns, bowel sounds, and motility
Stool for the presence of blood, mucus, or bile

PLANNING

The client will maintain a patent airway. The client demonstrates effective breathing patterns.

IMPLEMENTATION

Monitor vital signs. Monitor respiratory status. Encourage coughing and deep breathing and splinting procedures. Position client based on disorder for optimal breathing.

EVALUATION

Client's airway remains patent. Lung sounds remain clear. Respiratory status remains within normal limits.

PLANNING	IMPLEMENTATION	EVALUATION
The client will tolerate nutritional intake to meet body needs. The client describes components of a nutritionally adequate diet. The client verbalizes understanding of fluid and dietary restrictions.	Monitor food and fluid intake. Monitor for signs of dehydration such as dry mucous membranes, poor skin turgor, decreased urination, and increased pulse. Monitor weight. Develop meal plan with client. Instruct client in requirements and restrictions as prescribed based on GI disorder.	The client maintains adequate nutritional intake. The client maintains a stable weight. The client demonstrates the ability to select appropriate foods, based on restrictions or requirements.
PLANNING	IMPLEMENTATION	EVALUATION
The client passes stool of normal consistency for the disorder.	Monitor for and document the presence of bowel sounds and abdominal distention. Monitor stool patterns and consistency. Evaluate laboratory results of stool specimens.	The client verbalizes the presence of an optimal bowel pattern.
PLANNING	IMPLEMENTATION	EVALUATION
The client demonstrates optimal skin care routine.	Monitor skin integrity. Instruct client in the care of diversion, such as the colostomy/ileostomy if present. Establish a skin care routine and instruct client in measures to prevent skin breakdown.	Skin remains intact.
PLANNING	IMPLEMENTATION	EVALUATION
The client reports a decrease in reflux symptoms. The client demonstrates the use of nonpharmacological pain relief measures. The client verbalizes the need for pain medication and obtains relief from medication.	Monitor for pain. Demonstrate the use of nonpharmacological pain relief measures. Use comfort measures to assist in reducing pain. Administer pain medication as prescribed. Monitor for effectiveness of pain medication and document results.	The client uses pain-relief techniques. The client remains free of pain.
PLANNING	IMPLEMENTATION	EVALUATION
The client identifies personal strengths that may promote effective coping. Client identifies community resources and support systems that will assist in decreasing social isolation.	Assist client to identify personal strengths and methods of coping. Assist client to identify behaviors that contribute to feelings of social isolation. Provide information on community resources that may decrease social isolation after discharge.	The client uses support systems and community resources.
PLANNING	IMPLEMENTATION	EVALUATION
The client verbalizes knowledge of preventive health measures.	Instruct client in preventive health measures specific to needs, such as lifestyle plan, modifications, dietary changes, cessation of smoking, stress reduction, and exercise. Instruct client and family regarding measures to prevent disease transmission. Suggest consult with social service to plan for health maintenance needs at discharge.	The client follows prescribed treatment. The client implements preventive health measures.

◢ CLIENT NEEDS

SAFE, EFFECTIVE CARE ENVIRONMENT

Confidentiality issues related to GI disorder
Informed consent for treatments and surgical procedures
Consultation related to nutritional status
Referrals to home care and community services
Handling infectious drainage and secretions
Standard (universal) precautions
Preventing the transmission of disease

HEALTH PROMOTION AND MAINTENANCE

Health screening related to GI disorders
Health promotion programs related to GI disorders
Teaching related to prescribed dietary and other
  treatment measures
Teaching related to colostomy or ileostomy care
Teaching related to preventing the transmission of
  disease

PSYCHOSOCIAL INTEGRITY

Coping mechanisms
Support systems
Body image changes related to colostomy or ileostomy

PHYSIOLOGICAL INTEGRITY

Nutrition and oral hydration
Personal hygiene
Elimination
Nonpharmacological and pharmacological comfort
  measures
Medication therapy specific to GI disorder
Diagnostic tests related to GI system
Care of GI tubes
Monitoring for complications related to tests,
  procedures, and surgical interventions
Fluid and electrolyte imbalances
Infectious diseases of the GI tract

BIBLIOGRAPHY

deWit, S. (1998). *Essentials of medical-surgical nursing* (4th ed.). Philadelphia: W. B. Saunders.

Hill, S., & Howlett, H. (1997). *Success in practical nursing: Personal and vocational issues* (3rd ed.). Philadelphia: W. B. Saunders.

Leahy, J., & Kizilay, P. (1998). *Foundations of nursing practice: A nursing process approach*. Philadelphia: W. B. Saunders.

Luckmann, J. (1997). *Saunders manual of nursing care*. Philadelphia: W. B. Saunders.

National Council of State Boards of Nursing (1998). *National Council detailed test plan for the NCLEX-PN examination*. Chicago: Author.

O'Toole, M. (1997). *Miller-Keane encyclopedia & dictionary of medicine, nursing, & allied health* (6th ed.). Philadelphia: W. B. Saunders.

CHAPTER 44

Gastrointestinal System

I. Anatomy and Physiology

A. Functions of the gastrointestinal (GI) system
   1. Processes food substances
   2. Absorbs the products of digestion into the blood
   3. Excretes unabsorbed materials
   4. Provides an environment for microorganisms to synthesize nutrients such as vitamin K
   5. For risk factors associated with the GI system, see Box 44-1

B. Mouth
   1. Contains the lips, cheeks, palate, tongue, teeth (mastication), salivary glands (lubrication), muscles, and maxillary bones
   2. Saliva contains the amylase enzyme (ptyalin), which aids in digestion

C. Esophagus
   1. A collapsible muscular tube, about 10 inches long
   2. Carries food from the pharynx to the stomach

D. Stomach: contains the cardia, fundus, body, and pylorus

   1. Mucous glands
      a. Located in the mucosa
      b. Prevents autodigestion by providing an alkaline protective covering
   2. Cardiac opening: prevents reflux into the esophagus
   3. Pyloric sphincter: regulates the rate of stomach emptying into the small intestine
   4. Hydrochloric acid: kills microorganisms, breaks food into small particles, and provides a chemical environment that is required by the gastric enzymes
   5. Pepsin: the chief coenzyme of gastric juice that converts proteins into proteases and peptones
   6. Intrinsic factor: necessary for the absorption of vitamin B_{12}
   7. Gastrin: controls gastric acidity

E. Small intestine
   1. The small intestine terminates into the cecum
   2. Duodenum: contains the openings of the bile and pancreatic ducts
   3. Jejunum: approximately 8 feet long
   4. Ileum: approximately 12 feet long

F. Intestinal juice enzymes
   1. Amylase digests starch to maltose
   2. Maltase reduces maltose to monosaccharide glucose
   3. Lactase splits lactose into galactose and glucose
   4. Sucrase reduces sucrose to fructose and glucose
   5. Nucleoses split nucleic acids to nucleotides
   6. Enterokinase activates trypsinogen to trypsin

G. Large intestine
   1. Approximately 5 feet long
   2. Absorbs water and eliminates wastes
   3. Microbial production of vitamins K, B_{12}, riboflavin, and thiamine
   4. Colon
      a. Ascending
      b. Transverse
      c. Descending

BOX 44-1. Risk Factors Associated with the GI System

Family history of GI disorders
Chronic laxative use
Tobacco use
Chronic alcohol use
Chronic high stress levels
Allergic reactions to food or medications
Long-term GI conditions such as ulcerative colitis may predispose to colorectal cancer
Previous abdominal surgery or trauma may lead to adhesions
Neurological disorders can impair movement, particularly with chewing and swallowing
Cardiac, respiratory, and endocrine disorders may lead to constipation
Diabetes mellitus may predispose to oral candidal infections

---

d. Sigmoid

e. Rectum

5. Ileocecal valve: prevents contents of large intestine from entering ileum

6. Anal sphincters: guard the anal canal

H. Peritoneum

1. Lines the abdominal cavity

2. Forms the mesentery, which supports the intestines and blood supply

I. Liver

1. The largest gland in the body weighing 3 to 4 pounds

2. Contains Kupffer's cells, which remove bacteria in the portal venous blood

3. Removes excess glucose and amino acids from the portal blood

4. Synthesizes glucose, amino acids, and fats

5. Aids in the digestion of fats, carbohydrates, and proteins

6. Stores and filters blood (200 to 400 mL of blood stored)

7. Stores vitamins A, D, B_{12}, and iron

8. Secretes bile to emulsify fats (500 to 1000 mL bile a day)

9. Hepatic ducts

a. Deliver bile to the gallbladder via the cystic duct

b. Deliver bile to the duodenum via the common bile duct

c. The common bile duct opens into the duodenum with the pancreatic duct at the ampulla of Vater

d. The sphincter prevents the reflux of intestinal contents into the common bile duct and pancreatic duct

J. Gallbladder

1. Stores and concentrates bile

2. Contracts to force bile into the duodenum during the digestion of fats

3. The cystic duct joins the hepatic duct to form the common bile duct

4. The sphincter of Oddi guards the entrance into the duodenum

5. The presence of fatty materials in the duodenum stimulates the liberation of cholecystokinin, which causes contraction of the gallbladder and relaxation of the sphincter of Oddi

K. Pancreas

1. Exocrine gland

a. Secretes sodium bicarbonate to neutralize the acidity of the stomach contents as they enter the duodenum

b. Pancreatic juices contain enzymes for digesting carbohydrates, fats, and proteins

2. Endocrine gland

a. Insulin secretion is produced by the islets of Langerhans

b. Insulin is secreted into the bloodstream

c. Insulin is important for carbohydrate metabolism

II. Diagnostic Procedures

A. Upper GI (barium swallow)

1. Description: an examination of the upper GI tract under fluoroscopy after the client drinks barium sulfate

2. Preprocedure: instruct the client to fast from foods and fluids overnight prior to the study

3. Postprocedure

a. A laxative may be prescribed following the procedure

b. Instruct the client to drink six to eight glasses of water each day for 2 days to help pass the barium

c. Monitor stools for the passage of barium (stools will appear chalky white)

B. Lower GI (barium enema)

1. Description

a. A fluoroscopic and radiographic exam of the large intestine after rectal instillation of barium sulfate

b. May be done with or without air

2. Preprocedure

a. Laxatives on the day prior to and the morning of the test

b. Liquid diet 1 day prior to and on the morning of the test

3. Postprocedure

a. Increase fluid intake for 24 to 48 hours

b. Administer mild laxatives to facilitate emptying of the barium

c. Monitor stool for passage of barium

d. Notify the physician if a bowel movement does not occur within 2 days

C. Gastroscopy

1. Description: insertion of an endoscopic instrument through the esophagus into the stomach and upper portion of the small intestine to visualize the mucosal lining

2. Preprocedure

a. Obtain informed consent

b. Remove dentures

c. Administer sedative as required

d. Obtain baseline vital signs

e. Maintain NPO status for 12 hours prior to procedure

3. Postprocedure

a. Monitor vital signs, respiratory, cardiac, and neurological status

b. Monitor for return of gag reflex

c. Do not administer food or fluid until gag reflex returns

d. Monitor for signs of bleeding as evidenced by hypotension, pallor, and tachycardia

e. Monitor for perforation as evidenced by pain, tachypnea, and rales

D. Sigmoidoscopy

1. Description: endoscopic visualization of the sigmoid colon using a sigmoidoscope

2. Preprocedure

a. Obtain informed consent

b. A full liquid diet the evening before the test

c. Laxatives the evening before the test and an enema or suppository 1 hour prior to the test

3. Postprocedure
   a. Assess for side effects related to the sedative if administered
   b. Normal activities and diet may be resumed
   c. Notify the physician if temperature is higher than 101°F or if breathing difficulty, stomach pain, or bright red rectal bleeding occurs

E. Colonoscopy
   1. Description: a fiberoptic endoscopy study in which the lining of the large intestine is visually examined
   2. Preprocedure
      a. Obtain informed consent
      b. Clear liquid diet for 48 hours prior to the test
      c. Bowel preparation with laxatives on the evening prior to the test and an enema on the day of the test
   3. Postprocedure
      a. Monitor vital signs
      b. Monitor for side effects if sedation was administered
      c. A normal diet may be resumed
      d. Monitor for signs of colon perforation as evidenced by abdominal pain or distention malaise, fever, purulent rectal drainage, or lower GI bleeding

F. Gastric analysis
   1. Description: the passage of a nasogastric (NG) tube into the stomach to aspirate gastric contents for analysis of acidity, appearance, and volume
   2. Preprocedure
      a. Fast for 12 hours prior to the test
      b. Avoiding tobacco and chewing gum for 6 hours prior to the test
   3. Postprocedure
      a. May resume normal activities
      b. Refrigerate gastric samples if not tested within 4 hours

G. Gallbladder series
   1. Description: oral cholecystography to study the dye-filled gallbladder by radiographic film
   2. Preprocedure
      a. A low-fat meal on the evening prior to the test and then fasting at midnight the day before the test
      b. Administer six 0.5-g iopanoic acid (Telepaque) tablets 12 hours prior to the test
      c. Tablets should be taken with a large amount of water at 5-minute intervals
      d. Instruct the client to go to the emergency department if a rash, itching or hives, or difficulty in breathing occurs after taking the tablets

3. Postprocedure
   a. Inform the client that dysuria is common because the dye is excreted in the urine
   b. A normal diet may be resumed; however, a fatty meal may enhance dye excretion

H. Liver biopsy
   1. Description: a needle is inserted through the abdominal wall to the liver to obtain a tissue sample for biopsy and microscopic examination
   2. Preprocedure
      a. Obtained informed consent
      b. Assess hematological laboratory results
      c. Administer sedative as prescribed
      d. NPO after midnight on the day prior to the test
      e. Note that the client is placed in the supine or left lateral position during the procedure
   3. Postprocedure
      a. Assess vital signs frequently
      b. Assess the biopsy site for bleeding
      c. Monitor for peritonitis
      d. Maintain bed rest for 24 hour
      e. Place the client on the right side for 1 to 2 hours to decrease the risk of hemorrhage

I. Paracentesis
   1. Description: transabdominal removal of fluid from the peritoneal cavity for the analysis of electrolytes, red blood cells, white blood cells, bacterial and viral cultures, and cytology studies
   2. Preprocedure
      a. Obtain informed consent
      b. Have the client void prior to the start of procedure to empty the bladder and to move bladder out of the way of the paracentesis needle
      c. Measure abdominal girth, weight, and baseline vital signs
      d. Note that the client is positioned sitting on the edge of the bed with the back supported and the feet resting on a stool, or lying prone during the procedure
   3. Postprocedure
      a. Monitor vital signs
      b. Maintain bed rest
      c. Apply a dry sterile dressing to the insertion site
      d. Monitor the insertion site for bleeding
      e. Measure abdominal girth and weight
      f. Monitor for hematuria due to bladder trauma
      g. Instruct the client to notify the physician if the urine becomes bloody, pink, or red

J. Stool specimens
   1. Description: examination of stool by dipstick for the presence of bleeding
   2. Preprocedure: instruct the client to avoid aspirin, NSAIDs, red meat, poultry, and fish 3 days prior to the collection

K. Liver and pancreas laboratory studies
  1. Alkaline phosphatase
     a. Released during liver damage or biliary obstruction
     b. Normal value: 4.5 to 13 King-Armstrong U/dL
  2. Prothrombin time (PT)
     a. Prolonged with liver damage
     b. Normal value: 9.5 to 11.8 seconds
  3. Serum ammonia
     a. Assesses the ability of the liver to deaminate protein byproducts
     b. Normal value: 15 to 45 μ/dL
  4. Liver enzymes (transaminase studies)
     a. Elevated with liver damage
     b. SGOT: 10 to 50 IU/L
     c. SGPT: 5 to 35 IU/L
     d. LDH: 70 to 200 IU/L
  5. Cholesterol
     a. Increase indicates **pancreatitis** or biliary obstruction
     b. Normal value: 120 to 200 mg/dL
  6. Bilirubin
     a. Increase indicates liver damage or biliary obstruction
     b. Bilirubin direct: 0 to 0.3 mg/dL
     c. Bilirubin indirect: 0.1 to 1.0 mg/dL
     d. Bilirubin total: less than 1.5 mg/dL
  7. Amylase and lipase
     a. Elevations indicate **pancreatitis**
     b. Amylase: 50 to 180 Somogyi units/dL
     c. Lipase: 31–186 U/L

III. Data Collection

A. Abdominal assessment
  1. Inspect the skin for color, abnormalities, contour, and tautness and the abdomen for distention
  2. Auscultate for bowel sounds
  3. Percuss for air or solids
  4. Palpate for tenderness
B. Bowel sounds
  1. Auscultate bowel sounds before percussion and palpation
  2. Normal bowel sounds occur 5 to 34 times a minute or every 5 to 15 seconds
  3. Auscultate in all quadrants
  4. Listen at least 5 minutes in each quadrant before assuming sounds are absent

IV. Nasogastric, Esophageal, and Intestinal Tubes (refer to Chapter 18 regarding the descriptions and nursing care related to GI tubes)

V. Hiatus Hernia

A. Description
  1. Also known as esophageal or diaphragmatic hernia
  2. A portion of the stomach herniates through the diaphragm and into the thorax
  3. It results from weakening of the muscles of the diaphragm and is aggravated by factors that increase abdominal pressure such as pregnancy, **ascites**, obesity, tumors, and heavy lifting
  4. Complications include ulceration, hemorrhage, regurgitation and aspiration of stomach contents, and incarceration of the stomach in the chest with possible necrosis, peritonitis, and mediastinitis
B. Data collection
  1. Heartburn
  2. Feeling of fullness
  3. Discomfort or pain
  4. Regurgitation or vomiting
  5. Dysphagia
  6. Bleeding
C. Implementation
  1. Provide small, frequent meals and minimize the amount of liquids
  2. Elevate the head of the bed while eating and for 30 minutes after eating
  3. Administer antacids after meals and at bedtime as prescribed to relieve heartburn and to increase lower esophageal sphincter pressure
  4. Administer histamine H_2-receptor antagonists as prescribed to control esophageal reflux
  5. Avoid anticholinergics, which delay stomach emptying
  6. Instruct the client to avoid vigorous coughing
  7. Instruct the client to avoid constrictive clothing around waist
  8. Instruct clients to avoid sharp, forward bending
  9. Instruct clients to avoid highly seasoned and fatty foods
  10. Instruct the client to avoid alcohol, smoking, caffeine, chocolate, and carbonated and acidic beverages
  11. Instruct clients to avoid nighttime snacking to ensure that the stomach is empty
  12. Encourage weight reduction because obesity increases intra-abdominal pressure
D. Surgical implementation
  1. Indicated when the risk of complications such as aspiration exists and damage from chronic reflux is severe
  2. Surgical approaches include reinforcement of the lower esophageal sphincter (LES) to restore sphincter competence and prevent reflux
  3. Achieved by a procedure that involves wrapping of a portion of the stomach fundus around the distal esophagus to anchor it and reinforce the LES

VI. Esophageal Varices

A. Description
  1. Dilated and tortuous veins in the submucosa of the esophagus

2. They are caused by portal hypertension, are often associated with liver **cirrhosis**, and are at high risk for rupture if portal circulation pressure rises
3. Bleeding varices is an emergency
4. The goal of treatment is to control bleeding, prevent complications, and prevent the recurrence of a bleed

B. Data collection
   1. Hematemesis
   2. Melena
   3. Tarry stools
   4. **Ascites**
   5. Jaundice
   6. Hepatomegaly and splenomegaly
   7. Dilated abdominal veins
   8. Hemorrhoids
   9. Bleeding and shock

C. Implementation
   1. Monitor vital signs
   2. Elevate the head of the bed
   3. Monitor for orthostatic hypotension
   4. Monitor lung sounds and for the presence of respiratory distress
   5. Administer oxygen as prescribed to prevent tissue hypoxia
   6. Maintain NPO status
   7. Monitor LOC
   8. Monitor I&O
   9. Administer IV fluids as prescribed to restore fluid volume and electrolyte imbalances
   10. Monitor hemoglobin, hematocrit, and coagulation factors
   11. Blood or clotting factors are administered as prescribed
   12. Assist in inserting a nasogastric tube or a balloon tamponade as prescribed
   13. Assist with the administration of saline irrigation to the vasoconstrictor vessels as prescribed
   14. Prepare to assist with administering vasopressin (Pitressin) as prescribed to induce vasoconstriction and reduce bleeding
   15. Prepare to assist with administering nitroglycerin with the vasopressin (Pitressin), which produces a reduction in portal pressure
   16. Instruct the client to avoid activities that will initiate vasovagal responses
   17. Prepare the client for endoscopic procedures or surgical procedures as prescribed

D. Endoscopic injection (sclerotherapy)
   1. Injection of a sclerosing agent into and around bleeding varices
   2. Complications include chest pain, pleural effusion, aspiration pneumonia, esophageal stricture, and perforation of the esophagus

E. Endoscopic variceal ligation
   1. Ligation of the varices with an elastic rubber band
   2. Sloughing, followed by superficial ulceration,

occurs in the area of ligation within 3 to 7 days

F. Surgical shunt procedures
   1. Splenorenal: involves splenectomy with anastomosis of the splenic vein to the left renal vein
   2. Portacaval: shunting of the blood from the portal vein to the inferior vena cava
   3. Mesocaval: involves a side anastomosis of the superior mesenteric vein to the proximal end of the inferior vena cava
   4. Transjugular intrahepatic portal/systemic
      a. Uses the normal vascular anatomy of the liver to create a shunt with the use of a metallic stent
      b. The shunt is between the portal and systemic venous systems within the liver and is aimed at relieving portal hypertension

VII. Peptic Ulcer Disease

A. Description
   1. An ulceration in the mucosal wall of stomach, pylorus, or duodenum in portions that are accessible to gastric secretions
   2. Erosion may extend through the muscle to the peritoneum
   3. The most common peptic ulcers are gastric ulcers and duodenal ulcers

B. Gastric ulcers
   1. Description
      a. Involves ulceration of the mucosal lining that extends to the submucosal layer of the stomach
      b. Predisposing factors include stress, smoking, the use of steroids, NSAIDs, alcohol, a history of gastritis, or family history of gastric ulcers
      c. Complications include hemorrhage, perforation, and pyloric obstruction
   2. Data collection
      a. Gnawing, sharp pain in or left of the midepigastric region 1 to 2 hours after eating
      b. Nausea and vomiting
      c. Hematemesis
   3. Implementation
      a. Monitor vital signs
      b. Monitor for bleeding
      c. Administer small, frequent bland feedings during the active phase
      d. Administer histamine H_2-receptor antagonists as prescribed to decrease the secretion of gastric acid
      e. Administer antacids as prescribed to neutralize gastric secretions
      f. Administer anticholinergics as prescribed to reduce gastric motility
      g. Administer mucosal barrier protectants as prescribed 1 hour before each meal

h. Administer prostaglandins as prescribed for their protective and antisecretory actions

i. Instruct clients to avoid alcohol

j. Instruct clients to avoid caffeine and chocolate

k. Instruct clients to avoid smoking

l. Instruct the client to avoid aspirin or NSAIDs

m. Instruct the client to obtain adequate rest and reduce stress

4. Implementation during active bleeding

a. Monitor vital signs

b. Monitor for signs of dehydration, hypovolemic shock, sepsis, and respiratory insufficiency

c. Monitor I&O

d. Maintain NPO status and administer IV fluid replacement as prescribed

e. Monitor hemoglobin and hematocrit

f. Blood transfusions may be prescribed

g. Assist with insertion of an NG tube for decompression and for access for lavage

h. Assist with normal saline or tapwater lavage at room temperature to reduce active bleeding

i. Prepare to assist with administering vasopressin (Pitressin) by IV as prescribed to induce vasoconstriction and reduce bleeding

5. Estimating the amount of blood loss

a. Less than 500 mL: pulse rate begins to rise

b. 500 to 1000 mL: pulse increases to 100 to 110, BP begins to decrease, urine output declines, and signs of shock are present

c. 1000 to 2000 mL: pulse increases beyond 110 to 120 and BP continues to decrease

d. More than 2000 mL: pulse increases beyond 120 and BP and urine output decline significantly

6. Surgical implementation

a. Total **Gastrectomy**: also called esophagojejunostomy; removal of the stomach with attachment of the esophagus to the jejunum or duodenum

b. **Vagotomy**: surgical division of the vagus nerve to eliminate the vagal impulses that stimulate hydrochloric acid secretion in the stomach

c. **Gastric resection**: also called antrectomy; involves removal of the lower half of the stomach and usually includes a **vagotomy**

d. **Billroth I**: also called gastroduodenostomy; partial **gastrectomy** with the remaining segment anastomosed to the duodenum

e. **Billroth II**: also called gastrojejunostomy; partial **gastrectomy** with the remaining segment anastomosed to the jejunum

f. **Pyloroplasty**: Enlarges the pylorus to prevent or decrease pyloric obstruction, thereby enhancing gastric emptying

7. Postoperative implementation

a. Monitor vital signs

b. Position in Fowler's for comfort and to promote drainage

c. Monitor I&O

d. Administer fluids and electrolyte replacements IV as prescribed

e. Assess bowel sounds

f. Monitor nasogastric suction as prescribed

g. Do not irrigate NG tube or remove NG tube

h. Assist the physician with NG irrigation or removal of NG tube

i. Maintain NPO status as prescribed for 1 to 3 days until **peristalsis** returns

j. Progress the diet from NPO to sips of clear water to six small, bland meals a day as prescribed when bowel sounds return

k. Monitor for postoperative complications of hemorrhage, **dumping syndrome**, diarrhea, hypoglycemia, and vitamin B_{12} deficiency

VIII. Duodenal Ulcers

A. Description

1. A break in the mucosa of the duodenum

2. Risk factors and causes include alcohol intake, smoking, stress, caffeine, the use of aspirin, corticosteroids and NSAIDs, and infection with *Helicobacter pylori*

3. The goals of treatment are to eliminate the cause, decrease gastric acidity, and prevent complications

4. Complications include bleeding, perforation, gastric outlet obstruction, and intractable disease

B. Data collection

1. Burning pain in the midepigastric area 2 to 4 hours after eating and during the night

2. Pain that is often relieved by eating

3. Melena

C. Implementation

1. Monitor vital signs

2. Perform abdominal assessment

3. Instruct the client in a bland diet with small, frequent meals

4. Provide for adequate rest

5. Encourage the cessation of smoking

6. Instruct the client to avoid alcohol intake, caffeine, the use of aspirin, corticosteroids, and NSAIDs

7. Administer antacids as prescribed to neutralize acid secretions

8. Administer histamine H_2-receptor antagonists as prescribed to block the secretion of acid

D. Surgical implementation: surgery is performed only if the ulcer is unresponsive to medications or if hemorrhage, obstruction, or perforation occurs

IX. Dumping Syndrome

A. Description
1. Rapid emptying of the gastric contents into the small intestine
2. Occurs following **gastric resection**
B. Data collection
1. Symptoms occurring 30 minutes after eating
2. Nausea and vomiting
3. Abdominal cramping
4. Feelings of fullness
5. Diarrhea
6. Palpitation
7. Tachycardia
8. Perspiration
9. Weakness and dizziness
10. Borborygmi
C. Implementation
1. Instruct the client to eat a high-protein, high-fat, low-carbohydrate diet
2. Instruct the client to eat small meals and to avoid fluids with meals
3. Instruct clients to avoid sugar and salt
4. Instruct clients to lie down after meals
5. Instruct clients to take antiperistaltic and antispasmodic medications as prescribed to delay gastric emptying

X. Vitamin B_{12} Deficiency

A. Description
1. Results from either an inadequate intake of vitamin B_{12} or a lack of absorption of ingested vitamin B_{12} from the intestinal tract
2. Pernicious anemia results from a deficiency of intrinsic factor, which is necessary for intestinal absorption of vitamin B_{12}
B. Data collection
1. Severe pallor
2. Fatigue
3. Weight loss
4. Smooth, beefy red tongue
5. Slight jaundice
6. Paresthesias of the hands and feet
7. Disturbances with gait and balance
C. Implementation
1. Increase dietary intake of food rich in vitamin B_{12} if the anemia is the result of a dietary deficiency (Box 44–2)
2. Administer vitamin B_{12} injections as prescribed on a weekly basis initially and then monthly for maintenance (lifelong) if the

BOX 44–2. Foods Rich in Vitamin B_{12}	
Liver	Green, leafy vegetables
Organ meats	Citrus fruits
Dried beans	Brewer's yeast
Nuts	

BOX 44–3. Surgical Treatment for Gastric Cancer	
Total gastrectomy	Billroth I
Vagotomy	Billroth II
Gastric resection	Pyloroplasty

anemia is the result of a deficiency of the intrinsic factor

XI. Gastric Cancer

A. Description
1. An abnormal malignant growth in the abdomen
2. Risk factors include a diet high in complex carbohydrates, grains, and salt but low in animal fat; fresh, green leafy vegetables, fresh fruit; smoking; alcohol; and a history of gastric ulcers
3. Complications include hemorrhage, obstruction, metastasis, and **dumping syndrome**
4. The goal of treatment is to remove the tumor and provide a nutritional program
B. Data collection
1. Anorexia
2. Nausea and vomiting
3. Indigestion and epigastric discomfort
4. A sensation of pressure
5. Dysphagia
6. Weight loss
7. Palpable mass
8. Fatigue
9. Anemia
10. **Ascites**
C. Implementation
1. Monitor vital signs
2. Monitor nutritional status
3. Encourage small, bland, easily digestible meals with vitamin and mineral supplements
4. Monitor weight
5. Administer pain medication as prescribed
6. Monitor hemoglobin and hematocrit and monitor blood transfusion as prescribed
7. Provide emotional support
8. Prepare the client for chemotherapy or radiation therapy as prescribed
9. Prepare the client for surgical resection of the tumor as prescribed (Box 44–3)
D. Postoperative implementation
1. Monitor vital signs
2. Position in Fowler's for comfort and to promote drainage
3. Monitor I&O
4. Monitor fluids and electrolyte replacements IV as prescribed
5. Monitor bowel sounds
6. Monitor nasogastric suction as prescribed

7. Do not irrigate or remove the NG tube
8. Assist the physician with NG irrigation or removal of NG tube
9. Maintain NPO status as prescribed for 1 to 3 days until **peristalsis** returns
10. Progress the diet from NPO to sips of clear water to six small, bland meals a day as prescribed when bowel sounds return
11. Monitor for postoperative complications of hemorrhage, **dumping syndrome**, diarrhea, hypoglycemia, and vitamin B_{12} deficiency

XII. Ulcerative Colitis

A. Description
   1. Ulcerative and inflammatory disease of the bowel that results in poor absorption of nutrients
   2. Commonly begins in the rectum and spreads upward toward the cecum
   3. The colon becomes edematous and may develop bleeding lesions and ulcers
   4. The ulcers may lead to perforation
   5. Scar tissue develops and causes loss of elasticity and loss of ability to absorb nutrients
   6. Characterized by various periods of remission and exacerbation
   7. Acute **ulcerative colitis** results in vascular congestion, hemorrhage, edema, and ulceration of the bowel mucosa
   8. Chronic **ulcerative colitis** causes muscular hypertrophy, fat deposits, and fibrous tissue with bowel thickening, shortening, and narrowing
B. Data collection
   1. Anorexia
   2. Weight loss
   3. Malaise
   4. Abdominal tenderness and cramping
   5. Severe diarrhea that may contain blood and mucus
   6. Dehydration and electrolyte imbalances
   7. Anemia
   8. Vitamin K deficiency
C. Implementation
   1. Maintain NPO status and administer IVs and electrolytes as prescribed during the acute phase
   2. TPN may be prescribed during an acute phase
   3. Restrict the client's activity to reduce intestinal activity
   4. Monitor bowel sounds
   5. Monitor for abdominal tenderness and cramping
   6. Monitor stools, noting color, consistency, and the presence or absence of blood
   7. Monitor for perforation, peritonitis, and hemorrhage
   8. Following the acute phase, the diet progresses from clear liquids to low residue as tolerated
   9. Instruct the client to consume a low-roughage, low-residue diet and to avoid foods such as whole-wheat grains, nuts, raw fruits, and vegetables
   10. Instruct clients to avoid gas-forming foods and milk products
   11. Instruct the client to thoroughly chew solid foods
   12. Instruct the client to avoid caffeinated beverages, alcohol, and pepper
   13. Encourage clients to stop smoking
   14. Administer antidiarrheal medications as prescribed
   15. Administer antimicrobial, corticosteroids, and immunosuppressants as prescribed to prevent infection and reduce inflammation
D. Surgical implementation
   1. Total proctocolectomy with permanent ileostomy
      a. Involves removal of the colon, rectum, and anus with anal closure
      b. The end of the terminal ileum forms the stoma, which is located in the right lower quadrant
   2. Kock pouch (ileostomy)
      a. An intra-abdominal pouch is constructed from the terminal ileum
      b. The pouch is connected to the stoma with a nipplelike valve constructed from a portion of the ileum
      c. The stoma is flush with the skin
   3. Ileoanal reservoir
      a. A two-stage procedure that involves the excision of the rectal mucosa, abdominal colectomy, construction of the reservoir to the anal canal, and a temporary loop ileostomy
      b. The ileostomy is closed in approximately 4 months after the capacity of the reservoir is increased
   4. Preoperative colostomy/ileostomy
      a. Consult with an enterostomal therapist to assist in identifying optimal placement of the ostomy
      b. Instruct the client to eat a low-residue diet for a day or two prior to surgery as prescribed
      c. Administer intestinal antiseptics and antibiotics as prescribed to decrease bacterial content of the colon and to soften and decrease the bulk of the contents of the colon
      d. Administer laxatives and enemas as prescribed
   5. Postoperative colostomy
      a. Place a petroleum gauze over the stoma as prescribed to keep it moist, followed by a dry sterile dressing if a pouch system is not in place

b. Place a pouched system on the stoma as soon as possible
c. Monitor the stoma for size, unusual bleeding, or necrotic tissue
d. Monitor for color changes in the stoma
e. Note that the normal stoma color is red or pink, indicating high vascularity
f. Note that a pale pink stoma indicates low hemoglobin and hematocrit levels and a purple-black stoma indicates compromised circulation requiring physician notification
g. Assess the functioning of the colostomy
h. Expect that stool is liquid immediate postoperative but becomes more solid depending on the area of the colostomy; ascending colon—liquid stool; transverse colon—loose to semiformed; descending colon— close to normal
i. Monitor the pouch system for proper fit and signs of leakage
j. Empty pouch when one-third full
k. Fecal matter should not be allowed to remain on the skin
l. Administer analgesics and antibiotics as prescribed
m. Irrigate the perineal wound if present as prescribed and monitor for signs of infection
n. Instruct the client to avoid foods that cause excess gas formation and odor
o. Instruct the client on stoma care and irrigations as prescribed (Box 44–4)
p. Instruct clients that normal activities may be resumed when approved by the physician
6. Postoperative ileostomy
a. Note that the healthy stoma is red
b. Monitor for color change in the stoma to dark blue or black, and if it occurs, it should be reported to the physician

---

BOX 44–4. Colostomy Irrigation

DESCRIPTION

Instilling 500–1000 mL tepid H_2O through the stoma and allowing H_2O and stool to drain into collection bag

PROCEDURE

▲ If ambulatory, position client sitting on toilet
▲ If on bed rest, position client on side
▲ Hang irrigation bag so that bottom of bag is at the level of the client's shoulder or slightly higher
Insert irrigation tube carefully without force
Begin the flow of irrigation
Clamp tubing if cramping occurs; release tubing as cramping subsides
▲ Avoid frequent irrigations with H_2O, which can lead to loss of fluids and electrolytes
Perform irrigation around the same time each day
Perform irrigation preferably 1 hour after a meal

---

c. Note that normal stool is liquid
d. Monitor for dehydration and electrolyte imbalance
e. Do not give suppositories through the ileostomy

XIII. Crohn's Disease (Regional Enteritis)

A. Description
1. An inflammatory disease that can occur anywhere in the GI tract but most often affects the terminal ileum and leads to thickening and scarring, a narrowed lumen, fistulas, ulcerations, and abscesses
2. It is characterized by remissions and exacerbations
B. Data collection
1. Fever
2. Cramplike pain after meals
3. Diarrhea semisolid and may contain mucus, pus, and blood
4. Abdominal distention
5. Anorexia, nausea, and vomiting
6. Weight loss
7. Anemia
8. Dehydration
9. Electrolyte imbalances
C. Implementation: care is similar to the client with **ulcerative colitis**

XIV. Intestinal Tumors

A. Description
1. Malignant lesions that develop in the cells lining the bowel wall or develop as polyps in the colon or rectum
2. Complications include bowel perforation with peritonitis, abscess and/or fistula formation, frank hemorrhage, and complete intestinal obstruction
3. Metastasis occurs via the circulatory or lymphatic system or by direct extension to other areas in the colon or other organs
B. Data collection
1. Blood in stools
2. Abnormal stools
3. Anorexia
4. Vomiting
5. Weight loss
6. Malaise
7. Anemia
8. Ascending colon tumors—diarrhea
9. Descending colon tumor—constipation or some diarrhea, or flat ribbonlike stool due to a partial obstruction
10. Rectal tumor—alternating constipation and diarrhea
11. Guarding or abdominal distention
12. Abdominal mass (a late sign)
13. Cachexia (a late sign)
C. Implementation
1. Monitor for signs of complications, which

include bowel perforation with peritonitis, abscess and/or fistula formation, frank hemorrhage, and complete intestinal obstruction

2. Monitor for signs of intestinal perforation including low BP, rapid weak pulse, distended abdomen, and elevated temperature

3. Monitor for signs of intestinal obstruction, which may include vomiting (may be fecal contents), pain, constipation, and abdominal distention

4. Note that an early sign of intestinal obstruction includes increased peristaltic activity, which produces an increase in bowel sounds, and as the obstruction progresses, hypoactive sounds

D. Nonsurgical implementation
1. Radiation preoperatively to facilitate surgical resection and postoperatively to decrease the risk of recurrence or to reduce pain, hemorrhage, bowel obstruction, or metastasis

2. Chemotherapy used postoperatively to assist in the control of symptoms and spread of the disease

E. Surgical implementation: bowel resection and creation of colostomy or ileostomy

XV. Diverticulosis and Diverticulitis

A. Description
1. **Diverticulosis**
   a. Outpouching or herniations of the intestinal mucosa
   b. They can occur in any part of the intestine but are most common in the sigmoid colon
2. **Diverticulitis**
   a. Inflammation of one or more diverticuli
   b. Results when diverticulum perforates with local abscess formation
   c. A perforated diverticulum can progress to intra-abdominal perforation with generalized peritonitis

B. Data collection
1. Left lower quadrant abdominal pain that increases with coughing, straining, or lifting
2. Elevated temperature
3. Nausea and vomiting
4. Flatulence
5. Cramplike pain
6. Abdominal distention and tenderness
7. Palpable, tender rectal mass
8. Blood in stools

C. Implementation
1. Provide bed rest during the acute phase
2. Maintain NPO status or provide clear liquids during the acute phase as prescribed
3. Introduce a fiber-containing diet gradually when the inflammation is resolved
4. Instruct the client to refrain from lifting, straining, coughing, or bending to avoid increased intra-abdominal pressure

5. Administer antibiotics and pain medication as prescribed
6. Monitor for perforation, hemorrhage, fistulas, and abscesses
7. Instruct the client on the signs and symptoms of diverticular disease such as fever, abdominal pain, and bloody stools
8. Instruct clients to eat a diet high in cellulose such as wheat bran, whole grains, and cereals
9. Instruct clients to eat fruits and vegetables with a high fiber content and to avoid foods containing indigestible roughage or seeds
10. Instruct the client to avoid gas-forming foods, hot and cold liquids, and alcohol
11. Instruct the client to avoid enemas and laxatives other than bulk-forming products such as psyllium (Metamucil)

D. Surgical implementation
1. Colon resection with primary anastomosis
2. Temporary or permanent colostomy may be required for increased bowel inflammation

XVI. Hemorrhoids

A. Description
1. Dilated varicose veins of the anal canal
2. May be either internal, external, or prolapsed
3. Internal hemorrhoids lie above the anal sphincter and cannot be seen upon inspection of the perianal area
4. External hemorrhoids lie below the anal sphincter and can be seen on inspection
5. Prolapsed hemorrhoids can become thrombosed or inflamed
6. Hemorrhoids are caused from portal hypertension, straining, irritation, increased venous or abdominal pressure

B. Data collection
1. Bright red rectal bleeding
2. Pain associated with thrombosis
3. Rectal itching
4. Mucus rectal discharge

C. Implementation
1. Apply cold packs to the anal rectal area followed by sitzbaths as prescribed
2. Apply witch hazel soaks and topical anesthetics as prescribed
3. Encourage a high-fiber diet and fluids to promote bowel movements without straining
4. Administer stool softeners as prescribed

D. Endoscopic procedures
1. Sclerotherapy
2. Endoscopic ligation

E. Surgical procedures
1. Cryosurgery
2. Hemorrhoidectomy

F. Postoperative implementation
1. Assist the client to a prone or side-lying position to prevent bleeding
2. Maintain ice packs over the dressing as

prescribed until the packing is removed by the physician
3. Monitor for urinary retention
4. Administer stool softeners as prescribed
5. Instruct clients to increase fluids and fiber foods
6. Instruct clients to limit sitting to short periods
7. Instruct the client in the use of sitzbaths three to four times a day as prescribed

XVII. Appendicitis

A. Description
   1. Inflammation of the appendix
   2. When the appendix becomes inflamed or infected, rupture may occur within a matter of hours, leading to peritonitis and sepsis
B. Data collection
   1. Pain in periumbilical area that descends to right lower quadrant
   2. Abdominal pain that is most intense at McBurney's point
   3. Rebound tenderness and abdominal rigidity
   4. Low-grade fever
   5. Elevated WBC count
   6. Anorexia, nausea, and vomiting
   7. Client in side-lying position with abdominal guarding and legs flexed
   8. Constipation or diarrhea
C. Peritonitis: inflammation of the peritoneum
   1. Increased fever and chills
   2. Progressive abdominal distention and abdominal pain
   3. Right guarding of abdomen
   4. Tachycardia and tachypnea
   5. Pallor
   6. Restlessness
D. Appendectomy: surgical removal of the appendix
   1. Preoperative implementation
      a. Maintain NPO status
      b. Administer IV fluids to prevent dehydration as prescribed
      c. Monitor for changes in level of pain
      d. Monitor for signs of ruptured appendix and peritonitis
      e. Position right side lying or low to semi-Fowler's position to promote comfort
      f. Monitor bowel sounds
      g. Apply ice packs to the abdomen for 20 to 30 minutes every hour
      h. Administer antibiotics as prescribed
      i. Avoid application of heat to the abdomen
      j. Avoid laxatives or enemas
   2. Postoperative implementation
      a. Monitor temperature for signs of infection
      b. Assess incision for signs of infection such as redness, swelling, and pain
      c. Maintain NPO status until bowel function has returned
      d. Advance diet gradually as tolerated when bowel sounds return
      e. If rupture of the appendix has occurred,

expect a Penrose drain to be inserted or incision may be left open to heal from the inside out
   f. Expect that drainage from the Penrose may be profuse for the first 12 hours
   g. Position the client in a right side-lying or low to semi-Fowler's position with legs flexed to facilitate drainage
   h. Change the dressing as prescribed
   i. Record the type and amount of drainage
   j. Perform wound irrigations if prescribed
   k. Maintain NG suction and patency of the NG tube if present
   l. Administer antibiotics and analgesics as prescribed

XVIII. Cirrhosis (Box 44–5)

A. Description
   1. A chronic progressive disease of the liver characterized by diffuse damage to cells with fibrosis and nodular regeneration
   2. Repeated destruction of hepatic cells causes the formation of scar tissue
B. Complications
   1. Portal hypertension: a persistent increase in pressure within the portal vein that develops as a result of obstruction to flow
   2. **Ascites**
      a. The accumulation of fluid within the peritoneal cavity that results in venous congestion of the hepatic capillaries
      b. This leads to plasma leaking directly from the liver surface and portal vein
   3. Bleeding **esophageal varices:** fragile thin-walled distended esophageal veins that become irritated and rupture

---

BOX 44–5. Types of Cirrhosis

LAENNEC'S CIRRHOSIS
Alcohol-induced, nutritional, or portal cirrhosis
Cellular necrosis causes eventual widespread scar tissue with fibrotic infiltration of the liver

POSTNECROTIC CIRRHOSIS
Occurs after massive liver necrosis
Results as a complication of acute viral hepatitis or exposure to hepatotoxins
Scar tissue causes destruction of liver lobules and entire lobes

BILIARY CIRRHOSIS
Develops from chronic biliary obstruction, bile stasis, and inflammation resulting in severe obstructive jaundice

CARDIAC CIRRHOSIS
Associated with severe right-sided CHF and results in an enlarged edematous congested liver
The liver becomes anoxic, resulting in liver cell necrosis and fibrosis

4. Coagulation defects
   a. Decreased synthesis of bile fats in the liver prevent the absorption of fat-soluble vitamins
   b. Without vitamin K and clotting factors II, VII, IX and X, the client is prone to bleeding
5. Jaundice: occurs because the liver is unable to metabolize bilirubin and because the edema, fibrosis, and scarring of the hepatic bile ducts interfere with normal bile and bilirubin secretion
6. Portal systemic encephalopathy: end-stage hepatic failure and **cirrhosis** characterized by altered LOC, neurological symptoms, impaired thinking, and neuromuscular disturbances
7. Hepatorenal syndrome
   a. Progressive renal failure associated with hepatic failure
   b. Characterized by a sudden decrease in urinary output, elevated BUN and creatinine, decreased urine sodium excretion, and increased urine osmolarity

C. Data collection
   1. Anorexia and weight loss
   2. Early morning nausea and vomiting
   3. Dyspepsia
   4. Flatulence and changes in bowel habits
   5. Emaciation
   6. Fatigue
   7. Jaundice
   8. Abdominal pain or tenderness
   9. **Ascites**
   10. Peripheral edema
   11. Dry skin and rashes
   12. Petechiae or ecchymosis
   13. Spider angiomas on the nose, cheeks, upper thorax, and shoulders
   14. Hepatomegaly
   15. Protruding umbilicus
   16. Dilated abdominal veins
   17. Presence of blood in vomitus
   18. **Fetor hepaticus**, the fruity musty breath odor of chronic liver disease
   19. Amenorrhea and testicular atrophy
   20. Gynecomastia
   21. Impotence
   22. **Asterixis**, liver flap, a coarse tremor characterized by rapid nonrhythmic extension and flexions in the wrist and fingers
   23. Delirium

D. Implementation
   1. Elevate the head of the bed to minimize shortness of breath
   2. Provide a low-sodium diet initially, restricting sodium to 200 to 500 mg and restricting protein to 50 to 60 g (to reduce excess protein breakdown by intestinal bacteria) daily as prescribed
   3. Provide supplemental vitamins with thiamine, folate, and multivitamins as prescribed
   4. Total parenteral nutrition (TPN) may be prescribed
   5. Restrict fluid intake to 1500 mL daily as prescribed
   6. Administer diuretics as prescribed
   7. Monitor I&O
   8. Monitor electrolyte balance
   9. Weigh the client and measure abdominal girth daily
   10. Monitor LOC
   11. Monitor for precoma state (tremors, delirium)
   12. Monitor for **asterixis**
   13. Maintain gastric intubation to assess bleeding
   14. Maintain esophagogastric balloon tamponade to control bleeding varices if prescribed
   15. Blood products may be prescribed
   16. Monitor coagulation laboratory results
   17. Administer vitamin K if prescribed
   18. Avoid hepatotoxin intake
   19. Instruct the client to restrict alcohol
   20. Administer low-sodium antacids as prescribed
   21. Administer lactulose (Chronulac), which decreases the pH of the bowel, decreases production of ammonia by bacteria in the bowel, and facilitates the excretion of ammonia
   22. Administer neomycin (Mycifradin) as prescribed to inhibit protein synthesis in bacteria and decrease production of ammonia
   23. Avoid medications such as narcotics, sedatives, and barbiturates
   24. Prepare the client for paracentesis to remove abdominal fluid
   25. Prepare the client for surgical shunting procedures if prescribed

XIX. Cholecystitis

A. Description
   1. An inflammation of the gallbladder that may occur as an acute or chronic process
   2. Acute inflammation is associated with gallstones (cholelithiasis)
   3. Chronic **cholecystitis** results when inefficient bile emptying and gallbladder muscle wall disease cause a fibrotic and contracted gallbladder
   4. A calculous **cholecystitis** occurs in the absence of gallstones and is due to bacterial invasion via the lymphatic or vascular system

B. Data collection
   1. Nausea and vomiting
   2. Indigestion
   3. Belching
   4. Flatulence
   5. Epigastric pain that radiates to the scapula 2

to 4 hours after eating fatty foods and may persist for 4 to 6 hours

6. Pain is localized in the right upper quadrant
7. Guarding, rigidity, and rebound tenderness
8. Mass is palpated in the right upper quadrant
9. Murphy's sign (cannot take a deep breath when the examiner's fingers are passed below hepatic margin)
10. Elevated temperature
11. Tachycardia
12. Signs of dehydration

C. Biliary obstruction
1. Jaundice
2. Dark orange and foamy urine
3. Steatorrhea and clay-colored feces
4. Pruritus

D. Implementation
1. Maintain NPO status during nausea and vomiting episodes
2. Maintain nasogastric decompression as prescribed for severe vomiting
3. Administer analgesics as prescribed to relieve pain and reduce spasm (note: morphine or codeine may cause spasm of the sphincter of Oddi and increase pain)
4. Administer antispasmodic (anticholinergics) as prescribed to relax smooth muscles
5. Administer antiemetics as prescribed for nausea and vomiting
6. Instruct clients with chronic **cholecystitis** to eat low-fat meals more frequently in small amounts
7. Instruct clients to avoid gas-forming foods
8. Prepare the client for nonsurgical and surgical procedures as prescribed

E. Nonsurgical implementation
1. Dissolution therapy
   a. To remove cholesterol stones
   b. Chenodeoxycholic acid (Chenodiol) or ursodiol (Actigall) is administered PO to decrease size of stones or to dissolve small stones
   c. Direct contact with repeated injections and aspirations of a dissolution agent via percutaneous catheter may be performed
2. Extracorporeal shock wave lithotripsy
   a. Shock waves are administered that disintegrate stones in the biliary system
   b. Oral dissolution follows

F. Surgical implementation
1. **Cholecystectomy**: removal of the gallbladder
2. **Choledochotomy**: incision into the common bile duct to remove the stone

G. Postoperative implementation
1. Monitor for respiratory complications secondary to pain at the incision site
2. Encourage coughing and deep breathing
3. Encourage early ambulation
4. Instruct the client about splinting the abdomen to prevent discomfort during coughing

---

BOX 44–6. Care of a T Tube

DESCRIPTION

Surgically inserted to decompress biliary tree and maintain patency of the bile duct

IMPLEMENTATION

Position client in semi-Fowler's to facilitate drainage

Monitor the amount, color, consistency, and odor of drainage

Monitor for inflammation and protect the skin from irritation

Collect and administer excess bile output to the client via NG tube or administer synthetic bile salts as prescribed

Keep the drainage system below the level of the gallbladder

Report sudden increases in bile output to the physician

Monitor for foul odor and purulent drainage and report to the physician

Avoid irrigation, aspiration, or clamping of the T tube without a physician's order

As prescribed, clamp tube before eating and observe for abdominal discomfort and distention, nausea, chills, or fever

Unclamp tube if nausea or vomiting occurs

---

5. Administer antiemetics as prescribed for nausea and vomiting
6. Administer analgesics as prescribed for pain relief
7. Maintain NPO status as prescribed for 24 to 48 hours
8. Maintain NG tube suction as prescribed
9. Advance the diet from clear liquids to solids when prescribed and as tolerated by the client
10. Maintain a T tube (Box 44–6)

XX. Pancreatitis

A. Description
1. An acute or chronic inflammation of the pancreas with associated escape of pancreatic enzymes into surrounding tissue
2. Acute **pancreatitis** occurs suddenly as one attack or can be recurrent, but resolves
3. Chronic **pancreatitis** is a continual inflammation and destruction of the pancreas, with scar tissue replacing pancreatic tissue
4. Precipitating factors include trauma, the use of alcohol, biliary tract disease, viral or bacterial disease, hyperlipidemia, hypercalcemia, cholelithiasis, hyperparathyroidism, ischemic vascular disease, and peptic ulcer disease

B. Acute
1. Data collection
   a. Abdominal pain including a sudden onset,

midepigastric or left upper quadrant
location with radiation to the back
   b. Pain that is aggravated by a fatty meal,
      alcohol, or lying in a recumbent position
   c. Abdominal tenderness and guarding
   d. Nausea and vomiting
   e. Weight loss
   f. Cullen's sign (discoloration of the abdomen
      and periumbilical area)
   g. Turner's sign (bluish discoloration of the
      flanks)
   h. Absent or decreased bowel sounds
   i. Elevated temperature
   j. Hypotension
   k. Tachycardia
   l. Elevated WBC, glucose, bilirubin, alkaline
      phosphatase, and urinary amylase
   m. Elevated lipase and amylase
   n. Abnormally low calcium, sodium, and
      magnesium due to dehydration
2. Implementation
   a. Maintain NPO status and maintain
      hydration with IV fluids
   b. TPN is administered for severe nutritional
      depletion
   c. Provide small, frequent high-carbohydrate,
      high-protein, low-fat meals when
      prescribed and when tolerated by the client
   d. Administer supplemental preparations and
      vitamins and minerals to increase caloric
      intake if prescribed
   e. Maintain the NG tube to decrease gastric
      distention and suppress pancreatic
      secretion
   f. Administer meperidine hydrochloride
      (Demerol) as prescribed for pain because it
      causes less incidence of spasm of the
      smooth muscle of the pancreatic ducts and
      sphincter of Oddi (note: avoid morphine or
      codeine, which may cause spasms)
   g. Administer antacids as prescribed to
      neutralize gastric secretions
   h. Administer histamine-receptor-blocking
      medications as prescribed to decrease
      hydrochloric acid production so pancreatic
      enzymes are not activated
   i. Administer anticholinergics as prescribed to
      decrease vagal stimulation, decrease GI
      motility, and inhibit pancreatic enzyme
      secretion
   j. Instruct the client in the importance of
      avoiding alcohol
   k. Instruct the client in the importance of
      follow-up visits with the physician
   l. Instruct the client to notify the physician
      for acute abdominal pain, jaundice, clay-
      colored stools, and dark urine
C. Chronic
   1. Data collection
      a. Abdominal pain such as continuous
         burning or gnawing, and dullness with
         intense exacerbations

   b. Abdominal tenderness
   c. Left upper quadrant mass
   d. Steatorrhea and foul-smelling stools that
      may increase in volume as pancreatic
      insufficiency increases
   e. Weight loss
   f. Muscle wasting
   g. Jaundice
   h. Signs and symptoms of diabetes
2. Implementation
   a. Administer meperidine hydrochloride
      (Demerol) as prescribed for pain because it
      causes less incidence of spasm of the
      smooth muscle of the pancreatic ducts and
      sphincter of Oddi (note: avoid morphine or
      codeine, which may cause spasms)
   b. Maintain NPO status to avoid pain caused
      by eating
   c. TPN is administered for nutritional
      depletion as prescribed
   d. Provide small, frequent high-carbohydrate,
      high-protein, and low-fat meals when
      prescribed as tolerated by the client
   e. Provide supplemental preparations and
      vitamins and minerals to increase caloric
      intake
   f. Administer pancreatic enzymes as
      prescribed to aid in digestion and
      absorption of fat and protein
   g. Administer insulin or oral hypoglycemic
      medications as prescribed to control
      diabetes
   h. Instruct the client to avoid alcohol,
      caffeinated beverages, and rich fatty foods
   i. Instruct the clients in the use of pancreatic
      enzyme medications
   j. Instruct the client in the treatment plan for
      glucose management
   k. Instruct clients to notify the physician if
      increased steatorrhea occurs or if
      abdominal distention, cramping, and skin
      breakdown develops
   l. Instruct the client in the importance of
      follow-up visits

XXI. Hepatitis

A. Description
   1. An inflammation of the liver caused by a
      virus, bacteria, or exposure to drugs or
      hepatotoxins
   2. The goals of treatment include resting the
      inflamed liver to reduce metabolic demands
      and increase the blood supply, thus promoting
      cellular regeneration and preventing
      complications

XXII. Viral Hepatitis

A. Types of viral hepatitis
   1. Hepatitis A (HAV), infectious hepatitis
   2. Hepatitis B (HBV)

3. Hepatitis C (non-A, non-B)
4. Hepatitis D (delta agent hepatitis)
5. Hepatitis E (enterically transmitted non-A, non-B hepatitis)
B. Stages of viral hepatitis (Box 44–7)
C. Data collection
1. Preicteric stage
   a. Fatigue
   b. Malaise
   c. Headache
   d. Lethargy
   e. Increased temperature
   f. Anorexia
   g. Nausea and vomiting
   h. Abdominal tenderness
   i. Diarrhea or constipation
   j. Weight loss
   k. Dark-colored urine
   l. Joint pain
   m. Elevated AST, ALT, and bilirubin
2. Icteric stage
   a. Tea-colored urine
   b. Clay-colored stools
   c. Jaundice
   d. Pruritus
   e. Enlarged and tender liver
3. Posticteric stage
   a. Jaundice disappears
   b. Fatigue and malaise continues
   c. Appetite improves
   d. Stool and urine color returns to normal
   e. Liver remains enlarged
   f. Absence of clay-colored stools is an indication of resolution
D. Laboratory tests
1. ALT (alanine aminotransferase)
   a. Elevated to more than 1000 mU/mL and may rise to as high as 4000 mU/mL
   b. Normal adult blood value: 6 to 24 U/L depending on age
2. AST (aspartate aminotransferase)
   a. May rise to 1000 to 2000 mU/mL
   b. Normal adult blood value: 8 to 26 U/L

BOX 44–7. Stages of Viral Hepatitis

PREICTERIC STAGE

The first stage of hepatitis preceding the appearance of jaundice

ICTERIC STAGE

The second stage of hepatitis, which includes the appearance of jaundice and associated symptoms as elevated bilirubin levels, dark or tea-colored urine, and clay-colored stools

POSTICTERIC STAGE

The convalescent stage in which the jaundice decreases and the color of the urine and stool returns to normal

---

depending on age with highest normal value in the newborn
3. Alkaline phosphate levels
   a. May be normal or mildly elevated
   b. Normal: 30 to 90 IU/L or 4.5 to 13 King-Armstrong units/dL depending on age
4. Serum total bilirubin levels
   a. Elevated to greater than 2.5 mg/dL
   b. Normal: 0.3-1.0 mg/dL (less than 1.5 mg/dL)
   c. Elevated levels of bilirubin in the urine

XXIII. Hepatitis A (HAV), Infectious Hepatitis

A. Description
1. Commonly seen during the fall and winter
2. Is most prevalent in areas of poverty and areas with poor sanitation
3. Increased risk
   a. Contact with infected materials
   b. Handling contaminated feces
   c. Eating or drinking contaminated water, milk, or food
   d. Eating raw fish from contaminated water
B. Transmission
1. Fecal-oral route
2. Person-to-person contact
3. Parenteral
4. Contaminated uncooked shellfish, fruits, and vegetables
5. Contaminated water and milk
6. Poorly washed utensils
C. Incubation and infectious period
1. Incubation period is 15 to 50 days (2 to 6 weeks)
2. Infectious period is 2 to 3 weeks prior to, and 1 week after developing jaundice
D. Testing
1. Infection is established by the presence of hepatitis A virus (HAV) antibodies (anti-HAV) in the blood
2. IgM and IgG are normally present in the blood and increased levels indicate infection and inflammation
3. Ongoing inflammation of the liver is evidenced by the presence of elevated immunoglobulin M (IgM) antibodies, which persist in the blood for 4 to 6 weeks
4. Previous infection is indicated by the presence of elevated immunoglobulin G (IgG) antibodies
E. Complication: fulminant hepatitis
F. Prevention
1. Good handwashing
2. Stool and needle precautions
3. Treatment of municipal water supplies
4. Serologic screening of food handlers
5. Passive immunization
   a. Pre- and postexposure prophylaxis of immune globulin (IG)
   b. Immune globulin (IG) is not administered

postexposure if clinical manifestations have developed

    c. Clients who live in or visit high risk areas can be protected for up to 3 months following the administration of immune globulin (IG)

    d. The earlier in the incubation period that the immune globulin is given, the greater the protection

XXIV. Hepatitis B (HBV)

A. Description
1. Formerly called serum hepatitis
2. Is nonseasonal in nature
3. Prevalence increases in areas of overpopulation and poor hygiene
4. Increased-risk individuals
   a. Those who receive multiple blood transfusions
   b. Health care providers in contact with blood and blood products
   c. Hemodialysis clients
   d. Sexually active individuals with multiple partners
   e. Morticians
   f. Those undergoing tattooing
   g. Parenteral drug abusers
5. Sequelae of chronic hepatitis B infection may include chronic liver disease, cirrhosis, and primary liver cancer

B. Transmission
1. Blood or body fluid contact
2. Infected blood and blood products
3. Infected saliva or semen
4. Contaminated needles and equipment
5. Oral or sexual contact
6. Parenteral
7. Perinatal period
8. Blood or body fluid contact at birth or during early childhood

C. Incubation period: 40 to 180 days

D. Testing
1. Infection is established by the presence of hepatitis B antigen-antibody systems in the blood
2. Presence of hepatitis B surface antigens (HBsAG) is the serologic marker to establish the diagnosis of hepatitis B
3. The client is considered infectious if these antigens are present in the blood
4. If the serologic marker (HBsAG) is present after 6 months or longer, it indicates a carrier state or chronic hepatitis
5. Normally the serologic marker (HBsAG) level declines and disappears after the acute hepatitis B episode
6. The presence of antibodies to HBsAG (anti-HBS) indicates recovery and immunity to hepatitis B

7. Hepatitis B early antigen (HBeAG) is detected in the blood about 1 week after the appearance of HBsAG, and its presence determines the infective state of the client

E. Complications
1. Fulminant hepatitis
2. Chronic liver disease
3. Cirrhosis
4. Primary hepatocellular carcinoma

F. Prevention
1. Good handwashing
2. Screening blood donors
3. Testing of all pregnant women
4. Needle precautions
5. Instructing clients to avoid sharing personal items
6. Avoiding intimate sexual contact if hepatitis B surface antigen (HBsAG) is positive
7. Passive immunization
   a. Hepatitis B immune globulin involves three doses; an initial dose, a dose at 1 month, and a dose at 6 months
   b. Hepatitis B immune globulin may be given for postexposure prophylaxis when there has been percutaneous exposure to blood that contains HBsAg

XXV. Hepatitis C (Non-A, Non-B)

A. Description
1. Occurs year-round
2. Is common among drug abusers and is the major cause of post-transfusion hepatitis
3. Risk factors are similar to HBV because hepatitis C is also parenterally transmitted
4. Hepatitis C has been treated with interferon-alpha, which boosts the body's immune system
5. Increased-risk individuals
   a. Parenteral drug users
   b. Dialysis clients

B. Transmission
1. Same as HBV
2. Infected blood and blood products
3. Infected saliva or semen
4. Contaminated needles and equipment
5. Personal contact
6. Possibly by fecal-oral route
7. Parenteral

C. Incubation period: 14 to 180 days

D. Testing: there is no acceptable reliable serological screening test to detect hepatitis C

E. Complications
1. Chronic liver disease
2. Cirrhosis
3. Primary hepatocellular carcinoma

F. Prevention
1. Good handwashing
2. Stool and needle precautions
3. Screen blood donors

XXVI. Hepatitis D (Delta Agent Hepatitis, HDV)

A. Description
   1. Common in the Mediterranean and Middle Eastern areas
   2. Seen with hepatitis B and may cause infection only in the presence of active HBV infection
   3. Coinfection with the delta agent intensifies the acute symptoms of hepatitis B
   4. Transmission and risk of infection is the same as HBV, via contact with blood and blood products
   5. Prevention of HBV infection also prevents HDV infection, since HDV is dependent on HBV for replication

◆ B. Transmission
   1. Infected saliva or semen
   2. Parenteral
   3. Contaminated needles and equipment
   4. Oral or sexual contact
   5. Blood and blood products among persons already infected with HBV
   6. Perinatal period
   7. Via blood or body fluids contact at birth or during early childhood

C. Incubation period: 21 to 49 days

D. Testing
   1. Confirmed by the identification of intrahepatic delta antigen or a rise in the hepatitis D virus antibodies (anti-HD) titer
   2. Circulating hepatitis D antigen (HD Ag) is diagnostic of acute disease

E. Complications
   1. Chronic liver disease
   2. Fulminant hepatitis

◆ F. Prevention: because hepatitis D must coexist with hepatitis B, the precautions that help prevent hepatitis B are also useful in preventing delta hepatitis

XXVII. Hepatitis E (Enterically Transmitted Non-A, Non-B Hepatitis)

A. Description
   1. A water-borne virus
   2. Prevalent in areas where sewage disposal is inadequate or where communal bathing in contaminated rivers is practiced
   3. Risk of infection is the same as HAV
   4. Presents as a mild disease except in infected women in the third trimester of pregnancy, with whom the mortality rate is high
   5. Increased risk
      a. With travel to countries that have a high incidence of hepatitis E such as India, Burma, Afghanistan, Algeria, and Mexico
      b. Eating or drinking food or water contaminated with the virus

◆ B. Transmission
   1. Same as HAV
   2. Fecal-oral route

BOX 44–8. Client and Family Education for Hepatitis

Frequent handwashing

Do not share bathrooms unless the client strictly adheres to personal hygiene measures

Individual washcloths, towels, drinking and eating utensils, as well as toothbrushes and razors must be labeled and identified

The client must not prepare food for other family members

The client should avoid alcohol and over-the-counter medications, particularly acetaminophen (Tylenol) and sedatives, for 3 to 12 months because these medications are hepatotoxic

The client should increase activity gradually to prevent fatigue

The client should consume small, frequent, high-carbohydrate, low-fat foods

The client is not to donate blood

The client may maintain normal contact with people as long as proper personal hygiene is maintained

The client is to avoid sexual activity until hepatitis B surface antigen (HBsAg) results are negative

Close personal contact such as kissing should be discouraged until HBsAg test results are negative

If the client has hepatitis A and B, the family members should have immunoglobulin injections or vaccinations (Heptavax B)

The client needs to carry a Medic-Alert card noting the date of hepatitis onset

The client needs to inform other health care professionals, such as medical or dental personnel, of the onset of hepatitis

The client needs to keep follow-up appointments with the health care provider

---

3. Person-to-person contact
   4. Eating contaminated uncooked shellfish, fruits, and vegetables
   5. Drinking contaminated water and milk
   6. Poorly washed utensils
   7. Parenteral

C. Incubation period: 15 to 60 days

D. Testing: no available serological markers for hepatitis E

E. Complications
   1. High mortality rate in pregnant women
   2. Fetal demise

F. Prevention
   1. Good handwashing
   2. Good personal hygiene
   3. Treatment of water supplies
   4. Good sanitation measures

XXVIII. Instruction for Home Care for the Client and Family (Box 44–8)

PRACTICE QUESTIONS

1. The nurse is caring for a client receiving bolus feedings via a Levin-type nasogastric tube. As the nurse is finishing the feeding, the client asks for

the bed to be positioned flat to sleep. Which of the following positions is the most appropriate choice for this client at this time?

1 Head of the bed flat with the client in the supine position for at least 30 minutes

2 Head of the bed elevated 30 to 45 degrees with the client in the right lateral position for 60 minutes

3 Head of the bed elevated 45 to 60 degrees with the client in the supine position for 30 minutes

4 Head of the bed in semi-Fowler's with the client in the left lateral position for 60 minutes

2. Prior to administering an intermittent tube feeding through a nasogastric tube, the nurse checks for gastric residual. The nurse aspirates the stomach contents and withdraws 40 mL of undigested formula. What is the rationale for checking gastric residual prior to administering the tube feeding?

1 To confirm proper nasogastric tube placement

2 To observe the digestion of formula

3 To check fluid and electrolyte status

4 To evaluate absorption of the last feeding

3. A client presents to the emergency department with upper GI bleeding and is in moderate distress. In planning priorities for care, which nursing action is the first priority for this client?

1 Thorough investigation of precipitating events

2 Insertion of a nasogastric tube and Hematest of emesis

3 Complete abdominal physical examination

4 Determination of vital signs

4. The nurse is caring for a client with possible cholelithiasis who is being prepared for a cholangiogram. The nurse teaches the client about the procedure. Which of the following client statements indicates that the client understands the purpose of a cholangiogram?

1 "They are going to look at my gallbladder and ducts."

2 "This procedure will drain my gallbladder."

3 "My gallbladder will be irrigated."

4 "They will put medication in my gallbladder."

5. The nurse is caring for a client with acute pancreatitis and a history of alcoholism. Which of the following data is a sign of paralytic ileus?

1 Firm, nontender mass palpable at the lower right costal margin

2 Severe, constant pain with rapid onset

3 Inability to pass flatus

4 Loss of anal sphincter control

6. The nurse is caring for a client with a nasogastric tube connected to continuous gastric suction. The nurse observes that the client is mouth breathing, has dry mucous membranes, and the breath has a foul odor. In planning care, which of the following nursing orders is the most appropriate choice to maintain the integrity of this client's oral mucosa?

1 Offer small sips of water frequently

2 Encourage the client to suck on sour, hard candy

3 Brush teeth frequently; use mouthwash and water

4 Use lemon-glycerin swabs to provide oral hygiene

7. The nurse is caring for a client with a resolved intestinal obstruction who has a nasogastric tube in place. The client has tolerated the tube being clamped every 2 hours for 1 hour. The physician has now ordered the nasogastric tube to be discontinued. To determine if it is appropriate to discontinue the nasogastric tube, the nurse should check for

1 Proper nasogastric tube placement

2 The client's serum electrolyte levels

3 Presence of bowel sounds in all four quadrants

4 The pH of the gastric aspirate

8. The nurse has administered approximately half of a high-cleansing enema when the client complains of pain and cramping. Which of the following nursing actions is the most appropriate?

1 Raise the enema bag so that the solution can be completed quickly

2 Clamp the tubing for 30 seconds and restart the flow at a slower rate

3 Reassure the client and continue the flow

4 Discontinue the enema and notify the physician

9. The nurse is preparing to administer a high-cleansing enema. The nurse positions the client in the

1 Left lateral position with the right leg acutely flexed

2 Right Sims' position

3 Dorsal recumbent position

4 Right lateral position with the left leg acutely flexed

10. The nurse has aspirated 40 mL of undigested formula from the client's nasogastric tube before administering an intermittent tube feeding. The nurse understands that before administering the tube feeding, the 40 mL of gastric aspirate should be

1 Discarded properly and recorded as output on the client's I&O record

2 Poured into the nasogastric tube through a syringe with the plunger removed

3 Mixed with the formula and poured into the nasogastric tube through a syringe without a plunger

4 Diluted with water and injected into the na-

sogastric tube by putting pressure on the plunger

11. The nurse is participating in a health screening clinic, and is preparing teaching materials about colorectal cancer. The nurse plans to include which of the following in a list of risk factors for colorectal cancer?
   1 Age over 30 years
   2 High-fiber, low-fat diet
   3 Distant relative with colorectal cancer
   4 Personal history of ulcerative colitis or GI polyps

12. The hospitalized client with gastroesophageal reflux disease (GERD) is complaining of chest discomfort that feels like heartburn following a meal. After administering an ordered antacid, the nurse encourages the client to lie in which of the following positions?
   1 Supine with the head of bed flat
   2 On the stomach with the head flat
   3 On the left side with the head of bed elevated 30 degrees
   4 On the right side with the head of bed elevated 30 degrees

13. The nurse is planning to teach the client with gastroesophageal reflux disease (GERD) about substances that will increase the lower esophageal sphincter (LES) pressure. Which of the following items does the nurse include on this list?
   1 Fatty foods
   2 Nonfat milk
   3 Chocolate
   4 Coffee

14. The client has undergone esophagogastroduodenoscopy (EGD). The nurse places highest priority on which of the following items as part of the client's care plan?
   1 Checking for return of gag reflex
   2 Giving warm gargles for sore throat
   3 Monitoring temperature
   4 Monitoring complaints of heartburn

15. The nurse has taught the client about an upcoming endoscopic retrograde cholangiopancreatography (ERCP) procedure. The nurse evaluates that the client has not fully understood the information if the client makes which of the following statements?
   1 "I know I must sign the consent form."
   2 "I'm glad I don't have to lie still for this procedure."
   3 "I'm glad some medication will be given IV to relax me."
   4 "I hope the throat spray keeps me from gagging."

16. The client being seen in a physician's office has just been scheduled for a barium swallow (eso-phagography) the next day. The nurse writes down which of the following instructions for the client to follow before the test?
   1 Remove all metal and jewelry before the test
   2 Eat a regular supper and breakfast
   3 Continue to take all oral medications as scheduled
   4 Monitor own BM pattern for constipation

17. The nurse is teaching the client about an upcoming colonoscopy procedure. The nurse includes in the instructions that the client will be placed in which of the following positions for the procedure?
   1 Left Sims'
   2 Right Sims'
   3 Knee-chest
   4 Lithotomy

18. The nurse has given postprocedure instructions to a client who underwent colonoscopy. The nurse evaluates that the client did not fully understand the directions if the client states that
   1 "Intake should be light at first, then I can progress to regular intake."
   2 "It is normal to feel gassy or bloated after the procedure."
   3 "The abdominal muscles may be tender from stretching during the procedure."
   4 "It is all right to drive once I have been home for an hour or so."

19. The nurse is performing an abdominal assessment. The initial assessment is which of the following?
   1 Auscultation
   2 Inspection
   3 Palpation
   4 Percussion

20. The client is scheduled for an oral cholecystogram. The nurse plans to order what type of diet for the evening meal prior to the test?
   1 Low-protein
   2 High-carbohydrate
   3 Fat-free
   4 Liquid

21. Polyethylene glycol-electrolyte solution (Go-LYTELY) is prescribed for the client scheduled for a colonoscopy. The client begins to experience diarrhea following administration of the solution. What action by the nurse is most appropriate?
   1 Cancel the exam
   2 Prepare to start an IV
   3 Administer an enema
   4 Explain that diarrhea is expected

22. A nasogastric tube has been inserted into a client and the physician prescribes that the tube be attached to intermittent suction. The nurse atta-

ches the suction, noting that the pressure should not exceed
1   10 mmHg
2   20 mmHg
3   25 mmHg
4   30 mmHg

23. The nurse is caring for a client with a diagnosis of chronic gastritis. The nurse anticipates that this client is at risk for which of the following vitamin deficiencies?
1   Vitamin A
2   Vitamin B$_{12}$
3   Vitamin C
4   Vitamin E

24. The nurse is reviewing the medication record of a client with acute gastritis. Which of the following medications, if noted on the client's record, does the nurse question?
1   Digoxin (Lanoxin)
2   Indomethacin (Indocin)
3   Furosemide (Lasix)
4   Propranolol hydrochloride (Inderal)

25. The nurse is monitoring a client with a diagnosis of peptic ulcer. Which of the following findings most likely indicates perforation of the ulcer?
1   Bradycardia
2   Numbness in the legs
3   Nausea and vomiting
4   A rigid boardlike abdomen

26. The nurse provides medication instructions to a client with peptic ulcer disease. Which statement, if made by the client, indicates the best understanding of the medication therapy?
1   "The cimetidine (Tagamet) will cause me to produce less stomach acid."
2   "Sucralfate (Carafate) will change the fluid in my stomach."
3   "Antacids will coat my stomach."
4   "Omeprazole (Prilosec) will coat the ulcer and help it heal."

27. The client with peptic ulcer disease is scheduled for a pyloroplasty. The client asks the nurse about the procedure. The nurse bases the response on which of the following?
1   A pyloroplasty involves cutting the vagus nerve
2   A pyloroplasty involves removing the distal portion of the stomach
3   A pyloroplasty involves removal of the ulcer and a large portion of the cells that produce hydrochloric acid
4   A pyloroplasty involves an incision and resuturing of the pylorus to relax the muscle and enlarge the opening from the stomach to the duodenum

28. A client with a peptic ulcer is scheduled for a vagotomy. The client asks the nurse about the purpose of this procedure. The best nursing response is which of the following?
1   "It decreases food absorption in the stomach."
2   "It heals the gastric mucosa."
3   "It halts stress reactions."
4   "It reduces the stimulus to acid secretions."

29. The nurse is caring for a client following a Billroth II procedure. On review of the postoperative orders, which of the following, if prescribed, does the nurse question and verify?
1   Irrigating the NG tube
2   Coughing and deep-breathing exercises
3   Leg exercises
4   Early ambulation

30. The nurse is providing discharge instructions to a client following gastrectomy. Which of the following measures does the nurse instruct the client to follow to assist in preventing dumping syndrome?
1   Eat high-carbohydrate foods
2   Limit the fluids taken with meals
3   Ambulate following a meal
4   Sit in a high Fowler's position during meals

31. The nurse is monitoring a client for the early signs and symptoms of dumping syndrome. Which of the following symptoms indicates this occurrence?
1   Abdominal cramping and pain
2   Bradycardia and indigestion
3   Sweating and pallor
4   Double vision and chest pain

32. The nurse is instructing the male client who had a herniorrhaphy how to reduce postoperative swelling following the procedure. Which of the following does the nurse suggest to the client to prevent swelling?
1   Heat to the abdomen
2   Elevation of the scrotum
3   Limiting fluids
4   A low-fiber diet

33. A client is diagnosed as having irritable bowel syndrome. Which of the following instructions does the nurse not include in the plan of care?
1   Maintain a low-residue diet
2   Provide fiber and bulk in the diet
3   Eat regular meals
4   Drink 8 to 10 cups of liquid each day

34. The nurse is reviewing the record of a client with Crohn's disease. Which of the following stool characteristics does the nurse expect to note in this client?
1   Bloody stools
2   Diarrhea
3   Constipation alternating with diarrhea
4   Stool constantly oozing from the rectum

35. The nurse is performing a colostomy irrigation on a client. During the irrigation, the client begins to complain of abdominal cramps. Which of the following is the most appropriate nursing action?
    1 Notify the physician
    2 Increase the height of the irrigation
    3 Stop the irrigation temporarily
    4 Medicate for pain and resume irrigation

36. The nurse is teaching a client how to perform a colostomy irrigation. To enhance the effectiveness of the irrigation, what measure should the nurse instruct the client to do?
    1 Increase fluid intake
    2 Reduce the amount of irrigation solution
    3 Massage the abdomen gently
    4 Place heat on the abdomen

37. The nurse is reviewing the record of a client with a diagnosis of cirrhosis and notes that there is documentation of the presence of asterixis. To check for the presence of this sign, the nurse does which of the following?
    1 Ask the client to extend the arms
    2 Check for the presence of Homans' sign
    3 Instruct the client to lean forward
    4 Measure the abdominal girth

38. The client with ascites is scheduled for a paracentesis. The nurse is assisting the physician in performing the procedure. Which of the following positions does the nurse assist the client to assume for this procedure?
    1 Supine
    2 Left side-lying
    3 Right side-lying
    4 Upright position

39. The nurse is reviewing the laboratory results in a client with cirrhosis and notes that the ammonia level is elevated. Which of the following diets does the nurse anticipate will most likely be prescribed for this client?
    1 High-carbohydrate
    2 Moderate-fat
    3 High-protein
    4 Low-protein

40. Lactulose (Chronulac) is prescribed for a client with a diagnosis of hepatic encephalopathy. Which finding indicates that the client is responding to this medication therapy as anticipated?
    1 The fecal pH is acidic
    2 The client experiences diarrhea
    3 The client is able to tolerate a full diet
    4 Vomiting occurs

41. An ultrasound of the gallbladder is scheduled for the client with a suspected diagnosis of cholecystitis. The nurse explains to the client that this test

1 Requires the client to lie still for short intervals
2 Requires that the client be NPO
3 Is preceded by administration of an oral tablet
4 Is uncomfortable

42. The nurse is providing preoperative teaching to a client scheduled for a cholecystectomy. Which of the following interventions is of highest priority in the preoperative teaching plan?
    1 Teaching coughing and deep-breathing exercises
    2 Teaching leg exercises
    3 Instructions regarding fluid restrictions
    4 Checking the client's understanding of the surgical procedure

43. A Penrose drain is in place on the first postoperative day following a cholecystectomy. Serosanguineous drainage is noted on the dressing covering the drain. Which nursing intervention is most appropriate?
    1 Notify the physician
    2 Change the dressing
    3 Circle the amount on the dressing with a pen
    4 Continue to monitor the drainage

44. The client is admitted to the hospital for treatment of acute hepatitis B. Which activity order does the nurse expect to be prescribed?
    1 Bed rest
    2 Encourage ambulation
    3 Out of bed in a chair
    4 No activity restrictions

45. It had been determined that the client with hepatitis has contracted the infection from contaminated food. What type of hepatitis is this client most likely experiencing?
    1 Hepatitis A
    2 Hepatitis B
    3 Hepatitis C
    4 Hepatitis D

46. The nurse is reviewing the physician's orders written for a client admitted with acute pancreatitis. Which physician order does the nurse question if noted on the client's chart?
    1 NPO status
    2 Prepare for insertion of an NG tube
    3 An anticholinergic medication
    4 Morphine sulfate for pain

47. A client with peptic ulcer states that stress frequently causes exacerbation of the disease. The nurse interprets that which of the following items mentioned by the client is most likely responsible for the exacerbations?
    1 Sleeping 8 to 10 hours a night
    2 Eating five to six small meals per day
    3 Ability to work at home periodically

4 Frequent need to work overtime on short notice

48. The client with peptic ulcer disease (PUD) needs dietary modification to reduce episodes of epigastric pain. The nurse plans to teach the client that which of the following items does not need to be limited or eliminated with this disease?
    1 Wine
    2 Baked chicken
    3 Coffee
    4 Fresh fruit

49. The nurse instructs the ileostomy client to do which of the following as part of essential care of the stoma?
    1 Cleanse the peristomal skin meticulously
    2 Take in high-fiber foods such as nuts
    3 Massage the area below the stoma
    4 Limit fluid intake to prevent diarrhea

50. The client with hiatal hernia chronically experiences heartburn following meals. The nurse plans to teach the client to avoid which of the following, which is contraindicated with hiatal hernia?
    1 Taking in small, frequent, bland meals
    2 Lying recumbent following meals
    3 Raising the head of bed on 6-inch blocks
    4 Taking histamine-receptor-antagonist medication

51. The nurse is monitoring for stoma prolapse in a client with recent colostomy. The nurse observes to see if the stoma is
    1 Sunken and hidden
    2 Dark and bluish
    3 Narrowed and flattened
    4 Protruding and swollen

52. The client with a new colostomy is concerned about odor from stool in the ostomy drainage bag. The nurse teaches the client to include which of the following foods in the diet to reduce odor?
    1 Yogurt
    2 Broccoli
    3 Cucumbers
    4 Eggs

53. The nurse has given instructions to the client with an ileostomy about foods to eat to thicken the stool. The nurse evaluates that the client did not fully understand the instructions if the client states to eat which of the following foods to make the stool less watery?
    1 Pasta
    2 Boiled rice
    3 Bran
    4 Low-fat cheese

54. The nurse is doing preoperative teaching with the client who is about to undergo creation of a Kock

pouch. The nurse interprets that the client has the best understanding of the nature of the surgery if the client makes which of the following statements?
    1 "I will need to drain the pouch regularly with a catheter."
    2 "I will need to wear a drainage bag for the rest of my life."
    3 "The drainage from this type of ostomy will be formed."
    4 "I will be able to pass stool by the rectum eventually."

55. The client with chronic pancreatitis needs information on dietary modification to manage the health problem. The nurse plans to teach the client to limit which of the following items in the diet?
    1 Carbohydrate
    2 Protein
    3 Fat
    4 Water-soluble vitamins

56. The client with acute pancreatitis is experiencing severe pain from the disorder. The nurse teaches the client to avoid which of the following positions that could aggravate the pain?
    1 Sitting up
    2 Lying flat
    3 Leaning forward
    4 Flexing the left leg

57. The nurse is evaluating the effect of dietary counseling on the client with cholecystitis. The nurse evaluates that the client understands the instructions given if the client states that which of the following food items is acceptable in the diet?
    1 Baked scrod
    2 Sauces and gravies
    3 Fried chicken
    4 Fresh whipped cream

58. The client with cirrhosis is beginning to show signs of hepatic encephalopathy. The nurse plans a dietary consult to limit the amount of which of the following ingredients in the client's diet.
    1 Fat
    2 Carbohydrate
    3 Protein
    4 Minerals

59. The client with Crohn's disease has an order to begin taking antispasmodic medication. The nurse times the medication so that each dose is taken
    1 30 minutes before meals
    2 During meals
    3 60 minutes after meals
    4 Upon arising and at bedtime

60. A client is admitted to the hospital with acute viral hepatitis. Which of the following signs or

2

2

symptoms does the nurse expect based upon this diagnosis?

1 Spider angiomas
2 Fatigue
3 Pale urine
4 Weight gain

61. The client with viral hepatitis, in discussing with the nurse the need to avoid alcohol, states. "I'm not sure I can do that." The nurse responds by saying
1 "Everything will be all right."
2 "I think you should talk more with the doctor about this."
3 "I don't believe that."
4 "I'm not sure that I understand. Would you please explain?"

62. Of the following infection control methods, which is most appropriate to include in the plan of care to prevent hepatitis B in a client considered to be at high risk for exposure?
1 Correct handwashing technique
2 Hepatitis B (HBV) vaccine
3 Proper personal hygiene
4 Use of immune globulin

63. The nurse is caring for a client that is a hepatitis B carrier. Which statement made by the client indicates the best understanding of how to prevent transmission of the disease?
1 "I should be vaccinated as soon as possible."
2 "I never will share towels with anyone else."
3 "It is all right to kiss my wife."
4 "My wife should get the vaccine."

64. The client is admitted to the hospital with viral hepatitis, complaining of "no appetite" and "losing my taste for food." In order to provide adequate nutrition, the nurse teaches the client to
1 Eat a good supper when anorexia is not as severe
2 Eat less often, preferably only three large meals daily
3 Drink a lot of fluids, especially carbonated beverages
4 Select foods high in fat

65. The client, an African-American, has a diagnosis of acute viral hepatitis. Which of the following specific areas does the nurse inspect for jaundice in this client?

1 Flexor surfaces of the extremities
2 Hard palate of the mouth
3 Nailbeds
4 Skin

66. In planning care for a client with viral hepatitis who states, "I am so yellow," the nurse includes measures such as
1 Assisting the client in expressing feelings
2 Doing most ADLs for the client
3 Providing information to the client only when the client requests it
4 Restricting visitors until the jaundice subsides

67. After a liver biopsy, the client should be instructed to
1 Avoid alcohol for 8 hours
2 Save all stools to be checked for blood
3 Lie flat for 24 hours
4 Lie on the right side for 2 hours

68. A sexually active 20-year-old client has developed viral hepatitis. Which of the following statements if made by the client indicates a need for further teaching?
1 "A condom should be used for sexual intercourse."
2 "I can never drink alcohol again."
3 "I won't go back to work right away."
4 "My close friends should get the vaccine."

69. A client is admitted to the hospital with severe jaundice and is having diagnostic testing. With no complaints of fatigue, the client is encouraged to ambulate in the hall to maintain muscle strength. The client paces around the room, but will not enter the hallway. Which of the following problems most likely is the reason for the client's reluctance to walk in the hall?
1 Fear of catching another disease
2 Not wanting to overexert and get overly tired
3 Feeling self-conscious about self-image
4 Unfamiliarity with the hospital

70. A client with viral hepatitis has no appetite and food makes the client nauseated. Which of the following nursing interventions is appropriate?
1 Explain that high-fat diets are usually better tolerated
2 Encourage foods high in protein
3 Explain that the majority of calories need to be consumed in the evening hours
4 Monitor for fluid and electrolyte imbalance

ANSWERS

1. 2

RATIONALE: Aspiration is a possible complication associated with nasogastric tube feeding. The head of the bed is elevated 30 to 45 degrees for at least 30 minutes following bolus tube feeding to prevent vomiting and aspiration. The right lateral position uses gravity to facilitate gastric retention to prevent vomiting. The flat supine position is to be avoided for the first 30 minutes after a tube feeding.

TEST-TAKING STRATEGY: There are three components to each answer; the level of elevation of the head, the client's position, and the duration. The entire option needs to be correct. Option 1 can be eliminated immediately because this position could result in aspiration. Options 2 and 4 are the same elevation, but the right lateral position is the correct position and 60 minutes is the correct duration. Option 3 is ruled out because of the supine position and the longer duration.

LEVEL OF COGNITIVE ABILITY: Application
PHASE OF NURSING PROCESS: Implementation
CLIENT NEEDS: Physiological Integrity
CONTENT AREA: Adult Health/Gastrointestinal
REFERENCE
Monahan, F., & Neighbors, M. (1998). *Medical-surgical nursing: Foundations for clinical practice* (2nd ed.). Philadelphia: W. B. Saunders. p. 982.

2. 4

RATIONALE: All the stomach contents are aspirated and measured prior to administering a tube feeding. This procedure measures the gastric residual. The gastric residual is assessed in order to confirm whether undigested formula from a previous feeding remains and thereby evaluates absorption of the last feeding. It is important to assess gastric residual because administration of a tube feeding to a full stomach could result in overdistention, thus predisposing the client to regurgitation and possible aspiration.

TEST-TAKING STRATEGY: Note that the issue of the question is the purpose of assessing residual. Focusing on this issue should direct you to option 4. Review this procedure now if you had difficulty with this question.

LEVEL OF COGNITIVE ABILITY: Comprehension
PHASE OF NURSING PROCESS: Implementation
CLIENT NEEDS: Physiological Integrity
CONTENT AREA: Adult Health/Gastrointestinal
REFERENCE
Monahan, F., & Neighbors, M. (1998). *Medical-surgical nursing: Foundations for clinical practice* (2nd ed.). Philadelphia: W. B. Saunders. p. 982.

3. 4

RATIONALE: An initial nursing assessment should be performed while getting the client ready for treatment. The immediate determination of vital signs indicates whether the client is in shock from blood loss and also provides a baseline blood pressure and pulse by which to monitor the progress of treatment. Signs and symptoms of shock include low blood pressure; rapid, weak pulse; increased thirst; cold, clammy skin; and restlessness. Vital signs should be monitored every 10 to 15 minutes, and the physician should be informed of any significant changes. The client may not be able to provide subjective data until the immediate physical needs are met.

TEST-TAKING STRATEGY: Although all the options are important components of a complete nursing assessment for this client, use principles of prioritization when answering this question. A client with an acute upper GI bleed is at risk for shock. Monitoring vital signs is the nursing action that will assess circulation and provide information about the client's circulating volume status and alert the nurse to early stages of shock.

LEVEL OF COGNITIVE ABILITY: Application
PHASE OF NURSING PROCESS: Implementation
CLIENT NEEDS: Physiological Integrity
CONTENT AREA: Adult Health/Gastrointestinal
REFERENCE
Monahan, F., & Neighbors, M. (1998). *Medical-surgical nursing: Foundations for clinical practice* (2nd ed.). Philadelphia: W. B. Saunders. p. 964.

4. 1

RATIONALE: An IV cholangiogram is for diagnostic purposes. It outlines both the gallbladder and the ducts, so gallstones that have moved into the ductal system can be detected. X-rays are used to visualize biliary duct system after IV injection of radiopaque dye.

TEST-TAKING STRATEGY: Knowledge of the pathophysiology of cholelithiasis and the purpose of the cholangiogram will help in answering this question. Eliminate options 2, 3, and 4 because they are similar. If you are unfamiliar with this procedure, take time now to review.

LEVEL OF COGNITIVE ABILITY: Comprehension
PHASE OF NURSING PROCESS: Evaluation
CLIENT NEEDS: Physiological Integrity
CONTENT AREA: Adult Health/Gastrointestinal
REFERENCE
Monahan, F., & Neighbors, M. (1998). *Medical-surgical nursing: Foundations for clinical practice* (2nd ed.). Philadelphia: W. B. Saunders. p. 972.

5. 3

RATIONALE: An inflammatory reaction such as acute pancreatitis can cause paralytic ileus, the most common form of nonmechanical obstruction. Inability to pass flatus is a clinical manifestation of paralytic ileus. Option 1 is the description of the physical finding of liver enlargement. The liver is usually enlarged in cases of cirrhosis or hepatitis. Although this client may have an enlarged liver, this is not a sign of paralytic ileus or intestinal obstruction. Pain is associated with paralytic ileus, but the pain usually presents as a more constant generalized discomfort. Pain that is severe, constant, and rapid in onset is more likely caused by strangulation of the bowel. Loss of sphincter control is not a sign of paralytic ileus.

TEST-TAKING STRATEGY: Knowledge of the clinical manifestations and abdominal physical assessment findings of paralytic ileus will assist you in answering this question. Noting the word "paralytic" will assist in directing you to option 3. Review these clinical manifestations now if you had difficulty with this question.

LEVEL OF COGNITIVE ABILITY: Comprehension
PHASE OF NURSING PROCESS: Data Collection
CLIENT NEEDS: Physiological Integrity
CONTENT AREA: Adult Health/Gastrointestinal
REFERENCE
Monahan, F., & Neighbors, M. (1998). *Medical-surgical nursing: Foundations for clinical practice* (2nd ed.). Philadelphia: W. B. Saunders. p. 1076.

6. **3**

RATIONALE: After the nasogastric tube is in place, mouth care is extremely important. With one nare occluded, the client tends to mouth breathe, drying the mucous membranes. Previous vomiting will leave a bad taste in the client's mouth and a fecal odor may be present. Frequent small sips of water would be contraindicated when the client is on gastric suction. The hard candy would increase the salivation, but would not be useful in cleaning the oral cavity. Lemon-glycerin swabs have a drying or irritating effect on the mucous membranes.
TEST-TAKING STRATEGY: The issue of this question is a specific nursing action. It is important to know that a client on gastric suction will be NPO and swallowing water or other liquids is prohibited. The goal for this client is to maintain the integrity of the oral mucosa. Options 1, 2, and 4 are similar in that they provide moisture. Option 3 is the one that is different. It includes cleaning and providing moisture and these are the two key elements to maintaining mucosal integrity.
LEVEL OF COGNITIVE ABILITY: Application
PHASE OF NURSING PROCESS: Planning
CLIENT NEEDS: Physiological Integrity
CONTENT AREA: Adult Health/Gastrointestinal
REFERENCE
Monahan, F., & Neighbors, M. (1998). *Medical-surgical nursing: Foundations for clinical practice* (2nd ed.). Philadelphia: W. B. Saunders. p. 979.

7. **3**

RATIONALE: Distention, vomiting, and abdominal pain are a few of the symptoms associated with intestinal obstruction. Nasogastric tubes may be used to empty the stomach and relieve distention and vomiting. They are also used to treat partial or complete small bowel obstruction. The nurse may evaluate peristaltic movements by auscultating the abdomen. Bowel sounds return to normal as the obstruction is relieved and normal bowel function is restored. Discontinuing the nasogastric tube prior to normal bowel function may result in a return of the symptoms, necessitating reinsertion of the nasogastric tube. Serum electrolyte levels, tube placement, and pH of gastric aspirate are important assessments for the client with a nasogastric tube in place, but do not assist in determining the appropriateness of removing the nasogastric tube.
TEST-TAKING STRATEGY: Knowing the pathophysiology for intestinal obstruction and purpose of nasogastric tubes as a therapy, you will know that the tube is left in until normal bowel function returns. Checking for presence of bowel sounds is the assessment indicator for normal bowel function. It is not appropriate to discontinue the nasogastric tube until bowel sounds are present. Assessing the pH of gastric aspirate is one method of assessing tube placement. Checking tube placement is necessary routinely and prior to instilling substances through the tube, but not necessary prior to discontinuing the tube.
LEVEL OF COGNITIVE ABILITY: Comprehension
PHASE OF NURSING PROCESS: Implementation
CLIENT NEEDS: Physiological Integrity
CONTENT AREA: Adult Health/Gastrointestinal
REFERENCE
Monahan, F., & Neighbors, M. (1998). *Medical-surgical nursing: Foundations for clinical practice* (2nd ed.). Philadelphia: W. B. Saunders. p. 1074.

8. **2**

RATIONALE: The enema fluid should be administered slowly. If the client complains of fullness or pain, stop the flow for 30 seconds and restart at a slower rate. Slow enema administration and stopping the flow temporarily, if necessary, will decrease the likelihood of intestinal spasm and premature ejection of the solution. The higher the solution container is held above the rectum, the faster the flow and the greater the force in the rectum. Pain and cramping are usually due to intestinal spasm and will subside when the enema is stopped briefly, after which the enema may be resumed. There is no need to discontinue the enema and notify the physician at this time.
TEST-TAKING STRATEGY: Knowledge of the procedure for enema administration will assist you in answering this question. Noting the client's symptoms will assist in directing you to the correct option. Review this procedure now if you had difficulty with this question.
LEVEL OF COGNITIVE ABILITY: Application
PHASE OF NURSING PROCESS: Implementation
CLIENT NEEDS: Physiological Integrity
CONTENT AREA: Adult Health/Gastrointestinal
REFERENCE
Kozier, B., Erb, G., & Blais, K. (1998). *Fundamentals of nursing: Concepts, process, and practice* (5th ed.). Reading, MA: Addison-Wesley. pp. 1203, 1205.

9. **1**

RATIONALE: The sigmoid and descending colon are located on the left side. Therefore, the left lateral position uses gravity to facilitate the flow of solution into the sigmoid and descending colon. Acute flexion of the right leg allows for adequate exposure of the anus.
TEST-TAKING STRATEGY: Knowledge of anatomy of the rectum will assist in eliminating options 2 and 4. Attempt to visualize the remaining positions presented in options 1 and 3. By doing so, you should easily be able to eliminate option 3. Review this procedure now if you had difficulty with this question.
LEVEL OF COGNITIVE ABILITY: Application
PHASE OF NURSING PROCESS: Implementation
CLIENT NEEDS: Physiological Integrity
CONTENT AREA: Adult Health/Gastrointestinal
REFERENCE
Kozier, B., Erb, G., & Blais, K. (1998). *Fundamentals of nursing: Concepts, process, and practice* (5th ed.). Reading, MA: Addison-Wesley. p. 1204.

10. **2**

RATIONALE: After checking residual feeding contents, reinstill the gastric contents into the stomach by removing the syringe bulb or plunger, and pouring the gastric contents via the syringe into the nasogastric tube. Removal of the contents could disturb the client's electrolyte balance.
TEST-TAKING STRATEGY: Knowledge of the procedure for nasogastric intermittent tube feeding will assist you in answering this question. The question is asking you what should be done with aspirated gastric residual. It does not need to be mixed with water, nor should it be discarded. Gastric contents should be reinstilled in order to maintain the client's electrolyte balance. The gastric contents should be poured into the nasogastric tube through a syringe without a plunger and not injected by pushing on the plunger.
LEVEL OF COGNITIVE ABILITY: Comprehension
PHASE OF NURSING PROCESS: Planning

CLIENT NEEDS: Physiological Integrity
CONTENT AREA: Adult Health/Gastrointestinal
REFERENCE
Kozier, B., Erb, G., & Blais, K. (1998). *Fundamentals of nursing: Concepts, process, and practice* (5th ed.). Reading, MA: Addison-Wesley. p. 1050.

11. **4**

RATIONALE: Common risk factors for colorectal cancer include age over 40, first-degree relative with colorectal cancer; high-fat, low-fiber diet; and history of bowel problems such as ulcerative colitis or familial polyposis. Clients should be aware of risk factors as part of general health maintenance and primary disease prevention.
TEST-TAKING STRATEGY: Specific knowledge of risk factors related to colorectal cancer is needed to answer this question correctly. If needed, take a few moments to review this content area now.
LEVEL OF COGNITIVE ABILITY: Application
PHASE OF NURSING PROCESS: Planning
CLIENT NEEDS: Health Promotion and Maintenance
CONTENT AREA: Adult Health/Gastrointestinal
REFERENCE
Monahan, F., & Neighbors, M. (1998). *Medical-surgical nursing foundations for clinical practice* (2nd ed.). Philadelphia: W. B. Saunders. p. 969.

12. **3**

RATIONALE: The discomfort of reflux is aggravated by positions that compress the abdomen and the stomach. These include lying flat either on the back or stomach after a meal, or lying on the right side. The left side-lying position with the head of the bed elevated is most likely to give relief to the client.
TEST-TAKING STRATEGY: To answer this question correctly, evaluate each of the positions described in terms of their ability to put pressure on the stomach and cause reflux. Using knowledge of anatomy and these basic nursing positions, you should be able to eliminate each of the incorrect options systematically.
LEVEL OF COGNITIVE ABILITY: Application
PHASE OF NURSING PROCESS: Implementation
CLIENT NEEDS: Physiological Integrity
CONTENT AREA: Adult Health/Gastrointestinal
REFERENCE
Beare, P., & Myers, J. (1998). *Adult health nursing* (3rd ed.). St. Louis, MO: Mosby–Year Book. p. 1485.

13. **2**

RATIONALE: Foods that increase the LES pressure will decrease reflux, and lessen the symptoms of GERD. The food substance that will increase the LES pressure is nonfat milk. The other substances listed decrease the LES pressure, thus increasing reflux symptoms. Aggravating substances include chocolate, coffee, fatty foods, and alcohol.
TEST-TAKING STRATEGY: To answer this question accurately, it is necessary to understand the effect of various food substances on LES pressure and GERD. This will allow you to eliminate each of the incorrect options systematically. Review this now if you had difficulty with this question.
LEVEL OF COGNITIVE ABILITY: Application
PHASE OF NURSING PROCESS: Planning
CLIENT NEEDS: Health Promotion and Maintenance
CONTENT AREA: Adult Health/Gastrointestinal

REFERENCE
Beare, P., & Myers, J. (1998). *Adult health nursing* (3rd ed.). St. Louis, MO: Mosby–Year Book. p. 1484.

14. **1**

RATIONALE: The nurse places highest priority on assessing for return of the gag reflex and on managing the client's airway. The client's vital signs are monitored also; a sudden sharp increase in temperature could indicate perforation of the GI tract. This would be accompanied by other signs as well, such as pain. Monitoring for sore throat and heartburn are also important; the client's airway still takes priority, however.
TEST-TAKING STRATEGY: Remember the ABC, airway, breathing, and circulation. Note also that the question contains the key words "highest priority." This tells you that more than one or all of the options may be partially or totally correct. Use the ABCs to set your priorities.
LEVEL OF COGNITIVE ABILITY: Comprehension
PHASE OF NURSING PROCESS: Planning
CLIENT NEEDS: Physiological Integrity
CONTENT AREA: Adult Health/Gastrointestinal
REFERENCE
Beare, P., & Myers, J. (1998). *Adult health nursing* (3rd ed.). St. Louis, MO: Mosby–Year Book. p. 1465.

15. **2**

RATIONALE: The client does have to lie still for ERCP, which takes about an hour to perform. The client also has to sign a consent form. IV sedation is given to relax the client, and an anesthetic spray is used to help keep the client from gagging as the endoscope is passed.
TEST TAKING STRATEGY: Note the key words "has not fully understood." Invasive procedures require consent, so option 1 can be eliminated. Noting the name of the procedure and considering the anatomical location will assist in eliminating options 3 and 4. Review this procedure now if you had difficulty with this question.
LEVEL OF COGNITIVE ABILITY: Comprehension
PHASE OF NURSING PROCESS: Evaluation
CLIENT NEEDS: Physiological Integrity
CONTENT AREA: Adult Health/Gastrointestinal
REFERENCE
Beare, P., & Myers, J. (1998). *Adult health nursing* (3rd ed.). St. Louis, MO: Mosby–Year Book. p. 1472.

16. **1**

RATIONALE: A barium swallow, or esophagography, is an x-ray that uses a substance called barium for contrast to highlight abnormalities in the GI tract. The client is told to remove all jewelry before the test so it won't interfere with x-ray visualization of the field. The client should fast for 8 to 12 hours before the test, depending on the physician's instructions. Most oral medications are also withheld before the test. It is important after the procedure to monitor for constipation, which can occur as a result of the presence of barium in the GI tract.
TEST-TAKING STRATEGY: Note the key words "barium swallow" and "before." This tells you that the correct answer is an item that the client needs to comply with before the test is done. Eliminate option 4 first, because it is a part of aftercare. Knowing that the procedure is a type of x-ray that involves barium for contrast allows you to eliminate each of the incorrect options successfully.

LEVEL OF COGNITIVE ABILITY: Application
PHASE OF NURSING PROCESS: Implementation
CLIENT NEEDS: Physiological Integrity
CONTENT AREA: Adult Health/Gastrointestinal
REFERENCE
Beare, P., & Myers, J. (1998). *Adult health nursing* (3rd ed.). St. Louis, MO: Mosby–Year Book. p. 1465.

17. 1

RATIONALE: The client is placed in the left Sims' position for the procedure. This position takes the best advantage of the client's anatomy for ease in introducing the colonoscope. The other options are incorrect.
TEST-TAKING STRATEGY: Use concepts related to GI anatomy to answer this question. The answer would be the same as for giving the client an enema while lying down. When answering factual questions such as these, remember the guiding principles and attempt to visualize the procedure to help you select the correct option.
LEVEL OF COGNITIVE ABILITY: Application
PHASE OF NURSING PROCESS: Planning
CLIENT NEEDS: Physiological Integrity
CONTENT AREA: Adult Health/Gastrointestinal
REFERENCE
Monahan, F., & Neighbors, M. (1998). *Medical-surgical nursing: Foundations for clinical practice* (2nd ed.). Philadelphia: W. B. Saunders. p. 975.

18. 4

RATIONALE: The client should not drive for several hours after discharge because of receiving sedative medications during the procedure. Important decisions should also be delayed for at least 24 hours for the same reason. The client should resume intake slowly, and progress as tolerated. The client may experience gas or abdominal tenderness for a short while after the procedure, and this is normal.
TEST-TAKING STRATEGY: Note that the question contains the key words "did not fully understand." This tells you that the correct answer is an incorrect statement on the part of the client. Use knowledge of events during the procedure to choose the correct option. Knowledge that sedating medications are administered will direct you to option 4.
LEVEL OF COGNITIVE ABILITY: Comprehension
PHASE OF NURSING PROCESS: Evaluation
CLIENT NEEDS: Health Promotion and Maintenance
CONTENT AREA: Adult Health/Gastrointestinal
REFERENCE
Monahan, F., & Neighbors, M. (1998). *Medical-surgical nursing: Foundations for clinical practice* (2nd ed.). Philadelphia: W. B. Saunders. p. 976.

19. 2

RATIONALE: The appropriate technique for abdominal examination is inspection, auscultation, percussion, and palpation. Auscultation is performed after inspection to ensure that the motility of the bowel and bowel sounds are not altered. The sequence of maneuvers is inspect, auscultate, percuss, and palpate.
TEST-TAKING STRATEGY: Knowledge regarding the techniques used to assess the abdomen is required to answer the question. Remember that the sequence for abdominal assessment is different than the usual systematic approach. Review this technique now if you had difficulty with this question.

LEVEL OF COGNITIVE ABILITY: Application
PHASE OF NURSING PROCESS: Data Collection
CLIENT NEEDS: Physiological Integrity
CONTENT AREA: Adult Health/Gastrointestinal
REFERENCE
Monahan, F., & Neighbors, M. (1998). *Medical-surgical nursing: Foundations for clinical practice* (2nd ed.). Philadelphia: W. B. Saunders. p. 968.

20. 3

RATIONALE: Normal dietary intake of fat should be maintained during the days preceding the test in order to empty bile from the gallbladder. A fat-free diet is ordered on the evening before the test. The fat-free supper prevents contraction of the gallbladder and allows accumulation of the contrast substance needed for x-ray visualization.
TEST-TAKING STRATEGY: Knowledge that an oral cholecystogram is an x-ray of the gallbladder will assist in directing you to the correct option. Think about the function of the gallbladder to assist in selecting the correct option.
LEVEL OF COGNITIVE ABILITY: Application
PHASE OF NURSING PROCESS: Planning
CLIENT NEEDS: Physiological Integrity
CONTENT AREA: Adult Health/Gastrointestinal
REFERENCE
Monahan, F., & Neighbors, M. (1998). *Medical-surgical nursing: Foundations for clinical practice* (2nd ed.). Philadelphia: W. B. Saunders. p. 972.

21. 4

RATIONALE: The solution GoLYTELY is a bowel evacuant used in preparation for colonoscopy to cleanse the bowel. It is expected to cause a mild diarrhea and will clear the bowel in 4 to 5 hours.
TEST-TAKING STRATEGY: Knowledge regarding the purpose of this medication will assist in eliminating option 3 and easily direct you to option 4. Options 1 and 2 are not within the scope of nursing practice and should be eliminated.
LEVEL OF COGNITIVE ABILITY: Application
PHASE OF NURSING PROCESS: Implementation
CLIENT NEEDS: Physiological Integrity
CONTENT AREA: Adult Health/Gastrointestinal
REFERENCE
Hodgson, B., & Kizior, R. (2000). *Saunders nursing drug handbook 2000.* Philadelphia: W. B. Saunders. p. 841.

22. 3

RATIONALE: When GI tubes are attached to suction, it may be continuous or intermittent, with a pressure not exceeding 25 mmHg. The specific pressure and the intervals are prescribed by the physician.
TEST-TAKING STRATEGY: Knowledge regarding the restrictions related to the amount of pressure with suction on a GI tube is required to answer this question. Learn this now if you are unfamiliar with this procedure.
LEVEL OF COGNITIVE ABILITY: Comprehension
PHASE OF NURSING PROCESS: Implementation
CLIENT NEEDS: Physiological Integrity
CONTENT AREA: Adult Health/Gastrointestinal
REFERENCE
Monahan, F., & Neighbors, M. (1998). *Medical-surgical nursing: Foundations for clinical practice* (2nd ed.). Philadelphia: W. B. Saunders. p. 978.

23. 2

RATIONALE: Deterioration and atrophy of the lining of the stomach leads to the loss of function of the parietal cells. When the acid secretion decreases, the source of the intrinsic factor is lost, which results in the inability to absorb vitamin B_{12}. This leads to the development of pernicious anemia.
TEST-TAKING STRATEGY: Knowledge regarding the pathophysiology related to the lining of the stomach is required to answer this question. If you are unfamiliar with vitamin B_{12} deficiency and its relationship to gastric disorders, review now.
LEVEL OF COGNITIVE ABILITY: Comprehension
PHASE OF NURSING PROCESS: Data Collection
CLIENT NEEDS: Physiological Integrity
CONTENT AREA: Adult Health/Gastrointestinal
REFERENCE
Black, J., & Matassarin-Jacobs, E. (1997). *Medical-surgical nursing: Clinical management for continuity of care* (5th ed.). Philadelphia: W. B. Saunders. p. 1763.

24. 2

RATIONALE: Indomethacin is an NSAID and can cause ulceration of the esophagus, stomach, duodenum, or small intestine. It is contraindicated in a client with GI disorders. Furosemide is a loop diuretic. Digoxin is an antidysrhythmic. Propranolol is a beta-adrenergic blocker. Furosemide, digoxin, and propranolol are not contraindicated in clients with gastric disorders.
TEST-TAKING STRATEGY: Knowledge regarding the side effects associated with the medications identified in the options is required to answer this question. If you are unfamiliar with these medications, take time now to review them.
LEVEL OF COGNITIVE ABILITY: Comprehension
PHASE OF NURSING PROCESS: Implementation
CLIENT NEEDS: Safe, Effective Care Environment
CONTENT AREA: Adult Health/Gastrointestinal
REFERENCE
Hodgson, B., & Kizior, R. (2000). *Saunders nursing drug handbook 2000*. Philadelphia: W. B. Saunders. pp. 324–326, 452–454, 528–530, 877–880.

25. 4

RATIONALE: Perforation is a surgical emergency. It is characterized by sudden, sharp, intolerable severe pain beginning in the midepigastric area and spreading over the abdomen, which becomes rigid and boardlike. Nausea and vomiting may occur. Tachycardia may occur as hypovolemic shock develops. Numbness in the legs is not an associated finding.
TEST TAKING STRATEGY: Note the key words "most likely" in the stem of the question. Option 2 can be easily eliminated. Eliminate option 1 next because tachycardia rather than bradycardia develops if the client is bleeding. From the remaining two options, focusing on the key words will assist in directing you to option 4.
LEVEL OF COGNITIVE ABILITY: Comprehension
PHASE OF NURSING PROCESS: Data Collection
CLIENT NEEDS: Physiological Integrity
CONTENT AREA: Adult Health/Gastrointestinal
REFERENCE
Reference: Monahan, F., & Neighbors, M. (1998). *Medical-surgical nursing: Foundations for clinical practice* (2nd ed.). Philadelphia: W. B. Saunders. p. 1029.

26. 1

RATIONALE: Cimetidine, a histamine H_2-receptor antagonist, will decrease the secretion of gastric acid. Sucralfate promotes healing by coating the ulcer. Antacids neutralize acid in the stomach. Omeprazole inhibits gastric acid secretion.
TEST-TAKING STRATEGY: Knowledge regarding the actions of the medications used to treat peptic ulcers is required to answer this question. If you are unfamiliar with these medications or their actions, take time now to review them.
LEVEL OF COGNITIVE ABILITY: Comprehension
PHASE OF NURSING PROCESS: Evaluation
CLIENT NEEDS: Health Promotion and Maintenance
CONTENT AREA: Adult Health/Gastrointestinal
REFERENCE
Reference: Monahan, F., & Neighbors, M. (1998). *Medical-surgical nursing: Foundations for clinical practice* (2nd ed.). Philadelphia: W. B. Saunders. pp. 1027–1028.

27. 4

RATIONALE: Option 4 describes the procedure for a pyloroplasty. A vagotomy involves cutting the vagus nerve. A subtotal gastrectomy involves removing the distal portion of the stomach. A Billroth II procedure involves removal of the ulcer and a large portion of the cells that produce hydrochloric acid.
TEST-TAKING STRATEGY: Note the relationship between the words "pyloroplasty" and "pylorus" in the correct option. If you are unfamiliar with this procedure, take time now to review.
LEVEL OF COGNITIVE ABILITY: Comprehension
PHASE OF NURSING PROCESS: Planning
CLIENT NEEDS: Physiological Integrity
CONTENT AREA: Adult Health/Gastrointestinal
REFERENCE
Monahan, F., & Neighbors, M. (1998). *Medical-surgical nursing: Foundations for clinical practice* (2nd ed.). Philadelphia: W. B. Saunders. p. 1028.

28. 4

RATIONALE: A vagotomy, or cutting of the vagus nerve, is done to eliminate parasympathetic stimulation of gastric secretion. Options 1, 2, and 3 are incorrect descriptions of a vagotomy.
TEST-TAKING STRATEGY: Knowledge regarding the procedure and purpose of a vagotomy is required to answer this question. If you are unfamiliar with this procedure, take time now to review.
LEVEL OF COGNITIVE ABILITY: Comprehension
PHASE OF NURSING PROCESS: Implementation
CLIENT NEEDS: Physiological Integrity
CONTENT AREA: Adult Health/Gastrointestinal
REFERENCE
Monahan, F., & Neighbors, M. (1998). *Medical-surgical nursing: Foundations for clinical practice* (2nd ed.). Philadelphia: W. B. Saunders. p. 1028.

29. 1

RATIONALE: In a Billroth II resection, the proximal remnant of the stomach is anastamosed to the proximal jejunum. Patency of the NG tube is critical for preventing the retention of gastric secretions. The nurse, however, should never irrigate or reposition the gastric tube after gastric surgery unless specifically ordered by the physician. In this situation, the nurse should clarify the order. Options 2, 3, and 4 are appropriate postoperative interventions.

TEST-TAKING STRATEGY: Eliminate options 2, 3, and 4 because they are general postoperative measures. Consider the anatomical location of the surgical procedure to assist in directing you to option 1. Review postoperative measures now if you had difficulty with this question.
LEVEL OF COGNITIVE ABILITY: Comprehension
PHASE OF NURSING PROCESS: Implementation
CLIENT NEEDS: Safe, Effective Care Environment
CONTENT AREA: Adult Health/Gastrointestinal
REFERENCE
Monahan, F., & Neighbors, M. (1998). *Medical-surgical nursing: Foundations for clinical practice* (2nd ed.). Philadelphia: W. B. Saunders. p. 996.

30. **2**

RATIONALE: The client should be instructed to decrease the amount of fluid taken at meals. The client should also be instructed to avoid high-carbohydrate foods including fluids such as fruit nectars; to assume a low Fowler's position during meals; to lie down for 30 minutes after eating to delay gastric emptying; and to take antispasmodics as prescribed.
TEST-TAKING STRATEGY: Eliminate options 3 and 4 first because these measures will promote gastric emptying. From the remaining options, select option 2 because this measure will delay gastric emptying. If you are unfamiliar with this syndrome, take time now to review the important client teaching points.
LEVEL OF COGNITIVE ABILITY: Application
PHASE OF NURSING PROCESS: Implementation
CLIENT NEEDS: Health Promotion and Maintenance
CONTENT AREA: Adult Health/Gastrointestinal
REFERENCE
Monahan, F., & Neighbors, M. (1998). *Medical-surgical nursing: Foundations for clinical practice* (2nd ed.). Philadelphia: W. B. Saunders. p. 1000.

31. **3**

RATIONALE: Early manifestations occur 5 to 30 minutes after eating. Symptoms include vertigo, tachycardia, syncope, sweating, pallor, palpitations, and the desire to lie down.
TEST-TAKING STRATEGY: Knowledge regarding the early manifestations associated with dumping syndrome is required to answer this question. If you are unfamiliar with these manifestations, review them now.
LEVEL OF COGNITIVE ABILITY: Comprehension
PHASE OF NURSING PROCESS: Data Collection
CLIENT NEEDS: Physiological Integrity
CONTENT AREA: Adult Health/Gastrointestinal
REFERENCE
deWit, S. (1998). *Essentials of medical-surgical nursing* (4th ed.). Philadelphia: W. B. Saunders. p. 613.

32. **2**

RATIONALE: Following herniorrhaphy, the client should be instructed to elevate the scrotum and apply ice packs while in bed to decrease pain and swelling. Instruct the client to apply a scrotal support when out of bed.
TEST-TAKING STRATEGY: The issue of the question is to prevent swelling. Basic knowledge regarding the effects of heat and cold will assist in eliminating option 1. Options 3 and 4 can be eliminated next by focusing on the issue of

the question. Review postoperative care following herniorrhaphy now if you had difficulty with this question.
LEVEL OF COGNITIVE ABILITY: Application
PHASE OF NURSING PROCESS: Implementation
CLIENT NEEDS: Health Promotion and Maintenance
CONTENT AREA: Adult Health/Gastrointestinal
REFERENCE
Monahan, F., & Neighbors, M. (1998). *Medical-surgical nursing: Foundations for clinical practice* (2nd ed.). Philadelphia: W. B. Saunders. p. 1096.

33. **1**

RATIONALE: The client with irritable bowel syndrome should be encouraged to include fiber and bulk in the diet to help produce bulky soft stools and establish regular bowel habits. The client should ingest approximately 30 to 40 g of fiber each day. Eating regular meals, drinking 8 to 10 cups of liquids each day, and chewing food slowly promote normal bowel function.
TEST-TAKING STRATEGY: Note the key word "not" in the stem of the question. Also note that options 1 and 2 are opposite client instructions. This should indicate that one of these options is the correct one. Recalling that the goal is to establish regular bowel habits will assist in directing you to option 1.
LEVEL OF COGNITIVE ABILITY: Application
PHASE OF NURSING PROCESS: Planning
CLIENT NEEDS: Health Promotion and Maintenance
CONTENT AREA: Adult Health/Gastrointestinal
REFERENCE
deWit, S. (1998). *Essentials of medical-surgical nursing* (4th ed.). Philadelphia: W. B. Saunders. p. 619.

34. **2**

RATIONALE: Crohn's disease is characterized by nonbloody diarrhea of usually not more than four or five stools daily. Over time, the diarrhea episodes do increase in frequency, duration, and severity. Options 3 and 4 are not characteristics of Crohn's disease.
TEST-TAKING STRATEGY: Options 3 and 4 can be easily eliminated. From the remaining options, it is necessary to be familiar with the characteristics of Crohn's disease. If you are unfamiliar with this disorder, take time now to review.
LEVEL OF COGNITIVE ABILITY: Comprehension
PHASE OF NURSING PROCESS: Data Collection
CLIENT NEEDS: Physiological Integrity
CONTENT AREA: Adult Health/Gastrointestinal
REFERENCE
Monahan, F., & Neighbors, M. (1998). *Medical-surgical nursing: Foundations for clinical practice* (2nd ed.). Philadelphia: W. B. Saunders. p. 1067.

35. **3**

RATIONALE: If cramping occurs during colostomy irrigation, stop the irrigation flow temporarily and allow the client to rest. Cramping may occur from infusion that is too rapid or is causing too much pressure. Increasing the height of the irrigation will cause further discomfort. The physician does not need to be notified. Medicating the client for pain is not the most appropriate action.
TEST-TAKING STRATEGY: Focus on the issue of the question. This will assist in eliminating options 1, 2, and 4 and easily direct you to the correct option. If you had difficulty answering this question, take time now to review the procedure for colostomy irrigation.

LEVEL OF COGNITIVE ABILITY: Application
PHASE OF NURSING PROCESS: Implementation
CLIENT NEEDS: Physiological Integrity
CONTENT AREA: Adult Health/Gastrointestinal
REFERENCE
Ignatavicius, D., Workman, M., & Mishler, M. (1999). *Medical-surgical nursing across the health care continuum* (3rd ed.) Philadelphia: W. B. Saunders. p. 1417.

---

36. 3

RATIONALE: To enhance effectiveness of the irrigation, instruct the client to change position, ambulate, massage the abdomen gently, and to drink something warm. Options 1, 2, and 4 will not enhance the effectiveness of this procedure.
TEST-TAKING STRATEGY: Focus on the issue of the question, which is the measure that will enhance the effectiveness of the irrigation. This focus will assist in eliminating options 1, 2, and 4. If you are unfamiliar with this procedure, take time now to review.
LEVEL OF COGNITIVE ABILITY: Application
PHASE OF NURSING PROCESS: Implementation
CLIENT NEEDS: Health Promotion and Maintenance
CONTENT AREA: Adult Health/Gastrointestinal
REFERENCE
Ignatavicius, D., Workman, M., & Mishler, M. (1999). *Medical-surgical nursing across the health care continuum* (3rd ed.) Philadelphia: W. B. Saunders. p. 1417.

---

37. 1

RATIONALE: Asterixis is irregular flapping movements of the fingers and wrists when the hands and arms are outstretched, with the palms down, wrists bent up, and fingers spread. It is the most common and reliable sign that hepatic encephalopathy is developing.
TEST-TAKING STRATEGY: Knowledge regarding the procedure for this important assessment is required to answer this question. If you are unfamiliar with this assessment procedure, be sure to review now.
LEVEL OF COGNITIVE ABILITY: Application
PHASE OF NURSING PROCESS: Data Collection
CLIENT NEEDS: Physiological Integrity
CONTENT AREA: Adult Health/Gastrointestinal
REFERENCE
Monahan, F., & Neighbors, M. (1998). *Medical-surgical nursing: Foundations for clinical practice* (2nd ed.). Philadelphia: W. B. Saunders. p. 1150.

---

38. 4

RATIONALE: An upright position allows the intestine to float posteriorly and helps prevent intestinal laceration during catheter insertion.
TEST-TAKING STRATEGY: Attempt to visualize this procedure in selecting the correct option. Knowing that fluid will be aspirated from the abdominal cavity will assist in directing you to option 4. If you had difficulty with this question, review this procedure now.
LEVEL OF COGNITIVE ABILITY: Application
PHASE OF NURSING PROCESS: Implementation
CLIENT NEEDS: Physiological Integrity
CONTENT AREA: Adult Health/Gastrointestinal
REFERENCE
Monahan, F., & Neighbors, M. (1998). *Medical-surgical nursing: Foundations for clinical practice* (2nd ed.). Philadelphia: W. B. Saunders. p. 1144.

---

39. 4

RATIONALE: Most of the ammonia in the body is found in the GI tract. Protein provided by the diet is transported to the liver by the portal vein. The liver breaks down protein and this results in the formation of ammonia. A low-protein diet would be prescribed.
TEST-TAKING STRATEGY: Recall the physiology of the liver in answering this question. Note that the question stem states "most likely." You should be easily directed to option 4. Also note that options 3 and 4 are opposite, which should provide you with the clue that one of these options is correct.
LEVEL OF COGNITIVE ABILITY: Comprehension
PHASE OF NURSING PROCESS: Planning
CLIENT NEEDS: Physiological Integrity
CONTENT AREA: Adult Health/Gastrointestinal
REFERENCE
Monahan, F., & Neighbors, M. (1998). *Medical-surgical nursing: Foundations for clinical practice* (2nd ed.). Philadelphia: W. B. Saunders. pp. 1182–1183.

---

40. 1

RATIONALE: Lactulose is an osmotic laxative. The desired effect is two to three soft stools per day with an acid fecal pH. Lactulose creates an acid environment in the bowel, resulting in a fall of the colon's pH from 7 to 5. This causes ammonia to leave the circulatory system and move into the colon. Diarrhea may indicate excessive administration of the medication. Options 3 and 4 do not determine that a desired effect has occurred.
TEST-TAKING STRATEGY: Knowledge regarding the purpose and action of this medication is required to answer this question. Review this important medication now if you had difficulty with this question.
LEVEL OF COGNITIVE ABILITY: Comprehension
PHASE OF NURSING PROCESS: Evaluation
CLIENT NEEDS: Physiological Integrity
CONTENT AREA: Adult Health/Gastrointestinal
REFERENCE
Monahan, F., & Neighbors, M. (1998). *Medical-surgical nursing: Foundations for clinical practice* (2nd ed.). Philadelphia: W. B. Saunders. p. 1150.

---

41. 1

RATIONALE: Ultrasound of the gallbladder is a noninvasive procedure and is frequently used for emergency diagnosis of acute cholecystitis. The client does not need to be NPO but may be instructed to avoid carbonated beverages for 48 hours before the test to help decrease intestinal gas. It is a painless test and does not require the administration of oral tablets as preparation.
TEST-TAKING STRATEGY: Attempt to vizualize this procedure in selecting the correct option. This should be relatively easy; however, if you are unfamiliar with this test, take time now to review.
LEVEL OF COGNITIVE ABILITY: Application
PHASE OF NURSING PROCESS: Implementation
CLIENT NEEDS: Physiological Integrity
CONTENT AREA: Adult Health/Gastrointestinal
REFERENCE
Monahan, F., & Neighbors, M. (1998). *Medical-surgical nursing: Foundations for clinical practice* (2nd ed.). Philadelphia: W. B. Saunders. p. 976.

42. **1**

RATIONALE: After cholecystectomy, breathing tends to be shallow because deep breathing is painful as a result of the location of the incision. Teaching the importance of performing coughing and deep-breathing exercises is the priority.

TEST-TAKING STRATEGY: Use Maslow's hierarchy of needs theory to answer the question. Option 1 relates to airway. Additionally, recalling the anatomical location of the abdominal incision will assist in directing you to the correct option.

LEVEL OF COGNITIVE ABILITY: Application
PHASE OF NURSING PROCESS: Planning
CLIENT NEEDS: Physiological Integrity
CONTENT AREA: Adult Health/Gastrointestinal
REFERENCE
Monahan, F., & Neighbors, M. (1998). *Medical-surgical nursing: Foundations for clinical practice* (2nd ed.). Philadelphia: W. B. Saunders. p. 1116.

43. **2**

RATIONALE: Serosanguineous drainage with a small amount of bile is expected from the Penrose drain for the first 24 hours. Drainage then decreases and the drain is removed usually in 48 hours. The physician does not need to be notified. A sterile dressing covers the site and should be changed to prevent infection and skin excoriation.

TEST-TAKING STRATEGY: Eliminate options 3 and 4 first because they are similar. Knowledge of the normal expected findings following cholecystectomy will easily direct you to option 2.

LEVEL OF COGNITIVE ABILITY: Application
PHASE OF NURSING PROCESS: Implementation
CLIENT NEEDS: Physiological Integrity
CONTENT AREA: Adult Health/Gastrointestinal
REFERENCE
Monahan, F., & Neighbors, M. (1998). *Medical-surgical nursing: Foundations for clinical practice* (2nd ed.). Philadelphia: W. B. Saunders. p. 1114.

44. **1**

RATIONALE: Fatigue is a normal response to hepatic cellular damage. During the acute stage, rest is an essential intervention to reduce the liver's metabolic demands and increase its blood supply. Options 2, 3, and 4 are incorrect.

TEST-TAKING STRATEGY: Note the key word "acute" in the question. Knowing that the liver will need to rest in order to heal will easily assist you to option 1. If you are unfamiliar with the care of a client with hepatitis, take time now to review.

LEVEL OF COGNITIVE ABILITY: Comprehension
PHASE OF NURSING PROCESS: Planning
CLIENT NEEDS: Physiological Integrity
CONTENT AREA: Adult Health/Gastrointestinal
REFERENCE
Monahan, F., & Neighbors, M. (1998). *Medical-surgical nursing: Foundations for clinical practice* (2nd ed.). Philadelphia: W. B. Saunders. p. 1177.

45. **1**

RATIONALE: Hepatitis A is transmitted by the fecal-oral route via contaminated food or infected food handlers. Hepatitis B, C, and D is most commonly transmitted via infected blood or body fluids.

TEST-TAKING STRATEGY: Knowledge regarding the modes of transmission of the various types of hepatitis is required to answer this question. If you are unfamiliar with this important content area, take time now to review.

LEVEL OF COGNITIVE ABILITY: Comprehension
PHASE OF NURSING PROCESS: Data Collection
CLIENT NEEDS: Physiological Integrity
CONTENT AREA: Adult Health/Gastrointestinal
REFERENCE
Monahan, F., & Neighbors, M. (1998). *Medical-surgical nursing: Foundations for clinical practice* (2nd ed.). Philadelphia: W. B. Saunders. p. 1170.

46. **4**

RATIONALE: Meperidine (Demerol) rather than morphine is the medication of choice because morphine can cause spasms in the sphincter of Oddi. Options 1, 2, and 3 are appropriate interventions for the client with acute pancreatitis.

TEST-TAKING STRATEGY: Note the key word "acute" in the question. Knowledge regarding the treatment measures for acute pancreatitis is required to answer this question. Review this content now if you had difficulty with this question.

LEVEL OF COGNITIVE ABILITY: Comprehension
PHASE OF NURSING PROCESS: Implementation
CLIENT NEEDS: Safe, Effective Care Environment
CONTENT AREA: Adult Health/Gastrointestinal
REFERENCE
Monahan, F., & Neighbors, M. (1998). *Medical-surgical nursing: Foundations for clinical practice* (2nd ed.). Philadelphia: W. B. Saunders. p. 1118.

47. **4**

RATIONALE: Psychological or emotional stressors that exacerbate peptic ulcer disease may be found either at home or in the workplace. The frequent need to work overtime on short notice is the option that is potentially most stressful, since it is the item the client has least control over. An ability to work at home periodically is not necessarily stressful, because there is increased client control over timing of work and location. Adequate rest and proper dietary pattern (options 1 and 2) should alleviate symptoms, not worsen them.

TEST-TAKING STRATEGY: Begin to answer this question by eliminating options 1 and 2 because they are healthy living habits. Recall that psychological stress may be worsened in situations where there is little client control. This would help you to choose option 4 over option 3 as the correct answer, given the wording of the question.

LEVEL OF COGNITIVE ABILITY: Comprehension
PHASE OF NURSING PROCESS: Data Collection
CLIENT NEEDS: Physiological Integrity
CONTENT AREA: Adult Health/Gastrointestinal
REFERENCE
Monahan, F., & Neighbors, M. (1998). *Medical-surgical nursing: Foundations for clinical practice* (2nd ed.). Philadelphia: W. B. Saunders. p. 1027.

48. **2**

RATIONALE: Dietary modification for the client with PUD includes eliminating foods that are irritating to the client. Items that are generally eliminated or avoided are highly spiced foods, alcohol, caffeine, chocolate, and fresh fruits. Other foods may be taken according to the client's tolerance of that specific food.

TEST-TAKING STRATEGY: To answer this question accurately, it is necessary to understand which types of foods and beverages are irritating to the gastrointestinal mucosa. This will allow you to eliminate each of the incorrect options systematically. If this question was difficult, take a few moments to review this important content area now.
LEVEL OF COGNITIVE ABILITY: Application
PHASE OF NURSING PROCESS: Planning
CLIENT NEEDS: Health Promotion and Maintenance
CONTENT AREA: Adult Health/Gastrointestinal
REFERENCE

Monahan, F., & Neighbors, M. (1998). *Medical-surgical nursing: Foundations for clinical practice* (2nd ed.). Philadelphia: W. B. Saunders. p. 1027.

49. **1**

RATIONALE: The peristomal skin must receive meticulous cleansing because the ileostomy drainage has more enzymes and is more caustic to the skin than colostomy drainage. Foods such as nuts and those with seeds will pass through the ileostomy. The client should be taught that these foods will remain undigested. The area below the ileostomy may be massaged if needed if the ileostomy becomes blocked by high-fiber foods. Fluid intake should be maintained to at least 6 to 8 glasses of water per day to prevent dehydration.
TEST-TAKING STRATEGY: Note that the question contains the key words "essential care" and "stoma." This tells you that the correct answer will be the option that deals with the stoma directly. This helps you to eliminate each of the incorrect options easily.
LEVEL OF COGNITIVE ABILITY: Application
PHASE OF NURSING PROCESS: Implementation
CLIENT NEEDS: Health Promotion and Maintenance
CONTENT AREA: Adult Health/Gastrointestinal
REFERENCE

Monahan, F., & Neighbors, M. (1998). *Medical-surgical nursing: Foundations for clinical practice* (2nd ed.). Philadelphia: W. B. Saunders. p. 1014.

50. **2**

RATIONALE: Hiatal hernia is due to protrusion of a portion of the stomach above the diaphragm, where the esophagus usually is positioned. The client usually experiences pain due to reflux with ingestion of irritating foods, lying flat following meals or at night, and with large or fatty meals. Relief is obtained with intake of small, frequent, and bland meals; with use of histamine antagonists and antacids; and with elevation of the thorax following meals and during sleep.
TEST-TAKING STRATEGY: To answer this question accurately, it is necessary to know the aggravating factors for hiatal hernia and corrective actions. Note that the key word in the stem of the question is "contraindicated." This tells you that the correct answer will be the option that represents an aggravating factor for hiatal hernia discomfort.
LEVEL OF COGNITIVE ABILITY: Application
PHASE OF NURSING PROCESS: Planning
CLIENT NEEDS: Health Promotion and Maintenance
CONTENT AREA: Adult Health/Gastrointestinal
REFERENCE

Monahan, F., & Neighbors, M. (1998). *Medical-surgical nursing: Foundations for clinical practice* (2nd ed.). Philadelphia: W. B. Saunders. p. 1044.

51. **4**

RATIONALE: A prolapsed stoma is one in which bowel protrudes through the stoma, with an elongated and swollen appearance. A stoma retraction is characterized by sinking of the stoma. Ischemia of the stoma is associated with dusky or bluish color. A stoma with a narrowed opening either at the level of the skin or fascia is said to be stenosed.
TEST-TAKING STRATEGY: Focus on the key word "prolapse." To answer this question correctly, it is necessary to be familiar with the different complications that can occur with ostomy formation. If this question was difficult, take a few moments now to review these important items.
LEVEL OF COGNITIVE ABILITY: Comprehension
PHASE OF NURSING PROCESS: Data Collection
CLIENT NEEDS: Physiological Integrity
CONTENT AREA: Adult Health/Gastrointestinal
REFERENCE

Monahan, F., & Neighbors, M. (1998). *Medical-surgical nursing: Foundations for clinical practice* (2nd ed.). Philadelphia: W. B. Saunders. p. 1005.

52. **1**

RATIONALE: The client should be taught to include deodorizing foods in the diet, such as beet greens, parsley, buttermilk, and yogurt. Spinach also reduces odor, but is a gas-forming food as well. Broccoli, cucumbers, and eggs are gas-forming foods.
TEST-TAKING STRATEGY: To answer this question correctly, it is necessary to know the effect of various foods on the GI tract of the client with an ostomy. If this question was difficult, take a few moments to review which foods cause odor or gas, and those that have a deodorizing effect.
LEVEL OF COGNITIVE ABILITY: Application
PHASE OF NURSING PROCESS: Implementation
CLIENT NEEDS: Health Promotion and Maintenance
CONTENT AREA: Adult Health/Gastrointestinal
REFERENCE

Monahan, F., & Neighbors, M. (1998). *Medical-surgical nursing: Foundations for clinical practice* (2nd ed.). Philadelphia: W. B. Saunders. p. 1009.

53. **3**

RATIONALE: Foods that help to thicken the stool of the client with an ileostomy include pasta, boiled rice, and low-fat cheese. Bran is high in dietary fiber, and thus will increase output of watery stool by increasing propulsion through the bowel. Ileostomy output is liquid by nature. Addition or elimination of various foods can help to thicken or loosen this liquid drainage.
TEST-TAKING STRATEGY: To answer this question accurately, it is necessary to know that high-fiber foods such as bran can aggravate watery stools. This will help you to eliminate each of the incorrect options systematically. The wording of the question tells you that you are looking for an incorrect choice on the part of the client.
LEVEL OF COGNITIVE ABILITY: Comprehension
PHASE OF NURSING PROCESS: Evaluation
CLIENT NEEDS: Health Promotion and Maintenance
CONTENT AREA: Adult Health/Gastrointestinal
REFERENCE

Monahan, F., & Neighbors, M. (1998). *Medical-surgical nursing: Foundations for clinical practice* (2nd ed.). Philadelphia: W. B. Saunders. p. 1014.

54. 1

RATIONALE: A Kock pouch is a continent ileostomy. As the ileostomy begins to function, the client drains it every 3 to 4 hours, then decreasing to about three times a day or as needed when full. The client does not need to wear a drainage bag but should wear a dressing to absorb mucous drainage from the stoma. Ileostomy drainage is liquid in nature. The client would only be able to pass stool from the rectum if an ileal-anal pouch or anastomosis was created. This type of operation is a two-stage procedure.
TEST-TAKING STRATEGY: To answer this question accurately, it is necessary to understand the different surgical procedures that are performed with ileostomy, and their consequences on the bowel habits of the client. If this question was difficult, take a few moments to review this material at this time.
LEVEL OF COGNITIVE ABILITY: Comprehension
PHASE OF NURSING PROCESS: Evaluation
CLIENT NEEDS: Physiological Integrity
CONTENT AREA: Adult Health/Gastrointestinal
REFERENCE
Monahan, F., & Neighbors, M. (1998). *Medical-surgical nursing: Foundations for clinical practice* (2nd ed.). Philadelphia: W. B. Saunders. pp. 1012–1013.

55. 3

RATIONALE: The client should limit fat in the diet. The client should also take in small meals at each sitting. This will also reduce the amount of carbohydrate and protein that the client must digest at any one time. The client does not need to limit water-soluble vitamins in the diet.
TEST-TAKING STRATEGY: Note that the stem of the question contains the key word "limit." Use knowledge related to pancreatic function and dietary instructions to make your selection.
LEVEL OF COGNITIVE ABILITY: Application
PHASE OF NURSING PROCESS: Implementation
CLIENT NEEDS: Health Promotion and Maintenance
CONTENT AREA: Adult Health/Gastrointestinal
REFERENCE
Burrell, P., Gerlach, M., & Pless, B. (1997). *Adult nursing: Acute and community care* (2nd ed.). Stamford, CT: Appleton & Lange. p. 1548.

56. 2

RATIONALE: Positions such as sitting up, leaning forward, and flexing the legs (especially the left leg) may alleviate some of the pain associated with pancreatitis. The pain is aggravated by lying supine or walking. This is because the pancreas is located retroperitoneally, and the edema and inflammation intensify the irritation of the posterior peritoneal wall with these positions.
TEST-TAKING STRATEGY: Use your critical thinking skills to visualize the pancreas, and the potential effects from stretching associated with the various positions listed. This may help you to eliminate the incorrect options. Remember also that options that are similar are not likely to be correct. This will help you to eliminate at least options 1 and 3.
LEVEL OF COGNITIVE ABILITY: Application
PHASE OF NURSING PROCESS: Implementation
CLIENT NEEDS: Physiological Integrity
CONTENT AREA: Adult Health/Gastrointestinal

REFERENCE
Burrell, P., Gerlach, M., & Pless, B. (1997). *Adult nursing: Acute and community care* (2nd ed.). Stamford, CT: Appleton & Lange. p. 1545.

57. 1

RATIONALE: The client with cholecystitis should decrease overall intake of dietary fat. Foods that should be generally avoided to achieve this end include sauces and gravies, fatty meats, fried foods, products made with cream, and heavy desserts. The correct answer is baked scrod, which is low in fat.
TEST-TAKING STRATEGY: To answer this question correctly, it is necessary to know that clients with cholecystitis should decrease fat intake. Use knowledge of basic nutrition to make the selection accordingly.
LEVEL OF COGNITIVE ABILITY: Comprehension
PHASE OF NURSING PROCESS: Evaluation
CLIENT NEEDS: Health Promotion and Maintenance
CONTENT AREA: Adult Health/Gastrointestinal
REFERENCE
Monahan, F., & Neighbors, M. (1998). *Medical-surgical nursing: Foundations for clinical practice* (2nd ed.). Philadelphia: W. B. Saunders. p. 1111.

58. 3

RATIONALE: Ammonia is yielded as a product of protein metabolism. Clients with hepatic encephalopathy have high serum ammonia levels, which are responsible for the encephalopathy symptoms. Limiting protein intake will curb the elevation in serum ammonia, and prevent further deterioration of the client's mental status.
TEST-TAKING STRATEGY: To answer this question correctly, it is necessary to have an understanding of the relationships between cirrhosis, encephalopathy, and protein intake. If needed, take a few moments to review these key concepts at this time.
LEVEL OF COGNITIVE ABILITY: Application
PHASE OF NURSING PROCESS: Planning
CLIENT NEEDS: Health Promotion and Maintenance
CONTENT AREA: Adult Health/Gastrointestinal
REFERENCE
Monahan, F., & Neighbors, M. (1998). *Medical-surgical nursing: Foundations for clinical practice* (2nd ed.). Philadelphia: W. B. Saunders. p. 1183.

59. 1

RATIONALE: In order to be effective in decreasing bowel motility, antispasmodic medications should be administered 30 minutes before mealtimes. The other options are incorrect.
TEST-TAKING STRATEGY: Use concepts related to drug action to anticipate when the doses should be timed. Knowing that antispasmodics slow down gut motility, it can be reasoned that they should be taken before meals, an activity that normally stimulates increased GI motility.
LEVEL OF COGNITIVE ABILITY: Application
PHASE OF NURSING PROCESS: Planning
CLIENT NEEDS: Physiological Integrity
CONTENT AREA: Adult Health/Gastrointestinal
REFERENCE
Monahan, F., & Neighbors, M. (1998). *Medical-surgical nursing: Foundations for clinical practice* (2nd ed.). Philadelphia: W. B. Saunders. p. 1069.

60. **2**

RATIONALE: Common signs of acute viral hepatitis include weight loss, dark urine, and fatigue. The client is anorexic possibly from a toxin produced by the diseased liver, and finds food distasteful. The urine darkens because of excess bilirubin being excreted by the kidneys. Fatigue occurs during all phases of hepatitis. Spider angiomas, small, dilated blood vessels, are commonly seen in cirrhosis of the liver.

TEST-TAKING STRATEGY: Knowledge of thc signs and symptoms of viral hepatitis is needed to answer this question. Lethargy is a classic symptom associated with hepatitis. If you had difficulty with this question, take time now to review content associated with hepatitis.

LEVEL OF COGNITIVE ABILITY: Comprehension
PHASE OF NURSING PROCESS: Data Collection
CLIENT NEEDS: Physiological Integrity
CONTENT AREA: Adult Health/Gastrointestinal
REFERENCE
Lewis, S., Collier, I., & Heitkemper, M. (1996). *Medical-surgical nursing: Assessment and management of clinical problems* (4th ed.). St. Louis MO: Mosby–Year Book. p. 1261.

61. **4**

RATIONALE: Striving to explain that which is vague or clarifying the meaning of what has been said increases the understanding for both the client and the nurse. Giving false reassurance devalues the client's feelings. Telling the client what to do implies that the nurse knows what is best and discourages independent thinking. Refusing to consider the client's ideas may cause the client to discontinue interaction with the nurse for fear of further rejection. Placing the client's feelings on hold by referring the client to the doctor for further information is a block to communication.

TEST-TAKING STRATEGY: Knowledge about therapeutic communication techniques is helpful in answering this question. When answering communication questions, the use of communication tools indicates a correct answer. The use of communication blocks indicates an incorrect answer. Such blocks used are giving false reassurance in option 1, giving advice and placing the client's feelings on hold in option 2, and showing approval or disapproval in option 3. Remember to always focus on the client's feelings first.

LEVEL OF COGNITIVE ABILITY: Application
PHASE OF NURSING PROCESS: Implementation
CLIENT NEEDS: Psychosocial Integrity
CONTENT AREA: Adult Health/Gastrointestinal
REFERENCE
deWit, S. (1998). *Essentials of medical-surgical nursing* (4th ed.). Philadelphia: W. B. Saunders. pp. 652–653.

62. **2**

RATIONALE: Immunization is the most effective method of preventing HBV infection. Other general measures include handwashing. The use of immune globulin is to prevent hepatitis A and is indicated 1 to 2 weeks after exposure or for prophylaxis if traveling to endemic areas. Personal hygiene, such as handwashing after bowel movements and before eating, also helps prevent the transmission of hepatitis A.

TEST-TAKING STRATEGY: Knowledge regarding the transmission of hepatitis A and B will assist you in answering this question correctly. Although two of the options are correct for preventing transmission of hepatitis B, the best method in a high risk individual is immunization with hepatitis B vaccine according to the Centers for Disease Control and Prevention (CDC) guidelines. If you had diffi-

culty with this question, take time now to review content associated with hepatitis.

LEVEL OF COGNITIVE ABILITY: Application
PHASE OF NURSING PROCESS: Planning
CLIENT NEEDS: Safe, Effective Care Environment
CONTENT AREA: Adult Health/Gastrointestinal
REFERENCE
deWit, S. (1998). *Essentials of medical-surgical nursing* (4th ed.). Philadelphia: W. B. Saunders. p. 653.

63. **4**

RATIONALE: The vaccine is recommended for both sexual and household contacts of HBV carriers. Hepatitis B can be transmitted through intimate contact, such as kissing or sexual intercourse. The vaccine is used for prevention and is not given to carriers.

TEST-TAKING STRATEGY: It is important to look at the issue or specific subject content that the question is asking about. Also be alert to the key words. Note that the question addresses a client that is a hepatitis B carrier. Absolute terminology such as "never," "always," "must" tends to make a statement false. Therefore, eliminate option 2.

LEVEL OF COGNITIVE ABILITY: Comprehension
PHASE OF NURSING PROCESS: Evaluation
CLIENT NEEDS: Health Promotion and Maintenance
CONTENT AREA: Adult Health/Gastrointestinal
REFERENCE
deWit, S. (1998). *Essentials of medical-surgical nursing* (4th ed.). Philadelphia: W. B. Saunders. p. 653.

64. **3**

RATIONALE: Although no special diet is required in the treatment of viral hepatitis, it is generally recommended that clients have a diet with low fat content since fat may be poorly tolerated because of decreased bile production. Small, frequent meals are preferable and may even prevent nausea. Frequently, appetite is better in the morning so it is easier to eat a good breakfast. Carbonated beverages are used to counteract anorexia. An adequate fluid intake of 2500-3000 mL/day is also important.

TEST-TAKING STRATEGY: Knowledge of malnutritional needs during hepatitis is helpful in answering this question. Focus on key words in the stem of the question, such as "adequate." Use the process of elimination. This question is asking about adequate nutrition for a client with anorexia. Option 3 is the correct option. Options 1, 2, and 4 are incorrect with this situation.

LEVEL OF COGNITIVE ABILITY: Application
PHASE OF NURSING PROCESS: Implementation
CLIENT NEEDS: Physiological Integrity
CONTENT AREA: Adult Health/Gastrointestinal
REFERENCE
deWit, S. (1998). *Essentials of medical-surgical nursing* (4th ed.). Philadelphia: W. B. Saunders. p. 656.

65. **2**

RATIONALE: Jaundice occurs in the skin and mucous membranes. In light-skinned persons, it is first seen in the sclera of the eyes and later in the skin. In dark-skinned persons, jaundice is observed in the inner canthus of the eyes and hard palate of the mouth. Pallor is detected in the nailbeds, and flushing with increased body temperature, in the flexor surfaces of the extremities.

TEST-TAKING STRATEGY: Read all of the options very carefully before selecting an answer. Be alert to key words,

such as "African-American" and "specific." Review data collection procedures for jaundice now if you had difficulty with this question.
LEVEL OF COGNITIVE ABILITY: Comprehension
PHASE OF NURSING PROCESS: Data Collection
CLIENT NEEDS: Physiological Integrity
CONTENT AREA: Adult Health/Gastrointestinal
REFERENCE
deWit, S. (1998). *Essentials of medical-surgical nursing* (4th ed.). Philadelphia: W. B. Saunders. p. 652.

66. **1**

RATIONALE: To assist the client in adapting to changes in appearance, it is important for the nurse to encourage participation in self-care to foster independence and self-esteem. The client should be encouraged to ask questions in order to clarify misconceptions, learn ways to prevent the spread of hepatitis to reduce fear, and make good decisions. The client's feelings should be explored to discover how the client feels about the disease process and appearance so appropriate interventions can be planned.
TEST-TAKING STRATEGY: Use the process of elimination in answering the question. In order to promote coping and psychosocial adaptation, identify the use of therapeutic communication tools. When these are used, they indicate a correct answer. Giving information, clarifying, and focusing on the client's feelings are some of these tools. Always focus on the client's feelings first.
LEVEL OF COGNITIVE ABILITY: Application
PHASE OF NURSING PROCESS: Implementation
CLIENT NEEDS: Psychosocial Integrity
CONTENT AREA: Adult Health/Gastrointestinal
REFERENCE
deWit, S. (1998). *Essentials of medical-surgical nursing* (4th ed.). Philadelphia: W. B. Saunders. p. 653.

67. **4**

RATIONALE: In order to splint the puncture site, the client is kept on the right side for a minimum of 2 hours and should lie flat for 12 to 14 hours. Complications of the procedures include peritonitis, shock, or pneumothorax.
TEST-TAKING STRATEGY: Knowledge of care of a client undergoing a liver biopsy is needed to answer this question. Look for the specific subject content that the question is asking about. Read all of the options very carefully before selecting an answer, and eliminate the incorrect options. Use your knowledge of the anatomy of the body to assist you in selecting the correct option.
LEVEL OF COGNITIVE ABILITY: Application
PHASE OF NURSING PROCESS: Implementation
CLIENT NEEDS: Physiological Integrity
CONTENT AREA: Adult Health/Gastrointestinal
REFERENCE
deWit, S. (1998). *Essentials of medical-surgical nursing* (4th ed.). Philadelphia: W. B. Saunders. p. 646.

68. **2**

RATIONALE: To prevent transmission of hepatitis, a condom is advised during sexual intercourse as well as vaccina-

tion of the partner. Alcohol should be avoided for 1 year because it is detoxified in the liver and may interfere with recovery. Rest is especially important until laboratory studies show that the liver function has returned to normal. The client's activity is increased gradually.
TEST-TAKING STRATEGY: Note the key words "indicates a need for further teaching." Use the process of elimination and knowledge regarding hepatitis to answer the question.
LEVEL OF COGNITIVE ABILITY: Comprehension
PHASE OF NURSING PROCESS: Evaluation
CLIENT NEEDS: Health Promotion and Maintenance
CONTENT AREA: Adult Health/Gastrointestinal
REFERENCE
deWit, S. (1998). *Essentials of medical-surgical nursing* (4th ed.). Philadelphia: W. B. Saunders. p. 653.

69. **3**

RATIONALE: Clients frequently have a body image disturbance because of a change in appearance. This can be manifested in negative verbal or nonverbal behavior.
TEST-TAKING STRATEGY: The case situation gives you information you need in answering the question. Read all of the information. Look for key words in the question such as "severe jaundice" to focus your attention on the critical ideas in the case. A psychosocial issue is the concern in this question.
LEVEL OF COGNITIVE ABILITY: Comprehension
PHASE OF NURSING PROCESS: Data Collection
CLIENT NEEDS: Psychosocial Integrity
CONTENT AREA: Adult Health/Gastrointestinal
REFERENCE
deWit, S. (1998). *Essentials of medical-surgical nursing* (4th ed.). Philadelphia: W. B. Saunders. p. 652.

70. **4**

RATIONALE: If nausea persists, the client will need to be assessed for fluid and electrolyte imbalances. It is important to explain to the client that the majority of calories should be eaten in the morning hours because nausea occurs in the afternoon and evening. Clients should select a diet high in calories because energy is required for healing, and adequate carbohydrates can spare the protein. Changes in bilirubin interfere with fat absorption, so low-fat diets are better tolerated.
TEST-TAKING STRATEGY: Read all of the options very carefully before selecting an answer. Use the process of elimination and eliminate the incorrect options. Knowledge of the nutritional aspects of care for clients with acute hepatitis is helpful in answering this question. Review these concepts now if you had difficulty answering this question.
LEVEL OF COGNITIVE ABILITY: Application
PHASE OF NURSING PROCESS: Implementation
CLIENT NEEDS: Physiological Integrity
CONTENT AREA: Adult Health/Gastrointestinal
REFERENCE
Monahan, F., & Neighbors, M. (1998). *Medical-surgical nursing: Foundations for clinical practice* (2nd ed.). Philadelphia: W. B. Saunders. p. 1173.

BIBLIOGRAPHY

Beare, P., & Myers, J. (1998). *Adult health nursing* (3rd ed.). St. Louis, MO: Mosby–Year Book.

Black, J., & Matassarin-Jacobs, E. (1997). *Medical-surgical nursing: Clinical management for continuity of care* (5th ed.). Philadelphia: W. B. Saunders.

Burrell, P., Gerlach, M., & Pless, B. (1997). *Adult nursing: Acute and community care* (2nd ed.). Stamford, CT: Appleton & Lange.

Chernecky, C., & Berger, B. (1997). *Laboratory tests and diagnostic procedures* (2nd ed.). Philadelphia: W. B. Saunders.

deWit, S. (1998). *Essentials of medical-surgical nursing* (4th ed.). Philadelphia: W. B. Saunders.

Hodgson, B., & Kizior, R. (2000). *Saunders nursing drug handbook 2000*. Philadelphia: W. B. Saunders.

Ignatavicius, D., Workman, M., & Mishler, M. (1999). *Medical-surgical nursing across the health care continuum* (3rd ed.). Philadelphia: W. B. Saunders.

Kozier, B., Erb, G., & Blais, K. (1998). *Fundamentals of nursing: Concepts, process, and practice* (5th ed.). Reading, MA: Addison-Wesley.

Lehne, R. (1998). *Pharmacology for nursing care* (3rd ed.). Philadelphia: W. B. Saunders.

Leahy, J., & Kizilay, P. (1998). *Foundations of nursing practice: A nursing process approach*. Philadelphia: W. B. Saunders.

Lewis, S., Collier, I., & Heitkemper, M. (1996). *Medical-surgical nursing: Assessment and management of clinical problems* (4th ed.). St. Louis: Mosby–Year Book.

Luckmann, J. (1997). *Saunders manual of nursing care*. Philadelphia: W. B. Saunders.

Lutz, C., & Przytulski, K. (1997). *Nutrition and diet therapy* (2nd ed.). Philadelphia: F. A. Davis.

Monahan, F., & Neighbors, M. (1998). *Medical-surgical nursing: Foundations for clinical practice* (2nd ed.). Philadelphia: W. B. Saunders.

O'Toole, M. (1997). *Miller-Keane encyclopedia & dictionary of medicine, nursing, & allied health* (9th ed.). Philadelphia: W. B. Saunders.

CHAPTER 45

Gastrointestinal Medications

I. Antacids

A. Description
1. React with gastric acid to produce neutral salts or salts of low acidity
2. Inactivate pepsin and enhance mucosal protection
3. Used for peptic ulcer disease and gastroesophageal reflux disease
4. Should be taken on a regular schedule
5. Are usually administered seven times a day, 1 and 3 hours after each meal and at bedtime
6. To provide maximum benefit, treatment should elevate the gastric pH above 5
7. Antacid tablets should be chewed thoroughly and followed with a glass of water or milk
8. Liquid preparation should be shaken before dispensing
9. Interactions with other medications can be minimized by allowing 1 hour between antacid administration and the administration of other medications
10. Can interfere with the action of sucralfate (Carafate), and to minimize this interaction the medications should be administered 1 hour apart

B. Magnesium hydroxide
1. Rapid acting
2. Also referred to as milk of magnesia
3. Most prominent side effect is diarrhea
4. Usually administered in combination with aluminum hydroxide, an antacid that assists in preventing diarrhea
5. Contraindicated in clients with intestinal obstruction, appendicitis, or undiagnosed abdominal pain
6. In clients with renal impairment, magnesium can accumulate to high levels, causing signs of toxicity

C. Aluminum hydroxide (Amphojel, Alu-Cap, Dialume)

1. Slow acting
2. Contains significant amounts of sodium
3. Used with caution in clients with hypertension and heart failure
4. Most common side effect is constipation
5. Can reduce the effects of tetracyclines, warfarin sodium (Coumadin), and digoxin (Lanoxin)
6. Can reduce phosphate absorption and thereby cause hypophosphatemia

D. Calcium carbonate (Tums)
1. Rapid acting
2. Common side effect is constipation

E. Sodium bicarbonate
1. Rapid onset
2. Liberates carbon dioxide, increases intraabdominal pressure, and promotes flatulence
3. Used with caution in clients with hypertension and heart failure
4. Can cause systemic alkalosis in clients with renal impairment
5. Is useful for treating acidosis and elevating urinary pH to promote excretion of acidic medications following overdose

II. Histamine H$_2$ Inhibitors (Box 45–1)

A. Description
1. Suppress secretions of gastric acid
2. Alleviate symptoms of heartburn and assist in preventing complications of peptic ulcer disease
3. Prevent stress ulcers and reduce the recurrence of all ulcers

BOX 45–1. Histamine H$_2$ Inhibitors	
Cimetidine (Tagamet)	Nizatidine (Axid)
Famotidine (Pepcid)	Ranitidine (Zantac)

4. Promote healing in gastroesophageal reflux disease
5. Contraindicated in hypersensitivity
6. Used with caution in clients with impaired renal or hepatic function

B. Cimetidine (Tagamet)
1. Can be administered orally (PO), intramuscularly (IM), and intravenously (IV)
2. Food reduces the rate of absorption; if taken with meals, absorption will be slowed
3. Antacids can decrease the absorption of cimetidine
4. Cimetidine and antacids should be administered at least 1 hour apart from each other
5. Passes the blood-brain barrier, and central nervous system (CNS) side effects can occur
6. May cause mental confusion, agitation, psychosis, depression, anxiety, and disorientation
7. Dosage should be reduced in clients with renal impairment
8. If administered with warfarin sodium (Coumadin), phenytoin (Dilantin), theophylline, or lidocaine, the dosages of these medications should be reduced

C. Ranitidine (Zantac)
1. Can be administered PO, IM, or IV
2. Side effects are uncommon
3. It does not penetrate the blood-brain barrier as cimetidine does
4. Zantac is not affected by food

D. Famotidine (Pepcid) and nizatidine (Axid)
1. Similar to Zantac and Tagamet
2. Does not need to be administered with food

III. Proton Pump Inhibitors (Box 45–2)

A. Suppress gastric acid secretion
B. Used with active ulcer disease, erosive esophagitis, and pathological hypersecretory conditions
C. Contraindicated in hypersensitivity
D. Common side effects include headache, diarrhea, abdominal pain, and nausea

IV. Sucralfate (Carafate)

A. Creates a protective barrier against acid and pepsin
B. Administered PO; should be taken on an empty stomach
C. Administer at least 30 minutes apart from an antacid

D. May cause constipation
E. May impede absorption of warfarin sodium (Coumadin), phenytoin (Dilantin), theophylline, digoxin (Lanoxin), and some antibiotics and should be administered at least 2 hours apart from these medications

V. Misoprostol (Cytotec)

A. Used to prevent gastric ulcers caused by long-term therapy with nonsteroidal anti-inflammatory drugs (NSAIDs)
B. Suppresses secretion of gastric acid
C. Promotes secretion of bicarbonate and cytoprotective mucus
D. Maintains submucosal blood flow by promoting vasodilation
E. Administered with meals
F. Causes diarrhea and abdominal pain
G. Contraindicated for use in pregnancy

VI. Gastrointestinal Stimulants (Box 45–3)

A. Stimulate motility of the upper gastrointestinal (GI) tract and increases rate of gastric emptying without stimulating gastric, biliary, or pancreatic secretions
B. Used for gastroesophageal reflux
C. May cause restlessness, drowsiness, extrapyramidal reactions, dizziness, insomnia, headache
D. Contraindicated in clients with sensitivity
E. Contraindicated in clients with mechanical obstruction, perforation, or GI hemorrhage
F. Can precipitate hypertensive crisis in clients with pheochromocytoma
G. Safety in pregnancy is not established
H. Reglan can cause Parkinson-like reactions, and if this occurs the medication is discontinued
I. Propulsid may increase the absorption of cimetidine (Tagamet) and ranitidine (Zantac) when administered concurrently
J. Anticholinergics and narcotic analgesics antagonize the effects of Reglan
K. Alcohol, sedatives, cyclosporine (Sandimmune) increase medication effects

---

BOX 45–5. Medications for Cholelithiasis

Chenodiol (Chenix)
Monoctanoin (Moctanin)
Ursodiol (Actigall)

BOX 45–7. Bulk-Forming Laxatives

Methylcellulose (Citrucel)
Calcium polycarbophil (FiberCon)
Psyllium (Metamucil)

VII. Bile Acid Sequestrants (Box 45–4)

A. Description
1. Used to treat pruritus associated with biliary disease
2. Act by absorbing and combining with intestinal bile salts, which are then secreted in the feces, preventing intestinal reabsorption
3. May be used in the treatment of hypercholesterolemia in adults
4. Used cautiously in clients with bowel obstruction or severe constipation because of the adverse GI effects
5. Taste and palatability are often reasons for noncompliance and can be improved by the use of flavored products or mixing the medication with various juices
6. Stool softeners and other sources of fiber can be used to abate the GI side effects

B. Side effects
1. Constipation
2. Bloating and flatulence
3. Nausea
4. Fecal impaction and intestinal obstruction
5. Exacerbation of hemorrhoids
6. Hypoprothrombinemia
7. Decreased vitamin absorption

VIII. Medications for Cholelithiasis (Box 45–5)

A. Chenodiol (Chenix)
1. Decreases cholesterol production, lowering content of bile, thereby facilitating dissolution of gallstones
2. Can cause diarrhea and possible hepatotoxicity
3. Baseline liver functions should be performed
4. The client should be instructed to contact a physician if abdominal pain, sudden right upper quadrant pain, nausea, or vomiting occurs

B. Monoctanoin (Moctanin)
1. Used when stones made of calcium are resistant to dissolution by oral chenodiol
2. Administered through a T tube, nasal biliary catheter, or percutaneous transhepatic catheter

3. Effective only when in contact with the stone
4. Major side effects include diarrhea, nausea, and abdominal pain

C. Ursodiol (Actigall)
1. A naturally occurring bile salt
2. Suppresses hepatic synthesis and secretion of cholesterol and inhibits intestinal absorption of cholesterol
3. Requires months of therapy for dissolution of a gallstone to occur
4. Ultrasound images are obtained within 6 months to determine the effectiveness of the therapy
5. Clients should be instructed to report nausea, vomiting, diarrhea, or rash to the physician

IX. Medications to Treat Hepatic Encephalopathy (Box 45–6)

A. Lactulose (Cephulac)
1. Reduces ammonia levels
2. Improves protein tolerance in clients with advanced hepatic **cirrhosis**
3. Lowers the colonic pH from 7 to 5; this acidification pulls ammonia into the bowel to be excreted in the feces, thus lowering the ammonia level
4. Administered orally in the form of a syrup

B. Neomycin (Mycifradin)
1. Reduces the number of colonic bacteria that normally convert urea and amino acids into ammonia
2. Administered orally or via nasogastric (NG) tube
3. Used with caution in clients with kidney impairment

X. Laxatives

A. Bulk-forming laxatives (Box 45–7)
1. Description
   a. Absorb water into feces and increase bulk to produce large and soft stools
   b. For short-term use
   c. Contraindicated in bowel obstruction
2. Side effects

BOX 45–6. Medications to Treat Hepatic Encephalopathy

Lactulose (Cephulac)
Neomycin (Mycifradin)

BOX 45–8. Saline Cathartics

Magnesium hydroxide (milk of magnesia, MOM)
Magnesium sulfate (Epsom salt)
Phospho-Soda

BOX 45-9. Stool Softeners

Docusate calcium (Surfak)
Docusate sodium (Colace)
Docusate with casanthranol (Peri-Colace)

---

a. GI disturbances
b. Dehydration
c. Electrolyte imbalance
d. Dependency with chronic use
B. Stimulant cathartics
   1. Description: stimulate motility of the large intestine
   2. Bisacodyl (Dulcolax): do not administer within 60 minutes of an antacid or milk
   3. Cascara (castor oil): administer with juice; produces results in 2 to 6 hours
C. Saline cathartics (Box 45-8)
   1. Attract water into the large intestine to produce bulk
   2. Stimulate **peristalsis**
   3. Achieve results in 2 to 6 hours
D. Stool softeners (Box 45-9)
   1. Inhibit absorption of water so fecal mass remains large and soft
   2. Used to avoid straining
E. Lubricants
   1. Act to soften the feces
   2. Ease the strain of passing stool
   3. Lessen irritation to hemorrhoids
   4. Mineral oil
      a. Can cause lipid pneumonia if accidentally aspirated
      b. Interferes with absorption of fat-soluble vitamins A, D, E, and K
F. Opioids (Box 45-10)
   1. Decrease intestinal motility and **peristalsis**
   2. When poisons, infections, or bacterial toxins are the cause of diarrhea, opioids worsen the condition by delaying the elimination of toxins
   3. Tincture of opium has an unpleasant taste and can be diluted with 15 to 30 mL of water for administration
XI. Antispasmodics (Box 45-11)
A. Description: relax smooth muscle of GI tract
B. Side effects
   1. Constipation or diarrhea
   2. Rash
   3. Euphoria

BOX 45-10. Opioids

Codeine
Diphenoxylate hydrochloride with atropine (Lomotil)
Loperamide hydrochloride (Imodium)
Tincture of opium

BOX 45-11. Antispasmodics

Dicyclomine hydrochloride (Antispas)
Dicyclomine hydrochloride (Bentyl)

---

4. Weakness and dizziness
5. Drowsiness
6. Headache
7. Nausea

PRACTICE QUESTIONS

1. The client has been started on psyllium (Metamucil). The nurse teaches this client to take this medication with
   1 Gelatin, applesauce, or pudding
   2 A full glass of liquid, followed by a second
   3 A multivitamin and mineral supplement
   4 A dose of antacid

2. The client with gastroparesis has been given a prescription for metoclopramide (Reglan) four times a day. The nurse teaches the client to take the medication
   1 30 minutes before meals and at bedtime
   2 With each meal and at bedtime
   3 1 hour after each meal and at bedtime
   4 Every 6 hours spaced evenly around the clock

3. The nurse teaches the client taking metoclopramide (Reglan) to discontinue the medication immediately and call the physician if which of the following side effects occurs with long-term use?
   1 Anxiety or irritability
   2 Dry mouth not minimized by use of sugar-free hard candy
   3 Excessive excitability
   4 Uncontrolled rhythmic movements of the face or limbs

4. The client has just taken a dose of trimethobenzamide (Tigan). The nurse plans to monitor this client for relief of
   1 Nausea and vomiting
   2 Abdominal pain
   3 Heartburn
   4 Constipation

5. The client has a PRN order for ondansetron (Zofran). The nurse administers this medication to the postoperative client for relief of
   1 Urinary retention
   2 Incisional pain
   3 Nausea and vomiting
   4 Paralytic ileus

6. The client has an order to take magnesium citrate to prevent constipation following a barium study of the upper GI tract. The nurse plans to administer this medication

1 With a full glass of water
2 With fruit juice only
3 On ice
4 At room temperature

7. The nurse is administering a dose of prochlorperazine (Compazine) to a client for nausea and vomiting. The nurse monitors the client for which of the following frequent side effects of this medication?
   1 Diarrhea
   2 Drooling
   3 Excessive lacrimation
   4 Blurred vision

8. The client has begun medication therapy with pancrelipase (Pancrease). The nurse evaluates that the medication is having the optimal intended benefit if which of the following effects is observed?
   1 Reduction of steatorrhea
   2 Absence of abdominal pain
   3 Relief of heartburn
   4 Weight loss

9. The client asks the nurse why the medication cisapride (Propulsid) has been prescribed. The nurse incorporates which of the following in a reply?
   1 It is being used to relieve nighttime heartburn from gastroesophageal reflux
   2 It is used to prevent nausea and vomiting
   3 It can help to heal GI hemorrhage sites more quickly
   4 It may reverse a bowel obstruction, thus avoiding surgery

10. The nurse is giving the client directions for proper use of aluminum hydroxide tablets (Alu-Caps). The nurse tells the client to
    1 Chew the tablets thoroughly and follow with 4 oz of water
    2 Swallow whole with a full glass of water
    3 Take the tablet at the same time as other medications
    4 Take each dose with a laxative to prevent constipation

11. The client with a history of duodenal ulcer is taking calcium carbonate chewable tablets. The nurse evaluates that the client is experiencing optimal effects of the medication if
    1 Muscle twitching stops
    2 Heartburn is relieved
    3 Serum calcium levels rise
    4 Serum phosphorus levels decrease

12. The hospitalized client asks the nurse for sodium bicarbonate to relieve heartburn following a meal. The nurse determines that this client could not receive this medication if currently being treated for which of the following conditions?

1 Urinary calculi
2 Chronic bronchitis
3 Metabolic alkalosis
4 Respiratory acidosis

13. The client is complaining of gas pains following surgery and requests medication. The nurse selects which of the following medications from the PRN medication list to give to the client?
    1 Magnesium hydroxide (Milk of Magnesia [MOM])
    2 Droperidol (Inapsine)
    3 Acetaminophen (Tylenol)
    4 Simethicone (Mylicon)

14. The elderly client has recently been started on cimetidine (Tagamet). The nurse plans to monitor the client for which of the following most frequent central nervous system (CNS) side effects of this medication?
    1 Confusion
    2 Dizziness
    3 Tremors
    4 Hallucinations

15. The client with a gastric ulcer has an order for sucralfate (Carafate) 1g PO QID. The nurse schedules the medication for which of the following times?
    1 With meals and at bedtime
    2 1 hour before meals and at bedtime
    3 Every 6 hours around the clock
    4 1 hour after meals and at bedtime

16. The client who chronically uses nonsteroidal anti-inflammatory drugs (NSAIDs) has been taking misoprostol (Cytotec). The nurse evaluates that the medication is having the intended therapeutic effect if the client did not experience which of the following symptoms?
    1 Decreased platelet count
    2 Decreased white blood cell count
    3 Epigastric pain
    4 Diarrhea

17. The physician has written an order for ranitidine (Zantac) 300 mg once daily. The nurse schedules the medication for which of the following times?
    1 Before breakfast
    2 After lunch
    3 With supper
    4 At bedtime

18. The client is taking lansoprazole (Prevacid) for the chronic management of Zollinger-Ellison syndrome. The nurse instructs the client to take which of the following products if needed for headache?
    1 Acetaminophen (Tylenol)
    2 Ibuprofen (Motrin)
    3 Naprosyn (Aleve)
    4 Acetylsalicylic acid (aspirin)

19. The client has been taking omeprazole (Prilosec) for 4 weeks. The nurse evaluates that the client is receiving optimal intended effect of the medication if the client reports absence of which of the following symptoms?
    1 Constipation
    2 Heartburn
    3 Diarrhea
    4 Flatulence

20. The client is taking cascara sagrada and develops abdominal cramps. The nurse interprets that the client is most likely experiencing
    1 A common side effect of this medication
    2 Partial bowel obstruction
    3 A case of influenza
    4 Peptic ulcer disease

21. The physician prescribes bisacodyl (Dulcolax) for a client in preparation for a diagnostic test and wants to achieve a rapid effect from the medication. The nurse tells the client to take the medication
    1 With a large meal
    2 On an empty stomach
    3 At bedtime with a snack
    4 With two glasses of juice

22. The client who is advised to take senna (Senokot) for the treatment of constipation asks the nurse how this medication works. The nurse incorporates which of the following when formulating a response?
    1 It coats the bowel wall and makes it slippery
    2 It adds fiber and bulk to the stool
    3 It accumulates water and increases peristalsis
    4 It stimulates the vagus nerve to improve bowel tone

23. The client has a PRN order for loperamide (Imodium). The nurse plans to administer this medication if the client has
    1 Hematest-positive nasogastric tube drainage
    2 Abdominal pain
    3 Constipation
    4 An episode of diarrhea

24. The nurse has given instructions to the client who just received a prescription for diphenoxylate with atropine (Lomotil). The nurse evaluates that the client understands the use of the medication and its properties if the client states to
    1 Stay within the prescribed dose because it can be habit forming
    2 Take the medication with a bulk-forming laxative
    3 Expect increased salivation while taking the medication

    4 Anticipate side effects of nervous system excitability

25. The client has received a dose of dimenhydrinate (Dramamine). The nurse determines that the medication has been effective if the client states relief of
    1 Headache
    2 Chills
    3 Nausea and vomiting
    4 Buzzing sound in the ears

26. The nurse administers a dose of scopolamine to a preoperative client. The nurse tells the client to expect which of the following side effects of the medication?
    1 Excessive urination
    2 Diaphoresis
    3 Dry mouth
    4 Pupillary constriction

27. The nurse is preparing to administer a dose of hydroxyzine hydrochloride (Vistaril) to a client by the intramuscular route. The nurse tells the client to expect
    1 Pain at the injection site from the medication
    2 Relief from nausea within 5 minutes
    3 Excessive salivation as a side effect
    4 Increased alertness lasting generally 4 hours

28. The physician tells the nurse that a client can be given droperidol (Inapsine) for the relief of postoperative nausea. The nurse expects that the physician will order the medication by which of the following routes?
    1 Oral
    2 Intramuscular
    3 Subcutaneous
    4 Intranasally

29. The client is receiving propantheline (Pro-Banthīne) as adjunctive treatment for peptic ulcer disease. The nurse plans to administer this medication
    1 With meals
    2 Just after meals
    3 30 minutes before meals
    4 With antacids

30. The client is taking docusate sodium (Colace). The nurse monitors which of the following to determine whether the client is having a therapeutic effect from this medication?
    1 Abdominal pain
    2 Hematest-negative stools
    3 Reduction in steatorrhea
    4 Regular bowel movements

ANSWERS

1. 2

RATIONALE: Metamucil is a bulk-forming laxative. It should be taken with a full glass of water or juice, followed by another glass of liquid. This will help prevent impaction of the medication in the stomach or small intestine. The other options are incorrect.

TEST-TAKING STRATEGY: Use the process of elimination. Option 4 should be eliminated first because most medications are not taken with antacids. Eliminate options 1 and 3 next because they have no physiological benefit for medication effect. Review the administration of this medication now if you had difficulty with this question.

LEVEL OF COGNITIVE ABILITY: Application
PHASE OF NURSING PROCESS: Implementation
CLIENT NEEDS: Physiological Integrity
CONTENT AREA: Pharmacology
REFERENCE

Hodgson, B., & Kizior, R. (1999). *Saunders nursing drug handbook 1999*. Philadelphia: W. B. Saunders. p. 886.

2. 1

RATIONALE: The client should be taught to take this medication 30 minutes before meals and at bedtime. This allows the medication time to begin working before the client takes in food, which requires digestion and movement. The other options are incorrect.

TEST-TAKING STRATEGY: Remember that for an option to be correct, all of its parts must be correct. Eliminate option 4 first because it is the least plausible. Choose from among the remaining three choices by reasoning that if the medication is used to treat gastroparesis, it must be taken before meals to enhance digestion.

LEVEL OF COGNITIVE ABILITY: Application
PHASE OF NURSING PROCESS: Implementation
CLIENT NEEDS: Physiological Integrity
CONTENT AREA: Pharmacology
REFERENCE

Hodgson, B., & Kizior, R. (1999). *Saunders nursing drug handbook 1999*. Philadelphia: W. B. Saunders. p. 671.

3. 4

RATIONALE: If the client experiences tardive dyskinesia (rhythmic movements of the face or limbs), the client should stop the medication and call the physician. These side effects may be irreversible. Excitability is not a side effect of this medication. Anxiety, irritability, and dry mouth are side effects that are not so harmful to the client.

TEST-TAKING STRATEGY: To answer this question correctly, it is necessary to know that the medication can cause tardive dyskinesia, and to know what the signs and symptoms are. If needed, take a few moments to review the side effects of this medication now.

LEVEL OF COGNITIVE ABILITY: Application
PHASE OF NURSING PROCESS: Implementation
CLIENT NEEDS: Health Promotion and Maintenance
CONTENT AREA: Pharmacology
REFERENCE

Hodgson, B., & Kizior, R. (1999). *Saunders nursing drug handbook 1999*. Philadelphia: W. B. Saunders. p. 672.

4. 1

RATIONALE: Trimethobenzamide (Tigan) is an antiemetic agent that is used in the treatment of nausea and vomiting. The other options are incorrect.

TEST-TAKING STRATEGY: Recalling that trimethobenzamide is an antiemetic will easily direct you to option 1. If you are unfamiliar with this medication, take time now to review.

LEVEL OF COGNITIVE ABILITY: Comprehension
PHASE OF NURSING PROCESS: Evaluation
CLIENT NEEDS: Physiological Integrity
CONTENT AREA: Pharmacology
REFERENCE

Lehne, R. (1998). *Pharmacology for nursing care* (3rd ed.). Philadelphia: W. B. Saunders. p. 766.

5. 3

RATIONALE: Ondansetron is an antiemetic that is used in the treatment of postoperative nausea and vomiting, as well as nausea and vomiting associated with chemotherapy. The other options are incorrect.

TEST-TAKING STRATEGY: Recalling that ondansetron is an antiemetic will easily direct you to option 3. If you are unfamiliar with this medication, take time now to review.

LEVEL OF COGNITIVE ABILITY: Application
PHASE OF NURSING PROCESS: Implementation
CLIENT NEEDS: Physiological Integrity
CONTENT AREA: Pharmacology
REFERENCE

Lehne, R. (1998). *Pharmacology for nursing care* (3rd ed.). Philadelphia: W. B. Saunders. p. 794.

6. 3

RATIONALE: Magnesium citrate is available as an oral solution. It is used commonly as a laxative following certain studies of the GI tract. It should be served on ice, and should not be allowed to stand for prolonged periods. This would reduce the carbonation and make the solution even less palatable. Options 1, 2, and 4 are incorrect.

TEST-TAKING STRATEGY: Eliminate options 1 and 2 first, knowing that magnesium citrate is itself a liquid. To discriminate between the last two options, it is necessary to know it should be given cold to enhance palatability. Review this medication now if you had difficulty with this question.

LEVEL OF COGNITIVE ABILITY: Application
PHASE OF NURSING PROCESS: Planning
CLIENT NEEDS: Physiological Integrity
CONTENT AREA: Pharmacology
REFERENCE

Lehne, R. (1998). *Pharmacology for nursing care* (3rd ed.). Philadelphia: W. B. Saunders. pp. 792–793.

7. 4

RATIONALE: The nurse should monitor the client for blurred vision as a frequent side effect of prochlorperazine. Other frequent side effects of this phenothiazine-type antiemetic and antipsychotic are dry eyes, dry mouth, and constipation.

TEST-TAKING STRATEGY: To answer this question accurately, it is necessary to know the common side effects of phenothiazines. If you are unfamiliar with this medication, take time now to review.

LEVEL OF COGNITIVE ABILITY: Application
PHASE OF NURSING PROCESS: Data Collection
CLIENT NEEDS: Physiological Integrity
CONTENT AREA: Pharmacology
REFERENCE

Hodgson, B., & Kizior, R. (1999). *Saunders nursing drug handbook 1999*. Philadelphia: W. B. Saunders. p. 867.

8. 1

RATIONALE: Pancrease is a pancreatic enzyme used in clients with pancreatitis as a digestive aid. The medication should reduce the amount of fatty stools (steatorrhea). Another intended effect could be improved nutritional status. It is not used to treat abdominal pain or heartburn. It could result in weight gain, but should not result in weight loss if it is aiding in digestion.

TEST-TAKING STRATEGY: The name of the medication gives an indication of the possible uses of this medication. Use knowledge of physiology of the pancreas to assist in directing you to the correct option. Review this medication now if you had difficulty with this question.

LEVEL OF COGNITIVE ABILITY: Comprehension
PHASE OF NURSING PROCESS: Evaluation
CLIENT NEEDS: Physiological Integrity
CONTENT AREA: Pharmacology
REFERENCE

Hodgson, B., & Kizior, R. (1999). *Saunders nursing drug handbook 1999*. Philadelphia: W. B. Saunders. pp. 786–787.

9. 1

RATIONALE: Cisapride is a GI prokinetic agent that is often given to treat nighttime heartburn that is associated with gastroesophageal reflux disease. It is not used as an antiemetic. It is contraindicated in conditions where increased GI motility could cause harm, such as with GI hemorrhage, bowel perforation, or mechanical bowel obstruction.

TEST-TAKING STRATEGY: Familiarity with this medication is needed to answer this question correctly. If you had difficulty with this medication, take time now to review the use of this medication.

LEVEL OF COGNITIVE ABILITY: Comprehension
PHASE OF NURSING PROCESS: Implementation
CLIENT NEEDS: Physiological Integrity
CONTENT AREA: Pharmacology
REFERENCE

Hodgson, B., & Kizior, R. (1999). *Saunders nursing drug handbook 1999*. Philadelphia: W. B. Saunders. pp. 225–226.

10. 1

RATIONALE: Aluminum hydroxide tablets should be chewed thoroughly before swallowing. This prevents them from entering the small intestine undissolved. They should not be swallowed whole. Antacids should be taken at least 2 hours apart from other medications to prevent interactive effects. Constipation is a side effect of use of aluminum products, but it is not correct for the client to take a laxative with each dose. This promotes laxative abuse; the client should first try other means to prevent constipation.

TEST-TAKING STRATEGY: Eliminate option 4 first because this action does not promote healthy bowel function. Next eliminate option 3, using general knowledge of antacid interactive effects. Discriminate between the last two options using principles of digestion and medication use. Review the administration of this medication now if you had difficulty with this question.

LEVEL OF COGNITIVE ABILITY: Application
PHASE OF NURSING PROCESS: Implementation
CLIENT NEEDS: Health Promotion and Maintenance
CONTENT AREA: Pharmacology
REFERENCE

Hodgson, B., & Kizior, R. (1999) *Saunders nursing drug handbook 1999*. Philadelphia: W. B. Saunders. pp. 34–35.

11. 2

RATIONALE: Calcium carbonate is used as an antacid for the relief of heartburn and indigestion. It can also be used as a calcium supplement (option 3), or to bind phosphorus in the GI tract with renal failure (option 4). Option 1 is incorrect, although proper calcium levels are needed for proper neurological function.

TEST-TAKING STRATEGY: The key words in the stem are "duodenal ulcer" and "optimal effects." This tells you that more than one option may be correct, and that you must determine the correct therapeutic effect. Knowledge of concepts related to duodenal ulcer will allow you to eliminate each of the incorrect options easily. Review this medication now if you had difficulty with this question.

LEVEL OF COGNITIVE ABILITY: Analysis
PHASE OF NURSING PROCESS: Evaluation
CLIENT NEEDS: Physiological Integrity
CONTENT AREA: Pharmacology
REFERENCE

Deglin, J., & Vallerand, A. (1999). *Davis's drug guide for nurses* (6th ed.). Philadelphia: F. A. Davis. pp. 144–148.

12. 3

RATIONALE: Sodium bicarbonate is an electrolyte modifier and antacid. It would further aggravate metabolic alkalosis, which is the most difficult acid-base disturbance to correct. The other options are incorrect.

TEST-TAKING STRATEGY: Use knowledge of acid-base concepts to answer this question. This will allow you to immediately eliminate options 2 and 4 due to acidosis. Next eliminate option 1 as irrelevant. Review the contraindications associated with the use of this medication now if you had difficulty with this question.

LEVEL OF COGNITIVE ABILITY: Analysis
PHASE OF NURSING PROCESS: Data Collection
CLIENT NEEDS: Physiological Integrity
CONTENT AREA: Pharmacology
REFERENCE

Hodgson, B., & Kizior, R. (1999). *Saunders nursing drug handbook 1999*. Philadelphia: W. B. Saunders. p. 932.

13. 4

RATIONALE: Simethicone is an antiflatulent used in the relief of pain due to excessive gas in the GI tract. MOM is an antacid and laxative. Droperidol is used to treat postoperative nausea and vomiting. Acetaminophen is a nonnarcotic analgesic.

TEST-TAKING STRATEGY: The key words in this question are "gas pains." Knowledge of the classifications to which each of the medications belong is needed to answer this question. If this question was difficult, take time now to review this medication.

LEVEL OF COGNITIVE ABILITY: Application
PHASE OF NURSING PROCESS: Implementation
CLIENT NEEDS: Physiological Integrity
CONTENT AREA: Pharmacology
REFERENCE

Deglin, J., & Vallerand, A. (1999). *Davis's drug guide for nurses* (6th ed.). Philadelphia: F. A. Davis. p. 917.

14. 1

RATIONALE: Elderly clients are especially susceptible to CNS side effects of cimetidine. The most frequent of these is confusion. Less common CNS side effects include headache, dizziness, drowsiness, and hallucinations.

TEST-TAKING STRATEGY: Note the key words "most frequent." This tells you that more than one or all of the options may be partially or totally correct. Use your knowledge of the elderly and medication knowledge to choose correctly. Review this medication now if you had difficulty with this question.
LEVEL OF COGNITIVE ABILITY: Application
PHASE OF NURSING PROCESS: Planning
CLIENT NEEDS: Physiological Integrity
CONTENT AREA: Pharmacology
REFERENCE
Lehne, R. (1998). *Pharmacology for nursing care* (3rd ed.). Philadelphia: W. B. Saunders. p. 779.

15. **2**

RATIONALE: The medication should be scheduled for administration 1 hour before meals and at bedtime. The medication is timed to allow it to form a protective coating over the ulcer before food intake stimulates gastric acid production and mechanical irritation. The other options are incorrect.
TEST-TAKING STRATEGY: Specific knowledge of this medication and its timing is needed to answer this question. If needed, take a few moments to review this medication.
LEVEL OF COGNITIVE ABILITY: Application
PHASE OF NURSING PROCESS: Implementation
CLIENT NEEDS: Physiological Integrity
CONTENT AREA: Pharmacology
REFERENCE
Hodgson, B., & Kizior, R. (1999). *Saunders nursing drug handbook 1999*. Philadelphia: W. B. Saunders. p. 951.

16. **3**

RATIONALE: The client who chronically uses NSAIDs is prone to gastric mucosal injury. Misoprostol is specifically given to prevent this occurrence. Diarrhea can be a side effect of the medication, but is not an intended effect. Options 1 and 2 are incorrect.
TEST-TAKING STRATEGY: The key words are "intended therapeutic effect" and "did not experience." This tells you that the medication is being given to prevent the occurrence of specific symptoms. Knowledge of the medication's use is needed to correctly discriminate among the options. If you had difficulty with this question, take time now to review the actions of this medication.
LEVEL OF COGNITIVE ABILITY: Analysis
PHASE OF NURSING PROCESS: Evaluation
CLIENT NEEDS: Physiological Integrity
CONTENT AREA: Pharmacology
REFERENCE
Hodgson, B., & Kizior, R. (1999). *Saunders nursing drug handbook 1999*. Philadelphia: W. B. Saunders. p. 693.

17. **4**

RATIONALE: A single daily dose of ranitidine is scheduled to be given at bedtime. This allows for prolonged effect, and the greatest protection of gastric mucosa. The other options are incorrect.
TEST-TAKING STRATEGY: Specific knowledge of the timing of this medication is needed to answer this question. If you had difficulty with this question, take time now to review this medication.
LEVEL OF COGNITIVE ABILITY: Application
PHASE OF NURSING PROCESS: Implementation
CLIENT NEEDS: Physiological Integrity

CONTENT AREA: Pharmacology
REFERENCE
Hodgson, B., & Kizior, R. (1999). *Saunders nursing drug handbook 1999*. Philadelphia: W. B. Saunders. p. 901.

18. **1**

RATIONALE: Zollinger-Ellison syndrome is a hypersecretory condition of the stomach. The client should avoid taking medications that are irritating to the stomach lining. Irritants would include aspirin and nonsteroidal anti-inflammatory drugs (naprosyn and ibuprofen). The client should be advised to take acetaminophen for a headache.
TEST-TAKING STRATEGY: Remember that options that are similar are not likely to be correct. With this in mind, eliminate options 2 and 3 first. Choose acetaminophen over aspirin because it is least irritating to the stomach. Review this medication now if you had difficulty with this question.
LEVEL OF COGNITIVE ABILITY: Application
PHASE OF NURSING PROCESS: Implementation
CLIENT NEEDS: Health Promotion and Maintenance
CONTENT AREA: Pharmacology
REFERENCE
Hodgson, B., & Kizior, R. (1999). *Saunders nursing drug handbook 1999*. Philadelphia: W. B. Saunders. pp. 577–579.

19. **2**

RATIONALE: Omeprazole is a gastric pump inhibitor and is classified as an antiulcer agent. The intended effect of the medication is relief of pain from gastric irritation, often referred to as heartburn by clients.
TEST-TAKING STRATEGY: Specific knowledge of this medication and its uses is needed to answer this question. If needed, take a few moments to review this medication.
LEVEL OF COGNITIVE ABILITY: Analysis
PHASE OF NURSING PROCESS: Evaluation
CLIENT NEEDS: Physiological Integrity
CONTENT AREA: Pharmacology
REFERENCE
Hodgson, B., & Kizior, R. (1999). *Saunders nursing drug handbook 1999*. Philadelphia: W. B. Saunders. pp. 771–772.

20. **1**

RATIONALE: Cascara sagrada is a laxative that causes nausea and abdominal cramps as the most frequent side effects. Other health problems are not determined based on a single symptom.
TEST-TAKING STRATEGY: Remember that options that are similar are not likely to be correct. This will allow you to eliminate the two GI disorders (options 2 and 4). Choose option 1 over option 3, knowing that laxatives can cause abdominal cramping.
LEVEL OF COGNITIVE ABILITY: Comprehension
PHASE OF NURSING PROCESS: Data Collection
CLIENT NEEDS: Physiological Integrity
CONTENT AREA: Pharmacology
REFERENCE
Hodgson, B., & Kizior, R. (1999). *Saunders nursing drug handbook 1999*. Philadelphia: W. B. Saunders. pp. 157–158.

21. **2**

RATIONALE: Most rapid results from bisacodyl occur when it is taken on an empty stomach. It will not have a rapid effect if taken with a large meal. If it is taken at bedtime, the client will have a bowel movement in the morning. Taking the medication with two glasses of juice will not add to its effect.

TEST-TAKING STRATEGY: Focus on the key words "rapid effect." Recalling that food generally slows the absorption of medication will assist in directing you to option 2. If needed, take time now to review the administration of laxatives.
LEVEL OF COGNITIVE ABILITY: Application
PHASE OF NURSING PROCESS: Implementation
CLIENT NEEDS: Physiological Integrity
CONTENT AREA: Pharmacology
REFERENCE
Deglin, J., & Vallerand, A. (1999). *Davis's drug guide for nurses* (6th ed.). Philadelphia: F. A. Davis. pp. 108–110.

22. 3

RATIONALE: Senna works by changing the transport of water and electrolytes in the large intestine, which causes accumulation of water in the mass of stool and increased peristalsis. The other options are incorrect.
TEST-TAKING STRATEGY: Knowledge regarding the action of this medication is required to answer this question. If you answered incorrectly, take a few minutes to review this medication at this time.
LEVEL OF COGNITIVE ABILITY: Comprehension
PHASE OF NURSING PROCESS: Planning
CLIENT NEEDS: Physiological Integrity
CONTENT AREA: Pharmacology
REFERENCE
Deglin, J., & Vallerand, A. (1999). *Davis's drug guide for nurses* (6th ed.). Philadelphia: F. A. Davis. pp. 913–914.

23. 4

RATIONALE: Loperamide is an antidiarrheal agent. It is commonly administered after loose stools. It is used in the management of acute diarrhea, and also in chronic diarrhea such as with inflammatory bowel disease. It can also be used to reduce the volume of drainage from an ileostomy. The other options are incorrect.
TEST-TAKING STRATEGY: Knowledge that this medication is an antidiarrheal will easily direct you to the correct option. If needed, take a few moments to review the action of this medication now.
LEVEL OF COGNITIVE ABILITY: Application
PHASE OF NURSING PROCESS: Planning
CLIENT NEEDS: Physiological Integrity
CONTENT AREA: Pharmacology
REFERENCE
Lehne, R. (1998). *Pharmacology for nursing care* (3rd ed.). Philadelphia: W. B. Saunders. p. 799.

24. 1

RATIONALE: The client should not exceed the recommended dose because it may be habit forming. The medication is an antidiarrheal, and therefore should not be taken with a laxative. Side effects of the medication include dry mouth and drowsiness.
TEST-TAKING STRATEGY: To answer this question accurately, it is necessary to be familiar with this medication and its habit-forming properties. Familiarity with atropine as an ingredient may help you to eliminate options 3 and 4 immediately. Take a moment to review this medication if the question was difficult for you.
LEVEL OF COGNITIVE ABILITY: Comprehension
PHASE OF NURSING PROCESS: Evaluation
CLIENT NEEDS: Physiological Integrity
CONTENT AREA: Pharmacology

REFERENCE
Deglin, J., & Vallerand, A. (1999). *Davis's drug guide for nurses* (6th ed.). Philadelphia: F. A. Davis. pp. 293–295.

25. 3

RATIONALE: Dimenhydrinate is used to treat and prevent the symptoms of dizziness, vertigo, nausea, and vomiting that accompany motion sickness. The other options are incorrect.
TEST-TAKING STRATEGY: Knowledge that dimenhydrinate is used to treat motion sickness will easily direct you to option 3. If the medication is unfamiliar to you, take time now to review.
LEVEL OF COGNITIVE ABILITY: Comprehension
PHASE OF NURSING PROCESS: Evaluation
CLIENT NEEDS: Physiological Integrity
CONTENT AREA: Pharmacology
REFERENCE
Lehne, R. (1998). *Pharmacology for nursing care* (3rd ed.). Philadelphia: W. B. Saunders. p. 798.

26. 3

RATIONALE: Scopolamine is an anticholinergic medication that causes the frequent side effects of dry mouth, urinary retention, decreased sweating, and pupil dilation. The other options are incorrect.
TEST-TAKING STRATEGY: Recalling that this medication is an anticholinergic will easily direct you to option 3. If this medication is unfamiliar to you, take time now to review the side effects associated with anticholinergics.
LEVEL OF COGNITIVE ABILITY: Application
PHASE OF NURSING PROCESS: Implementation
CLIENT NEEDS: Physiological Integrity
CONTENT AREA: Pharmacology
REFERENCE
Lehne, R. (1998). *Pharmacology for nursing care* (3rd ed.). Philadelphia: W. B. Saunders. p. 798.

27. 1

RATIONALE: Hydroxyzine hydrochloride is an antiemetic and sedative/hypnotic. It is often used in conjunction with narcotic analgesics for added effect. Medications administered by the IM route generally take 20 to 30 minutes to become effective. Hydroxyzine hydrochloride causes dry mouth and drowsiness as side effects.
TEST-TAKING STRATEGY: Begin to answer this question by eliminating option 2, since IM medications do not work that rapidly. Use knowledge regarding the medication to assist in directing you to option 1. If you had difficulty with this medication, take time now to review.
LEVEL OF COGNITIVE ABILITY: Application
PHASE OF NURSING PROCESS: Implementation
CLIENT NEEDS: Physiological Integrity
CONTENT AREA: Pharmacology
REFERENCE
Hodgson, B., & Kizior, R. (1999). *Saunders nursing drug handbook 1999*. Philadelphia: W. B. Saunders. p. 508.

28. 2

RATIONALE: Droperidol may be administered by the intramuscular or intravenous routes. It is not administered subcutaneously or orally. Additionally, oral medications are not well tolerated by the client who is experiencing nausea.
TEST-TAKING STRATEGY: Focus on the client's problem and use knowledge regarding the routes of administration

of this medication to answer the question. If this medication is unfamiliar to you, review it now.

LEVEL OF COGNITIVE ABILITY: Comprehension
PHASE OF NURSING PROCESS: Planning
CLIENT NEEDS: Physiological Integrity
CONTENT AREA: Pharmacology
REFERENCE
Hodgson, B., & Kizior, R. (1999). *Saunders nursing drug handbook 1999*. Philadelphia: W. B. Saunders. p. 358.

29. **3**

RATIONALE: Propantheline is an antimuscarinic anticholinergic medication that decreases GI secretions. It should be administered 30 minutes prior to meals. The other options are incorrect.

TEST-TAKING STRATEGY: Use the process of elimination. Option 4 can be eliminated immediately since most medications cannot be administered with antacids due to interactive effects. Next, eliminate options 1 and 2 because they are similar. If this medication is unfamiliar to you, take time now to review.

LEVEL OF COGNITIVE ABILITY: Application
PHASE OF NURSING PROCESS: Planning
CLIENT NEEDS: Physiological Integrity
CONTENT AREA: Pharmacology

REFERENCE
Deglin, J., & Vallerand, A. (1999). *Davis's drug guide for nurses* (6th ed.). Philadelphia: F. A. Davis. pp. 857–859.

30. **4**

RATIONALE: Docusate sodium is a stool softener that promotes absorption of water into the stool, producing a softer consistency of stool. The intended effect is relief or prevention of constipation. The medication does not relieve abdominal pain, stop GI bleeding, or decrease the amount of fat in the stools.

TEST-TAKING STRATEGY: Knowledge that docusate is a stool softener will easily direct you to option 4. If you are unfamiliar with the action of this medication, take time now to review.

LEVEL OF COGNITIVE ABILITY: Application
PHASE OF NURSING PROCESS: Data Collection
CLIENT NEEDS: Physiological Integrity
CONTENT AREA: Pharmacology
REFERENCE
Hodgson, B., & Kizior, R. (1999). *Saunders nursing drug handbook 1999*. Philadelphia: W. B. Saunders. pp. 344–345.

BIBLIOGRAPHY

Chernecky, C., & Berger, B. (1997). *Laboratory tests and diagnostic procedures* (2nd ed.). Philadelphia: W. B. Saunders.

Deglin, J., & Vallerand, A. (1999). *Davis's drug guide for nurses* (6th ed.). Philadelphia: F. A. Davis.

Hodgson, B., & Kizior, R. (1999). *Saunders nursing drug handbook 1999*. Philadelphia: W. B. Saunders.

Kuhn, M. (1998). *Pharmacotherapeutics: A nursing process approach* (4th ed.). Philadelphia: F. A. Davis.

Lehne, R. (1998). *Pharmacology for nursing care* (3rd ed.). Philadelphia: W. B. Saunders.

Luckmann, J. (1997). *Saunders manual of nursing care*. Philadelphia: W. B. Saunders.

Monahan, F., & Neighbors, M. (1998). *Medical-surgical nursing: Foundations for clinical practice* (2nd ed.). Philadelphia: W. B. Saunders.

O'Toole, M. (1997). *Miller-Keane encyclopedia & dictionary of medicine, nursing, & allied health* (6th ed.). Philadelphia: W. B. Saunders.

UNIT XII

The Adult Client with a Respiratory Disorder

PYRAMID TERMS

Bacille Calmette-Guérin (BCG) Vaccine—A vaccine containing attenuated tubercle bacilli that may be given to people in foreign countries or to those traveling to foreign countries, to produce increased resistance to TB.

Chest Tubes—Placed in the pleural space to remove air or fluid from the chest and thus restore negative pressure to reexpand the lung.

Chronic Airflow Limitation (CAL), Chronic Obstructive Lung Disease (COLD), Chronic Obstructive Pulmonary Disease (COPD)—A group of diseases that includes emphysema, asthma, bronchiectasis, and bronchitis. Characterized by progressive airflow limitations into and out of the lungs, elevated airway resistance, irreversible lung distention, and arterial blood gas imbalance.

Emphysema—A chronic pulmonary disease marked by a narrowing of the small airways and the trapping of air, with destructive changes in their walls. Also known as chronic obstructive pulmonary disease (COPD). In emphysema, the stimulus to breathe is a low PO_2 instead of increased PCO_2.

Endotracheal Tube—A large-bore catheter inserted into the trachea through either the nose or the mouth. Used to maintain a patent airway and indicated when the client needs mechanical ventilation. The tube isolates the airway, provides access for suctioning secretions from the large airways of the pulmonary tree, and allows delivery of specific concentrations of oxygen up to 100%.

Mantoux Test—The most reliable determinant of infection with tuberculosis (TB). A small amount (0.1 mL) of intermediate-strength purified protein derivative (PPD) containing 5 tuberculin units is given intradermally in the forearm. An area of induration measuring 10 mm or more in diameter 48 to 72 hours after injection indicates the individual has been exposed to TB.

Mechanical Ventilation—The use of a ventilator if the client is unable to ventilate enough to maintain proper levels of oxygen and carbon dioxide in the blood.

Multidrug-Resistant Tuberculosis (MDRTB)—A multidrug-resistant strain of TB can occur as a result of improper or noncompliant use of treatment programs and the development of mutations in the tubercle bacilli.

Mycobacterium tuberculosis—The causative organism (bacillus) of tuberculosis.

Suctioning—A sterile procedure that involves the removal of respiratory secretions that accumulate in the tracheal bronchial airway when the client is unable to expectorate secretions. Performed to maintain a patent airway.

Tracheostomy—An artificial opening into the trachea created to establish an airway. It may be temporary or permanent. Provides a patent airway by bypassing complete upper airway obstruction, as from pharyngeal tumors or laryngeal edema, by facilitating the removal of secretions, or by preventing aspiration of gastric contents.

Tuberculosis—A highly communicable disease caused by *Mycobacterium tuberculosis*. It is transmitted by the airborne route via droplet infection.

▶ PYRAMID TO SUCCESS

The Pyramid to Success focuses on maintaining a patent airway. Pyramid points also focus on infectious diseases, particularly tuberculosis, respiratory care in relation to oxygen delivery systems, the client with pneumonia, or the client with chronic obstructive pulmonary disease. The Pyramid to Success includes the care to the client with tuberculosis, especially with regard to the importance of the medication regimen, providing adequate nutrition and adequate rest to promote the healing process, and the prevention of the progression of the disease. Focus on assisting the client to cope with the social isolation issues that exist during the period of illness and on teaching the client and family the critical measures of screening and of preventing respiratory disease and the transmission of disease.

NURSING PROCESS

DATA COLLECTION

Risk factors related to respiratory disorders
Exposure to respiratory irritants, infectious disease, or TB
Fatigue and lethargy
Anorexia and weight loss
Chills or fever
Changes in pattern of respirations and dyspnea
Cough, sputum production, and hemoptysis
Chest tightness and a dull, aching chest pain that may accompany the cough
Voice changes
Night sweats
Skin color changes
Changes in mentation

PLANNING	IMPLEMENTATION	EVALUATION
Client consumes adequate fluids. Client expectorates sputum. Client performs respiratory treatments as prescribed.	Monitor vital signs. Monitor sputum production, noting color, amount, consistency, and odor. Provide adequate fluids and hydration to prevent retention of thick secretions. Position client for comfort and ease of respiration. Instruct client in the use of incentive spirometry and breathing exercises. Suction PRN.	Airway remains patent.
PLANNING	IMPLEMENTATION	EVALUATION
The client exhibits normal breathing patterns.	Monitor vital signs. Monitor respirations and breathing patterns. Monitor for signs of altered respirations. Monitor for changes in skin color, altered mentation, and cyanosis.	Respirations remain normal in rate and depth.
PLANNING	IMPLEMENTATION	EVALUATION
The client exhibits signs of adequate gas exchange.	Monitor respiratory status, noting skin color. Monitor for changes in mental status. Monitor for cardiac irregularities. Monitor peripheral vascular status. Administer oxygen as prescribed. Provide several periods of rest during the day.	Airway remains patent and the client does not exhibit signs of cyanosis.

PLANNING

Client identifies signs of infection. The client verbalizes actions to prevent the transmission of the disease.

IMPLEMENTATION

Monitor temperature. Monitor for signs of infection. Monitor sputum culture and sensitivity results and chest x-ray results. Provide respiratory isolation during infectious stage of respiratory disease until treatment is well established. Instruct the client to cover the mouth and nose when coughing, sneezing, and laughing. Instruct client how to properly dispose of used tissues. Educate the client, family, and close contacts about transmission and prevention.

EVALUATION

Temperature remains within normal limits. Client complies with the treatment regimen. Demonstrates behaviors that will prevent the transmission of the disease.

PLANNING

The client complies with increased nutritional intake. The client maintains prescribed daily calorie requirements.

IMPLEMENTATION

Perform and offer mouth care. Assess the client's food likes and dislikes. Provide foods rich in iron, protein, and vitamin C. Increase fluid intake. Monitor body weight. Plan meal and snack times after rest periods.

EVALUATION

Client maintains body weight through adequate nutritional intake. Maintains the optimal intake of nutrients and calories to promote tissue healing and to prevent infection.

PLANNING

The client describes the treatment plan. The client describes the importance of adequate rest periods. The client alternates rest periods with activity. The client verbalizes the need for follow-up care.

IMPLEMENTATION

Instruct client regarding prescribed treatment plan and the importance of compliance. Instruct client in the importance of adequate rest and activity. Instruct client in breathing techniques. Instruct client regarding administration of prescribed medications. Instruct client and family in prescribed respiratory treatments, care to tracheostomy site if present, and suctioning techniques. Identify support systems. Assist to mobilize home care and community resources as appropriate. Instruct client in the importance of follow-up care and sputum culture testing if prescribed.

EVALUATION

Client complies with treatment plan. Client demonstrates performance of prescribed respiratory treatments. Client complies with seeking medical help for routine follow-up and laboratory analysis. Client uses appropriate community resources.

PLANNING

The client verbalizes appropriate diversional activities. Client identifies support systems.

IMPLEMENTATION

Encourage diversional activities on the basis of the client's interests. Encourage family members to visit during hospitalization for short periods, maintaining respiratory precautions if prescribed.

EVALUATION

Client participates in appropriate diversional activities. Client uses support systems.

◆ CLIENT NEEDS

SAFE, EFFECTIVE CARE ENVIRONMENT

- Client rights
- Confidentiality related to the respiratory disorder
- Informed consent related to diagnostic and surgical procedures
- Consultations and referrals related to respiratory disorder
- Handling infectious materials such as sputum or body fluids
- Respiratory precautions
- Standard (universal) precautions
- Asepsis when caring for wounds and when performing suctioning

HEALTH PROMOTION AND MAINTENANCE

- Prevention of respiratory disorders and infectious diseases
- Health promotion programs
- Health screening related to risks for respiratory disorders
- Instructions related to the prevention of transmission of infection
- Instructions related to medication administration
- Instructions related to breathing exercises, respiratory therapy, and care
- Instructions related to adequate fluid and nutritional intake
- Instructions related to need for follow-up care

PSYCHOSOCIAL INTEGRITY

Religious and spiritual influences
Coping mechanisms
Grief and loss
Situational role changes
Body image changes
Support systems
Community resources

PHYSIOLOGICAL INTEGRITY

Nutrition and oral hygiene
Personal hygiene and rest and sleep
Comfort interventions
Medication administration
Alterations in body systems
Infectious diseases
Respiratory care
Oxygen delivery systems
Pneumonia
Chronic obstructive pulmonary disease
Tuberculosis

BIBLIOGRAPHY

de Wit, S. (1998). *Essentials of medical-surgical nursing* (4th ed.). Philadelphia: W. B. Saunders.

Hill, S., & Howlett, H. (1997). *Success in practical nursing: Personal and vocational issues* (3rd ed.). Philadelphia: W. B. Saunders.

Leahy, J., & Kizilay, P. (1998). *Foundations of nursing practice: A nursing process approach*. Philadelphia: W. B. Saunders.

Luckmann, J. (1997). *Saunders manual of nursing care*. Philadelphia: W. B. Saunders.

Monahan, F., & Neighbors, M. (1998). *Medical-surgical nursing: Foundations for clinical practice* (2nd ed.). Philadelphia: W. B. Saunders.

National Council of State Boards of Nursing. (1998). *National Council detailed test plan for the NCLEX-PN examination*. Chicago: Author.

O'Toole, M. (1997). *Miller-Keane encyclopedia & dictionary of medicine, nursing, & allied health* (6th ed.). Philadelphia: W. B. Saunders.

CHAPTER 46

Respiratory System

· ·

I. Anatomy and Physiology

A. Primary Functions
   1. Provides oxygen for metabolism in the tissues
   2. Removes carbon dioxide, the waste product of metabolism
B. Secondary functions
   1. Facilitates sense of smell
   2. Produces speech
   3. Maintains acid-base balance
   4. Maintains body water levels
   5. Maintains heat balance
C. Upper respiratory tract
   1. Nose: humidifies, warms, and filters inspired air
   2. Sinuses
      a. Air-filled cavities within the hollow bones that surround the nasal passages
      b. Provide resonance during speech
   3. Pharynx
      a. Located behind the oral and nasal cavities
      b. Divided into the nasopharynx, oropharynx, and laryngopharynx
      c. Passageway for both the respiratory and digestive tracts
   4. Larynx
      a. Located above the trachea and just below the pharynx at the root of the tongue
      b. Commonly called the voice box
      c. Contains two pairs of vocal cords, the false and true cords
      d. The opening between the true vocal cords is the glottis
      e. The glottis plays an important role in coughing, which is the most fundamental defense mechanism of the lungs
   5. Epiglottis
      a. Leaf-shaped elastic structure that is attached along one end to the top of the larynx
      b. It prevents food from entering the tracheobronchial tree by closing over the glottis during swallowing
D. Lower respiratory tract
   1. Trachea

   a. Located in front of the esophagus
   b. Branches into the right and left main-stem bronchi at the carina
   2. Main-stem bronchi
      a. Begins at the carina
      b. The right bronchus is slightly wider, shorter, and more vertical than the left bronchus
      c. The main-stem bronchi divide into five secondary or lobar bronchi that enter each of the five lobes of the lung
      d. The bronchi are lined with cilia, which propel mucus up and away from the lower airway to the trachea where it can be expectorated or swallowed
   3. Bronchioles
      a. Branch from the secondary bronchi and subdivide into the small terminal and respiratory bronchioles
      b. They contain no cartilage and depend on the elastic recoil of the lung for patency
      c. The terminal bronchioles contain no cilia and do not participate in gas exchange
   4. Alveolar ducts and alveoli
      a. Acinus is a term used to indicate all structures distal to the terminal bronchiole
      b. Alveolar ducts branch from the respiratory bronchioles
      c. Alveolar sacs that arise from the ducts contain clusters of alveoli, which are the basic units of gas exchange
      d. Cells in the walls of the alveoli secrete surfactant, a phospholipid protein that reduces the surface tension in the alveoli
      e. Without surfactant, collapse of the alveoli occurs
   5. Lungs
      a. Located in the pleural cavity in the thorax
      b. Extend from just above the clavicles to the diaphragm, the major muscle of inspiration
      c. The right lung, which is larger than the left, is divided into three lobes, the upper, middle, and lower lobe
      d. The left lung, which is somewhat narrower

than the right lung to accommodate the heart, is divided into two lobes

e. Innervation of the respiratory structures is accomplished by the phrenic nerve, vagus nerve, and thoracic nerves

f. The parietal pleura lines the inside of the thoracic cavity, including the upper surface of the diaphragm

g. The visceral pleura covers the pulmonary surfaces

h. A thin fluid layer that is produced by the cells lining the pleura, lubricates the visceral and parietal pleura, allowing them to glide smoothly and painlessly during respiration

i. Blood flow through the lungs occurs via the pulmonary system and the bronchial system

6. Accessory muscles of respiration: include the scalene muscles, which elevate the first two ribs; the sternocleidomastoid muscles, which raise the sternum; and the trapezius and pectoralis muscles, which fix the shoulders

7. The respiratory process

a. The diaphragm descends into the abdominal cavity during inspiration, causing negative pressure in the lungs

b. The negative pressure draws air from the area of greater pressure, the atmosphere, into the area of lesser pressure, the lungs

c. In the lungs, air passes through the terminal bronchioles into the alveoli to oxygenate the body tissues

d. At the end of inspiration, the diaphragm and intercostal muscles relax and the lungs recoil

e. As the lungs recoil, pressure within the lungs becomes greater than atmospheric pressure, causing the air that now contains the cellular waste products of carbon dioxide and water to move from the alveoli in the lungs to the atmosphere

f. Expiration is a passive process

II. Risk Factors for Respiratory Disease

A. Smoking
B. Use of chewing tobacco
C. Allergies
D. Frequent respiratory illnesses
E. Chest injury
F. Surgery
G. Exposure to chemicals and environmental pollutants
H. Crowded living conditions
I. Family history of infectious disease
J. Geographic residence and travel to foreign countries

III. Diagnostic Tests

A. Chest x-ray (CXR)
1. Description: used to provide information regarding the anatomic location and appearance of the lungs

2. Preprocedure
a. Remove all jewelry and other metal objects from the chest area
b. Assess the ability to inhale and hold the breath
c. Question females regarding pregnancy or the possibility of pregnancy

3. Postprocedure: assist the client to dress

B. Sputum specimen
1. Description: a specimen obtained by expectoration or tracheal **suctioning** to assist in the identification of organisms or abnormal cells

2. Preprocedure
a. Determine specific purpose of the collection and check the institutional policy for appropriate collection of specimen
b. Obtain an early morning sterile specimen from **suctioning** or expectoration after a respiratory treatment, if a treatment is prescribed
c. Obtain 15 mL of sputum
d. Instruct the client to rinse the mouth with water prior to collection
e. Instruct the client to take several deep breaths and then cough deeply to obtain sputum
f. Always collect the specimen before starting antibiotics

3. Postprocedure
a. If culture of the sputum is prescribed, transport to the lab immediately
b. Assist the client with mouth care

C. Bronchoscopy
1. Description: direct visual examination of the larynx, trachea, and bronchi with a fiberoptic bronchoscope

2. Preprocedure
a. Obtain informed consent
b. NPO from midnight prior to the procedure
c. Obtain vital signs
d. Monitor coagulation studies
e. Remove dentures or eyeglasses
f. Prepare suction equipment
g. Administer medication for sedation as prescribed
h. Have emergency resuscitation equipment readily available

3. Postprocedure
a. Monitor vital signs
b. Maintain a semi-Fowler's position
c. Assess for gag reflex
d. Maintain NPO status until the gag reflex returns
e. Have an emesis basin readily available for client to expectorate saliva
f. Monitor for bloody sputum
g. Monitor respiratory status particularly if sedation was administered
h. Monitor for complications such as bronchospasm, bacteremia, bronchial

perforation indicated by facial or neck crepitus, dysrhythmias, fever, hemorrhage, hypoxemia, and pneumothorax

   i. Notify the physician if fever or difficulty in breathing occurs following the procedure

D. Pulmonary angiography

  1. Description: an invasive fluoroscopic procedure following injection of iodine, radiopaque, or contrast material through a catheter inserted through the antecubital or femoral vein into the pulmonary artery or one of its branches

  2. Preprocedure

    a. Obtain informed consent

    b. Assess for allergies to iodine, seafood, and other radiopaque dyes

    c. Maintain NPO status for 8 hours prior to the procedure

    d. Monitor vital signs

    e. Monitor coagulation studies

    f. Establish an IV access

    g. Administer sedation as prescribed

    h. Instruct clients that they must lie still during the procedure

    i. Instruct clients that they may feel an urge to cough, flushing, nausea, or a salty taste following injection of the dye

    j. Have emergency resuscitation equipment available

  3. Postprocedure

    a. Monitor vital signs

    b. Avoid taking blood pressures in the extremity used for injection for 24 hours

    c. Monitor peripheral neurovascular status

    d. Assess the insertion site for bleeding

    e. Monitor for delayed reaction to the dye

E. Thoracentesis

  1. Description: removal of fluid or air from the pleural space via a transthoracic aspiration

  2. Preprocedure

    a. Obtain informed consent

    b. Obtain baseline vital signs

    c. Prepare the client for ultrasound or chest x-ray if prescribed prior to the procedure

    d. Assess coagulation studies

    e. Note that the client is positioned sitting upright with arms and head supported by a table at the bedside during the procedure

    f. If the client cannot sit up, the client is placed lying in bed on the unaffected side with the head of the bed elevated 45 degrees

    g. Inform the client not to cough, breathe deeply, or move during the procedure

  3. Postprocedure

    a. Monitor vital signs

    b. Monitor respiratory status

    c. Apply a pressure dressing and assess the puncture site for bleeding and crepitus

    d. Monitor for signs of pneumothorax, air embolism, and pulmonary edema

F. Pulmonary function test (PFTs)

  1. Description: include a number of different tests used to evaluate lung mechanics, gas exchange and acid-base disturbance through spirometric measurements, lung volumes, and arterial blood gases

  2. Preprocedure

    a. Determine if an analgesic that may depress the respiratory function is being administered

    b. Consult with the physician regarding holding bronchodilators prior to testing

    c. Instruct the client to void prior to the procedure and to wear loose clothing

    d. Remove dentures

    e. Instruct the client to refrain from smoking or eating a heavy meal for 4 to 6 hours prior to the test

  3. Postprocedure: resume normal diet and any bronchodilators and respiratory treatments that were held prior to procedure

G. Lung biopsy

  1. Description

    a. A percutaneous lung biopsy is performed to obtain tissue for analysis by culture or cytologic examination

    b. A needle biopsy is done to identify pulmonary lesions, changes in lung tissue, and the cause of pleural effusion

  2. Preprocedure

    a. Obtain informed consent

    b. Maintain NPO status prior to the procedure

    c. Inform the client that a local anesthetic will be used but that a sensation of pressure during needle insertion and aspiration may be felt

    d. Administer analgesics and sedatives as prescribed

  3. Postprocedure

    a. Monitor vital signs

    b. Apply a dressing to the biopsy site and monitor for drainage or bleeding

    c. Monitor for signs of respiratory distress and notify the physician if they occur

    d. Monitor for signs of pneumothorax and air emboli and notify the physician if they occur

    e. Prepare the client for chest x-ray if prescribed

H. Ventilation-perfusion lung scan

  1. Description

    a. In the perfusion scan, blood flow to the lungs is evaluated

    b. The ventilation scan determines the patency of the pulmonary airways and detects abnormalities in ventilation

    c. A radionuclide may be injected for the procedure

  2. Preprocedure

    a. Obtain informed consent

    b. Assess for allergies to dye, iodine, or seafood

    c. Remove jewelry around the chest area

d. Review breathing methods that may be required during testing
e. Establish an IV access
f. Administer sedation if prescribed
g. Have emergency resuscitation equipment available

3. Postprocedure
   a. Monitor the client for reaction to the radionuclide
   b. For 24 hours following the procedure, rubber gloves are worn when urine is being discarded; they should be washed with soap and water before removing; then, the hands should be washed after the gloves are removed
   c. Instruct the client to wash hands carefully with soap and water for 24 hours following the procedure

I. Bronchography
   1. Description
      a. A liquid contrast medium is instilled into the trachea followed by chest x-rays of the bronchial tree
      b. It is performed to diagnose abnormalities of the bronchi such as narrowing, dilation, and obstruction
   2. Preprocedure
      a. Obtain informed consent
      b. Assess for allergies to iodine, shellfish, and contrast media
      c. Maintain NPO status for several hours prior to the test to prevent postprocedure aspiration
      d. Administer sedation as prescribed
   3. Postprocedure
      a. Assess vital signs
      b. Assess for dyspnea or bleeding
      c. Encourage coughing and deep breathing
      d. Maintain NPO status until the gag reflex returns
      e. Encourage fluid intake when the gag reflex returns

J. Arterial blood gases (ABGs) (refer to Chapter 9 for information on ABGs)

K. Pulse oximetry
   1. Description
      a. A noninvasive test that registers how saturated the client's hemoglobin is with oxygen
      b. This arterial oxygen saturation (SaO_2) is recorded as a percentage
      c. The normal value is 95% to 100%
      d. After a hypoxic client uses up the readily available oxygen (measured as the arterial oxygen pressure, PaO_2, on arterial blood gas testing), the reserve oxygen, that oxygen attached to the hemoglobin (SaO_2), is drawn on to provide oxygen to the tissues
      e. A pulse oximeter reading can alert the nurse to hypoxemia before clinical signs occur

2. Procedure
   a. A sensor is placed on the client's finger, toe, nose, earlobe, or forehead to measure oxygen saturation, which is then displayed on a monitor
   b. Maintain transducer at heart level
   c. Do not select an extremity with an impediment to blood flow
   d. Results lower than 91% necessitate immediate treatment
   e. If the SaO_2 is below 85%, the body's tissues have a difficult time becoming oxygenated; an SaO_2 of less than 70% is life-threatening

IV. Procedures
A. Incentive spirometry (Box 46–1)
B. **Suctioning**
   1. Aseptic technique
   2. Hyperoxygenate by Ambu, increasing flow rate or by deep breaths
   3. Lubricate the catheter with sterile water
   4. Tracheal **suctioning**—insert the catheter 4 inches
   5. Nasotracheal **suctioning**—insert the catheter to induce the cough reflex
   6. Do not apply suction while inserting the catheter
   7. Apply suction intermittently for 10 to 15 seconds; rotate the catheter and withdraw
   8. Hyperoxygenate and encourage deep breaths
C. Chest physiotherapy (CPT)
   1. Description: percussion and vibration over the thorax to loosen secretions in the affected area of the lungs
   2. Implementation
      a. A layer of material (gown or pajamas) is placed between the hands and the client's skin
      b. Best time is in the morning upon rising, 1 hour before meals or 2 to 3 hours after meals
      c. Stop if pain occurs
      d. Dispose of sputum properly
      e. Provide mouth care after procedure
   3. Contraindications
      a. When bronchospasm is increased by its use
      b. History of pathological fractures
      c. Rib fractures

BOX 46–1. Client Instructions for Incentive Spirometry

Use lips to form seal around mouthpiece
Inspire deeply
Hold inspiration for a few seconds
Forcefully exhale
Avoid use of spirometry at mealtimes as it may produce nausea

d. Chest incisions
D. Postural drainage
  1. Description
    a. Use of gravity to drain secretions from segments of the lungs
    b. May be combined with CPT
  2. Implementation
    a. Position the client properly (the lung segment to be drained is uppermost)
    b. Best time is in the morning upon arising, 1 hour before or 2 to 3 hours after meals
    c. Stop if cyanosis or exhaustion is increased
    d. Maintain the position 5 to 20 minutes after procedure
    e. Dispose of sputum properly
    f. Provide mouth care after the procedure
  3. Contraindications
    a. Unstable vital signs
    b. Increased intracranial pressure

V. Oxygen

A. Implementation
  1. Assess color and vital signs prior to and during treatment
  2. Place a "No Smoking" sign at the client's bedside
  3. Assess for presence of chronic lung problems
  4. Humidify the oxygen
B. Nasal cannula (nasal prongs) (Box 46–2)
  1. Description
    a. Used at flow rates of 1 to 6 L/minute providing approximate oxygen concentrations of 24% (at 1 L/minute) to 44% (at 6 L/minute)
    b. Flow rates higher than 6 L/minute do not significantly increase oxygenation because the anatomic reserve or dead space (oral and nasal cavities) is full
    c. Used for the client with **chronic airflow limitation** (**CAL**, **COPD**) and for long-term oxygen use; however, the **CAL** client who retains carbon dioxide should never receive oxygen at a rate higher than 2 to 3 L/minute unless on a mechanical ventilator because of the potential for apnea or respiratory arrest
    d. Effective oxygen concentration can be delivered to both nose breathers and mouth breathers with the use of a nasal cannula
  2. Implementation
    a. Place the nasal prongs in the nostrils with the openings facing the client

---

BOX 46–2. FIO$_2$ Delivered via Nasal Cannula

24% at 1 L/minute	36% at 4 L/minute
28% at 2 L/minute	40% at 5 L/minute
32% at 3 L/minute	44% at 6 L/minute

BOX 46–3. FIO$_2$ Delivered via Simple Face Mask

Flow rate must be set to at least 5 L/minute to flush the mask of carbon dioxide
40% at 5 L/minute
45%–50% at 6 L/minute
55%–60% at 8 L/minute

---

    b. Add humidification as prescribed when a flow rate higher than 2 L/minute is prescribed
    c. Check the water level and change the humidifier as needed
    d. Monitor the client for changes in respiratory rate or depth
    e. Assess the mucosa because high flow rates have a drying effect and increase mucosal irritation
    f. Monitor skin integrity because the oxygen tubing can irritate the skin
    g. Provide water-soluble jelly to the nares PRN
C. Simple face mask (Box 46–3)
  1. Description
    a. A face mask used to deliver oxygen concentrations of 40% to 60% for short-term oxygen therapy or in an emergency
    b. A minimal flow rate of 5 L/minute is needed to prevent the rebreathing of exhaled air
  2. Implementation
    a. Be sure mask fits securely over nose and mouth as a poorly fitting mask reduces the FIO$_2$ delivered
    b. Monitor the skin and provide skin care to the area covered by the mask because pressure and moisture under the bag may cause skin breakdown
    c. Monitor the client closely for risk of aspiration because the mask limits the client's ability to clear the mouth, especially if vomiting occurs
    d. Provide emotional support to decrease anxiety to the client who feels claustrophobic
    e. Consult with the physician regarding switching the client from a mask to a nasal cannula during eating
D. Partial rebreather mask
  1. Description
    a. A partial rebreather mask consists of a mask with a reservoir bag that provides an oxygen concentration of 70% to 90%, with flow rates of 6 to 15 L/minute
    b. The client rebreathes one-third of the exhaled tidal volume, which is high in oxygen, thus providing a high FIO$_2$
  2. Implementation
    a. Make sure that the reservoir does not twist or kink, which results in a deflated bag

b. Adjust the flow rate to keep the reservoir bag inflated two-thirds full during inspiration because deflation results in decreased oxygen delivered and rebreathing of exhaled air

E. Non-rebreather mask
1. Description
   a. A non-rebreather mask provides the highest concentration of the low-flow systems and can deliver an FIO_2 greater than 90%, depending on the client's ventilatory pattern
   b. It is most frequently used in the client with deteriorating respiratory status who might require intubation
   c. The non-rebreather mask has a one-way valve between the mask and the reservoir and two flaps over the exhalation ports
   d. The valve allows the client to draw his or her entire oxygen from the reservoir bag
   e. The flaps prevent room air from entering through the exhalation ports
   f. During exhalation air leaves through these exhalation ports while the one-way valve prevents exhaled air from reentering the reservoir bag
2. FIO_2 Delivered: 60% to 100% FIO_2 at a liter flow that maintains the bag two-thirds full
3. Implementation
   a. Remove mucus or saliva from the mask
   b. Monitor the client closely
   c. Ensure that the valve and flaps are intact and functional during each breath
   d. Valves should open during expiration and close during inhalation
   e. Suffocation can occur if the reservoir bag kinks or if the oxygen source disconnects

F. High-flow oxygen delivery systems
1. A high-flow system provides oxygen concentrations of 24% to 100% at 8 to 15 L/minute
2. Hi-flow systems include the Venturi mask, aerosol mask, face tent, **tracheostomy** collar, and T-piece
3. These devices, when properly fitted, deliver a consistent and accurate oxygen concentration that meets the client's inspiratory effort

G. Venturi mask
1. Description
   a. The Venturi mask delivers the most accurate oxygen concentration
   b. Its operation is based on a mechanism that pulls in a specific proportional amount of room air for each liter flow of oxygen
   c. An adapter is located between the bottom of the mask and the oxygen source and contains holes of different sizes, which allows only specific amounts of air to mix with the oxygen
   d. The adapter allows selection of the amount of oxygen desired

2. FIO_2 delivered: 24% to 55% FIO_2 with flow rates of 4 to 10 L/minute
3. Implementation
   a. Monitor closely to ensure an accurate flow rate for specific FIO_2
   b. Keep the orifice for the Venturi adapter open and uncovered to ensure adequate oxygen delivery
   c. Ensure that the mask fits snugly and the tubing is free of kinks because the FIO_2 is altered if kinking occurs or if the mask fits poorly
   d. Monitor the client for dry mucous membranes because humidity or aerosol can be added to the system

H. Face tent, aerosol mask, **tracheostomy** collar and T-piece
1. Face tent
   a. Fits over the client's chin, with the top extending halfway across the face
   b. The oxygen concentration varies, but the face tent is useful instead of a tight-fitting mask for the client who has facial trauma and burns
2. Aerosol mask: an aerosol mask is used for the client who requires high humidity after extubation or upper airway surgery or for the client who has thick secretions
3. **Tracheostomy** collar and T-piece
   a. The **tracheostomy** collar can be used to deliver high humidity and the desired oxygen to the client with a **tracheostomy**
   b. A special adapter called the T-piece, can be used to deliver any desired FIO_2 to the client with a **tracheostomy**, laryngectomy, or **endotracheal tube**
4. FIO_2 delivered: 24% to 100% FIO_2 with flow rates at least 10 L/minute
5. Implementation
   a. Change delivery system to a nasal cannula during mealtimes
   b. Ensure that aerosol mist escapes from the vents of the delivery system during inspiration and expiration
   c. Empty condensation from the tubing to prevent the client from being lavaged with water and promote an adequate flow rate
   d. Ensure that there is sufficient water in the canister and change the aerosol water container as needed
   e. Keep the exhalation port on the T-piece open and uncovered (if the port is occluded, the client can suffocate)
   f. Position the T-piece so that it does not pull on the **tracheostomy** or **endotracheal tube** and cause erosion of skin at the **tracheostomy** insertion site
   g. Make sure the humidifier creates enough mist; a mist should be seen during inspiration and expiration

VI. Endotracheal Tubes

A. Description
1. Used to maintain a patent airway
2. Indicated when the client needs **mechanical ventilation**
3. If the client requires an artificial airway for longer than 10 to 14 days, a **tracheostomy** may be created to avoid mucosal and vocal cord damage that can be caused by the **endotracheal tube**
4. The cuff (located at the distal end of the tube) when inflated, produces a seal between the trachea and the cuff to prevent aspiration and ensure delivery of a set tidal volume when **mechanical ventilation** is used; an inflated cuff also prevents air from passing to the vocal cords, nose, or mouth
5. The pilot balloon permits air to be inserted into the cuff, prevents air from escaping, and is used as a guideline for determining the presence or absence of air in the cuff
6. The universal adapter enables attachment of the tube to **mechanical ventilation** tubing or other types of oxygen delivery systems

B. Orotracheal
1. Allows use of a larger-diameter tube and reduces the work of breathing
2. Indicated when the client has a nasal obstruction or a predisposition to epistaxis
3. Uncomfortable and can be manipulated by the tongue causing airway obstruction; an oral airway may be needed to keep the client from biting on the tube

C. Nasotracheal
1. Smaller-sized tube increases resistance and increases the client's work of breathing
2. Discouraged in clients with bleeding disorders
3. More comfortable for the client and the client is unable to manipulate with the tongue

D. Implementation
1. Placement is confirmed by chest x-ray (correct placement is 1 to 2 cm above the carina)
2. Placement is assessed by auscultating both sides of chest while manually ventilating with a resuscitation bag
3. If breath sounds and chest wall movement are absent of the left side, the tube may be in the right main stem bronchus
4. Auscultation over the stomach is performed to rule out esophageal intubation
5. If the tube is in the stomach, louder breath sounds will be heard over the stomach than over the chest, and abdominal distention will be present
6. Secure the tube immediately after intubation with adhesive tape
7. Monitor position of tube at the lip or nose
8. Monitor the skin and mucous membranes
9. Suction only when needed
10. The oral tube needs to be moved to the opposite side of the mouth daily to prevent pressure and necrosis of the lip and mouth area, prevent nerve damage, and facilitate inspection and cleaning of the mouth; moving the tube to the opposite side of the mouth should be done by two health care providers
11. Prevent pulling or tugging on the tube to prevent dislodgment; suction, coughing, and speaking attempts by the client place extra stress on the tube and can cause dislodgment
12. Keep a resuscitation (Ambu) bag at the bedside at all times
13. Assess the pilot balloon to ensure the cuff is inflated

E. Extubation
1. Hyperoxygenate the client and suction the **ET** tube and the oral cavity
2. Place the client in semi-Fowler's position
3. The cuff is deflated and the tube is removed at peak inspiration
4. Instruct the client to cough and deep breathe to assist in removing accumulated secretions in the throat after removal
5. Apply oxygen therapy as prescribed
6. Monitor respiratory status for signs of obstruction and notify the physician if they occur
7. Inform the client that hoarseness or a sore throat is normal and to limit talking if hoarseness or a sore throat occurs

VII. Tracheostomy

A. Description
1. A tracheotomy is a surgical incision into the trachea for the purpose of establishing an airway
2. A **tracheostomy** is the stoma or opening that results from the tracheotomy
3. The **tracheostomy** can be temporary or permanent

B. Implementation
1. Monitor respirations
2. Monitor ABGs and pulse oximetry
3. Encourage coughing and deep breathing
4. Maintain a semi- to high Fowler's position
5. Monitor for bleeding, difficulty breathing, absence of breath sounds, and crepitus, which are indications of hemorrhage, pneumothorax, and subcutaneous **emphysema**
6. Provide respiratory treatments as prescribed
7. Suction PRN; hyperoxygenate the client before **suctioning**
8. If client is allowed to eat, sit the client up for meals and ensure that the cuff is inflated (if tube is not capped) for meals, and for 1 hour after meals
9. Assess the stoma and secretions for blood or purulent drainage
10. Follow the physician's orders and agency

BOX 46–4. Complications of a Tracheostomy

Tube obstruction
Tube dislodgment
Pneumothorax
Subcutaneous emphysema
Bleeding
Infection
Tracheomalacia
Tracheal stenosis
Tracheoesophageal fistula
Trachea–innominate fistula

policy for cleaning the **tracheostomy** site and inner cannula; usually half-strength hydrogen peroxide is used

11. Administer humidified oxygen as prescribed because the normal humidification process is bypassed in a client with a **tracheostomy**
12. Obtain assistance in changing **tracheostomy** ties; cut and remove old ties after placing new ties holding the **tracheostomy** in place
13. Keep a resuscitation (Ambu) bag, obturator, clamps, and a tracheotomy set at the bedside

C. Complications (Box 46–4)

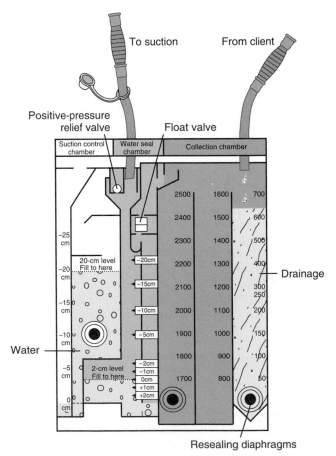

To suction   From client

Positive-pressure
relief valve   Float valve

Suction control | Water seal | Collection chamber
chamber | chamber |

–25 cm

20-cm level
Fill to here   –20cm

–20 cm

–15cm

–15 cm

–10cm

–10 cm

–5cm

Water

–5 cm

2-cm level
Fill to here   –2cm
–1cm
0cm
+1cm
+2cm

0 cm

2500 1600 700
2400 1500 600
2300 1400 500
2200 1300 400
2100 1200 300 250
2000 1100 200
1900 1000 150
1800 900 100
1700 800 50

Drainage

Resealing diaphragms

FIGURE 46–1. A commonly used disposable chest drainage system that combines the three bottles into a single device. (Courtesy of Deknatel, Fall River, MA.)

VIII. Chest Tube Drainage System (Fig. 46–1)

A. Description
   1. Returns negative pressure to the intrapleural space
   2. Used to remove abnormal accumulations of air and fluids from the pleural space
B. Collection chamber
   1. Where the **chest tube** from the client connects to the system
   2. Drainage from the tube drains into and collects in a series of calibrated columns in this chamber
C. Water seal chamber
   1. Establishes 2 cm of water pressure
   2. If positive pressure is greater than 2 cm, air or fluid is expelled into the drainage system
   3. Allows for air to move from the pleural space into the drainage system but not back into the chest
   4. Water oscillates (moves up as the client inhales and moves down as the client exhales)
   5. Bubbling indicates an air leak from the lung or bronchus
D. Suction control chamber
   1. Provides the suction, which can be controlled to provide negative pressure to the chest
   2. This chamber is filled with various levels of water to achieve the desired level of suction; without this control lung tissue could be sucked into the **chest tube**
   3. Bubbling in this chamber indicates that there is suction and it does not indicate that air is escaping from the pleural space
E. Implementation
   1. An occlusive sterile dressing is maintained at the insertion site
   2. A chest x-ray assesses the position of the tube and determines whether the lung has reexpanded
   3. Monitor respiratory status and breath sounds
   4. Keep the drainage system below the level of the chest, free of kinks, dependent loops, or other obstructions
   5. Ensure all connections are secure
   6. Monitor drainage; it should not exceed 200 mL/hour for 2 consecutive hours
   7. Monitor for fluctuation of the fluid level in the water seal chamber
   8. Fluctuation in the water seal chamber stops if the tube is obstructed, if a dependent loop exists, if suction is not working properly, or if the lung has reexpanded
   9. If the client has a known pneumothorax, intermittent bubbling in the water seal chamber is expected as air is drained from the chest, but constant bubbling is indicative of an air leak in the system
   10. Encourage coughing and deep breathing
   11. Change the client's position frequently to promote drainage and ventilation
   12. Keep a clamp and a sterile occlusive dressing at the bedside at all times

13. Mark the **chest tube** drainage in the collection chamber at 1- to 4-hour intervals using a piece of tape
14. Notify a registered nurse if any alterations in the functioning of the drainage system occur
15. When the **chest tube** is removed, the client is asked to perform the Valsalva maneuver; an airtight dressing is taped in place after removal of the **chest tube**

IX. Mechanical Ventilation

A. Description
   1. Used to overcome the client's inability to ventilate or oxygenate adequately
   2. It may be intermittent or continuous, short term, or long term
B. Implementation
   1. Assess the client first and the ventilator second
   2. Assess vital signs, respiratory status, and breathing patterns
   3. Monitor color, particularly in the lips and nailbeds
   4. Monitor the chest for bilateral expansion
   5. Obtain a pulse oximetry reading
   6. Assess the need for **suctioning** and observe the type, color, and amount of secretions
   7. Ensure that the alarms are set
   8. If the cause of an alarm cannot be determined, ventilate the client manually with a resuscitation bag until the problem is corrected
   9. Empty ventilator tubing when moisture collects
   10. Turn the client at least every 2 hours or get the client out of bed as prescribed to prevent complications of immobility
   11. Have resuscitation equipment available at the bedside
C. Causes of alarms
   1. High-pressure alarm
      a. Increased secretions in the airway
      b. Wheezing or bronchospasm causing decreased airway size
      c. Displacement of the **ET** tube
      d. Obstructed **ET** tube due to water or a kink in the tubing
      e. Client coughs, gags, or bites on the oral **ET**
      f. Client is anxious or fights the ventilator
   2. Low-pressure alarm
      a. Disconnection or leak in the ventilator or in the client's airway cuff
      b. The client stops spontaneous breathing
D. Complications
   1. Hypotension caused by the application of positive pressure, which increases intrathoracic pressure and inhibits blood return to the heart
   2. Respiratory complications such as pneumothorax or subcutaneous **emphysema** due to positive pressure
   3. Gastrointestinal alterations such as stress ulcers

   4. Malnutrition
   5. Infections
   6. Muscular deconditioning
   7. Ventilator dependence or inability to wean
E. Weaning: the process of going from ventilator dependence to spontaneous breathing

X. Chest Injuries

A. Rib fracture
   1. Description
      a. Results from direct blunt chest trauma and causes a potential for intrathoracic injury such as pneumothorax or pulmonary contusion
      b. Pain with movement and chest splinting result in impaired ventilation and inadequate clearance of secretions
   2. Data collection
      a. Pain at injury site that increases with inspiration
      b. Tenderness at site
      c. Shallow respirations
      d. Client splints the chest
      e. Fractures noted on chest x-ray
   3. Implementation
      a. Note that ribs usually unite spontaneously
      b. Position client in high Fowler's
      c. Administer pain medication as prescribed to maintain adequate ventilatory status
      d. Monitor for increased respiratory distress
      e. Instruct the client to self-splint with hands and arms
B. Flail chest
   1. Description
      a. A blunt chest trauma associated with accidents that may result in hemothorax and rib fractures
      b. The loose segment of the chest wall becomes paradoxical to the expansion and contraction of the rest of the chest wall
   2. Data collection
      a. Paradoxical respirations (the inward movement of the thorax during inspiration with outward movement during expiration)
      b. Severe pain in the chest
      c. Dyspnea
      d. Cyanosis
      e. Tachycardia
      f. Hypotension
      g. Shallow respirations
      h. Tachypnea
   3. Implementation
      a. Position client in high Fowler's
      b. Administer humidified oxygen as prescribed
      c. Monitor for increased respiratory distress
      d. Encourage coughing and deep breathing
      e. Administer pain medication as prescribed
      f. Maintain bed rest and limit activity to reduce O_2 demands

g. Prepare for intubation with **mechanical ventilation** as prescribed

C. Pulmonary contusion
   1. Description
      a. Characterized by interstitial hemorrhage associated with intra-alveolar hemorrhage, resulting in decreased pulmonary compliance
      b. The major complication is adult respiratory distress syndrome (ARDS)
   2. Data collection
      a. Dyspnea
      b. Hypoxemia
      c. Increased bronchial secretions
      d. Hemoptysis
      e. Restlessness
      f. Decreased breath sounds
      g. Rales and wheezes
   3. Implementation
      a. Maintain airway and ventilation
      b. Position client in high Fowler's
      c. Administer oxygen as prescribed
      d. Monitor for increased respiratory distress
      e. Maintain bed rest and limit activity to reduce O_2 demands
      f. Prepare for **mechanical ventilation** as prescribed

D. Pneumothorax
   1. Description
      a. The accumulation of atmospheric air in the pleural space, which results in a rise in intrathoracic pressure and reduced vital capacity
      b. The loss of negative intrapleural pressure results in collapse of the lung
      c. Diagnosis of pneumothorax is made by chest x-ray
   2. Data collection
      a. Dyspnea
      b. Tachycardia
      c. Tachypnea
      d. Sharp chest pain
      e. Absent breath sounds on the affected side
      f. Decreased chest expansion unilaterally
      g. Cyanosis
      h. Hypotension
      i. Subcutaneous **emphysema**
      j. Sucking sound with open chest wound
      k. Tracheal deviation to the unaffected side with tension pneumothorax
   3. Implementation
      a. Apply pressure dressing over the open chest wound
      b. Administer oxygen as prescribed
      c. Position client in high Fowler's
      d. Prepare for **chest tube** placement with underwater seal drainage until the lung has fully expanded
      e. Monitor the **chest tube** drainage system
      f. Monitor for subcutaneous **emphysema**

XI. Respiratory Failure

A. Description
   1. Occurs when the client cannot eliminate carbon dioxide from the alveoli
   2. The carbon dioxide retention results in hypoxemia
   3. Oxygen reaches the alveoli but cannot be absorbed or used properly
   4. The lungs can move air sufficiently but cannot oxygenate the pulmonary blood properly
   5. Respiratory failure occurs as a result of a mechanical abnormality of the lungs or chest wall, a defect in the respiratory control center in the brain, or an impairment in the function of the respiratory muscles

B. Data collection
   1. Dyspnea
   2. Headache
   3. Confusion
   4. Restlessness
   5. Tachycardia
   6. Cyanosis
   7. Dysrhythmias
   8. Decreased level of consciousness
   9. Alterations in respirations and breath sounds

C. Implementation
   1. Identify and treat the cause of respiratory failure
   2. Administer oxygen as prescribed to maintain the PaO_2 level above 60 mmHg
   3. Position the client in high Fowler's
   4. Encourage deep breathing
   5. Administer bronchodilators as prescribed
   6. Prepare the client for **mechanical ventilation** if supplemental oxygen cannot maintain acceptable PaO_2 levels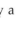

XII. Adult Respiratory Distress Syndrome (ARDS)

A. Description
   1. A form of acute respiratory failure caused by a diffuse lung injury leading to extravascular lung fluid
   2. The interstitial edema causes compression and obliteration of the terminal airways and leads to reduced lung volume and compliance
   3. The ABGs identify respiratory acidosis and hypoxemia that does not respond to an increased percentage of oxygen, and the chest x-ray shows interstitial edema
   4. Some of the causes include sepsis, fluid overload, shock, trauma, neurological injuries, burns, disseminated intravascular coagulation (DIC), drug ingestion, and the inhalation of toxic substances

B. Data collection
   1. Tachypnea
   2. Dyspnea
   3. Decreased breath sounds

4. Deteriorating blood gas levels
5. Hypoxemia despite high concentrations of delivered oxygen
6. Decreased pulmonary compliance
7. Pulmonary infiltrates

C. Implementation
1. Identify and treat the cause of the ARDS
2. Administer oxygen as prescribed
3. Position client in high Fowler's
4. Restrict fluid intake as prescribed
5. Provide respiratory treatments as prescribed
6. Administer diuretics, anticoagulants, or steroids as prescribed
7. Prepare the client for intubation and **mechanical ventilation**

XIII. Chronic Obstructive Pulmonary Disease (COPD)

A. Description
1. Also known as **chronic obstructive lung disease (COLD)** and **chronic airflow limitation (CAL)**
2. A group of diseases that include **emphysema**, asthma, bronchiectasis, and bronchitis
3. Characterized by progressive airflow limitations into and out of the lungs, elevated airway resistance, irreversible lung distention, and arterial blood gas imbalance
4. **COPD** leads to pulmonary insufficiency, pulmonary hypertension, and cor pulmonale
5. In **emphysema**, the stimulus to breathe is low PO_2 instead of increased PCO_2

B. Data collection
1. Cough
2. Exertional dyspnea
3. Wheezing and crackles
4. Sputum production
5. Weight loss
6. Barrel chest **(emphysema)**
7. Use of accessory muscles
8. Cyanosis
9. Clubbing of fingers
10. Orthopnea
11. Cardiac dysrhythmias
12. Congestion and hyperinflation on chest x-ray
13. ABGs indicate respiratory acidosis and hypoxemia
14. Pulmonary function tests (PFTs) demonstrate decreased vital capacity

C. Implementation
1. Monitor vital signs
2. Administer oxygen as prescribed at 2 to 3 L/minute
3. Monitor pulse oximetry
4. Provide respiratory treatments and chest physical therapy
5. Reposition the client for breathing comfort and to mobilize secretions
6. Instruct the client in diaphragmatic or abdominal and pursed-lip breathing techniques
7. Record the color, amount, and consistency of sputum
8. Suction the client if necessary to clear the airway and prevent infection
9. Monitor weight
10. Encourage small, frequent meals to prevent dyspnea
11. Encourage fluids up to 3000 mL/day to keep secretions thin unless contraindicated
12. Position in high Fowler's and leaning forward to aid in breathing
13. Provide a high-calorie, high-protein, and high-carbohydrate diet with vitamin C and nitrogen
14. Allow activity as tolerated
15. Administer bronchodilators as prescribed and instruct the client in the use of both oral and inhalant medications
16. Administer steroids as prescribed to reduce inflammation
17. Administer mucolytics as prescribed to thin secretions
18. Administer antibiotics for infection if prescribed

D. Client education
1. Stop smoking
2. Recognize the signs and symptoms of respiratory infection and hypoxia
3. Adhere to activity limitations, alternating rest periods with activity
4. Avoid exposure to individuals with infections and avoid crowds
5. Demonstrate pursed-lip and diaphragmatic or abdominal breathing
6. Instruct in the use of medications and inhalers
7. Instruct in the use of oxygen therapy
8. Instruct the client in nutritional requirements
9. Avoid eating gas-producing foods, spicy foods, and extremely hot or cold foods
10. Instruct in the importance of receiving the influenza vaccine as recommended
11. When dusting, use a wet cloth
12. Avoid powerful odors
13. Avoid extremes in temperature
14. Avoid fireplaces, pets, and feather pillows

XIV. Pneumonia

A. Description
1. An infection of the pulmonary tissue including the interstitial spaces, the alveoli, and the bronchioles
2. The edema associated with inflammation stiffens the lung, decreases compliance in vital capacity, and causes hypoxemia
3. Can be community acquired or hospital acquired

4. The chest x-ray presents as diffuse patches throughout the lungs or consolidates in a lobe
5. A sputum culture identifies the organism
6. The WBCs and erythrocyte sedimentation rate (ESR) are elevated

B. Data collection
1. Chills
2. Elevated temperature
3. Pleuritic pain
4. Rales, rhonchi, and wheezes
5. Use of accessory muscles
6. Cyanosis
7. Mental status changes
8. Sputum production
   a. Rusty, green, or bloody (pneumococcal pneumonia)
   b. Yellow-green (bronchopneumonia)

C. Implementation
1. Administer oxygen as prescribed
2. Monitor respiratory status
3. Monitor for labored respirations, cyanosis, and cold and clammy skin
4. Encourage coughing and deep breathing and use of incentive spirometer
5. Position in semi-Fowler's to facilitate breathing and lung expansion
6. Change positions frequently and ambulate as tolerated to mobilize secretions
7. Provide chest physical therapy
8. Perform nasotracheal **suctioning** if the client is unable to clear secretions
9. Monitor pulse oximetry
10. Monitor and record color, consistency, and amount of sputum
11. Provide a high-calorie, high-protein diet with small, frequent meals
12. Encourage fluids to 3 liters a day to liquefy secretions unless contraindicated
13. Provide a balance of rest and activity, increasing activity gradually
14. Administer antibiotics as prescribed
15. Administer antipyretics, bronchodilators, cough suppressants, mucolytic agents, and expectorants as prescribed
16. Prevent the spread of infection by handwashing and the proper disposal of secretions

D. Client education
1. The importance of rest, proper nutrition, and adequate fluid intake
2. Avoid chilling and exposure to individuals with respiratory infections or viruses
3. Instruct regarding medications and the use of inhalants as prescribed
4. Instruct to notify the physician if chills, fever, dyspnea, hemoptysis, or increased fatigue occurs
5. Instruct in the importance of receiving the influenza vaccine as recommended

XV. Pleural Effusion

A. Description
1. The collection of fluid in the pleural space
2. Any condition that interferes with either secretion or drainage of this fluid will lead to pleural effusion

B. Data collection
1. Pleuritic pain that is sharp and increases with inspiration
2. Dyspnea on exertion
3. Dry, nonproductive cough caused by bronchial irritation or mediastinal shift
4. Malaise
5. Tachycardia
6. Elevated temperature
7. Decreased breath sounds
8. Chest x-ray (CXR) shows pleural effusion and a mediastinal shift away from the fluid

C. Implementation
1. Identify and treat underlying cause
2. Monitor vital signs
3. Monitor breath sounds
4. Position the client in high Fowler's
5. Encourage coughing and deep breathing
6. Prepare the client for thoracentesis
7. If pleural effusion is recurrent, prepare the client for pleurectomy or pleurodesis

D. Pleurectomy
1. Consists of surgically stripping the parietal pleura away from the visceral pleura
2. This produces an intense inflammatory reaction that promotes adhesion formation between the two layers during healing

E. Pleurodesis
1. Involves the instillation of a sclerosing substance into the pleural space via a thorocotomy tube
2. This creates an inflammatory response that scleroses tissues together

XVI. Empyema

A. Description
1. The collection of pus within the pleural cavity
2. The fluid is thick, opaque, and foul smelling
3. The most common cause is pulmonary infection and lung abscess caused by thoracic surgery or chest trauma, where bacteria are introduced directly into the pleural space
4. Treatment focuses on emptying the empyema cavity, reexpanding the lung, and controlling the infection

B. Data collection
1. Recent febrile illnesses or trauma
2. Chest pain
3. Cough
4. Dyspnea
5. Anorexia and weight loss
6. Malaise
7. Elevated temperature and chills
8. Night sweats
9. Diminished chest wall movement on the affected side
10. Pleural exudate on CXR

C. Implementation
1. Monitor vital signs

2. Monitor breath sounds
3. Position the client in semi- or high Fowler's
4. Encourage coughing and deep breathing
5. Administer antibiotics as prescribed
6. Instruct the client to splint chest as necessary
7. Assist with **chest tube** insertion to promote drainage and lung expansion
8. If marked pleural thickening occurs, prepare the client for decortication, a surgical procedure that involves removal of the restrictive mass of fibrin and inflammatory cells if prescribed

XVII. Pleurisy

A. Description
1. Inflammation of the visceral and parietal membranes
2. These membranes rub together during respiration and cause pain
3. May be caused by pulmonary infarction or pneumonia
4. It usually occurs on one side of the chest in the lower lateral portions in the chest wall
B. Data collection
1. Knifelike pain that is aggravated on deep breathing and coughing
2. Dyspnea
3. Pleural friction rub heard on auscultation
4. Apprehension
C. Implementation
1. Monitor vital signs
2. Administer analgesics as prescribed
3. Apply hot or cold applications as prescribed
4. Encourage coughing and deep breathing
5. Instruct the client to lie on the affected side to splint the chest

XVIII. Pulmonary Embolism

A. Description
1. Occurs when a thrombus that forms in a deep vein detaches and travels to the right side of the heart and then lodges in a branch of the pulmonary artery
2. Clients prone to pulmonary embolism are those at risk for deep vein thrombosis including prolonged immobilization, surgery, obesity, pregnancy, CHF, advanced age, and prior history of thromboembolism
3. Fat emboli can occur as a complication following a fracture of a flat long bone
4. Treatment is aimed at preventing venous stasis and includes range of motion (ROM) exercises and early ambulation following surgery, the use of antiembolism or pneumatic compression stockings, and preventing pressure under the popliteal space
B. Data collection
1. Dyspnea accompanied by anginal and pleuritic pain exacerbated by inspiration
2. Cough

3. Blood-tinged sputum
4. Tachycardia
5. Chest pain
6. Tachypnea
7. Hypotension
8. Shallow respirations
9. Rales on auscultation
10. Low-grade fever
11. Distended neck veins
12. Cyanosis
13. Positive Homans' sign
C. Implementation
1. Monitor vital signs
2. Administer oxygen as prescribed
3. Position client in high Fowler's
4. Maintain bed rest and active and passive ROM exercises as prescribed
5. Encourage the use of incentive spirometry as prescribed
6. Monitor pulse oximetry
7. Prepare for intubation and **mechanical ventilation** for severe hypoxemia
8. Prepare for the administration of anticoagulants such as heparin sodium (Liquaemin) or warfarin sodium (Coumadin)
9. Prepare the client for embolectomy, vein ligation, or insertion of an umbrella filter as prescribed

XIX. Lung Cancer (refer to Chapter 40 for information on lung cancer)

A. Surgical Implementation
1. Laser therapy: to relieve endobronchial obstruction
2. Thoracotomy with pneumonectomy: surgical removal of a lung for bronchiogenic carcinoma
3. Thoracotomy with lobectomy: surgical removal of one lobe of the lung for tumors confined to a single lobe
4. Thoracotomy with segmental resection: surgical removal of a lobe segment for clients unable to tolerate lobectomy or pneumonectomy
B. Preoperative implementation
1. Explain the potential postoperative need for **chest tubes**
2. Note that a **chest tube** is not inserted for a pneumonectomy, and the serum fluid that accumulates in the empty thoracic cavity eventually consolidates, preventing shifts of the mediastinum, heart, and remaining lung
C. Postoperative implementation
1. Monitor vital signs
2. Monitor cardiac and respiratory status
3. Maintain the **chest tube** drainage system, which will drain air and/or blood that accumulates in the pleural space
4. Monitor the **chest tube** insertion site for subcutaneous air and drainage
5. Administer oxygen as prescribed

6. Monitor pulse oximetry
7. Provide activity as tolerated
8. Encourage active ROM exercises to the operative shoulder as prescribed
9. Maintain the client's position based on the procedure performed

D. Pneumonectomy
1. Avoid complete lateral positioning because the mediastinum is no longer held in place on both sides by lung tissue
2. Extreme turning may cause mediastinum shift and compression of the remaining lung

E. Segmental (wedge) resection: elevate the head of the bed 30 to 45 degrees and avoid positioning the client on the operative side as prescribed

XX. Laryngeal Cancer (refer to Chapter 40 for information on laryngeal cancer)

A. Surgical implementation
1. Small tumor excision or total laryngectomy: performed for infiltrate tumors that involve vocal cord paralysis and for tumors that do not respond to radiation therapy
2. Radical neck dissection
    a. Involves a laryngectomy and **tracheostomy**
    b. Performed when lymph node involvement is present

B. Preoperative implementation
1. Establish methods of communication for the client
2. Encourage the client to express feelings about changes in body image and loss of voice
3. Describe the rehabilitation program and information about the tracheotomy and **suctioning**

C. Postoperative implementation
1. Monitor vital signs
2. Assess respiratory status
3. Position the client in high Fowler's position
4. Monitor airway patency and provide frequent **suctioning** to remove bloody secretions
5. Maintain mechanical ventilator support or a **tracheostomy** collar with humidification as prescribed
6. Maintain surgical drains in the neck area if present
7. Observe for hemorrhage and edema in the neck
8. Administer oxygen via a high humidity **tracheostomy** mask as prescribed
9. Monitor pulse oximetry
10. Monitor the color, amount, and consistency of sputum
11. Monitor IV fluids or TPN until nutrition is administered via an nasogastric, gastrostomy, or jejunostomy tube
12. Assess gag and cough reflexes and ability to swallow
13. Provide oral hygiene

14. Provide stoma and laryngectomy care
15. Increased intake in fluids
16. Increase activity, as tolerated
17. Provide consultation with a speech and language pathologist as prescribed
18. Prepare the client for rehabilitation and speech therapy through the use of an artificial larynx followed by esophageal speech
19. Reinforce the method of communication established preoperatively

D. Client education
1. Teach the clean **suctioning** technique
2. Instruct the client how to clean the incision and provide stoma care
3. Protect the neck from injury
4. Avoid swimming, showering, and using aerosol sprays
5. Demonstrate ways to prevent debris from entering the stoma
6. Instruct the client to wear a stoma guard to shield the stoma
7. Advise the client to wear loose-fitting, high-collared clothing to hide the stoma
8. Advise the client to increase humidity in the home
9. Instruct in ROM exercises for arms, shoulders, and neck daily
10. Avoid exposure to people with infections
11. Alternate rest periods with activity
12. Increase fluid intake to 3000 mL/day
13. Advise the client to obtain a Medic-Alert bracelet

XXI. Carbon Monoxide Poisoning (refer to Chapter 38 for information on carbon monoxide poisoning)

XXII. Histoplasmosis

A. Description
1. A pulmonary fungal infection caused by spores of *Histoplasma capsulatum*
2. Transmission occurs by the inhalation of spores that are commonly located in contaminated soil
3. Spores are also usually found in bird droppings

B. Data collection
1. Dyspnea
2. Chills
3. Chest pain
4. Elevated temperature
5. Pulmonary infiltrates on CXR
6. Elevated WBC
7. Positive skin test
8. Positive agglutination test
9. Splenomegaly
10. Hepatomegaly

C. Implementation
1. Administer oxygen as prescribed
2. Administer antiemetics, antihistamines, antipyretics, and steroids as prescribed

3. Administer fungicidal medications as prescribed
4. Encourage coughing and deep breathing
5. Position the client in semi-Fowler's
6. Monitor vital signs
7. Monitor respiratory status
8. Monitor for nephrotoxicity from fungicidal medications
9. Instruct the client to spray the area with water before sweeping barn and chicken coops

XXIII. Sarcoidosis

A. Description
1. Epitheloid cell tubercles in the lung
2. Cause is unknown
3. High titer of Epstein-Barr may be identified
4. Virus incidence is highest in blacks and young adults
B. Data collection
1. Night sweats
2. Fever
3. Weight loss
4. Cough
5. Nodules on the face
6. Polyarthritis
7. Kveim test: Sarcoid node antigen is injected intradermally and causes local nodular lesion in approximately 1 month
C. Implementation
1. Administer corticosteroids as prescribed to control symptoms
2. Monitor temperature
3. Increase fluid intake
4. Provide frequent periods of rest
5. Provide small nutritious meals

XXIV. Occupational Lung Disease (Silicosis)

A. Description
1. Known as asbestosis and coal workers' pneumoconiosis
2. Fibrotic disease of lungs caused by inhalation of inorganic dusts over long periods
3. Common in miners and sandblasters
4. **Tuberculosis** is a frequent complication
B. Data collection
1. Frequent respiratory infections
2. Blood-streaked sputum
3. Cough
4. Chest x-ray for nodular lesions of lungs
C. Implementation
1. Administer antitussive as prescribed for cough
2. Administer medications for TB as prescribed
3. Eliminate toxic substances
4. Administer oxygen as prescribed
5. Encourage coughing and deep breathing

XXV. Tuberculosis

A. Description
1. A highly communicable disease caused by *Mycobacterium tuberculosis*
2. *M. tuberculosis* is a nonmotile, nonsporulating, acid-fast rod that secretes niacin, and when the bacillus reaches a susceptible site, it multiplies freely
3. Because *M. tuberculosis* is an aerobic bacterium, it primarily affects the pulmonary system, especially the upper lobes where the oxygen content is greatest, but can also affect other areas of the body such as the brain, intestines, peritoneum, kidney, joints, and liver
4. An exudative-type response causes a nonspecific pneumonitis and the development of granulomas in the lung tissue
5. **Tuberculosis (TB)** has an insidious onset, and many clients are not aware of symptoms until the disease is well advanced
6. **A multidrug-resistant tuberculosis (MDRTB)** can exist as a result of improper or noncompliant use of treatment programs and the development of mutations in the tubercle bacilli
7. The goal of treatment is to prevent transmission, control symptoms, and prevent progression of the disease
B. Risk factors
1. Alcoholism
2. Intravenous drug use
3. Malnutrition
4. Infection
5. The elderly
6. The homeless
7. Refugees
8. Minority groups
9. Individuals from a lower socioeconomic group
10. Children younger than 5 years of age
11. Individuals living in crowded areas, such as long-term care facilities, prisons, and mental health facilities
12. Individuals in constant, frequent contact with an untreated or undiagnosed individual
13. Individuals with immune dysfunction, HIV, or immunosuppression from medication therapy
14. Drinking unpasteurized milk if cows are infected with bovine **TB**
C. Transmission
1. Via aerosolization or airborne route by droplet infection
2. When an infected individual coughs, laughs, sneezes, or sings, droplet nuclei containing **TB** bacteria enter the air and may be inhaled by others
3. Identification of those individuals in close contact with the infected individual is important so that they can be tested and treated as necessary
4. When contacts have been identified, these people are assessed with a tuberculin test and chest x-ray to determine infection with **TB**
5. After the infected individual has received **TB**

medication for 2 to 3 weeks, the risk of transmission is greatly reduced

D. Disease progression
1. Droplets enter the lungs and the bacteria form a tubercle lesion
2. With the development of acquired immunity, further multiplication of the bacilli may be controlled and the defense systems encapsulate the tubercle, leaving a scar
3. If encapsulation does not occur, bacteria may enter the lymph system, travel to the lymph nodes, and cause an inflammatory response called granulomatous inflammation
4. Other bacilli are attacked and primary lesions (primary infection) form
5. The primary lesions may become dormant, but can be reactivated and become a secondary infection when reexposed to the bacterium
6. In an active phase, **TB** can cause necrosis and cavitation in the lesions, leading to rupture and the spread of necrotic tissue and damage to various parts of the body

E. Diagnostic findings
1. Past exposure to **TB**
2. The client's country of origin and travel to foreign countries in which there is a high incidence of **TB**
3. Recent history of influenza, pneumonia, febrile illness, cough, and foul-smelling sputum production
4. Previous tests for **TB**
5. Recent **bacille Calmette-Guérin (BCG) vaccine** (a vaccine containing attenuated tubercle bacilli that may be given in foreign countries or if traveling to foreign countries to produce increased resistance to **TB**)
6. An individual who has received **BCG** will have a positive skin test and should be evaluated for **TB** with a chest x-ray

F. Clinical manifestations
1. Early detection of **TB** depends on subjective findings rather than presentation of symptoms
2. Fatigue
3. Lethargy
4. Anorexia
5. Weight loss
6. Low-grade fever
7. Chills
8. Night sweats
9. Persistent cough and the production of mucoid and mucopurulent sputum, which is occasionally streaked with blood
10. Chest tightness and a dull, aching chest pain may accompany the cough

G. Chest assessment
1. A physical examination of the chest does not provide conclusive evidence of **TB**
2. Chest x-ray is not definitive but the presence of multinodular infiltrates with calcification in the upper lobes suggests **TB**

3. If the disease is active, caseation and inflammation may be seen on the chest x-ray
4. Advanced disease
   a. Dullness with percussion over involved parenchymal areas, bronchial breath sounds, rhonchi, and/or crackles
   b. Partial obstruction of a bronchus, caused by endobronchial disease or compression by lymph nodes, may produce localized wheezing and dyspnea

H. Sputum cultures
1. Sputum specimens are obtained for an acid-fast smear
2. A sputum culture identifying *Mycobacterium tuberculosis* confirms the diagnosis
3. After medications are started, sputum samples are obtained again to determine the effectiveness of therapy
4. Most clients have negative cultures after 3 months of compliance to medication therapy

I. Mantoux Test
1. The most reliable determinant of infection with **TB**
2. A positive reaction does not mean that active disease is present but indicates exposure to **TB** or the presence of inactive (dormant) disease
3. Once the test result is positive, it will be positive in any future tests
4. A small amount (0.1 mL) of intermediate-strength purified protein derivative (PPD) containing 5 tuberculin units is administered intradermally in the forearm
5. An area of induration measuring 10 mm or more in diameter, 48 to 72 hours after injection, indicates the individual has been exposed to **TB**
6. For individuals with HIV infection or who are immunosuppressed, a reaction of 5 mm or greater is considered positive
7. Once an individual's skin test is positive, a chest x-ray is necessary to rule out active **TB** or to detect old, healed lesions

J. The hospitalized client
1. The client with active **TB** is placed in respiratory isolation precautions in a well-ventilated room
2. The room should have at least six exchanges of fresh air per hour and should be ventilated to the outside environment if possible
3. The nurse wears a particulate respirator (a special individually fitted mask) when caring for the client and a gown when there is a possibility of contamination of clothing
4. Hands are always thoroughly washed before and after caring for the client
5. If the client needs to leave the room for a test or procedure, the client is required to wear a mask
6. Isolation is discontinued when the client is no longer considered infectious
7. After the infected individual has received **TB**

medication for 2 to 3 weeks, the risk of transmission is greatly reduced

8. When the results of two sputum cultures are negative, the client is no longer considered infectious

K. The client at home
1. Provide the client and family with information about **TB** and allay concerns about the contagious aspect of the infection
2. Instruct the client to follow the medication regimen exactly as prescribed and always to have a supply of the medication on hand
3. Advise the client of the side effects of the medication and ways of minimizing them to ensure compliance
4. Reassure the client that after 2 to 3 weeks of medication therapy, it is unlikely that the client will infect anyone
5. Inform the client that activities should be resumed gradually
6. Instruct the client about the need for adequate nutrition and a well-balanced diet to promote healing and to prevent recurrence of infection
7. Instruct the client to increase foods rich in iron, protein, and vitamin C
8. Inform the client and family that respiratory isolation is not necessary because family members have already been exposed
9. Instruct the client to cover the mouth and nose when coughing or sneezing and to dispose of used tissues in plastic bags
10. Instruct the client and family about thorough handwashing
11. Inform the client that examination of the sputum is needed every 2 to 4 weeks once medication therapy is initiated
12. Inform clients that when the results of two sputum cultures are negative, clients are no longer considered infectious and can usually return to their former employment
13. Advise the client to avoid excessive exposure to silicone or dust because these substances can cause further lung damage
14. Instruct the client regarding the importance of compliance to treatment, follow-up care, and sputum cultures as prescribed

L. Medications
1. The most effective method for treating the disease and preventing transmission
2. Treatment of identified lesions depends on whether the individual has active disease or has been exposed to the disease
3. Treatment is difficult because the bacterium has a waxy substance on the capsule, which makes penetration and destruction difficult
4. The use of a multiple medication regimen destroys organisms as quickly as possible and minimizes the emergence of medication-resistant organisms
5. Active **TB** is treated with a combination of

medications to which the organism is susceptible
6. Individuals with active **TB** are treated for 6 to 9 months; however, clients with HIV infection will be treated for a longer period
7. After the infected individual has received medication for 2 to 3 weeks, the risk of transmission is greatly reduced
8. Most clients have negative sputum cultures after 3 months with compliance to medication therapy
9. Individuals who have been exposed to active **TB** are treated with preventive isoniazid (INH) for 9 to 12 months

M. First-line or second-line medications
1. First-line medications provide the most effective antituberculosis activity with an acceptable degree of toxicity
2. Second-line medications provide adequate antimicrobial activity but have excessive toxicities
3. Current infecting organisms are proving resistant to standard first-line medications, and the resistant organisms develop because individuals with the disease fail to complete the course of treatment; surviving bacteria adapt to the drug and become resistant
4. Multidrug therapies are instituted because of the resistant bacteria

N. **Multidrug-Resistant Tuberculosis (MDRTB)**
1. Occurs when a client receiving two medications (first- and second-line medications) discontinues one of the medications without the physician's knowledge
2. The client briefly experiences some response from the single medication, but then large numbers of resistant organisms begin to grow
3. The client, infectious again, transmits the drug-resistant organism to other individuals
4. As this event is repeated, an organism develops that is resistant to many of the first-line tuberculosis medications

XXVI. First-Line Medications for TB (Table 46–1)

A. Isoniazid (INH)
1. Description
a. Bactericidal

Table 46–1. First-Line and Second-Line Medications

First-Line	Second-Line
Isoniazid (INH)	Capreomycin (Capastat Sulfate)
Rifampin (Rifadin)	Kanamycin sulfate (Kantrex)
Ethambutol (Myambutol)	Ethionamide (Trecator-SC)
Streptomycin	Aminosalicylate sodium
Pyrazinamide (Tebrazid)	(Sodium para-aminosalicylic acid [PAS])
	Cycloserine (Seromycin)

b. Inhibits synthesis of mycolic acids and acts to kill actively growing organisms in the extracellular environment

c. Inhibits growth of dormant organisms in the macrophages and caseating granulomas

d. Active only during cell division

e. Used in combination with other antitubercular medications

2. Contraindications and cautions

a. Contraindicated in clients with hypersensitivity or with acute liver disease

b. Use with caution in clients with chronic liver disease, alcoholism, or renal impairment

c. Use with caution in clients taking niacin, nicotinic acid (Nicobid)

d. Use with caution in clients taking hepatotoxic medications because the risk for hepatotoxicity increases

e. Alcohol increases the risk of hepatotoxicity

f. Isoniazid (INH) may increase the risk of toxicity of carbamazepine (Tegretol) and phenytoin (Dilantin)

g. Isoniazid (INH) may decrease ketoconazole (Nizoral) concentrations

3. Side effects

a. Peripheral neuritis

b. Neurotoxicity

c. Irritation at the injection site with IM administration

d. Nausea and vomiting

e. Dry mouth

f. Pyridoxine (vitamin B_6) deficiency

g. Dizziness

h. Hyperglycemia

i. Increased liver function tests

j. Hepatotoxicity

k. Hepatitis

l. Hypersensitivity reactions

4. Implementation

a. Monitor for hypersensitivity

b. Monitor for hepatic dysfunction

c. Monitor for sensitivity to niacin, nicotinic acid (Nicobid)

d. Monitor liver function tests

e. Monitor for signs of hepatitis such as anorexia, nausea, vomiting, weakness, fatigue, dark urine or jaundice, and if these symptoms occur, hold medication and notify the physician

f. Monitor for tingling, numbness, or burning of the extremities

g. Assess mental status

h. Monitor for visual changes and notify the physician if they occur

i. Assess for dizziness and initiate safety precautions

j. Monitor CBC and blood glucose results

k. Administer 1 hour before or 2 hours after a meal because food may delay absorption

l. Administer at least 1 hour before antacids, especially those that contain aluminum

5. Client education

a. Instruct the client not to skip doses and to take medication for the full length of the prescribed therapy

b. Instruct the client not to take any other medication without consulting the physician

c. Advise the client of the importance of follow-up physician visits, vision testing, and lab tests

d. Instruct the client to avoid alcohol

e. Advise the client to take medication on an empty stomach with 8 oz of water 1 hour before or 2 hours after meals and to avoid taking antacids with the medication

f. Instruct the client to avoid tyramine-containing foods because they may cause a reaction such as red and itching skin, a pounding heartbeat, light-headedness, a hot or clammy feeling, or a headache, and if this does occur, to notify the physician

g. Instruct the client in the signs of neurotoxicity, hepatitis, and hepatotoxicity

h. Instruct client to notify physician if signs of neurotoxicity, hepatitis and hepatotoxicity, or visual changes occur

B. Rifampin (Rifadin)

1. Description

a. Inhibits bacterial RNA synthesis

b. Binds to DNA-dependent RNA polymerase

c. Blocks RNA transcription

d. Used in conjunction with at least one other antitubercular medication

2. Contraindications and cautions

a. Contraindicated in clients with hypersensitivity

b. Use with caution in clients with hepatic dysfunction or alcoholism

c. Use of alcohol or hepatotoxic medications may increase the risk of hepatotoxicity

3. Side effects

a. Heartburn

b. Nausea

c. Vomiting

d. Diarrhea

e. Hypersensitivity reaction including fever, chills, shivering, headache, muscle and bone pain, and dyspnea

f. Increased liver function tests

g. Hepatotoxicity

h. Hepatitis-increased uric acid levels

i. Blood dyscrasias

j. Colitis

4. Implementation

a. Assess for hypersensitivity

b. Evaluate CBC, uric acid, and liver function tests

c. Assess for signs of hepatitis, and if they occur, hold medication and notify the physician

d. Monitor stools for signs of colitis

e. Monitor mental status

f. Assess for visual changes

5. Client education

   a. Instruct the client not to skip doses and to take medication for the full length of the prescribed therapy

   b. Instruct the client not to take any other medication without consulting the physician

   c. Advise the client of the importance of follow-up physician visits and lab tests

   d. Instruct clients to avoid alcohol

   e. Advise clients to take medication on an empty stomach with 8 oz of water 1 hour before or 2 hours after meals and to avoid taking antacids with the medication

   f. Instruct the client that urine, feces, sweat, and tears will be red-orange and that soft contact lens can become permanently discolored

   g. Instruct the client to notify the physician if yellow eyes or skin develops or if weakness, fatigue, nausea, vomiting, sore throat, fever, or unusual bleeding occurs

C. Ethambutol (Myambutol)

   1. Description

      a. Bacteriostatic

      b. Interferes with cell metabolism and multiplication by inhibiting one or more metabolites in susceptible bacteria

      c. Inhibits bacterial RNA synthesis

      d. Active only during cell division

      e. It is slow acting and must be used in combination with other bactericidal agents

   2. Contraindications and cautions

      a. Contraindicated in clients with hypersensitivity, optic neuritis, and in children under 13 years of age

      b. Use with caution in clients with renal dysfunction, gout, ocular defects, diabetic retinopathy, cataracts, and ocular inflammatory conditions

      c. Use with caution in the client taking neurotoxic medications because the risk for neurotoxicity increases

   3. Side effects

      a. Anorexia

      b. Nausea

      c. Vomiting

      d. Dizziness

      e. Malaise

      f. Mental confusion

      g. Joint pain

      h. Dermatitis

i. Optic neuritis

j. Peripheral neuritis

k. Thrombocytopenia

l. Increased uric acid levels

m. Anaphylactoid reaction

4. Implementation

   a. Assess for hypersensitivity

   b. Evaluate results of CBC, renal, and liver function tests

   c. Obtain baseline visual acuity and color discrimination, especially to the color green

   d. Monitor for visual changes such as altered color perception and decreased visual acuity, and if changes occur, discontinue medication and notify the physician

   e. Administer once every 24 hours with food to decrease GI upset

   f. Monitor uric acid concentrations and monitor for painful or swollen joints or signs of gout

   g. Monitor I&O and for adequate renal function

   h. Assess mental status

   i. Monitor for dizziness and initiate safety precautions

   j. Assess for peripheral neuritis (numbness, tingling, or burning of the extremities), and if it occurs, notify the physician

5. Client education

   a. Inform clients that they can prevent nausea related to the medications by taking the daily dose at bedtime or take prescribed antinausea medications

   b. Instruct the client not to skip doses and to take the medication for the full length of the prescribed therapy

   c. Instruct clients not to take any other medication without consulting the physician

   d. Advise clients of the importance of follow-up physician visits, vision testing, and lab tests

   e. Instruct the client to notify the physician immediately if visual problems, a rash, swelling and pain in the joints, or numbness, tingling, or burning in the hands or feet occurs

D. Streptomycin (Box 46–5)

   1. Description

      a. An aminoglycoside antibiotic that is used in conjunction with at least one other antitubercular medication

      b. Bactericidal because of receptor binding action, interfering with protein synthesis in susceptible microorganisms

   2. Contraindications and cautions

      a. Contraindicated in clients with hypersensitivity, myasthenia gravis, parkinsonism, or eighth cranial nerve damage

      b. Use with caution in the elderly, in

BOX 46–5. Toxic Effects of Streptomycin

NEPHROTOXICITY	NEUROTOXICITY
Changes in urine output	Muscle numbness
Increased thirst	Tingling
Decreased appetite	Twitching
Nausea/vomiting	Seizures

VESTIBULAR OTOTOXICITY	AUDITORY OTOTOXICITY
Dizziness	Ringing in the ears
Clumsiness	Loss of hearing
Unsteadiness	A full feeling in the ears

neonates because of renal insufficiency and immaturity, and in young infants because it may cause CNS depression
   c. The risk of toxicity increases when taken with other aminoglycosides, or nephrotoxic- or ototoxic-producing medications
3. Side effects
   a. Hypersensitivity
   b. Loss of vision
   c. Neuromuscular blockade
   d. Increased liver and renal function tests
   e. Signs of peripheral neuritis such as burning of the face or mouth
4. Implementation
   a. Assess for hypersensitivity
   b. Monitor liver and renal function tests
   c. Obtain baseline audiometric test and repeat every 1 to 2 months because the medication impairs the eighth cranial nerve
   d. Monitor for ototoxic, neurotoxic, and nephrotoxic reactions
   e. Assess hearing acuity
   f. Monitor for visual changes
   g. Assess hydration status and maintain adequate hydration during therapy
   h. Monitor I&O
   i. Assess urinalysis
   j. Monitor for superinfections
   k. Monitor for signs of peripheral neuritis
5. Client education
   a. Instruct the client not to skip doses and to take medication for the full length of the prescribed therapy
   b. Instruct clients not to take any other medication without consulting the physician
   c. Advise clients of the importance of follow-up physician visits and lab tests
   d. Instruct the client to notify the physician if hearing loss, changes in vision, or urinary problems occur
E. Pyrazinamide (Tebrazid)
  1. Description

   a. Exact mechanism of action is unknown
   b. May be bacteriostatic or bactericidal depending on its concentration at the infection site and susceptibility of infecting bacteria
   c. Used in conjunction with at least one other antitubercular medication after failure or ineffectiveness of the primary medications occurs
2. Contraindications and cautions
   a. Contraindicated in clients with hypersensitivity
   b. Use with caution in clients with diabetes mellitus, renal impairment, gout, and in children
   c. May decrease the effects of allopurinol (Zyloprim), colchicine, probenecid (Benemid), sulfinpyrazone (Anturane)
   d. Cross-sensitivity is possible with isoniazid (INH), ethionamide (Trecator-SC) or niacin, nicotinic acid (Nicobid)
3. Side effects
   a. Increases liver function and uric acid levels
   b. Arthralgia
   c. Myalgia
   d. Photosensitivity
   e. Hepatotoxicity
   f. Thrombocytopenia
4. Implementation
   a. Assess for hypersensitivity
   b. Evaluate CBC, liver function tests, and uric acid levels
   c. Observe for hepatotoxic effects, and if they occur hold medication and notify the physician
   d. Assess for painful or swollen joints
   e. Evaluate blood glucose and diabetic status because diabetes may be difficult to control while on medication
5. Client education
   a. Instruct clients to take the medication with food to reduce GI distress
   b. Instruct the client to avoid sunlight or ultraviolet light until photosensitivity is determined
   c. Instruct clients to notify the physician if any side effects occur
   d. Instruct clients not to skip doses and to take medication for the full length of the prescribed therapy
   e. Instruct clients not to take any other medication without consulting the physician
   f. Advise the client of the importance of follow-up physician visits and lab tests

XXVII. Second-Line Medications

A. Capreomycin sulfate (Capastat Sulfate)
  1. Description
   a. Mechanism of action is unknown

b. Used to treat **MDRTB** when significant resistance to other medications is expected

c. Must be given IM

2. Contraindications and cautions
   a. The risk of nephrotoxicity, ototoxicity, and neuromuscular blockade is increased with the use of aminoglycosides or loop diuretics
   b. Use with caution in clients with renal insufficiency, acoustic nerve impairment, hepatic disorder, myasthenia gravis, and parkinsonism
   c. Do not administer to the client receiving streptomycin

3. Side effects
   a. Nephrotoxicity
   b. Ototoxicity
   c. Neuromuscular blockade

4. Implementation
   a. Perform baseline audiometric testing
   b. Monitor renal and hepatic electrolyte levels prior to administration
   c. Monitor I&O
   d. Reconstitute medication with 2 mL 0.9% isotonic NaCl injection or sterile water for IM injection; allow 2 to 3 minutes for the medication to dissolve
   e. Reconstituted medication may be stored for 48 hours at room temperature
   f. Administer deep IM in a large muscle mass
   g. Rotate injection sites
   h. Observe injection site for redness, excessive bleeding, and inflammation

5. Client education
   a. Instruct clients not to perform tasks that require mental alertness
   b. Instruct the client to report any hearing loss, balance disturbances, respiratory difficulty, weakness, or signs of hypersensitivity reactions

B. Kanamycin (Kantrex)
1. Description
   a. An aminoglycoside antibiotic that is used in conjunction with at least one other antitubercular medication
   b. Bactericidal because of receptor binding action, interfering with protein synthesis in susceptible microorganisms

2. Contraindications and cautions
   a. Contraindicated in clients with hypersensitivity, neuromuscular disorders, or eighth cranial nerve damage
   b. Use with caution in the elderly, in neonates because of renal insufficiency and immaturity, and in young infants because it may cause CNS depression
   c. The risk of toxicity increases when taken with other aminoglycosides, or nephrotoxic- or ototoxic-producing medications

3. Side effects
   a. Hypersensitivity
   b. Pain and irritation at the injection site
   c. Nephrotoxicity as evidenced by increased BUN and serum creatinine
   d. Ototoxicity as evidenced by tinnitus, dizziness, ringing/roaring in the ears, and reduced hearing
   e. Neurotoxicity as evidenced by headache, dizziness, lethargy, tremors, and visual disturbances
   f. Superinfections

4. Implementation
   a. Monitor for hypersensitivity
   b. Monitor liver and renal function tests
   c. Obtain baseline audiometric test and repeat every 1 to 2 months because the medication impairs the eighth cranial nerve
   d. Monitor for ototoxic, neurotoxic, and nephrotoxic reactions
   e. Monitor hearing acuity
   f. Monitor for visual changes
   g. Monitor hydration status and maintain adequate hydration during therapy
   h. Monitor I&O
   i. Monitor urinalysis
   j. Monitor for superinfections

5. Client education
   a. Instruct the client not to skip doses and to take medication for the full length of the prescribed therapy
   b. Instruct the client not to take any other medication without consulting the physician
   c. Advise clients of the importance of follow-up physician visits and lab tests
   d. Instruct clients to notify physician if hearing loss, changes in vision, or urinary problems occur

C. Ethionamide (Trecator-SC)
1. Description
   a. Mechanism of action is unknown
   b. Used to treat **(MDRTB)** when significant resistance to other medications is expected

2. Contraindications and cautions
   a. Contraindicated in clients with hypersensitivity
   b. Use with caution in clients with diabetes mellitus or renal dysfunction

3. Side effects
   a. Anorexia
   b. Nausea
   c. Vomiting
   d. Metallic taste in the mouth
   e. Orthostatic hypotension
   f. Jaundice
   g. Mental changes
   h. Peripheral neuritis
   i. Rash

4. Implementation

a. Monitor liver and renal function tests
b. Monitor glucose levels in the diabetic client
c. Administer pyridoxine as prescribed to reduce the risk of neurotoxicity
5. Client education
   a. Instruct clients to take medication with food or meals to minimize GI irritation
   b. Instruct clients to change positions slowly
   c. Instruct clients to report signs of a rash, which can progress to exfoliative dermatitis if the medication is not discontinued
   d. Instruct the client to avoid alcohol
   e. Instruct the client to report signs of jaundice
   f. Instruct clients to report side effects of the medication if they occur
D. Aminosalicylate sodium (sodium para-aminosalicylic acid [PAS])
   1. Description
      a. Inhibits folic acid metabolism in mycobacteria
      b. Used to treat **MDRTB** when significant resistance to other medications is expected
   2. Contraindications and cautions
      a. Contraindicated with hypersensitivity to aminosalicylates, salicylates, or compounds containing para-aminophenyl group
      b. Aminobenzoates block the absorption of aminosalicylate sodium (sodium para-aminosalicylic acid [PAS])
   3. Side effects
      a. Bitter taste in the mouth
      b. GI tract irritation
      c. Allergic reactions
      d. Exfoliative dermatitis
      e. Blood dyscrasias
      f. Crystalluria
      g. Changes in thyroid function
   4. Implementation
      a. Monitor for hypersensitivity
      b. Offer clear water to rinse the mouth; chewing gum or sucking on hard candy will alleviate the bitter taste
      c. Encourage fluid intake to prevent crystalluria
      d. Monitor I&O
   5. Client education
      a. Instruct the client to discard the medication if a purplish brown discoloration occurs
      b. Instruct clients to take medication with food or antacids
      c. Inform clients that urine may turn red on contact with hypochlorite bleach if the bleach was used to clean a toilet
      d. Instruct the client not to take aspirin or over-the-counter medications without the physician's approval

e. Inform diabetic clients that a false-positive result can occur in glucose monitoring
f. Instruct clients to report signs of blood dyscrasia such as sore throat or mouth, malaise, fatigue, bruising, or bleeding
E. Cycloserine (Seromycin)
   1. Description
      a. Interferes with cell wall biosynthesis
      b. Used to treat **(MDRTB)** when significant resistance to other medications is expected
   2. Contraindications and cautions
      a. Use of alcohol or ethionamide (Trecator-SC) increases the risk of seizures
      b. Use with caution in clients with epilepsy, depression, severe anxiety, psychosis, renal insufficiency, or the client who uses alcohol
   3. Side effects
      a. Hypersensitivity
      b. CNS reactions
      c. Neurotoxicity
      d. Seizures
      e. CHF
      f. Headache
      g. Vertigo
      h. Altered LOC
      i. Anxiety
      j. Confusion
      k. Depression
      l. Irritability
      m. Nervousness
      n. Mood changes
      o. Thoughts of suicide
   4. Implementation
      a. Monitor LOC
      b. Monitor for changes in mental status
      c. Monitor renal and hepatic function tests
      d. Monitor serum drug level to avoid the risk of neurotoxicity; peak concentrations, measured 2 hours after dosing, should be 25 to 35 μg/ml
   5. Client education
      a. Instruct the client to take the medication after meals to prevent GI upset
      b. Instruct the client to avoid alcohol
      c. Instruct the client to report signs of a rash or signs of CNS toxicity
      d. Instruct clients to avoid driving or performing tasks that require alertness until the reaction to the medication has been determined
      e. Advise clients of the need for weekly serum drug levels

PRACTICE QUESTIONS

1. The nurse is assisting in planning care for a client scheduled for insertion of a tracheostomy. What equipment does the nurse plan to have at the bedside when the client returns from surgery?

1 Oral airway
2 Epinephrine
3 Obturator
4 Tracheostomy set with the next larger size

2. The nursing instructor is observing a nursing student suctioning a client through a tracheostomy tube. Which of the following observations, if made by the nursing instructor, indicates an inappropriate action?
   1 Hyperventilating the client with 100% oxygen prior to suctioning
   2 Instilling 3 to 5 mL normal saline in the tracheotomy tube to loosen secretions
   3 Suctioning the client every hour
   4 Applying suction only during withdrawal of the catheter

3. The nurse is caring for a client with an endotracheal tube attached to a ventilator. The high-pressure alarm sounds on the ventilator. The nurse prepares to perform which of the following most appropriate nursing interventions?
   1 Check for a disconnection
   2 Evaluate the cuff for a leak
   3 Notify the respiratory therapist
   4 Suction the client

4. The nurse is preparing to obtain a sputum specimen from the client. Which of the following nursing actions facilitates obtaining the specimen?
   1 Limiting fluids
   2 Having the client take three deep breaths
   3 Ask the client to spit into the collection container
   4 Ask the client to obtain the specimen after eating

5. The nurse is caring for a client following a bronchoscopy and biopsy. Which of the following signs if noted in the client should be reported immediately?
   1 Blood-streaked sputum
   2 Dry cough
   3 Hematuria
   4 Laryngeal stridor

6. The nurse is suctioning a client via a tracheostomy tube. When suctioning, the nurse must limit the suctioning to a maximum of
   1 5 seconds
   2 15 seconds
   3 30 seconds
   4 1 minute

7. The nurse is suctioning a client through an endotracheal tube. During the suctioning procedure the nurse notes cardiac irregularities on the monitor. Which of the following is the most appropriate nursing intervention?
   1 Continue to suction

2 Ensure that the suction is limited to 15 seconds
3 Stop the procedure and reoxygenate the client
4 Notify the physician immediately

8. The nurse is preparing for removal of an endotracheal tube (ET) from a client. In preparing to assist the physician in this procedure, which of the following initial nursing actions is most appropriate?
   1 Suction the ET tube
   2 Deflate the cuff
   3 Turn the ventilator to the off position
   4 Obtain a code cart and place it at the bedside

9. The nurse is preparing to care for a client who will be weaned from a tracheostomy tube. The nurse is planning to use a tracheostomy plug and to insert it into the opening in the outer cannula. Which of the following nursing interventions is required prior to plugging the tube?
   1 Suction the client
   2 Deflate the cuff
   3 Ensure that the client is able to swallow
   4 Ensure that the client is able to speak

10. The nurse is caring for a client with a chest tube drainage system. The nurse notes a fluctuating water level on inspiration and expiration in the submerged tube in the water seal chamber of the chest tube system. Which nursing action is most appropriate?
    1 No action is necessary
    2 Encourage coughing and deep breathing
    3 Suction the client
    4 Increase the suction

11. The emergency room nurse is caring for a client who sustained a blunt injury to the chest wall. Which of the following signs if noted in the client indicates the presence of a pneumothorax?
    1 A sucking sound at the site of injury
    2 Diminished breath sounds
    3 A low respiratory rate
    4 The presence of a barrel chest

12. The nurse is caring for a client hospitalized with acute exacerbation of chronic obstructive pulmonary disease (COPD). Which of the following does the nurse expect to note in evaluating this client?
    1 Increased oxygen saturation with exercise
    2 A shortened expiratory phase of respiration
    3 A hyperinflated chest on x-ray
    4 A widened diaphragm noted on chest x-ray

13. An oxygen delivery system is prescribed for the client with chronic airflow limitation (CAL) in order to deliver a precise oxygen concentration. Which of the following types of oxygen delivery systems does the nurse anticipate to be prescribed?

1 Venturi mask
2 Aerosol mask
3 Face tent
4 Tracheostomy collar

14. Theophylline (Theo-Dur) tablets are prescribed for the client with chronic airflow limitation (CAL). The nurse reinforces instructions with the client about the medication. Which of the following nursing statements is not a component of the teaching plan?
    1 "Take the medication on an empty stomach."
    2 "Take the medication with food."
    3 "Continue to take the medication even if you are feeling better."
    4 "Periodic blood levels will need to be obtained."

15. The nurse is reinforcing instructions with the hospitalized client with emphysema, measures that will enhance the effectiveness of breathing during dyspneic periods. Which of the following positions does the nurse instruct the client to assume?
    1 Side lying in bed
    2 Sitting in a recliner chair
    3 Sitting up in bed
    4 Sitting on the side of the bed leaning on an overbed table

16. The nurse is gathering data on a client with a diagnosis of tuberculosis (TB). The nurse reviews the results of which of the following diagnostic tests that will confirm this diagnosis?
    1 Bronchoscopy
    2 Chest x-ray
    3 Sputum culture
    4 Tuberculin skin test

17. The nursing instructor asks the nursing student to describe the route of transmission of tuberculosis (TB). The nursing instructor evaluates that the student understands this route of transmission if the student states that TB is transmitted by
    1 The airborne route
    2 Blood and body fluids
    3 Fomites
    4 Hand to mouth

18. The nurse is caring for a client with emphysema. The client is receiving oxygen. The nurse checks the oxygen flow rate to ensure that it does not exceed
    1 1 L/minute
    2 1 to 3 L/minute
    3 6 L/minute
    4 10 to 12 L/minute

19. The nurse instructs the client in pursed-lip breathing. The client asks the nurse about the purpose of this type of breathing. The nurse tells the client that the primary purpose of pursed-lip breathing is to
    1 Promote oxygen intake
    2 Strengthen the diaphragm
    3 Strengthen the intercostal muscles
    4 Promote carbon dioxide elimination

20. The low-pressure alarm sounds on the ventilator. The nurse checks the client and then attempts to determine the cause of the alarm. The nurse cannot determine the cause of the alarm. Which of the following initial actions does the nurse take?
    1 Check the client's vital signs
    2 Ventilate the client manually
    3 Administer oxygen
    4 Start cardiopulmonary resuscitation (CPR)

21. The client is receiving isoetharine hydrochloride (Bronkosol) using a nebulizer. The nurse monitors for which of the following as a side effect of this medication?
    1 Constipation
    2 Diarrhea
    3 Bradycardia
    4 Tachycardia

22. The nurse is caring for a client who is on strict bed rest. The nurse assists in developing a plan of care and suggests goals related to the prevention of deep vein thrombosis (DVT) and pulmonary emboli. Which of the following nursing actions is most helpful to prevent these disorders from developing?
    1 Applying a heating pad to the lower extremities
    2 Encouraging active ROM exercises
    3 Placing a pillow under the knees
    4 Restricting fluids

23. A client is suspected of having pulmonary emboli (PE). The nurse understands that which of the following is not a common clinical manifestation of PE?
    1 Decreased respirations
    2 Tachypnea
    3 Dyspnea
    4 Chest pain

24. The nurse is planning to teach a client about the use of a respiratory inhaler. Which of the following is not a component of the teaching plan?
    1 Remove the cap and shake the inhaler well before use
    2 Press the canister down with your finger as you breathe in
    3 Inhale the mist and quickly exhale
    4 Wait 1 minute between puffs if more than one puff has been prescribed

25. The nurse is assigned to care for a client following a left pneumonectomy. The nurse avoids positioning this client
    1 On the side
    2 Semi-Fowler's
    3 Low Fowler's
    4 With the head of the bed elevated 40 degrees

26. The nurse is performing nasotracheal suctioning on a client. The nurse interprets that the client is adequately tolerating the procedure if which of the following observations is made?
    1 Secretions are becoming bloody
    2 Heart rate decreases from 78 to 54
    3 Coughing occurs with suctioning
    4 Skin color becomes cyanotic

27. The nurse is monitoring the function of a client's chest tube. The chest tube is attached to a Pleurevac drainage system. The nurse notes that the fluid in the water seal chamber rises with inspiration and falls with expiration. The nurse interprets that
    1 The client has residual pneumothorax
    2 The system is patent
    3 Suction should be added to the system
    4 There is a leak in the system

28. The client has a chest tube attached to a Pleurevac drainage system. As part of routine nursing care, the nurse ensures that
    1 The connection between the chest tube and the drainage system is taped, and that an occlusive dressing is maintained at the insertion site
    2 The amount of drainage into the chest tube is noted and recorded every 24 hours in the client's record
    3 The suction control chamber has sterile water added every shift, and that the system is kept below waist level
    4 The water seal chamber has continuous bubbling, and that monitoring for crepitus is done once a shift

29. A female client is scheduled to have a chest x-ray. Which of the following questions is of most importance to the nurse during data collection with this client?
    1 "Is there any possibility that you could be pregnant?"
    2 "Are you wearing any metal chains or jewelry?"
    3 "Can you hold your breath easily?"
    4 "Are you able to hold your arms above your head?"

30. The nurse is caring for the client after pulmonary angiography with catheter insertion via the left groin. The nurse monitors for an allergic reaction to the contrast medium by noting the presence of

    1 Hematoma in the left groin
    2 Discomfort in the left groin
    3 Stridor
    4 Hypothermia

31. An elderly client hospitalized with a rib fracture asks the nurse why the nurse is not strapping the ribs. Which of the following responses by the nurse is the most appropriate?
    1 "That isn't done anymore because people often develop pneumonia from the constricting effect on the lungs."
    2 "That might help you breathe better, but this facility does not carry rib straps in the stockroom. When you get home, you can purchase a rib strap at the medical supply store."
    3 "Rib straps are only useful if the ribs are fractured in several places at once."
    4 "That's a good idea. I'll ask the physician for an order for a rib strap this afternoon."

32. The nurse is teaching the client with chronic respiratory failure how to use a metered dose inhaler correctly. The nurse instructs the client to
    1 Inhale through the nose
    2 Inhale quickly
    3 Take two inhalations during one breath
    4 Hold the breath after inhalation

33. The nurse is caring for the client who is suspected of having lung cancer. The nurse monitors the client for which of the following frequent early symptoms of lung cancer?
    1 Hemoptysis
    2 Cough
    3 Hoarseness
    4 Pleuritic pain

34. The nurse is caring for the client who has had a pulmonary resection. The nurse avoids which of the following as the least effective method of splinting the client's incision for coughing and deep breathing?
    1 Apply firm, even pressure to the site after a deep breath and before a cough
    2 Apply firm pressure with the hands before the client takes a deep breath to cough
    3 Have the client hold a pillow firmly against the incision during a cough.
    4 Put support under the incision and push down on the shoulder during a cough.

35. The client has had radical neck dissection and begins to hemorrhage at the incision site. Which of the following actions by the nurse is contraindicated?
    1 Lowering the head of bed to a flat position
    2 Applying manual pressure over the site
    3 Monitoring the client's airway
    4 Calling the physician immediately

36. The nurse is reinforcing discharge instructions to the client with pulmonary sarcoidosis. The nurse evaluates that the client understands the information if the client verbalizes to report which of the following early signs of exacerbation?
    1 Fever
    2 Weight loss
    3 Fatigue
    4 Shortness of breath

37. The nurse working on a medical respiratory nursing unit is caring for several clients with respiratory disorders. The nurse identifies which of the following clients on the nursing unit as being at the least risk for infection with tuberculosis?
    1 A woman newly immigrated from Korea
    2 An uninsured man who is homeless
    3 An elderly woman admitted from a long-term care facility
    4 A man who is an inspector for the U.S. Postal Service

38. The nurse is reading the PPD skin test results for a client with no documented health problems. The site has no induration and a l-mm area of ecchymosis. The nurse interprets that the result is
    1 Positive
    2 Negative
    3 Uncertain
    4 Borderline

39. The nurse reads the client's Mantoux skin test as positive. The nurse notes that previous tests were negative. The client becomes upset and asks the nurse what this means. The nurse's response is based on the understanding that the client has
    1 No evidence of tuberculosis
    2 Systemic tuberculosis
    3 Pulmonary tuberculosis
    4 Exposure to tuberculosis

40. The nurse is caring for the client who had a PPD skin test planted 48 hours ago upon admission to the nursing unit. The nurse reads the result as positive. Which of the following actions by the nurse has the highest priority?
    1 Report the findings to the physician
    2 Call the radiology department for a chest x-ray
    3 Document the finding in the client's record
    4 Call the employee health service department

41. The nurse is caring for the client with tuberculosis who is fearful of the disease and anxious about prognosis. In planning nursing care, the nurse incorporates which of the following as the best strategy to assist the client in coping with the illness?
    1 Encourage the client to visit with the pastoral care department chaplain
    2 Ask family members if they wish a psychiatric consult

3 Provide reassurance that continued compliance with medication therapy is the most proactive way to cope with the disease
    4 Allow the client to deal with the disease individually

42. The nurse has instructed the client diagnosed with tuberculosis about how to prevent the spread of infection after discharge. The nurse evaluates that the client needs further reinforcement of information if the client makes which of the following statements?
    1 "It's very important to wash my hands after I touch my mask, tissues, or body fluids."
    2 "I should cough into tissues and throw them away carefully."
    3 "It's important to cover my mouth if I laugh, sneeze, or cough."
    4 "I should use disposable plates, forks, and knives."

43. The nurse is caring for the client diagnosed with tuberculosis. Which of the following findings, if made by the nurse, is not consistent with the usual clinical presentation of tuberculosis?
    1 Nonproductive or productive cough
    2 Anorexia and weight loss
    3 Chills and night sweats
    4 High-grade fever

44. The client is being discharged to home after 2 weeks of hospitalization for a diagnosis of tuberculosis (TB), and is worried about the possibility of infecting family and others. The nurse interprets that the client would get the most reassurance from the knowledge that
    1 The family does not need therapy, and the client will not be contagious after 1 month of drug therapy
    2 The family does not need therapy, and the client will not be contagious after 6 consecutive weeks of drug therapy
    3 The family will receive prophylactic therapy, and the client will not be contagious after 1 continuous week of drug therapy
    4 The family will be treated prophylactically, and the client will not be contagious after 2 to 3 consecutive weeks of drug therapy

45. The client diagnosed with tuberculosis is distressed over the loss of physical stamina and fatigue. The nurse plans to teach the client that
    1 This is a short-lived problem, which should be gone within 1 week of drug therapy
    2 This is an unexpected finding with TB, but it should resolve within a month or so
    3 This is expected, and the client should very gradually increase activity as tolerated
    4 This is expected, and will last for at least a year

46. The nurse is teaching the client with tuberculosis (TB) about dietary elements that should be increased in the diet. The nurse suggests that the client increase intake of
    1 Meats and citrus fruits
    2 Grains and broccoli
    3 Eggs and spinach
    4 Potatoes and fish

47. The nurse has reinforced discharge teaching with the client who was diagnosed with tuberculosis. The client has been on medication for a week and a half. The nurse evaluates that the client has understood the information if the client makes which of the following statements?
    1 "I need to continue drug therapy for 2 months."
    2 "I should not be contagious after 2 to 3 weeks of medication therapy."
    3 "I can't shop at the mall for the next 6 months."
    4 "I can return to work if a sputum culture comes back negative."

48. The client with tuberculosis asks the nurse about precautions to take after discharge to prevent infection of others. The nurse responds to the client's question based on the understanding that
    1 The client should maintain enteric precautions only
    2 The disease is transmitted by droplet nuclei
    3 Clothing and sheets should be bleached after each use
    4 Deep-pile carpet should be removed from the home

49. The nurse is preparing to give a bed bath to the immobilized client with tuberculosis. The nurse plans to wear which of the following items when performing this care?
    1 Particulate respirator, gown, and gloves
    2 Particulate respirator and protective eyewear
    3 Surgical mask and gloves
    4 Surgical mask, gown, and protective eyewear

50. The client with tuberculosis, whose status is being monitored in an ambulatory care clinic, asks the nurse when it is permissible to return to work. The nurse replies that the client may resume employment when
    1 Two sputum cultures are negative
    2 Five sputum cultures are negative
    3 A sputum culture and a chest x-ray are negative
    4 A sputum culture and a PPD test are negative

51. The nurse has given the client with tuberculosis instructions for proper handling and disposal of respiratory secretions. The nurse evaluates that the client understands the instructions if the client verbalizes to
    1 Wash hands at least four times a day
    2 Turn the head to the side if coughing or sneezing
    3 Discard used tissues in a plastic bag
    4 Brush the teeth and rinse the mouth once a day

52. The client has been taking isoniazid (INH) for a month and a half. The client complains to the nurse about numbness, paresthesias, and tingling in the extremities. The nurse interprets that the client is experiencing
    1 Small blood vessel spasm
    2 Impaired peripheral circulation
    3 Hypercalcemia
    4 Peripheral neuritis

53. The client is to begin a 6-month course of therapy with isoniazid (INH). The nurse plans to teach the client to
    1 Use alcohol in small amounts only
    2 Report yellow eyes or skin immediately
    3 Increase the intake of Swiss or aged cheeses
    4 Avoid vitamin supplements during therapy

54. The client has been started on long-term therapy with rifampin (Rifadin). The nurse teaches the client that the medication
    1 Should be double dosed if one dose is forgotten
    2 May be discontinued independently if symptoms are gone in 3 months
    3 Causes orange discoloration of sweat, tears, urne, and feces
    4 Should always be taken with food or antacids

55. The nurse has given the client taking ethambutol (Myambutol) information about the medication. The nurse evaluates that the client understands the instructions if the client states to immediately report
    1 Distressing GI side effects
    2 Impaired sense of hearing
    3 Orange-red discoloration of body secretions
    4 Difficulty discriminating the color red from green

ANSWERS

1. **3**

RATIONALE: A replacement tube of the same size and an obturator is kept at the bedside at all times in case the tracheostomy tube is dislodged. Additionally, a curved hemostat that could be used to hold the trachea open if dislodgment occurs should also be kept at the bedside. Oral airway and epinephrine are not needed.

TEST-TAKING STRATEGY: Eliminate option 4 first because a tracheostomy set of the next larger size is not appropriate for the client. Next eliminate option 2 because it is unrelated to the issue of the question. From the remaining options, recall that the airway has been altered because of the tracheostomy, so an oral airway is not necessary. Remember that a replacement tube and an obturator should be kept at the bedside of a client with a tracheostomy, along with a curved hemostat, at all times.

LEVEL OF COGNITIVE ABILITY: Application
PHASE OF NURSING PROCESS: Planning
CLIENT NEEDS: Physiological Integrity
CONTENT AREA: Adult Health/Respiratory
REFERENCE
Monahan, F., & Neighbors, M. (1998). *Medical-surgical nursing: Foundations for clinical practice* (2nd ed.). Philadelphia: W. B. Saunders. p. 566.

2. **3**

RATIONALE: The client should be suctioned as needed. Suctioning unnecessarily needs to be avoided because it can increase secretions and cause mechanical trauma to the tissues. The client should be hyperoxygenated with 100% oxygen prior to suctioning and if tracheal secretions are thick and not easily removed, directly instill 3 to 5 mL of sterile normal saline into the trachea to try to reduce the viscosity of the secretions and stimulate coughing. Suction is not applied during insertion of the catheter, and intermittent suction and a twirling motion of the catheter are used during withdrawal.

TEST-TAKING STRATEGY: Note the key word "inappropriate" in the question, then carefully read each option attempting to visualize the procedure. Note the key words in option 3, "every hour." This should assist in directing you in selecting this option. The client should be suctioned as needed, not on a preset scheduled time unless specifically required and indicated by the physician.

LEVEL OF COGNITIVE ABILITY: Comprehension
PHASE OF NURSING PROCESS: Evaluation
CLIENT NEEDS: Physiological Integrity
CONTENT AREA: Adult Health/Respiratory
REFERENCE
Monahan, F., & Neighbors, M. (1998). *Medical-surgical nursing: Foundations for clinical practice* (2nd ed.). Philadelphia: W. B. Saunders. p. 566.

3. **4**

RATIONALE: When the high-pressure alarm sounds on a ventilator, it is most likely due to an obstruction. The obstruction can be caused by the client biting on the tube, kinking of the tubing, or mucus plugging requiring suctioning. It is also important to assess the tubing for the presence of any water and determine if the client is out of rhythm with breathing with the ventilator.

TEST-TAKING STRATEGY: Note the key words "high-pressure alarm" in the question. Recalling that that the high-pressure alarm indicates a possible obstruction will assist in directing you to the correct option. Review nursing interventions related to care of a client on a ventilator now if you had difficulty with this question.

LEVEL OF COGNITIVE ABILITY: Application
PHASE OF NURSING PROCESS: Planning
CLIENT NEEDS: Physiological Integrity
CONTENT AREA: Adult Health/Respiratory
REFERENCE
Black, J., & Matassarin-Jacobs, E. (1997). *Medical-surgical nursing: Clinical management for continuity of care* (5th ed.). Philadelphia: W. B. Saunders. p. 1186.

4. **2**

RATIONALE: To obtain a sputum specimen, the client should brush the teeth to reduce contamination then cough into a sputum specimen container. The client should be encouraged to cough and not spit so as to obtain sputum. Sputum can be thinned by fluids or by a respiratory treatment such as inhalation of nebulized saline or water. The optimal time to obtain a specimen is upon arising in the morning.

TEST-TAKING STRATEGY: Read each option carefully using the process of elimination. Option 1 can be eliminated first because general principles indicate that fluids assist in loosening or thinning secretions. Eliminate option 3 because of the word "spit." Spit is very different from saliva. Next eliminate option 4 because of the words "after eating."

LEVEL OF COGNITIVE ABILITY: Application
PHASE OF NURSING PROCESS: Planning
CLIENT NEEDS: Physiological Integrity
CONTENT AREA: Adult Health/Respiratory
REFERENCE
Black, J., & Matassarin-Jacobs, E. (1997). *Medical-surgical nursing: Clinical management for continuity of care* (5th ed.). Philadelphia: W. B. Saunders. p. 1063.

5. **4**

RATIONALE: If a biopsy was performed during a bronchoscopy, blood-streaked sputum is expected for several hours. Frank blood is indicative of hemorrhage. A dry cough may be expected. The client should be assessed for signs of complications, which would include cyanosis, dyspnea, stridor, hemoptysis, hypotension, tachycardia, and dysrhythmias. Hematuria is unrelated to this procedure.

TEST-TAKING STRATEGY: Eliminate option 3 first because it is unrelated to the procedure. Next eliminate option 2 because a dry cough may be expected. Noting that a biopsy has been performed will assist in eliminating option 1, as pink-tinged sputum would be expected. Note that option 4, the correct option, relates to airway. If you had difficulty with this question, review postprocedure care following bronchoscopy with biopsy.

LEVEL OF COGNITIVE ABILITY: Application
PHASE OF NURSING PROCESS: Data Collection
CLIENT NEEDS: Physiological Integrity
CONTENT AREA: Adult Health/Respiratory
REFERENCE
Monahan, F., & Neighbors, M. (1998). *Medical-surgical nursing: Foundations for clinical practice* (2nd ed.). Philadelphia: W. B. Saunders. p. 549.

6. **2**

RATIONALE: Hypoxemia can be caused by prolonged suctioning from stimulation of the pacemaker cells within the

heart. A vasovagal response may occur, causing bradycardia. Limit suctioning pass to 15 seconds and preoxygenate the client prior to suctioning.
TEST-TAKING STRATEGY: Knowledge regarding the procedure for suctioning is required to answer this question. Recall that during suctioning the client's airway is blocked; therefore, you should be able to eliminate options 3 and 4 readily easily. From the remaining 2 options, eliminate option 1 because of the very short time frame. It does not seem reasonable that 5 seconds would achieve removal of secretions. Review the procedure for suctioning now if you had difficulty with this question.
LEVEL OF COGNITIVE ABILITY: Application
PHASE OF NURSING PROCESS: Implementation
CLIENT NEEDS: Physiological Integrity
CONTENT AREA: Adult Health/Respiratory
REFERENCE
Black, J., & Matassarin-Jacobs, E. (1997). *Medical-surgical nursing: Clinical management for continuity of care* (5th ed.). Philadelphia: W. B. Saunders. p. 1175.

7. **3**

RATIONALE: During suctioning, the nurse should monitor the client closely for side effects including hypoxemia, cardiac irregularities due to vagal stimulation, mucosal trauma, hypotension, and paroxysmal coughing. If side effects develop, especially cardiac irregularities, stop the procedure and reoxygenate the client.
TEST-TAKING STRATEGY: Use the process of elimination, recalling that suction can cause cardiac irregularities. This principle should easily direct you to option 3. If you had difficulty with this question, review the complications and interventions associated with suctioning procedure.
LEVEL OF COGNITIVE ABILITY: Application
PHASE OF NURSING PROCESS: Implementation
CLIENT NEEDS: Physiological Integrity
CONTENT AREA: Adult Health/Respiratory
REFERENCE
Black, J., & Matassarin-Jacobs, E. (1997). *Medical-surgical nursing: Clinical management for continuity of care* (5th ed.). Philadelphia: W. B. Saunders. p. 1176.

8. **1**

RATIONALE: Once the client has been weaned successfully and has achieved an acceptable level of consciousness to sustain spontaneous respiration, an ET tube may be removed. The ET tube is suctioned first and then the cuff is deflated and the tube is removed. There is no reason to have a code cart placed at the bedside, as this may cause alarm and concern in the client. Additionally, resuscitative equipment should have already been at the client's bedside.
TEST-TAKING STRATEGY: Note the key word "initial" in the stem of the question. Use the ABCs, airway, breathing, and circulation. Remember airway is the first priority.
LEVEL OF COGNITIVE ABILITY: Application
PHASE OF NURSING PROCESS: Planning
CLIENT NEEDS: Physiological Integrity
CONTENT AREA: Adult Health/Respiratory
REFERENCE
Black, J., & Matassarin-Jacobs, E. (1997). *Medical-surgical nursing: Clinical management for continuity of care* (5th ed.). Philadelphia: W. B. Saunders. p. 1184.

9. **2**

RATIONALE: Plugging a tracheostomy tube is usually done by inserting the tracheostomy plug (decannulation stopper) into the opening of the outer cannula. This closes off the tracheostomy, and airflow and respiration occur normally through the nose and mouth. When plugging a cuffed tracheostomy tube, the cuff must be deflated. If it remains inflated, ventilation cannot occur and respiratory arrest could result.
TEST-TAKING STRATEGY: Note the key word "required" in the question. This should assist in directing you to the option that addresses a priority physiological need. Use the process of elimination and you should easily be directed to option 2, as an inflated cuff would cause airway obstruction.
LEVEL OF COGNITIVE ABILITY: Comprehension
PHASE OF NURSING PROCESS: Planning
CLIENT NEEDS: Physiological Integrity
CONTENT AREA: Adult Health/Respiratory
REFERENCE
Black, J., & Matassarin-Jacobs, E. (1997). *Medical-surgical nursing: Clinical management for continuity of care* (5th ed.). Philadelphia: W. B. Saunders. p. 1071.

10. **1**

RATIONALE: With normal breathing, the water level rises with inspiration and falls with expiration. The opposite occurs when the client is on positive-pressure mechanical ventilation. This is an expected normal occurrence in a chest tube drainage system; therefore, no action is necessary.
TEST-TAKING STRATEGY: Knowledge regarding the normal expected findings in monitoring a chest tube drainage system is required to answer this question. Knowing that the fluctuating water level is expected will assist in directing you easily to option 1. Review chest tube drainage systems now if you had difficulty with this question.
LEVEL OF COGNITIVE ABILITY: Application
PHASE OF NURSING PROCESS: Implementation
CLIENT NEEDS: Physiological Integrity
CONTENT AREA: Adult Health/Respiratory
REFERENCE
Monahan, F., & Neighbors, M. (1998). *Medical-surgical nursing: Foundations for clinical practice* (2nd ed.). Philadelphia: W. B. Saunders. p. 578.

11. **2**

RATIONALE: This client has sustained a blunt or a closed-chest injury. Basic symptoms of a closed pneumothorax are shortness of breath and chest pain. A larger pneumothorax may present with tachypnea, cyanosis, diminished breath sounds, and subcutaneous emphysema. There may also be hyperresonance on the affected side.
TEST-TAKING STRATEGY: Note the key word "blunt" in the question. This will assist in eliminating option 1, sucking chest wound injury. Knowing that in a respiratory injury increased respirations will occur will assist in eliminating option 3. Option 4 can be eliminated because a barrel chest is a characteristic finding in a client with COPD.
LEVEL OF COGNITIVE ABILITY: Comprehension
PHASE OF NURSING PROCESS: Data Collection
CLIENT NEEDS: Physiological Integrity
CONTENT AREA: Adult Health/Respiratory
REFERENCE
Monahan, F., & Neighbors, M. (1998). *Medical-surgical nursing: Foundations for clinical practice* (2nd ed.). Philadelphia: W. B. Saunders. pp. 692–693.

12. 3

RATIONALE: Clinical manifestations of COPD include hypoxemia, hypercapnia, dyspnea on exertion and at rest, oxygen desaturation with exercise, use of accessory muscles of respirations, and a prolonged expiratory phase of respiration. Chest x-ray will reveal a hyperinflated chest and a flattened diaphragm if the disease is advanced.

TEST-TAKING STRATEGY: Use the process of elimination, reading each option carefully. Eliminate option 1 because oxygen desaturation rather than saturation would occur. Next eliminate option 2 because in the client with COPD, a prolonged expiratory phase would be noted. From the remaining options, reading carefully will assist in directing you to option 3, the correct option. If you are unfamiliar with the manifestations associated with COPD, take time now to review.

LEVEL OF COGNITIVE ABILITY: Comprehension
PHASE OF NURSING PROCESS: Data Collection
CLIENT NEEDS: Physiological Integrity
CONTENT AREA: Adult Health/Respiratory
REFERENCE
Monahan, F., & Neighbors, M. (1998). *Medical-surgical nursing: Foundations for clinical practice* (2nd ed.). Philadelphia: W. B. Saunders. p. 668.

13. 1

RATIONALE: The Venturi mask is the best oxygen delivery system for the client with CAL because it delivers a precise oxygen concentration. The face tent, aerosol mask, and tracheostomy collar are also high-flow oxygen delivery systems but are most often used to administer high humidity.

TEST-TAKING STRATEGY: Note the key words "precise oxygen concentration." Knowledge regarding the various types of oxygen delivery systems will assist in answering this question. Eliminate options 2, 3, and 4 because they are similar in that they are used to provide humidity.

LEVEL OF COGNITIVE ABILITY: Comprehension
PHASE OF NURSING PROCESS: Planning
CLIENT NEEDS: Physiological Integrity
CONTENT AREA: Adult Health/Respiratory
REFERENCE
deWit, S. (1998). *Essentials of medical-surgical nursing* (4th ed.). Philadelphia: W. B. Saunders. p. 452

14. 1

RATIONALE: The medication should be administered with food such as milk and crackers to prevent GI irritation. Options 2, 3, and 4 are appropriate instructions regarding the use of this medication.

TEST-TAKING STRATEGY: Noting that options 1 and 2 are opposite in terms of administering the medication should alert you that one of these options is the correct answer. Knowledge regarding the administration of this medication is required to answer correctly. If you are unfamiliar with this important medication, take time now to review.

LEVEL OF COGNITIVE ABILITY: Application
PHASE OF NURSING PROCESS: Planning
CLIENT NEEDS: Health Promotion and Maintenance
CONTENT AREA: Pharmacology
REFERENCE
Hodgson, B., & Kizior, R. (2000). *Saunders nursing drug handbook 2000.* W. B. Saunders. p. 44

15. 4

RATIONALE: Positions that will assist the client with breathing include sitting up and leaning on an overbed table, sitting up and resting with elbows on the knees, or standing and leaning against a wall.

TEST-TAKING STRATEGY: Eliminate options 2 and 3 first because they are similar. Next eliminate option 1 because this position will not enhance breathing. If you had difficulty with this question, take time now to review the positions that will decrease the work of breathing in a client with emphysema.

LEVEL OF COGNITIVE ABILITY: Application
PHASE OF NURSING PROCESS: Implementation
CLIENT NEEDS: Physiological Integrity
CONTENT AREA: Adult Health/Respiratory
REFERENCE
Monahan, F., & Neighbors, M. (1998). *Medical-surgical nursing: Foundations for clinical practice.* (2nd ed.). Philadelphia: W. B. Saunders. p. 677.

16. 3

RATIONALE: Definitive diagnosis of TB is confirmed through culture and isolation of *Mycobacterium tuberculosis*. A presumptive diagnosis is made on the basis of a tuberculin skin test, a sputum smear that is positive for acid-fast bacteria, a chest x-ray, and histologic evidence of granulomatous disease on biopsy.

TEST-TAKING STRATEGY: Note the key word "confirm" in the stem of the question. Confirmation is made by identifying *Mycobacterium tuberculosis*. If you had difficulty with this question, take time now to review diagnostic procedures related to TB.

LEVEL OF COGNITIVE ABILITY: Comprehension
PHASE OF NURSING PROCESS: Data Collection
CLIENT NEEDS: Physiological Integrity
CONTENT AREA: Adult Health/Respiratory
REFERENCE
Monahan, F., & Neighbors, M. (1998). *Medical-surgical nursing: Foundations for clinical practice* (2nd ed.). Philadelphia: W. B. Saunders. p. 652.

17. 1

RATIONALE: Tuberculosis is an infectious disease caused by the bacillus *Mycobacterium tuberculosis* and spread primarily by the airborne route. Options 2, 3, and 4 are incorrect.

TEST-TAKING STRATEGY: Knowledge that TB is a respiratory disease should easily direct you to option 1. If you had difficulty with this question, take time now to review the transmission of this important disease.

LEVEL OF COGNITIVE ABILITY: Comprehension
PHASE OF NURSING PROCESS: Evaluation
CLIENT NEEDS: Physiological Integrity
CONTENT AREA: Adult Health/Respiratory
REFERENCE
Monahan, F., & Neighbors, M. (1998). *Medical-surgical nursing: Foundations for clinical practice* (2nd ed.). Philadelphia: W. B. Saunders. p. 650.

18. 2

RATIONALE: One to 3 liters of oxygen by nasal cannula may be required to raise the PaO_2 to 60 to 80 mmHg. However, oxygen is used cautiously and should not exceed 3 liters. Because of the long-standing hypercapnia, the respiratory drive is triggered by low oxygen levels rather than increased carbon dioxide levels, as is the case in a normal respiratory system.

TEST-TAKING STRATEGY: Knowledge regarding the physiology associated with emphysema is required to answer this question. If you are unfamiliar with this important concept, take time now to review.
LEVEL OF COGNITIVE ABILITY: Comprehension
PHASE OF NURSING PROCESS: Data Collection
CLIENT NEEDS: Physiological Integrity
CONTENT AREA: Adult Health/Respiratory
REFERENCE
Black, J., & Matassarin-Jacobs, E. (1997). *Medical-surgical nursing: Clinical management for continuity of care* (5th ed.). Philadelphia: W. B. Saunders. p. 1117.

19. 4

RATIONALE: Pursed-lip breathing facilitates maximal expiration for clients with obstructive lung disease. This type of breathing allows better expiration by increasing airway pressure that keeps air passages open during exhalation. Options 1, 2, and 3 are not the purposes of this type of breathing.
TEST-TAKING STRATEGY: Attempt to visualize the use of this procedure to assist you in answering correctly. Knowledge regarding the respiratory conditions in which this type of breathing is helpful will also assist in directing you to option 4. Review the purpose of this procedure now if you had difficulty with this question.
LEVEL OF COGNITIVE ABILITY: Application
PHASE OF NURSING PROCESS: Implementation
CLIENT NEEDS: Health Promotion and Maintenance
CONTENT AREA: Adult Health/Respiratory
REFERENCE
Monahan, F., & Neighbors, M. (1998). *Medical-surgical nursing: Foundations for clinical practice* (2nd ed.). Philadelphia: W. B. Saunders. p. 676.

20. 2

RATIONALE: If at any time an alarm is sounding and the nurse cannot quickly ascertain the problem, the client is disconnected from the ventilator and manual resuscitation is used to support respirations until the problem can be corrected. There is no reason to begin CPR. Checking vital signs is not the initial action. Although oxygen is helpful, it will not provide ventilation to the client.
TEST-TAKING STRATEGY: Read the question carefully and note that the issue relates to adequate ventilation of the client. Focusing on this issue will easily direct you to option 2. If you are unfamiliar with management of ventilators and alarms, take time now to review.
LEVEL OF COGNITIVE ABILITY: Application
PHASE OF NURSING PROCESS: Implementation
CLIENT NEEDS: Physiological Integrity
CONTENT AREA: Adult Health/Respiratory
REFERENCE
Black, J., & Matassarin-Jacobs, E. (1997). *Medical-surgical nursing: Clinical management for continuity of care* (5th ed.). Philadelphia: W. B. Saunders. p. 1186.

21. 4

RATIONALE: Side effects that can occur from the use of this medication include tremors, nausea, nervousness, palpitations, tachycardia, peripheral vasodilation, and dryness of the mouth or throat.
TEST-TAKING STRATEGY: Knowledge that this medication causes sympathomimetic stimulation will easily direct you to option 4. If you are unfamiliar with the side effects related to this medication, take time now to review.

LEVEL OF COGNITIVE ABILITY: Application
PHASE OF NURSING PROCESS: Data Collection
CLIENT NEEDS: Physiological Integrity
CONTENT AREA: Pharmacology,
REFERENCE
Hodgson, B., & Kizior, R. (2000). *Saunders nursing drug handbook 2000*. Philadelphia: W. B. Saunders. pp. 548–550.

22. 2

RATIONALE: Persons at greatest risk for pulmonary emboli are immobilized clients. Basic preventive measures include early ambulation, leg elevation, active leg exercises, elastic stockings, and intermittent pneumatic calf compression. Keeping the client well hydrated is essential because dehydration predisposes to clotting. A pillow under the knees may cause venous stasis. Heat should not be applied without a physicians, prescription.
TEST-TAKING STRATEGY: Knowledge regarding preventive measures related to preventing DVT and pulmonary emboli is required to answer this question. Use basic principles related to care of the immobile client to assist in answering this question. If you are unfamiliar with these basic measures, it is important that you review now.
LEVEL OF COGNITIVE ABILITY: Application
PHASE OF NURSING PROCESS: Planning
CLIENT NEEDS: Physiological Integrity
CONTENT AREA: Adult Health/Respiratory
REFERENCE
Monahan, F., & Neighbors, M. (1998). *Medical-surgical nursing: Foundations for clinical practice* (2nd ed.). Philadelphia: W. B. Saunders. p. 682.

23. 1

RATIONALE: The most common clinical manifestations of PE are tachypnea, dyspnea, and chest pain.
TEST-TAKING STRATEGY: Note the key word "not" in the stem of the question. Knowledge regarding the most common clinical manifestations of PE are required to answer this question. Note, however, that options 1 and 2 address a similar issue but opposite effects. This may provide you with the clue that one of these options is the correct one. You would expect an increased respiratory rate in PE; therefore, select option 1.
LEVEL OF COGNITIVE ABILITY: Comprehension
PHASE OF NURSING PROCESS: Data Collection
CLIENT NEEDS: Physiological Integrity
CONTENT AREA: Adult Health/Respiratory
REFERENCE
Black, J., & Matassarin-Jacobs, E. (1997). *Medical-surgical nursing: Clinical management for continuity of care* (5th ed.). Philadelphia: W. B. Saunders. p. 1127.

24. 3

RATIONALE: The client should be instructed to hold the breath at least 5 to 10 seconds before exhaling the mist. Options 1, 2, and 4 are accurate instructions regarding the use of the inhaler.
TEST-TAKING STRATEGY: Knowledge regarding the use of the inhaler is required to answer this question. If you are unfamiliar with the client teaching points related to the use of an inhaler, take time now to review.
LEVEL OF COGNITIVE ABILITY: Application
PHASE OF NURSING PROCESS: Planning
CLIENT NEEDS: Health Promotion and Maintenance
CONTENT AREA: Adult Health/Respiratory

REFERENCE
Black J., & Matassarin-Jacobs, E. (1997). *Medical-surgical nursing: Clinical management for continuity of care* (5th ed.). Philadelphia: W. B. Saunders. p. 1112.

25. 1

RATIONALE: Complete lateral positioning should be avoided following pneumonectomy. Because the mediastinum is no longer held in place on both sides by lung tissue, extreme turning may cause mediastinal shift and compression of the remaining lung.
TEST-TAKING STRATEGY: Eliminate options 2, 3, and 4 because they are similar. Additionally, option 4 describes semi-Fowler's position. If you had difficulty with this question, take time now to review care to the client following pneumonectomy.
LEVEL OF COGNITIVE ABILITY: Application
PHASE OF NURSING PROCESS: Implementation
CLIENT NEEDS: Physiological Integrity
CONTENT AREA: Adult Health/Respiratory
REFERENCE
Black, J., & Matassarin-Jacobs, E. (1997). *Medical-surgical nursing: Clinical management for continuity of care* (5th ed.). Philadelphia: W. B. Saunders. p. 1161.

26. 3

RATIONALE: The nurse monitors for adverse effects of suctioning, which include cyanosis, excessively rapid or slow heart rate, or sudden development of bloody secretions. If they occur, the nurse stops suctioning and reports these signs to the physician immediately. Coughing is a normal response to suctioning for the client with an intact cough reflex, and does not indicate that the client cannot tolerate the procedure.
TEST-TAKING STRATEGY: The wording of the question asks you to select an option that would be a normal or expected finding while suctioning a client. Cyanosis and bradycardia are abnormal findings, and are eliminated first. Of the two remaining choices, the use of the word "becoming" in association with bloody secretions tells you that this has not been an ongoing problem, making this an incorrect option also. Since the cough reflex is normally present, and suction triggers coughing, this is the preferable one of the two remaining options.
LEVEL OF COGNITIVE ABILITY: Comprehension
PHASE OF NURSING PROCESS: Evaluation
CLIENT NEEDS: Physiological Integrity
CONTENT AREA: Adult Health/Respiratory
REFERENCE
Taylor, C., Lillis, C., & LeMone, P. (1997). *Fundamentals of nursing: The art and science of nursing care* (3rd ed.). Philadelphia: Lippincott-Raven. p. 1348.

27. 2

RATIONALE: When the chest tube is patent, the water in the water seal chamber rises with inspiration and falls with expiration. This is referred to as tidaling, and indicates proper function of the system.
TEST-TAKING STRATEGY: Knowing that there is negative pressure (pulling pressure) with inspiration, it is natural that the fluid level in the water seal chamber would rise on inspiration. It is also a natural consequence that with exhalation the fluid level falls. This makes options 3 and 4 incorrect. Choose option 2 over option 1 because there is no mention of bubbling in the water seal chamber. This occurs if the client has pneumothorax, even though the fluid still rises and falls. Review the important measures required in the care of a client with a chest tube now if you had difficulty with this question.
LEVEL OF COGNITIVE ABILITY: Analysis
PHASE OF NURSING PROCESS: Data Collection
CLIENT NEEDS: Physiological Integrity
CONTENT AREA: Adult Health/Respiratory
REFERENCE
Black J., & Matassarin-Jacobs, E. (1997). *Medical-surgical nursing: Clinical management for continuity of care* (5th ed.). Philadelphia: W. B. Saunders. p. 1163.

28. 1

RATIONALE: The nurse ensures that all system connections are securely taped to prevent accidental disconnection, and that an occlusive dressing is maintained at the chest tube insertion site. Drainage is noted and recorded every hour in the first 24 hours after insertion and every 8 hours thereafter. The system is kept below the level of the waist. Monitoring for crepitus is done once every 8 hours. Sterile water is added to the suction control chamber only as needed to replace evaporation losses. Continuous bubbling in the water seal chamber indicates an air leak in the system and requires immediate investigation and correction.
TEST-TAKING STRATEGY: Note that each option has two parts. In order for the option to be correct, both parts of the answer must be correct. Knowing this, eliminate options 3 and 4 first. Water needs to be added only as needed and there should not be continuous bubbling in the water seal. Knowing that chest tube assessment is done every 8 hours at least, helps you to choose option 1 over option 2. Review the important measures required in the care of a client with a chest tube now if you had difficulty with this question.
LEVEL OF COGNITIVE ABILITY: Application
PHASE OF NURSING PROCESS: Implementation
CLIENT NEEDS: Physiological Integrity
CONTENT AREA: Adult Health/Respiratory
REFERENCE
Black, J., & Matassarin-Jacobs, E. (1997). *Medical-surgical nursing: Clinical management for continuity of care* (5th ed.). Philadelphia: W. B. Saunders. pp. 1163–1165.

29. 1

RATIONALE: The most important item to ask about is the client's pregnancy status, because pregnant women should not be exposed to radiation. Clients are also asked to remove any chains or metal objects that could interfere with obtaining an adequate film. A chest x-ray is most often done at full inspiration, which gives optimal lung expansion. If a lateral view of the chest is ordered, the client is asked to raise the arms above the head. Most films are done in posterior-anterior (PA) view.
TEST-TAKING STRATEGY: This question asks which is of "most importance." This implies that more than one or all of the options are correct. Eliminate options 3 and 4 first, because they can be determined by the radiologic technologist. Option 1 is a higher priority than option 2, because of potential negative teratogenic consequences to the fetus.
LEVEL OF COGNITIVE ABILITY: Comprehension
PHASE OF NURSING PROCESS: Data Collection
CLIENT NEEDS: Physiological Integrity
CONTENT AREA: Adult Health/Respiratory

REFERENCE

Black, J., & Matassarin-Jacobs, E. (1997). *Medical-surgical nursing: Clinical management for continuity of care* (5th ed.). Philadelphia: W. B. Saunders. pp. 1059–1060.

30. **3**

RATIONALE: Signs of allergic reaction to the contrast dye include early signs such as localized itching and edema, which are then followed by more severe symptoms such as respiratory distress, stridor, and decreased blood pressure.

TEST-TAKING STRATEGY: Hypothermia is an unrelated event and is eliminated first. Discomfort is expected, and is eliminated next. Hematoma formation is a complication of the procedure, but does not indicate allergic reaction, and is therefore eliminated. The remaining option is stridor, which is a sign of severe allergic reaction, and possible anaphylaxis. Review the signs of an allergic reaction to the contrast medium now if you had difficulty with this question.

LEVEL OF COGNITIVE ABILITY: Comprehension

PHASE OF NURSING PROCESS: Data Collection

CLIENT NEEDS: Physiological Integrity

CONTENT AREA: Adult Health/Respiratory

REFERENCE

Black, J., & Matassarin-Jacobs, E. (1997). *Medical-surgical nursing: Clinical management for continuity of care* (5th ed.). Philadelphia: W. B. Saunders. pp. 638, 1062.

31. **1**

RATIONALE: Strapping the ribs is an outmoded therapy. Strapping the ribs has a constricting effect on the ribs and deep breathing, and can actually increase the risk of atelectasis and pneumonia.

TEST-TAKING STRATEGY: This question can be answered by logically thinking through the physiologic effects of restricting lung mobility. This will help to eliminate each of the incorrect responses. Review interventions for rib fractures now if you had difficulty with this question.

LEVEL OF COGNITIVE ABILITY: Application

PHASE OF NURSING PROCESS: Implementation

CLIENT NEEDS: Physiological Integrity

CONTENT AREA: Adult Health/Respiratory

REFERENCE

Black, J., & Matassarin-Jacobs, E. (1997). *Medical-surgical nursing: Clinical management for continuity of care* (5th ed.). Philadelphia: W. B. Saunders. p. 2526.

32. **4**

RATIONALE: Instructions for using a metered-dose inhaler include to shake the canister; hold it right side up; inhale slowly and evenly through the mouth; deliver one spray per breath; and hold the breath after inhalation.

TEST-TAKING STRATEGY: This question is straightforward and tests a fundamental concept of medication administration using inhalers. If you selected an incorrect option, review the key principles of this medication therapy now.

LEVEL OF COGNITIVE ABILITY: Application

PHASE OF NURSING PROCESS: Implementation

CLIENT NEEDS: Health Promotion and Maintenance

CONTENT AREA: Adult Health/Respiratory

REFERENCE

Taylor, C., Lillis, C., & LeMone, p. (1997). *Fundamentals of nursing: The art and science of nursing care* (3rd ed.). Philadelphia: Lippincott-Raven. p. 1335.

33. **2**

RATIONALE: Cough is the most frequent early symptom of lung cancer, which begins as nonproductive and hacking, and progresses to productive. In the smoker who already has a cough, a change in the character and frequency of cough usually occurs. Hoarseness and blood-streaked sputum are later signs. Pain is a very late sign, and is usually pleuritic in nature.

TEST-TAKING STRATEGY: Begin to answer this question by eliminating pain and hemoptysis, because it is reasonable that these would be later signs. To discriminate between cough and hoarseness, think about location. Hoarseness indicates that the affected tissue is the upper airway, whereas cough indicates lower airway. Since the question is asking about lung cancer, which is lower airway, the answer must be cough. Review the common early signs of lung cancer now if you had difficulty with this question.

LEVEL OF COGNITIVE ABILITY: Comprehension

PHASE OF NURSING PROCESS: Data Collection

CLIENT NEEDS: Physiological Integrity

CONTENT AREA: Adult Health/Respiratory

REFERENCE

Monahan, F., & Neighbors, M. (1998). *Medical-surgical nursing: Foundations for clinical practice* (2nd ed.). Philadelphia: W. B. Saunders. p. 696.

34. **2**

RATIONALE: The nurse avoids interventions that will place pressure on the chest during inspiration, as it interferes with lung expansion. Acceptable methods of splinting include the use of the hands, a pillow, or a towel or drawsheet during a forced expiratory cough.

TEST-TAKING STRATEGY: Note the key words "least effective." Option 3 is obviously correct and is eliminated. Option 4 is not as widely used but is a technique that supports the area above and below an incision. Since this option is also correct, it is eliminated next. Options 1 and 2 seem to oppose each other. To choose correctly, you need to know that applying pressure to the chest before the breath interferes with lung expansion, and is not as helpful to the client overall. This would guide you to choose option 2 as the answer to the question according to the way it is worded.

LEVEL OF COGNITIVE ABILITY: Application

PHASE OF NURSING PROCESS: Implementation

CLIENT NEEDS: Physiological Integrity

CONTENT AREA: Adult Health/Respiratory

REFERENCE

Black, J., & Matassarin-Jacobs, E. (1997). *Medical-surgical nursing: Clinical management for continuity of care* (5th ed.). Philadelphia: W. B. Saunders. p. 1157.

35. **1**

RATIONALE: If the client begins to hemorrhage from the surgical site following radical neck dissection, the nurse elevates the head of the bed to maintain airway patency and prevent aspiration. The nurse applies pressure over the bleeding site, and calls the physician immediately.

TEST-TAKING STRATEGY: This question is very straightforward. Options 2 and 3 are obviously indicated, and are eliminated immediately as possible options. Calling the physician is also indicated immediately, while lowering the head of bed does not help with airway maintenance. Thus, option 1 is the contraindicated action, and is the answer to the question.

LEVEL OF COGNITIVE ABILITY: Application
PHASE OF NURSING PROCESS: Implementation
CLIENT NEEDS: Physiological Integrity
CONTENT AREA: Adult Health/Respiratory
REFERENCE
Monahan, F., & Neighbors, M. (1998). *Medical-surgical nursing: Foundations for clinical practice* (2nd ed.). Philadelphia: W. B. Saunders. p. 410.

36. **4**

RATIONALE: Dry cough and dyspnea are indicative of an exacerbation of pulmonary sarcoidosis. Others include chest pain, hemoptysis, and pneumothorax. Systemic signs and symptoms include weakness and fatigue, malaise, fever, and weight loss.
TEST-TAKING STRATEGY: Note the key word "early" in the stem of the question. Since sarcoidosis is a pulmonary problem, eliminate options 1 and 2 first. Choose option 4 over option 3 since the shortness of breath (and impaired ventilation) appears first, and would cause the fatigue as a secondary symptom.
LEVEL OF COGNITIVE ABILITY: Comprehension
PHASE OF NURSING PROCESS: Evaluation
CLIENT NEEDS: Health Promotion and Maintenance
CONTENT AREA: Adult Health/Respiratory
REFERENCE
Black, J., & Matassarin-Jacobs, E. (1997). *Medical-surgical nursing: Clinical management for continuity of care* (5th ed.). Philadelphia: W. B. Saunders. p. 1150.

37. **4**

RATIONALE: People at high risk for acquiring tuberculosis include immigrants from Asia, Africa, Latin America, and Oceania; medically underserved populations (ethnic minorities, homeless); those with HIV or other immunosuppressive disorders; residents in group settings (long-term care, correctional facilities); and health care workers.
TEST-TAKING STRATEGY: The question asks for the client at least risk. Begin to answer this question by eliminating options 1 and 2, since immigrants and the medically underserved are more frequently affected by the disease. To discriminate between the last two, the postal inspector, option 4, may or may not come in contact with many people, depending on job description. The client from the long-term care facility, however, lives in a group setting, where a large number of people share a common environment 24 hours a day. This makes option 4 the correct answer, as the postal worker is at less overall risk than any of the others in the options.
LEVEL OF COGNITIVE ABILITY: Comprehension
PHASE OF NURSING PROCESS: Data Collection
CLIENT NEEDS: Physiological Integrity
CONTENT AREA: Adult Health/Respiratory
REFERENCE
Black, J., & Matassarin-Jacobs, E. (1997). *Medical-surgical nursing: Clinical management for continuity of care* (5th ed.). Philadelphia: W. B. Saunders. p. 1140.

38. **2**

RATIONALE: A positive PPD reading has induration measuring 10 mm or more. A small area of ecchymosis is insignificant, and is probably related to injection technique.
TEST-TAKING STRATEGY: To answer this question accurately, it is necessary to know that induration is necessary for a positive result. Since the client in this question has no induration, the result can only be negative. Take time to review PPD skin testing results, if you had difficulty with this question.
LEVEL OF COGNITIVE ABILITY: Comprehension
PHASE OF NURSING PROCESS: Data Collection
CLIENT NEEDS: Physiological Integrity
CONTENT AREA: Adult Health/Respiratory
REFERENCE
Black, J., & Matassarin-Jacobs, E. (1997). *Medical-surgical nursing: Clinical management for continuity of care* (5th ed.). Philadelphia: W. B. Saunders. p. 720.

39. **4**

RATIONALE: A client who tests positive on a Mantoux skin test has either been exposed to tuberculosis or has inactive (dormant) tuberculosis. The client must then undergo chest x-ray and sputum culture to confirm the diagnosis.
TEST-TAKING STRATEGY: It is necessary to be familiar with the concept and possible results of a Mantoux skin testing to be able to answer this question correctly. Use the process of elimination, eliminating options 2 and 3 first, because they both indicate the presence of TB. In selecting between options 1 and 4, review the case of the question, noting that the Mantoux skin test is positive. From this information, it is best to eliminate option 1. Because of the importance of this content, be sure to review this area now if the question was difficult for you.
LEVEL OF COGNITIVE ABILITY: Comprehension
PHASE OF NURSING PROCESS: Evaluation
CLIENT NEEDS: Psychosocial Integrity
CONTENT AREA: Adult Health/Respiratory
REFERENCE
Black, J., & Matassarin-Jacobs, E. (1997). *Medical-surgical nursing: Clinical management for continuity of care* (5th ed.). Philadelphia: W. B. Saunders. p. 1142.

40. **1**

RATIONALE: The nurse who notes a positive PPD reading calls the physician immediately. The physician would order a chest x-ray to rule out whether the client has clinically active tuberculosis (TB), or old, healed lesions. Sputum culture is done next as indicated to confirm the diagnosis of active TB. The client can be placed on TB precautions prophylactically until a final diagnosis is made.
TEST-TAKING STRATEGY: The question asks for the highest priority action, which implies that one or all of the responses may be correct. Since the nurse may not order diagnostic tests, eliminate option 2 first. Likewise, option 4 can be eliminated, since calling employee health service is of no benefit to the client. To discriminate between the last two options, notifying the physician should have a higher priority than the documentation, even though they may both be done in the same narrow time period. Note that the question asks for the highest priority, not the first nursing action.
LEVEL OF COGNITIVE ABILITY: Application
PHASE OF NURSING PROCESS: Implementation
CLIENT NEEDS: Safe, Effective Care Environment
CONTENT AREA: Adult Health/Respiratory
REFERENCE
deWit, S. (1998). *Essentials of medical-surgical nursing.* (4th ed.). Philadelphia: W. B. Saunders. p. 437.

41. 3

RATIONALE: A primary role of the nurse in working with the client with tuberculosis is to teach the client about medication therapy. The anxious client may not absorb information optimally. The nurse continues to reinforce teaching using a variety of methods (repetition, teaching aids), and teaches the family about the medications as well. The most effective way of coping with the disease is to learn about the therapy that will eradicate it. This gives the client a measure of power over the situation and outcome.
TEST-TAKING STRATEGY: The question asks for the best strategy for coping with anxiety about the disease and its prognosis. This implies that more than one or all responses are partially or completely true. Options 2 and 4 are the least useful of the four choices, and may be eliminated first. Option 2 does not involve the client, and option 4 gives no active assistance to the client. The two remaining alternatives are both viable, but option 3 is the better of the two choices. TB is a controllable disease, not necessarily a fatal one, which may help to discriminate between these plausible options.
LEVEL OF COGNITIVE ABILITY: Application
PHASE OF NURSING PROCESS: Planning
CLIENT NEEDS: Psychosocial Integrity
CONTENT AREA: Adult Health/Respiratory
REFERENCE
deWit, S. (1998). *Essentials of medical-surgical nursing.* (4th ed.). Philadelphia: W. B. Saunders. p. 438.

42. 4

RATIONALE: Since tuberculosis is transmitted by droplet, it cannot be carried on clothing, eating utensils, or other possessions. It is not necessary to discard any of these. It is important to perform proper handwashing after contact with body substances, tissues, or face masks. The client should cover the mouth with a tissue when laughing, coughing, or sneezing, and dispose of tissues carefully. The client may also need to wear a tight-fitting mask as advised by the physician.
TEST-TAKING STRATEGY: Use the process of elimination to answer the question. Options 2 and 3 are obvious correct actions on the part of the client, and are therefore eliminated according to the way this question is worded. To discriminate between the last two options, you need to recall that TB is an airborne disease, so the organisms cannot be carried on inanimate objects. Using this knowledge, choose option 4 as the answer to the question as it is stated. Review client teaching points related to the prevention of the spread of TB now if you had difficulty with this question.
LEVEL OF COGNITIVE ABILITY: Comprehension
PHASE OF NURSING PROCESS: Evaluation
CLIENT NEEDS: Health Promotion and Maintenance
CONTENT AREA: Adult Health/Respiratory
REFERENCE
Black, J., & Matassarin-Jacobs, E. (1997). *Medical-surgical nursing: Clinical management for continuity of care* (5th ed.). Philadelphia: W. B. Saunders. p. 1146.

43. 4

RATIONALE: The client with tuberculosis usually experiences cough (either productive or nonproductive), fatigue, anorexia, weight loss, dyspnea, hemoptysis, chest discomfort or pain, chills and sweats (which may occur at night), and a low-grade fever.

TEST-TAKING STRATEGY: Knowledge of the usual signs and symptoms of TB is needed to answer this question correctly. Options 1 and 2 may be eliminated first, because they are symptoms that are common in the client with TB. To discriminate between the last two, you need to know either that the client may get night sweats or that the fever is low grade. Take time to review the clinical manifestations associated with TB now if you had difficulty with this question.
LEVEL OF COGNITIVE ABILITY: Comprehension
PHASE OF NURSING PROCESS: Data Collection
CLIENT NEEDS: Physiological Integrity
CONTENT AREA: Adult Health/Respiratory
REFERENCE
Black, J., & Matassarin-Jacobs, E. (1997). *Medical-surgical nursing: Clinical management for continuity of care* (5th ed.). Philadelphia: W. B. Saunders. p. 1141.

44. 4

RATIONALE: Family members or others who have been in close association with a client diagnosed with TB are placed on prophylactic therapy with isoniazid (INH) for 6 to 12 months. The client is usually not communicable after taking medication for 2 to 3 consecutive weeks. However, the client must take the full course of therapy (for 6 months or longer) to prevent reinfection or drug-resistant TB.
TEST-TAKING STRATEGY: Each of the options for this question has two parts. Remember that in order for the option to be correct, both of the parts must also be correct. Knowing that the family requires prophylactic therapy allows you to eliminate options 1 and 2. In order to discriminate between options 3 and 4, you need to recall that the client is not contagious after 2 to 3 weeks of therapy. Take time now to review the concepts related to the prevention of the spread of TB if you had difficulty with this question.
LEVEL OF COGNITIVE ABILITY: Comprehension
PHASE OF NURSING PROCESS: Planning
CLIENT NEEDS: Psychosocial Integrity
CONTENT AREA: Adult Health/Respiratory
REFERENCE
Black, J., & Matassarin-Jacobs, E. (1997). *Medical-surgical nursing: Clinical management for continuity of care* (5th ed.). Philadelphia: W. B. Saunders. p. 1143.

45. 3

RATIONALE: The client with TB has significant fatigue and loss of physical stamina. This can be very frightening for the client. The nurse teaches the client that this will resolve as the therapy progresses, and that the client should gradually increase activity as energy levels permit.
TEST-TAKING STRATEGY: A helpful concept to remember in answering this question is that fatigue due to respiratory problems may not resolve easily, and is an expected occurrence, due to tissue hypoxia. Knowing this, you can eliminate options 1 and 2 first. Discriminate between options 3 and 4 in this way: since the client is on medication therapy for 6 to 9 months, or even up to 12 months, it is not reasonable that the fatigue would last for "at least a year." Thus, option 3 is more plausible than option 4, and is the correct response.
LEVEL OF COGNITIVE ABILITY: Application
PHASE OF NURSING PROCESS: Planning
CLIENT NEEDS: Health Promotion and Maintenance
CONTENT AREA: Adult Health/Respiratory
REFERENCE
deWit, S. (1998). *Essentials of medical-surgical nursing.* (4th ed.). Philadelphia: W. B. Saunders. p. 438.

46. 1

RATIONALE: The nurse teaches the client with TB to increase intake of protein, iron, and vitamin C. Foods rich in vitamin C include citrus fruits, berries, melons, pineapple, broccoli, cabbage, green peppers, tomatoes, potatoes, chard, kale, asparagus, and turnip greens. Food sources that are rich in iron include liver and other meats, from which 10% to 30% of available iron is absorbed. Less than 10% of iron is absorbed from eggs, and less than 5% is absorbed from grains and vegetables.

TEST-TAKING STRATEGY: This question is difficult. To answer it correctly, you must recall that the diet in tuberculosis should be high in protein, vitamin C, and calories. It is then necessary to know which types of foods contain these various nutrients. If you had difficulty with this question, take a few moments to review these nutritional concepts.

LEVEL OF COGNITIVE ABILITY: Application
PHASE OF NURSING PROCESS: Implementation
CLIENT NEEDS: Health Promotion and Maintenance
CONTENT AREA: Adult Health/Respiratory
REFERENCE
deWit, S. (1998). *Essentials of medical-surgical nursing.* (4th ed.). Philadelphia: W. B. Saunders. p. 436.

47. 2

RATIONALE: The client is continued on medication therapy for 6 to 12 months, depending on the situation. The client is generally considered to be not contagious after 2 to 3 weeks of medication therapy. The client is instructed to wear a mask if there will be exposure to crowds until the medication is effective in preventing transmission. The client is allowed to return to employment when the results of two sputum cultures are negative.

TEST-TAKING STRATEGY: This question is worded to make you look for a correct statement. Knowing that the drug therapy lasts for at least 6 months helps you to eliminate option 1 first. Knowing that two sputum cultures must be negative helps you to eliminate option 4 next. To discriminate between the remaining choices, knowing that the client is not contagious after 2 to 3 weeks of therapy helps you to choose option 2 and eliminate option 3, since they basically oppose each other. If you had difficulty with this question, take time now to review the infectious period of TB.

LEVEL OF COGNITIVE ABILITY: Comprehension
PHASE OF NURSING PROCESS: Evaluation
CLIENT NEEDS: Physiological Integrity
CONTENT AREA: Adult Health/Respiratory
REFERENCE
deWit, S. (1998). *Essentials of medical-surgical nursing* (4th ed.). Philadelphia: W. B. Saunders. p. 438.

48. 2

RATIONALE: Tuberculosis is spread by droplet nuclei, or the airborne route. The disease is not carried on objects such as clothing, eating utensils, linens, or furniture. Bleaching of clothing and linens is unnecessary, although the client and family members should use good handwashing technique. It is unnecessary to remove carpeting from the home.

TEST-TAKING STRATEGY: Knowing that TB is not carried on inanimate objects helps you to eliminate options 3 and 4 first. To discriminate between options 1 and 2, you must be able to recall that the disease is transmitted by the airborne route. If you had difficulty with this question, take time now to review the transmission mode of TB.

LEVEL OF COGNITIVE ABILITY: Comprehension
PHASE OF NURSING PROCESS: Planning
CLIENT NEEDS: Health Promotion and Maintenance
CONTENT AREA: Adult Health/Respiratory
REFERENCE
Black, J., & Matassarin-Jacobs, E. (1997). *Medical-surgical nursing: Clinical management for continuity of care* (5th ed.). Philadelphia: W. B. Saunders. p. 1146.

49. 1

RATIONALE: The nurse who is in contact with a client with TB should wear an individually fitted particulate respirator. The nurse would also wear gloves as per universal precautions. The nurse wears a gown when there is a possibility that the clothing could become contaminated, such as when giving a bed bath.

TEST-TAKING STRATEGY: Knowing that the nurse should wear a particulate respirator helps you to eliminate options 3 and 4 first. Knowledge of basic universal precautions forces you to choose option 1 over option 2. In this nursing situation, option 1 is the best option.

LEVEL OF COGNITIVE ABILITY: Application
PHASE OF NURSING PROCESS: Planning
CLIENT NEEDS: Safe, Effective Care Environment
CONTENT AREA: Adult Health/Respiratory
REFERENCE
deWit, S. (1998). *Essentials of medical-surgical nursing* (4th ed.). Philadelphia: W. B. Saunders. p. 438.

50. 1

RATIONALE: The client must have sputum cultures performed every 2 to 4 weeks after initiation of antituberculosis drug therapy. The client may return to work when the results of two sputum cultures are negative, because the client is considered noninfectious at that point.

TEST-TAKING STRATEGY: Use the process of elimination to answer the question. Knowing that a positive PPD never reverts to negative helps you to automatically eliminate option 4 as a possible answer. To discriminate among the other three options, it is necessary to know that two negative sputum cultures are required. If this question was difficult, review these key points now.

LEVEL OF COGNITIVE ABILITY: Application
PHASE OF NURSING PROCESS: Implementation
CLIENT NEEDS: Health Promotion and Maintenance
CONTENT AREA: Adult Health/Respiratory
REFERENCE
deWit, S. (1998). *Essentials of medical-surgical nursing* (4th ed.). Philadelphia: W. B. Saunders. p. 438.

51. 3

RATIONALE: The client with tuberculosis should wash the hands carefully after each contact with respiratory secretions. The client should cover the mouth and nose when laughing, sneezing, or coughing. Used tissues are discarded in a plastic bag. Oral care is done as for any other client.

TEST-TAKING STRATEGY: Note that the question specifically asks for information about handling and disposal of secretions. The only options that address this topic directly are options 2 and 3, so options 1 and 4 are eliminated. Since turning the head to the side for coughing and sneezing does not specifically address the handling of secretions, eliminate that option. Disposal of tissues in a plastic bag is correct, and is therefore chosen as the more correct response.

LEVEL OF COGNITIVE ABILITY: Comprehension
PHASE OF NURSING PROCESS: Evaluation
CLIENT NEEDS: Health Promotion and Maintenance
CONTENT AREA: Adult Health/Respiratory
REFERENCE
deWit, S. (1998). *Essentials of medical-surgical nursing* (4th ed.). Philadelphia: W. B. Saunders. p. 440.

52. **4**

RATIONALE: A common side effect of INH is peripheral neuritis. This is manifested by numbness, tingling, and paresthesias in the extremities. This side effect can be minimized with pyridoxine (vitamin B_6) intake.
TEST-TAKING STRATEGY: Options 1 and 2 do not relate to the symptoms presented in the question. Thus, these two may be eliminated first. To discriminate between the last two, you should know either that peripheral neuritis is a side effect of the medication or that these signs and symptoms do not correlate with hypercalcemia. Take time now to review the side effects associated with INH if you had difficulty with this question.
LEVEL OF COGNITIVE ABILITY: Comprehension
PHASE OF NURSING PROCESS: Data Collection
CLIENT NEEDS: Physiological Integrity
CONTENT AREA: Adult Health/Respiratory
REFERENCE
Hodgson, B., & Kizior, R. (2000). *Saunders nursing drug handbook 2000*. Philadelphia: W. B. Saunders. p. 551.

53. **2**

RATIONALE: INH is hepatotoxic, and therefore the client is taught to report signs and symptoms of hepatitis immediately (which includes yellow skin and sclera). For the same reason, alcohol should be avoided during therapy. The client should avoid intake of Swiss cheese, fish such as tuna, and foods containing tyramine because they may cause a reaction characterized by redness and itching of the skin, flushing, sweating, fast heartbeat, headache, or light-headedness. The client can avoid developing peripheral neuritis by increasing intake of pyridoxine (vitamin B_6) during the course of INH therapy.
TEST-TAKING STRATEGY: Use the process of elimination to answer the question. Since alcohol intake is prohibited with many medications, option 1 should be eliminated first. Because the client receiving this medication typically is supplemented with vitamin B_6, option 4 is incorrect and is eliminated next. Knowing that the medication is hepatotoxic allows you to choose option 2 over option 3. If you had difficulty with this question, take time now to review this important medication.
LEVEL OF COGNITIVE ABILITY: Application
PHASE OF NURSING PROCESS: Planning
CLIENT NEEDS: Health Promotion and Maintenance
CONTENT AREA: Adult Health/Respiratory

REFERENCE
Hodgson, B., & Kizior, R. (2000). *Saunders nursing drug handbook 2000*. Philadelphia: W. B. Saunders. p. 551.

54. **3**

RATIONALE: Rifampin should be taken exactly as directed. Doses should not be doubled or skipped. The client should not stop therapy until directed to do so by a physician. The medication should be administered on an empty stomach unless it causes GI upset, and then it may be taken with food. Antacids, if prescribed, should be taken at least 1 hour prior to the medication. Rifampin causes orange-red discoloration to body secretions and will permanently stain soft contact lenses.
TEST-TAKING STRATEGY: Options 1 and 2 are examples of poor medication advice in general, and are eliminated first. Knowing that this medication causes discoloration of body secretions helps you to choose option 3 over option 4. You may also choose option 3 by noting the word "always" in option 4. It is not often that a distracter containing such an absolute descriptor is correct. If you had difficulty with this question, take time now to review the side effects associated with this medication.
LEVEL OF COGNITIVE ABILITY: Application
PHASE OF NURSING PROCESS: Implementation
CLIENT NEEDS: Physiological Integrity
CONTENT AREA: Adult Health/Respiratory
REFERENCE
Hodgson, B., & Kizior, R. (2000). *Saunders nursing drug handbook 2000*. Philadelphia: W. B. Saunders. p. 906.

55. **4**

RATIONALE: Ethambutol causes optic neuritis, which decreases visual acuity and the ability to discriminate between red and green. This poses a potential safety hazard when driving a motor vehicle. The client is taught to report this symptom immediately. The client is also taught to take the medication with food if GI upset occurs. Impaired hearing results from antitubercular therapy with streptomycin. Orange-red discoloration of secretions occurs with rifampin.
TEST-TAKING STRATEGY: Option 1 is the least likely symptom to report; rather, it should be managed by taking the medication with food. Thus, this option may be eliminated first. To discriminate among the other options, it is necessary to know that this medication causes optic neuritis, and causing difficulty with red-green discrimination. If this question was difficult, take a moment to review antitubercular medications because the incorrect options for this question are typical side effects of other antitubercular medications.
LEVEL OF COGNITIVE ABILITY: Comprehension
PHASE OF NURSING PROCESS: Evaluation
CLIENT NEEDS: Health Promotion and Maintenance
CONTENT AREA: Adult Health/Respiratory
REFERENCE
Hodgson, B., & Kizior, R. (2000). *Saunders nursing drug handbook 2000*. Philadelphia: W. B. Saunders. p. 391.

BIBLIOGRAPHY

Black, J., and Matassarin-Jacobs, E. (1997). *Medical-surgical nursing: Clinical management for continuity of care* (5th ed.). Philadelphia: W. B. Saunders.

Burrell, P., Gerlach, M., & Pless, B. (1997). *Adult nursing: Acute and community care* (2nd ed.). Stamford, CT: Appleton & Lange.

Chernecky, C., & Berger, B. (1997). *Laboratory tests and diagnostic procedures* (2nd ed.). Philadelphia: W. B. Saunders.

Deglin, J., & Vallerand, A. (1999). *Davis's drug guide for nurses* (6th ed.). Philadelphia: F. A. Davis.

deWit, S. (1998). *Essentials of medical-surgical nursing* (4th ed.). Philadelphia: W. B. Saunders.

Hodgson, B., & Kizior, R. (2000). *Saunders nursing drug handbook 2000*. Philadelphia: W. B. Saunders.

Ignatavicius, D., Workman, M., & Mishler, M. (1999). *Medical-surgical nursing: Across the health care continuum* (3rd ed.). Philadelphia: W. B. Saunders.

Leahy, J., & Kizilay, P. (1998). *Foundations of nursing practice: A nursing process approach*. Philadelphia: W. B. Saunders.

Lehne, R. (1998). *Pharmacology for nursing care* (3rd ed.). Philadelphia: W. B. Saunders.

Luckmann, J. (1997). *Saunders manual of nursing care*. Philadelphia: W. B. Saunders.

Lutz, C., & Przytulski, K. (1997). *Nutrition and diet therapy* (2nd ed.). Philadelphia: F. A. Davis.

Monahan, F., & Neighbors, M. (1998). *Medical-surgical nursing: Foundations for clinical practice* (2nd ed.). Philadelphia: W. B. Saunders.

O'Toole, M. (1997). *Miller-Keane encyclopedia & dictionary of medicine, nursing, & allied health* (6th ed.). Philadelphia: W. B. Saunders.

Taylor, C., Lillis, C., & LeMone, P. (1997). *Fundamentals of nursing: The art and science of nursing care* (3rd ed.). Philadelphia: Lippincott-Raven.

CHAPTER 47

Respiratory Medications

I. Bronchodilators (Box 47–1)

A. Description
1. Dilate the airways of the respiratory tree, thereby making air exchange and respiration easier for the client
2. Relax the smooth muscle of the bronchi
3. Stimulate the central nervous system (CNS) and respiration, dilate coronary and pulmonary vessels, and cause diuresis
4. Used to treat allergic rhinitis and sinusitis, acute bronchospasm, acute and chronic asthma, bronchitis, **chronic obstructive pulmonary disease,** and **emphysema**
5. Contraindicated in individuals with hypersensitivity, peptic ulcer disease, severe cardiac disease and cardiac dysrhythmias, hyperthyroidism, and uncontrolled seizure disorders
6. Used cautiously with clients with hypertension and diabetes mellitus
7. Used with caution in clients with narrow-angle glaucoma
8. Theophylline increases the risk of digitalis toxicity, decreases the effects of lithium, and decreases theophylline levels when administered with phenytoin (Dilantin)
9. Beta blockers, cimetidine (Tagamet), and erythromycin increase the effects of theophylline
10. Barbiturate and carbamazepine (Tegretol) decrease the effects of theophylline

B. Side effects
1. Palpitations and tachycardia
2. Dizziness and headaches
3. May increase blood glucose levels
4. Nausea and vomiting
5. Restlessness, irritability, and insomnia
6. Tremors and nervousness
7. Muscle cramping in extremities
8. Mouth dryness and throat irritation with inhalers
9. Tolerance and bronchoconstriction with inhalers

C. Implementation
1. Monitor vital signs
2. Monitor for cardiac irregularities
3. Monitor for wheezing, cough, and sputum production
4. Monitor for confusion and restlessness
5. Provide adequate fluids for hydration and instruct the client to increase fluid intake
6. Administer oral medications with food to decrease gastrointestinal (GI) upset
7. Instruct the client in the side effects of bronchodilators
8. Instruct clients how to monitor pulse and to report any abnormalities to the physician

---

BOX 47–1. Bronchodilators

ADRENERGICS
Ephedrine sulfate
Epinephrine (Adrenalin)
Albuterol (Proventil, Ventolin)
Bitolterol mesylate (Tornalate)
Isoetharine HCl (Bronkosol)
Isoproterenol (Isuprel)
Metaproterenol sulfate (Alupent, Metaprel)
Pirbuterol acetate (Maxair)
Salmeterol (Serevent)
Terbutaline sulfate (Brethine, Bricanyl)

ANTICHOLINERGIC
Ipratropium bromide (Atrovent)

METHYLXANTHINE (XANTHINE) DERIVATIVES
Aminophylline (Truphylline)
Theophylline
Theophylline (Aerolate, Slo-phyllin, Theolair)
Theophylline (Theo-Dur, Slo-bid, Theo-24, Uni-Dur, Uniphyl)
Oxtriphylline (Choledyl)

BOX 47–2. Glucocorticoids (Steroids)

Beclomethasone (Vanceril, Beclovent)
Triamcinolone (Amcort, Aristocort, Azmacort)
Fluticasone (Flonase, Flovent)
Dexamethasone (Decadron)
Hydrocortisone (Cortef)
Prednisone (Deltasone)

---

9. Instruct clients not to crush enteric-coated or sustained-release tablets or capsules
10. Administer medication at regular intervals around the clock to maintain a sustained therapeutic level
11. Monitor for a therapeutic serum theophylline level of 10 to 20 μg/mL. Note that toxicity is likely to occur when the serum level is greater than 20 μg/mL
12. Instruct the client how to use an inhaler or nebulizer and how to monitor the amount of medication remaining in an inhaler canister
13. Instruct the client to avoid caffeine products such as coffee, tea, cola, and chocolate
14. Instruct the client to avoid over-the-counter medications
15. Instruct clients to avoid smoking because it decreases the effectiveness of the medication
16. Instruct the diabetic client to monitor blood glucose levels
17. Instructs clients with asthma to wear Medic-Alert bracelets

II. Glucocorticoids (Steroids) (Box 47–2)

A. Description
   1. Anti-inflammatory
   2. Reduce inflammation and edema of the airway passages in client with **chronic obstructive pulmonary disease (COPD),** asthma, chronic bronchitis, and **emphysema**
B. Side effects and implementation: refer to Chapter 43 for information regarding the side effects and implementation measures for the client taking a glucocorticoid (steroid)

III. Mast-Cell Stabilizer (Box 47–3)

A. Description
   1. An antiasthmatic, antiallergic, and a mast-cell stabilizer that inhibits mast-cell release after exposure to antigens
   2. Cromolyn sodium (Intal) is not an antihistamine but is used for the treatment of allergic rhinitis, bronchial asthma, and exercised-induced bronchospasm

---

BOX 47–3. Mast-Cell Stabilizer

Cromolyn sodium (Intal)

BOX 47–4. Leukotriene Receptor Antagonist

Zafirlukast (Accolate)

---

   3. Cromolyn sodium (Intal) is contraindicated in clients with known hypersensitivity
   4. Oral cromolyn sodium (Intal) is used with caution in clients with impaired hepatic or renal function
B. Side effects
   1. Cough or bronchospasm following inhalation
   2. Nasal sting or sneezing following inhalation.
   3. Bad taste in the mouth
C. Implementation
   1. Monitor vital signs
   2. Monitor respirations and monitor for signs of wheezing
   3. Instruct the client to drink a few sips of water before and after inhalation to prevent cough and bad taste in the mouth
   4. Administer oral capsules at least 30 minutes before meals
   5. Instruct the client not to discontinue medication abruptly because a rebound asthmatic attack can occur

IV. Leukotriene Receptor Antagonist
(Box 47–4)

A. Description
   1. Used in the prophylaxis and chronic treatment of bronchial asthma
   2. Not used for acute asthma episodes
   3. Prevents bronchoconstriction caused by specific antigens
   4. Reduces airway edema and smooth muscle constriction
   5. Contraindicated with hypersensitivity and in breast-feeding mothers
   6. Used with caution in clients with impaired hepatic function
   7. Coadministration of inhaled corticosteroids increases the risk of upper respiratory infection
B. Side effects
   1. Dizziness, headache
   2. Nausea, vomiting, and diarrhea
   3. Dyspepsia
   4. Generalized pain and myalgia
   5. Fever
C. Implementation
   1. Monitor liver function laboratory values
   2. Monitor vital signs
   3. Monitor respirations and for signs of wheezing
   4. Instruct the client to take medication 1 hour before or 2 hours after meals
   5. Instruct the client to increase fluid intake
   6. Instruct the client not to discontinue medication and to take as prescribed even during symptom-free periods

---

BOX 47-5. Antihistamines

Chlorpheniramine maleate (Chlor-Trimeton)
Diphenhydramine (Benadryl)
Promethazine HCl (Phenergan)
Trimeprazine tartrate (Temaril)
Hydroxyzine (Atarax, Vistaril)
Terfenadine (Seldane)
Clemastine fumarate (Tavist)
Tripelenamine HCl (Pelamine)
Azatadine maleate (Optimine)
Cyproheptadine HCl (Periactin)
Brompheniramine maleate (Dimetane)
Dexchlorpheniramine maleate (Polaramine)
Triprolidine and pseudoephedrine (Actifed)
Triprolidine HCl (Alleract)
Astemizole (Hismanal)
Cetirizine (Zyrtec)
Loratadine (Claritin)
Methdilazine HCl (Tacaryl)

V. Antihistamines (Box 47–5)

A. Description
1. Called histamine antagonists or H_1 blockers; these medications compete with histamine for receptor sites, thus preventing a histamine response
2. When the H_1 receptor is stimulated, the smooth muscles, including those lining the nasal cavity, are constricted
3. Decrease nasopharyngeal secretions by blocking the H_1 receptor and decrease nasal itching that causes sneezing
4. Used for the common cold, rhinitis, nausea and vomiting, motion sickness, urticaria, and as a sleep aid
5. Diphenhydramine (Benadryl) has an anticholinergic effect and should be avoided in clients with narrow-angle glaucoma
6. Can cause CNS depression if taken with alcohol, narcotics, hypnotics, or barbiturates
7. Used with caution in clients with **chronic obstructive pulmonary disease (COPD)** because these medications have a drying effect
B. Side effects
1. Drowsiness and sedation
2. Dizziness
3. Nervousness and irritability
4. Palpitations and tachycardia
5. Hypotension or hypertension
6. Blurred vision
7. Urinary retention
8. Constipation
9. Dry mouth
C. Implementation
1. Monitor vital signs
2. Monitor for signs of urinary dysfunction
3. Administer with food or milk and instruct the client to take at bedtime to avoid daytime sedation
4. Instruct the client to avoid hazardous activities
5. Instruct the client to avoid over-the-counter medications, alcohol, and other CNS depressants
6. Instruct clients taking medication for motion sickness to take the medication 30 minutes before the event, and then before meals and at bedtime during the event
7. Instruct the client to take hard candy or ice chips for a dry mouth

VI. Nasal and Systemic Decongestants
(Box 47–6)

A. Description
1. Produces vasoconstriction of the capillaries within the nasal mucosa, shrinks nasal mucosal membranes, and reduces fluid secretion
2. Used for allergic rhinitis, hay fever, and acute coryza (profuse nasal discharge)
3. Contraindicated or used with extreme caution in clients with hypertension, cardiac disease, hyperthyroidism, and diabetes mellitus
4. Nasal decongestants can cause tolerance and rebound nasal congestion (vasodilation), caused by irritation of the nasal mucosa, and should not be used for more than 48 hours
B. Side effects
1. Frequent use of decongestants, especially nasal sprays or drops, can result in tolerance and rebound nasal congestion (vasodilation), caused by irritation of the nasal mucosa
2. Nervousness, restlessness, and tremors
3. Tachycardia and hypertension
4. Hyperglycemia
C. Implementation
1. Monitor for blood pressure changes and cardiac irregularities
2. Instruct the client to monitor blood glucose levels
3. Instruct the client to avoid caffeine-containing products because they can increase restlessness and palpitations
4. Instruct clients in the importance of limiting the use of nasal sprays and drops to prevent rebound nasal congestion

---

BOX 47-6. Nasal and Systemic Decongestants

Ephedrine
Naphazoline HCl (Allerest)
Oxymetazoline HCl (Afrin)
Phenylephrine HCl (Neo-Synephrine)
Phenylpropanolamine HCl (Dimetapp)
Pseudoephedrine (Sudafed)
Tetrahydrozoline HCl (Tyzine)
Xylometazoline HCl (Otrivin)

BOX 47–7. Mucolytic Agents (Expectorants)

Guaifenesin (glyceryl guaiacolate) (Glycotuss, Humibid, Robitussin)
Iodinated glycerol (Iophen)
Potassium iodide (SSKI)
Acetylcysteine (Mucomyst)
Guaifenesin and dextromethorphan (Robitussin-DM)

VII. Mucolytic Medications (Expectorants)
(Box 47–7)

A. Description
   1. Loosen bronchial secretions so that they can be eliminated with coughing
   2. Used for dry, unproductive cough and to stimulate bronchial secretions
   3. Guaifenesin and dextromethorphan (Robitussin-DM) are both an antitussive and expectorant
   4. Mucolytic agents with dextromethorphan should not be used with clients with **COPD** because they suppress the cough
   5. Acetylcysteine (Mucomyst) can increase airway resistance and should not be used in clients with asthma
B. Side effects
   1. GI irritation
   2. Skin rash
   3. Oropharyngeal irritation

C. Implementation
   1. Instruct the client to take the medication with a full glass of water to loosen mucus and to maintain an adequate fluid intake
   2. Instruct the client to drink the diluted liquid form of saturated solution of potassium iodide (SSKI) through a straw to avoid discoloration of tooth enamel
   3. Avoid the administration of potassium iodide (SSKI) if hyperkalemia is present
   4. Encourage client to cough and deep breathe
   5. Acetylcysteine (Mucomyst), administered by nebulization, should not be mixed with another medication
   6. If acetylcysteine is administered with a bronchodilator, the bronchodilator should be administered 5 minutes before the acetylcysteine
   7. Monitor for side effects of acetylcysteine such as nausea and vomiting, stomatitis, and runny nose

VIII. Antitussives (Cough Suppressants)
(Box 47–8)

A. Description
   1. Act on the cough control center in the medulla to suppress the cough reflex
   2. Used for a cough that is nonproductive and irritating

BOX 47–8. Antitussives

NARCOTICS
Codeine
Guaifenesin and codeine (Cheracol Cough, Robitussin A-C)
Hydrocodone bitartrate (Hycodan)

NONNARCOTICS
Benzonatate (Tessalon)
Diphenhydramine HCl (Benadryl)
Promethazine with dextromethorphan

B. Side effects
   1. Drowsiness and sedation
   2. GI irritation
   3. Nausea
   4. Dizziness
   5. Dry mouth
   6. Constipation
   7. Respiratory depression
C. Implementation
   1. Instruct the client that if the cough lasts longer than 1 week and a fever or rash occurs, the physician should be notified
   2. Encourage clients to take adequate fluids with the medication
   3. Encourage clients to sleep with the head of the bed elevated
   4. Instruct the client to avoid hazardous activities
   5. Note that drug dependency can occur
   6. Avoid administration in the client with a head injury or postoperative cranial surgery
   7. Avoid administering to client using narcotics, sedative hypnotics, barbiturates, or antidepressants, as CNS depression can occur
   8. Instruct clients to avoid the use of alcohol

IX. Narcotic Antagonist (Box 47–9)

A. Description
   1. Reverses respiratory depression in narcotic overdose
   2. Use of the medication is avoided in nonnarcotic respiratory depression
B. Side effects
   1. CNS depression
   2. Nausea and vomiting
   3. Sweating and tremors
   4. Tachycardia and increased blood pressure
C. Implementation
   1. Monitor vital signs, especially respirations
   2. Have oxygen and resuscitative equipment available during administration

---

BOX 47–9. Narcotic Antagonist

Naloxone HCl (Narcan)

▶ **X. Instructing the Client to Use an Inhaler**

A. Shake inhaler well before using
B. Remove cap from inhaler
C. Breathe deeply in and out through the mouth
D. Insert the mouthpiece into the mouth or in front of the open mouth, holding the inhaler upright
E. If a spacer is used, attach the spacer to the inhaler and place the end of the spacer in the mouth, passing the teeth and above the tongue
F. With the index finger on the top of the canister, depress the top while inhaling slowly
G. Remove the inhaler and hold the breath for as long as possible, then exhale slowly
H. Wait 1 to 2 minutes before the next dose
I. If two different inhalers are prescribed and one of the medications contains a steroid, administer the bronchodilator first and the steroid second
J. Wait 5 minutes following the bronchodilator before inhaling the steroid
K. Clean the mouthpiece following use

PRACTICE QUESTIONS

1. The nurse is preparing to administer albuterol (Proventil) to a client. The nurse checks for which of the following parameters before and during therapy?
   1 Increased urine output
   2 Nausea and vomiting
   3 Respiratory distress
   4 Complaints of headache

2. The nurse is administering a dose of isoproterenol HCl (Isuprel) to a client. The nurse plans to monitor for which of the following side effects of this medication?
   1 Increased pulse and blood pressure
   2 Drowsiness
   3 Hyperglycemia
   4 Hypokalemia

3. The nurse has an order to give the client metaproterenol sulfate (Alupent) two puffs and beclamethasone (Vanceril) two puffs by metered-dose inhaler. The nurse administers the medication by giving the
   1 Beclomethasone first and then the metaproterenol
   2 Metaproterenol first and then the beclomethasone
   3 Alternating a single puff of each, beginning with the beclomethasone
   4 Alternating a single puff of each, beginning with the metaproterenol

4. The client has begun therapy with oxtriphylline (Choledyl). The nurse plans to tell the client to limit the intake of which of the following while taking this medication?
   1 Oysters, lobster, and shrimp
   2 Coffee, cola, and chocolate
   3 Cottage cheese, cream cheese, and dairy creamers
   4 Grapefruit, oranges, and pineapple

5. The client with an order to take theophylline (Slo-Bid) daily has been given medication instructions by the nurse. The nurse evaluates that the client needs further information about the medication if the client states to
   1 Avoid changing brands of the medication without physician approval
   2 Avoid over-the-counter (OTC) cough and cold medications unless approved by physician
   3 Drink at least 2 liters of fluid per day
   4 Take the daily dose at bedtime

6. The client is taking brompheniramine maleate (Dimetane). The nurse checks for which of the following side effects of this medication?
   1 Excitability
   2 Drowsiness
   3 Excess salivation
   4 Diarrhea

7. The client taking brompheniramine maleate (Dimetane) is scheduled for allergy skin testing, and tells the nurse in the physician's office that a dose was taken this morning. The nurse determines that
   1 A lower dose of allergen will need to be injected
   2 A higher dose of allergen will need to be injected
   3 The client should have the skin test read a day later than usual
   4 The client should reschedule the appointment

8. The client is receiving acetylcysteine (Mucomyst) 20% solution diluted in 0.9% NS by nebulizer. The nurse should have which of the following items available for possible use after giving this medication?
   1 Suction equipment
   2 Nasogastric tube
   3 Intubation tray
   4 Ambu bag

9. The nurse is assisting to administer acetylcysteine (Mucomyst) to a client admitted with acetaminophen (Tylenol) overdose. Before giving this medication, the nurse ensures that the
   1 Client knows how to use a nebulizer
   2 Antidote to acetaminophen is readily available
   3 Stomach is empty from emesis or lavage
   4 Solution is given full strength

10. The client has an order to take guaifenesin (Humibid) every 4 hours as needed. The nurse evaluates that the client understands the most effective use of this medication if the client states to
   1 Take the tablet with a full glass of water

2 Take an extra dose if the cough is accompanied by fever

3 Beware of irritability as a side effect

4 Crush the sustained-release tablet if immediate relief is needed

11. The postoperative client has received a dose of naloxone HCl (Narcan) for respiratory depression shortly after transfer to the nursing unit from the postanesthesia care unit. Following administration of the medication, the nurse checks the client for

1 Pupillary changes

2 Sudden episodes of vomiting

3 Sudden increase in pain

4 Scattered lung wheezes

12. The client with suspected narcotic overdose has received a dose of naloxone HCl (Narcan). The client subsequently becomes restless, starts to vomit, and complains of abdominal cramping. The blood pressure increases from 110/72 to 160/86. The nurse provides emotional support and reassurance while administering care to the client, knowing that

1 These effects will only last a few moments

2 These are signs of opioid withdrawal

3 The client may otherwise sign out against medical advice

4 The client may next become suicidal

13. The nurse is assisting in caring for a client who is receiving a dose of naloxone HCl (Narcan) intravenously to treat narcotic overdose. The nurse plans to have which of the following available as supportive equipment in case it is needed?

1 Nasogastric tube

2 Paracentesis tray

3 Central line insertion tray

4 Resuscitation equipment

14. The nurse is reinforcing instructions to the client about the effects of diphenhydramine HCl (Benadryl), which has been ordered as a cough suppressant. The nurse does not include which of the following items in the instructions?

1 Avoid driving or other activities requiring mental alertness while taking this medication

2 Use sugarless gum, candy, or oral rinses to decrease dry mouth

3 Avoid using alcohol while taking this medication

4 Administer on an empty stomach

15. The client has been prescribed a cough formula containing codeine. The nurse has given the cli-

ent instructions for its use. The nurse evaluates that the client understands the instructions if the client verbalizes to self-check for

1 Excitability

2 Constipation

3 Rapid pulse

4 Excessive urination

16. The nurse is caring for the client who has been taking hydrocodone bitartrate (Hycodan) for the past 3 months. The nurse checks the client for which of the following side effects of this medication?

1 Psychological and physical dependence

2 Tachycardia and hypertension

3 Diarrhea and abdominal cramping

4 Increased respiratory rate and bronchospasm

17. Cromolyn sodium (Intal) is prescribed for the client with allergic asthma. The nurse tells the client about this medication, knowing that it acts to

1 Inhibit the release of mediators from mast cells after exposure to an antigen

2 Promote the migration of eosinophils into the inflammatory site

3 Increase the number of eosinophils

4 Dilate the bronchi

18. Cromolyn sodium (Intal) inhaler is prescribed for the client with allergic asthma. The nurse reinforces instructions regarding the side effects of this medication, knowing that which undesirable side effect is associated with this medication?

1 Constipation

2 Hypotension

3 Insomnia

4 Cough

19. Terbutaline sulfate (Brethine) is prescribed for the client with bronchitis. This medication should be used with caution if which of the following existing medical conditions is present in the client?

1 Hypothyroidism

2 Polycystic disease

3 Osteoarthritis

4 Diabetes mellitus

20. Zafirlukast (Accolate) is prescribed for the client with bronchial asthma. Which of the following laboratory tests does the nurse expect to be prescribed prior to the administration of this medication?

1 Platelet count

2 Complete blood cell count

3 Liver function tests

4 Neutrophil count

ANSWERS

1. **3**

RATIONALE: Albuterol is a bronchodilator of the adrenergic type. The nurse checks the respiratory pattern, pulse, and blood pressure prior to and during therapy. The color, character, and amount of sputum are also noted.
TEST-TAKING STRATEGY: Use the ABCs, airway, breathing, and circulation, to answer the question. Option 3 is the only option that addresses airway. Review this medication now if you had difficulty with this question.
LEVEL OF COGNITIVE ABILITY: Application
PHASE OF NURSING PROCESS: Data Collection
CLIENT NEEDS: Physiological Integrity
CONTENT AREA: Pharmacology
REFERENCE
Deglin, J., & Vallerand, A. (1999). *Davis's drug guide for nurses* (6th ed.). Philadelphia: F. A. Davis. p. 16.

2. **1**

RATIONALE: Isoproterenol is an adrenergic bronchodilator. Side effects can include tachycardia, hypertension, chest pain, dysrhythmias, nervousness, restlessness, and headache, among others. The nurse monitors for these effects during therapy.
TEST-TAKING STRATEGY: To answer this question accurately it is necessary to understand that this medication is a bronchodilator. Thus, it causes bronchodilation but also increases pulse and blood pressure due to its cardiovascular effects. Remembering that tachycardia is a side effect should assist in selecting the option that identifies an increased pulse, option 1.
LEVEL OF COGNITIVE ABILITY: Application
PHASE OF NURSING PROCESS: Planning
CLIENT NEEDS: Physiological Integrity
CONTENT AREA: Pharmacology
REFERENCE
Hodgson, B., & Kizior, R. (1999). *Saunders nursing drug handbook 1999.* Philadelphia: W. B. Saunders. p. 554.

3. **2**

RATIONALE: Metaproterenol is a bronchodilator. Beclomethasone is a glucocorticoid. Bronchodilators are always administered before glucocorticoids, when both are to be given on the same time schedule. This allows for widening of the air passages by the bronchodilator, which then makes the glucocorticoid more effective.
TEST-TAKING STRATEGY: To answer this question correctly, it is necessary to know two different things. First you must know that a bronchodilator is always given before a glucocorticoid. This would allow you to eliminate options 3 and 4, since you would not alternate the medications. Second, to discriminate between options 1 and 2, it is necessary to know that metaproterenol is a bronchodilator, whereas beclomethasone is a glucocorticoid.
LEVEL OF COGNITIVE ABILITY: Application
PHASE OF NURSING PROCESS: Implementation
CLIENT NEEDS: Physiological Integrity
CONTENT AREA: Pharmacology
REFERENCE
deWit, S. (1998). *Essentials of medical-surgical nursing* (4th ed.). Philadelphia: W. B. Saunders. p. 448.

4. **2**

RATIONALE: Oxtriphylline is a xanthine bronchodilator. The nurse teaches the client to limit the intake of xanthine-containing foods while taking this medication. These include coffee, cola, and chocolate.
TEST-TAKING STRATEGY: To answer this question correctly, it is necessary to understand that oxtriphylline is a xanthine bronchodilator and to know which food items are naturally high in xanthines. Take time now to review the foods naturally high in xanthines, if you had difficulty with this question.
LEVEL OF COGNITIVE ABILITY: Application
PHASE OF NURSING PROCESS: Planning
CLIENT NEEDS: Health Promotion and Maintenance
CONTENT AREA: Pharmacology
REFERENCE
Deglin, J., & Vallerand, A. (1999). *Davis's drug guide for nurses* (6th ed.). Philadelphia: F. A. Davis. p. 124.

5. **4**

RATIONALE: The client taking a single daily dose of theophylline, a xanthine bronchodilator, should take the medication early in the morning. This enables the client to have maximal benefit from the medication during daytime activities. Additionally, this medication causes insomnia. The client should take in at least 2 liters of fluid per day to decrease viscosity of secretions. The client should check with the physician before changing brands of the medication. The client also checks with the physician before taking OTC cough, cold, or other respiratory preparations with theophylline because they could have interactive effects, increasing the side effects of theophylline and causing dysrhythmias.
TEST-TAKING STRATEGY: Note the key words "needs further information." General principles related to medication therapy will assist in eliminating options 1 and 2. Additionally, recalling that option 3 is an important measure to thin secretions will direct you to option 4. Review this medication now if you had difficulty with this question.
LEVEL OF COGNITIVE ABILITY: Comprehension
PHASE OF NURSING PROCESS: Evaluation
CLIENT NEEDS: Health Promotion and Maintenance
CONTENT AREA: Pharmacology
REFERENCE
Lehne, R. (1998). *Pharmacology for nursing care.* (3rd ed.). Philadelphia: W. B. Saunders. pp. 755–756.

6. **2**

RATIONALE: A frequent side effect of brompheniramine (Dimetane), an antihistamine, is drowsiness or sedation. Others include blurred vision, hypertension (and sometimes hypotension), dry mouth, constipation, urinary retention, and sweating.
TEST-TAKING STRATEGY: Recall that antihistamines typically cause drowsiness. To answer this question correctly, it is necessary to know that this medication is an antihistamine. Take time now to review the side effects of antihistamines if you had difficulty with this question.
LEVEL OF COGNITIVE ABILITY: Application
PHASE OF NURSING PROCESS: Data Collection
CLIENT NEEDS: Physiological Integrity
CONTENT AREA: Pharmacology
REFERENCE
Asperheim, M. K. (1996). *Pharmacology: An introductory text* (8th ed.). Philadelphia: W. B. Saunders. p. 106.

7. **4**

RATIONALE: Brompheniramine is an antihistamine, which provides relief of symptoms caused by allergy. Antihistamines should be discontinued for at least 3 days (72 hours) before allergy skin testing to avoid false negative readings. This client should have the appointment rescheduled for 3 days after discontinuing the medication.
TEST-TAKING STRATEGY: To answer this question correctly, it is necessary to know that this medication is an antihistamine. It is also necessary to know that antihistamines reduce the allergic response. With this in mind, option 1 is eliminated first, since it makes no sense. Options 2 and 3 are also eliminated, because the medication would still interfere with the test results.
LEVEL OF COGNITIVE ABILITY: Comprehension
PHASE OF NURSING PROCESS: Planning
CLIENT NEEDS: Physiological Integrity
CONTENT AREA: Pharmacology
REFERENCE
Hodgson, B., & Kizior, R. (1999). *Saunders nursing drug handbook 1999*. Philadelphia: W. B. Saunders. p. 125.

8. **1**

RATIONALE: Acetylcysteine can be given orally or by nasogastric tube to treat acetaminophen overdose, or it may be given by inhalation for use as a mucolytic. The nurse administering this medication as a mucolytic should have suction equipment available in case the client cannot manage to clear the increased volume of liquefied secretions.
TEST-TAKING STRATEGY: To answer this question, it is necessary to know that acetylcysteine may be given for either acetaminophen overdose or as a mucolytic agent. It is also necessary to know that the inhalation route is used only for mucolytic effects. With this in mind, options 3 and 4 are eliminated, because the client does not need resuscitation. Option 2 is eliminated also, since this medication is being administered by nebulizer. If you had difficulty with this question, take time now to review the purpose of this medication and the related nursing interventions.
LEVEL OF COGNITIVE ABILITY: Application
PHASE OF NURSING PROCESS: Planning
CLIENT NEEDS: Safe, Effective Care Environment
CONTENT AREA: Pharmacology
REFERENCE
Deglin, J., & Vallerand, A. (1999). *Davis's drug guide for nurses* (6th ed.). Philadelphia: F. A. Davis. p. 6.

9. **3**

RATIONALE: Acetylcysteine can be given orally or by nasogastric tube to treat acetaminophen overdose, or it may be given by inhalation for use as a mucolytic. Prior to giving the medication as an antidote to acetaminophen, the nurse ensures that the client's stomach is empty through emesis or gastric lavage. The solution is diluted in cola, water, or juice to make the solution more palatable. It is then administered orally or by nasogastric tube.
TEST-TAKING STRATEGY: Begin to answer this question by eliminating options 1 and 2. This medication is not given by the inhalation route to treat acetaminophen overdose, and acetylcysteine is the antidote (to acetaminophen). To discriminate between the last two options, it is necessary to know two things: first, the solution must be diluted, which forces you to choose option 3 as correct and second, knowing that the stomach must be emptied for maximal effect of the antidote also forces you to choose option 3 as correct.

LEVEL OF COGNITIVE ABILITY: Application
PHASE OF NURSING PROCESS: Implementation
CLIENT NEEDS: Physiological Integrity
CONTENT AREA: Pharmacology
REFERENCE
Deglin, J., & Vallerand, A. (1999). *Davis's drug guide for nurses* (6th ed.). Philadelphia: F. A. Davis. p. 6.

10. **1**

RATIONALE: Guaifenesin is an expectorant. It should be taken with a full glass of water to decrease viscosity of secretions. Sustained-release preparations should not be broken open, crushed, or chewed. The medication may occasionally cause dizziness, headache, or drowsiness as side effects. The client should contact the physician if the cough lasts longer than 1 week, or is accompanied by fever, rash, sore throat, or persistent headache.
TEST-TAKING STRATEGY: Begin to answer this question by eliminating option 4 first. Sustained-relief preparations are not crushed or broken. Option 2 is eliminated next because fever indicates infection, and an "extra dose" of an expectorant is not helpful in treating infection. To discriminate between the last two options, knowing that increased fluids helps to liquefy secretions for more effective coughing allows you to choose option 1 as correct. If you had difficulty with this question, take time now to review this medication.
LEVEL OF COGNITIVE ABILITY: Comprehension
PHASE OF NURSING PROCESS: Evaluation
CLIENT NEEDS: Health Promotion and Maintenance
CONTENT AREA: Pharmacology
REFERENCE
Hodgson, B., & Kizior, R. (1999). *Saunders nursing drug handbook 1999*. Philadelphia: W. B. Saunders. p. 482.

11. **3**

RATIONALE: Naloxone is an antidote to opioids, and it may also be given to the postoperative client to treat respiratory depression. When given to the postoperative client for respiratory depression, it may also reverse the effects of analgesics. Therefore, the nurse must check the client for a sudden increase in the level of pain experienced.
TEST-TAKING STRATEGY: To answer this question correctly, it is necessary to know that this medication is an antidote to narcotic analgesics, and that it would likely cause sudden pain in the postoperative client, or return of pain in clients who receive narcotic analgesics. If you had difficulty with this question, take time now to review this medication.
LEVEL OF COGNITIVE ABILITY: Comprehension
PHASE OF NURSING PROCESS: Data Collection
CLIENT NEEDS: Physiological Integrity
CONTENT AREA: Pharmacology
REFERENCE
Hodgson, B., & Kizior, R. (1999). *Saunders nursing drug handbook 1999*. Philadelphia: W. B. Saunders. p. 719.

12. **2**

RATIONALE: Signs of opioid withdrawal include increased temperature and blood pressure, abdominal cramping, vomiting, and restlessness. They can occur anywhere from a few minutes to a few hours after administration of naloxone, depending on the opioid involved, the degree of dependence, and the dose of naloxone.

TEST-TAKING STRATEGY: Eliminate option 1 first as the least plausible, since these types of symptoms identified in the question are not likely to disappear in a few moments. Option 4 is eliminated next, because there is no supporting information in the stem. To discriminate between the remaining two, knowing that the client with narcotic overdose may well have a history of prior chronic use would cause you to choose option 2 over option 3.
LEVEL OF COGNITIVE ABILITY: Comprehension
PHASE OF NURSING PROCESS: Implementation
CLIENT NEEDS: Psychosocial Integrity
CONTENT AREA: Pharmacology
REFERENCE
Hodgson, B., & Kizior, R. (1999). *Saunders nursing drug handbook 1999*. Philadelphia: W. B. Saunders. pp. 719–720.

13. **4**

RATIONALE: The nurse should have resuscitation equipment readily available to support naloxone therapy if it is needed. Other adjuncts that may be needed include oxygen, a mechanical ventilator, and available medications such as vasopressors.
TEST-TAKING STRATEGY: Note the key words "narcotic overdose." Knowing the effects of these medications, you would want to have other resuscitation equipment available. Option 4 is also the most global response.
LEVEL OF COGNITIVE ABILITY: Application
PHASE OF NURSING PROCESS: Planning
CLIENT NEEDS: Safe, Effective Care Environment
CONTENT AREA: Pharmacology
REFERENCE
Deglin, J., & Vallerand, A. (1999). *Davis's drug guide for nurses* (6th ed.). Philadelphia: F. A. Davis. p. 700.

14. **4**

RATIONALE: Diphenhydramine has several uses, including antihistamine, antitussive, antidyskinetic, and sedative/hypnotic. Instructions for use include to take with food or milk to decrease GI upset, and to use oral rinses or sugarless gum or hard candy to minimize dry mouth. Because the medication causes drowsiness, the client should avoid use of alcohol or CNS depressants, operating a car, or engaging in other activities requiring mental acuity during use.
TEST-TAKING STRATEGY: Note the key word "not." Knowing that the medication has a sedative effect helps you to eliminate options 1 and 3 first. Knowing that the medication causes dry mouth helps you choose option 4. If you had difficulty with this question, take time now to review client education related to this medication.
LEVEL OF COGNITIVE ABILITY: Application
PHASE OF NURSING PROCESS: Implementation
CLIENT NEEDS: Health Promotion and Maintenance
CONTENT AREA: Pharmacology
REFERENCE
Deglin, J., & Vallerand, A. (1999). *Davis's drug guide for nurses* (6th ed.). Philadelphia: F. A. Davis. p. 291.

15. **2**

RATIONALE: The client is taught about side effects that could occur with use of codeine. The most common include drowsiness, confusion, hypotension, nausea and vomiting, and constipation. Others include bradycardia, respiratory depression, and urinary retention.
TEST-TAKING STRATEGY: This question tests the concept that narcotic analgesics cause constipation as a side effect. Knowing that the medication causes drowsiness helps you to eliminate option 1 first. Knowing that the medication causes a decreased pulse helps you to eliminate option 3 next. Remember, codeine causes constipation.
LEVEL OF COGNITIVE ABILITY: Comprehension
PHASE OF NURSING PROCESS: Evaluation
CLIENT NEEDS: Health Promotion and Maintenance
CONTENT AREA: Pharmacology
REFERENCE
Eckler, J., & Fair, J. (1996). *Pharmacology essentials*. Philadelphia: W. B. Saunders. p. 207.

16. **1**

RATIONALE: Hydrocodone is an opioid analgesic that also has antitussive properties. Side effects of this medication include physical and psychological dependence, bradycardia and hypotension, respiratory depression, nausea, vomiting, constipation, sedation, and confusion.
TEST-TAKING STRATEGY: Use the process of elimination recalling that hydrocodone is an opioid analgesic that causes physical and psychological dependence. If this question was difficult, review information on the implications of opioid use and its side effects now.
LEVEL OF COGNITIVE ABILITY: Application
PHASE OF NURSING PROCESS: Data Collection
CLIENT NEEDS: Physiological Integrity
CONTENT AREA: Pharmacology
REFERENCE
Hodgson, B., & Kizior, R. (1999). *Saunders nursing drug handbook 1999*. Philadelphia: W. B. Saunders. p. 497.

17. **1**

RATIONALE: Cromolyn sodium is an antiasthmatic, antiallergic, and a mast-cell stabilizer that inhibits the release of mediators from mast cells after exposure to an antigen. It can also interrupt the migration of eosinophils into the inflammatory site and decrease the number of eosinophils. These actions decrease airway hyperresponsiveness in some clients with asthma. It has no bronchodilating action.
TEST-TAKING STRATEGY: Eliminate options 2 and 3 first because they are similar. To select between the remaining options, it is helpful to know that cromolyn sodium (Intal) has no bronchodilating action. Also, note the relationship between the words "antigen" in the correct option and "allergic" in the question.
LEVEL OF COGNITIVE ABILITY: Comprehension
PHASE OF NURSING PROCESS: Implementation
CLIENT NEEDS: Physiological Integrity
CONTENT AREA: Pharmacology
REFERENCE
Hodgson, B., & Kizior, R. (1999). *Saunders nursing drug handbook 1999*. Philadelphia: W. B. Saunders. p. 265.

18. **4**

RATIONALE: The most common undesired clinical responses associated with inhalation therapy of cromolyn sodium are bronchospasm, cough, nasal congestion, throat irritation, and wheezing. Clients receiving this medication orally may experience pruritus, nausea, diarrhea, and myalgia.
TEST-TAKING STRATEGY: Note the key word "undesirable." Use the ABCs, airway, breathing, and circulation, to select the correct option. Option 4 addresses airway.

LEVEL OF COGNITIVE ABILITY: Application
PHASE OF NURSING PROCESS: Implementation
CLIENT NEEDS: Physiological Integrity
CONTENT AREA: Pharmacology
REFERENCE
Hodgson, B., & Kizior, R. (1999). *Saunders nursing drug handbook 1999*. Philadelphia: W. B. Saunders. pp. 266–267.

19. 4

RATIONALE: Terbutaline sulfate (Brethine) is contraindicated in clients with hypersensitivity to sympathomimetics. It should be used with caution in clients with impaired cardiac function, diabetes mellitus, hypertension, hyperthyroidism, and clients with a history of seizures. The medication may increase blood glucose levels.
TEST-TAKING STRATEGY: This is a difficult question and knowledge regarding this medication is required to answer correctly. Take time now to review the contraindications associated with this medication if you had difficulty with this question.
LEVEL OF COGNITIVE ABILITY: Analysis
PHASE OF NURSING PROCESS: Planning
CLIENT NEEDS: Physiological Integrity
CONTENT AREA: Pharmacology

REFERENCE
Hodgson, B., & Kizior, R. (1999). *Saunders nursing drug handbook 1999*. Philadelphia: W. B. Saunders. pp. 969–970.

20. 3

RATIONALE: Zafirlukast (Accolate) is a leukotriene receptor antagonist that is used in the prophylaxis and chronic treatment of bronchial asthma. It is used with caution in clients with impaired hepatic function. Liver function laboratory values should be obtained as a baseline and should be monitored during administration of the medication.
TEST-TAKING STRATEGY: Use the process of elimination, eliminating options 2 and 4 first, because a complete blood count would include a neutrophil count. From this point, you need to know that this medication affects hepatic function. If you had difficulty with this question, take time now to review this medication.
LEVEL OF COGNITIVE ABILITY: Comprehension
PHASE OF NURSING PROCESS: Planning
CLIENT NEEDS: Physiological Integrity
CONTENT AREA: Pharmacology
REFERENCE
Hodgson, B., & Kizior, R. (1999). *Saunders nursing drug handbook 1999*. Philadelphia: W. B. Saunders. pp. 1064–1065.

BIBLIOGRAPHY

Asperheim, M. K. (1996). *Pharmacology: An introductory text* (8th ed.). Philadelphia: W. B. Saunders.

Deglin, J., & Vallerand, A. (1999). *Davis's drug guide for nurses* (6th ed.). Philadelphia: F. A. Davis.

deWit, S. (1998). *Essentials of medical-surgical nursing* (4th ed.). Philadelphia: W. B. Saunders.

Eckler, J., & Fair, J. (1996). *Pharmacology essentials*. Philadelphia: W. B. Saunders.

Hodgson, B., & Kizior, R. (1999). *Saunders nursing drug handbook 1999*. Philadelphia: W. B. Saunders.

Lehne, R. (1998). *Pharmacology for nursing care* (3rd ed.). Philadelphia: W. B. Saunders.

UNIT XIII

···

The Adult Client with a Cardiovascular Disorder

PYRAMID TERMS

Arterial Anastomosis—Ensures that when one of the blood-supplying arteries is damaged, flow is maintained from the other arteries. Blood flow to the hands, feet, brain, and other organs is protected by arterial anastomosis.

Blood Pressure (BP)—Measures the force exerted by the blood against the walls of the blood vessels. If the BP falls too low, blood flow to the tissues, heart, brain, and other organs becomes inadequate. If the BP becomes too high, the risk of vessel rupture and damage increases.

Cardiac Output—The total volume of blood pumped through the heart in 1 minute.

Diastole—The phase of the cardiac cycle in which the heart relaxes between contractions. It represents the period when the two ventricles are dilated by the blood flowing into them.

Diastolic Pressure—The force of the blood exerted against the artery walls when the heart relaxes or fills. Normal diastolic pressure is 60 to 90 mmHg.

Postural (Orthostatic) Hypotension—A blood pressure fall of more than 10 to 15 mmHg of the systolic pressure or a fall of more than 10 mmHg of the diastolic pressure and a 10% to 20% increase in heart rate. Occurs when the client's blood pressure is not adequately maintained when moving from a lying to a sitting or standing position.

Pulse Pressure—The difference between the systolic pressure and diastolic pressure. Normal pulse pressure is 30 to 40 mmHg.

Systole—The phase of contraction of the heart, especially of the ventricles, during which blood is forced into the aorta and pulmonary artery.

Systolic Pressure—The maximum pressure of blood exerted against the artery walls when the heart contracts. Normal systolic pressure is 100 to 140 mmHg.

◢ PYRAMID TO SUCCESS

Pyramid points focus on data collection related to cardiovascular risks, health screening and promotion, complications of the various cardiovascular disorders, emergency implementation measures, and client education. Focus on the findings in angina, myocardial infarction (MI), congestive heart failure (CHF) and pulmonary edema, hypertension, and arterial and vascular disorders. Focus on the care of the client following diagnostic treatments and surgical procedures. Note appropriate and therapeutic client positions, particularly with arterial and venous disorders of the extremities. Focus on treatments and medications prescribed for the various cardiovascular disorders, and client teaching related to prescribed treatment plans. Be familiar with the components related to cardiac rehabilitation.

NURSING PROCESS

DATA COLLECTION

- Demographic data, including age, sex, and cultural background
- Lifestyle habits; dietary and activity patterns
- Characteristics of chest pain
- Dyspnea—exertional, paroxysmal nocturnal, and orthopnea
- Altered level of consciousness, syncope, or fainting
- Palpitations
- Respiratory distress, cough, or blood-tinged sputum
- An increase or decrease in heart rate, blood pressure, or respirations
- Weight gain and edema
- Fatigue and weakness
- Extremity pain
- Skin color and temperature changes
- Capillary filling time and peripheral pulses
- Cardiac enzymes, electrocardiography (ECG), and laboratory and diagnostic tests
- Psychosocial data

PLANNING	IMPLEMENTATION	EVALUATION
The client verbalizes chest discomfort. The client describes measures to relieve chest discomfort including medication and activity restrictions.	Assess characteristics of pain. Determine precipitants of pain. Identify measures that relieve the pain. Administer nitroglycerin or pain medication as prescribed. Document the effectiveness of the medication.	The client obtains relief of chest discomfort.
PLANNING	IMPLEMENTATION	EVALUATION
The client maintains adequate cardiac output.	Monitor vital signs. Monitor for cardiac irregularities. Administer oxygen as prescribed. Monitor for the presence of cyanosis. Monitor for fluid overload and the presence of edema. Monitor weight. Monitor level of consciousness. Monitor extremities for color, temperature, and sensation. Instruct the client in measures to avoid circulatory compromise.	The client maintains adequate circulatory status.
PLANNING	IMPLEMENTATION	EVALUATION
Client describes barriers to compliance with treatment plan and identifies methods to modify barriers.	Assess client's understanding of illness. Assist client to explore denial. Engage client in discussion about anxiety, fears, symptoms, and impact of illness. Assist with initiating support services and resources for the client.	The client acknowledges cardiovascular symptoms.

PLANNING

The client describes the required diet, medications, activity, and limitations. The client verbalizes reportable signs and symptoms of activity worsening the condition. The client verbalizes the significance of symptoms. The client reports significant symptoms.

IMPLEMENTATION

Instruct client in the correct procedure for taking nitroglycerin and other prescribed medications. Instruct client in diet and prescriptions. Instruct client regarding signs and symptoms requiring notifying health care provider. Assist with initiating home care and community support.

EVALUATION

Client verbalizes accurate information regarding medications, diet, and the modification of risk factors associated with cardiovascular disorders. Client remains asymptomatic and implements appropriate treatments to alter the atherosclerotic progression. The client uses resources in the community.

◢ CLIENT NEEDS

SAFE, EFFECTIVE CARE ENVIRONMENT

Informed consent related to treatments and procedures
Cardiovascular consultations and referrals
Standard (universal) precautions

HEALTH PROMOTION AND MAINTENANCE

Prevention of cardiovascular disease
Health screening and health promotion programs
Alterations in lifestyle
Teaching related to diet therapy, exercise, and the administration of medications
Assisting with the mobilization of appropriate community resources
Cardiac rehabilitation

PSYCHOSOCIAL INTEGRITY

Fear, anxiety, and denial
Accepting lifestyle changes
Body image changes
Coping mechanisms
Support systems

PHYSIOLOGICAL INTEGRITY

Nonpharmacological and pharmacological comfort interventions
Assisting with basic care measures
Activity limitations and rest and sleep
Monitoring cardiac enzymes and laboratory values related to the cardiovascular system
Monitoring for complications related to cardiovascular disorders
Interventions required in emergencies

BIBLIOGRAPHY

deWit, S. (1998). *Essentials of medical-surgical nursing* (4th ed.). Philadelphia: W. B. Saunders.

Hill, S., & Howlett, H. (1997). *Success in practical nursing: Personal and vocational issues* (3rd ed.). Philadelphia: W. B. Saunders.

Leahy, J., & Kizilay, P. (1998). *Foundations of nursing practice: A nursing process approach*. Philadelphia: W. B. Saunders.

Luckmann, J. (1997). *Saunders manual of nursing care*. Philadelphia: W. B. Saunders.

Monahan, F., & Neighbors, M. (1998). *Medical-surgical nursing: Foundations for clinical practice* (2nd ed.). Philadelphia: W. B. Saunders.

National Council of State Boards of Nursing (1998). *National Council detailed test plan for the NCLEX-PN examination*. Chicago: Author.

O'Toole, M. (1997). *Miller-Keane encyclopedia & dictionary of medicine, nursing, & allied health* (6th ed.). Philadelphia: W. B. Saunders.

CHAPTER 48

Cardiovascular System

···

I. Anatomy and Physiology

A. Heart and heart layers
1. The heart is located in the left side of the mediastinum
2. The epicardium covers the outer surface of the heart
3. The myocardium is the middle layer and is the actual contracting muscle of the heart
4. The endocardium is the innermost layer and lines the inner chambers and the heart valves

B. Pericardium
1. The pericardium encases and protects the heart from trauma and infection
2. The parietal pericardium is the tough, fibrous outer membrane that is attached anteriorly to the lower half of the sternum, posteriorly to the thoracic vertebrae and inferiorly to the diaphragm
3. The visceral pericardium is the thin inner layer that closely adheres to the heart
4. The pericardial space is between the parietal and visceral layers; it holds 5 to 20 mL of pericardial fluid that lubricates the pericardial surfaces and cushions the heart

C. Heart chambers
1. The right atrium receives deoxygenated blood from the body via the superior and inferior venae cavae
2. The right ventricle receives blood from the right atrium and pumps it to the lungs via the pulmonary artery
3. The left atrium receives oxygenated blood from the lungs via four pulmonary veins
4. The left ventricle is the largest and most muscular chamber; it receives oxygenated blood from the lungs via the left atrium and pumps blood into the systemic circulation via the aorta

D. Heart valves
1. The atrioventricular valves lie between the atria and the ventricles
2. The atrioventricular valves close at the beginning of ventricular contraction and prevent blood from flowing back into the atria

from the ventricles; these valves open when the ventricle relaxes
3. The bicuspid or mitral valve is located on the left side of the heart
4. The tricuspid valve is located on the right side of the heart
5. The pulmonic semilunar valve lies between the right ventricle and the pulmonary artery
6. The aortic semilunar valve lies between the left ventricle and the aorta
7. The semilunar valves prevent blood from flowing back into the ventricles during relaxation; they open during ventricular contraction and close when the ventricles begin to relax

E. Atrioventricular node (AV)
1. The AV node is located in the lower aspect of the atrial septum
2. The AV node receives electrical impulses from the sinoatrial (SA) node

F. The bundle of His (AV bundle)
1. The bundle of His fuses with the AV node to form another pacemaker site
2. It branches into the right bundle branch (RBB), which branches down the right side of the interventricular septum, and the left bundle branch (LBB), which extends into the left ventricle
3. The right and left bundle branches terminate into Purkinje's fibers
4. If the SA node fails, the bundle of His can initiate and sustain a heart rate at 40 to 60 beats per minute (bpm)

G. Purkinje's fibers
1. Purkinje's fibers are a diffuse network of conducting strands located beneath the ventricular endocardium
2. These fibers spread the wave of depolarization through the ventricles

H. Coronary arteries
1. The coronary arteries supply the capillaries of the myocardium with blood
2. The right coronary artery (RCA) supplies the right atrium and ventricle, the inferior portion

663

of the left ventricle, the posterior septal wall, and the sinoatrial and the atrioventricular nodes

3. The left coronary artery (LCA) consists of two major branches, the left anterior descending (LAD) and the circumflex arteries
4. The LAD supplies blood to the anterior wall of the left ventricle, the anterior ventricular septum, and the apex of the left ventricle
5. The circumflex artery supplies blood to the left atrium and the lateral and posterior surfaces of the left ventricle

I. Sinoatrial node (SA)
1. The SA node or pacemaker initiates each heart beat
2. Its location is at the junction of the superior vena cava and the right atrium
3. It generates electrical impulses at approximately 60 to 100 times per minute and is controlled by the sympathetic and parasympathetic systems

J. Heart sounds
1. The first heart sound (S_1) is heard as the AV valves close
2. The second heart sound (S_2) is heard when the semilunar valves close

K. Heart rate
1. The faster the heart rate, the less time the heart has for filling, and the **cardiac output** decreases
2. An increase in heart rate increases oxygen consumption
3. The normal heart rate is 60 to 100 bpm
4. Sinus tachycardia is a rate of more than 100 bpm
5. Sinus bradycardia is a rate of less than 60 bpm

L. Autonomic nervous system
1. Stimulation of sympathetic nerve fibers releases the neurotransmitter norepinephrine, producing an increased heart rate, increased conduction speed through the AV node, increased atrial and ventricular contractility, and peripheral vasoconstriction; stimulation occurs when a decrease in pressure is detected
2. Stimulation of the parasympathetic nerve fibers releases the neurotransmitter acetylcholine, which decreases the heart rate and lessens atrial and ventricular contractility and conductivity; stimulation occurs when an increase in pressure is detected

M. Blood pressure control
1. Baroreceptors, also called pressoreceptors, are located in the walls of the aortic arch and carotid sinuses
2. Baroreceptors are specialized nerve endings that are affected by changes in the arterial **blood pressure**
3. Increases in arterial pressure stimulate baroreceptors, and the heart rate and arterial pressure decrease
4. Decreases in arterial pressure lead to a lessened stimulation of the baroreceptors,

and vasoconstriction occurs as does an increase in heart rate
5. Stretch receptors, located in the vena cava and the right atrium, respond to pressure changes that affect circulatory blood volume
6. When the **blood pressure** decreases due to hypovolemia, a sympathetic response occurs, causing an increased heart rate and blood vessel constriction; when the **blood pressure** increases due to hypervolemia, the opposite effect occurs
7. The antidiuretic hormone (ADH) influences **blood pressure** indirectly by regulating vascular volume
8. Increases in blood volume result in decreased ADH release, increasing diuresis, decreasing blood volume, and thus **blood pressure**
9. Decreases in blood volume result in increased ADH release; this promotes an increase in blood volume and thus **blood pressure**
10. Renin, a potent vasoconstrictor, causes the **blood pressure** to increase
11. Renin converts angiotensinogen to angiotensin I; angiotensin I is then converted to angiotensin II in the lungs
12. Angiotensin II stimulates the release of aldosterone, which promotes water and sodium retention by the kidneys; this action increases blood volume and **blood pressure**

N. The vascular system
1. The arteries are vessels through which the blood passes away from the heart to various parts of the body; they convey blood with high concentrations of oxygen from the left side of the heart to the tissues
2. The arterioles control the blood flow into the capillaries
3. The capillaries allow the exchange of fluid and nutrients between the blood and the interstitial spaces
4. Venules receive blood from the capillary bed and move it into the veins
5. Veins transport deoxygenated blood from the tissues back toward the heart and lungs for oxygenation
6. Valves help return blood to the heart against the force of gravity
7. The lymphatics drain the tissues and return the tissue fluid to the blood

II. **Diagnostic Tests and Procedures**
(refer to Chapter 10 for normal laboratory values)

A. Cardiac enzymes
1. CK-MB (creatine kinase, myocardial muscle)
   a. An elevation in value indicates myocardial damage
   b. An elevation occurs within 4 to 6 hours

and peaks 18 to 24 hours following the acute ischemic attack

    c. Normal value in conventional units is 0 to 7 U/L

  2. LDH (lactic acid dehydrogenase)

    a. Elevations in LDH occur within 48 hours following myocardial infarction

    b. When the serum concentration of LDH 1 is higher than LDH 2, the pattern is indicated as "flipped," signifying myocardial necrosis

    c. Normal value in conventional units is 70 to 200 IU/L

B. CBC (complete blood cell) count

  1. The red blood cell count decreases in rheumatic heart disease and infective endocarditis and increases in conditions characterized by inadequate tissue oxygenation

  2. The white blood cell (WBC) count increases in infectious and inflammatory diseases of the heart and following myocardial infarction because large numbers of WBCs are required to dispose of the necrotic tissue resulting from the infarction

  3. An elevated hematocrit can result from vascular volume depletion

  4. A decrease in hematocrit and hemoglobin can indicate anemia

C. Blood coagulation factors: an increase in coagulation factors can occur during and after a myocardial infarction, which places the client at greater risk of thrombophlebitis and extension of clots in the coronary artery

D. Serum lipids

  1. The lipid profile measures serum cholesterol, triglycerides, and lipoprotein levels

  2. The lipid profile is used to assess the risk of developing coronary artery disease

E. Electrolytes

  1. Potassium level

    a. Hypokalemia causes increased cardiac electrical instability, ventricular dysrhythmias, and increased risk of digitalis toxicity.

    b. In hypokalemia, the ECG shows flattening and inversion of the T wave, the appearance of a U wave, and depression of the ST segment

    c. Hyperkalemia causes asystole and ventricular dysrhythmias

  2. Sodium level

    a. The serum sodium level decreases with the use of diuretics

    b. The serum sodium level decreases in congestive heart failure, indicating water excess

F. Calcium level

  1. Hypocalcemia can cause ventricular dysrhythmias, prolonged QT interval, and cardiac arrest

  2. Hypercalcemia can cause a shortened QT

interval, AV block, tachycardia or bradycardia, digitalis hypersensitivity, and cardiac arrest

G. Phosphorus level; phosphorus levels should be interpreted with calcium levels because the kidneys retain or excrete one electrolyte in an inverse relationship to the other

H. Magnesium level

  1. A low magnesium level can cause ventricular tachycardia and fibrillation

  2. A high magnesium level can cause muscle weakness, hypotension, bradycardia, and a prolonged PR interval and wide QRS complex

I. Blood urea nitrogen (BUN): the BUN is elevated in heart disorders such as congestive heart failure and cardiogenic shock, which adversely affects renal circulation

J. Blood glucose: an acute cardiac episode can elevate the blood glucose

K. Chest x-ray

  1. Description

    a. Done to determine the size, silhouette, and position of the heart

    b. Specific pathologic changes are difficult to determine via x-ray, but anatomic changes can be seen

  2. Implementation

    a. Prepare the client for x-ray by explaining the purpose of the procedure

    b. Remove jewelry

L. ECG (electrocardiogram)

  1. Description: a noninvasive common diagnostic test that evaluates the heart's function by recording electrical activity

  2. Implementation

    a. Advise the client to lie still, breathe normally, and refrain from talking during the test

    b. Reassure the client that an electrical shock will not occur

    c. Document any cardiac medications the client is taking

M. Holter monitoring

  1. Description

    a. A noninvasive test in which the client wears a Holter monitor and an ECG tracing is recorded continuously over 24 or more hours

    b. It identifies dysrhythmias if they occur and evaluates the effectiveness of antidysrhythmics or pacemaker therapy

  2. Implementation: instruct the client to resume normal daily activities and to maintain a diary documenting activities and any symptoms that may develop

N. Echocardiogram

  1. Description

    a. A noninvasive procedure based on the principles of ultrasound

    b. It evaluates structural and functional changes in the heart

  2. Implementation: advise the client to lie still,

breathe normally, and refrain from talking during the test

O. Exercise testing (stress)
  1. Description
     a. A noninvasive test that studies the heart during activity and detects and evaluates coronary artery disease
     b. The treadmill testing is the most commonly used mode of stress testing
     c. Stress testing may be used in conjunction with myocardial radionuclide testing at which point the procedure becomes invasive because a radionuclide must be injected
     d. A consent form is required if a radionuclide is injected
  2. Preprocedure implementation
     a. Obtain informed consent if required
     b. Provide adequate rest the night before the procedure
     c. Instruct the client to eat a light meal 1 to 2 hours before the procedure
     d. Instruct the client to avoid smoking, alcohol, and caffeine prior to the procedure
     e. Ask the physician about taking prescribed medication on the day of the procedure
     f. Instruct the client to wear nonconstrictive, comfortable clothing and supportive shoes
  3. Postprocedure implementation
     a. Instruct the client to notify the physician if any chest pain, dizziness, or shortness of breath occurs
     b. Instruct the client to avoid taking a hot bath or shower for at least 1 to 2 hours

P. Digital subtraction angiography
  1. Description
     a. Combines x-ray techniques and a computerized subtraction technique with fluoroscopy for visualization of the cardiovascular system
     b. A contrast medium (dye) is injected
  2. Preprocedure implementation
     a. Assess the client for allergy to contrast medium (dye), iodine, or seafood
     b. Obtain informed consent
  3. Postprocedure implementation
     a. Monitor vital signs
     b. Assess the injection site for bleeding or discomfort

Q. Nuclear cardiology
  1. Description
     a. The use of radionuclide techniques and scanning in cardiovascular assessment
     b. The most common tests include technetium pyrophosphate scanning, thallium imaging, and multigated angiogram (MUGA) scan
  2. Preprocedure implementation
     a. Obtain informed consent
     b. Inform the client that a small amount of radioisotope will be injected and that the radiation exposure and risks are minimal

  3. Postprocedure implementation
     a. Assess vital signs
     b. Assess injection site for bleeding or discomfort
     c. Inform clients that they may feel fatigued

R. Cardiac catheterization
  1. Description
     a. Involves insertion of a catheter into the heart and surrounding vessels
     b. Obtains information about the structure and performance of the heart valves and circulatory system
  2. Preprocedure implementation
     a. Obtain informed consent form
     b. Assess for allergies to seafood, iodine, or radiopaque dyes
     c. Withhold solid food for 6 to 8 hours and liquids for 4 hours to prevent vomiting and aspiration during the procedure
     d. Document the client's height and weight because these data will be needed to determine the amount of dye to be administered
     e. Document baseline vital signs and note the quality and presence of peripheral pulses for postprocedure comparison
     f. Inform the client that a local anesthetic will be administered prior to catheter insertion
     g. Inform clients that they may feel fatigued because they must lie still and quiet on a relatively hard table for up to 2 hours
     h. Inform clients that they may feel a fluttery feeling as the catheter passes through the heart; a flushed, warm feeling when the dye is injected; a desire to cough; and palpitations caused by heart irritability
     i. Prepare the insertion site by shaving and cleaning with an antiseptic solution if prescribed
     j. Administer preprocedure medications if prescribed
     k. Prepare for IV insertion
  3. Postprocedure implementation
     a. Monitor vital signs and cardiac rhythm every 30 minutes for 2 hours initially for dysrhythmias
     b. Monitor for chest pain and if dysrhythmias or chest pain occurs, notify the physician
     c. Monitor peripheral pulses and the color, warmth, and sensation of the extremity distal to the insertion site every 30 minutes for 2 hours initially
     d. Notify the physician if the client complains of numbness and tingling; if the extremity becomes cool, pale, or cyanotic; or if sudden loss of peripheral pulses occurs
     e. Monitor the pressure dressing for bleeding or hematoma formation
     f. Apply a sandbag to the insertion site to provide additional pressure if required
     g. Monitor for bleeding and if bleeding

occurs, apply pressure immediately and notify the physician

h. Monitor for hematoma and if a hematoma develops, notify the physician

i. Keep the extremity extended for 4 to 6 hours, keeping the leg straight to prevent arterial occlusion

j. Maintain strict bed rest for 6 to 12 hours; however, the client may turn from side to side; do not elevate the head of the bed more than 15 degrees

k. If the antecubital vessel was used, immobilize the arm on an armboard

l. Encourage fluids if not contraindicated to promote renal excretion of the dye

m. Monitor for nausea, vomiting, and rash or other signs of hypersensitivity to the dye

III. Therapeutic Management

A. Percutaneous transluminal coronary angioplasty (PTCA)

1. Description

   a. One or more arteries are dilated with a balloon catheter to open the vessel lumen and improve arterial blood flow

   b. Clients can experience reocclusion after the procedure, and the procedure may need to be repeated

   c. Complications can include arterial dissection or rupture, immobilization of plaque fragments, spasm, and acute MI

   d. Firm commitment is needed on the part of the client to stop smoking, lose weight, exercise, and stop any behaviors that lead to progression of artery occlusion

2. Preprocedure implementation

   a. Maintain NPO status after midnight

   b. Prepare the groin area with antiseptic soap and shave per institutional procedure and as prescribed

   c. Assess baseline vital signs and peripheral pulses

3. Postprocedure implementation

   a. Monitor vital signs closely

   b. Monitor distal pulses in both extremities

   c. Maintain bed rest as prescribed, keeping the limb straight for 6 to 8 hours

   d. Administer anticoagulants and antiplatelets as prescribed to prevent thrombus formation

   e. Monitor IV nitroglycerin if prescribed to prevent coronary spasm

   f. Instruct the client in the administration of nitrates, calcium channel blockers, antiplatelets, and anticoagulants as prescribed

   g. Instruct the client to take daily aspirin permanently if prescribed

   h. Assist the client with planning lifestyle modifications

B. Laser-assisted angioplasty

1. Description

   a. A laser probe is advanced through a cannula similar to that used for PTCA

   b. Used for clients with small occlusions in the distal superficial femoral, proximal popliteal, and common iliac arteries

   c. Heat from the laser vaporizes the plaque to open the occluded artery

2. Preprocedure and postprocedure care

   a. Similar to the PTCA

   b. Monitor for complications of coronary dissection, acute occlusion, perforation, embolism, and MI

C. Coronary artery stents

1. Description

   a. Used instead of PTCA to eliminate the risk of acute coronary vessel closure and to improve long-term patency of the vessel

   b. A balloon catheter bearing the stent is inserted into the coronary artery and positioned at the site of occlusion

   c. When placed in the coronary artery, the stent reopens the blocked artery

2. Postprocedure implementation

   a. Acute thrombosis is a major concern following the procedure and the client is placed on antiplatelet and anticoagulation therapy for several months following the procedure

   b. Monitor for complications of the procedure such as stent migration or occlusion, coronary artery dissection, and bleeding due to anticoagulation

D. Atherectomy

1. Description

   a. Removes plaque from an artery by the use of a cutting chamber on the inserted catheter or a rotating blade that pulverizes the plaque

   b. Used to improve blood flow to ischemic limbs in individuals with peripheral arterial disease

2. Postprocedure implementation: monitor for complications of perforation, embolus, and restenosis

E. Transmyocardial revascularization

1. Used for clients with widespread atherosclerosis involving vessels that are too small and numerous for replacement or balloon catheterization

2. Uses a high-powered laser that creates 15 to 30 holes (channels) in the heart

3. Blood enters these small channels providing the affected region of the heart with oxygenated blood

4. Performed through a small chest incision

5. The opening on the heart's surface heals over; however, the main channels remain and perfuse the myocardium

F. Arterial revascularization

1. Description

a. Performed to increase arterial blood flow to the affected limb

b. Inflow procedures involve bypassing arterial occlusion above the superficial femoral arteries

c. Outflow procedures involve surgical bypassing of arterial occlusions at or below the superficial femoral arteries

d. Graft material is sutured above and below the occlusion to facilitate blood flow around the occlusion

2. Preoperative implementation

a. Assess baseline vital signs and peripheral pulses

b. Prepare for IV insertion and urinary catheter as prescribed

3. Postoperative implementation

a. Assess vital signs

b. Monitor **blood pressure** and notify the physician if changes occur

c. Monitor for hypotension, which may indicate hypovolemia

d. Monitor for hypertension, which may place stress on the graft and facilitate clot formation

e. Maintain bed rest for 24 hours as prescribed

f. Instruct the client to keep affected extremity straight, limit movement, and avoid bending the knee and hip

g. Monitor for warmth, redness, and edema, which are often expected outcomes as a result of increased blood flow

h. Monitor for graft occlusion, which often occurs within the first 24 hours

i. Assess peripheral pulses and for changes in color and temperature of the extremity

j. Monitor for a sharp increase in pain because pain is frequently the first indicator of postoperative graft occlusion

k. If signs of graft occlusion occur, notify the physician immediately

l. Encourage coughing and deep breathing and the use of incentive spirometry

m. Maintain NPO status and progress to clear liquids as prescribed

n. Use strict aseptic technique when in contact with the incision

o. Assess incision for drainage, warmth, or swelling

p. Monitor for excessive bleeding (a small amount of bloody drainage is expected)

q. Monitor the area over the graft for hardness, tenderness, and warmth, which may indicate infection; if this occurs, notify the physician immediately

r. Instruct the client about proper foot care and measures to prevent ulcer formation

s. Instruct clients to take medications as prescribed

t. Instruct clients how to care for incision

u. Assist clients in modifying lifestyle to prevent further plaque formation

G. Coronary artery bypass graft (CABG)

1. Description

a. The occluded coronary arteries are bypassed with the client's own venous or arterial blood vessels

b. The saphenous vein or internal mammary artery is used to bypass lesions in the coronary arteries

c. Performed when the client does not respond to medical management of coronary artery disease (CAD) or when disease progression is evident

2. Preoperative implementation

a. Familiarize the client and family with the cardiac surgical critical care unit

b. Instruct the client how to splint a chest incision, cough and deep breathe and perform arm and leg exercises

c. Instruct the client to inform the nurse of any postoperative pain, as pain medication will be available

d. Inform the client to expect a sternal incision, possibly a leg incision, one or two chest tubes, a Foley catheter, and several IV fluid catheters

e. Inform the client that an endotracheal tube will be in place and connected to a ventilator for 6 to 24 hours

f. Advise clients that they should breathe with the ventilator and not fight it

g. Inform the family that the client will not be able to talk while the endotracheal tube is in place

h. Encourage the client and family to discuss anxieties and fears related to surgery

i. Note that prescribed medications are to be discontinued preoperatively (diuretics 2 to 3 days prior to surgery, digitalis 12 hours prior to surgery, and aspirin and anticoagulants 1 week prior to surgery)

j. Administer medications as prescribed, which may include potassium chloride, antihypertensives, antidysrhythmics, and antibiotics

3. Transfer from the cardiac surgical unit

a. Monitor vital signs, level of consciousness, and peripheral perfusion

b. Monitor for dysrhythmias

c. Auscultate lungs and assess respiratory status

d. Encourage the client to splint, cough and deep breathe and use an incentive spirometer to raise secretions and prevent atelectasis

e. Monitor temperature and WBC count, which if elevated after 3 to 4 days, indicates infection

f. Provide adequate fluids and hydration as prescribed to liquefy secretions

g. Assess suture line and chest tube insertion

sites for redness, purulent discharge, and signs of infection
    h. Assess the sternal suture line for instability, which may indicate an infection
    i. Guide the client in a gradual resumption of activity
    j. Assess the client for tachycardia, **orthostatic hypotension**, and fatigue before, during, and after activity
    k. Discontinue activities if **BP** drops more than 10 to 20 mmHg or pulse increases more than 10 beats per minute
    l. Monitor episodes of pain closely
    m. See Box 48–1 for home care instructions
H. Heart transplant
  1. A donor heart from an individual with a comparable body weight and ABO compatibility is transplanted into a recipient in less than 6 hours of procurement
  2. The surgeon removes the diseased heart, leaving the posterior portion of the atria, which serves as an anchor for the new heart
  3. Because a remnant of the client's atria remains, two unrelated P waves are noted on the ECG
  4. The transplanted heart is denervated and unresponsive to vagal stimulation; because the heart is denervated, clients do not experience angina
  5. Symptoms of heart rejection include hypotension, dysrhythmias, weakness, fatigue, and dizziness
  6. Endomyocardial biopsies are performed at regular scheduled intervals and whenever rejection is suspected
  7. Clients require immunosuppressive therapy for the rest of their lives

---

BOX 48–1. Home Care Instructions Following Cardiac Surgery

Instruct client on how to progress with activities at home

Inform client to limit pushing or pulling activities for 6 weeks following discharge

Instruct client about incisional care and to record signs of redness, swelling, or drainage

Inform clients that sternotomy heals in about 6 to 8 weeks

Instruct client to avoid crossing legs, to wear elastic hose as prescribed until edema subsides, and to elevate surgical limb when sitting in a chair

Instruct client in the use of prescribed medications

Instruct client in dietary measures including the avoidance of saturated fats and cholesterol and the use of salt

Instruct client that sexual intercourse can be resumed on the advice of the physician after exercise tolerance is assessed; if the client can walk one block or climb two flights of stairs without symptoms, the client can safely resume sexual activity

---

  8. The heart rate approximates 100 bpm and responds slowly with increases in heart rate, contractility and **cardiac output**, and to exercise and stress

IV. Management of Dysrhythmias

A. Vagal maneuvers
  1. Description: induce vagal stimulation of the cardiac conduction system and are used to terminate supraventricular tachydysrhythmias
  2. Carotid sinus massage
    a. The physician instructs the client to turn the head away from the side to be massaged
    b. The physician massages over the carotid artery for 6 to 8 seconds until there is a change in cardiac rhythm
    c. Observe the cardiac monitor for a change in rhythm
    d. Record an ECG rhythm strip before, during, and after the procedure
    e. Have a defibrillator and resuscitative equipment available
    f. Monitor vital signs, cardiac rhythm, and LOC following the procedure
  3. Valsalva maneuvers
    a. The physician instructs the client to bear down or induces a gag reflex in the client, both of which stimulate a vagal reflex
    b. Monitor the heart rate, rhythm, and **BP**
    c. Observe the cardiac monitor for a change in rhythm
    d. Record an ECG rhythm strip before, during, and after the procedure
    e. Provide an emesis basin if the gag reflex is stimulated, and initiate precautions to prevent aspiration
    f. Have a defibrillator and resuscitative equipment available

B. Cardioversion
  1. Description
    a. Synchronized countershock to convert an undesirable rhythm to a stable rhythm
    b. An elective procedure done by the physician
    c. A lower wattage of energy is used than with defibrillation
    d. The defibrillator is synchronized to the client's R wave to avoid discharging the shock during the vulnerable period (T wave)
    e. If the defibrillator is not synchronized, it will discharge on the T wave and cause ventricular fibrillation (VF)
  2. Preprocedure Implementation
    a. Obtain informed consent
    b. Administer sedation as prescribed
    c. Hold digoxin (Lanoxin) 48 hours preprocedure as prescribed to prevent postcardioversion ventricular irritability
  3. During the procedure

    a. Ensure the skin is clean and dry in the area where the electrode paddles will be placed

    b. Oxygen is stopped during the procedure to avoid hazard of fire

    c. Be sure no one is touching the bed or the client when delivering the countershock

  4. Postprocedure implementation

    a. Maintain airway patency

    b. Administer oxygen as prescribed

    c. Assess vital signs

    d. Assess level of consciousness

    e. Monitor cardiac rhythm

    f. Monitor for indications of successful response such as conversion to sinus rhythm, strong peripheral pulses, and an adequate **BP**

C. Defibrillation

  1. Description

    a. An asynchronous countershock used to terminate pulseless ventricular tachycardia (VT) or VF

    b. Three rapid consecutive shocks are delivered with the first at an energy of 200 joules

    c. If unsuccessful, the shock is repeated at 200 to 300 joules

    d. The third and subsquent shock will be at 360 joules

  2. During the procedure

    a. Oxygen is stopped during the procedure to avoid hazard of fire

    b. Be sure no one is touching the bed or the client when delivering the countershock

D. Use of paddle electrodes

  1. Apply conductive pads

  2. Place one paddle over the pad on the upper right chest to the right of the sternum, and the other on the lower left chest with the center in the midaxillary line

  3. Apply firm pressure with the paddles

  4. Be sure no one is touching the bed or the client when delivering the countershock

E. Automatic external defibrillator (AED)

  1. Used by laypersons and emergency medical technicians for prehospital cardiac arrest

  2. Place the client on a firm, dry surface

  3. Stop CPR

  4. Ensure that no one is touching the client to avoid motion artifact during rhythm analysis

  5. Place the electrode paddles in the correct position on the client's chest

  6. Press the analyzer button, and when the rhythm is analyzed, which may take 30 seconds, the machine will advise whether a shock is necessary

  7. Shocks are recommended for pulseless VF only

  8. If shock is recommended, the shock is delivered with the first at an energy of 200 joules

  9. If unsuccessful, the shock is repeated at 200 to 300 joules

  10. The third and subsequent shock will be at 360 joules

  11. If unsuccessful, CPR is continued for 1 minute, and then another series of three shocks are delivered each at 360 joules of energy

F. Implantable cardioverter defibrillator (ICD)

  1. Description

    a. Monitors cardiac rhythm and detects and terminates episodes of VT and VF

    b. It senses VT or VF and delivers 25 to 30 joules up to four times if necessary

    c. Used in clients with a history of VF or in unstable VT that is unresponsive to medication

    d. Electrodes are placed in the right atrium and ventricle and apical pericardium

    e. The generator is implanted in the abdomen

  2. Client education

    a. Basic functioning of the ICD

    b. How to perform cough CPR

    c. How to take the pulse and to take it daily and maintain a diary of pulse rates

    d. Wear loose-fitting clothing

    e. Avoid contact sports and strenuous activities

    f. Report any fever, redness, swelling, or drainage from the insertion site

    g. Report symptoms of fainting, nausea, weakness, blackouts, and rapid pulse rates to the physician

    h. During shock discharge the client may feel faint or short of breath

    i. Instruct clients to sit or lie down if they feel a shock and to notify the physician

    j. Instruct clients and family how to access the emergency medical system

    k. Encourage the family to learn CPR

    l. Advise the client to maintain a diary of any shocks that are delivered including the date, preceding activity, the number of shocks, and if the shocks were successful

    m. Instruct the client to avoid electromagnetic fields directly over the ICD because they can inactivate the device

    n. Instruct the client that if beeping tones are heard, to move away from the magnetic field immediately and notify the physician

    o. Keep pacemaker ID in a wallet and obtain and wear a Medic-Alert bracelet

    p. Inform all health care providers that an ICD is inserted

V. Pacemakers (Box 48–2)

A. Description: a temporary or permanent device that provides electrical stimulation and maintains the heart rate when the client's intrinsic pacemaker fails to provide a perfusing rhythm

B. Settings

BOX 48–2. Pacemakers: Client Education

Instruct client about the pacemaker including the programmed rate

Instruct client in the signs of battery failure and when to notify the physician

Instruct client to report any fever, redness, swelling, or drainage from the insertion site

Report signs of dizziness, weakness or fatigue, swelling of the ankles or legs, chest pain, or shortness of breath

Keep pacemaker ID in wallet and wear a Medic-Alert bracelet

Instruct client how to take a pulse, to take the pulse daily, and maintain a diary of pulse rates

Wear loose-fitting clothing

Avoid contact sports

Inform all health care providers that a pacemaker is inserted

Instruct clients to inform airport security that they have a pacemaker because it may set off the security detector

Instruct client that most electrical appliances can be used without any interference with the functioning of the pacemaker; however, advise the client not to operate electrical appliances directly over the pacemaker site

Avoid transmitter towers and antitheft devices in stores

Instruct client that if any unusual feelings occur when near any electrical devices, to move 5 to 10 feet away and to check the pulse

Emphasize the importance of follow-up with the physician

1. Synchronous or demand: sense the client's rhythm and paces only if the client's intrinsic rate falls below the set pacemaker rate
2. Asynchronous or fixed rate: pace at a preset rate regardless of the client's intrinsic rhythm
3. Overdrive pacing: suppresses the underlying rhythm in tachydysrhythmias so that the sinus node will regain control of the heart

C. Spikes
1. When a pacing stimulus is delivered to the heart, a spike (straight vertical line) is seen on the monitor or ECG strip
2. Also referred to as "capture," meaning that the pacemaker successfully depolarized or captured the chamber
3. The spike should be followed by a P wave, indicating atrial depolarization, or a QRS complex indicating ventricular depolarization
4. If the electrode is in the ventricle, the spike is in front of the QRS complex; if the electrode is in the atria, the spike is before the P wave
5. If the electrode is in both the atria and ventricle, the spike is before both the QRS complex and P wave

D. Temporary pacemakers
1. Noninvasive temporary pacing (NTP)
   a. Used as an emergency measure or when a client is transported and the risk of bradydysrhythmia exists in the client
   b. A large electrode patch is placed on the chest and back
   c. Wash skin with soap and water prior to applying electrodes
   d. Do not shave the hair or apply alcohol or tinctures to the skin
   e. The posterior electrode is placed between the spine and left scapula behind the heart, avoiding placement over bone
   f. The anterior electrode is placed between V2 and V5 position over the heart
   g. Do not place the anterior electrode over female breast tissue; rather, displace breast tissue and place under the breast
   h. Do not assess pulse or take the **BP** on the left side, because the results will not be accurate due to the muscle twitching and electrical current
   i. Ensure that electrodes are in good contact with the skin
   j. If loss of capture occurs, assess the skin contact of the electrodes; the current is increased until capture is regained
2. Transvenous invasive temporary pacing
   a. A pacing lead wire is placed through the antecubital, femoral, jugular, or subclavian vein into the right atrium for atrial pacing, or the right ventricle and positioned in contact with the endocardium
   b. Monitor cardiac rhythm continuously
   c. Monitor vital signs
   d. Monitor pacemaker insertion site
   e. Restrict client movement to prevent lead wire displacement
3. Epicardial invasive temporary pacing: applied by a transthoracic approach and the lead wires are loosely threaded on the epicardial surface of the heart after open heart surgery
4. Reducing the risk of microshock
   a. Use only inspected and approved equipment
   b. Insulate exposed portion of wires with plastic or rubber material (fingers of rubber gloves) when wires are not attached to the pulse generator, and cover with nonconductive tape
   c. Ground all electrical equipment using a three-pronged plug
   d. Wear gloves when handling exposed wires
   e. Keep dressings dry

E. Permanent pacemakers
1. A pulse generator is internal and surgically implanted in a subcutaneous pocket under the clavicle or abdominal wall
2. The leads are passed transvenously via the cephalic or subclavian vein to the endocardium on the right side of the heart
3. May be single chambered in which the lead wire is placed in the chamber to be paced, or

may be dual chambered with lead wires placed in the atrium and right ventricle
4. It is programmed when inserted and can be reprogrammed if necessary by noninvasive transmission from the external programmer to the implanted generator
5. Pacemakers are powered by either a lithium battery that has an average life span of 10 years, nuclear powered with a life span of 20 years or longer, or designed to be recharged externally

VI. Coronary Artery Disease
A. Description
1. A narrowing or obstruction of the coronary arteries due to atherosclerosis, an accumulation of fatty plaques made of lipids in the arteries
2. Causes a decreased perfusion of myocardial tissue and inadequate myocardial oxygen supply
3. Leads to hypertension, angina, dysrhythmias, myocardial infarction, congestive heart failure, and death
4. Collateral circulation, more than one artery supplying a muscle with blood, is normally present in the coronary arteries, especially in older people
5. The development of collateral circulation takes time and happens when chronic ischemia occurs to meet the metabolic demands; therefore, an occlusion of a coronary artery in a younger individual is more likely to be lethal than in an older individual
6. Symptoms occur when the coronary artery is occluded to the point that inadequate blood supply to the muscle occurs, causing ischemia
7. Coronary artery narrowing is significant if the lumen diameter of the left main artery is reduced at least 50%, or if any major branch is reduced at least 75%
8. The goal of treatment is to alter the atherosclerotic progression
B. Data collection
1. Findings may be normal during asymptomatic periods
2. Chest pain
3. Palpitations
4. Dyspnea
5. Syncope
6. Cough or hemoptysis
7. Excessive fatigue
C. Diagnostic studies
1. ECG
   a. When blood flow is reduced and ischemia occurs, ST segment depression or T wave inversion is noted; the ST segment returns to normal when the blood flow returns
   b. With infarction, cell injury results in ST segment elevation followed by T wave inversion

2. Cardiac catheterization
   a. Provides the most definitive source for diagnosis
   b. Would show the presence of atherosclerotic lesions
3. Blood lipid levels
   a. Blood lipid levels may be elevated
   b. Cholesterol-lowering medications may be prescribed to reduce the development of atherosclerotic plaques
D. Implementation
1. Instruct the client regarding the purpose of diagnostic medical and surgical procedures and the expected preprocedure and postprocedure activities
2. Assist the client to identify risk factors that can be modified
3. Assist clients to set goals that will promote changes in lifestyle to reduce the impact of risk factors
4. Assist clients to identify barriers to compliance with the therapeutic plan and to identify methods to overcome barriers
5. Instruct the client regarding a low-calorie, low-sodium, low-cholesterol, and low-fat diet with an increase in dietary fiber
6. Stress to the client that dietary changes are not temporary and must be maintained for life; instruct the client regarding prescribed medications
7. Provide community resources to the client regarding exercise, smoking reduction, and stress reduction
E. Surgical procedures
1. Percutaneous transluminal coronary angioplasty (PTCA) to compress the plaque against the walls of the artery and dilate the vessel
2. Laser angioplasty to vaporize the plaque
3. Atherectomy to remove the plaque from the artery
4. Vascular stent to prevent the artery from closing and prevent restenosis
5. Coronary artery bypass graft to improve blood flow to the myocardial tissues that are at risk for ischemia or infarction due to the occluded artery
F. Medications
1. Nitrates to dilate the coronary arteries and to decrease preload and afterload
2. Calcium channel blockers to dilate coronary arteries and reduce vasospasm
3. Cholesterol-lowering medications may be prescribed to reduce the development of atherosclerotic plaques
4. Beta blockers to reduce **blood pressure** in those individuals who are hypertensive

VII. Angina
A. Description
1. Chest pain resulting from myocardial ischemia

caused by inadequate myocardial blood and oxygen supply
2. Caused by an imbalance between oxygen supply and demand
3. Causes include obstruction of coronary blood flow due to atherosclerosis, coronary artery spasm, and conditions that increase myocardial oxygen consumption
4. The goal of treatment is to provide relief of an acute attack, correct the imbalance between myocardial oxygen supply and demand, and to prevent the progression of the disease and further attacks to reduce the risk of MI

B. Patterns of angina
  1. Stable angina
    a. Also called exertional angina
    b. Occurs with activities such as exertion or emotional stress; the pain is relieved with rest or nitroglycerin
    c. It usually has a stable pattern of onset, duration, severity, and relieving factors
  2. Unstable angina
    a. Also called preinfarction angina
    b. Occurs with an unpredictable degree of exertion or emotion and increases in occurrence, duration, and severity over time
    c. Pain may not be relieved with nitroglycerin
  3. Variant angina
    a. Also called Prinzmetal's or vasoplastic angina
    b. Results from coronary artery spasm, is similar to classic angina, but lasts longer
    c. It may occur at rest
    d. Attacks may be associated with elevation of the ST segment on the ECG
  4. Intractable angina: a chronic incapacitating angina that is unresponsive to interventions
  5. Preinfarction angina
    a. Associated with acute coronary insufficiency
    b. Angina that lasts longer than 15 minutes
    c. A symptom of worsening cardiac ischemia
  6. Postinfarction angina: occurs after an MI when residual ischemia may cause episodes of angina

C. Data collection
  1. Pain
    a. Can develop slowly or quickly
    b. Usually described as mild or moderate pain
    c. Substernal, crushing, or squeezing pain
    d. May radiate to the shoulders, arms, jaw, neck, and back
    e. Usually lasts less than 5 minutes; however, can last up to 15 to 20 minutes
    f. Relieved by nitroglycerin or rest
  2. Dyspnea
  3. Pallor
  4. Sweating
  5. Palpitations and tachycardia
  6. Dizziness and faintness
  7. Hypertension
  8. Digestive disturbances

D. Diagnostic studies
  1. ECG: normal during rest, with ST depression or elevation and/or T wave inversion during an episode of pain
  2. Stress test: chest pain or changes in the ECG or vital signs during testing may indicate ischemia
  3. Cardiac enzymes: normal findings in angina
  4. Cardiac catheterization: provides a definitive diagnosis by providing information about the patency of the coronary arteries

E. Implementation
  1. Immediate management
    a. Assess pain
    b. Provide bed rest
    c. Administer oxygen at 3 liters nasal cannula as prescribed
    d. Administer nitroglycerin as prescribed to dilate the coronary arteries, reduce the oxygen requirements of the myocardium, and relieve the chest pain
    e. Obtain a 12-lead ECG
    f. Provide continuous cardiac monitoring
  2. Following acute episode
    a. Instruct the client regarding purpose of diagnostic medical and surgical procedures and the expected preprocedure and postprocedure expectations
    b. Assist the client to identify angina-precipitating events
    c. Instruct the client that if chest pain occurs, to stop activity and rest and take nitroglycerin as prescribed
    d. Instruct the client that if the pain persists, to seek medical attention
    e. Instruct clients regarding prescribed medications
    f. Provide diet instruction to clients, stressing that dietary changes are not temporary and must be maintained for life
    g. Assist the client to identify risk factors that can be modified
    h. Assist the client to set goals that will promote changes in lifestyle to reduce the impact of risk factors
    i. Assist clients to identify barriers to compliance with therapeutic plan and to identify methods to overcome barriers
    j. Provide community resources to clients regarding exercise, smoking cessation, and stress reduction

F. Surgical procedures
  1. Percutaneous transluminal coronary angioplasty (PTCA) to assess the condition of the coronary arteries and to compress the plaque, if present, against the walls of the artery and dilate the vessel
  2. Laser angioplasty to vaporize the plaque if present

3. Atherectomy to remove the plaque, if present, from the artery
4. Vascular stent to prevent the artery from closing and prevent restenosis
5. Coronary artery bypass graft to improve blood flow to the myocardial tissues that are at risk for ischemia or infarction due to the occluded artery

G. Medications
   1. Vasodilators to maintain coronary artery vasodilation and promote a greater flow of blood and oxygen to the heart
   2. Calcium channel blockers to dilate coronary arteries and reduce vasospasm
   3. Beta blockers to reduce the oxygen requirements of the heart and reduce **blood pressure** in those individuals who are hypertensive
   4. Antiplatelet therapy to inhibit platelet aggregation and reduce the risk of developing an acute MI

VIII. Myocardial Infarction (MI)

A. Description
   1. Occurs when myocardial tissue is abruptly and severely deprived of oxygen
   2. Ischemia can lead to necrosis of myocardial tissue if blood flow is not restored
   3. Infarction does not occur instantly, but evolves over several hours
   4. Obvious physical changes do not occur in the heart until 6 hours after the infarction when the infarcted area appears blue and swollen
   5. After 48 hours, the infarct turns gray with yellow streaks as neutrophils invade the tissue
   6. By 8 to 10 days after infarction, granulation tissue forms
   7. Over 2 to 3 months, the necrotic area develops into a scar; scar tissue permanently changes the size and shape of the entire left ventricle

B. Location of MI
   1. Obstruction of the LAD artery results in anterior or septal MIs or both
   2. Obstruction of the circumflex artery results in posterior wall MI or lateral wall MI
   3. Obstruction of the right coronary artery results in inferior wall MI

C. Risk factors
   1. Atherosclerosis
   2. CAD
   3. Elevated cholesterol levels
   4. Smoking
   5. Hypertension
   6. Obesity
   7. Physical inactivity
   8. Impaired glucose tolerance
   9. Stress

D. Diagnostic studies
   1. Total CK levels
      a. Rise within 3 hours after the onset of chest pain

b. Peak within 24 hours after damage and death of cardiac tissue
   2. CK-MB isoenzyme
      a. Peak elevation occurs 12 to 24 hours after the onset of chest pain
      b. Levels return to normal 48 to 72 hours later
   3. LDH levels
      a. Rise within 12 to 24 hours after MI
      b. Peak between 40 and 72 hours and fall to normal in 7 days
      c. Serum levels of LDH_1 isoenzyme rise higher than serum levels of LDH_2
   4. WBC count: an elevated count of 10,000 to 20,000 cells/mm^3 appears on the second day post-MI and lasts up to a week
   5. ECG
      a. ST segment elevation, T wave inversion, abnormal Q wave
      b. Hours to days after the MI, ST and T wave changes will return to normal but the Q wave usually remains permanently
   6. Diagnostic tests following the acute stage
      a. Exercise tolerance test or stress test may be prescribed to assess for ECG changes and ischemia and to evaluate for medical therapy or identify clients who may need invasive therapy
      b. Thallium scans may be prescribed to assess for ischemia or necrotic muscle tissue
      c. MUGA scans: may be used to evaluate left ventricular function
      d. Cardiac catheterization: performed to determine the extent and location of obstructions of the coronary arteries

E. Data collection
   1. Pain
      a. Crushing substernal pain
      b. Radiates to the jaw, back, and left arm
      c. Occurs without cause, primarily early in the morning
      d. Is unrelieved by rest or nitroglycerin; relieved only by opioids
      e. Pain lasts 30 minutes or more
   2. Nausea and vomiting
   3. Diaphoresis
   4. Dyspnea
   5. Dysrhythmias
   6. Feelings of fear and anxiety
   7. Pallor, cyanosis, and coolness of extremities

F. Complications of MI
   1. Dysrhythmias
   2. Heart failure
   3. Pulmonary edema
   4. Cardiogenic shock
   5. Thrombophlebitis
   6. Pericarditis
   7. Mitral valve insufficiency
   8. Postinfarction angina
   9. Ventricular rupture
   10. Dressler's syndrome (a combination of pericarditis, pericardial effusion, and pleural

effusion, which can occur several weeks to months following an MI)

G. Implementation acute stage
1. Obtain a description of the chest discomfort
2. Assess vital signs
3. Assess cardiovascular status and maintain cardiac monitoring
4. Obtain a 12-lead ECG
5. Administer nitroglycerin as prescribed
6. Administer morphine sulfate as prescribed to relieve chest discomfort that is unresponsive to nitroglycerin
7. Administer oxygen at 2 to 4 liters by nasal cannula as prescribed
8. Position the client in semi-Fowler's position to enhance comfort and tissue oxygenation
9. Establish an IV access route
10. Administer IV nitroglycerin and antidysrhythmics as prescribed
11. Monitor thrombolitic therapy, which may be prescribed within the first 6 hours of the coronary event
12. Monitor for signs of bleeding if the client is receiving thrombolytics
13. Monitor lab values as prescribed
14. Administer beta blockers to slow the heart rate and increase myocardial perfusion while reducing the force of myocardial contraction as prescribed
15. Monitor for complications related to MI
16. Monitor for cardiac dysrhythmias because tachycardia and PVCs frequently occur in the first few hours after MI
17. Assess distal peripheral pulses and skin temperature because poor **cardiac output** may be identified by cool, diaphoretic skin and diminished or absent pulses
18. Monitor I&O
19. Assess respiratory rate and breath sounds for signs of heart failure, as indicated by the presence of crackles or wheezes or dependent edema
20. Monitor **blood pressure** closely after the administration of medications, and if the **BP** is less than 100 systolic or 25 mmHg lower than the previous reading, lower the head of the bed and notify the physician
21. Provide reassurance to the client and family

H. Implementation following acute episode
1. Maintain bed rest for the first 24 to 36 hours
2. Allow the client to stand to void or use a bedside commode if prescribed
3. Provide range of motion exercises to prevent thrombus formation and maintain muscle strength
4. Progress to dangling at the side of the bed or out of bed to the chair for 30 minutes three times a day as prescribed
5. Progress to ambulation in the client's room and to the bathroom, then in the hallway three times a day
6. Monitor for complications

7. Encourage the client to verbalize feelings regarding the MI

I. Cardiac rehabilitation: process of actively assisting the client with cardiac disease to achieve and maintain a vital and productive life within the limitations of the heart disease

IX. Heart Failure

A. Description
1. The inability of the heart to maintain adequate circulation to meet the metabolic needs of the body due to an impaired pumping capability
2. **Cardiac output** is diminished and peripheral tissue is not adequately perfused
3. Congestion of the lungs and periphery may occur

B. Classification
1. Acute: occurs suddenly
2. Chronic: develops over time; however, a client with chronic heart failure can develop an acute episode

C. Types of heart failure
1. Right-sided heart failure/left-sided heart failure
   a. Because the two ventricles of the heart represent two separate pumping systems, it is possible for one to fail alone for a short period
   b. Most heart failure begins with left ventricular failure and progresses to failure of both ventricles
   c. Acute pulmonary edema, a medical emergency, results from left ventricular failure
   d. If pulmonary edema is not treated, death will occur from suffocation because the client literally drowns in his or her own fluids
2. Forward failure/backward failure
   a. In forward failure, an inadequate output of the affected ventricle causes decreased perfusion to vital organs
   b. In backward failure, blood backs up behind the affected ventricle, causing increased pressure in the atrium behind the affected ventricle
3. Low output/high output
   a. In low-output failure, not enough **cardiac output** is available to meet the demands of the body
   b. High-output failure occurs when a condition causes the heart to work harder to meet the demands of the body
4. Systolic failure/diastolic failure
   a. Systolic failure leads to problems with contraction and the ejection of blood
   b. Diastolic failure leads to problems with the heart relaxing and filling with blood

D. Compensatory mechanisms
1. Act to restore **cardiac output** to near normal levels

2. Initially these mechanisms increase **cardiac output**; however, they eventually have a damaging effect on pump action
3. Contribute to an increase in myocardial oxygen consumption and when this occurs, myocardial reserve is exhausted and clinical manifestations of heart failure develop
4. Include increased heart rate, improved stroke volume, arterial vasoconstriction, sodium and water retention, and myocardial hypertrophy

E. Data collection
   1. Right-sided heart failure
      a. Signs of right-sided failure will be evident in the systemic circulation
      b. Pitting, and dependent edema in the feet, legs, sacrum, back, and buttocks
      c. Ascites from portal hypertension
      d. Tenderness of right upper quadrant; organomegaly
      e. Distended neck veins
      f. Pulsus alternans (regular alteration of weak and strong beats noted in the pulse)
      g. Abdominal pain and bloating
      h. Anorexia and nausea
      i. Fatigue
      j. Weight gain
      k. Nocturnal diuresis
   2. Left-sided heart failure
      a. Signs of the left-sided failure will be evident in the pulmonary system
      b. Cough, which may become productive with frothy sputum
      c. Dyspnea upon exertion
      d. Orthopnea
      e. Paroxysmal nocturnal dyspnea
      f. Presence of rales or crackles on auscultation
      g. Tachycardia
      h. Pulsus alternans
      i. Fatigue
      j. Pallor
      k. Cyanosis
      l. Confusion and disorientation
      m. Signs of cerebral anoxia
   3. Acute pulmonary edema
      a. Severe dyspnea and orthopnea
      b. Pallor
      c. Tachycardia
      d. Expectoration of large amounts of blood-tinged, frothy sputum
      e. Wheezing and rales
      f. Bubbling respirations
      g. Acute anxiety, apprehension, and restlessness
      h. Profuse sweating
      i. Cold, clammy skin
      j. Cyanosis
      k. Nasal flaring
      l. Use of accessory breathing muscles
      m. Tachypnea
      n. Hypocapnia evidenced by muscle cramps, weakness, dizziness, and paresthesias

F. Immediate management
   1. Place client in high Fowler's with legs in a dependent position to reduce pulmonary congestion and relieve edema
   2. Administer oxygen in high concentrations by mask or cannula as prescribed by the physician to improve gas exchange and pulmonary function
   3. Prepare for intubation and ventilator support if required; monitor lung sounds for rales and decreased breath sounds
   4. Suction as needed to maintain a patent airway
   5. Assess level of consciousness
   6. Provide reassurance to the client
   7. Monitor vital signs closely, noting tachycardia or pulsus alternans
   8. Monitor for hypotension due to decreased tissue perfusion, or hypertension due to anxiety or history of hypertension
   9. Monitor heart rate on a cardiac monitor for dysrhythmias
   10. Assess for edema in dependent areas and in the sacral, lumbar, and posterior thigh region with the client in bed
   11. Insert a Foley catheter as prescribed and monitor urine output closely following administration of a diuretic
   12. Monitor I&O
   13. The administration of unnecessary IV fluids is avoided
   14. Morphine is administered as prescribed to provide sedation and vasodilation; monitor for respiratory depression or hypotension after administration
   15. Diuretics are administered as prescribed to reduce preload, enhance renal excretion of sodium and water, reduce circulating blood volume, and reduce pulmonary congestion
   16. Digitalis is administered as prescribed to increase ventricular contractility and improve **cardiac output**
   17. Bronchodilators are administered as prescribed for severe bronchospasm or bronchoconstriction
   18. Vasodilators are administered as prescribed to reduce afterload, increase the capacity of the systemic venous bed, and decrease venous return to the heart
   19. Monitor weight to determine a response to treatment
   20. Assess for hepatomegaly and ascites and measure and record abdominal girth
   21. Monitor peripheral pulses
   22. Monitor blood gas results and evaluate electrolyte values for imbalances
   23. Monitor potassium level closely, which may decrease due to the diuretic, and administer potassium supplements as prescribed to prevent digitalis toxicity

G. Following the acute episode
   1. Encourage client to verbalize feelings about

the necessary lifestyle changes that are required as a result of the heart failure
2. Assist the client to identify precipitating risk factors of heart failure and methods of eliminating these risk factors
3. Instruct the client in the prescribed medication regimen which may include digoxin (Lanoxin), a diuretic, and vasodilators
4. Advise the client to notify the physician if side effects occur from the medications
5. Advise the client to avoid over-the-counter medications
6. Instruct clients to contact the physician if they are unable to take medications due to illness
7. Instruct the client to avoid large amounts of caffeine found in coffee, tea, cocoa, chocolate, and some carbonated beverages
8. Instruct clients on following a low-sodium, low-fat, low-cholesterol diet as prescribed
9. Provide the client with a list of potassium-rich foods because diuretics will cause hypokalemia (except for potassium-sparing diuretics)
10. Instruct the client regarding fluid restriction if prescribed, advising the client to spread out the fluid throughout the day and to suck on hard candy to reduce thirst
11. Instruct the client to space periods of activity and rest
12. Advise the client to avoid isometric activities that increase pressure in the heart
13. Instruct clients to monitor weight
14. Instruct the client to report signs of fluid retention such as edema or weight gain

X. Cardiogenic Shock

A. Failure of the heart to pump adequately, thereby reducing **cardiac output** and compromising tissue perfusion
B. Necrosis of more than 40% of the left ventricle occurs, usually as a result of occlusions of major coronary vessels
C. The goal of treatment is to relieve pain and decrease myocardial oxygen requirements through preload, and possibly afterload reduction

XI. Inflammatory Diseases of the Heart

A. Pericarditis
1. Description
   a. An acute or chronic inflammation of the pericardium
   b. Chronic pericarditis, a chronic inflammatory thickening of the pericardium, constricts the heart, causing compression
   c. The pericardial sac becomes inflamed
   d. Can result in loss of pericardial elasticity or an accumulation of fluid within the sac

   e. Heart failure or cardiac tamponade may result
2. Data collection
   a. Precordial pain in the anterior chest that radiates to the left side of the neck, shoulder, or back
   b. Pain that is aggravated by breathing (particularly inspiration), coughing, and swallowing
   c. Pain is worse when in the supine position and may be relieved by leaning forward
   d. Pericardial friction rub (scratchy, high-pitched sound) heard on auscultation produced by the rubbing of the inflamed pericardial layers
   e. Fever and chills
   f. Fatigue and malaise
   g. Elevated WBC count
   h. ECG changes
   i. Signs of right-sided heart failure in clients with chronic constrictive pericarditis
3. Implementation
   a. Assess the nature of the pain
   b. Position the client side-lying, high Fowler's, or upright and leaning forward
   c. Administer analgesics, NSAIDs, or steroids as prescribed for pain
   d. Avoid the administration of aspirin and anticoagulants because they increase the risk of cardiac tamponade
   e. Auscultate for a pericardial friction rub
   f. Evaluate blood culture report
   g. Administer antibiotics for bacterial infection as prescribed
   h. Administer diuretics and digoxin (Lanoxin) as prescribed to the client with chronic constrictive pericarditis
   i. Monitor for signs of cardiac tamponade including pulsus paradoxus, jugular vein distention with clear lung sounds, muffled heart sounds, and decreased **cardiac output**
   j. The physician is notified if signs of cardiac tamponade occur
B. Myocarditis
1. Description: an acute or chronic inflammation of the myocardium due to pericarditis, systemic infection, or allergic response
2. Data collection
   a. Fever
   b. Pericardial friction rub
   c. A gallop rhythm
   d. A murmur that sounds like fluid passing an obstruction
   e. Pulsus alternans
   f. Signs of heart failure
   g. Fatigue
   h. Dyspnea
   i. Tachycardia
   j. Chest pain
3. Implementation

a. Assist the client to a position of comfort such as sitting up and leaning forward
b. Administer analgesics, salicylates, or NSAIDs as prescribed to reduce fever and pain
c. Administer oxygen as prescribed
d. Provide adequate rest periods
e. Limit activities to avoid overexertion and to decrease the workload of the heart
f. Administer digoxin (Lanoxin) as prescribed and monitor for signs of digoxin toxicity
g. Administer antidysrhythmics as prescribed
h. Administer antibiotics as prescribed to treat the causative organism
i. Monitor for complications, which can include thrombus, CHF, or cardiomyopathy

C. Endocarditis
1. Description
   a. An inflammation of the inner lining of the heart and valves
   b. Occurs primarily in clients who are IV drug abusers, have had valve replacements, or have mitral valve prolapse or other structural defects
   c. Ports of entry for the infecting organism include the oral cavity (especially if the client had a dental procedure in the previous 3 to 6 months), cutaneous invasion, infections, or by invasive procedures or surgery
2. Data collection
   a. Fever
   b. Anorexia
   c. Weight loss
   d. Fatigue
   e. Cardiac murmurs
   f. Heart failure
   g. Embolic complications from vegetation fragments traveling through the circulation
   h. Petechiae
   i. Splinter hemorrhages in the nailbeds
   j. Osler's nodes (reddish, tender lesions) on the pads of the fingers, hands, and toes
   k. Janeway's lesions (nontender hemorrhagic lesions) on the fingers, toes, nose, or earlobes
   l. Splenomegaly
   m. Clubbing of the fingers
3. Implementation
   a. Provide adequate rest balanced with activity to prevent thrombus formation
   b. Maintain antiembolism stockings
   c. Monitor cardiovascular status
   d. Monitor for signs of heart failure
   e. Monitor for signs of emboli
   f. Monitor for splenic emboli as evidenced by sudden abdominal pain radiating to the left shoulder, and the presence of rebound abdominal tenderness on palpation
   g. Monitor for renal emboli as evidenced by flank pain radiating to the groin, hematuria, and pyuria
   h. Monitor for confusion, aphasia, or dysphagia, which may be indicative of central nervous system (CNS) emboli
   i. Monitor for pulmonary emboli as evidenced by pleuritic chest pain, dyspnea, and cough
   j. Assess skin, mucous membranes, and conjunctivae for petechiae
   k. Assess nailbeds for splinter hemorrhages
   l. Assess for Osler's nodes on the pads of the fingers, hands, and toes
   m. Assess for Janeway's lesions on the fingers, toes, nose, or earlobes
   n. Assess for clubbing of the fingers
   o. Evaluate blood culture results
   p. IV antibiotics are administered as prescribed
   q. Plan and arrange for discharge, providing resources required for the continued administration of IV antibiotics
4. Client education
   a. Instruct the client regarding the signs and symptoms of complications and to notify the physician if they occur
   b. Inform clients about the importance of good oral hygiene
   c. Instruct clients to brush teeth twice daily with a soft toothbrush followed by oral rinses
   d. Instruct the client to avoid irrigation devices, electric toothbrushes, and flossing because these activities can cause the gums to bleed, allowing the entrance of bacteria into the mucous membranes and bloodstream
   e. Advise clients of the importance of prophylactic antibiotics prior to any invasive procedure and the importance of informing all health care professionals of their disease history

XII. Cardiac Tamponade

A. A pericardial effusion occurs when the space between the parietal and visceral layers of the pericardium fills with fluid
B. Pericardial effusion places the client at risk for cardiac tamponade, an accumulation of fluid in the pericardial cavity
C. Tamponade restricts ventricular filling and **cardiac output** drops
D. Acute tamponade occurs when small volumes (20 to 50 mL) of fluid accumulate in the pericardium

XIII. Valvular Heart Disease

A. Description
1. Occurs when the heart valves cannot fully

open (stenosis) or close completely (insufficiency or regurgitation)
2. Prevents efficient blood flow through the heart

B. Types
1. Mitral stenosis: valvular tissue thickens and narrows valve opening
2. Mitral insufficiency/regurgitation: valve is incompetent and prevents complete valve closure
3. Mitral valve prolapse: valve leaflets protrude into left atrium during **systole**
4. Aortic stenosis: valvular tissue thickens and narrows valve opening
5. Aortic insufficiency: valve is incompetent and prevents complete valve closure

C. Repair procedures
1. Balloon valvuloplasty
   a. An invasive nonsurgical procedure
   b. The passage of a balloon catheter from the femoral vein through the atrial septum, to the mitral valve or through the femoral artery to the aortic valve
   c. The balloon is inflated to enlarge the orifice
   d. Institute precautions for arterial puncture if appropriate
   e. Monitor for bleeding from the catheter insertion site
   f. Monitor for signs of systemic emboli
   g. Monitor for signs of a regurgitant valve by monitoring cardiac rhythm, heart sounds, and **cardiac output**
2. Mitral annuloplasty: tightening and suturing the malfunctioning valve annulus to eliminate or markedly reduce regurgitation
3. Commissurotomy/valvotomy
   a. Accomplished with cardiopulmonary bypass during open heart surgery
   b. The valve is visualized, thrombi are removed from the atria, fused leaflets are incised, and calcium is debrided from the leaflets, thus widening the orifice

D. Valve replacement procedures (Box 48–3)
1. Mechanical prosthetic valves
   a. Prosthetic valves are very durable but can fail
   b. Thromboembolism is a problem following the valve replacement, and anticoagulant therapy is required over a lifetime
2. Bioprosthetic valves
   a. Biological grafts are xenografts (valves from other species), porcine valves (pig), bovine valves (cow), or homografts (human cadavers)
   b. Little risk of clot formation; therefore, long-term anticoagulation is not indicated
3. Preoperative implementation: consult with the physician regarding discontinuing anticoagulants 72 hours prior to surgery
4. Postoperative implementation
   a. Monitor closely for signs of bleeding

BOX 48–3. Client Instruction Following Valve Replacement

Instruct clients that adequate rest is important and that they will easily become fatigued

Instruct client in the need for anticoagulant therapy if a mechanical prosthetic valve was inserted

Instruct client in the hazards related to anticoagulant therapy and to notify the physician if bleeding or excessive bruising occurs

Inform client about the importance of good oral hygiene to reduce the risk of infective endocarditis

Instruct client to brush teeth twice daily with a soft toothbrush followed by oral rinses

Instruct client to avoid irrigation devices, electric toothbrushes, and flossing because these activities can cause the gums to bleed, allowing bacteria into the mucous membranes and bloodstream

Instruct the client to monitor incision and to report any drainage or redness

Inform clients that they should avoid any dental procedures for 6 months

Inform client that heavy lifting (greater than 10 lb) is to be avoided and to exercise caution when in an automobile to prevent injury to the sternal incision

Inform client with a prosthetic valve that a soft audible clicking may be heard

Advise clients of the importance of prophylactic antibiotics prior to any invasive procedure and the importance of informing all health care professionals of the valvular disease history

Advise client to wear a Medic-Alert bracelet

b. Monitor **cardiac output** and for signs of heart pump failure
c. Administer digoxin (Lanoxin) as prescribed to maintain **cardiac output** and prevent atrial fibrillation

XIV. Cardiomyopathy

A. Description
1. A subacute or chronic disorder of the heart muscle
2. Treatment is palliative, not curative, and clients need to deal with numerous lifestyle changes and a shortened life span

B. Dilated cardiomyopathy (DCM)
1. Description
   a. Most common type
   b. Heart ejects less than 40% of the blood in the left ventricle (normal is 70%) and reduced **cardiac output** leads to heart failure
2. Data collection
   a. Symptoms of left ventricular heart failure
   b. Weakness and fatigue
   c. Activity intolerance
   d. Chest pain
   e. Dysrhythmias

f. Eventually signs of right-sided heart failure

3. Implementation
   a. Symptomatic treatment of heart failure
   b. Diuretics, cardiac glycosides, and vasodilators to increase **cardiac output**
   c. Antidysrhythmics to control dysrhythmias
   d. Instruct clients to report any signs of dizziness or fainting, which may indicate a dysrhythmia
   e. Instruct clients to avoid ingestion of alcohol because of its cardiac depressant effect
   f. Heart transplant

C. Hypertrophic cardiomyopathy (HCM)
   1. Description
      a. Characterized by massive ventricular hypertrophy leading to hypercontraction of the left ventricle and rigid ventricle walls
      b. Causes obstruction in the left ventricular outflow
   2. Data collection
      a. Exertional dyspnea
      b. Syncope
      c. Chest pain that occurs at rest, is prolonged, has no relation to exertion, and is not relieved by nitrates
      d. Dysrhythmias
   3. Implementation
      a. Symptomatic treatment of symptoms similar to the care of a client with MI
      b. Conversion of atrial fibrillation if it occurs
      c. Instruct the client to report any signs of dizziness or fainting, which may indicate a dysrhythmia
      d. Instruct clients to avoid ingestion of alcohol because of its cardiac depressant effect
      e. Beta blockers and calcium antagonists to decrease the outflow obstruction and decrease heart rate
      f. Vasodilators and cardiac glycosides are contraindicated because vasodilating and positive inotropic effects augment the obstruction
      g. Ventriculomyotomy or muscle resection with mitral valve replacement

D. Restrictive cardiomyopathy
   1. Description: characterized by restriction of filling of the ventricles
   2. Data collection
      a. Exertional dyspnea
      b. Weakness
   3. Implementation
      a. Symptomatic treatment of heart failure
      b. Exercise restriction
      c. Diuretics, cardiac glycosides, and vasodilators to increase **cardiac output**
      d. Antidysrhythmics to control dysrhythmias
      e. Instruct the client to report any signs of

dizziness or fainting, which may indicate a dysrhythmia
f. Instruct client to avoid ingestion of alcohol because of its cardiac depressant effect

XV. Vascular Disorders

A. Venous thrombosis
   1. Description
      a. Thrombus can be associated with an inflammatory process
      b. When a thrombus develops, inflammation occurs, thickening the vein wall leading to embolization
   2. Types
      a. Thrombophlebitis: a thrombus associated with inflammation
      b. Phlebothrombus: a thrombus without inflammation
      c. Phlebitis: vein inflammation associated with invasive procedures such as IVs
      d. Deep vein thrombophlebitis (DVT): more serious than a superficial thrombophlebitis because of the risk for pulmonary embolism
   3. Risks factors for thrombus formation
      a. Venous stasis from varicose veins, congestive heart failure (CHF), immobility
      b. Hypercoagulability disorders
      c. Injury to the venous wall from IV injections, fractures, and trauma
      d. Following surgery, particularly hip surgery and open prostate surgery
      e. Pregnancy
      f. Ulcerative colitis
      g. Use of oral contraceptives

B. Phlebitis
   1. Data collection
      a. Red, warm area radiating up an extremity
      b. Pain and soreness
      c. Swelling
   2. Implementation
      a. Apply warm moist soaks as prescribed to dilate the vein and promote circulation
      b. Assess temperature of soak prior to applying
      c. Assess for signs of complications, such as tissue necrosis, infection, or pulmonary embolus

C. Deep vein thrombophlebitis (DVT) (Box 48–4)
   1. Data collection
      a. Calf or groin tenderness or pain with or without swelling
      b. Positive Homans' sign
      c. Warm skin that is tender to touch
   2. Implementation
      a. Provide bed rest
      b. Elevate the affected extremity above the level of the heart as prescribed
      c. Avoid using the knee gatch or a pillow under knees

BOX 48–4. Instructions for the Client with DVT

Educate the client regarding the hazards of anticoagulation therapy

Instruct the client to recognize the signs and symptoms of bleeding

Instruct client to avoid prolonged sitting or standing, constrictive clothing, or crossing legs when seated

Instruct client to elevate legs for 10 to 20 minutes every few hours each day

Plan a progressive walking program with the client as prescribed

Instruct client how to inspect legs for edema and how to measure circumference of legs

Instruct the client about antiembolism stockings as prescribed

Advise the client to avoid smoking

Advise the client to avoid any medications unless they are prescribed by the physician

Emphasize the importance of follow-up physician visits and laboratory studies

Advise client to wear a Medic-Alert bracelet

---

    d. Do not massage the extremity

    e. Provide thigh-high compression or antiembolism stockings as prescribed to reduce venous stasis and to assist in the venous return of blood to the heart

    f. Administer intermittent or continuous warm, moist compresses as prescribed

    g. Palpate the site gently, monitoring for warmth and edema

    h. Measure and record the circumference of the thighs and calves

    i. Monitor for shortness of breath and chest pain because it may be indicative of pulmonary emboli

    j. Thrombolytic therapy (t-PA, tissue plasminogen activator) may be prescribed, and needs to be initiated within 5 days after the onset of symptoms

    k. Heparin therapy may be prescribed to prevent enlargement of the existing clot and prevent the formation of new clots

    l. Monitor activated partial thromboplastin time (APTT) during heparin therapy

    m. Administer warfarin (Coumadin) as prescribed when the symptoms of DVT have resolved

    n. Monitor PT and international normalized ratio (INR) during warfarin (Coumadin) therapy

    o. Monitor for the hazards and side effects associated with anticoagulant therapy

    p. Administer analgesics as prescribed to reduce pain

    q. Administer diuretics as prescribed to reduce lower extremity edema

D. Venous insufficiency

  1. Description

    a. Occurs as a result of prolonged venous hypertension, which stretches the veins and damages the valves

    b. The resultant edema and venous stasis causes venous stasis ulcers, swelling, and cellulitis

    c. Treatment focuses on decreasing edema and promoting venous return from the affected extremity

    d. Treatment for venous stasis ulcers focuses on healing the ulcer and preventing stasis and ulcer recurrence

  2. Data collection

    a. Stasis dermatitis or discoloration along the ankles extending up to the calf

    b. Edema

    c. The presence of ulcer formation

  3. Implementation

    a. Instruct the client to wear elastic or compression stockings during the day and evening as prescribed

    b. Instruct clients to put elastic stockings on upon awakening and before getting out of bed

    c. Advise clients to put on a clean pair of elastic stockings each day and that they will probably need to wear the stockings for the rest of their life

    d. Instruct clients to avoid prolonged sitting or standing, constrictive clothing, or crossing the legs when seated

    e. Instruct the client to elevate the legs for 10 to 20 minutes every few hours each day

    f. Instruct the client that when in bed to elevate the legs above the level of the heart

    g. Instruct the client in the use of an intermittent sequential pneumatic compression system if prescribed; instruct the client to apply the compression system twice daily for 1 hour in the morning and evening

    h. Advise clients with an open ulcer that the compression system is applied over a dressing

  4. Wound care

    a. Provide care to the wound as prescribed by the physician

    b. Assess the client's ability to care for the wound and initiate home care resources as necessary

    c. If an Unna boot (a dressing constructed of gauze moistened with zinc oxide) is prescribed, it will be changed by the physician weekly

    d. The wound is cleansed with normal saline prior to application of the Unna boot; povidone-iodine (Betadine) or hydrogen peroxide is not used because it destroys granulation tissue

    e. The Unna boot is covered with an elastic

wrap that hardens to promote venous return and prevent stasis

f. Monitor for signs of arterial occlusion from an Unna boot that may be too tight

g. Keep tape off the client's skin

5. Medications

a. Apply topical agents to the wound as prescribed to debride the ulcer, eliminate necrotic tissue, and promote healing

b. When applying topical agents, apply an oil-based agent such as petroleum jelly (Vaseline) on the surrounding skin because debriding agents can injure healthy tissue

c. Administer antibiotics as prescribed if infection or cellulitis occurs

E. Varicose veins

1. Description

a. Distended, protruding veins that appear darkened and tortuous

b. Vein walls weaken and dilate, and valves become incompetent

2. Data collection

a. Pain in the legs that is dull and aching after standing

b. A feeling of fullness in the legs

c. Ankle edema

3. Trendelenburg test

a. Place the client in a supine position with the legs elevated

b. When the client sits up, if varicosities are present, veins fill from the proximal end; veins normally fill from the distal end

4. Implementation

a. Assist with the Trendelenburg test by placing the client in a supine position with legs elevated

b. Emphasize the importance of antiembolism stockings as prescribed

c. Instruct clients to elevate legs as much as possible

d. Instruct clients to avoid constrictive clothing and pressure on the legs

e. Prepare the client for sclerotherapy or vein stripping as prescribed

5. Sclerotherapy

a. A solution is injected into the vein followed by the application of a pressure dressing

b. An incision and drainage of the trapped blood in the sclerosed vein is performed 14 to 21 days after the injection, followed by the application of a pressure dressing for 12 to 18 hours

6. Vein stripping

a. Varicose veins are removed if they are larger than 4 mm in diameter or if they are in clusters

b. Preoperatively assist the physician with vein marking

c. Evaluate pulses as a baseline for comparison postoperatively

d. Maintain elastic (Ace) bandages on the client's legs postoperatively

e. Monitor the groin and leg for bleeding through the elastic bandages

f. Monitor the extremity for edema, warmth, color, and pulses

g. Elevate the legs above the level of the heart postoperatively

h. Encourage range of motion exercises of the legs

i. Instruct clients to avoid leg dangling or chair sitting

j. Instruct clients to elevate legs when sitting

k. Emphasize the importance of wearing elastic stockings after bandage removal

XVI. Arterial Disorders

A. Peripheral arterial disease (PAD)

1. Description

a. A chronic disorder in which partial or total arterial occlusion deprives the lower extremities of oxygen and nutrients

b. Tissue damage occurs below the arterial occlusion

c. Atherosclerosis is the most common cause of PAD

2. Data collection

a. Intermittent claudication

b. Rest pain characterized by numbness, burning, or aching in the distal portion of the lower extremities that awakens the client at night and is relieved by placing the extremity in a dependent position

c. Lower back or buttock discomfort

d. Loss of hair and dry, scaly skin on lower extremities

e. Thickened toenails

f. Cold and gray-blue or darkened color of skin in lower extremities

g. Elevational pallor and dependent rubor in lower extremities

h. Decreased or absent peripheral pulses

i. Signs of arterial ulcer formation characterized as painful, and occurring on or between the toes, or on the upper aspect of the foot

j. **Blood pressure** measurements at the thigh, calf, and ankle are lower than the brachial pressure (normally **BP** readings in the thigh and calf are higher than those in the upper extremities)

3. Implementation

a. Assess pain

b. Monitor the extremities for color, motion and sensation, and pulses

c. Obtain **blood pressure** measurements

d. Assess for signs of ulcer formation or signs of gangrene

e. Assist in developing an individualized

exercise program that is initiated gradually and slowly increased

f. Encourage prescribed exercise that will improve arterial flow through the development of collateral circulation

g. Instruct the client to walk to the point of claudication, stop and rest, then walk a little farther

h. Because swelling in the extremities prevents arterial blood flow, instruct clients to elevate their feet at rest but to refrain from elevating them above the level of the heart because extreme elevation slows arterial blood flow to the feet

i. In severe cases of PAD, clients with edema may sleep with the affected limb hanging from the bed or they may sit upright in a chair for comfort

j. Instruct all clients with PAD to avoid crossing their legs, which interferes with blood flow

k. Instruct clients to avoid exposure to cold (causes vasoconstriction to the extremities) and to wear socks or insulated shoes for warmth at all times

l. Instruct the client to never apply direct heat to the limb, such as with a heating pad or hot water, because the decreased sensitivity in the limb will cause burning

m. Instruct the client to inspect skin on the extremities daily and to report any signs of skin breakdown

n. Instruct the client to avoid tobacco and caffeine because of their vasoconstrictive effects

o. Instruct clients in the use of hemorrheologic and antiplatelet medications as prescribed

p. Inform clients of the importance of taking all medications prescribed by the physician

4. Procedures to improve arterial blood flow
   a. Percutaneous transluminal angioplasty
   b. Laser-assisted angioplasty
   c. Atherectomy
   d. Bypass surgery

B. Raynaud's disease
1. Description
   a. Vasospasms of the arterioles and arteries of the upper and lower extremities
   b. Vasospasm causes constriction of the cutaneous vessels
   c. Attacks are intermittent and occur with exposure to cold or stress
   d. Affects primarily the fingers, toes, ears, and cheeks

2. Data collection
   a. Blanching of the extremity followed by cyanosis during vasoconstriction
   b. Reddened tissue when the vasospasm is relieved

   c. Numbness, tingling, swelling, and a cold temperature at the affected body part

3. Implementation
   a. Monitor pulses
   b. Administer vasodilators as prescribed
   c. Instruct the client regarding medication therapy
   d. Assist the client to identify and avoid precipitating factors such as cold and stress
   e. Instruct clients to avoid smoking
   f. Instruct clients to wear warm clothing, socks, and gloves in cold weather
   g. Advise clients to try to avoid injuries to the fingers and hands

C. Buerger's disease
1. Description
   a. Also known as thromboangiitis obliterans
   b. An occlusive disease of the median and small arteries and veins
   c. The distal upper and lower limbs are most commonly affected

2. Data collection
   a. Intermittent claudication (pain in the muscles resulting from an inadequate blood supply)
   b. Ischemic pain occurring in the digits while at rest
   c. Aching pain that is more severe at night
   d. Cool, numb, or tingling sensation
   e. Diminished pulses in the distal extremities
   f. Extremities are cool and red in the dependent position
   g. Development of ulcerations in the extremities

3. Implementation
   a. Instruct the client to stop smoking
   b. Monitor pulses
   c. Instruct the client to avoid injury to upper and lower extremities
   d. Administer vasodilators as prescribed
   e. Instruct clients regarding medication therapy

XVII. Aortic Aneurysms

A. Description
1. Abnormal dilation of the arterial wall caused by localized weakness and stretching in the medial layer or wall of an artery
2. The aneurysm can be located anywhere along the abdominal aorta
3. The goal of treatment is to limit the progression of the disease by modifying risk factors, controlling the **BP** to prevent strain on the aneurysm, recognizing symptoms early, and preventing rupture

B. Types
1. Fusiform: diffuse dilation that involves the entire circumference of the arterial segment
2. Saccular: distinct, localized outpouching of the artery wall

3. Dissecting: created when blood separates the layers of the artery wall forming a cavity between them
4. False (pseudoaneurysm)
   a. Occurs when the clot and connective tissue are outside the arterial wall
   b. Formed after complete rupture and subsequent formation of a scar sac
C. Data collection
   1. Thoracic
      a. Pain extending to the neck, shoulders, lower back, or abdomen
      b. Syncope
      c. Dyspnea
      d. Increased pulse
      e. Cyanosis
      f. Weakness
   2. Abdominal
      a. Prominent pulsating mass in the abdomen at or above the umbilicus
      b. Systolic bruit over the aorta
      c. Tenderness on deep palpation
      d. Abdominal or lower back pain
   3. Rupturing aneurysm
      a. Severe abdominal or back pain
      b. Lumbar pain radiating to the flank and groin
      c. Hypotension
      d. Increased pulse rate
      e. Signs of shock
   4. Diagnostic tests
      a. Done to confirm the presence of an aneurysm
      b. Done to confirm the size and location of the aneurysm
      c. Includes abdominal ultrasound, CT scan, and arteriography
   5. Implementation
      a. Monitor vital signs
      b. Assess risk factors for arterial disease process
      c. Obtain information regarding back or abdominal pain
      d. Question the client regarding the sensation of palpation in the abdomen
      e. Inspect the skin for the presence of vascular disease or breakdown
      f. Check peripheral circulation including pulses, temperature, and color
      g. Observe for signs of rupture
      h. Note any tenderness over the abdomen
      i. Monitor for abdominal distention
   6. Nonsurgical implementation
      a. Modify risk factors
      b. Instruct the client regarding the procedure for monitoring **BP**
      c. Instruct the client on the importance of regular physician visits to monitor the size of the aneurysm
      d. Instruct the client that if severe back or abdominal pain or fullness, soreness over the umbilicus, sudden development of

discoloration in the extremities, or a persistent elevation of **blood pressure** occurs, to notify the physician immediately
      e. Instruct the client with a thoracic aneurysm to immediately report the occurrence of chest or back pain, shortness of breath, difficulty swallowing, or hoarseness
D. Pharmacological implementation
   1. Administer antihypertensives to maintain **BP** within normal limits and prevent strain on the aneurysm
   2. Instruct the client in the purpose of the medications
   3. Instruct the client about the side effects and schedule of the medication
E. Abdominal aneurysm resection
   1. Description: surgical resection or excision of the aneurysm; the excised section is replaced with a graft that is sewn end to end
   2. Preoperative implementation
      a. Assess all peripheral pulses as a baseline for postoperative comparison
      b. Instruct clients on coughing and deep-breathing exercises
      c. Administer bowel preparation as prescribed
   3. Postoperative implementation
      a. Monitor vital signs
      b. Monitor peripheral pulses distal to the graft site
      c. Monitor for signs of graft occlusion including changes in pulses, cool to cold extremities below the graft, white or blue extremities or flanks, severe pain, or abdominal distention
      d. Limit elevation of the head of the bed to 45 degrees to prevent flexion of the graft
      e. Monitor for hypovolemia and renal failure due to the large amount of blood loss during surgery
      f. Monitor urine output hourly, and if it is less than 50 mL per hour, notify the physician
      g. Monitor serum creatinine and BUN daily
      h. Monitor respiratory status and auscultate breath sounds to identify respiratory complications
      i. Encourage turning, coughing, and deep breathing, while splinting the incision
      j. Ambulate as prescribed
      k. Maintain nasogastric tube to low suction until bowel sounds return
      l. Assess for bowel sounds and report their return to the physician
      m. Monitor for pain and administer medication as prescribed
      n. Assess the incision site for bleeding or signs of infection
      o. Prepare the client for discharge by providing instructions regarding pain

management, wound care, and activity restrictions

p. Instruct clients not to lift objects greater than 15 to 20 lb for 6 to 12 weeks

q. Advise clients to avoid activities requiring pushing, pulling, or straining

r. Instruct clients not to drive a vehicle until approved by the physician

F. Thoracic aneurysm repair
1. Description
   a. A thoracotomy or median sternotomy approach is used to enter the thoracic cavity
   b. The aneurysm is exposed, excised, and a graft or prosthesis is sewn onto the aorta
   c. Total cardiopulmonary bypass is necessary for excision of aneurysms in the ascending aorta
   d. Partial cardiopulmonary bypass is used for clients with an aneurysm in the descending aorta
2. Postoperative implementation
   a. Monitor vital signs
   b. Monitor for signs of hemorrhage such as a drop in **blood pressure**, increased pulse rate, and respirations and report to the physician immediately
   c. Monitor chest tubes for an increase in chest drainage, which may indicate bleeding or separation at the graft site
   d. Assess sensation and motion of all extremities, and if deficits occur, which can be due to a lack of blood supply during surgery, notify the physician
   e. Monitor respiratory status and auscultate breath sounds to identify respiratory complications
   f. Encourage turning, coughing, and deep breathing, while splinting the incision
   g. Monitor cardiac status for dysrhythmias
   h. Monitor for pain and administer medication as prescribed
   i. Assess the incision site for bleeding or signs of infection
   j. Prepare the client for discharge by providing instructions regarding pain management, wound care, and activity restrictions
   k. Instruct clients not to lift objects greater than 15 to 20 lb for 6 to 12 weeks
   l. Advise clients to avoid activities requiring pushing, pulling, or straining
   m. Instruct clients not to drive a vehicle until approved by the physician

XVIII. Hypertension

A. Description (Table 48–1)
1. Persistent elevation of the systolic **blood pressure (BP)** above 140 mmHg and the diastolic **blood pressure** above 90 mmHg

Table 48–1. Hypertension

Organ Involvement	Complications
Eyes	Visual changes
Brain	Cerebrovascular accident (CVA)
Cardiovascular system	CHF, hypertensive crisis
Kidneys	Renal failure

2. Most significant predictor of developing coronary artery disease
3. Major risk factor for coronary, cerebral, renal, and peripheral vascular disease
4. The disease is initially asymptomatic
5. The goals of treatment include to reduce **BP** and to prevent or lessen the extent of organ damage
6. Nonpharmacological approaches, such as lifestyle changes, may be initially prescribed and if the **BP** cannot be decreased after a reasonable time period (1 to 3 months), then the client may require pharmacological treatment

B. Primary or essential hypertension
1. No known etiology
2. Risk factors
   a. Aging
   b. Family history
   c. Black race with higher prevalence in males
   d. Obesity
   e. Smoking
   f. Stress

C. Secondary hypertension
1. Treatment depends on the cause and the organs involved
2. Occurs as a result of other disorders or conditions
3. Precipitating disorders or conditions
   a. Cardiovascular disorders
   b. Renal disorders
   c. Endocrine system disorders
   d. Pregnancy
   e. Medications

D. Data collection
1. May be asymptomatic
2. Headache
3. Visual disturbances
4. Dizziness
5. Chest pain
6. Tinnitus
7. Flushed face
8. Epistaxis

E. Implementation
1. Goals
   a. To reduce **BP**
   b. To prevent or lessen the extent of organ damage
2. Question the client regarding signs and symptoms indicative of hypertension
3. Obtain **BP** two or more times on both arms with the client supine and standing

4. Compare **BP** with prior documentation
5. Determine family history
6. Identify current medication therapy
7. Obtain weight
8. Evaluate dietary patterns and sodium intake of client
9. Monitor for visual changes or retinal damage
10. Monitor for cardiovascular changes, such as distended neck veins, increased heart rate, and dysrhythmias
11. Evaluate chest x-ray for heart enlargement
12. Monitor the neurological system
13. Evaluate renal function
14. Evaluate results of diagnostic and laboratory studies

F. Nonpharmacological implementation
1. Weight reduction if necessary or maintenance of ideal weight
2. Dietary sodium restriction to 2 g daily as prescribed
3. Moderate intake of alcohol and caffeine-containing products
4. Initiation of a regular exercise program
5. Avoidance of smoking
6. Relaxation techniques and biofeedback therapy
7. Elimination of unnecessary medications that may contribute to the hypertension

G. Stepped-care approach
1. Description
   a. If a pharmacological approach to treating hypertension is required, a single medication is prescribed and monitored for its effectiveness (Box 48–5)
   b. Medications are added to the treatment regimen until the **BP** is controlled
2. Step 1: a single medication is prescribed, which may be a diuretic, beta blocker, calcium channel blocker, or ACE inhibitor
3. Step 2
   a. Step 1 therapy is evaluated after 1 to 3 months
   b. If the response is not adequate, compliance is evaluated
   c. The medication may be increased or a new medication prescribed, or a second medication added to the treatment plan
4. Step 3
   a. Compliance is evaluated
   b. Further evaluation of step 2
   c. If a therapeutic response is not adequate, a second medication is substituted or a third medication is added to the treatment plan

5. Step 4
   a. Compliance is evaluated
   b. Careful data collection of factors limiting the antihypertensive response is done
   c. A third or fourth medication may be added to the treatment plan
H. See Box 48–6 for client education

BOX 48–6. Client Education for Hypertension

Educate client to prevent noncompliance with the treatment plan
Describe the disease process, explaining that symptoms usually do not develop until organs have suffered damage
Initiate and assist the client in planning a regular exercise program, avoiding heavy weight lifting and isometric exercises
Emphasize the importance of beginning the exercise program gradually
Encourage client to express feelings about daily stress
Assist client to identify ways to reduce stress
Teach relaxation techniques
Instruct clients how to incorporate relaxation techniques into their daily living pattern
Instruct client and family in the technique for monitoring blood pressure
Instruct client to maintain a diary of blood pressure readings
Emphasize the importance of lifelong medication and the need for follow-up treatment
Emphasize the importance of medications and instruct client not to stop the medication without consulting physician
Instruct client and family on the dietary restriction, which may include sodium, fat, calories, and cholesterol
Instruct client how to shop for and prepare low-sodium meals
Provide a list of products that contain sodium
Instruct client to read labels of products to determine sodium content, focusing on substances listed such as sodium, NaCl and MSG
Instruct client to bake, roast, or boil foods, avoid salt in preparation of foods, and avoid salt at the table
Instruct client that fresh foods are best to consume and to avoid canned foods
Instruct client about the action, side effects, and scheduling of medications
Advise client if uncomfortable side effects occur to contact physician and not stop the medication
Instruct client to avoid over-the-counter medication
Stress the importance of follow-up care

XIX. Hypertensive Crisis

A. Description
1. Any clinical condition requiring immediate reduction in **blood pressure**
2. An acute and life-threatening condition

BOX 48–5. Antihypertensive Medications

Diuretics	Vasodilators
ACE inhibitors	Beta blockers
Calcium channel blockers	Sympatholytics

3. The accelerated hypertension requires emergency treatment because target organ damage (brain, heart, retina) can occur quickly
4. Death can be caused by stroke, renal failure, or cardiac disease

B. Data collection
1. A **diastolic pressure** above 120 mmHg
2. Headache
3. Drowsiness
4. Confusion
5. Changes in neurological status
6. Tachycardia and tachypnea
7. Dyspnea
8. Cyanosis
9. Seizures

C. Implementation
1. Maintain a patent airway
2. IV antihypertensive medications are prescribed, which may include nitroprusside (Nipride), diazoxide (Hyperstat), or trimethaphan camsylate (Arfonad) (see Box 48–5)
3. Monitor vital signs, assessing **BP** every 5 minutes
4. Monitor for hypotension during the administration of antihypertensives
5. Place client in supine position if hypotension occurs
6. Have emergency medications and resuscitation equipment readily available
7. Maintain bed rest with the head of the bed at 45 degrees
8. Monitor IV therapy, assessing for fluid overload
9. Monitor I&O
10. Insert a Foley catheter as prescribed
11. Monitor urinary output, and if oliguria or anuria occurs, notify the physician

PRACTICE QUESTIONS

1. A client is scheduled for a cardiac catheterization using a radiopaque dye. Which of the following assessments is most critical before the procedure?
   1 Intake and output prior to procedure
   2 Baseline peripheral pulse rates
   3 Height and weight
   4 Allergy to iodine or shellfish

2. The client is scheduled for a dipyridamole (Persantine) thallium 201 scan. The nurse checks to make sure that the client has not had which of the following prior to the procedure?
   1 Milk products
   2 Caffeine
   3 Excess sugar
   4 A fatty meal

3. A client with no history of cardiovascular disease presents to the ambulatory clinic with flulike symptoms. The client suddenly complains of chest pain. Which of the following questions best helps the nurse to discriminate pain due to a noncardiac problem?
   1 "Have you ever had this pain before?"
   2 "Can you describe the pain to me?"
   3 "Does the pain get worse when you breathe in?"
   4 "Can you rate the pain on a scale of 1 to 10, with 10 being the worst?"

4. The client with myocardial infarction (MI) has been transferred from the coronary care unit (CCU) to the general medical unit with cardiac monitoring via telemetry. The nurse plans to allow for which of the following client activities?
   1 Strict bed rest for 24 hours after transfer
   2 Bathroom privileges and self-care activities
   3 Unsupervised hallway ambulation with distances under 200 feet
   4 Ad lib activities because the client is monitored

5. The nurse notes bilateral 2+ edema in the lower extremities of a client with myocardial infarction admitted 2 days ago. The nurse plans to do which of the following next?
   1 Review the intake and output records for the last 2 days
   2 Change the time of diuretic administration from morning to evening
   3 Request a sodium restriction of 1 g/day from the physician
   4 Order daily weights starting on the following morning

6. The nurse is collecting data from a client with a primary diagnosis of heart failure. Which of the following disorders reported by the client does not play a role in exacerbating the heart failure?
   1 Recent upper respiratory infection
   2 Nutritional anemia
   3 Peptic ulcer disease
   4 Atrial fibrillation

7. The nurse is admitting a client with heart failure who was being sent directly to the hospital from the physician's office. The nurse plans on having which of the following medications readily available for use?
   1 Diltiazem (Cardizem)
   2 Digoxin (Lanoxin)
   3 Propranolol (Inderal)
   4 Metoprolol (Lopressor)

8. The nurse assesses the sternotomy incision of a client on the third postoperative day after cardiac surgery. The incision shows some slight "puffiness" along the edges, is nonreddened, and has no apparent drainage. Temperature is 99° oral. The WBC count is 7500/mm³. The nurse interprets that the incision line

1 Is slightly edematous but shows no active signs of infection
2 Shows no sign of infection although the WBC count is elevated
3 Shows early signs of infection although the temperature is near normal
4 Shows early signs of infection supported by an elevated WBC count

9. The client who is 24 hours' postcardiac surgery has a urine output averaging 20 mL/hour for 2 hours. The client received a single infusion of 500 mL of intravenous fluid. Urine output for the subsequent hour was 25 mL. Daily laboratory results indicate the BUN is 45 mg/dL and the serum creatinine is 2.2 mg/dL. The nurse interprets that the client is at risk for
1 Hypovolemia
2 Urinary tract infection
3 Glomerulonephritis
4 Acute renal failure

10. The nurse is preparing to ambulate the client on the third postoperative day following cardiac surgery. The nurse plans to do which of the following to enable the client to best tolerate the ambulation?
1 Encourage the client to cough and deep breathe
2 Premedicate the client with an analgesic
3 Provide the client with a walker
4 Remove telemetry equipment

11. The client is wearing a continuous cardiac monitor, which begins to sound its alarm. The nurse sees no ECG complexes (cardiac rhythm) on the screen. The first action of the nurse is to
1 Check the client's status and lead placement
2 Press the recorder button on the ECG console
3 Call the physician
4 Call a code blue

12. The client with rapid rate atrial fibrillation asks the nurse why the physician is going to perform carotid massage. The nurse responds that this procedure may stimulate the
1 Vagus nerve to slow the heart rate
2 Vagus nerve to increase the heart rate, overdriving the rhythm
3 Diaphragmatic nerve to slow the heart rate
4 Diaphragmatic nerve to overdrive the rhythm

13. The nurse is caring for a monitored client alone in a room at the end of the hall. The client has a short burst of ventricular tachycardia followed by ventricular fibrillation (VF). The client immediately loses consciousness. The nurse
1 Calls for help and initiates cardiopulmonary resuscitation (CPR)
2 Starts oxygen by cannula at 10 L/minute and lowers the head of the bed

3 Goes to the nurses' station quickly and calls a code
4 Runs to get a defibrillator from an adjacent nursing unit

14. The nurse is evaluating the client's response to cardioversion. Which of the following observations is of highest priority to the nurse?
1 Oxygen flow rate
2 Status of airway
3 Blood pressure
4 Level of consciousness

15. An automatic external defibrillator (AED) is available to treat the client who goes into cardiac arrest. The nurse assesses the cardiac rhythm by
1 Applying standard ECG monitoring leads to the client and observing the rhythm
2 Holding the defibrillator paddles firmly against the chest
3 Applying the adhesive patch electrodes to the skin and moving away from the client
4 Connecting standard ECG electrodes to a transtelephonic monitoring device

16. The nurse is caring for the client immediately after insertion of a permanent demand pacemaker via the right subclavian vein. The nurse takes care not to dislodge the pacing catheter by
1 Limiting movement and abduction of the right arm
2 Limiting movement and abduction of the left arm
3 Assisting the client to get out of bed and ambulate with a walker
4 Having the physical therapist do active range of motion to the right arm

17. The client diagnosed with thrombophlebitis 1 day ago suddenly complains of chest pain and shortness of breath, and is visibly anxious. The nurse immediately assesses the client for other signs and symptoms of
1 Myocardial infarction
2 Pneumonia
3 Pulmonary embolism
4 Pulmonary edema

18. A client seeks treatment in the physician's office for unsightly varicose veins, and sclerotherapy is recommended. Before leaving the examining room, the client says to the nurse, "Can you tell me again how this sclerotherapy is done?" In formulating a response, the nurse incorporates the knowledge that sclerotherapy consists of
1 Injecting an agent into the vein to damage the vein wall and close the vein off
2 Tying off the vein at the upper end to prevent stasis from occurring
3 Tying off the vein at the lower end to prevent stasis from occurring
4 Surgical removal of the varicosity

19. The client is having a follow-up physician office visit after vein ligation and stripping. The client describes a sensation of "pins and needles" in the affected leg. Based on evaluation of this comment, the nurse
    1 Reassures the client that this is only temporary
    2 Advises the client to take acetaminophen (Tylenol) until it is gone
    3 States that warm packs should help
    4 Reports the complaint to the physician

20. A 24-year-old male seeks medical attention for complaints of claudication in the arch of the foot. The nurse also notes superficial thrombophlebitis of the lower leg. The nurse next assesses the client for
    1 Familial tendency toward peripheral vascular disease
    2 Smoking history
    3 Recent exposure to allergens
    4 History of recent insect bites

21. The nurse has given instructions to the client with Raynaud's disease about self-management of the disease process. The nurse evaluates that the client needs further reinforcement if the client states that
    1 Smoking cessation is very important
    2 Sources of caffeine should be eliminated from the diet
    3 Taking nifedipine (Procardia) as prescribed will decrease vessel spasm
    4 Moving to a warmer climate should help

22. The nurse is checking the blood pressure of a client diagnosed with primary hypertension. The nurse ensures accurate measurement by avoiding which of the following?
    1 Seating the client with arm bared, supported, and at heart level
    2 Measuring the blood pressure after the client is seated quietly for 5 minutes
    3 Using a cuff with a rubber bladder that encircles at least 80% of the limb
    4 Taking the blood pressure within 30 minutes following nicotine or caffeine ingestion

23. The client is at risk for pulmonary embolism, and is on anticoagulant therapy with warfarin (Coumadin). The client's prothrombin time is 20 seconds with a control of 11 seconds. The nurse determines that this result is
    1 The same as the client's own baseline level
    2 Lower than the needed therapeutic level
    3 Within the therapeutic range
    4 Higher than the therapeutic range

24. The client who has been receiving heparin therapy is also started on warfarin (Coumadin). The client asks the nurse why both medications are being administered. In formulating a response, the nurse incorporates the understanding that warfarin
    1 Stimulates breakdown of specific clotting factors by the liver, and it takes 2 to 3 days for this to exert an anticoagulant effect
    2 Inhibits synthesis of specific clotting factors in the liver, and it takes 3 to 4 days for this medication to exert an anticoagulant effect
    3 Stimulates production of the body's own thrombolytic substances, but it takes 2 to 4 days for this to begin
    4 Has the same mechanism of action as heparin, and the crossover time is needed for the serum level of warfarin to be therapeutic

25. The nurse has an order to begin administering warfarin sodium (Coumadin) to a client. While implementing this order, the nurse ensures that which of the following medications is available on the nursing unit as the antidote for warfarin?
    1 Vitamin K (AquaMEPHYTON)
    2 Aminocaproic acid (Amicar)
    3 Potassium chloride (KCl injection)
    4 Protamine sulfate (protamine injection)

26. The client is admitted with an arterial ischemic leg ulcer. The nurse assesses the ulcer expecting to note that it
    1 Has a pink-colored base
    2 Is superficial, with uneven edges
    3 Has little granulation tissue
    4 Has brown pigmentation surrounding it

27. The nurse is assessing the neurovascular status of the client who returned to the surgical nursing unit 4 hours ago after undergoing aortoiliac bypass graft. The affected leg is warm, and the nurse notes redness and edema. The pedal pulse is palpable and unchanged from admission. The nurse interprets that the neurovascular status is
    1 Normal, due to increased blood flow through the leg
    2 Slightly deteriorating and should be monitored for another hour
    3 Moderately impaired, and the surgeon should be called
    4 Adequate from an arterial approach, but venous complications are arising

28. A client is admitted with possible rheumatic endocarditis. The nurse checks the client for signs and symptoms of concurrent
    1 Viral infection
    2 Yeast infection
    3 Staphylococcal infection
    4 Streptococcal infection

29. The client with an abdominal aortic aneurysm (AAA) is not a candidate for surgery because the aneurysm is not yet large enough. The client is fearful that the aneurysm will rupture, causing death. The nurse plans to assist the client in cop-

ing with this fear by emphasizing what the client can do for self-monitoring. Which of the following items is unnecessary for the nurse to include in discussions with the client?
1 Antibiotic prophylaxis before invasive procedures
2 Importance of follow-up CT scans
3 Management of hypertension
4 Reporting abdominal or back pain

30. The client is admitted with a venous stasis leg ulcer. The nurse assesses the ulcer, expecting to note that it
1 Has a pale-colored base
2 Is deep, with even edges
3 Has little granulation tissue
4 Has brown pigmentation surrounding it

31. The client has an Unna boot applied for treatment of venous stasis leg ulcer. The nurse notes that the client's toes are mottled and cool, and the client verbalizes some numbness and tingling of the foot. The nurse interprets that the boot
1 Is controlling leg edema
2 Has been applied too tightly
3 Is impairing venous return
4 Has not yet dried

32. The nurse is planning care for an ambulatory client with a venous stasis leg ulcer. The nurse anticipates that which type of dressing will be used in the care of this client?
1 Damp to dry isotonic saline dressings
2 One-half strength Betadine dressings
3 Dry, sterile dressings
4 Zinc oxide dressings (Unna boot)

33. The nurse is caring for a client receiving digoxin (Lanoxin) in the treatment of heart failure. The nurse monitors the client for
1 Thrombocytopenia and weight gain
2 Anorexia, nausea, and yellow vision
3 Diarrhea and hypotension
4 Fatigue and muscle twitching

34. The nurse has reinforced instructions to the client who is beginning therapy with digitalis (Digoxin). The nurse evaluates that the client needs reinforcement if the client makes which of the following statements?
1 "I should call the doctor if my daily pulse rate is under 60 or over 100."
2 "If I miss a dose, I should just take two the next day."
3 "I shouldn't change brands without asking the doctor first."
4 "The pills should be kept in their original container, so they don't get mixed up with my other medicines."

35. The client with angina complains that the anginal pain is prolonged and severe, and occurs at the same time each day, most often in the morning. On further data collection, the nurse notes that that the pain occurs in the absence of precipitating factors. This type of anginal pain is best described as
1 Stable angina
2 Unstable angina
3 Variant angina
4 Nonanginal pain

36. The client is taking hydrochlorothiazide (hydroDIURIL, HCTZ) without taking any form of electrolyte supplement. The nurse encourages intake of which of the following foods?
1 Canned pears
2 Oranges
3 Cranberry juice
4 Applesauce

37. The client taking hydrochlorothiazide (hydroDIURIL, HCTZ) has been started on triamterene (Dyrenium) as well. The client asks the nurse why both medications are required. The nurse formulates a response based on the understanding that
1 Triamterene is a potassium-sparing diuretic, while HCTZ is a potassium-losing diuretic
2 HCTZ is a potassium-sparing diuretic, whereas triamterene is a potassium-losing diuretic
3 Both are weak potassium-losing diuretics
4 Both are weak potassium-sparing diuretics

38. The diabetic client who has been controlled with daily insulin has been placed on atenolol (Tenormin) for control of angina pectoris. Due to the effects of the medication, the nurse checks that which of the following signs or symptoms is the most reliable indicator of hypoglycemia?
1 Tachycardia
2 Sweating
3 Low blood glucose level
4 Anxiety

39. The hypertensive client who has been taking metoprolol (Lopressor) has been instructed to decrease the dose of the medication. The client asks the nurse why this must be done over a period of 1 to 2 weeks. In formulating a response, the nurse incorporates the understanding that abrupt withdrawal could
1 Give the client insomnia
2 Cause enhanced side effects of other prescribed medications
3 Result in hypoglycemia
4 Precipitate rebound hypertension

40. The nurse is administering medications to a client newly admitted to the nursing unit with a history of cardiac disease. The client has an order for propranolol (Inderal) 20 mg PO, and albuterol (Proventil, Ventolin) two puffs by inhalation. The nurse should

1 Administer the propranolol first, followed by the albuterol

2 Administer the albuterol first, followed by the propranolol

3 Let the client decide which to take first, according to preference

4 Call the physician to verify the order

41. The client who has begun taking fosinopril (Monopril) is very distressed, telling the nurse that the client cannot taste food normally since beginning the medication 2 weeks ago. The nurse provides the best support to the client by

1 Requesting that the physician change the order to another brand of ACE inhibitor

2 Reassuring the client that this is expected, and generally disappears in 2 to 3 months

3 Telling the client not to take the medication with food

4 Suggesting that the client taper the dose until taste returns to normal

42. The nurse is caring for the client with a history of mild heart failure who is receiving diltiazem (Cardizem) for hypertension. The nurse checks the client for

1 Tachycardia and rebound hypertension

2 Wheezing and shortness of breath

3 Bradycardia, weight gain, and peripheral edema

4 Chest pain and tachycardia

43. The client receiving nifedipine (Procardia) for angina complains of feeling listless, with generalized weakness and no energy. In order to support the client most effectively, the nurse must understand that these symptoms

1 Are unrelated to taking the medication

2 Are an expected effect of the medication

3 Indicate toxic reaction to the medication

4 Indicate underdosing of the medication

44. The nurse is planning to administer amlodipine (Norvasc) to a client. The nurse plans to do which of the following before giving the medication?

1 Check blood pressure and heart rate

2 Check respiratory rate

3 Check heart rate and respiratory rate

4 Check level of consciousness and blood pressure

45. The client taking nitroglycerin sublingually PRN for control of episodes of chest pain says to the nurse that perhaps the medication shouldn't be used unless absolutely necessary for pain. On further data collection, the nurse determines that the client knows the reasons for taking the medication, and that the client can afford to pay for the medication. The nurse next explores with the client any concerns about

1 Status of the heart disease

2 Potential myocardial infarction

3 Developing tolerance to the medication

4 Inconvenience of the medication schedule

46. The client has been prescribed a transdermal nitroglycerin system (Nitrodisc, Nitro-Dur) for the management of angina pectoris. The client asks the nurse why the patch must be removed at bedtime each night. In formulating a reply, the nurse incorporates the understanding that

1 Lack of pain relief (tolerance) occurs when worn continuously for 24 hours

2 Hypotension occurs frequently at night unless removed

3 The system is too irritating to the skin to be worn for 24 hours

4 The patch usually falls off from friction with the bedclothes anyway

47. The nurse has an order to administer a dose of nitroglycerin ointment (Nitro-Bid, Nitrostat) to a client. The nurse avoids doing which of the following in preparing the medication for administration?

1 Using the manufacturer's papers

2 Using the fingers to spread the ointment

3 Applying the dose in an even layer

4 Washing off the previous application

48. The nurse is giving the client instructions about the use of a transdermal nitroglycerin system (Nitro-Dur, Transderm-Nitro). The nurse would not include which of the following points?

1 Apply the patch with very light pressure to avoid rapid absorption

2 Units are waterproof, so bathing and showering are allowed

3 Do not change brands because the dosages may not be equivalent

4 Do not cut or trim the patch to adjust dosage

49. A hypertensive client with target organ renal damage has been prescribed minoxidil (Loniten). The client asks the nurse why the physician has also prescribed propranolol for concurrent use. The nurse's response is based on the understanding that propranolol

1 Is used to get better control of hypertension than with minoxidil alone

2 Prevents reflex tachycardia that is caused by the minoxidil

3 Exerts a protective effect on the kidneys

4 Prevents fluid retention and weight gain

50. The client has begun antidysrhythmic therapy with esmolol HCl (Brevibloc). Knowing the side effects that could affect the client's psychosocial well-being, the nurse does anticipatory counseling about the possibility of

1 Anxiety and confusion

2 Anxiety and pain

3 Paranoia

4 Decreased libido and impotence

51. The nurse has given medication instructions to the client receiving disopyramide (Norpace). The nurse evaluates that the client needs clarification of the information if the client states to
    1 Change position slowly
    2 Avoid extreme heat
    3 Keep tissues nearby for excessive salivation
    4 Use caution with driving

52. The client has begun taking quinidine gluconate (Duraquin, Quinalan). The nurse checks for which of the following most frequent side effects of this medication?
    1 Constipation and dehydration
    2 Diarrhea, nausea, and cramping
    3 Tachycardia and hypertension
    4 Bleeding tendencies

53. The client is beginning amiodarone (Cordarone) therapy while in the hospital. To minimize gastrointestinal side effects, the nurse provides the client with

1 Antidiarrheal agents
2 Antacids
3 Increased fiber and fluids
4 Soft diet

54. The nurse is reinforcing instructions to the client receiving colestipol hydrochloride (Colestid). The nurse advises the client to increase intake of
    1 Carbohydrates
    2 Fats
    3 Fiber and fluids
    4 Protein

55. The client had an aortic valve replacement 2 days ago. This morning the client says to the nurse, "I don't feel any better than I did before surgery." The most appropriate response by the nurse is
    1 "It's only the second day post-op. Cheer up."
    2 "This is a normal frustration, it'll get better."
    3 "You are concerned that you don't feel any better after surgery."
    4 "You will feel better in a week or two."

ANSWERS

1. **4**

RATIONALE: This procedure requires a signed consent, because it involves injection of a radiopaque dye into the blood vessel. The risk of allergic reaction and possible anaphylaxis is serious, and must be assessed before the procedure.
TEST-TAKING STRATEGY: The question asks you for the "most critical" assessment, implying several options may be plausible. Using the concept of criticality, eliminate options 1 and 3. The remaining options compete for priority, but the risk of anaphylaxis makes option 4 the correct choice. Review preprocedure interventions for a cardiac catheterization now if you had difficulty with this question.
LEVEL OF COGNITIVE ABILITY: Application
PHASE OF NURSING PROCESS: Data Collection
CLIENT NEEDS: Physiological Integrity
CONTENT AREA: Adult Health/Cardiovascular
REFERENCE
Monahan, F., & Neighbors, M. (1998). *Medical-surgical nursing: Foundations for clinical practice* (2nd ed.). Philadelphia: W. B. Saunders. p. 203.

2. **2**

RATIONALE: This test is an alternative to the exercise thallium 201 scan. The dipyridamole (Persantine) dilates the coronary arteries as exercise would. Before the procedure, any form of caffeine should be withheld, as well as aminophylline or theophylline. Aminophylline is the antagonist to dipyridamole.
TEST-TAKING STRATEGY: The question is looking for an incorrect item, evidenced by the word "not" in the stem. Factors that put a strain on the heart, such as nicotine and caffeine, can interfere with cardiac diagnostic test results. Look for items such as these in similarly worded questions.
LEVEL OF COGNITIVE ABILITY: Comprehension
PHASE OF NURSING PROCESS: Data Collection

CLIENT NEEDS: Physiological Integrity
CONTENT AREA: Adult Health/Cardiovascular
REFERENCE
Black, J., & Matassarin-Jacobs, E. (1997). *Medical-surgical nursing: Clinical management for continuity of care* (5th ed.). Philadelphia: W. B. Saunders. p. 1230.

3. **3**

RATIONALE: Chest pain is assessed using the standard pain assessment parameters (e.g., characteristics, location, intensity, duration, precipitating and alleviating factors, and associated symptoms). Options 1, 2, and 4 may help discriminate the origin of pain. Pain of pleuropulmonary origin usually worsens on inspiration.
TEST-TAKING STRATEGY: This question is looking for a method of discriminating among causes of pain. The three incorrect responses, although appropriate to use in practice, are general assessment questions only. Option 3 will discriminate between a cardiac and noncardiac cause of pain.
LEVEL OF COGNITIVE ABILITY: Analysis
PHASE OF NURSING PROCESS: Data Collection
CLIENT NEEDS: Physiological Integrity
CONTENT AREA: Adult Health/Cardiovascular
REFERENCE
Monahan, F., & Neighbors, M. (1998). *Medical-surgical nursing: Foundations for clinical practice* (2nd ed.). Philadelphia: W. B. Saunders. p. 188.

4. **2**

RATIONALE: Upon transfer from CCU, the client is allowed self-care activities and bathroom privileges. Supervised ambulation in the hall for brief distances is encouraged, with distances gradually increased (50, 100, 200 feet).
TEST-TAKING STRATEGY: Eliminate options 3 and 4 first because they are excessive, given that the client has just transferred from CCU. Option 1 is not viable since the client would be doing less activity than in CCU prior to transfer. Review activity prescriptions for the client with an MI now if you had difficulty with this question.

LEVEL OF COGNITIVE ABILITY: Application
PHASE OF NURSING PROCESS: Planning
CLIENT NEEDS: Physiological Integrity
CONTENT AREA: Adult Health/Cardiovascular
REFERENCE
Black, J., & Matassarin-Jacobs, E. (1997). *Medical-surgical nursing: Clinical management for continuity of care* (5th ed.). Philadelphia: W. B. Saunders. p. 1264.

5. 1

RATIONALE: Edema, the accumulation of excess fluid in the interstitial spaces, can be measured by intake greater than output, and by a sudden increase in weight. Diuretics should be given in the morning whenever possible to avoid nocturia. Strict sodium restrictions are reserved for clients with severe symptoms.
TEST-TAKING STRATEGY: The question asks what the nurse should do next. Options 2 and 3 can be eliminated immediately. Options 1 and 4 are both correct choices, but option 1 can give the nurse immediate information about fluid balance.
LEVEL OF COGNITIVE ABILITY: Application
PHASE OF NURSING PROCESS: Planning
CLIENT NEEDS: Physiological Integrity
CONTENT AREA: Adult Health/Cardiovascular
REFERENCE
Monahan, F., & Neighbors, M. (1998). *Medical-surgical nursing: Foundations for clinical practice* (2nd ed.). Philadelphia: W. B. Saunders. pp. 89–90.

6. 3

RATIONALE: Heart failure is precipitated or exacerbated by physical or emotional stress, dysrhythmias, infections, anemia, thyroid disorders, pregnancy, Paget's disease, nutritional deficiencies (thiamine, alcoholism), pulmonary disease, and hypervolemia.
TEST-TAKING STRATEGY: The question asks for an item that is not related to the heart failure. Since heart failure is exacerbated by factors that increase the workload of the heart, options 1, 2, and 4 can be eliminated systematically. Review the precipitating factors associated with heart failure now if you had difficulty with this question.
LEVEL OF COGNITIVE ABILITY: Comprehension
PHASE OF NURSING PROCESS: Data Collection
CLIENT NEEDS: Health Promotion and Maintenance
CONTENT AREA: Adult Health/Cardiovascular
REFERENCE
Black, J., & Matassarin-Jacobs, E. (1997). *Medical-surgical nursing: Clinical management for continuity of care* (5th ed.). Philadelphia: W. B. Saunders. p. 1278.

7. 2

RATIONALE: Digoxin exerts a positive inotropic effect on the heart, while slowing the overall rate through a variety of mechanisms. It is the medication of choice used to treat heart failure. Diltiazem (calcium channel blocker), propranolol, and metoprolol (beta-adrenergic blockers) have a negative inotropic effect and would worsen the failing heart.
TEST-TAKING STRATEGY: Medication knowledge is necessary to answer this question. Review these medications if necessary at this time. Similarities exist between options 3 and 4, thus they can be eliminated first.
LEVEL OF COGNITIVE ABILITY: Comprehension
PHASE OF NURSING PROCESS: Planning
CLIENT NEEDS: Physiological Integrity
CONTENT AREA: Pharmacology

REFERENCE
Black, J., & Matassarin-Jacobs, E. (1997). *Medical-surgical nursing: Clinical management for continuity of care* (5th ed.). Philadelphia: W. B. Saunders. p. 1283.

8. 1

RATIONALE: Sternotomy incision sites are assessed for signs and symptoms of infection, such as redness, swelling, induration, and "bogginess," or "stepping." An elevated temperature and WBC count after 3 to 4 days usually indicate infection.
TEST-TAKING STRATEGY: Rule out options 2 and 4 because the WBC count is normal. The lack of drainage, redness, or "bogginess" helps you choose option 1 over 4.
LEVEL OF COGNITIVE ABILITY: Comprehension
PHASE OF NURSING PROCESS: Evaluation
CLIENT NEEDS: Physiological Integrity
CONTENT AREA: Adult Health/Cardiovascular
REFERENCE
Monahan, F., & Neighbors, M. (1998) *Medical-surgical nursing: Foundations for clinical practice* (2nd ed.). Philadelphia: W. B. Saunders. p. 996.

9. 4

RATIONALE: The client who undergoes cardiac surgery is at risk for renal injury from poor perfusion, hemolysis, low cardiac output, or vasopressor drug therapy. Renal insult is signaled by decreased urine output and increased BUN and creatinine. The client may need medications such as dopamine to increase renal perfusion, and could possibly need peritoneal dialysis or hemodialysis.
TEST-TAKING STRATEGY: The question gives no evidence of any infection, so eliminate options 2 and 3 first. Hypovolemia is ruled out next because of the high BUN and creatinine values, and the poor response to fluid administration. Review laboratory values and postcardiac surgery complications now if you had difficulty with this question.
LEVEL OF COGNITIVE ABILITY: Analysis
PHASE OF NURSING PROCESS: Data Collection
CLIENT NEEDS: Physiological Integrity
CONTENT AREA: Adult Health/Cardiovascular
REFERENCE
Monahan, F., & Neighbors, M. (1998). *Medical-surgical nursing: Foundations for clinical practice* (2nd ed.). Philadelphia: W. B. Saunders. p. 202.

10. 2

RATIONALE: The nurse should encourage regular use of pain medication for the first 48 to 72 hours after cardiac surgery, because analgesia will promote rest, decrease myocardial oxygen consumption due to pain, and allow better participation in activities such as coughing, deep breathing, and ambulation.
TEST-TAKING STRATEGY: The question asks for the best action of the nurse to help a client tolerate ambulation. Coughing and deep breathing will not actively help endurance, so eliminate that first, as well as removal of telemetry equipment, which is contraindicated unless ordered. Options 2 and 3 are both helpful, but 2 is better, for the reasons stated above.
LEVEL OF COGNITIVE ABILITY: Application
PHASE OF NURSING PROCESS: Planning
CLIENT NEEDS: Physiological Integrity
CONTENT AREA: Adult Health/Cardiovascular

REFERENCE
Monahan, F., & Neighbors, M. (1998) *Medical-surgical nursing: Foundations for clinical practice* (2nd ed.). Philadelphia: W. B. Saunders. p. 202.

11. 1

RATIONALE: Sudden loss of ECG complexes indicates either ventricular asystole, or possibly electrode displacement. Accurate assessment of the client and equipment is necessary to determine the cause, and provide an appropriate response.
TEST-TAKING STRATEGY: Options 3 and 4 are incorrect because you are calling for assistance when you don't know what the problem is. Option 2 may sound reasonable, but the ECG monitor automatically starts recording when an alarm sounds. Option 1 is the best option because you should always assess the client directly before taking any action.
LEVEL OF COGNITIVE ABILITY: Application
PHASE OF NURSING PROCESS: Implementation
CLIENT NEEDS: Physiological Integrity
CONTENT AREA: Adult Health/Cardiovascular
REFERENCE
Black, J., & Matassarin-Jacobs, E. (1997). *Medical-surgical nursing: Clinical management for continuity of care* (5th ed.). Philadelphia: W. B. Saunders. p. 1310.

12. 1

RATIONALE: Carotid sinus massage is one of maneuvers used for vagal stimulation to decrease a rapid heart rate and possibly terminate a tachydysrhythmia. The others are the Valsalva maneuvers of inducing the gag reflex, and asking the client to strain or bear down. Medication therapy is often needed as an adjunct to keep the rate down or maintain the normal rhythm.
TEST-TAKING STRATEGY: Knowledge of anatomy and physiology alone may be sufficient to guide you through this question. A rapid rate dysrhythmia would need to be slowed, which is the function of the vagus nerve. The diaphragmatic nerve affects respiration. If you are unfamiliar with the functions of these nerves, take time now to review.
LEVEL OF COGNITIVE ABILITY: Comprehension
PHASE OF NURSING PROCESS: Implementation
CLIENT NEEDS: Physiological Integrity
CONTENT AREA: Adult Health/Cardiovascular
REFERENCE
Monahan, F., & Neighbors, M. (1998). *Medical-surgical nursing: Foundations for clinical practice* (2nd ed.). Philadelphia: W. B. Saunders. p. 176.

13. 1

RATIONALE: When VF occurs, the nurse remains with the client and initiates CPR until a defibrillator is available and attached to the client.
TEST-TAKING STRATEGY: Eliminate options 3 and 4 first because you would never leave the client alone. Of the remaining two options, lowering the head of the bed is appropriate (for resuscitation), but the oxygen by cannula at 10 liters is incorrect. Option 1 is the correct option.
LEVEL OF COGNITIVE ABILITY: Application
PHASE OF NURSING PROCESS: Implementation
CLIENT NEEDS: Physiological Integrity
CONTENT AREA: Adult Health/Cardiovascular

REFERENCE
Black, J., & Matassarin-Jacobs, E. (1997). *Medical-surgical nursing: Clinical management for continuity of care* (5th ed.). Philadelphia: W. B. Saunders. p. 1305.

14. 2

RATIONALE: Nursing responsibilities after cardioversion include maintenance of a patent airway, oxygen administration, assessment of vital signs and level of consciousness, and dysrhythmia detection.
TEST-TAKING STRATEGY: There is more than one correct answer, as evidenced by the phrase "highest priority" in the stem. This question is easy, though, since it follows the ABCs of life support. Airway comes first.
LEVEL OF COGNITIVE ABILITY: Comprehension
PHASE OF NURSING PROCESS: Data Collection
CLIENT NEEDS: Physiological Integrity
CONTENT AREA: Adult Health/Cardiovascular
REFERENCE
Monahan, F., & Neighbors, M. (1998). *Medical-surgical nursing: Foundations for clinical practice* (2nd ed.). Philadelphia: W. B. Saunders. p. 259.

15. 3

RATIONALE: The nurse or rescuer puts two large adhesive patch electrodes on the client's chest in the usual defibrillator position. The nurse stops CPR and orders anyone near the client to move away and not touch the client. The defibrillator then analyzes the rhythm, which may take up to 30 seconds. The machine then indicates if it is necessary to defibrillate.
TEST-TAKING STRATEGY: If you are not familiar with this piece of equipment, look first at the word "automatic" in the name. This implies that a person is not as involved in the process as with a conventional defibrillator, and may help you eliminate option 2. Since standard ECG monitoring leads do not play an active role once a resuscitation is under way (options 1 and 4), you can eliminate these other two similar, but incorrect, responses. Option 4 is especially tricky because automatic external defibrillation can be done transtelephonically, but it is done through the use of patch electrodes that interact via telephone lines to a base station, which controls any actual defibrillation.
LEVEL OF COGNITIVE ABILITY: Comprehension
PHASE OF NURSING PROCESS: Data Collection
CLIENT NEEDS: Physiological Integrity
CONTENT AREA: Adult Health/Cardiovascular
REFERENCE
Monahan, F., & Neighbors, M. (1998). *Medical-surgical nursing: Foundations for clinical practice* (2nd ed.). Philadelphia: W. B. Saunders. p. 262.

16. 1

RATIONALE: In the first several hours after insertion of either a permanent or temporary pacemaker, the most common complication is pacing electrode dislodgment. The nurse helps prevent this complication by limiting the client's activities.
TEST-TAKING STRATEGY: The stem of the question tells you that the pacemaker was inserted on the right side. Therefore, to prevent pacing electrode dislodgment, motion must be limited on that side. Options 3 and 4 involve movement of the right arm. Limiting the movement of the left arm (option 2) is of no benefit to the client. Thus, option 1 is the clear choice.

LEVEL OF COGNITIVE ABILITY: Application
PHASE OF NURSING PROCESS: Implementation
CLIENT NEEDS: Physiological Integrity
CONTENT AREA: Adult Health/Cardiovascular
REFERENCE
Monahan, F., & Neighbors, M. (1998). *Medical-surgical nursing: Foundations for clinical practice* (2nd ed.). Philadelphia: W. B. Saunders. p. 256.

17. **3**

RATIONALE: Pulmonary embolism is a life-threatening complication of deep vein thrombosis and thrombophlebitis. Chest pain is the most common symptom, which is sudden in onset, and may be aggravated by breathing. Other signs and symptoms include dyspnea, cough, diaphoresis, and apprehension.
TEST-TAKING STRATEGY: This question tests your ability to analyze signs and symptoms of pulmonary embolism in a client at risk. Each of the incorrect options should be ruled out because myocardial infarction and pulmonary edema are cardiac-related problems and are therefore similar, and pneumonia is an infectious process. Review these concepts if needed.
LEVEL OF COGNITIVE ABILITY: Analysis
PHASE OF NURSING PROCESS: Data Collection
CLIENT NEEDS: Physiological Integrity
CONTENT AREA: Adult Health/Cardiovascular
REFERENCE
Black, J., & Matassarin-Jacobs, E. (1997). *Medical-surgical nursing: Clinical management for continuity of care* (5th ed.). Philadelphia: W. B. Saunders. p. 1435.

18. **1**

RATIONALE: Sclerotherapy is the injection of a sclerosing agent into a varicosity. The agent damages the vessel and causes aseptic thrombosis, which results in vein closure. With no blood flow through the vessel, there is no distention. The surgical procedure for varicose veins is vein ligation and stripping. This procedure involves tying off the varicose vein and large tributaries, and then removal of the vein with the use of hook and wires via multiple small incisions in the leg.
TEST-TAKING STRATEGY: If you are uncertain of the answer to this question, look at the word "sclerotherapy." A vessel that is sclerosed is blocked. This may help you to select the correct option. At the very least, you should be able to eliminate options 2 and 3 readily, because neither of these makes sense using principles of blood flow and gravity. Also, they are very similar, and so are likely to be incorrect. Review this procedure now if you had difficulty with this question.
LEVEL OF COGNITIVE ABILITY: Comprehension
PHASE OF NURSING PROCESS: Planning
CLIENT NEEDS: Physiological Integrity
CONTENT AREA: Adult Health/Cardiovascular
REFERENCE
Black, J., & Matassarin-Jacobs, E. (1997). *Medical-surgical nursing: Clinical management for continuity of care* (5th ed.). Philadelphia: W. B. Saunders. p. 1439.

19. **4**

RATIONALE: Hypersensitivity or a sensation of "pins and needles" in the surgical limb may indicate temporary or permanent nerve injury following surgery. The saphenous vein and the saphenous nerve run close together in the distal third of the leg. Since complications from this surgery are relatively rare, this symptom should be reported.
TEST-TAKING STRATEGY: Pins-and-needles sensations usually indicate nerve irritation or damage. Knowing this, options 2 and 3 can be eliminated as the least likely correct choices. Reassuring the client about something being "only temporary" is not often a good choice, unless this is known to be absolutely true. By the process of elimination, then, the physician should be notified.
LEVEL OF COGNITIVE ABILITY: Comprehension
PHASE OF NURSING PROCESS: Implementation
CLIENT NEEDS: Physiological Integrity
CONTENT AREA: Adult Health/Cardiovascular
REFERENCE
Black, J., & Matassarin-Jacobs, E. (1997). *Medical-surgical nursing: Clinical management for continuity of care* (5th ed.). Philadelphia: W. B. Saunders. p. 1439.

20. **2**

RATIONALE: The mixture of arterial and venous manifestations (claudication and phlebitis, respectively) in the young male client suggests thromboangiitis obliterans (Buerger's disease). This is a relatively uncommon disorder that is characterized by inflammation and thrombosis of smaller arteries and veins. This disorder is typically found in young adult males who smoke. The cause is unknown, but is suspected to have an autoimmune component.
TEST-TAKING STRATEGY: A basic knowledge of this disorder is really needed to answer this question. You can first eliminate options 3 and 4 because they would most likely cause local skin reactions. The question asks which item you should assess "next." It is often better to assess a modifiable factor before a nonmodifiable one. This may help you prioritize your answer.
LEVEL OF COGNITIVE ABILITY: Comprehension
PHASE OF NURSING PROCESS: Data Collection
CLIENT NEEDS: Health Promotion and Maintenance
CONTENT AREA: Adult Health/Cardiovascular
REFERENCE
Monahan, F., & Neighbors, M. (1998). *Medical-surgical nursing: Foundations for clinical practice* (2nd ed.). Philadelphia: W. B. Saunders. p. 351.

21. **4**

RATIONALE: The disorder responds favorably to removal of nicotine and caffeine. Medications such as calcium channel blockers may inhibit vessel spasm and prevent symptoms. Avoiding exposure to cold is very important. However, moving to a warmer climate may not necessarily be beneficial because the symptoms could still occur with the use of air conditioning, and during periods of cooler weather.
TEST-TAKING STRATEGY: Note the key words "needs further reinforcement." All of the options look good on first reading. However, when you analyze each of them, you realize that relocation is the least favorable of all the choices, from the viewpoints of practicality, and encountering new environmental concerns.
LEVEL OF COGNITIVE ABILITY: Comprehension
PHASE OF NURSING PROCESS: Evaluation
CLIENT NEEDS: Health Promotion and Maintenance
CONTENT AREA: Adult Health/Cardiovascular
REFERENCE
Monahan, F., & Neighbors, M. (1998). *Medical-surgical nursing: Foundations for clinical practice* (2nd ed.). Philadelphia: W. B. Saunders. p. 355.

22. 4

RATIONALE: Blood pressure should be taken with the client seated with the arm bared, positioned with support and at heart level. The client should sit with legs on floor, feet uncrossed, and not speak during the recording. The client should not have smoked tobacco or taken in caffeine in the 30 minutes preceding the measurement. The client should rest quietly for 5 minutes before the reading is taken. The cuff bladder should encircle at least 80% of the limb being measured. Gauges other than a mercury sphygmomanometer should be calibrated every 6 months to ensure accuracy. Finally, two or more readings should be averaged.

TEST-TAKING STRATEGY: Since blood pressure measurement is a finely honed skill, this should be fairly easy to answer. If you had difficulty answering, however, remember in questions worded such as these, variables that interfere with accuracy (such as caffeine and nicotine in this instance) are likely to be the correct choice.

LEVEL OF COGNITIVE ABILITY: Application
PHASE OF NURSING PROCESS: Implementation
CLIENT NEEDS: Physiological Integrity
CONTENT AREA: Adult Health/Cardiovascular
REFERENCE
Black, J. & Matassarin-Jacobs, E. (1997). *Medical-surgical nursing: Clinical management for continuity of care* (5th ed.). Philadelphia: W. B. Saunders. p. 1399.

23. 3

RATIONALE: The therapeutic range for prothrombin time (PT) is 1.5 to 2 times the control for clients at high risk for thrombus. Based on the client's control value, the therapeutic range for this individual would be 16.5 to 22 seconds.

TEST-TAKING STRATEGY: A key to answering this question as stated is in the control value. If you know that the purpose of anticoagulant therapy is to prolong clotting times, then you can immediately eliminate options 1 and 2. Since the PT value in the question is not even double the control, option 3 is your best choice.

LEVEL OF COGNITIVE ABILITY: Analysis
PHASE OF NURSING PROCESS: Evaluation
CLIENT NEEDS: Physiological Integrity
CONTENT AREA: Pharmacology
REFERENCE
Hodgson, B., & Kizior, R. (2000). *Saunders nursing drug handbook 2000.* Philadelphia: W. B. Saunders. pp. 1062–1064.

24. 2

RATIONALE: Warfarin works in the liver. It inhibits synthesis of four vitamin K–dependent clotting factors (X, IX, VII, and II), but it takes 3 to 4 days before the therapeutic effect of warfarin is exhibited.

TEST-TAKING STRATEGY: Heparin and warfarin do not act in the same way, so eliminate option 4 first. Warfarin is an anticoagulant, not a thrombolytic, so option 3 is incorrect. Recalling that the liver synthesizes clotting factors helps you to choose option 2 over option 1.

LEVEL OF COGNITIVE ABILITY: Comprehension
PHASE OF NURSING PROCESS: Planning
CLIENT NEEDS: Physiological Integrity
CONTENT AREA: Pharmacology
REFERENCE
Hodgson, B., & Kizior, R. (2000). *Saunders nursing drug handbook 2000.* Philadelphia: W. B. Saunders. pp. 1062–1063.

25. 1

RATIONALE: The antidote to warfarin is vitamin K, and should be readily available for use if excessive bleeding or hemorrhage should occur.

TEST-TAKING STRATEGY: This is an example of an item that must be memorized. It is a critical concept, and is a likely area for testing. Take the time to learn this now if needed.

LEVEL OF COGNITIVE ABILITY: Application
PHASE OF NURSING PROCESS: Implementation
CLIENT NEEDS: Physiological Integrity
CONTENT AREA: Pharmacology
REFERENCE
Hodgson, B., & Kizior, R. (2000). *Saunders nursing drug handbook 2000.* Philadelphia: W. B. Saunders. pp. 1062–1064.

26. 3

RATIONALE: Arterial leg ulcers tend to be deep and pale, with uneven edges and little granulation tissue. The client usually has rest pain, and the ulcer site is painful. Surrounding skin has coloration consistent with peripheral arterial disease.

TEST-TAKING STRATEGY: This question is asking you to discriminate between signs and symptoms of arterial and venous leg ulcers. Since arterial ulcers are caused by marked reduction in blood flow and tissue malnutrition, you can eliminate options 1 and 2. Brown discoloration (option 4) indicates clogging of peripheral tissue with waste products of metabolism, and indicates a venous problem. The answer is option 3, which is also consistent with tissue malnutrition.

LEVEL OF COGNITIVE ABILITY: Comprehension
PHASE OF NURSING PROCESS: Data Collection
CLIENT NEEDS: Physiological Integrity
CONTENT AREA: Adult Health/Cardiovascular
REFERENCE
Monahan, F., & Neighbors, M. (1998). *Medical-surgical nursing: Foundations for clinical practice* (2nd ed.). Philadelphia: W. B. Saunders. p. 333.

27. 1

RATIONALE: An expected outcome of surgery is warmth, redness, and edema in the surgical extremity, due to increased blood flow.

TEST-TAKING STRATEGY: Option 3 can be easily eliminated because the pedal pulse is unchanged. Venous complications from immobilization due to surgery would not be apparent within 4 hours, so eliminate option 4 next. To help you choose between options 1 and 2, think about the effects of sudden reperfusion in an ischemic limb. There would be redness from new blood flow, and edema from the sudden change in pressure in the blood vessels. Thus option 1 is better than option 2.

LEVEL OF COGNITIVE ABILITY: Analysis
PHASE OF NURSING PROCESS: Data Collection
CLIENT NEEDS: Physiological Integrity
CONTENT AREA: Adult Health/Cardiovascular
REFERENCE
Ignatavicius, D., Workman, M., & Mishler, M. (1999). *Medical-surgical nursing across the health care continuum* (3rd ed.). Philadelphia: W. B. Saunders. p. 857–859.

28. **4**

RATIONALE: Rheumatic endocarditis is a major indicator of rheumatic fever, which is a complication of infection with group A beta-hemolytic streptococcal infections. It is frequently triggered by streptococcal pharyngitis.
TEST-TAKING STRATEGY: Streptococcal infections are largely responsible for rheumatic heart disease. Remembering this concept should help you answer questions in this area.
LEVEL OF COGNITIVE ABILITY: Comprehension
PHASE OF NURSING PROCESS: Data Collection
CLIENT NEEDS: Physiological Integrity
CONTENT AREA: Adult Health/Cardiovascular
REFERENCE
Monahan, F., & Neighbors, M. (1998) *Medical-surgical nursing: Foundations for clinical practice* (2nd ed.). Philadelphia: W. B. Saunders. p. 233.

29. **1**

RATIONALE: Psychosocial care of the client with medical management of an AAA includes listening to the client's concerns, and reinforcing the rationales for ongoing medical surveillance. This includes periodic CT scans to monitor the size of the aneurysm, and careful adherence to medication and diet therapy for hypertension. The client is instructed to report any sensation of abdominal fullness, or complaints of abdominal or back pain to the physician without delay.
TEST-TAKING STRATEGY: This question is worded to make you look for an option that is not part of routine management for the client with unrepaired AAA. Options 2 and 4 can be eliminated quickly, because they are obviously good actions. If you have any difficulty with the last two, remember that increased blood pressure (option 3) could cause strain and rupture, which leaves option 1 as the correct answer.
LEVEL OF COGNITIVE ABILITY: Comprehension
PHASE OF NURSING PROCESS: Planning
CLIENT NEEDS: Physiological Integrity
CONTENT AREA: Adult Health/Cardiovascular
REFERENCE
Monahan, F., & Neighbors, M. (1998). *Medical-surgical nursing: Foundations for clinical practice* (2nd ed.). Philadelphia: W. B. Saunders. p. 367.

30. **4**

RATIONALE: Venous leg ulcers, also called stasis ulcers, tend to be more superficial than arterial ulcers, and the ulcer bed is pink. The edges of the ulcer are uneven, and there is evidence of granulation tissue. There is a brown pigmentation to the skin, from accumulation of metabolic waste products due to venous stasis. The client also exhibits peripheral edema.
TEST-TAKING STRATEGY: This question is asking you to discriminate between signs and symptoms of arterial and venous leg ulcers. Knowing that the information in options 1, 2, and 3 is due to tissue malnutrition (and thus an arterial problem), you can easily select the correct answer.
LEVEL OF COGNITIVE ABILITY: Comprehension
PHASE OF NURSING PROCESS: Data Collection
CLIENT NEEDS: Physiological Integrity
CONTENT AREA: Adult Health/Cardiovascular
REFERENCE
Monahan, F., & Neighbors, M. (1998). *Medical-surgical nursing: Foundations for clinical practice* (2nd ed.). Philadelphia: W. B. Saunders. p. 332.

31. **2**

RATIONALE: An Unna boot that is applied too tightly can cause signs of arterial occlusion. The nurse assesses the circulation to the foot and teaches the client to do the same.
TEST-TAKING STRATEGY: The symptoms described in the question are signs of arterial compromise. Option 2 is the only choice that is consistent with this circumstance. Whenever you have a question with this much information, it is there for a purpose; read it carefully and think about the message it is telling you.
LEVEL OF COGNITIVE ABILITY: Comprehension
PHASE OF NURSING PROCESS: Data Collection
CLIENT NEEDS: Physiological Integrity
CONTENT AREA: Adult Health/Cardiovascular
REFERENCE
Monahan, F., & Neighbors, M. (1998). *Medical-surgical nursing: Foundations for clinical practice* (2nd ed.). Philadelphia: W. B. Saunders. p. 390.

32. **4**

RATIONALE: Therapy for venous stasis ulcers consists of oxygen-permeable polyethylene film (Op Site) or oxygen-impermeable hydrocolloid dressing (DuoDerm). Opinions vary as to whether oxygen-permeable or oxygen-impermeable is better. For the ambulatory client, the physician may apply a gauze dressing moistened with zinc oxide to the leg, which hardens like a cast (Unna boot). This dressing then prevents venous stasis and provides a sterile environment for the wound. The dressing is changed on a weekly basis. Betadine is not used; it is a strong agent that could cause further damage to friable tissues. Dry, sterile dressings do not keep the wound moist. Damp to dry dressings are not as effective.
TEST-TAKING STRATEGY: This question is a classic example of your ability to discriminate among the uses of different types of dressings. Review the purpose of each of them now if needed.
LEVEL OF COGNITIVE ABILITY: Comprehension
PHASE OF NURSING PROCESS: Planning
CLIENT NEEDS: Physiological Integrity
CONTENT AREA: Adult Health/Cardiovascular
REFERENCE
Monahan, F., & Neighbors, M. (1998) *Medical-surgical nursing: Foundations for clinical practice* (2nd ed.). Philadelphia: W. B. Saunders. p. 390.

33. **2**

RATIONALE: The first signs and symptoms of digitalis toxicity in adults include abdominal pain, nausea, vomiting, visual disturbances (blurred, yellow or green vision, halos around lights), bradycardia, and other dysrhythmias.
TEST-TAKING STRATEGY: Medication side effects and toxicities are a difficult area to learn, simply because there are so many of them. This one is a classic, though; take the time to learn this if you have the need.
LEVEL OF COGNITIVE ABILITY: Application
PHASE OF NURSING PROCESS: Data Collection
CLIENT NEEDS: Physiological Integrity
CONTENT AREA: Pharmacology
REFERENCE
Hodgson, B., & Kizior, R. (2000). *Saunders nursing drug handbook 2000.* Philadelphia: W. B. Saunders. pp. 324–326.

34. 2

RATIONALE: Client teaching includes taking the dose exactly as prescribed each day. If more than 12 hours go by, the client should omit that dose until the next scheduled one; the client should not double dose. A daily pulse check is imperative, and the client should know parameters for which the physician should be called. Clients are advised not to mix digoxin in pill boxes with other medications, because they may be similar in appearance. The physician should be consulted before changing brands, because the bioavailability of the drug may be different.

TEST-TAKING STRATEGY: This question is worded to make you look for an incorrect statement. Option 2 is a red flag, not just for this medication, but many others as well. It is not good practice to double dose any prescribed medications.

LEVEL OF COGNITIVE ABILITY: Comprehension
PHASE OF NURSING PROCESS: Evaluation
CLIENT NEEDS: Health Promotion and Maintenance
CONTENT AREA: Pharmacology
REFERENCE
Hodgson, B., & Kizior, R. (2000). *Saunders nursing drug handbook 2000.* Philadelphia: W. B. Saunders. pp. 324–326.

35. 3

RATIONALE: Stable angina is induced by exercise and relieved by rest or nitroglycerin tablets. Unstable angina occurs at lower and lower levels of activity, or at rest, is less predictable, and is often a precursor of myocardial infarction. Variant angina, or Prinzmetal's angina, is prolonged and severe, and occurs at the same time each day, most often in the morning.

TEST-TAKING STRATEGY: Eliminate option 4 first. Evaluate the data presented in the question to determine the correct option. If you had difficulty with this question, review the characteristics of the various types of angina.

LEVEL OF COGNITIVE ABILITY: Comprehension
PHASE OF NURSING PROCESS: Data Collection
CLIENT NEEDS: Physiological Integrity
CONTENT AREA: Adult Health/Cardiovascular
REFERENCE
Monahan, F., & Neighbors, M. (1998). *Medical-surgical nursing: Foundations for clinical practice* (2nd ed.). Philadelphia: W. B. Saunders. p. 286.

36. 2

RATIONALE: HCTZ is a potassium-losing diuretic, and clients are at risk for hypokalemia. Potassium is found in many foods, especially unprocessed foods, many vegetables, fruits, and fresh meats. Since potassium is very water-soluble, foods that are prepared in water are often lower in potassium than the same foods cooked another way (boiled vs. baked potato). Clients who need potassium added to the diet are encouraged to take in these foods. Many salt substitutes are also high in potassium.

TEST-TAKING STRATEGY: Evaluating food choices in terms of their water content and according to how highly processed they are may be a helpful approach for some questions related to potassium. In this question you will see that each of the incorrect options is processed to some degree and has a high water content.

LEVEL OF COGNITIVE ABILITY: Application
PHASE OF NURSING PROCESS: Implementation
CLIENT NEEDS: Physiological Integrity
CONTENT AREA: Adult Health/Cardiovascular

REFERENCE
Lutz, C., & Przytulski, K. (1997). *Nutrition and diet therapy* (2nd ed.). Philadelphia: F. A. Davis. pp. 390–391.

37. 1

RATIONALE: Distal tubule and potassium-sparing diuretics include amiloride (Midamor), spironolactone (Aldactone), and triamterene (Dyrenium). They are weak diuretics that are of particular use when combined with potassium-losing diuretics. This is especially useful when medication and dietary supplement of potassium are not appropriate.

TEST-TAKING STRATEGY: From the construct of this question, the options are visually divided into two sets: options 1 and 2, and 3 and 4. Neither 3 nor 4 makes sense, so eliminate these first. Of the remaining two, it is especially helpful to remember that HCTZ (a common diuretic) is potassium-losing. This will help you answer correctly using the process of elimination.

LEVEL OF COGNITIVE ABILITY: Comprehension
PHASE OF NURSING PROCESS: Planning
CLIENT NEEDS: Physiological Integrity
CONTENT AREA: Pharmacology
REFERENCE
Hodgson, B., & Kizior, R. (2000). *Saunders nursing drug handbook 2000.* Philadelphia: W. B. Saunders. pp. 494–496, 1021–1022.

38. 3

RATIONALE: Beta-adrenergic blocking agents, such as atenolol, inhibit the appearance of warning signs and symptoms of acute hypoglycemia, which would include anxiety, increased heart rate, and sweating. Therefore, the client receiving this medication should adhere to the therapeutic regimen, and monitor blood glucose levels carefully.

TEST-TAKING STRATEGY: Note the use of the words "most reliable" in the question. This indicates that more than one response could be partially or completely correct. Each of the options is, in fact, a sign or symptom of hypoglycemia. Knowledge of the masking effects of beta-adrenergic blocking agents helps you to choose the blood glucose level as the most reliable indicator.

LEVEL OF COGNITIVE ABILITY: Comprehension
PHASE OF NURSING PROCESS: Data Collection
CLIENT NEEDS: Physiological Integrity
CONTENT AREA: Pharmacology
REFERENCE
Hodgson, B., & Kizior, R. (2000). *Saunders nursing drug handbook 2000.* Philadelphia: W. B. Saunders. pp. 78–81.

39. 4

RATIONALE: Beta-adrenergic blocking agents should be tapered slowly. This will avoid abrupt withdrawal syndrome, characterized by headache, malaise, palpitations, tremors, sweating, rebound hypertension, dysrhythmias, and possibly myocardial infarction (in clients with cardiac disorders including angina pectoris).

TEST-TAKING STRATEGY: This question is fairly straightforward. To answer it correctly, you need to know that all beta-adrenergic blocking agents should be tapered slowly to prevent the effects noted above, as well as a return of the symptoms for which the medication was prescribed. The question guides you in the right direction by telling you the client was taking this medication for hypertension. Remember, read the question carefully. All information is there for a reason.

LEVEL OF COGNITIVE ABILITY: Comprehension
PHASE OF NURSING PROCESS: Planning
CLIENT NEEDS: Physiological Integrity
CONTENT AREA: Pharmacology
REFERENCE
Hodgson, B., & Kizior, R. (2000). *Saunders nursing drug handbook 2000.* Philadelphia: W. B. Saunders. pp. 677–679.

40. **4**

RATIONALE: Propranolol is a noncardioselective beta-adrenergic blocking agent. It blocks stimulation of beta$_1$ (myocardial) and beta$_2$ (pulmonary, vascular, and uterine) receptor sites. Albuterol is a sympathomimetic bronchodilator with relatively high beta$_2$ selectivity. The effects of the albuterol could be blocked by the action of propranolol. The nurse should verify the order with the physician.
TEST-TAKING STRATEGY: In order to answer this question successfully, you must know the basic actions of each of these medications, and to know that propranolol is a noncardioselective beta blocker. Because they oppose each other, they should be used cautiously together. The only option that indicates use of caution by the nurse is the one that verifies the order for the concurrent use of these two medications.
LEVEL OF COGNITIVE ABILITY: Comprehension
PHASE OF NURSING PROCESS: Implementation
CLIENT NEEDS: Safe, Effective Care Environment
CONTENT AREA: Pharmacology
REFERENCE
Hodgson, B., & Kizior, R. (2000). *Saunders nursing drug handbook 2000.* Philadelphia: W. B. Saunders. pp. 877–880.

41. **2**

RATIONALE: ACE inhibitors, such as fosinopril, cause temporary impairment of taste (dysgeusia). The nurse can tell the client that this effect usually disappears in 2 to 3 months even with continued therapy, and provide nutritional counseling if appropriate to avoid weight loss.
TEST-TAKING STRATEGY: Eliminate option 4 first as a poor nursing action. The nurse does not encourage dosage changes on any prescribed medication. Taking the drug with food is not going to change the taste of the food, so that can be eliminated next. Of the remaining two options, you need to know that this effect occurs with all medications in the ACE inhibitor group. Thus, you are left with the correct option, which is supporting the client through teaching.
LEVEL OF COGNITIVE ABILITY: Application
PHASE OF NURSING PROCESS: Implementation
CLIENT NEEDS: Psychosocial Integrity
CONTENT AREA: Pharmacology
REFERENCE
Hodgson, B., & Kizior, R. (2000). *Saunders nursing drug handbook 2000.* Philadelphia: W. B. Saunders. pp. 449–450.

42. **3**

RATIONALE: Calcium channel blocking agents, such as diltiazem, are used cautiously in clients with conditions that could be worsened by the medication, such as aortic stenosis, bradycardia, heart failure, acute myocardial infarction, and hypotension. The nurse assesses for signs and symptoms that indicate worsening of these underlying disorders. In this question, the nurse assesses for signs and symptoms indicating heart failure.
TEST-TAKING STRATEGY: To answer this question, you must know that diltiazem is a calcium channel blocker, and

that these medications decrease the rate and force of cardiac contraction. This helps you to eliminate options 1 and 4, because bradycardia is expected. Option 2 is eliminated because these signs could indicate bronchoconstriction, which does not occur with calcium channel blockers, but rather with some beta-adrenergic blockers.
LEVEL OF COGNITIVE ABILITY: Comprehension
PHASE OF NURSING PROCESS: Data Collection
CLIENT NEEDS: Physiological Integrity
CONTENT AREA: Pharmacology
REFERENCE
Hodgson, B., & Kizior, R. (2000). *Saunders nursing drug handbook 2000.* Philadelphia: W. B. Saunders. pp. 327–329.

43. **2**

RATIONALE: The client receiving a calcium channel blocking agent such as nifedipine may develop weakness and lethargy as an expected effect of the medication. Options 1, 3, and 4 are incorrect.
TEST-TAKING STRATEGY: To answer this question, you need to know that nifedipine is a calcium channel blocking agent, and that this medication decreases the rate and force of cardiac contraction, lowering the oxygen demand and also the cardiac output. By thinking through this process, you can reach the conclusion that decreased energy would then be an expected effect of the medication.
LEVEL OF COGNITIVE ABILITY: Comprehension
PHASE OF NURSING PROCESS: Data Collection
CLIENT NEEDS: Physiological Integrity
CONTENT AREA: Pharmacology
REFERENCE
Hodgson, B., & Kizior, R. (2000). *Saunders nursing drug handbook 2000.* Philadelphia: W. B. Saunders. pp. 744–745.

44. **1**

RATIONALE: Prior to administering a calcium channel blocking agent, the nurse should check the blood pressure and heart rate, which could both decrease in response to the action of this medication.
TEST-TAKING STRATEGY: To answer this question, you must know that amlodipine is a calcium channel blocker, and that this group of medications decreases the rate and force of cardiac contraction. This in turn lowers the heart rate and blood pressure. Option 2 can be eliminated easily because it is irrelevant. With options 3 and 4, note that only half of the option is correct. When answering questions such as these, with two items per option, both of the items must be correct for that option to be correct.
LEVEL OF COGNITIVE ABILITY: Application
PHASE OF NURSING PROCESS: Planning
CLIENT NEEDS: Physiological Integrity
CONTENT AREA: Pharmacology
REFERENCE
Hodgson, B., & Kizior, R. (2000). *Saunders nursing drug handbook 2000.* Philadelphia: W. B. Saunders. pp. 51–52.

45. **3**

RATIONALE: Tolerance to nitrates can develop over time. Some clients confuse tolerance with addiction. The nurse needs to explore the client's concerns and offer accurate information and support to help the client adapt to the illness and prescribed therapy.
TEST-TAKING STRATEGY: The question tells you that the client is hesitant about taking the medication and that the nurse has ruled out lack of knowledge or financial

barriers. Options 1 and 2 can be eliminated first because they are not reasons to stop taking the medication. Because the schedule is PRN for chest pain, there can be no inconvenience (option 4). Thus, you are left with the psychosocial concerns of the client to explore.
LEVEL OF COGNITIVE ABILITY: Comprehension
PHASE OF NURSING PROCESS: Data Collection
CLIENT NEEDS: Health Promotion and Maintenance
CONTENT AREA: Pharmacology
REFERENCE
Lehne, R. (1998). *Pharmacology for nursing care* (3rd ed.). Philadelphia: W. B. Saunders. pp. 465–469.

46. 1

RATIONALE: Clients have developed tolerance when wearing a transdermal system or using nitropaste continuously for 24 hours. This is manifested by lack of pain relief from the medication. This can be avoided by having the client wear the nitrate for 12 hours, leaving 12 hours "nitrate free."
TEST-TAKING STRATEGY: Option 4 should be eliminated first as the least plausible of all the options. Hypotension (option 2) is least likely to occur at night when the client is supine. Of the two remaining options, option 1 is more plausible than option 3; the product is not very marketable if it is too irritating.
LEVEL OF COGNITIVE ABILITY: Comprehension
PHASE OF NURSING PROCESS: Planning
CLIENT NEEDS: Physiological Integrity
CONTENT AREA: Pharmacology
REFERENCE
Lehne, R. (1998). *Pharmacology for nursing care* (3rd ed.). Philadelphia: W. B. Saunders. pp. 465–469.

47. 2

RATIONALE: The ointment is readily absorbed through the skin, so using the fingers will result in the nurse becoming hypotensive. Proper administration of nitroglycerin ointment involves the use of the dose-measuring applicator paper supplied by the manufacturer, applying in a thin, uniform layer, and applying to a nonhairy area of the chest, abdomen, anterior thigh, or forearm. The previous dose is removed before applying, and sites are rotated to avoid inflammation.
TEST-TAKING STRATEGY: This question tests fundamental principles of medication administration for nitroglycerin ointment. Review these principles now if needed.
LEVEL OF COGNITIVE ABILITY: Application
PHASE OF NURSING PROCESS: Planning
CLIENT NEEDS: Physiological Integrity
CONTENT AREA: Pharmacology
REFERENCE
Hodgson, B., & Kizior, R. (2000). *Saunders nursing drug handbook 2000*. Philadelphia: W. B. Saunders. pp. 750–753.

48. 1

RATIONALE: Transdermal patches can be applied to a hairless site using firm pressure to ensure good contact with skin, especially at the edges. The units are waterproof, but should not be trimmed to adjust the dose, because that will interfere with the absorption rate. Brands should not be switched back and forth because they may not be equivalent in dose. If the client becomes loose or falls off, it should be replaced.

TEST-TAKING STRATEGY: Note the key word "not" in the question. Each of the incorrect options listed is a standard administration technique. If you are unfamiliar with this medication, take a moment to review it now.
LEVEL OF COGNITIVE ABILITY: Application
PHASE OF NURSING PROCESS: Implementation
CLIENT NEEDS: Health Promotion and Maintenance
CONTENT AREA: Pharmacology
REFERENCE
Lehne, R. (1998). *Pharmacology for nursing care* (3rd ed.). Philadelphia: W. B. Saunders. pp. 465–469.

49. 2

RATIONALE: Minoxidil is a direct-acting peripheral vasodilator that acts on arterioles, with little effect on veins. It is used in severe hypertension with target organ damage, such as the kidneys. It causes reflex tachycardia, so a beta-adrenergic blocking agent must be prescribed for use at the same time. A diuretic is also needed to correct sodium and water retention that will occur.
TEST-TAKING STRATEGY: To answer this question, you must know that minoxidil is a vasodilator and that propranolol is a beta-adrenergic blocker. Option 1 is incorrect because minoxidil is not a first-line agent to use against hypertension. Propranolol exerts no protective effect on the kidney, so is eliminated next. Knowing that beta blockers can cause fluid retention, this option is also discarded, leaving reflex tachycardia.
LEVEL OF COGNITIVE ABILITY: Comprehension
PHASE OF NURSING PROCESS: Planning
CLIENT NEEDS: Physiological Integrity
CONTENT AREA: Pharmacology
REFERENCE
Hodgson, B., & Kizior, R. (2000). *Saunders nursing drug handbook 2000*. Philadelphia: W. B. Saunders. pp. 689–691.

50. 4

RATIONALE: Esmolol HCl is an antidysrhythmic and has some of the same side effects experienced when taking other beta-adrenergic blocking agents. That is, fatigue, decreased libido, and impotence may result. For the total well-being of the client, medication instructions should address this aspect of therapy.
TEST-TAKING STRATEGY: This side effect may occur with other beta-adrenergic blockers as well. This may be helpful to remember if questions arise on psychosocial aspects of care with these medications.
LEVEL OF COGNITIVE ABILITY: Comprehension
PHASE OF NURSING PROCESS: Planning
CLIENT NEEDS: Psychosocial Integrity
CONTENT AREA: Pharmacology
REFERENCE
Hodgson, B., & Kizior, R. (2000). *Saunders nursing drug handbook 2000*. Philadelphia: W. B. Saunders. pp. 939–941.

51. 3

RATIONALE: Disopyramide is an antidysrhythmic that is used in the treatment of atrial and ventricular tachydysrhythmias. It has fewer side effects than other antidysrhythmics, but does exert an anticholinergic effect. For that reason, clients should be cautioned about dry mouth, and to keep sugarless hard candy or gum nearby, or perform frequent oral rinses. Because of reduced perspiration, clients may develop heat intolerance, and should avoid extremely warm weather. The possibility of dizziness and blurred vision indicates the use of caution when driving. Another possible side effect includes hypotension, so clients should change position slowly if this occurs.

TEST-TAKING STRATEGY: If you know that this medication is an antidysrhythmic, you can anticipate that this medication will have cardiovascular effects. This might help you eliminate options 1 and 2 because these options are cardiovascular in nature. You would need to know that this medication has an anticholinergic effect to discriminate between options 3 and 4.
LEVEL OF COGNITIVE ABILITY: Comprehension
PHASE OF NURSING PROCESS: Evaluation
CLIENT NEEDS: Health Promotion and Maintenance
CONTENT AREA: Pharmacology
REFERENCE
Hodgson, B., & Kizior, R. (2000). *Saunders nursing drug handbook 2000*. Philadelphia: W. B. Saunders. pp. 337–339.

52. 2

RATIONALE: Quinidine is an antidysrhythmic, which decreases myocardial excitability and slows the velocity of conduction through the heart. The most common side effects relate to the GI system, and include diarrhea, cramping, nausea, and anorexia. Hypotension, tachycardia, and dysrhythmias are less frequent side effects that relate to the cardiovascular system.
TEST-TAKING STRATEGY: Note the key phrase "most frequent side effects." If you know that quinidine is an antidysrhythmic you may be able to eliminate option 3 as an unlikely combination. Options 1 and 2 seem to oppose each other, so it is likely that one of these is correct. In fact, quinidine causes the distressing GI side effects noted above.
LEVEL OF COGNITIVE ABILITY: Comprehension
PHASE OF NURSING PROCESS: Data Collection
CLIENT NEEDS: Physiological Integrity
CONTENT AREA: Pharmacology
REFERENCE
Hodgson, B., & Kizior, R. (2000). *Saunders nursing drug handbook 2000*. Philadelphia: W. B. Saunders. pp. 894–896.

53. 3

RATIONALE: Gastrointestinal side effects occur in up to 25% of clients taking amiodarone. The nurse can minimize these effects by providing a diet high in fiber, and by increasing fluids, unless contraindicated. This will minimize the risk of constipation.
TEST-TAKING STRATEGY: You can begin by eliminating a soft diet, as the client does not demonstrate difficulty chewing or swallowing. Since GI side effects are generally of two types, irritation/diarrhea or constipation, examine the remaining options. Antacids and antidiarrheals are similar in that they represent treatment of irritation, while the only other option is for constipation. In this case, you should select the option that is different from the other two.
LEVEL OF COGNITIVE ABILITY: Application
PHASE OF NURSING PROCESS: Implementation
CLIENT NEEDS: Physiological Integrity
CONTENT AREA: Pharmacology
REFERENCE
Hodgson, B., & Kizior, R. (2000). *Saunders nursing drug handbook 2000*. Philadelphia: W. B. Saunders. pp. 47–49.

54. 3

RATIONALE: Colestipol hydrochloride is a bile acid sequestrant useful in lowering serum cholesterol levels. The drug causes constipation in 10% to 50% of clients, with possible fecal impaction. Because of this, clients are advised to carefully monitor their elimination patterns, increase intake of fiber and fluids, and to take stool softeners or possibly laxatives if needed.
TEST-TAKING STRATEGY: If you look at the way this question is written, you will notice that each of the incorrect options represents a major type of food (e.g., carbohydrate, fat, protein). In this question, the correct option is the one that is different from the others, that is, fiber and fluids.
LEVEL OF COGNITIVE ABILITY: Application
PHASE OF NURSING PROCESS: Implementation
CLIENT NEEDS: Health Promotion and Maintenance
CONTENT AREA: Pharmacology
REFERENCE
Hodgson, B., & Kizior, R. (2000). *Saunders nursing drug handbook 2000*. Philadelphia: W. B. Saunders. pp. 253, 1116.

55. 3

RATIONALE: Paraphrasing is restating the client's message in the nurse's own words. Option 3 uses the therapeutic communication technique of paraphrasing. The client is frustrated and is searching for understanding.
TEST-TAKING STRATEGY: Therapeutic communication techniques are the answers to your questions regarding responses to a client. Therapeutic communication techniques enhance communication. Always select responses that will enhance communication. Option 1 belittles the client's concerns and feelings. Options 2 and 4 are offering false reassurance by the nurse.
LEVEL OF COGNITIVE ABILITY: Application
PHASE OF NURSING PROCESS: Implementation
CLIENT NEEDS: Psychosocial Integrity
CONTENT AREA: Adult Health/Cardiovascular
REFERENCE
Leahy, J., & Kizilay, P. (1998). *Foundations of nursing practice: a nursing process approach*. Philadelphia: W. B. Saunders. pp. 227–231.

BIBLIOGRAPHY

Black, J., & Matassarin-Jacobs, E. (1997). *Medical-surgical nursing: Clinical management for continuity of care* (5th ed.). Philadelphia: W. B. Saunders.

Burrell, L., Gerlach, M., & Pless, B. (1997). *Adult nursing: Acute and community care* (2nd ed.). Stamford, CT: Appleton & Lange.

Chernecky, C., & Berger, B. (1997). *Laboratory tests and diagnostic procedures* (2nd ed.). Philadelphia: W. B. Saunders.

Hodgson, B., & Kizior, R. (2000). *Saunders nursing drug handbook 2000.* Philadelphia: W. B. Saunders.

Ignatavicius, D., Workman, M., & Mishler, M. (1999). *Medical-surgical nursing across the health care continuum* (3rd ed.). Philadelphia: W. B. Saunders.

Leahy, J., & Kizilay, P. (1998). *Foundations of nursing practice: A nursing process approach.* Philadelphia: W. B. Saunders.

Lehne, R. (1998). *Pharmacology for nursing care* (3rd ed.). Philadelphia: W. B. Saunders.

Luckmann, J. (1997). *Saunders manual of nursing care.* Philadelphia: W. B. Saunders.

Lutz, C., & Przytulski, K. (1997). *Nutrition and diet therapy* (2nd ed.). Philadelphia: F. A. Davis.

Monahan, F., & Neighbors, M. (1998). *Medical-surgical nursing: Foundations for clinical practice* (2nd ed.). Philadelphia: W. B. Saunders.

O'Toole, M. (1997). *Miller-Keane encyclopedia & dictionary of medicine, nursing & allied health* (6th ed.). Philadelphia: W. B. Saunders.

Paul, S., & Hebra, J. (1998). *The nurse's guide to cardiac rhythm interpretation.* Philadelphia: W. B. Saunders.

CHAPTER 49

Cardiovascular Medications

I. **Anticoagulants** (Box 49–1)

A. Description
1. Prevents the extension and formation of clots by inhibiting factors in the clotting cascade and decreasing blood coagulability
2. Used for thrombosis, pulmonary embolism, and myocardial infarction (MI)
3. Contraindicated with active bleeding, except for disseminated intravascular coagulation (DIC), bleeding disorders or blood dyscrasias, ulcers, liver and kidney disease, and spinal cord or brain injuries

B. Side effects (Box 49–2)
1. Bleeding
2. Hypotension

C. Heparin sodium (Liquaemin)
1. Description
   a. Prevents thrombin from converting fibrinogen to fibrin
   b. Prevents thromboembolism
   c. The therapeutic dose does not dissolve clots, but prevents new thrombus formation
2. Blood levels (refer to Chapter 10 for information on therapeutic blood levels)
3. Implementation
   a. Monitor clotting time and activated partial thromboplastin time (APTT)
   b. Monitor platelet count
   c. Observe for bleeding gums, bruises, nosebleeds, hematuria, hematemesis, occult blood in the stools, and petechiae
   d. When administering heparin subcutaneously, inject into the abdomen

using a small needle at a 90-degree angle and do not aspirate or rub the injection site
   e. Antidote: protamine sulfate

D. Warfarin sodium (Coumadin)
1. Description
   a. Decreases prothrombin activity and prevents the use of vitamin K by the liver
   b. Used for long-term anticoagulation
   c. Prolongs clotting time and is monitored by the prothrombin time (PT) and international normalized ratio (INR)
   d. Used mainly to prevent thromboembolitic conditions such as thrombophlebitis, pulmonary embolism, and embolism formation caused by atrial fibrillation, thrombosis, MI, or heart valve damage
   e. Usually given for 2 to 3 months after an MI to decrease the incidence of deep vein thrombosis and thromboembolism
2. Blood levels (refer to Chapter 10 for information on therapeutic blood levels)
3. Implementation
   a. Monitor PT and INR
   b. Avoid the administration of salicylates
   c. Observe for bleeding gums, bruises, nosebleeds, tarry stools, hematuria, hematemesis, and petechiae
   d. Teach the client to use a soft toothbrush and electric razor
   e. Antidote: vitamin K, phytonadione (AquaMEPHYTON)

II. **Thrombolytic Medications** (Box 49–3)

A. Description
1. Activates plasminogen, leading to its conversion to plasma, a substance that degrades clots and dissolves formed blood clots
2. Plasminogen generates plasmin (the enzyme that dissolves clots)

BOX 49–1. Anticoagulants
Heparin sodium (Liquaemin)
Warfarin sodium (Coumadin)

BOX 49-2. Substances to Avoid with Anticoagulants

Green, leafy vegetables and foods high in vitamin K
Salicylates
Steroids
Nonsteroidal anti-inflammatory drugs (NSAIDs)
Sulfonamides
Phenytoin (Dilantin)
Cimetidine (Tagamet)
Allopurinol (Zyloprim)
Oral hypoglycemic agents

---

3. Used early in the course of myocardial infarct, (within 4 to 6 hours of the onset of the infarct), to restore blood flow, limit myocardial damage, preserve left ventricular function, and prevent death
B. Contraindications
   1. Active internal bleeding
   2. History of cerebrovascular accident (CVA)
   3. Intracranial problems
   4. Intracranial surgery or trauma within the previous 2 months
   5. History of thoracic, pelvic, or abdominal surgery in the previous 10 days
   6. History of hepatic or renal disease
   7. Uncontrolled hypertension
   8. Recently required, prolonged cardiopulmonary resuscitation (CPR)
C. Side effects
   1. Bleeding
   2. Dysrhythmias
   3. Fever
   4. Allergic reactions
D. Implementation
   1. Obtain thrombin time (TT), APTT, PT, fibrinogen level, hematocrit, and platelet count
   2. Monitor vital signs
   3. Monitor for hypotension and tachycardia
   4. Monitor for bleeding

BOX 49-3. Thrombolytic Medications

Alteplase (Activase, t-PA, Tissue Plasminogen Activator)
   Clot-specific and activates only fibrin-bound plasminogen; promotes the conversion of plasminogen to plasmin
Anistreplase (Eminase)
   Clot-specific and activates only fibrin-bound plasminogen; promotes the conversion of plasminogen to plasmin
Streptokinase (Kabikinase, Streptase)
   Acts systemically and converts plasminogen to plasmin
Urokinase (Abbokinase)
   Acts systemically and converts plasminogen to plasmin

BOX 49-4. Antiplatelet Medications

Aspirin (acetylsalicylic acid, ASA)
Dipyridamole (Persantine)
Ticlopidine HCl (Ticlid)
Sulfinpyrazone (Anturane)

---

5. Monitor all excretions for occult blood
6. Monitor for neurological changes such as slurred speech, lethargy, confusion, and hemiparesis
7. Avoid injections and apply direct pressure over a puncture sites for 20 to 30 minutes
8. Handle the client as little as possible when moving
9. If bleeding develops, the physician is notified and medication is discontinued
10. Antidote is aminocaproic acid (Amicar); used only in acute, life-threatening conditions

III. Antiplatelet Medications (Box 49–4)

A. Description
   1. Inhibits the aggregation of platelets in the clotting process, thereby prolonging the bleeding time
   2. May be used in conjunction with anticoagulants
   3. Used in the prophylaxis of long-term complications following MI, coronary revascularization, and cerebrovascular accidents
   4. Sulfinpyrazone (Anturane) is also used for treating gout and may be used in atrioventricular (AV) shunts for hemodialysis to prevent clotting
   5. Contraindicated in bleeding disorders and known sensitivity
B. Side effect: bleeding
C. Implementation
   1. Determine sensitivity prior to administration
   2. Monitor vital signs
   3. Instruct client to take medication with food if GI upset occurs
   4. Monitor bleeding time
   5. Monitor for side effects related to bleeding
   6. Instruct the client in the use of the medication and to monitor for side effects related to bleeding

IV. Cardiac Glycosides (Box 49–5)

A. Description
   1. Causes the heart muscle fibers to contract more efficiently, thus increases the force of myocardial contractions
   2. The increase in myocardial contractility increases cardiac, peripheral, and kidney

BOX 49–5. Cardiac Glycosides

Digoxin (Lanoxicaps, Lanoxin)
Digitoxin (Crystodigin)

BOX 49–6. Classifications of Diuretics

Thiazide Diuretics
Loop Diuretics
Osmotic Diuretics
Potassium-Sparing Diuretics
Carbonic Anhydrase Inhibitors

function by increasing **cardiac output**, decreasing preload, improving blood flow to the periphery and kidneys, decreasing edema, and increasing fluid excretion; as a result, fluid retention in the lungs and extremities is decreased
3. Used for congestive heart failure, atrial tachycardia, atrial fibrillation, and atrial flutter
4. Use with caution in clients with renal disease, hypothyroidism, and hypokalemia
B. Side effects
1. Anorexia, nausea, and vomiting
2. Headache
3. Blurred vision, diplopia, and photophobia
4. Yellow-green halos
5. Bradycardia
6. Drowsiness
7. Fatigue and weakness
C. Implementation
1. Monitor for toxicity as evidenced by anorexia, nausea, vomiting, visual disturbances, confusion, and bradycardia
2. Monitor serum digoxin level, electrolyte levels, and renal function tests
3. Therapeutic digoxin range is 0.5 to 2.0 ng/mL and levels above 2.0 ng/mL are toxic
4. An increased risk of toxicity exists in clients with hypercalcemia, hypokalemia, hypomagnesemia, or hypothyroidism
5. Monitor potassium level and if hypokalemia occurs (K below 3.5 mEq/L), the physician is notified
6. Instruct client to avoid over-the-counter medications
7. Monitor the client taking a potassium-wasting diuretic or cortisone medications closely for hypokalemia, because the hypokalemia can cause digoxin toxicity
8. Note that elderly clients are more sensitive to toxicity
9. Advise the client to eat foods high in potassium such as fresh and dried fruits, fruit juices, vegetables, and potatoes
10. Monitor apical pulse; if apical pulse rate is below 60, medication should be held and the physician notified
11. Teach the client how to measure the pulse and to notify the physician if the pulse rate is below 60 or above 100
12. Teach the client signs and symptoms of toxicity
13. Antidote: digoxin immune Fab (Digibind) used in extreme toxicity

V. Antihypertensive Medications (Box 49–6)

A. Thiazide diuretics (Box 49–7)
1. Description
   a. Increases sodium and water excretion by inhibiting sodium reabsorption in the distal tubule of the kidney
   b. Used for hypertension and peripheral edema
   c. Used in clients with normal renal function
   d. Not effective for immediate diuresis
   e. Contraindicated in renal failure
   f. Use with caution in the client taking lithium because lithium toxicity can occur
   g. Use with caution in clients taking digoxin, corticosteroids, and hypoglycemic medications
2. Side effects
   a. Electrolyte imbalances such as hypokalemia and hyponatremia
   b. Hyperglycemia
   c. Hyperuricemia
   d. Hypovolemia and hypotension
   e. Headaches
   f. Nausea, vomiting, and constipation
   g. Photosensitivity
3. Implementation
   a. Monitor vital signs
   b. Monitor weight and urine output
   c. Monitor electrolyte levels, glucose, and uric acid levels
   d. Check the peripheral extremities for edema

BOX 49–7. Thiazide and Thiazide-like Diuretics

THIAZIDE DIURETICS

Hydrochlorothiazide (Esidrex, Oretic, Hydro-DIURIL)
Chlorothiazide (Diuril)
Bendroflumethiazide (Naturetin)
Benzthiazide (Aquatag, Hydrex)
Hydroflumethiazide (Saluron, Diucardin)
Methyclothiazide (Aquatensen, Enduron)
Polythiazide (Renese-R)
Thichlormethiazide (Metahydrin, Naqua)

THIAZIDE-LIKE DIURETICS

Chlorthalidone (Hygroton)
Indapamide (Lozol)
Metolazone (Zaroxolyn)
Quinethazone (Hydromox)

BOX 49–8. Loop Diuretics

Furosemide (Lasix)
Bumetanide (Bumex)
Ethacrynic acid (Edecrine)
Torsemide (Demadex)

---

e. Monitor for signs of digitalis or lithium toxicity if the client is on these medications
f. Instruct the client to take medication in the morning to avoid nocturia and sleep interruption
g. Instruct the client how to record **blood pressure**
h. Instruct the client to eat foods rich in potassium and how to take potassium supplements if prescribed
i. Instruct the client to take medication with food to avoid GI upset
j. Instruct the client to change positions slowly to prevent **orthostatic hypotension**
k. Instruct the client to use sunscreen when in direct sunlight
l. Instruct the diabetic client to have blood glucose checked periodically

B. Loop diuretics (Box 49–8)
  1. Description
    a. Inhibits sodium and chloride reabsorption from the loop of Henle and the distal tubule
    b. They have little effect on the blood glucose; however, they cause marked depletion of water and electrolytes, increased uric acid levels, and cause the excretion of calcium
    c. Are more potent than the thiazide diuretics causing rapid diuresis
    d. Used for hypertension, edema associated with congestive heart failure (CHF), hypercalcemia, and renal disease
    e. Use with caution in clients taking digoxin or lithium
    f. Can cause ototoxicity, deafness, and thiamine deficiency
  2. Side effects: similar to the thiazide diuretics
  3. Implementation: similar to the thiazide diuretics

C. Osmotic diuretics (Box 49–9)
  1. Description
    a. Increases osmotic pressure of the glomerular filtrate, inhibiting reabsorption of water and electrolytes

---

BOX 49–9. Osmotic Diuretics

Mannitol (Osmitrol)
Urea (Ureaphil)

---

b. Used for oliguria and to prevent renal failure
c. Used to decrease intracranial pressure
d. Used to decrease intraocular pressure in narrow-angle glaucoma
e. Mannitol is used with chemotherapy to induce diuresis
  2. Side effects
    a. Fluid and electrolyte imbalances
    b. Pulmonary edema from the rapid shifts of fluid
    c. Nausea and vomiting
    d. Tachycardia from the rapid fluid loss
    e. Dehydration
  3. Implementation
    a. Monitor vital signs
    b. Monitor weight and urine output
    c. Monitor electrolyte levels
    d. Monitor for signs of pulmonary edema
    e. Monitor for signs of dehydration
    f. Monitor neurological status
    g. Change client's position slowly to prevent **orthostatic hypotension**

D. Carbonic anhydrase inhibitors (Box 49–10)
  1. Description
    a. Blocks the action of the enzyme carbonic anhydrase needed to maintain the acid-base balance
    b. Inhibition of this enzyme, carbonic anhydrase, causes increased sodium, potassium, and bicarbonate excretion
    c. Metabolic acidosis can occur with prolonged use (used to treat metabolic alkalosis)
    d. Used to decrease intraocular pressure in open-angle (chronic) glaucoma, to produce diuresis, manage epilepsy, treat high-altitude sickness
    e. Contraindicated in narrow-angle or acute glaucoma
  2. Side effects: similar to thiazide diuretics
  3. Implementation: similar to thiazide diuretics

E. Potassium-sparing diuretics (Box 49–11)
  1. Description
    a. Act on the distal tubule to promote sodium and water excretion and potassium retention
    b. Used for edema and hypertension, to increase urine output, to treat fluid retention and overload associated with CHF, hepatic cirrhosis, or nephrotic syndrome, and for diuretic-induced hypokalemia

---

BOX 49–10. Carbonic Anhydrase Inhibitors

Acetazolamide (Diamox)
Dichlorphenamide (Daranide)
Methazolamide (Neptazane)

BOX 49-11. **Potassium-Sparing Diuretics**

Spironolactone (Aldactone)
Amiloride HCl (Midamor)
Triamterene (Dyrenium)
Amiloride HCl and hydrochlorothiazide (Moduretic)
Spironolactone and hydrochlorothiazide (Aldactazide)
Triamterene and hydrochlorothiazide (Dyazide, Maxzide)

BOX 49-12. **Peripherally Acting Alpha-Adrenergic Blockers**

Doxazosin mesylate (Cardura)
Prazosin (Minipress)
Terazosin (Hytrin)
Guanadrel sulfate (Hylorel)
Guanethidine (Ismelin)
Reserpine (Serpasil)
Phenoxybenzamine (Dibenzyline)
Phentolamine (Regitine)
Tolazoline (Priscoline)

   c. Contraindicated in severe kidney or hepatic disease or in severe hyperkalemia
   d. Use with caution in clients with diabetes
   e. Use with caution in clients taking antihypertensives and lithium
   f. Use with caution in clients taking angiotensin-converting enzyme (ACE) inhibitors because hyperkalemia can result
   g. Use with caution in clients taking potassium supplements
  2. Side effects
   a. Hyperkalemia
   b. Nausea, vomiting, diarrhea
   c. Weakness, dizziness
   d. Photosensitivity
  3. Implementation
   a. Monitor vital signs
   b. Monitor urine output
   c. Monitor for signs and symptoms of hyperkalemia such as nausea, diarrhea, abdominal cramps, tachycardia followed by bradycardia, or oliguria
   d. Monitor for a potassium level greater than 5.3 mEq/L, which indicates hyperkalemia
   e. Instruct the client to avoid foods high in potassium
   f. Instruct the client to avoid exposure to direct sunlight
   g. Instruct the client to monitor for signs of hyperkalemia
   h. Instruct the client to avoid salt substitutes because they contain potassium
   i. Instruct the client to take with or after meals to decrease GI irritation

VI. Peripherally Acting Alpha-Adrenergic Blockers (Box 49-12)

A. Description
  1. Decreases sympathetic vasoconstriction by reducing the effects of norepinephrine at peripheral nerve endings, resulting in vasodilation and decreased **blood pressure**
  2. Used to maintain renal blood flow
  3. Used to treat hypertension
B. Side effects
  1. **Orthostatic hypotension**
  2. Reflex tachycardia

  3. GI disturbances
  4. Drowsiness
  5. Nasal congestion
  6. Edema and weight gain
  7. Reserpine (Serpasil) can cause depression, GI irritation, and impotence
C. Implementation
  1. Monitor vital signs
  2. Monitor for fluid retention and edema
  3. Instruct the client to change positions slowly to prevent **orthostatic hypotension**
  4. Instruct the client how to monitor **blood pressure**
  5. Instruct the client to monitor for edema
  6. Instruct clients to decrease salt intake
  7. Instruct clients to avoid over-the-counter medications

VII. Centrally Acting Sympatholytics (Adrenergic Blockers) (Box 49-13)

A. Description
  1. Stimulates alpha-receptors in the central nervous system (CNS) to inhibit vasoconstriction, thus reducing peripheral resistance
  2. Used to treat hypertension
  3. Contraindicated in impaired liver function
B. Side effects
  1. Sodium and water retention
  2. Drowsiness and dizziness
  3. Hypotension
  4. Bradycardia
  5. Dry mouth
  6. Impotence
  7. Depression
C. Implementation
  1. Monitor vital signs
  2. Instruct the client not to discontinue

BOX 49-13. **Centrally Acting Sympatholytics**

Clonidine (Catapres)
Methyldopa (Aldomet)
Guanabenz acetate (Wytensin)
Guanfacine (Tenex)

medication because abrupt withdrawal can cause severe rebound hypertension
3. Monitor liver function tests

VIII. ACE Inhibitors (Box 49–14)

A. Description
   1. Prevents peripheral vasoconstriction by blocking conversion of angiotensin I to angiotensin II
   2. Used to treat hypertension
   3. Avoid use with potassium supplements and potassium-sparing diuretics
B. Side effects
   1. Nausea, vomiting, and diarrhea
   2. Persistent cough
   3. Hypotension
   4. Tachycardia
   5. Hyperkalemia
   6. Headache and dizziness
   7. Fatigue and insomnia
   8. Hypoglycemic reaction in diabetics
   9. Bruising, petechiae, and bleeding
   10. Diminished taste
C. Implementation
   1. Monitor vital signs
   2. Monitor potassium levels
   3. Monitor for hypoglycemic reaction in diabetics
   4. Instruct the client to take captopril (Capoten) 20 minutes to 1 hour before a meal
   5. Monitor for bruising, petechiae, or bleeding with captopril (Capoten)
   6. Instruct the client not to discontinue captopril (Capoten) because rebound hypertension can occur
   7. Instruct the client not to take over-the-counter medications
   8. Instruct the client how to take **blood pressure**
   9. Instruct the client if dizziness occurs and persists to notify the physician
   10. Inform the client that the taste of food may be diminished during the first month of therapy

IX. Antianginal Medications (Box 49–15)

A. Nitrates
   1. Description

BOX 49–14. ACE Inhibitors

Captopril (Capoten)
Enalapril maleate (Vasotec)
Benazepril (Lotensin)
Fosinopril (Monopril)
Lisinopril (Prinivil, Zestril)
Quinapril HCL (Accupril)
Ramipril (Altace)

BOX 49–15. Antianginal Medications

Nitroglycerin (Nitro-Bid, Nitrostat, Transderm-Nitro Patch)
Isosorbide mononitrate (Imdur)
Isosorbide dinitrate (Isordil, Sorbitrate)
Pentaerythritol tetranitrate (Peritrate)
Amyl nitrite

   a. Produce vasodilation
   b. Reduce myocardial oxygen consumption
   c. Contraindicated in clients with marked hypotension, increased intracranial pressure (ICP), or severe anemia
   d. Use with caution with severe renal or hepatic disease
   e. Avoid abrupt withdrawal of long-acting preparations to prevent the rebound effect of severe pain due to myocardial ischemia
   2. Side effects
   a. Headache
   b. **Orthostatic hypotension**
   c. Dizziness and weakness
   d. Nausea and vomiting
   e. Flushing or pallor
   3. Sublingual medications
   a. Monitor vital signs
   b. Offer sips of water before giving because dryness may inhibit medication absorption
   c. Instruct the client to place under the tongue and leave until fully dissolved
   d. Instruct the client not to swallow the medication
   e. Instruct the client to take 1 tablet for pain, and repeat every 5 minutes for a total of three doses
   f. Instruct the client to seek medical help immediately if pain is not relieved in 15 minutes, following the three doses
   g. Inform the client that a stinging or biting sensation may indicate that the tablet is fresh
   h. Instruct the client to store medication in a dark, tightly closed bottle
   i. Instruct the client to check expiration date on the medication bottle because expiration may occur within 6 months of obtaining medication
   j. Instruct the client to take acetaminophen (Tylenol) for headache
   4. Translingual medications
   a. Instruct the client to direct the spray against the oral mucosa
   b. Instruct clients to avoid inhaling the spray
   5. Sustained-released medications: instruct the client to swallow and not to chew or crush the medication
   6. Transmucosal-buccal medications
   a. Instruct the client to place between the

BOX 49–16. Beta-Adrenergic Blockers

Propranolol HCl (Inderal)
Metoprolol tartrate (Lopressor)
Acebutolol (Sectral)
Atenolol (Tenormin)
Betaxolol (Kerlone)
Bisoprolol fumarate (Zebeta)
Nadolol (Corgard)
Penbutolol (Levatol)
Pindolol (Visken)
Timolol maleate (Blocadren)
Carteolol HCl (Cartrol)
Labetalol HCl (Normodyne, Trandate)
Carvedilol (Coreg)
Esmolol (Brevibloc)
Levbunolol HCl (Betagan)
Metipranolol HCl (OptiPranolol)
Sotalol (Betapace)

upper lip and gum or in the buccal area between the cheek and gum
  b. Inform the client that the medication will adhere to the oral mucosa and slowly dissolve
7. Transdermal patch
  a. Instruct the client to apply the patch to a hairless area, using a new patch and different site each day
  b. As prescribed, instruct the client to remove patch after 12 to 14 hours allowing 10 to 12 "patch-free" hours each day to prevent tolerance
8. Topical ointments
  a. Instruct the client to remove ointment on the skin from previous dose
  b. Instruct the client to squeeze a ribbon of ointment of the prescribed length onto the applicator paper
  c. Instruct the client to spread the ointment over a 6- $\times$ -6-inch area using the chest, back, abdomen, upper arm, or anterior thigh (avoiding hairy areas), and cover with plastic wrap
  d. Instruct the client to rotate sites and to avoid touching the ointment when applying

X. Beta-Adrenergic Blockers (Box 49–16)

A. Description
  1. Decreases **cardiac output**, heart rate, and **blood pressure**
  2. Decreases the workload of the heart and decreases oxygen demands
  3. Used for angina, dysrhythmias, hypertension, migraine headaches, and prevention of MI and glaucoma
  4. Contraindicated in clients with asthma, bradycardia, CHF, severe renal or hepatic disease, hyperthyroidism, and CVA

  5. Use with caution in clients with diabetes because it may mask symptoms of hypoglycemia
  6. Use with caution in clients on antihypertensives
B. Side effects
  1. Bradycardia
  2. Bronchospasm
  3. Hypotension
  4. Fatigue, dizziness, and weakness
  5. Nausea and vomiting
  6. Hypoglycemia
  7. Depression
  8. Nightmares
C. Implementation
  1. Monitor vital signs
  2. Hold medication if pulse or **blood pressure** is not within prescribed parameters
  3. Monitor for signs of CHF
  4. Monitor for respiratory distress and for signs of wheezing and dyspnea
  5. Instruct the client to report dizziness, light-headedness, or nasal congestion
  6. Instruct the client not to stop medication because rebound hypertension, rebound tachycardia, or an anginal attack can occur
  7. Advise the clients on insulin that early signs of hypoglycemia such as tachycardia and nervousness can be masked by the beta-blocker
  8. Instruct clients on insulin to monitor their blood glucose
  9. Instruct the client and family how to take a pulse and **blood pressure**
  10. Instruct the client to change positions slowly to prevent **orthostatic hypotension**
  11. Instruct clients to avoid over-the-counter cold medications and nasal decongestants

XI. Calcium Channel Blockers (Box 49–17)

A. Description
  1. Decreases cardiac contractility and the workload of the heart, thus decreasing the need for oxygen
  2. Promotes vasodilatation of the coronary and peripheral vessels
  3. Used for angina, dysrhythmias, and hypertension

BOX 49–17. Calcium Channel Blockers

Diltiazem (Cardizem)
Nifedipine (Procardia)
Verapamil HCl (Calan)
Nicardipine (Cardene)
Amlodipine (Norvasc)
Bepridil (Vascor)
Felodipine (Plendil)
Isradipine (DynaCirc)

BOX 49-18. Peripheral Vasodilators

Alpha-adrenergic Blocker
Tolazoline (Priscoline)

Beta-adrenergic Agonist
Isoxsuprine (Vasodilan)

Direct-acting Peripheral Vasodilators
Cyclandelate (Cyclan, Cyclospasmol)
Ergoloid mesylates (Hydergine)
Nicotinyl alcohol

Alpha Blocker
Prazosin HCl (Minipress)

Calcium Channel Blocker
Nifedipine (Procardia)

Hemorrheologic
Pentoxifylline (Trental)
Increases microcirculation and tissue perfusion

4. Used with caution in clients with CHF or bradycardia
B. Side effects
   1. Bradycardia
   2. Hypotension
   3. Reflex tachycardia as a result hypotension
   4. Headache
   5. Dizziness and fatigue
   6. Peripheral edema
   7. Constipation
   8. Flushing of the skin
   9. Changes in liver and kidney function
C. Implementation
   1. Monitor vital signs
   2. Monitor for signs of CHF
   3. Monitor liver enzymes and kidney function tests
   4. Instruct the client not to discontinue medication
   5. Instruct the client how to take a pulse
   6. Instruct clients to notify the physician if dizziness or fainting occurs
   7. Instruct clients not to crush or chew sustained-released tablets

XII. Peripheral Vasodilators (Box 49-18)

A. Description
   1. Decreases peripheral resistance by exerting a direct action on the arteries or on both the arteries and veins
   2. Increases blood flow to the extremities
   3. Used in peripheral vascular disorders of venous and arterial vessels
   4. Most effective for disorders resulting from vasospasm (Raynaud's disease)
   5. These medications may decrease some of the symptoms of cerebral vascular insufficiency
B. Side effects
   1. Dizziness
   2. **Orthostatic hypotension**
   3. Palpitations and tachycardia

4. Flushing
5. GI distress
C. Implementation
   1. Monitor vital signs especially **blood pressure** and heart rate
   2. Monitor for **orthostatic hypotension** and tachycardia
   3. Monitor for signs of inadequate blood flow to the extremities such as pallor, coldness of the extremities, and pain
   4. Instruct the client that it may take up to 3 months for a desired therapeutic response
   5. Advise the client not to smoke because smoking increases vasospasm
   6. Instruct the client to avoid aspirin or aspirin-like compounds unless approved by the physician
   7. Instruct the client to take the medication with meals if GI disturbances occur
   8. Instruct the client to avoid alcohol because it may cause a hypotensive reaction
   9. Encourage the client to change positions slowly to avoid **orthostatic hypotension**

XIII. Antihyperlipidemic Medications

A. Description
   1. Reduces serum levels of cholesterol, triglycerides, or low-density lipoprotein (LDL)
   2. When cholesterol, triglycerides, and LDL are elevated, the client is at increased risk for coronary artery disease
   3. In many cases diet alone will not lower blood lipid levels; therefore, antilipemic medications will be prescribed
B. Bile acid sequestrants (Box 49-19)
   1. Description
      a. Binds with acids in the intestines
      b. Bile acid sequestrants should not be used as the only therapy in clients with elevated triglycerides because they typically raise triglyceride levels
   2. Side effects
      a. Constipation
      b. Peptic ulcer
   3. Implementation
      a. Cholestyramine resin (Questran) comes in a gritty powder that must be mixed thoroughly in juice or water prior to administration
      b. Monitor the client for early signs of peptic ulcer such as nausea and abdominal discomfort followed by abdominal pain and distention
      c. Instruct the client that the medication

BOX 49-19. Bile Acid Sequestrants

Cholestyramine resin (Questran)
Colestipol (Colestid)

BOX 49–20. HMG-CoA Reductase Inhibitors

Pravastatin (Pravachol)
Lovastatin (Mevacor)

must be taken with and followed by sufficient fluids
C. HMG-CoA reductase inhibitors (Box 49–20)
  1. Description
    a. Lovastatin (Mevacor) is highly protein-bound and should not be administered with anticoagulants
    b. Lovastatin (Mevacor) should not be administered with gemfibrozil (Lopid)
    c. Administer lovastatin (Mevacor) with caution to clients on immunosuppressive medications
  2. Side effects
    a. Dizziness
    b. Headache
    c. Blurred vision
    d. Rash and pruritus
    e. Elevated liver enzymes
    f. Causes GI disturbances, headaches, muscle cramps, and fatigue
  3. Implementation
    a. Monitor serum liver enzymes
    b. Instruct the client to receive an annual eye examination because the medication causes cataract formation
    c. If lovastatin (Mevacor) is not effective in lowering the lipid level after 3 months, it should be discontinued
D. Other antihyperlipidemic medications (Box 49–21)
  1. Description
    a. Gemfibrozil (Lopid) should not be taken with anticoagulants because they compete for protein sites, and if the client is on an anticoagulant, the anticoagulant dose should be reduced during antilipemic therapy and the INR monitored closely
    b. Do not administer gemfibrozil (Lopid) with lovastatin (Mevacor)
    c. Clofibrate (Atromid-S) should not be used long term because of its side effects such as

dysrhythmias, angina, thromboembolism, and gallstones
  2. Implememation
    a. Monitor vital signs
    b. Monitor liver enzyme levels
    c. Monitor serum cholesterol and triglyceride levels
    d. Instruct the client to restrict intake of fats, cholesterol, carbohydrates, and alcohol
    e. Instruct the client to stop smoking
    f. Instruct the client to follow an exercise program
    g. Instruct the client that it will take several weeks before the lipid level declines
    h. Instruct the client to have an annual eye examination and to report any changes in vision
    i. Instruct the diabetic client taking gemfibrozil (Lopid) to monitor blood glucose levels regularly
    j. Instruct the client to increase fluid intake
    k. Note that niacin, nicotinic acid (Nicobid) has numerous side effects, which include GI disturbances, flushing of the skin, elevated liver enzymes, hyperglycemia, and hyperuricemia
    l. Instruct the client that aspirin may assist in reducing the side effects of niacin, nicotinic acid (Nicobid)
    m. Instruct the client to take niacin, nicotinic acid (Nicobid), with meals to reduce GI discomfort

PRACTICE QUESTIONS

1. The nurse reinforces discharge instructions to the postoperative client taking warfarin sodium (Coumadin). Which statement, if made by the client, reflects the need for further teaching?
   1 "I will take Ecotrin for my headaches because it is coated."
   2 "I will be certain to limit my alcohol consumption."
   3 "I will take my pills every day at the same time."
   4 "I have already called my family to pick up a Medic-Alert bracelet."

2. The client taking digoxin (Lanoxin) has a serum potassium (K^+) of 3 mEq/L and is complaining of anorexia. The physician orders a digoxin level to rule out digoxin toxicity. The nurse checks the results of the test, knowing that the therapeutic serum level for digoxin is which of the following?
   1 3.5 ng/mL
   2 2 to 4 ng/mL
   3 3 ng/mL
   4 0.5 to 2.0 ng/mL

BOX 49–21. Other Antihyperlipidemic Medications

Clofibrate (Atromid-S)
Gemfibrozil (Lopid)
Niacin, nicotinic acid (Nicobid)
Simvastatin (Zocor)
Fluvastatin (Lescol)
Atorvastatin (Lipitor)

3. Heparin sodium (Liquaemin) by subcutaneous (SC) injection is prescribed for the client. When administering the medication, the nurse
   1 Administers with a 23- to 25-gauge, 1-inch needle
   2 Aspirates before injection
   3 Applies heat after the injection
   4 Administers with a 25- to 27-gauge, 5/8-inch needle

4. The client with a cardiac irregularity is being treated with procainamide (Pronestyl). The client complains of dizziness and tells the nurse that this has been occurring for the past few days. The initial nursing action is to
   1 Administer PRN nitroglycerin tablets
   2 Auscultate the client's apical pulse and obtain a blood pressure
   3 Contact the physician
   4 Tell the client that this is an expected side effect

5. A 51-year-old client is admitted with a diagnosis of myocardial infarction. The client is started on streptokinase (Streptase) therapy. The nurse knows that teaching has been effective when the client's wife states that the purpose of the medication is
   1 To thin the blood
   2 To slow the clotting of the blood
   3 To dissolve any clots in the coronary arteries
   4 To prevent further clots from forming in coronary arteries

6. The client is being treated for moderate hypertension and has been taking diltiazem (Cardizem) for several months. The client is seen by the physician, and Prinzmetal's angina is diagnosed. The nurse planning care for the client understands that which action of the medication provides a therapeutic effect for this new diagnosis?
   1 Increases oxygen demands within the myocardium
   2 Prevents influx of calcium ions in vascular smooth muscle
   3 Leads to an increase in calcium absorption in the vascular smooth muscle
   4 Increases the force of contraction of ventricular tissues

7. The nurse is caring for a client who is taking propranolol (Inderal). Which of the following data indicates a potential serious complication associated with this medication?
   1 A baseline blood pressure of 150/80 mmHg followed by a blood pressure of 138/72 mmHg after two doses of the medication
   2 A baseline resting heart rate of 88 beats/minute followed by a resting heart rate of 72 beats/minute after two doses of the medication
   3 The development of audible expiratory wheezes
   4 The development of complaints of insomnia

8. The client is admitted to the emergency department with an acute anterior wall myocardial infarction. Streptokinase (Streptase) therapy is prescribed. The spouse is concerned about the dangers of this treatment. Which of the following statements by the nurse is most appropriate?
   1 "Your loved one is very ill. The physician has made the best decision for you."
   2 "There is no reason to worry. We use this medication all the time."
   3 "I'm certain you made the correct decision to use this medication."
   4 "You have concerns about whether this treatment is the best option."

9. The physician prescribed digoxin (Lanoxin) 0.25 mg for a client with atrial fibrillation. The medication is available as 0.125-mg tablets. The nurse calculates that the client will receive two tablets of digoxin. When the nurse administers the medication, the client looks at the medication and states, "Every time I get chest pain, I will take one of these heart pills." After double-checking the dosage calculation the nurse decides to
   1 Not administer the medication as prescribed and calculated
   2 Administer one-half tablet of the medication instead of the dosage calculated
   3 Administer the medication as prescribed and calculated, and monitor for untoward effects such as seizures
   4 Administer the medication as prescribed and calculated and proceed with further client teaching

10. The nurse is caring for an elderly client who will be discharged home. Furosemide (Lasix) is prescribed for the client. The nurse reinforces instructions to the client about the medication. Which of the following statements, if made by the client, indicates the need for further teaching?
    1 "I will take my medication every morning with breakfast."
    2 "I will call my doctor if my ankles swell or my rings get tight."
    3 "I need to drink lots of coffee and tea to keep myself healthy."
    4 "I will sit up slowly before standing each morning."

11. Isosorbide mononitrate (Imdur) is prescribed for a client with angina pectoris. The client tells the nurse that the medication is causing a chronic headache. The nurse most appropriately suggests that the client
    1 Contact the physician
    2 Discontinue the medication
    3 Cut the dose in half
    4 Take the medication with food

12. The client is being discharged with a prescription for propranolol (Inderal). When reinforcing instruction to the client about the medication, the nurse includes which of the following?
    1 Gentle exercising will prevent orthostatic hypotension
    2 Hot baths and showers are advised to increase vasodilation
    3 Medication should be taken on an empty stomach to enhance absorption
    4 Medication should be withheld if the pulse rate drops below 60 beats/minute

13. Heparin sodium (Liquaemin) is prescribed for the client. The nurse expects that the physician will order which of the following to monitor for a therapeutic effect of the medication?
    1 Prothrombin time (PT)
    2 Activated partial thromboplastin time (APTT)
    3 Hematocrit (HCT)
    4 Hemoglobin (HgB)

14. The client has suffered an acute myocardial infarction and is receiving tissue plasminogen activator (t-PA). Which of the following is a priority nursing intervention while caring for the client?
    1 Have heparin sodium (Liquaemin) available
    2 Monitor for renal failure
    3 Monitor for signs of bleeding
    4 Monitor psychosocial status

15. The nurse is reinforcing instructions to the client about the use of a nitrate patch for the treatment of angina pectoris. Which of the following does the nurse include in the instructions to prevent client tolerance to nitrates?
    1 Do not remove the patches
    2 Have a 12-hour "no nitrate" time
    3 Have a 24-hour "no nitrate" time
    4 Keep nitrates on 24 hours, then off 24 hours

16. The client was admitted to the medical unit with nausea and bradycardia. The family handed the nurse a small white envelope labeled "heart pill." The envelope is sent to pharmacy and reveals digoxin (Lanoxin). The family states, "That doctor doesn't know how to take care of my family." The most therapeutic response by the nurse is
    1 "You are concerned that your loved one receives the best care."
    2 "You're right! I've never seen a doctor put pills in an envelope."
    3 "I think you're wrong. That physician has been in practice over 30 years."
    4 "Don't worry about this. I'll take care of everything."

17. The client with a diagnosis of congestive heart failure is seen in the clinic. The client is being treated with a variety of medications including digoxin (Lanoxin) and furosemide (Lasix). Which of the following findings on data collection leads

the nurse to suspect that the client is hypokalemic?
    1 Diarrhea
    2 Intermittent intestinal colic
    3 Muscle weakness and leg cramps
    4 Tingling of fingers and toes

18. The nurse is reinforcing dietary instructions to a client who is taking triamterene (Dyrenium). The nurse instructs the client that it is appropriate to consume which of the following food items daily?
    1 Avocado
    2 Banana
    3 Baked potato
    4 Apple

19. Hydrochlorothiazide (HydroDIURIL) is prescribed for the client. The nurse checks the client's record for documentation of which of the following prior to administering the medication?
    1 Penicillin allergy
    2 Hyperkalemia
    3 Sulfa allergy
    4 History of osteoporosis

20. Cholestyramine resin (Questran) is prescribed for a client with elevated triglycerides and a serum cholesterol of 398 mg/dL. The nurse reinforces instructions to the client about the medication. Which of the following statements, if made by the client, indicates the need for further education?
    1 "Constipation and bloating might be a problem."
    2 "I'll continue to watch my diet and reduce my fats."
    3 "I'll continue my nicotinic acid from the health food store."
    4 "Walking a mile each day will help the whole process."

21. The client is experiencing impotence after taking guanfacine (Tenex). The client states, "I would sooner have a stroke than keep living with the side effects of this medication." The most appropriate response by the nurse is
    1 "I can understand completely."
    2 "The doctor should change your prescription."
    3 "You wouldn't really want to have a stroke."
    4 "You are concerned about the side effects of your medication."

22. The physician tells the nurse that a potassium-sparing diuretic is being prescribed for the client with congestive heart failure. The nurse reviews the physician's orders, expecting that which of the following medications will be prescribed?
    1 Spironolactone (Aldactone)
    2 Furosemide (Lasix)
    3 Ethacrynic acid (Edecrin)
    4 Hydrochlorothiazide (HydroDIURIL)

23. A client with coronary artery disease complains of substernal chest pain. After checking the client's heart rate and blood pressure, the nurse administers nitroglycerin 0.4 mg sublingually. After 5 minutes the client states, "My chest still hurts." If the vital signs have remained stable, the nurse
    1 Waits another 10 minutes and then administers a second nitroglycerin tablet
    2 Applies 10 liters of oxygen via nasal cannula
    3 Administers another nitroglycerin tablet
    4 Calls the resuscitation team immediately

24. The client is admitted to the hospital with a diagnosis of paroxysmal nocturnal dyspnea (PND). The nurse reviews the physician's orders, expecting that which of the following medications will be prescribed for this condition?
    1 Lidocaine (Xylocaine)
    2 Propranolol (Inderal)
    3 Bumetanide (Bumex)
    4 Urokinase (Abbokinase)

25. The client arrives in the emergency department after complaining of unrelieved chest pain for 2 days. The pain has subsided slightly but never disappeared. When the nurse approaches the client with a nitroglycerin sublingual tablet, the client states, "I don't need that. My dad takes that for his heart. There's nothing wrong with my heart." Which of the following best describes the client's response?
    1 Obsessive-compulsive behavior
    2 Denial
    3 Phobic behavior
    4 Anger

26. The nurse is collecting data from a client being admitted to the nursing unit with a diagnosis of syncope. The client tells the nurse that he or she has been taking enalapril (Vasotec), atenolol (Tenormin), and aspirin (ASA) daily. The client admits that the medications were prescribed by different physicians. The admitting physician wrote in the client's order sheet "administer medications as taken at home." Which of the following is the most appropriate action for the nurse to take?
    1 Give the medications as ordered by the physician
    2 Send the client's medication bottles to the pharmacy for identification and then administer the medications as ordered
    3 Contact the physician, describe the medications, and request order clarification
    4 Refuse to give any medications and wait until the physician makes rounds to clarify the orders

27. A 66-year-old client is seen in the clinic complaining of not feeling well. The client is taking several medications for the control of heart disease and hypertension. These medications include atenolol (Tenormin), digoxin (Lanoxin), and chlorothiazide (Diuril). A tentative diagnosis of digoxin toxicity is made. The nurse collects data from the client, knowing that which of the following supports this diagnosis?
    1 Chest pain, hypotension, and paresthesias
    2 Constipation, dry mouth, and sleep disorder
    3 Double vision, loss of appetite, and nausea
    4 Dyspnea, edema, and palpitations

28. A 79-year-old client is being treated for congestive heart failure with bumetanide (Bumex). The vital signs are blood pressure 100/60 mmHg, pulse 96, and respirations 24. The nurse checks which of the following priority items prior to administering the medication?
    1 Blood pressure
    2 Weight
    3 Urine output
    4 Temperature

29. Atorvastatin (Lipitor) has been prescribed for a client with an elevated cholesterol level. The nurse collects a health history from the client, knowing that the medication is contraindicated in which of the following conditions?
    1 Cirrhosis
    2 Coronary artery disease
    3 Diabetes mellitus
    4 Hypothyroidism

30. Warfarin sodium (Coumadin) is prescribed for the client. The nurse expects that the physician will order which of the following to monitor for a therapeutic effect of the medication?
    1 Prothrombin time (PT)
    2 Activated partial thromboplastin time (APTT)
    3 Red blood cell (RBC) count
    4 Platelet count

ANSWERS

1. **1**

RATIONALE: Ecotrin is an aspirin-containing product and should be avoided. Excessive alcohol consumption should be avoided when taking warfarin. Taking prescribed medication at the same time increases client compliance. The Medic-Alert bracelet provides health care personnel with emergency information.
TEST-TAKING STRATEGY: Note the key words "need for further teaching." Recalling that warfarin is an anticoagulant and that Ecotrin is an aspirin-containing product will easily direct you to option 1. Review client teaching points related to warfarin now if you had difficulty with this question.
LEVEL OF COGNITIVE ABILITY: Comprehension
PHASE OF NURSING PROCESS: Evaluation
CLIENT NEEDS: Health Promotion and Maintenance
CONTENT AREA: Pharmacology
REFERENCE
Hodgson, B., & Kizior, R. (2000). *Saunders nursing drug handbook 2000.* Philadelphia: W. B. Saunders. pp. 1062–1064.

2. **4**

RATIONALE: Therapeutic levels for digoxin range from 0.5 to 2.0 ng/mL. Options 1, 2, and 3 identify toxic levels.
TEST-TAKING STRATEGY: Knowledge of normal serum levels for digoxin is necessary to answer the question. It is important to be aware of the reason for concern. The client's potassium was low, which increases the likelihood of digitalis toxicity. If you had difficulty with this question, take time now to learn the therapeutic level for digoxin.
LEVEL OF COGNITIVE ABILITY: Comprehension
PHASE OF NURSING PROCESS: Data Collection
CLIENT NEEDS: Physiological Integrity
CONTENT AREA: Pharmacology
REFERENCE
Hodgson, B., & Kizior, R. (2000). *Saunders nursing drug handbook 2000.* Philadelphia: W. B. Saunders. p. 326.

3. **4**

RATIONALE: For SC heparin sodium injection, a 25- to 27-gauge, 3/8- to 5/8-inch needle is used to prevent tissue trauma and inadvertent intramuscular injection. A 1-inch needle would inject the heparin sodium into the muscle. The application of heat may vary the absorption of the heparin. Aspiration prior to injection is avoided with heparin sodium.
TEST-TAKING STRATEGY: Recalling the anatomy of muscle and subcutaneous layers of tissue will assist in directing you to option 4. If you had difficulty with this question, take time now to review the principles related to heparin administration
LEVEL OF COGNITIVE ABILITY: Application
PHASE OF NURSING PROCESS: Implementation
CLIENT NEEDS: Physiological Integrity
CONTENT AREA: Pharmacology
REFERENCE
Hodgson, B., & Kizior, R. (2000). *Saunders nursing drug handbook 2000.* Philadelphia: W. B. Saunders. p. 489.

4. **2**

RATIONALE: Dizziness is a sign of toxicity. Additional signs of toxicity from procainamide include confusion, drowsiness, decreased urination, nausea, vomiting, and tachydysrhythmias. The initial nursing action is to auscultate the client's apical pulse and obtain a blood pressure. The physician may need to be notified but data collection is necessary first. Options 1 and 4 are incorrect actions.
TEST-TAKING STRATEGY: Note the key word "initial." Use the steps of the nursing process and note that option 2 is the only option that addresses data collection. Review the toxic effects of this medication now if you had difficulty with this question.
LEVEL OF COGNITIVE ABILITY: Comprehension
PHASE OF NURSING PROCESS: Implementation
CLIENT NEEDS: Physiological Integrity
CONTENT AREA: Pharmacology
REFERENCE
Deglin, J., & Vallerand, A. (1999). *Davis's drug guide for nurses* (6th ed.). Philadelphia: F. A. Davis. pp. 842–843.

5. **3**

RATIONALE: Streptokinase converts plasminogen in the blood to plasmin. Plasmin is an enzyme that digests or dissolves fibrin clots wherever they exist. Options 1, 2, and 4 describe mechanisms of action of heparin sodium and warfarin sodium.
TEST-TAKING STRATEGY: Knowledge regarding the action of streptokinase is required to answer this question. Remember that streptokinase dissolves clots. Review this medication now if you had difficulty with this question.
LEVEL OF COGNITIVE ABILITY: Comprehension
PHASE OF NURSING PROCESS: Evaluation
CLIENT NEEDS: Physiological Integrity
CONTENT AREA: Pharmacology
REFERENCE
Lehne, R. (1998). *Pharmacology for nursing care* (3rd ed.). Philadelphia: W. B. Saunders. p. 544.

6. **2**

RATIONALE: Diltiazem is a calcium channel blocker that inhibits calcium influx through the slow channels of the membrane of smooth muscle cells. Calcium channel blockers decrease myocardial oxygen demands and block calcium channels, thereby decreasing the force of contraction of the ventricular tissue.
TEST-TAKING STRATEGY: Knowledge of the mechanisms involved in Prinzmetal's angina (coronary artery spasm) is required to understand why calcium channel blockers would be prescribed. Review the action of calcium channel blockers now if you had difficulty with this question.
LEVEL OF COGNITIVE ABILITY: Analysis
PHASE OF NURSING PROCESS: Planning
CLIENT NEEDS: Physiological Integrity
CONTENT AREA: Pharmacology
REFERENCE
Hodgson, B., & Kizior, R. (2000). *Saunders nursing drug handbook 2000.* Philadelphia: W. B. Saunders. pp. 327–329.

7. **3**

RATIONALE: Audible expiratory wheezes may indicate a serious adverse reaction, bronchospasm. Beta-blockers may induce this reaction particularly in clients with chronic obstructive pulmonary disease (COPD) or asthma. A normal decrease in blood pressure and heart rate is expected. Insomnia is a frequent mild side effect and should be monitored.

TEST-TAKING STRATEGY: Knowledge regarding the side effects and adverse effects of propranolol is required to answer this question. Use the process of elimination, eliminating options 1 and 2, as these are expected responses from the medication. Noting the key words "serious complication" will assist in directing you to option 3. Review the adverse effects of this medication now if you had difficulty with this question.
LEVEL OF COGNITIVE ABILITY: Comprehension
PHASE OF NURSING PROCESS: Data Collection
CLIENT NEEDS: Physiological Integrity
CONTENT AREA: Pharmacology
REFERENCE

Hodgson, B., & Kizior, R. (2000). *Saunders nursing drug handbook 2000*. Philadelphia: W. B. Saunders. pp. 877–880.

8. **4**

RATIONALE: Paraphrasing is restating the client's or family member's own words. Option 1 represents a communication block that denies the person's right to an opinion. Option 2 is offering a false reassurance. In option 3 the nurse is expressing approval, which can be harmful to the client-nurse or family-nurse relationship.
TEST-TAKING STRATEGY: Use therapeutic communication techniques. Remembering to address client feelings first will easily direct you to option 4. Review these therapeutic techniques now if you had difficulty with this question.
LEVEL OF COGNITIVE ABILITY: Application
PHASE OF NURSING PROCESS: Implementation
CLIENT NEEDS: Psychosocial Integrity
CONTENT AREA: Pharmacology
REFERENCE

Leahy, J., & Kizilay, P. (1998). *Foundations of nursing practice: A nursing process approach*. Philadelphia: W. B. Saunders. pp. 226–229.

9. **4**

RATIONALE: It is appropriate to treat atrial fibrillation with the prescribed and calculated dose of digoxin as indicated in the question. The issue of the question is that the client verbalizes inaccurate and unsafe knowledge regarding this medication and the treatment for chest pain. This client needs further education regarding the safe administration of medications for episodes of chest pain.
TEST-TAKING STRATEGY: Knowledge regarding the use of this medication is required to answer this question. Perform the calculation first and determine that the dose that the nurse is to give is correct. Then eliminate options 1 and 2. Note the issue of the question, the need for client teaching. This should direct you to option 4.
LEVEL OF COGNITIVE ABILITY: Comprehension
PHASE OF NURSING PROCESS: Planning
CLIENT NEEDS: Health Promotion and Maintenance
CONTENT AREA: Pharmacology
REFERENCE

Hodgson, B., & Kizior, R. (2000). *Saunders nursing drug handbook 2000*. Philadelphia: W. B. Saunders. pp. 324–326.

10. **3**

RATIONALE: Tea and coffee are stimulants as well as mild diuretics. These are a poor choice for hydration. Taking the medication at the same time each day improves compliance. Because furosemide is a diuretic, morning is the best time to take the medication so as not to interrupt sleep. Notification of the health care provider is appropriate if edema is

noticed in the hands, feet, face, or if the client is short of breath. Sitting up slowly prevents postural hypotension.
TEST-TAKING STRATEGY: Note the key words "need for further teaching." Use the process of elimination. Tea and coffee are stimulants, and diuretics that can potentially worsen dehydration. Additionally, coffee and tea are not healthy items. This should alert you that this is the correct option for this question, as stated. Review client teaching points related to this medication now if you had difficulty with this question.
LEVEL OF COGNITIVE ABILITY: Comprehension
PHASE OF NURSING PROCESS: Evaluation
CLIENT NEEDS: Health Promotion and Maintenance
CONTENT AREA: Pharmacology
REFERENCE

Hodgson, B., & Kizior, R. (2000). *Saunders nursing drug handbook 2000*. Philadelphia: W. B. Saunders. pp. 452–454.

11. **4**

RATIONALE: Headache is a frequent side effect of isosorbide mononitrate and usually disappears during continued therapy. If a headache occurs during therapy, the client should be instructed to take the medication with food or meals. It is not necessary to contact the physician unless the headaches persist with therapy. It is not appropriate to instruct the client to discontinue therapy or adjust the dosages.
TEST-TAKING STRATEGY: Use the process of elimination. Eliminate options 2 and 3 first because it is not within the scope of nursing responsibilities to instruct a client to discontinue or adjust dosages. Knowing that the headache can be relieved with the administration of food with the medication will assist in directing you to option 4. Review this medication now if you had difficulty with this question.
LEVEL OF COGNITIVE ABILITY: Application
PHASE OF NURSING PROCESS: Implementation
CLIENT NEEDS: Health Promotion and Maintenance
CONTENT AREA: Pharmacology
REFERENCE

Hodgson, B., & Kizior, R. (2000). *Saunders nursing drug handbook 2000*. Philadelphia: W. B. Saunders. pp. 556–557.

12. **4**

RATIONALE: Most beta-blockers may be administered with food or on an empty stomach but propranolol is best absorbed if taken with meals or directly after eating. Exercise will not prevent orthostatic hypotension. Hot showers and baths are not advised because of their vasodilating effect. The client needs to be instructed how to take the pulse rate and to notify the physician if the heart rate falls below 60 beats/minute.
TEST-TAKING STRATEGY: Use the process of elimination. Recalling that bradycardia can occur with propranolol will easily direct you to option 4. If you had difficulty with this question, take time now to review this medication.
LEVEL OF COGNITIVE ABILITY: Application
PHASE OF NURSING PROCESS: Implementation
CLIENT NEEDS: Health Promotion and Maintenance
CONTENT AREA: Pharmacology
REFERENCE

Deglin, J., & Vallerand, A. (1999). *Davis's drug guide for nurses* (6th ed.). Philadelphia: F. A. Davis. p. 865.

13. **2**

RATIONALE: The PT assesses for the therapeutic effect of warfarin sodium and the APTT assesses the therapeutic

effect of heparin sodium. HCT and HgB assess red blood cell concentrations. Baseline assessment including an APTT value should be completed, as well as ongoing daily APTT values while the client is on heparin sodium therapy. Heparin sodium doses are determined based on these laboratory results.
TEST-TAKING STRATEGY: Use the process of elimination. Eliminate options 3 and 4 because these laboratory values are unrelated to heparin sodium therapy. Knowledge of the appropriate test for monitoring therapeutic values of both heparin sodium and warfarin sodium is required to answer this question. Learn them now.
LEVEL OF COGNITIVE ABILITY: Comprehension
PHASE OF NURSING PROCESS: Data Collection
CLIENT NEEDS: Physiological Integrity
CONTENT AREA: Pharmacology
REFERENCE
Lehne, R. (1998). *Pharmacology for nursing care* (3rd ed.). Philadelphia: W. B. Saunders. pp. 534–539.

14. 3

RATIONALE: t-PA is a thrombolytic. Hemorrhage is a complication of any type of thrombolytic medication. The client should be monitored for bleeding. Monitoring for renal failure and the client's psychosocial status is important; however, it is not the most critical. Heparin sodium is given following thrombolytic therapy, but the question is not asking for the associated medications following t-PA therapy.
TEST-TAKING STRATEGY: Note the key word "priority." Use the principles of prioritizing and knowledge regarding this medication to direct you to option 3. Additionally, remember that bleeding is a priority.
LEVEL OF COGNITIVE ABILITY: Comprehension
PHASE OF NURSING PROCESS: Data Collection
CLIENT NEEDS: Physiological Integrity
CONTENT AREA: Pharmacology
REFERENCE
Lehne, R. (1998). *Pharmacology for nursing care* (3rd ed.). Philadelphia: W. B. Saunders. p. 546.

15. 2

RATIONALE: To help prevent tolerance, clients need a 12-hour "no nitrate" time, sometimes referred to as a pharmacological vacation away from the medication. In addition to having a 12-hour "no nitrate" vacation, clients must rotate the nitrate patch and wash their hands to prevent topical absorption through the fingers. Options 1, 3, and 4 are incorrect.
TEST-TAKING STRATEGY: Knowledge of the absorption and distribution of nitrates is necessary to answer this question. Option 1 can be easily eliminated based on the issue of the question. Eliminate options 3 and 4 next because they are similar. Review the administration of nitrate patches now if you had difficulty with this question.
LEVEL OF COGNITIVE ABILITY: Application
PHASE OF NURSING PROCESS: Implementation
CLIENT NEEDS: Health Promotion and Maintenance
CONTENT AREA: Pharmacology
REFERENCE
Lehne, R. (1998). *Pharmacology for nursing care* (3rd ed.). Philadelphia: W. B. Saunders. p. 468.

16. 1

RATIONALE: Option 1 is a therapeutic nonjudgmental response. Option 2 creates doubt about the physician's practice without actually knowing the circumstances. Option 3 is argumentative and nontherapeutic. Option 4 dismisses the family's concerns and disempowers the family.
TEST-TAKING STRATEGY: Use therapeutic communication techniques to answer the question. Remember that reflection of the client's or family's concerns is the most therapeutic. Review therapeutic communication techniques now if you had difficulty with this question.
LEVEL OF COGNITIVE ABILITY: Application
PHASE OF NURSING PROCESS: Implementation
CLIENT NEEDS: Psychosocial Integrity
CONTENT AREA: Pharmacology
REFERENCE
Leahy, J., & Kizilay, P. (1998). *Foundations of nursing practice: A nursing process approach.* Philadelphia: W. B. Saunders. pp. 226–229.

17. 3

RATIONALE: Clients on potassium-wasting diuretics are at high risk of hypokalemia. Clinical manifestations of hypokalemia include fatigue, anorexia, nausea, vomiting, muscle weakness, leg cramps, decreased bowel motility, paresthesias, and dysrhythmias.
TEST-TAKING STRATEGY: Use the process of elimination and knowledge regarding the signs of electrolyte imbalances to answer the question. Diarrhea and intestinal colic are signs of hyperkalemia. Tingling of the fingers and toes are signs of hypocalcemia. If you had difficulty with this question, take time now to review the signs of electrolyte imbalances.
LEVEL OF COGNITIVE ABILITY: Comprehension
PHASE OF NURSING PROCESS: Data Collection
CLIENT NEEDS: Physiological Integrity
CONTENT AREA: Pharmacology
REFERENCE
deWit, S. (1998). *Essentials of medical-surgical nursing* (4th ed.). Philadelphia: W. B. Saunders. p. 110.

18. 4

RATIONALE: Triamterene is a potassium-sparing diuretic, which means that the client must avoid foods high in potassium. Options 1, 2, and 3 are high-potassium foods.
TEST-TAKING STRATEGY: Knowledge that triamterene is a potassium-sparing diuretic and knowledge of those food items high in potassium is required to answer this question. If you are unfamiliar with this medication and those foods high in potassium, take time now to review.
LEVEL OF COGNITIVE ABILITY: Application
PHASE OF NURSING PROCESS: Implementation
CLIENT NEEDS: Physiological Integrity
CONTENT AREA: Pharmacology
REFERENCE
deWit, S. (1998). *Essentials of medical-surgical nursing* (4th ed.). Philadelphia: W. B. Saunders. p. 108.

19. 3

RATIONALE: Thiazide diuretics like hydrochlorothiazide are sulfa-based medications, and a client with a sulfa allergy is at risk for an allergic reaction. Options 1, 2, and 4 are incorrect. Thiazide diuretics have been useful in reducing the incidence of osteoporosis in postmenopausal women by normalizing parathyroid function and calcium absorption.
TEST-TAKING STRATEGY: Knowledge of the chemical makeup of thiazide diuretics is necessary to answer this question. Recalling that these medications contain a sulfa ring in their makeup will easily direct you to option 3.

Review the contraindications associated with the thiazide diuretics now if you had difficulty with this question.
LEVEL OF COGNITIVE ABILITY: Application
PHASE OF NURSING PROCESS: Planning
CLIENT NEEDS: Safe, Effective Care Environment
CONTENT AREA: Pharmacology
REFERENCE
Hodgson, B., & Kizior, R. (2000). *Saunders nursing drug handbook 2000.* Philadelphia: W. B. Saunders. pp. 494–496.

20. **3**

RATIONALE: Nicotinic acid should be avoided because it may lead to liver abnormalities. All lipid-lowering medications can also cause liver abnormalities, so a combination of nicotinic acid and cholestyramine is to be avoided. Constipation and bloating are the two most common side effects. Both walking and the reduction of fats in the diet are therapeutic measures to reduce cholesterol and triglyceride levels.
TEST-TAKING STRATEGY: Use the process of elimination and knowledge regarding the therapies prescribed to lower the triglyceride and cholesterol levels. Recalling that over-the-counter medications should be avoided when a client is taking a prescription medication will easily direct you to option 3. Review client teaching points related to cholestyramine now if you had difficulty with this question.
LEVEL OF COGNITIVE ABILITY: Comprehension
PHASE OF NURSING PROCESS: Evaluation
CLIENT NEEDS: Health Promotion and Maintenance
CONTENT AREA: Pharmacology
REFERENCE
Hodgson, B., & Kizior, R. (2000). *Saunders nursing drug handbook 2000.* Philadelphia: W. B. Saunders. pp. 215–217.

21. **4**

RATIONALE: Reflection of the client's own comment lets the client know that you are hearing his or her concerns without judging. The nurse cannot understand what the client is experiencing. Option 2 devalues the physician's judgment. Option 3 is confrontative and unsupportive.
TEST-TAKING STRATEGY: Use therapeutic communication techniques. Select nonjudgmental responses that reflect the fact you are listening to the client's concerns. Review these techniques now if you had difficulty with this question.
LEVEL OF COGNITIVE ABILITY: Application
PHASE OF NURSING PROCESS: Implementation
CLIENT NEEDS: Psychosocial Integrity
CONTENT AREA: Pharmacology
REFERENCE
Leahy, J., & Kizilay, P. (1998). *Foundations of nursing practice: A nursing process approach.* Philadelphia: W. B. Saunders. pp. 226–229.

22. **1**

RATIONALE: Spironolactone is a potassium-sparing diuretic that promotes sodium excretion while conserving potassium. Options 2, 3, and 4 identify diuretics that do not conserve potassium.
TEST-TAKING STRATEGY: Knowledge that spironolactone is a potassium-sparing diuretic is required to answer this question. Take time now to review the potassium-sparing diuretics if you are unfamiliar with them and had difficulty with this question.
LEVEL OF COGNITIVE ABILITY: Comprehension
PHASE OF NURSING PROCESS: Planning

CLIENT NEEDS: Physiological Integrity
CONTENT AREA: Pharmacology
REFERENCE
Hodgson, B., & Kizior, R. (2000). *Saunders nursing drug handbook 2000.* Philadelphia: W. B. Saunders. p. 942.

23. **3**

RATIONALE: Nitroglycerin tablets are usually ordered one every 5 minutes PRN for chest pain for a total dose of 3 tablets. Waiting 10 minutes is inappropriate if the client is having chest pain. Oxygen at 10 liters is an unsafe dose. There is no need to call the resuscitation team at this time.
TEST-TAKING STRATEGY: Focus on the information provided in the question and use knowledge regarding the administration of nitroglycerin for chest pain. Recalling that a nitroglycerin tablet can be administered for three doses 5 minutes apart if the vital signs remain stable will easily direct you to option 3. Review the administration of nitroglycerin now if you had difficulty with this question.
LEVEL OF COGNITIVE ABILITY: Application
PHASE OF NURSING PROCESS: Implementation
CLIENT NEEDS: Physiological Integrity
CONTENT AREA: Pharmacology
REFERENCE
Hodgson, B., & Kizior, R. (2000). *Saunders nursing drug handbook 2000.* Philadelphia: W. B. Saunders. p. 752.

24. **3**

RATIONALE: The PND may be due to increased venous return when lying in bed. When this occurs, a diuretic is prescribed. Bumetanide is a diuretic. Propranolol is a beta-blocker. Lidocaine is an antidysrhythmic, and urokinase is a thrombolytic.
TEST-TAKING STRATEGY: Knowledge of the pathophysiology associated with PND and the classifications of the medications in each of the options will easily direct you to option 3. Review PND and the actions of the medications identified in the options now if you had difficulty with this question.
LEVEL OF COGNITIVE ABILITY: Application
PHASE OF NURSING PROCESS: Planning
CLIENT NEEDS: Physiological Integrity
CONTENT AREA: Pharmacology
REFERENCE
Hodgson B., & Kizior, R. (2000). *Saunders nursing drug handbook 2000.* Philadelphia: W. B. Saunders. pp. 126, 591, 877, 1034.

25. **2**

RATIONALE: Denial is the most common reaction when a client has a myocardial infarction or anginal pain. No angry behavior was identified in the question. Phobias and obsessive-compulsive disorders are mental health diagnoses.
TEST-TAKING STRATEGY: Use the process of elimination. Eliminate options 1 and 3 first because these are medical diagnoses. Recalling that denial is the most common reaction when a person has chest pain will easily direct you to option 2. Review psychosocial responses in the client experiencing chest pain now if you had difficulty with this question.
LEVEL OF COGNITIVE ABILITY: Comprehension
PHASE OF NURSING PROCESS: Data Collection
CLIENT NEEDS: Psychosocial Integrity
CONTENT AREA: Pharmacology
REFERENCE
Black, J., & Matassarin-Jacobs, E. (1997). *Medical-surgical nursing: Clinical management for continuity of care* (5th ed.). Philadelphia: W. B. Saunders. p. 1266.

26. 3

RATIONALE: The nurse is ultimately responsible for giving the correct medication. When medication orders are vague, the nurse must contact the physician. Often the physician is unaware of other medications prescribed by other physicians. The nurse never administers the medication without verification. Waiting until the physician makes rounds delays necessary treatment.
TEST-TAKING STRATEGY: Use the process of elimination. Options 1 and 2 are easily eliminated because they are similar. Eliminate option 4 because it is not appropriate to wait to clarify an unclear physician's order. Review the safeguards related to the physician's orders now if you had difficulty with this question.
LEVEL OF COGNITIVE ABILITY: Application
PHASE OF NURSING PROCESS: Implementation
CLIENT NEEDS: Safe, Effective Care Environment
CONTENT AREA: Pharmacology
REFERENCE
Lehne, R. (1998). *Pharmacology for nursing care* (3rd ed.). Philadelphia: W. B. Saunders. p. 70.

27. 3

RATIONALE: Double vision, loss of appetite, and nausea are signs of digoxin toxicity. Additional signs of digoxin toxicity include bradycardia; difficulty reading; visual alterations such as green and yellow vision and seeing spots or halos; confusion; vomiting; diarrhea; decreased libido; and impotence.
TEST-TAKING STRATEGY: Knowledge regarding the signs of digoxin toxicity is required to answer the question. Remember GI and visual disturbances. If you had difficulty with this question, take time now to review digoxin toxicity.
LEVEL OF COGNITIVE ABILITY: Comprehension
PHASE OF NURSING PROCESS: Data Collection
CLIENT NEEDS: Physiological Integrity
CONTENT AREA: Pharmacology
REFERENCE
Hodgson, B., & Kizior, R. (2000). *Saunders nursing drug handbook 2000.* Philadelphia: W. B. Saunders. pp. 324–326.

28. 1

RATIONALE: Hypotension is a common side effect with this medication and an increased risk exists in an elderly client. Options 2 and 3 will also require monitoring but are not the priority. The temperature is unrelated to administering this medication.
TEST-TAKING STRATEGY: Focus on key word "priority."

Blood pressure is mentioned in the question and also in option 1. Also, remember the ABCs. Blood pressure reflects circulation.
LEVEL OF COGNITIVE ABILITY: Comprehension
PHASE OF NURSING PROCESS: Data Collection
CLIENT NEEDS: Physiological Integrity
CONTENT AREA: Pharmacology
REFERENCE
Hodgson, B., & Kizior, R. (2000). *Saunders nursing drug handbook 2000.* Philadelphia: W. B. Saunders. pp. 126–128.

29. 1

RATIONALE: Lipitor is an antihyperlipidemic medication. It is contraindicated in pregnancy, lactation, liver disease, biliary cirrhosis or obstruction, severe renal dysfunction, and in clients who are hypersensitive to the medication. Options 2, 3, and 4 are not contraindications to the use of this medication.
TEST-TAKING STRATEGY: Knowledge regarding the contraindications associated with use of this medication is required to answer this question. If you are unfamiliar with this medication, take time now to review.
LEVEL OF COGNITIVE ABILITY: Comprehension
PHASE OF NURSING PROCESS: Data Collection
CLIENT NEEDS: Physiological Integrity
CONTENT AREA: Pharmacology
REFERENCE
Hodgson, B., & Kizior, R. (2000). *Saunders nursing drug handbook 2000.* Philadelphia: W. B. Saunders. pp. 1115–1116.

30. 1

RATIONALE: The PT will assess for the therapeutic effect of warfarin sodium and the APTT will assess the therapeutic effect of heparin sodium. The RBC and platelet count will assess red blood cell concentrations and the client's potential for bleeding, respectively. Warfarin doses are determined based on this laboratory result.
TEST-TAKING STRATEGY: Use the process of elimination. Eliminate options 3 and 4 because these laboratory values are unrelated to warfarin therapy. Knowledge of the appropriate test for monitoring therapeutic values of both heparin sodium and warfarin sodium is required to answer this question. Learn them now.
LEVEL OF COGNITIVE ABILITY: Comprehension
PHASE OF NURSING PROCESS: Data Collection
CLIENT NEEDS: Physiological Integrity
CONTENT AREA: Pharmacology
REFERENCE
Lehne, R. (1998). *Pharmacology for nursing care* (3rd ed.). Philadelphia: W. B. Saunders. pp. 534–539.

BIBLIOGRAPHY

Black, J., & Matassarin-Jacobs, E. (1997). *Medical-surgical nursing: Clinical management for continuity of care* (5th ed.). Philadelphia: W. B. Saunders.
Deglin, J., & Vallerand, A. (1999). *Davis's drug guide for nurses* (6th ed.). Philadelphia: F. A. Davis.

deWit, S. (1998). *Essentials of medical-surgical nursing* (4th ed.). Philadelphia: W. B. Saunders.
Hodgson, B., & Kizior, R. (2000). *Saunders nursing drug handbook 2000.* Philadelphia: W. B. Saunders.
Leahy, J., & Kizilay, P. (1998). *Foundations of nursing practice: A nursing process approach.* Philadelphia: W. B. Saunders.
Lehne, R. (1998). *Pharmacology for nursing care* (3rd ed.). Philadelphia: W. B. Saunders.

UNIT XIV

....

The Adult Client with a Renal System Disorder

PYRAMID TERMS

Anuria—Urine output of less than 100 mL a day.

Hemodialysis—The process of cleansing the client's blood. The diffusion of dissolved particles from one fluid compartment into another across a semipermeable membrane. The client's blood flows through one fluid compartment and the dialysate is in another fluid compartment.

Internal Arteriovenous Fistula (AV Fistula)—Access of choice for chronic dialysis clients. Created surgically by which an artery in the arm is anastomosed to a vein. This creates an opening, or fistula, between a large artery and a large vein. The flow of arterial blood into the venous system causes the veins to become engorged (maturity). It requires 1 to 2 weeks to mature before they can be used. Maturity is necessary so that the engorged vein can be punctured for the dialysis procedure, using a large-bore needle.

Nephrolithiasis—Refers to the formation of kidney stones, which are formed in the renal parenchyma.

Oliguria—Urine output of less than 400 mL a day.

Peritoneal Dialysis—The peritoneum is the dialyzing membrane (semipermeable membrane) and substitutes for kidney function during renal failure. Works on the principles of diffusion and osmosis, and the dialysis occurs via the transfer of fluid and solute from the bloodstream through the peritoneum.

Renal Failure—The loss of kidney function. The types of renal failure are acute renal failure or chronic renal failure. The signs and symptoms of renal failure are caused by the retention of wastes, the retention of fluids, and the inability of the kidneys to regulate electrolytes.

Urolithiasis—Refers to the formation of urinary stones or calculi. Urinary calculi are formed in the ureter.

PYRAMID TO SUCCESS

Pyramid points focus on the preprocedure and postprocedure care to the client undergoing diagnostic tests and procedures related to the renal system. Be familiar with renal failure, dialysis procedures such as hemodialysis and continuous ambulatory peritoneal dialysis (CAPD), dialysis access devices, urinary diversions, and postoperative care to the client following urinary or renal surgery. Focus on the care to the client following prostatectomy and the treatment measures for the client with urinary or renal calculi. Additionally, pyramid points address measures that promote urinary elimination, prevent infection, and the maintenance of skin integrity.

NURSING PROCESS

DATA COLLECTION

Medications client is presently taking
Associated medical conditions
Family history
Trauma and injury
Changes in pattern of urination such as frequency, nocturia, hesitancy, urgency, dribbling, incontinence, and retention
Urine output as polyuria, oliguria, and anuria
Changes in appearance of urine such as dilute, concentrated, hematuria, and pyuria

Proteinuria
Dysuria or flank pain
Fever and chills
Hypertension
Periorbital and peripheral edema
Weight changes
Level of consciousness (LOC)
Laboratory values

PLANNING	IMPLEMENTATION	EVALUATION
The client maintains adequate urinary output.	Obtain client data noting family history, history of trauma and injury, associated medical conditions, and current medication therapy. Monitor vital signs. Monitor urinary patterns. Monitor characteristics of urine. Monitor input and output (I&O). Maintain patency of urinary catheter and tubes if present. Prepare client for dialysis procedure if prescribed.	The client is free of urinary obstruction.
The client verbalizes the need to implement pain-control measures. The client describes methods of promoting comfort.	Obtain data regarding the presence and characteristics of pain. Provide comfort measures to relieve discomfort. Administer pain medication as prescribed. Document effectiveness of pain-relief measures.	Client obtains relief from pain and is comfortable.
The client consumes fluids as prescribed. Laboratory values remain within normal range.	Monitor vital signs. Monitor LOC. Monitor for cardiac irregularities. Monitor weight, noting changes or fluctuations. Monitor for periorbital or peripheral edema. Monitor for signs of dehydration. Evaluate results of electrolyte and laboratory values.	An acceptable fluid balance is maintained. Laboratory values remain within a safe range. Risks of complications related to fluid imbalances are minimized.
The client verbalizes the signs and symptoms of infection.	Monitor for signs of infection. Monitor for fever or alterations in blood pressure. Monitor incision site for drainage and infection. Monitor dialysis access site for signs of infection. Instruct client to monitor for signs and symptoms of infection.	The client does not exhibit signs of infection. The client is free of previous infection.
The client monitors skin integrity and implements measures to prevent alteration in skin integrity.	Monitor skin integrity. Monitor dressings, wound, and stoma sites. Change wound dressings as necessary. Initiate measures as prescribed to prevent skin breakdown. Instruct client in measures to prevent skin breakdown.	Skin integrity remains intact.
The client implements measures to prevent injury.	Monitor for risks related to potential for injury. Monitor LOC. Provide a safe, hazard-free environment. Note nephrotoxic medications that may be prescribed. Monitor dialysis access device for patency. Monitor for complications associated with dialysis.	The client remains free from injury.

PLANNING

The client describes the prescribed diet and fluid intake plan. The client performs self-care activities and prescribed exercises. The client obtains adequate sleep and rest. The client demonstrates the ability to apply an external pouch, provide skin care, empty a pouch, and self-catheterize correctly if a urinary diversion is present. The client describes the correct procedure for the administration of prescribed medications. The client describes the plan for post-treatment follow-up, including knowledge regarding medications and the need for physician notification.

IMPLEMENTATION

Instruct client in adequate diet related to disorder. Instruct client in the need for increased fluids unless contraindicated. Instruct client to obtain adequate rest and to avoid fatigue. Encourage and instruct client to perform bladder-training exercises as appropriate. Instruct client with urinary diversion how to apply an external pouch, provide skin care, empty a pouch, and self-catheterize. Instruct client in home care procedures. Instruct client in measures to reduce the risk of bleeding that may be associated with certain renal disorders. Instruct client in signs of complications and the need to notify the physician. Instruct client regarding the importance of medications and follow-up care.

EVALUATION

Complies with prescribed diet and fluid prescription. The client achieves a state of nutrition that promotes healing and prevents further deterioration. The client explains preventive health actions related to diet modification and fluid intake. The client demonstrates the use of selected exercises related to bladder-training programs. The client demonstrates appropriate procedure for caring for urinary diversion if present. The client explains the correct procedure regarding the administration of medications. The client keeps follow-up appointments and seeks medical care if signs of complications arise.

PLANNING

The client participates in social interactions and avoids self-isolation.

IMPLEMENTATION

Encourage client to verbalize feelings related to altered body image. Assist client in identifying coping mechanisms. Assist with mobilizing support services and community services as necessary.

EVALUATION

Demonstrates effective coping mechanisms related to limitations to personal lifestyle. Uses community and support services.

◆ CLIENT NEEDS

SAFE, EFFECTIVE CARE ENVIRONMENT

Client rights
Confidentiality related to renal disorder
Informed consent related to diagnostic and surgical procedures
Renal organ donation
Consultations and referrals related to renal disorder
Accident prevention related to complications associated with disorder
Asepsis related to wound care
Standard (universal) precautions related to care of the client

HEALTH PROMOTION AND MAINTENANCE

Instructions regarding the prevention of the recurrence of a urinary and renal disorder
Instructions regarding prescribed treatments related to urinary or renal disorder
Instructions regarding postoperative management
Instructions regarding home care measures

PSYCHOSOCIAL INTEGRITY

Religious and spiritual influences
Body image disturbances
Loss of function of a body part that occurs in clients with a renal disorder
Coping mechanisms
Support systems
Community resources

PHYSIOLOGICAL INTEGRITY

Elimination measures
Comfort interventions
Prescribed nutrition and fluid measures
Skin integrity
Personal hygiene
Adequate rest and sleep
Medication administration
Diagnostic tests and laboratory results
Fluid and electrolyte disorders
Care related to dialysis access devices
Urinary diversions
Care to the client following prostatectomy
Treatment measures for the client with urinary or renal calculi

BIBLIOGRAPHY

deWit, S. (1998). *Essentials of medical-surgical nursing* (4th ed.). Philadelphia: W. B. Saunders.

Hill, S. & Howlett, H. (1997). *Success in practical nursing: Personal and vocational issues* (3rd ed.). Philadelphia: W. B. Saunders.

Leahy, J., & Kizilay, P. (1998). *Foundations of nursing practice: A nursing process approach*. Philadelphia: W. B. Saunders.

Luckmann, J. (1997). *Saunders manual of nursing care*. Philadelphia: W. B. Saunders.

Monahan, F., & Neighbors, M. (1998). *Medical-surgical nursing: Foundations for clinical practice* (2nd ed.). Philadelphia: W. B. Saunders.

National Council of State Boards of Nursing (1998). *National Council detailed test plan for the NCLEX-PN examination*. Chicago: Author.

O'Toole, M. (1997). *Miller-Keane encyclopedia & dictionary of medicine, nursing, & allied health* (6th ed.). Philadelphia: W. B. Saunders.

CHAPTER 50

Renal System

· ·

I. Anatomy and Physiology

A. Kidneys
1. Attached to the abdominal wall at the level of the last thoracic and first three lumbar vertebrae
2. Enclosed in the renal capsule
3. The cortex is the outer layer of the renal capsule
4. The medulla is surrounded by cortex
· 5. The nephron makes up the functional unit of the kidney
6. Functions of kidneys
   a. Maintain homeostasis of the blood
   b. Excrete end products of body metabolism
   c. Control fluid and electrolyte balance
   d. Excrete bacterial toxins, water-soluble drugs, and drug metabolites
   e. Secrete renin and erythropoietin, which play a role in the function of the parathyroid hormones and vitamin D
7. Nephron
   a. Functional renal unit
   b. Composed of glomerulus and tubules
8. Glomerulus
   a. Is encased in Bowman's capsule
   b. Filters the fluid out of blood
9. Tubules
   a. Includes proximal, distal, and Henle's loop
   b. Fluid is converted to urine in the tubules and then moves to the pelvis of the kidney
   c. Fluid moves to the pelvis of the kidney, flows through the ureter, and empties into the bladder
B. Bladder
1. The ureterovesical sphincter prevents the reflux of urine from the bladder to the ureter
2. The total capacity of the bladder is 1 liter
C. Prostate gland
1. Surrounds the male urethra
2. Contains a duct that opens into the prostatic portion of the urethra and secretes the alkaline portion of seminal fluid
D. Urine production

1. As fluid flows through the proximal tubules, water and solutes are reabsorbed
2. Water and solutes that are not reabsorbed become urine
3. The process of selective reabsorption determines the amount of water and solutes to be secreted
E. Homeostasis of water
1. Antidiuretic hormone (ADH) is primarily responsible for the reabsorption of water by the kidneys
2. ADH is produced by the hypothalamus and secreted from the posterior lobe of the pituitary gland
3. Secretion of ADH is stimulated by dehydration or high sodium intake and by a fall in blood volume
4. ADH increases the permeability to water of the distal convoluted tubules and collecting duct
5. Water is drawn out of the tubules by osmosis into a high salt concentration of fluid in the medulla and its capillaries; water returns to the blood, and concentrated urine remains in the tubule to be excreted
6. When clients lack ADH, they develop diabetes insipidus
7. Clients with diabetes insipidus produce very large amounts of dilute urine and without treatment have difficulty drinking sufficient water to survive
F. Homeostasis of sodium
1. When the amount of sodium increases, extra water is retained to preserve osmotic pressure
2. An increase in sodium and water produces an increase in the blood volume and blood pressure (BP)
3. When the BP increases, glomerular filtration increases and extra water and salt are lost; blood volume is reduced and returns the BP to normal
4. Reabsorption of sodium in the distal convoluted tubules is controlled by the hormones of the renin-angiotensin system

5. Renin is secreted when the BP or concentration of fluid in the distal convoluted tubule is low
6. Renin is an enzyme and splits angiotensin I from angiotensinogen and converts to angiotensin II as blood flows through the lung
7. Angiotensin II, a potent vasoconstrictor, stimulates the secretion of aldosterone
8. Aldosterone stimulates the distal convoluted tubules to reabsorb more sodium and excrete more potassium
9. The additional sodium increases water reabsorption and increases blood volume and the BP, returning it to normal; the stimulus for the secretion of renin is then removed

G. Homeostasis of potassium
1. Increases in potassium stimulate the secretion of aldosterone
2. Aldosterone stimulates the distal convoluted tubules to secrete potassium; this acts to return the potassium concentration to normal

H. Homeostasis of acidity (pH)
1. Blood pH is controlled by maintaining the concentration of buffer systems
2. Carbonic acid and sodium bicarbonate form the most important buffer for neutralizing acids in the plasma
3. The concentration of carbonic acid is controlled by the respiratory system
4. The concentration of sodium bicarbonate is controlled by the kidneys
5. Normal pH is 7.35 to 7.45, maintained by keeping the ratio of concentrations of sodium bicarbonate to carbon dioxide constant at 20:1
6. Strong acids are neutralized by sodium bicarbonate to produce carbonic acid and the sodium salts of the strong acid; this process quickly restores the ratio and thus blood pH
7. The carbonic acid produced dissociates into carbon dioxide and water and because the concentration of carbon dioxide is maintained at a constant level by the respiratory system, the excess carbonic acid is rapidly excreted
8. Sodium combined with the strong acid is actively reabsorbed in the distal convoluted tubules in exchange for hydrogen or potassium ions; the strong acid is neutralized by the secretion of ammonia and is excreted as ammonia or potassium salts

---

BOX 50–1. Risk Factors Associated with Renal Disorders

Frequent urinary tract infections
High-sodium diet
Contact sports
Trauma and injury
History of hypertension
Family history of renal disease
Medication use
Associated medical conditions

BOX 50–2. Normal Renal Function Tests

BUN (blood urea nitrogen), 5–20 mg/dL
Serum creatinine, 0.6–1.3 mg/dL
Creatinine clearance, 100–120 mL/minute
Uric acid serum, 2.5–8.0 mg/dL
Uric acid urine, 250–750 mg/24 hours

II. **Diagnostic Tests** (Boxes 50–1; 50–2)
A. Urinalysis
1. Description: a urine test for evaluation of the renal system and for determining renal disease
2. Implementation
   a. Wash perineal area
   b. Use a clean container
   c. Obtain 10 to 15 mL of the first morning sample
   d. Note that refrigerated samples may alter the specific gravity
   e. If the client is menstruating, indicate on the laboratory requisition form

B. Specific gravity
1. Description: a urine test that measures the specific gravity of the urine
2. Implementation
   a. Obtain a freshly voided specimen
   b. Fill the specific gravity container one-half to two-thirds full
   c. Place the hydrometer (urinometer) in the urine and spin gently
   d. Read the scale at the level of the meniscus

C. Urine culture and sensitivity
1. Description: a urine test that identifies the presence of microorganisms and determines the specific antibiotics that will appropriately treat the existing microorganism
2. Implementation
   a. Clean the perineal area and urinary meatus with bacteriostatic solution
   b. Collect a midstream sample in a sterile container
   c. Send the collected specimen to the laboratory immediately
   d. Note that urine from clients who forced fluids may be too dilute to provide a positive culture
   e. Identify any sources of potential contaminants during the collection of the specimen such as the hands, skin, clothing, hair, or vaginal or rectal secretions

D. Creatinine clearance
1. Description
   a. A blood and timed urine specimen that evaluates kidney function
   b. Blood is drawn at the start of the test and the morning of the day that the 24-hour urine specimen collection is complete
2. Implementation
   a. Encourage adequate fluids before and during the test

b. Instruct the client as prescribed to avoid tea, coffee, and medications during testing

c. If the client is taking adrenocorticotropic hormone (ACTH), cortisone, or thyroxine, check with the physician regarding administration of these medications during testing

d. place the urine specimen on ice or refrigerate and check with the laboratory regarding the addition of a preservative to the specimen during collection

E. VMA (vanillylmandelic acid)
   1. Description
      a. A 24-hour urine collection to diagnose pheochromocytoma, a tumor of the adrenal gland
      b. The test identifies an assay of catecholamines in the urine
   2. Implementation
      a. Instruct the client to avoid caffeine, cocoa, vanilla, cheese, gelatin, licorice, and fruits for at least 2 days prior to beginning the urine collection and during the collection, and to avoid taking medications for 2 to 3 days prior to beginning the test as prescribed
      b. Instruct the client to avoid stress and to maintain adequate food and fluids during the test
      c. Save all urine, label the container, add a preservative, and place specimen on ice or refrigerate
      d. Check with the laboratory regarding medication restrictions

F. 17-Ketosteroids
   1. Description: a 24-hour urine collection to diagnose endocrine imbalances of adrenal glands, ovaries, and testes
   2. Implementation
      a. Encourage fluids and a normal diet during testing
      b. Add a preservative and place the specimen collection on ice or refrigerate
      c. Note that obesity and severe mental and physical stress may affect the test results
      d. Note that levels may increase during the third trimester of pregnancy

G. Uric acid
   1. Description: a 24-hour urine collection to diagnose gout and kidney disease
   2. Implementation
      a. Encourage fluids and a regular diet during testing
      b. Place the specimen on ice or refrigerate and check with the laboratory regarding the addition of a preservative

H. KUB (kidneys, ureters, and bladder)
   1. Description: an x-ray film that views the urinary system and adjacent structures; used to detect urinary calculi
   2. Implementation: there is no specific preparation

I. Intravenous pyelogram (IVP)
   1. Description
      a. The injection of a radiopaque dye that outlines the renal system
      b. Performed to identify abnormalities in the system
   2. Implementation preprocedure
      a. Obtain informed consent
      b. Assess the client for allergies to iodine, seafood, and radiopaque dyes
      c. Withhold food and fluids after midnight on the night before the test
      d. Administer laxatives as prescribed
      e. Inform the client about possible throat irritation, flushing of the face, warmth, or a salty taste that may be experienced during the test
   3. Implementation postprocedure
      a. Monitor vital signs
      b. Instruct the client to drink at least 1 liter of fluids unless contraindicated
      c. Monitor the venipuncture site for bleeding
      d. Monitor urinary output

J. Renal angiography
   1. Description: the injection of a radiopaque dye through a catheter for examination of the renal arterial supply
   2. Implementation preprocedure
      a. Obtain informed consent
      b. Assess the client for allergies to iodine, seafood, and radiopaque dyes
      c. Inform the client about the possible burning feeling or the feeling of heat along the vessel after the dye is injected
      d. Withhold food and fluids after midnight on the night before the test
      e. Instruct the client to void immediately before the procedure
      f. Administer enemas as prescribed
      g. Shave the injection sites as prescribed
      h. Assess and mark the peripheral pulses
   3. Implementation postprocedure
      a. Assess vital signs and peripheral pulses
      b. Provide bed rest and use of a sandbag at insertion site for 4 to 8 hours
      c. Assess the color and temperature of the involved extremity
      d. Inspect the catheter insertion site for bleeding or swelling
      e. Force fluids unless contraindicated
      f. Monitor urinary output

K. Renal scan
   1. Description: an IV injection of a radioisotope for visual imaging of renal blood flow
   2. Implementation preprocedure
      a. Obtain informed consent
      b. Assess for allergies
      c. Assist with administering radioisotope as necessary
      d. Instruct clients that they will be required to remain motionless
      e. Instruct the client that imaging may be

repeated at various intervals before the test is complete

3. Implementation postprocedure
   a. Encourage fluids unless contraindicated
   b. Assess the client for signs of delayed allergic reaction, such as itching and hives
   c. Note that the radioactivity is eliminated in 24 hours
   d. Follow standard precautions when caring for incontinent clients and double-bag client linens per agency policy

L. Cystometrogram (CMG)
   1. Description: a graphic recording of the pressures exerted at varying filling phases of the bladder
   2. Implementation preprocedure: inform the client about the voiding requirements during the procedure
   3. Implementation postprocedure: monitor the client's voiding after the procedure

M. Cystoscopy
   1. Description: the bladder mucosa is examined for inflammation, calculi, or tumors by means of a cystoscope
   2. Implementation preprocedure
      a. Obtain informed consent
      b. Withhold food and fluids after midnight on the night before the test
      c. Administer enemas and medications as prescribed
   3. Implementation postprocedure
      a. Monitor vital signs
      b. Monitor for postural hypotension
      c. Force fluids as prescribed
      d. Monitor I&O
      e. Encourage deep-breathing exercises to relieve bladder spasms
      f. Administer analgesics as prescribed
      g. Administer sitz baths for back and abdominal pain
      h. Note that leg cramps are common due to the lithotomy position maintained during the procedure
      i. Assess urine for color and consistency
      j. Note that pink-tinged or tea-colored urine is common
      k. Monitor for bright red urine or clots and notify the physician if this occurs

N. Renal biopsy
   1. Description: insertion of a needle into the kidney to obtain a sample of tissue for examination
   2. Implementation preprocedure
      a. Assess vital signs
      b. Assess baseline clotting studies
      c. Obtain informed consent
      d. Withhold food and fluids after midnight on the night before the test
   3. Implementation during the procedure: position the client prone with a pillow under the abdomen and shoulders
   4. Implementation postprocedure

      a. Monitor vital signs
      b. Monitor hemoglobin and hematocrit
      c. Place the client in the supine position and on bed-rest for 8 hours as prescribed
      d. Provide pressure to the biopsy site for 30 minutes
      e. Check the biopsy site for bleeding
      f. Force fluids, 1500 to 2000 mL, as prescribed
      g. Instruct the client to avoid heavy lifting and strenuous activity for 2 weeks

III. Renal Failure

A. Description
   1. The loss of kidney function
   2. The types of **renal failure** include acute **renal failure** or chronic **renal failure**
   3. The signs and symptoms of **renal failure** are caused by the retention of wastes, the retention of fluids, and the inability of the kidneys to regulate electrolytes

B. Acute **Renal Failure** (ARF)
   1. Description
      a. The sudden loss of kidney function caused by renal cell damage from ischemia or toxic substances
      b. ARF occurs abruptly and can be reversible
      c. It leads to hypoperfusion, cell death, and decompensation in renal function
      d. The prognosis is dependent on the cause and the condition of the client
      e. Near normal or normal kidney function may resume gradually
   2. Causes
      a. Infection
      b. Renal artery occlusion
      c. Obstruction
      d. Acute kidney disease
      e. Dehydration
      f. Diuretic therapy
      g. Ischemia from hypovolemia, heart failure, septic shock, and blood loss
      h. Toxic substances such as medications, particularly antibiotics
   3. Oliguric phase
      a. Duration is 8 to 15 days; and the longer the duration, the less chance of recovery
      b. Sudden drop in urine output; urine output less than 400 mL/day
      c. Urine specific gravity of 1.010 to 1.016
      d. Anorexia, nausea, and vomiting
      e. Hypertension
      f. Decreased skin turgor
      g. Pruritus
      h. Tingling of the extremities
      i. Drowsiness progressing to disorientation to coma
      j. Edema
      k. Dysrhythmias
      l. Signs of congestive heart failure (CHF) and pulmonary edema

m. Signs of pericarditis

n. Signs of acidosis

4. Diuretic phase

   a. Urine output rises slowly and then diuresis occurs (4 to 5 liters/day)

   b. Excessive urine output indicates recovery of damaged nephrons

   c. Hypotension

   d. Tachycardia

   e. Improvement in LOC

5. Recovery phase

   a. A slow process; complete recovery may take 1 to 2 years

   b. Urine volume is normal

   c. Increase in strength

   d. Increase in LOC

6. Convalescent phase

   a. May take months to recover fully and for blood urea nitrogen (BUN) to return to normal

   b. Client can develop chronic **renal failure** (CRF)

C. Chronic **renal failure** (CRF)

1. Description

   a. The progressive loss and ongoing deterioration in kidney function that occurs slowly over time

   b. It occurs in four stages, is irreversible, and results in uremia or end-stage renal disease

   c. CRF requires dialysis or kidney transplant to maintain life

   d. Hypervolemia can occur due to the inability of the kidneys to excrete sodium and water, or hypovolemia can occur due to the inability of the kidneys to conserve sodium and water

2. Causes

   a. May follow ARF

   b. Renal artery occlusion

   c. Chronic urinary obstruction

   d. Recurrent infections

   e. Hypertension

   f. Metabolic disorders

   g. Diabetes mellitus

   h. Autoimmune disorders

3. Data collection

   a. Anorexia and nausea

   b. Headache

   c. Weakness and fatigue

   d. Hypertension

   e. Confusion and lethargy followed by convulsions and coma

   f. Kussmaul's respirations

   g. Diarrhea or constipation

   h. Muscle twitching and numbness of extremities

   i. Decreased urine output

   j. Decreased urine-specific gravity

   k. Proteinuria

   l. Anemia

   m. Azotemia

   n. Fluid overload and signs of heart failure

o. Uremic frost

D. Implementation

1. Monitor vital signs

2. Monitor intake and urine output (hourly in ARF)

3. Monitor weight, noting that an increase of 1/2 to 1 lb daily indicates fluid retention

4. Monitor BUN, creatinine, and electrolyte values

5. Monitor for acidosis and treat with sodium bicarbonate as prescribed

6. Assess urinalysis for protein, hematuria, casts, and specific gravity

7. Monitor LOC

8. Assess for signs of infection because client may not demonstrate a temperature or demonstrate an increased white blood cell count

9. Assess for dysrhythmias because a potassium level above 6 mEq/L will cause peaked T waves and widened QRS complex

10. Monitor for fluid overload; assess lung for rales and rhonchi

11. Monitor for edema

12. Administer prescribed diet of moderate protein to decrease the workload on the kidneys; high carbohydrate and low potassium and phosphorus

13. Restrict sodium intake as prescribed based on the electrolyte level

14. Restrict fluids to equal urinary output as prescribed, which is usually 400 mL of intake allowed over the previous day's output

15. Administer sodium polystyrene sulfonate (Kayexalate) to lower the potassium level as prescribed

16. Be alert to nephrotoxic medications, such as antibiotics that may be prescribed

17. Prepare the client for dialysis if prescribed

E. Special problems in **renal failure**

1. Hypertension

   a. Failure of the kidneys to maintain homeostasis of the blood pressure

   b. Monitor vital signs

   c. Maintain fluid and sodium restrictions as prescribed

   d. Administer diuretics and antihypertensives as prescribed

   e. Administer propranolol (Inderal), a beta-adrenergic antagonist, as prescribed, which decreases renin release (renin causes vasoconstriction)

2. Hypervolemia

   a. Monitor vital signs

   b. Monitor I&O and weight

   c. Monitor for edema

   d. Monitor electrolytes

   e. Monitor for hypertension

   f. Monitor for CHF and pulmonary edema

   g. Administer diuretics as prescribed

   h. Instruct the client to avoid salty foods

i. Instruct clients to avoid antacids or cold remedies containing sodium bicarbonate

3. Hypovolemia
   a. Monitor vital signs
   b. Monitor I&O
   c. Monitor electrolytes
   d. Monitor for hypotension
   e. Monitor for dehydration
   f. Provide replacement therapy based on electrolyte results as prescribed
   g. Provide sodium supplements as prescribed depending on electrolyte value

4. Potassium retention
   a. Monitor vital signs and apical rate
   b. Monitor potassium level
   c. Monitor for dysrhythmias (peaked T waves and widened QRS complex), indicating hyperkalemia
   d. Provide a low-potassium diet
   e. Administer medication as prescribed to lower the potassium
   f. Prepare the client for dialysis

5. Phosphorus retention
   a. Phosphorus rises and calcium drops, which leads to stimulation of parathyroid hormone causing bone demineralization
   b. Treatment is aimed at lowering serum phosphorus levels
   c. Administer aluminum hydroxide preparations as prescribed (usually 1 to 5 g/day) that bind phosphorus in the intestine and allow the phosphorus to be eliminated
   d. Administer aluminum hydroxide preparations at meals and not with other medications because they bind medications in the intestinal tract
   e. Administer stool softeners and laxatives as prescribed to prevent constipation because aluminum hydroxide preparations are constipating

6. Low calcium
   a. Occurs because of the high phosphorus level and because of the inability of the diseased kidney to activate vitamin D
   b. The absence of vitamin D causes a poor absorption of calcium from the intestinal tract
   c. Monitor calcium level
   d. Administer calcium supplements as prescribed
   e. Administer activated vitamin D as prescribed

7. Metabolic acidosis
   a. The kidneys are unable to excrete hydrogen ions and manufacture bicarbonate, and acidosis occurs
   b. Administer alkalyzers such as sodium bicarbonate as prescribed
   c. Note that clients with CRF adjust to low bicarbonate levels and do not become acutely ill

8. Anemia
   a. A decreased rate of production of red blood cells (RBCs) occurs as a result of the diseased kidney and the decreased secretion of erythropoietin
   b. Monitor hemoglobin and hematocrit
   c. Administer epoetin alfa (Epogen) as prescribed to stimulate the production of RBCs
   d. Administer folic acid (vitamin B$_9$) as prescribed instead of oral iron because oral iron is not well absorbed by the GI tract in CRF and causes nausea and vomiting
   e. Administer blood transfusions if prescribed, but blood transfusions are prescribed only when necessary because they decrease the stimulus to produce RBCs
   f. Monitor bleeding
   g. Provide a soft toothbrush
   h. Administer stool softeners as prescribed
   i. Avoid the administration of acetylsalicylic acid (aspirin) because the medication is excreted by the kidneys and if administered, high toxic levels will occur and prolong bleeding time

9. GI bleeding
   a. Urea is broken down to ammonia by the intestinal bacteria, and ammonia is a mucosal irritant that causes ulceration and bleeding
   b. Monitor hemoglobin and hematocrit
   c. Monitor stools for occult blood

10. Infection and injury
    a. Infection and injury need to be monitored and avoided because tissue breakdown causes increased potassium levels
    b. Monitor for signs of infection
    c. Avoid urinary catheters and provide strict asepsis during insertion and catheter care
    d. Instruct the client to avoid fatigue, which decreases body resistance
    e. Instruct the client to avoid people with infections
    f. Administer antibiotics as prescribed monitoring for nephrotoxic effects

11. Pruritus
    a. Urate crystals are excreted through the skin to get rid of excess wastes
    b. Uremic frost is seen in advanced stages of **renal failure**
    c. Monitor for skin breakdown, rash, and uremic frost
    d. Provide good skin care and oral hygiene
    e. Avoid the use of soaps
    f. Administer antipruritics as prescribed

12. Muscle cramps
    a. Occur in the extremities and hands and can be due to the low sodium level
    b. Monitor electrolytes

   c. Administer electrolyte replacements as prescribed
   d. Administer heat and massage as prescribed
13. Ocular irritation
   a. Calcium deposits in the conjunctiva cause burning and watering of the eyes
   b. Administer medications to control phosphate level as prescribed
   c. Administer lubricating eye drops
14. Insomnia and fatigue
   a. The diseased kidneys cause a buildup of wastes, causing fatigue in the client
   b. Provide adequate rest periods
   c. Administer mild CNS depressants as prescribed
15. Neurological changes
   a. The buildup of active particles and fluids causes changes in the brain cells and leads to confusion and impairment in the decision-making ability
   b. Monitor for confusion and monitor LOC
   c. Protect the client from injury
   d. Provide a safe and hazard-free environment
   e. Use side rails as needed
   f. Provide a calm and restful environment
   g. Provide comfort measures and backrubs
16. Psychosocial problems: monitor the client for psychosocial problems such as depression, anxiety, suicidal behavior, denial, dependency/independence conflict, and changes in body image

IV. Hemodialysis

A. Description
   1. The diffusion of dissolved particles from one fluid compartment into another across a semipermeable membrane
   2. The client's blood flows through one fluid compartment and the dialysate is in another fluid compartment
B. Functions of **hemodialysis**
   1. Cleanses the blood of accumulated waste products
   2. Removes the byproducts of protein metabolism such as urea, creatinine, and uric acid
   3. Removes excessive fluids
   4. Maintains or restores the body's buffer system
   5. Maintains or restores electrolyte levels
C. Principles of **hemodialysis**
   1. The semipermeable membrane is made of a thin, porous cellophane
   2. The pore size of the membrane allows small particles to pass through such as urea, creatinine, uric acid, and water molecules
   3. Proteins, bacteria, and blood cells are too large to pass through the membrane; the client's blood flows into the dialyzer

   4. The movement of substances occurs from the blood to the dialysate
   5. Diffusion: the movements of particles from an area of greater concentration to lesser concentration
   6. Osmosis: the movement of fluids across a semipermeable membrane from an area of lesser to an area of greater concentration
   7. Ultrafiltration: the movement of fluid across a semipermeable membrane as a result of an artificially created pressure gradient
D. Dialysate bath
   1. Composed of water and major electrolytes
   2. The dialysate bath need not be sterile because bacteria are too large to pass through
E. Implementation
   1. Monitor vital signs
   2. Monitor laboratory values before, during, and after dialysis
   3. Assess the client for fluid overload prior to the procedure
   4. Assess patency of blood access device
   5. Weigh the client before and after the procedure to determine fluid loss
   6. Hold antihypertensives and sedatives prior to the procedure as prescribed
   7. Monitor for shock and hypovolemia during the procedure
   8. Provide adequate nutrition (client may eat prior to the procedure)

V. Complications of Hemodialysis
(Box 50–3)

A. Disequilibrium syndrome
   1. Description
      a. A rapid change in the composition of the extracellular fluid (ECF) occurs during hemodialysis
      b. Solutes are removed from the blood faster than from the cerebrospinal fluid (CSF) and brain; fluid is pulled into the brain, causing cerebral edema
   2. Data collection
      a. Nausea
      b. Vomiting
      c. Headache
      d. Hypertension
      e. Restlessness and agitation
      f. Confusion
      g. Seizures

BOX 50–3. Complications of Hemodialysis
Hypotension and shock
Muscle cramping
Electrolyte changes
Sepsis
Loss of blood
Hepatitis
Disequilibrium syndrome
Dialysis encephalopathy

3. Implementation
   a. Monitor for signs of disequilibrium syndrome
   b. Notify the physician if signs of disequilibrium syndrome occur
   c. Prepare to dialyze the client for a shorter period at reduced blood flow rates to prevent occurrence
B. Dialysis encephalopathy
   1. Description: an aluminum toxicity that occurs as a result of aluminum in the H_2O sources used in the dialysate bath and the ingestion of aluminum-containing antacids (phosphate binders)
   2. Data collection
      a. Progressive neurological impairment
      b. Mental cloudiness
      c. Speech disturbances
      d. Dementia
      e. Muscle incoordination
      f. Bone pain
      g. Seizures
   3. Implementation
      a. Monitor for signs of dialysis encephalopathy
      b. Notify the physician if signs of dialysis encephalopathy occur
      c. Administer aluminum chelating agents as prescribed so that the aluminum is freed up and dialyzed from the body

VI. Access for Hemodialysis

A. Subclavian and femoral catheter (Fig. 50–1)
   1. Description
      a. A subclavian (subclavian vein) or femoral (femoral vein) catheter may be inserted for short-term or temporary use in ARF
      b. May be used until a fistula or graft matures, or when the client has fistula or graft access failure due to infection or clotting
   2. Implementation
      a. Monitor the insertion site for hematoma, bleeding, dislodging, and infection
      b. Do not use these catheters for any other reason other than dialysis

3. Subclavian vein catheter
   a. Is usually filled with 10,000 units of heparin and capped to maintain patency between dialysis treatments
   b. The catheter should not be uncapped
   c. The catheter may be left in place for up to 6 weeks if complications do not occur
4. Femoral vein catheter
   a. The client should not sit up more than 45 degrees, or the catheter may kink and occlude
   b. Monitor extremity for circulation, temperature, and pulse
   c. Prevent pulling or disconnecting of the catheter when giving care
   d. Maintain an IV of 250 mL of normal saline with 1250 units heparin at 10 to 20 gtt/minute as prescribed to maintain the line
   e. Use an IV control pump with microdrip tubing if the heparin infusion is prescribed
B. External arteriovenous shunt (AV shunt) (Fig. 50–2)
   1. Description
      a. Access is formed by the surgical insertion of two Silastic cannulas into an artery and a vein in the forearm or leg, to form an external blood path
      b. The cannulas are connected to form a U shape; blood flows from the client's artery through the shunt into the vein
      c. A tube leading to the membrane compartment is connected to the arterial cannula
      d. Blood fills the membrane compartment and flows back to the client by way of a tube connected to the venous cannula
      e. When dialysis is complete, the cannulas are clamped and reattached to form their U shape
   2. Advantages
      a. Can be used immediately following creation
      b. No venipuncture is necessary for dialysis
   3. Disadvantages
      a. External danger of disconnecting or dislodging
      b. Risk of hemorrhage, infection, or clotting

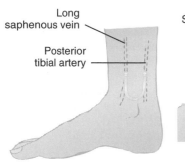

Long saphenous vein
Posterior tibial artery
Lower leg shunt

Subclavian vein
Clavicle
Subclavian cannula

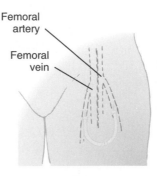

Femoral artery
Femoral vein
Femoral catheter

FIGURE 50–1. Alternative access areas for hemodialysis: ankle, clavicle, and thigh. (From Black, J., & Matassarin-Jacobs, E. [1997]. *Medical-surgical nursing: A nursing process approach* [5th ed.]. Philadelphia: W. B. Saunders. p. 1653.)

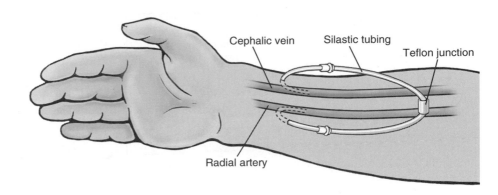

FIGURE 50–2. An external arteriovenous shunt provides access to blood for hemodialysis. The arterial cannula is connected to the dialyzer. Blood returns through the venous cannula. When not connected to the hemodialyzer, the arterial cannula is connected to the venous cannula. (From Monahan, F., & Neighbors, M. [1998]. *Medical-surgical nursing: Foundations for Clinical practice* [2nd ed.]. Philadelphia: W. B. Saunders. p. 1405.)

In the figure: Cephalic vein, Silastic tubing, Teflon junction, Radial artery

c. Skin erosion around the catheter site can occur

4. Implementation
   a. Avoid wetting the shunt
   b. A dressing is completely wrapped around the shunt and kept dry and intact
   c. Cannula clamps need to be available at the client's bedside
   d. Do not take a blood pressure, draw blood, place an IV, or administer injections in the shunt extremity
   e. Monitor for hemorrhage, infection, and clotting
   f. Monitor skin integrity around the insertion site
   g. Note that the shunt is patent if it is warm
   h. Auscultate and palpate for a bruit, although a bruit may not be heard and is not always felt with the shunt
   i. Notify the physician immediately if signs of clotting, hemorrhage, or infection occur

5. Signs of clotting
   a. Fold back Ace wrap to expose Silastic tubing and assess for signs of clotting
   b. Fibrin-white flecks noted in the tubing
   c. The separation of serum and cells
   d. The absence of a previously heard bruit
   e. Coolness of the tubing or extremity
   f. Client complaints of a tingling sensation

C. **Internal arteriovenous fistula (AV fistula)** (Fig. 50–3)
   1. Description
      a. Access of choice for chronic dialysis clients
      b. Created surgically in which an artery in the arm is anastomosed to a vein; this creates an opening or fistula between a large artery and a large vein
      c. The flow of arterial blood into the venous system causes the veins to become engorged (maturity)
      d. Maturity takes about 1 to 2 weeks and is required before the fistula can be used, so that the engorged vein can be punctured for the dialysis procedure using a large-bore needle
      e. Subclavian or femoral catheters, peritoneal dialysis, or an external AV shunt can be used for dialysis while the fistula is maturing

   2. Advantages
      a. Since the fistula is internal, there is less danger of clotting and bleeding
      b. The fistula can be used indefinitely
      c. Decreased incidence of infection
      d. No external dressing is required
      e. Allows freedom of movement

   3. Disadvantages
      a. Cannot be used immediately after insertion
      b. Needle insertions are required for dialysis
      c. Infiltration of the needles during dialysis can occur and cause hematomas
      d. An aneurysm can form in the fistula
      e. Arterial steal syndrome can develop (too much blood is diverted to the vein and arterial perfusion to the hand is compromised)
      f. CHF can occur from the increased blood flow in the venous system

D. Internal arteriovenous graft (AV graft)
   1. Description
      a. The internal graft is used primarily for chronic dialysis clients who do not have adequate blood vessels for the creation of a fistula
      b. An artificial graft made of Gore-Tex or a bovine (cow) carotid artery is used to create an artificial vein for blood flow
      c. The procedure involves the anastomosis of the graft to the artery, a tunneling under the skin, and anastomosis to a vein
      d. The graft can be used 2 weeks after insertion
      e. Complications of the graft include clotting, aneurysms, and infection

   2. Advantages
      a. Since the graft is internal, there is less danger of clotting and bleeding
      b. The graft can be used indefinitely
      c. Decreased incidence of infection
      d. No external dressing is required
      e. Allows freedom of movement

   3. Disadvantages
      a. Cannot be used immediately after insertion
      b. Needle insertions are required for dialysis

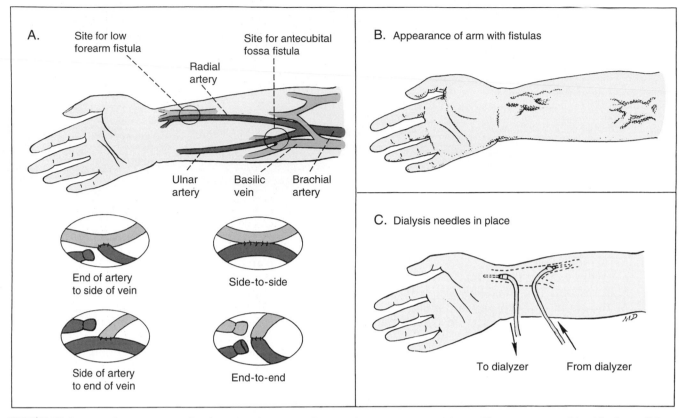

FIGURE 50–3. Internal arteriovenous fistula. Surgical creation of an arteriovenous anastomosis provides easy access to blood for hemodialysis. This method reduces the risk of infection and makes external shunts unnecessary except during hemodialysis. The internal fistula must be created 2 to 6 weeks before it can be used. Note that in this illustration, arteries, not veins, are toned. *A*, Types of fistulas. *B*, Appearance of arm with fistula. *C*, Dialysis needles in place. (From Black, J., & Matassarin-Jacobs, E. [1997]. *Medical-surgical nursing: A nursing process approach* [5th ed.]. Philadelphia: W. B. Saunders. p. 1652.)

c. Infiltration of the needles during dialysis can occur and cause hematomas
d. An aneurysm can form in the fistula
e. Arterial steal syndrome can develop (too much blood is diverted to the vein and arterial perfusion to the hand is compromised)
f. CHF can occur from the increased blood flow in the venous system
E. Implementation of **AV fistula** and AV graft
1. Do not take a blood pressure, draw blood, place an IV, or administer injections in the fistula or graft extremity
2. Monitor for clotting
a. Complaints of tingling or discomfort in the extremity
b. Inability to palpate or auscultate a bruit or thrill over the fistula or graft
c. Monitor for arterial steal syndrome
e. Palpate or auscultate for bruit or thrill over the fistula or graft
f. Palpate pulses below the fistula or graft and monitor for hand swelling as an indication of ischemia
g. Monitor for infection
h. Monitor lung and heart sounds for signs of CHF
i. Notify the physician immediately if signs of

clotting, infection, or arterial steal syndrome occur

VII. Peritoneal Dialysis

A. Description
1. The peritoneum is the dialyzing membrane (semipermeable membrane) and substitutes for kidney function during kidney failure
2. Works on the principles of diffusion and osmosis; the dialysis occurs via the transfer of fluid and solute from the bloodstream through the peritoneum
3. The peritoneum membrane is large and porous, allowing solutes and fluid to move via an osmotic gradient from an area of higher concentration in the body to lower concentration in the dialyzing fluid
4. The peritoneal cavity is rich in capillaries; therefore, it provides a ready access to blood supply
B. Contraindications for **peritoneal dialysis**
1. Peritonitis
2. Recent abdominal surgery
3. Abdominal adhesions
4. Impending renal transplant
C. Dialysate solution
1. Solution is sterile

2. Electrolytes
   a. Sodium, 140 to 145 mEq
   b. Chloride, 101 to 110 mEq
   c. Calcium, 3.5 to 4.0 mEq
   d. Magnesium, 1.5 mEq
   e. Lactate/acetate (base) 43 to 45 mEq
3. Osmolarity
   a. 1.5% = 365 mOsm
   b. 4.25% = 504 mOsm
4. Glucose concentrations
   a. 1.5%
   b. 2.5%
   c. 4.25%
   d. The higher the glucose concentration, the greater the amount of fluid removed during an exchange
   e. Increasing the glucose concentration increases the concentration of active particles that cause osmosis, and increases the rate of ultrafiltration and the amount of fluid removed
5. Potassium: if hyperkalemia is not a problem, 4 mEq of potassium may be added to each bag of solution
6. Heparin: added to the dialysate solution to prevent clotting of the catheter
7. Antibiotics: prophylactic antibiotics may be added to dialysate to prevent peritonitis
8. Insulin: may be added to the dialysate for the diabetic client

VIII. Access for Peritoneal Dialysis (Fig. 50–4)

A. Description
   1. A surgical insertion of a siliconized rubber catheter into the abdominal cavity is required to allow infusion of dialysis fluid
   2. The preferred insertion site is 3 to 5 cm below the umbilicus because this area is relatively avascular and has less fascial resistance

3. The catheters are tunneled under the skin to stabilize the catheter and reduce the risk of infection
4. Over a period of 1 to 2 weeks following insertion, there is an ingrowth of fibroblasts and blood vessels into the cuffs of the catheter, which fix the catheter in place and provide an extra barrier against dialysate leakage and bacterial invasion

B. Types of **peritoneal dialysis**
   1. Continuous ambulatory **peritoneal dialysis** (CAPD)
      a. Closely resembles renal function because it is a continuous process
      b. Does not require a machine for the procedure
      c. Promotes client independence
      d. The client performs self-dialysis 24 hours a day, 7 days a week
      e. Four dialysis cycles are administered in 24 hours, including an 8-hour dwell overnight
      f. 1.5 to 3.0 liters of dialysate is instilled into the abdomen four times daily and left in place for 4 to 10 hours
      g. The dialysis bag, attached to the catheter, is folded and carried in the client's clothing until time for outflow
      h. After dwell, the bag is placed lower than the insertion site so fluid drains by gravity flow
      i. When full, the bag is changed and new dialysate is instilled into the abdomen and the process continues
   2. Automated **peritoneal dialysis** (APD)
      a. Similar to CAPD in that it is a continuous dialysis process
      b. Requires a peritoneal cycling machine
      c. Can be done as intermittent peritoneal dialysis (IPD), continuous cycling peritoneal dialysis (CCPD), or nightly peritoneal dialysis (NPD)

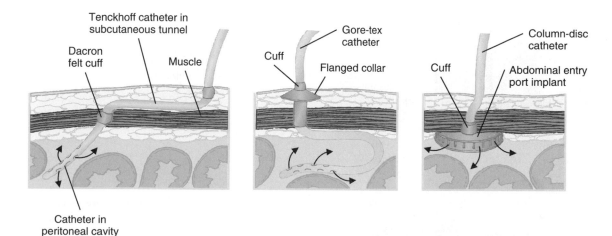

FIGURE 50–4. Three types of peritoneal dialysis catheter. The Tenckhoff catheter has two Dacron felt cuffs that hold the catheter in place and prevent dialysate leakage and bacterial invasion; a subcutaneous tunnel also helps to prevent infection. The Gore-Tex catheter has a Dacron cuff above a flanged collar. The column-disk catheter has a cuff and a large abdominal entry port implant. (From Black, J., & Matassarin-Jacobs, E. [1997]. *Medical-surgical nursing: A nursing process approach* [5th ed.]. Philadelphia: W. B. Saunders.)

C. **Peritoneal dialysis** infusion (Fig. 50–5)
  1. Description
    a. One infusion (inflow), dwell, and outflow is considered one exchange
    b. Uses an open system, which presents a risk of infection
    c. Inflow: the infusion of 1 to 2 liters of dialysate is infused by gravity into the peritoneal space, which usually takes approximately 20 minutes
    d. Dwell time: the amount of time that the dialysate solution remains in the peritoneal space; prescribed by the physician
    e. Outflow: fluid drains out of body by gravity into the drainage bag
  2. Implementation before treatment
    a. Monitor vital signs
    b. Obtain weight
    c. Have the client void if possible
    d. Assess electrolyte and glucose levels
  3. Implementation during treatment
    a. Monitor vital signs
    b. Monitor for signs of infection
    c. Monitor for respiratory distress, pain, or discomfort
    d. Monitor for signs of pulmonary edema
    e. Monitor for hypotension and hypertension
    f. Monitor for malaise, nausea, and vomiting

  g. Assess the catheter site dressing for wetness or bleeding
  h. Monitor dwell time as prescribed by the physician, and initiate outflow
  i. Do not allow dwell time to extend beyond the physician's order because this increases the risk for hyperglycemia
  j. Turn the client from side to side or have the client sit upright if flow is slow to start
  k. Monitor outflow, which should be a continuous stream after the clamp is opened
  l. Monitor outflow for color and clarity
  m. Monitor I&O accurately
  n. If outflow is less than inflow, the difference is equal to the amount absorbed or retained by the client during dialysis and should be counted as intake

IX. Complications of Peritoneal Dialysis

A. Peritonitis
  1. Maintain meticulous sterile technique with hooking up or clamping off bags, and when caring for catheter insertion site
  2. Follow institutional procedure for hooking up or clamping off bags, which may include

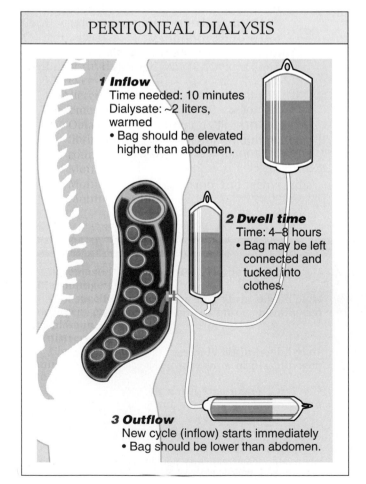

PERITONEAL DIALYSIS

1 Inflow
Time needed: 10 minutes
Dialysate: ~2 liters, warmed
• Bag should be elevated higher than abdomen.

2 Dwell time
Time: 4–8 hours
• Bag may be left connected and tucked into clothes.

3 Outflow
New cycle (inflow) starts immediately
• Bag should be lower than abdomen.

FIGURE 50–5. Components of long-term peritoneal dialysis system. (From Luckmann, J. [1997]. *Saunders manual of nursing care.* Philadelphia: W. B. Saunders. p. 1191.)

scrubbing the connection sites with an antiseptic
3. Monitor temperature closely
4. Monitor for fever, cloudy outflow, and rebound abdominal tenderness
5. If peritonitis is suspected, obtain a culture of the outflow to determine the infective organism
6. Administer antibiotics as prescribed

B. Abdominal pain
1. Pain during inflow is common during the first few exchanges and is caused by peritoneal irritation and usually disappears after a week or two
2. The cold temperature of dialysate aggravates the discomfort, and the dialysate should be warmed before use only with a special dialysate warmer pad
3. Place a heating pad on the abdomen during the inflow to relieve discomfort

C. Insufficient outflow
1. May be caused by catheter migration out of the peritoneal area and if this occurs, it must be repositioned by the physician
2. Insufficient outflow can also be caused by a full colon
3. Maintain drainage bag below the client's abdomen
4. Change the client's position during outflow by turning or ambulating
5. Check for kinks in the tubing
6. Encourage a high-fiber diet
7. Administer stool softeners as prescribed

D. Leakage around the catheter site
1. Over a period of 1 to 2 weeks following insertion of the catheter, an ingrowth of fibroblasts and blood vessels into the cuffs of the catheter occurs, which fix the catheter in place and provide an extra barrier against dialysate leakage and bacterial invasion
2. It may take up to 2 weeks for the client to tolerate a full exchange without leaking around the catheter site

E. Characteristics of outflow
1. During the first or initial exchanges, the outflow may be bloody; outflow should be clear and colorless thereafter
2. A brown outflow indicates bowel perforation
3. If the outflow is the same color as urine, it indicates bladder perforation
4. Cloudy outflow indicates peritonitis

X. Uremic Syndrome

A. Description
1. The accumulation of nitrogenous waste products in the blood due to the inability of the kidneys to filter out these waste products
2. It may occur as a result of ARF or CRF

B. Data collection
1. **Oliguria**

2. The presence of protein, red blood cells, and casts in the urine
3. A urine-specific gravity of 1.010
4. Elevated levels of urea, uric acid, potassium, and magnesium in the urine
5. Hypotension or hypertension
6. Alterations in level of consciousness
7. Electrolyte imbalances
8. Stomatitis
9. Nausea or vomiting
10. Diarrhea or constipation

C. Implementation
1. Monitor vital signs
2. Monitor electrolyte values
3. Monitor I&O
4. Provide a diet low in protein unless the client is on **peritoneal dialysis**
5. Limit sodium, nitrogen, potassium, and phosphate intake as prescribed

XI. Cystitis/Urinary Tract Infections (UTI)
(Box 50–4)

A. Description
1. Inflammation of the bladder from infection or obstruction of the urethra
2. The most common causative organisms are *Escherichia coli*, *Enterobacter*, *Pseudomonas*, and *Serratia*
3. More common in females because females have a shorter urethra than males, and the location of the urethra in the female is close to the rectum
4. Sexually active and pregnant women are most vulnerable to cystitis

B. Data collection
1. Frequency and urgency
2. Burning on urination
3. Voiding in small amounts
4. Inability to void
5. Incomplete emptying of the bladder

BOX 50–4. Causes of Cystitis

Hormonal changes influencing alterations in vaginal flora
Loss of bactericidal properties of prostatic secretions in the male
Sexual intercourse
Poor-fitting diaphragms
Use of spermicides
Synthetic underwear and pantyhose
Wet bathing suits
Allergens or irritants such as soaps, sprays, bubble bath, and perfumed sanitary napkins
Invasive urinary tract procedures
Indwelling urethral catheters
Bladder distention
Urinary stasis
Calculus

6. Lower abdominal discomfort or back discomfort
7. Cloudy, dark, foul-smelling urine
8. Hematuria
9. Bladder spasms
10. Malaise, chills, and fever
11. Nausea and vomiting

C. Implementation
1. Obtain a urine specimen for culture and sensitivity to identify bacterial growth prior to administering prescribed antibiotics
2. Instruct the client to force fluids up to 3000 mL a day, especially if the client is taking a sulfonamide because these medications can form crystals in concentrated urine
3. Maintain acid urine pH (5.5) by an acid ash diet; instruct the client about foods to consume on an acid ash diet
4. Use a strict aseptic technique when inserting a urinary catheter
5. Maintain closed urinary drainage systems for clients with indwelling catheters
6. Provide meticulous perineal care for clients with indwelling catheters
7. Administer medications as prescribed, which may include analgesics, antiseptics, antispasmodics, antibiotics, and antimicrobials
8. Note that if the client is prescribed an aminoglycoside, a sulfonamide, or nitrofurantoin (Macrodantin), that the actions of these medications are diminished by acidic urine
9. Discourage caffeine products such as coffee, tea, and cola
10. Instruct the client to avoid alcohol
11. Provide heat to the abdomen or sitz baths for complaints of discomfort
12. Instruct client to take medications as prescribed
13. Instruct the client to take antibiotics on schedule and to take the entire course of medications as prescribed, which may be a course of 10 to 14 days
14. Instruct the client in the importance of follow-up urine culture following treatment
15. Preventive measures are listed in Box 50–5

XII. Urosepsis

A. Description
1. A gram-negative bacteremia originating in the urinary tract
2. The most common organism responsible is *Escherichia coli*
3. The most common cause is the presence of an indwelling catheter or an untreated UTI in a client that is medically compromised
4. The major problem is the ability of the bacterium to develop resistant strains

---

BOX 50–5. Prevention of Cystitis

Teach the female client good perineal care and to wipe from front to back
Instruct client to avoid bubble baths and tub baths and avoid vaginal deodorants
Instruct client to void every 2–3 hours
Instruct client to void and drink a glass of water after intercourse
Instruct women to wear cotton pants, to avoid wearing pantyhose with slacks, to avoid tight clothes and sitting around in a wet bathing suit
Teach pregnant women to void every 2 hours
Encourage menopausal women to use estrogen vaginal creams to restore pH
Instruct women to use water-soluble lubricants for coitus, especially after menopause

---

5. Urosepsis can lead to septic shock if not treated aggressively
B. Data collection: fever is the most common and earliest manifestation
C. Implementation
1. Obtain a urine specimen for urine culture and sensitivity
2. IV antibiotics are usually prescribed until the client has been afebrile for 3 to 5 days
3. Administer oral antibiotics as prescribed after the 3- to 5-day afebrile period

XIII. Urethritis

A. Description
1. An inflammation of the urethra that is commonly associated with sexually transmitted diseases (STD) and may be seen with cystitis
2. In men it is most often caused by gonorrhea and chlamydial infection
3. In women it is most often caused by feminine hygiene sprays, perfumed toilet paper and sanitary napkins, spermicidal jellies, UTIs, and changes in the vaginal mucosal lining
B. Data collection
1. Males
   a. Burning on urination
   b. Frequency
   c. Urgency
   d. Nocturia
   e. Difficulty voiding
   f. Discharge from the penis
2. Females
   a. Frequency
   b. Urgency
   c. Nocturia
   d. Painful urination
   e. Difficulty voiding
   f. Lower abdominal discomfort
C. Implementation
1. Encourage fluids

2. Prepare the client for testing to determine if an STD is present
3. Administer antibiotics as prescribed
4. Instruct the client in the administration of sitz baths
5. If stricture occurs, prepare the client for dilation of the urethra and instillation of an antiseptic solution
6. Instruct the client to avoid intercourse until the symptoms subside or the treatment of the STD is complete
7. Instruct women to avoid the use of perfumed toilet paper and sanitary napkins and feminine hygiene sprays

XIV. Ureteritis and Pyelonephritis

A. Ureteritis
   1. An inflammation of the ureter that is commonly associated with pyelonephritis
   2. Chronic pyelonephritis causes the ureter to become fibrotic and narrowed by strictures
B. Pyelonephritis
   1. An inflammation of the renal pelvis and the parenchyma commonly caused by bacterial invasion
   2. Acute pyelonephritis often occurs after bacterial contamination of the urethra or following an invasive procedure of the urinary tract
   3. Chronic pyelonephritis most commonly occurs following chronic obstruction with reflux or chronic disorders
   4. *Escherichia coli* is the most common bacterial organism
C. Acute pyelonephritis
   1. Usually a short course that recurs as a relapse of a previous infection or as a new infection
   2. Can progress to bacteremia or chronic pyelonephritis
   3. Data collection
      a. Fever and chills
      b. Nausea
      c. Flank pain on the affected side
      d. Costovertebral angle (CVA) tenderness
      e. Headache
      f. Muscular pain
      g. Dysuria
      h. Frequency and urgency
      i. Cloudy, bloody, or foul-smelling urine
      j. Increased white blood cells in the urine
D. Chronic pyelonephritis
   1. A slow, progressive disease that is usually associated with recurrent acute attacks
   2. Causes contraction of the kidney and dysfunctioning of the nephrons, which are replaced by scar tissue
   3. Can lead to **renal failure**
   4. Data collection
      a. It is frequently diagnosed incidentally when a client is being evaluated for hypertension

b. Poor urine concentrating ability
c. Pyuria
d. Azotemia
e. Proteinuria
f. Anemia
g. Acidosis
E. Implementation
   1. Monitor vital signs
   2. Monitor I&O
   3. Monitor weight
   4. Encourage fluids up to 3000 mL a day
   5. Encourage adequate rest
   6. Instruct the client in a high-calorie, low-protein diet
   7. Provide warm moist compresses to the flank area
   8. Encourage the client to take warm baths
   9. Administer analgesics, antipyretics, and antiemetics as prescribed
   10. Administer antibiotics as prescribed
   11. Administer urinary antiseptics as prescribed
   12. Monitor for signs of **renal failure**

XV. Glomerulonephritis

A. Description
   1. A term that includes a variety of disorders, most of which are caused by an immunological reaction
   2. It results in proliferative and inflammatory changes within the glomerular structure
   3. Destruction, inflammation, and sclerosis of the glomeruli of both kidneys occur
   4. The inflammation of the glomeruli results from an antigen-antibody reaction produced from an infection elsewhere in the body
   5. Loss of kidney function develops
B. Causes
   1. Immunologic diseases
   2. Streptococcal infection group A beta-hemolytic
   3. History of pharyngitis or tonsillitis 2 to 3 weeks prior to symptoms
   4. Autoimmune diseases
C. Types
   1. Acute: occurs 2 to 3 weeks after a streptococcal infection
   2. Chronic: can occur after the acute phase or slowly over time
D. Complications
   1. Heart failure
   2. Hypertensive encephalopathy
   3. Pulmonary edema
   4. Renal failure
E. Data collection
   1. Gross hematuria
   2. Dark, smoky, cola-colored or red-brown urine
   3. Proteinuria that produces a persistent and excessive foam in the urine
   4. Urinary debris
   5. Mid- to high specific gravity

6. Low urinary pH
7. **Oliguria** or **anuria**
8. Headache
9. Chills and fever
10. Fatigue and weakness
11. Anorexia, nausea, and vomiting
12. Pallor
13. Edema in the face and periorbital area, feet, or generalized edema
14. Shortness of breath, ascites, pleural effusion, and CHF
15. Abdominal or flank pain
16. Hypertension
17. Reduced visual acuity
18. Increased BUN and creatinine
19. Increased antistreptolysin O titer (used to diagnosis disorders caused by streptococcal infections)

F. Implementation
1. Monitor vital signs
2. Monitor I&O and urine closely
3. Monitor weight daily
4. Monitor for edema
5. Monitor for fluid overload, ascites, pulmonary edema, and CHF
6. Restrict fluid intake as prescribed
7. Provide a high-calorie, low-protein diet
8. Restrict sodium intake as prescribed if edema is present
9. Provide bed rest and limited activity
10. Instruct the client to obtain treatment for infections, specifically sore throats and upper respiratory infections
11. Administer diuretics, antihypertensives, and antibiotics as prescribed
12. Monitor for signs of **renal failure**, cardiac failure, and hypertensive encephalopathy
13. Initiate seizure precautions as indicated and provide safety measures
14. Instruct the client to report signs of bloody urine, headache, or edema

XVI. Nephrotic Syndrome

A. Description: a set of clinical manifestations arising from protein wasting secondary to diffuse glomerular damage

B. Data collection
1. Proteinuria
2. Hypoalbuminemia
3. Edema
4. Hyperlipidemia
5. Waxy pallor to the skin
6. Anemia
7. Anorexia
8. Malaise
9. Irritability
10. Amenorrhea or abnormal menses
11. Hematuria may be present
12. Hypertension

C. Implementation
1. Monitor vital signs

2. Monitor I&O
3. Bed rest if severe edema is present
4. Normal to low-protein diet as prescribed with adequate carbohydrate and calorie intake
5. Monitor weight daily
6. Provide a mild sodium restriction as prescribed
7. Monitor potassium level because potassium may be restricted from the diet if the potassium rises
8. Administer diuretics as prescribed
9. Administer steroids and cytotoxic medications as prescribed
10. Administer plasma volume expanders such as albumin, plasma, and dextran to raise the osmotic pressure
11. Administer anticoagulants as prescribed for those clients who develop renal vein thrombosis

XVII. Hydronephrosis

A. Description
1. Distention of the renal pelvis and calices caused by an obstruction of normal urine flow
2. The urine becomes trapped proximal to the obstruction
3. The causes include calculus, tumors, scar tissue, or kinks in the ureter

B. Data collection
1. Hypertension
2. Headache
3. Flank pain
4. Electrolyte imbalances

C. Implementation
1. Monitor vital signs frequently
2. Monitor for fluid and electrolyte imbalances, including dehydration after the obstruction is relieved
3. Monitor for diuresis, which can lead to fluid depletion
4. Monitor weights daily
5. Monitor urine for specific gravity, albumin, and glucose
6. Administer fluid replacement as prescribed

XVIII. Genitourinary Tuberculosis

A. Description
1. Usually a late manifestation of tuberculosis caused by the spread of *Mycobacterium tuberculosis* from the lungs through the bloodstream
2. *M. tuberculosis* is the cause of tuberculosis and is most often seen in the poor, the malnourished, those living in close housing, and in the immunosuppressed

B. Data collection
1. Frequency and pain on urination
2. Bladder spasms
3. Fatigue

4. Weight loss
5. Tubercle bacilli in urine culture
6. Lesions noted on x-ray
7. Tuberculosis nodules noted on the prostate

C. Implementation
   1. Administer antitubercular medications as prescribed
   2. Use precautions when handling urine specimens because the bacillus in the urine is infectious
   3. Instruct the client to use precautions to prevent the spread of the disease
   4. Instruct the client to use condoms during intercourse to prevent the spread of the disease

XIX. Polycystic Disease

A. Description
   1. A cystic formation and hypertrophy of the both kidneys that leads to cystic rupture, infection, the formation of scar tissue, and damaged nephrons
   2. There is no know way to arrest the progress of the destructive cysts
   3. The ultimate result of this disease is **renal failure**

B. Types
   1. Infantile polycystic disease: an inherited autosomal recessive trait that results in the death of the infant within a few months after birth
   2. Adult polycystic disease: autosomal dominant trait that results in end-stage renal disease

C. Data collection
   1. Flank, lumbar, or abdominal pain
   2. Fever and chills
   3. UTIs
   4. Hematuria, proteinuria, and pyuria
   5. Calculi
   6. Hypertension
   7. Palpable abdominal masses and enlarged kidneys

D. Implementation
   1. Monitor for gross hematuria, which indicates cyst rupture
   2. Increase sodium and water because waste, rather than retention, of sodium occurs
   3. Provide bed rest if ruptured cysts and bleeding occur
   4. Prepare the client for percutaneous cyst puncture for relief of obstruction, or for draining an abscess
   5. Prepare the client for dialysis or renal transplantation
   6. Encourage the client to seek genetic counseling

XX. Urolithiasis and Nephrolithiasis

A. Description
   1. Calculi or stones can form anywhere in the urinary tract; however, the most frequent site is the kidney
   2. The problems that can occur as a result of calculi are pain, obstruction, and tissue trauma with secondary hemorrhage and infection
   3. Kidney, ureters, and bladder (KUB) film, intravenous pyelogram (IVP), computed tomography (CT) scan, and renal ultrasonography will determine the stone location
   4. A stone analysis will be done after passage to determine the type of stone and assist in determining treatment
   5. **Urolithiasis** refers to the formation of urinary stones; urinary calculi are formed in the ureter
   6. **Nephrolithiasis** refers to the formation of kidney stones; kidney stones are formed in the renal parenchyma
   7. When a calculus occludes the ureter and blocks the flow of urine, the ureter dilates; this is known as hydroureter
   8. If the obstruction is not removed, urinary stasis results in infection, impairment of renal function on the side of the blockage, and resultant hydronephrosis and irreversible kidney damage

B. Causes
   1. Family history of stone formation
   2. Diet high in calcium, vitamin D, milk, protein, oxalate, purines, or alkali
   3. A high intake of purine-rich food
   4. Obstruction and urinary stasis
   5. Dehydration
   6. Use of diuretics, which can cause volume depletion
   7. UTIs and prolonged urinary catheterization
   8. Immobilization
   9. Hypercalcemia and hyperparathyroidism
   10. Elevated uric acid as in gout

C. Data collection
   1. Renal colic originates in the lumbar region and radiates around the side and down toward the testicle in the male, and to the bladder in the female
   2. Ureteral colic radiates toward the genitalia and thigh
   3. Sharp, severe pain of sudden onset
   4. Dull, aching kidney
   5. Nausea and vomiting, pallor, and diaphoresis during acute pain
   6. Urinary frequency with alternating retention
   7. Signs of UTI
   8. Low-grade fever
   9. RBCs, WBCs, and bacteria in urinalysis
   10. Hematuria

D. Implementation
   1. Monitor vital signs
   2. Monitor I&O
   3. Assess for fever, chills, and infection
   4. Monitor for nausea, vomiting, and diarrhea

BOX 50–6. Alkaline Ash Diet

OUTCOME

Increases the pH
Reduces the acidity of the urine

FOODS TO INCLUDE

Milk
Fruits except cranberries, plums, and prunes
Rhubarb
Most vegetables
Small amounts of beef, halibut, veal, trout, and salmon allowed

---

5. Force fluids up to 3000 mL/day unless contraindicated to facilitate the passage of the stone and prevent infection
6. Strain all urine for the presence of stones
7. Send stones to the laboratory for analysis
8. Provide warm baths and heat to the flank area
9. Administer analgesics at regularly scheduled intervals as prescribed to relieve pain
10. Assess the client's response to pain medication
11. Administer IV fluids as prescribed to increase the flow of urine and facilitate the passage of the stone
12. Assist the client in performing relaxation techniques to assist in relieving pain
13. Instruct the client in the diet specific to the stone composition
14. Maintain urinary pH depending on the type of stone
15. Turn and reposition immobilized clients
16. Prepare the client for surgical procedures if prescribed

E. Stone composition (Boxes 50–6 and 50–7)
   1. Calcium phosphate stones

BOX 50–7. Acid Ash Diet

OUTCOME

Decreases pH
Makes the urine more acid

FOODS TO INCLUDE

Cheese and eggs
Meat, fish, oysters, and poultry
Bread, cereal, and whole grains
Pastries
Cranberries, prunes, plums, and tomatoes
Peas

FOODS TO AVOID

Carbonated beverages
Baking soda or powder
All vegetables except corn and legumes
Olives and pickles
Nuts other than peanuts

---

   a. Caused by supersaturation of urine with calcium and phosphate
   b. Diet includes acid ash foods because calcium stones have an alkaline chemistry
   c. Dietary prescription may include to decrease intake of foods high in calcium and phosphate to reduce urinary calcium content, and to avoid excess vitamin D intake to prevent stones from forming
2. Calcium oxalate stones
   a. Caused by supersaturation of urine with calcium and oxalate
   b. Diet includes acid ash foods because calcium stones have alkaline chemistry
   c. Dietary prescription may include decreasing intake of foods high in calcium
   d. Dietary prescription may include avoiding oxalate food sources to reduce urinary oxalate content and the formation of stones
   e. Oxalate-rich food sources include tea, almonds, cashews, chocolate, cocoa, beans, spinach, and rhubarb
3. Struvite stones
   a. Also called triple phosphate stones and are made of magnesium and ammonium phosphate
   b. Caused by urea splitting by bacteria
   c. Struvite stones tend to form in alkaline urine
   d. Diet includes acid ash foods
   e. Dietary prescription includes to limit high-phosphate foods such as dairy products, red and organ meats, and whole grains to reduce urinary phosphate content
4. Uric acid stones
   a. Caused by excess dietary purine or gout
   b. Uric acid stones tend to form in acidic urine
   c. Dietary prescription may include alkaline ash foods and decreased intake of purine sources such as organ meats, gravies, red wines, and sardines to reduce urinary purine content
   d. Allopurinol (Zyloprim) may be prescribed to lower uric acid levels
5. Cystine stones
   a. Caused by cystine crystal formation
   b. Cystine stones tend to form in acidic urine
   c. Diet includes alkaline ash foods
   d. Dietary prescription may also include a low intake of methionine, an essential amino acid that forms cystine; the client is instructed to avoid meat, milk, cheese, and eggs
   e. Dietary measures also focus on encouraging fluids up to 3 liters a day unless contraindicated, to help dilute the urine and prevent cystine crystals from forming

XXI. Surgical Management of Kidney Stones

A. Cystoscopy
1. May be done for stones located in the bladder or lower ureter
2. There is no incision
3. One or two ureteral catheters are inserted past the stone
4. The stone may be manipulated and dislodged by the procedure
5. The catheters may mechanically guide the stones downward as they are removed
6. Catheters are left in place for 24 hours to drain the urine trapped proximal to the stone and to dilate the ureter
7. A continuous chemical irrigation may be prescribed to dissolve the stone

B. Extracorporeal shock wave lithotripsy (ESWL)
1. Noninvasive mechanical procedure for breaking up stones that are located in the kidney or upper ureter so that they can pass spontaneously or be removed by other methods
2. Fluoroscopy is used to visualize the stone
3. There is no incision or drain
4. Ultrasonic waves are delivered through a bath of warm water to the areas of the stone to disintegrate it
5. Stones are passed in the urine within a few days
6. Preprocedure: NPO for 8 hours prior to procedure
7. Postprocedure
   a. Monitor vital signs
   b. Monitor I&O
   c. Monitor for bleeding
   d. Monitor for pain and signs of urinary obstruction
   e. Instruct the client to increase fluid intake to wash out the stone fragments
   f. Inform the client that ambulation is important

C. Percutaneous lithotripsy
1. Performed for stones in the bladder, ureter, or kidney
2. An invasive procedure in which a guide is inserted under fluoroscopy near the area of the stone
3. An ultrasonic wave is aimed at the stone to break it into fragments
4. May be performed via cystoscopy or nephroscopy
5. No incision is required for cystoscopy; however, a small flank incision is needed for nephrostomy
6. The client may possibly have an indwelling catheter
7. A nephrostomy tube may be placed to administer chemical irrigations to break up the stone; the nephrostomy tube may remain in place for 1 to 5 days
8. Encourage the client to drink 3000 to 4000 mL of fluid per day following the procedure as prescribed
9. Monitor for and instruct the client to monitor for complications of infection, hemorrhage, and extravasation of fluid into the retroperitoneal cavity

D. Ureterolithotomy
1. An open surgical procedure; performed if lithotripsy is not effective
2. Performed if the location of the stone is in the ureter
3. Incision into the ureter is made through the lower abdomen or flank to remove the stone
4. The client may have a Penrose drain, ureteral stent catheter, and an indwelling bladder catheter

E. Pyelolithotomy
1. A flank incision into the kidney is made to remove stones from the renal pelvis
2. A large flank incision is required
3. The client will have a Penrose drain and indwelling catheter

F. Nephrolithotomy
1. Incision into the kidney is made to remove the stone
2. A large flank incision is required
3. The client may have a nephrostomy tube and an indwelling catheter

G. Partial or total nephrectomy
1. Performed if there is extensive kidney damage, renal infection, or severe obstruction and to prevent stone recurrence
2. Implementation postoperative
   a. The plan of care will be based on the incision location and the type of drainage tubes present
   b. Monitor incision particularly if a Penrose drain is in place, as it will drain large amounts of urine
   c. Protect the skin from urinary drainage
   d. Place an ostomy pouch over the Penrose drain to protect the skin if urinary drainage is excessive
   e. Monitor nephrostomy tube, which may be attached to a drainage bag for a free flow of urine
   f. If urethral catheters are in place, do not irrigate
   g. Monitor indwelling Foley catheter for drainage
   h. Encourage fluid intake to ensure 2500 to 3000 mL or more of urine output per day
   i. Monitor I&O closely
   j. Determine composition of stone from laboratory analysis
   k. Instruct the client in dietary restrictions if required
   l. Instruct clients about medications that may be needed long-term to reduce the development of calculi

m. Medications prescribed for calcium stones may include phosphates, thiazide diuretics, and allopurinol (Zyloprim)

n. Vitamin B$_6$ or magnesium oxide may be prescribed for clients with oxalate stones

o. Allopurinol (Zyloprim) may be prescribed for oxalate and uric acid stones

p. Long-term antibiotics may be prescribed for struvite or cystine stones

XXII. Kidney Tumors

A. Description
1. May be benign or malignant, bilateral or unilateral
2. Common sites of metastasis include bone, lungs, liver, spleen, or other kidney
3. The exact cause of renal carcinoma is unknown

B. Data collection
1. Dull flank pain
2. Palpable renal mass
3. Painless gross hematuria

C. Radical nephrectomy
1. Description
   a. Removal of the entire kidney, adjacent adrenal gland, and renal artery and vein
   b. Radiation therapy and possibly chemotherapy may follow radical nephrectomy
2. Implementation postoperative
   a. Monitor vital signs
   b. Monitor abdomen for distention caused by bleeding
   c. Observe bed linens under the client for bleeding
   d. Monitor for hypotension, decreases in urinary output, and alterations in level of consciousness as indicating signs of hemorrhage
   e. Monitor for signs of adrenal insufficiency
   f. In clients with adrenal insufficiency, a large urinary output followed by hypotension and subsequent **oliguria** occurs
   g. IV fluids and packed red blood cells may be prescribed
   h. Monitor I&O and daily weight
   i. Monitor for a urinary output of 30 to 50 mL/hour to ensure adequate renal perfusion
   j. Monitor urine for specific gravity
   k. Maintain semi-Fowler's position
   l. Monitor for signs of respiratory complications related to surgery
   m. Encourage coughing and deep-breathing exercises
   n. Monitor bowel sounds for paralytic ileus
   o. Apply antiembolism stockings as prescribed
   p. Do not irrigate or manipulate the nephrostomy tube if in place
   q. Administer pain medications as prescribed

XXIII. Bladder Trauma

A. Description
1. Occurs following a blunt or penetrating injury to the lower abdomen
2. Penetrating wounds occur as a result of a stabbing, gunshot wound, or from other objects piercing the abdominal wall
3. A fractured pelvis that causes bone fragments to puncture the bladder is the most common cause of bladder trauma
4. When a blunt trauma occurs, it causes compression of the abdominal wall and the bladder

B. Data collection
1. **Anuria**
2. Hematuria
3. Pain over costovertebral angle (CVA)
4. Nausea and vomiting

C. Implementation
1. Monitor vital signs
2. Monitor for hematuria, hemorrhage, and signs of shock
3. Promote bed rest
4. Monitor pain level
5. Prepare the client for insertion of a suprapubic catheter to aid in urinary drainage if prescribed
6. Prepare the client for surgical repair of the laceration if prescribed

XXIV. Epididymitis

A. Description
1. An acute or chronic inflammation of the epididymis that occurs as a result of a UTI, sexually transmitted disease, prostatitis, or as a result of long-term use of a Foley catheter
2. The infective organism passes upward through the urethra and ejaculatory duct and along the vas deferens to the epididymis

B. Data collection
1. Scrotal pain
2. Groin pain
3. Swelling in scrotum and groin
4. Pus and bacteria in the urine
5. Fever and chills
6. Abscess development

C. Implementation
1. Encourage fluid intake
2. Encourage bed rest with the scrotum elevated to prevent traction on the spermatic cord, to facilitate drainage and to relieve pain
3. Instruct the client in the intermittent application of cold compresses to the scrotum
4. Instruct the client in the use of sitz baths
5. Instruct the client in the administration of antibiotics for self and sexual partner if chlamydia or gonorrhea is the cause
6. Instruct the client to avoid lifting, straining, and sexual contact until the infection subsides

XXV. Prostatitis

A. Description
1. An inflammation of the prostate gland that can be caused by an infectious agent (bacterial) or by tissue hyperplasia (abacterial)
2. Bacterial prostatitis occurs as a result of the organism reaching the prostate via the urethra or bloodstream
3. Abacterial prostatitis usually occurs following a viral illness or a decrease in sexual activity

B. Data collection
1. Bacterial
   a. Fever and chills
   b. Dysuria
   c. Urethral discharge
   d. Boggy, tender prostate
   e. Urethral discharge on palpation of prostrate
   f. White blood cells (WBCs) found in prostatic secretions
2. Abacterial
   a. Backache
   b. Dysuria
   c. Perineal pain
   d. Frequency
   e. Hematuria
   f. Irregularly enlarged, firm and tender prostate

C. Implementation
1. Encourage adequate fluid intake
2. Instruct client in the use of sitz baths to promote comfort
3. Administer antibiotics, analgesics, antispasmodics, and stool softeners as prescribed
4. Inform the client of activities to drain the prostate such as intercourse, masturbation, and prostatic massage
5. Instruct the client to avoid spicy foods, coffee, alcohol, prolonged auto rides, and sexual intercourse during an acute inflammation

XXVI. Benign Prostatic Hypertrophy (BPH)

A. Description
1. A slow enlargement of the prostate gland with hypertrophy and hyperplasia of normal tissue
2. The enlargement causes narrowing of the urethra and results in partial or complete obstruction
3. The cause is unknown and the disorder usually occurs in men older than 50 years

B. Data collection
1. Urgency, frequency, and hesitancy
2. Changes in size and force of urinary stream
3. Retention
4. Dribbling
5. Nocturia
6. Hematuria
7. Urinary stasis
8. Urinary tract infections

C. Implementation
1. Encourage fluids of up to 2000 to 3000 mL/day unless contraindicated
2. Prepare for bladder drainage via urinary catheterization for distention
3. Avoid administering medications that cause urinary retention such as anticholinergics
4. Administer androgen-depriving agents such as finasteride (Proscar) as prescribed
5. Prepare the client for surgery as prescribed (Box 50–8)

D. Transurethral resection (TUR)
1. Insertion of a scope into the urethra to excise prostatic tissue
2. Bleeding is common following TUR and monitoring for hemorrhage is an important nursing intervention
3. A continuous bladder irrigation (CBI) will be prescribed postoperatively to maintain the urine at a pink color
4. Bladder spasms are common following surgery and antispasmodics may be prescribed
5. Dribbling or incontinence may occur postoperatively, and it is important for the nurse to instruct the client to monitor for recurrence
6. Sterility may or may not occur following the surgical procedure

E. Suprapubic prostatectomy
1. Removal of the prostate via an abdominal approach and an opening into the bladder
2. The client will have an abdominal dressing that may drain copious amounts of urine, and the abdominal dressing will need to be changed frequently
3. Severe hemorrhage is possible, and monitoring for blood loss is an important nursing intervention
4. Bladder spasms are common, and antispasmodics may be prescribed for the bladder spasms
5. CBI will be prescribed and administered to keep the urine pink in color
6. A longer healing process is involved compared with the TUR
7. Sterility occurs with this procedure

F. Retropubic prostatectomy
1. Removal of the prostate gland by a low abdominal incision without opening the bladder
2. Less bleeding occurs with this procedure, and the client experiences fewer bladder spasms
3. There is minimal abdominal drainage

BOX 50–8. Surgical Interventions for BPH

Transurethral resection (TUR)
Retropubic prostatectomy
Suprapubic prostatectomy
Perineal prostectomy

4. CBI may be used
5. Sterility occurs with this procedure
G. Perineal prostatectomy
1. The prostate gland is removed through an incision made between the scrotum and anus
2. Minimal bleeding occurs with this procedure
3. The client needs to be monitored closely for infection because the risk of infection is increased with this type of prostatectomy
4. Urinary incontinence is common
5. The procedure causes sterility
6. It is important to teach the client how to perform perineal exercises
7. It is important to avoid inserting rectal tubes and taking the temperature rectally
8. Avoid administration of enemas
H. Postoperative implementation
1. Monitor vital signs
2. Monitor urinary output
3. Increase fluids to 2400 to 3000 mL/day unless contraindicated
4. Ambulate the client as early as possible and as soon as the urine begins to clear
5. Monitor urine for hemorrhage and clots
6. Monitor for arterial bleeding as evidenced by bright red urine with numerous clots, and if it occurs, increase CBI and notify the physician immediately
7. Monitor for venous bleeding as evidenced by burgundy-colored urine output, and if it occurs, inform the physician, who may apply traction on the catheter
8. Monitor hemoglobin and hematocrit levels
9. Expect red to light pink urine for 24 hours, turning to amber in 3 days
10. Inform the client that a continuous feeling of the urge to void is normal
11. Instruct the client to avoid attempts to void around the catheter because it will cause bladder spasms
12. Administer antibiotics, analgesics, stool softeners, and antispasmodics as prescribed
13. Monitor three-way Foley catheter, which will have a 30- to 45-mL retention balloon
14. Maintain CBI with normal saline or prescribed solution to keep the catheter free of obstruction
I. Postoperative suprapubic prostatectomy
1. Monitor suprapubic and Foley catheter drainage
2. Monitor CBI if prescribed
3. Note that the Foley catheter will be removed 2 to 4 days' postoperatively if the client has a suprapubic catheter
4. Clamp the suprapubic catheter after the Foley catheter is removed and instruct the client to attempt to void
5. After the client has voided, assess residual urine in the bladder by unclamping the suprapubic tube
6. Prepare for removal of the suprapubic catheter when the client consistently empties the bladder and residual urine is 75 mL or less

7. Monitor the suprapubic incision dressing, which may become saturated with urine until the incision heals
J. Postoperative retropubic prostatectomy
1. Note that because the bladder is not entered, there is no urinary drainage on the abdominal dressing
2. Monitor for infection
3. Assess for urinary or purulent drainage on the dressing, and if this occurs notify the physician
4. Monitor for fever and increased pain, which may indicate an infection
K. Postoperative perineal prostatectomy
1. Note that the client will have an incision that may or may not have a drain
2. Avoid rectal thermometers, rectal tubes, and enemas because they may cause trauma and bleeding

XXVII. Kidney Transplantation

A. Description
1. Implantation of a human kidney from a compatible donor into a recipient
2. Performed for irreversible kidney failure
3. Immunosuppressive medications must be taken by the recipient for life
B. Living related donors
1. The most desirable source of kidneys for transplant is living related donors who match the client closely
2. Screened for ABO blood group, tissue-specific antigen, human leukocyte antigen (HLA) suitability, and mixed lymphocyte culture index (histocompatibility)
3. Donor must be in excellent health with two properly functioning kidneys
4. The emotional well-being of the donor is determined
5. Complete understanding of the donation process and outcome is necessary
C. Cadaver donors
1. Must meet criteria of brain death
2. Must be under 60 years of age
3. Must have normal renal function
4. No malignant disease outside of the CNS can be present
5. No generalized infection can be present
6. No abdominal or renal trauma can be present
7. Normal BP must be present
8. The potential donor must have a negative hepatitis B antigen and negative HIV antibody
9. Continuous ventilation and heartbeat is maintained until the kidneys are surgically removed
10. Once the potential donor has demonstrated cerebral death, it is crucial to restore intravascular volume, wean from vasopressors, and establish diuresis

D. Warm ischemic time
1. The time elapsed between cessation, perfusion, and cooling of the kidney, and the time required for anastomosis of kidney
2. Maximal allowable warm ischemic time is 30 to 60 minutes
3. The kidney can be cooled and then the maximum time for transplantation is increased to 24 to 48 hours

E. Implementation preoperative
1. Verify histocompatability tests of identical twin or family member
2. Administer immunosuppressive medications to the recipient as prescribed, for 2 days before the transplantation
3. Maintain protective isolation
4. Verify that **hemodialysis** of the recipient was completed 24 hours before the transplant
5. Ensure the client is free of any infections
6. Assess renal function studies
7. Encourage discussion of feelings of both donor and recipient

F. Implementation postoperative
1. The kidney begins to function immediately or may be delayed a few days
2. **Hemodialysis** is performed until adequate kidney function is established
3. Monitor vital signs
4. Monitor I&O
5. Monitor urine output every hour
6. Monitor daily laboratory studies, urine for blood and specific gravity, daily weight, pulse oximetry, and BUN and creatinine levels
7. Maintain client in semi-Fowler's position
8. Monitor for patency of Foley catheter
9. Note that urine is pink and bloody initially but gradually returns to normal within several days to weeks
10. Monitor for gross hematuria and clots, which are not expected, and notify the physician if they occur
11. Monitor three-way Foley irrigation if prescribed, to prevent blood clot formation
12. Note that Foley should be removed as soon as possible to prevent infection
13. Maintain protective isolation precautions and monitor for infection
14. Monitor IV fluids closely and for fluid overload
15. Begin oral fluids in 24 hours as prescribed
16. Monitor for bowel sounds and initiate diet as prescribed when bowel sounds return
17. Maintain good oral hygiene, monitoring for stomatitis and bacterial and fungal infections
18. Encourage coughing and deep-breathing exercises
19. Maintain strict aseptic technique with wound care
20. Administer medications as prescribed, which may include antifungal medications, antibiotics, immunosuppressive agents, and corticosteroids
21. Assess for organ rejection (Box 50–9)

BOX 50–9. Client Instructions Following Kidney Transplant

Instruct client to avoid prolonged periods of sitting
Instruct client to recognize the signs and symptoms of infection and rejection
Instruct client to avoid contact sports
Instruct client to avoid exposure to people with infections
Instruct client in the signs and symptoms of infection and to monitor for infection
Instruct client in the use of medications as prescribed and in the importance of maintenance of immunosuppressive therapy for life

---

22. Promote live donor and recipient relationship
23. Monitor the client and recipient for depression

G. Graft rejection: except for identical twin donor and recipient, the major postoperative complication is graft rejection
1. Data collection
   a. Fever
   b. Malaise
   c. Elevated WBC
   d. Graft tenderness
   e. Signs of deteriorating renal function
   f. Acute hypertension
   g. Anemia
2. Hyperacute rejection
   a. Occurs immediately after surgery to 48 hours' postoperatively
   b. Implementation: removal of rejected kidney
3. Acute rejection
   a. Occurs within 6 weeks but can occur as late as 2 years
   b. Potentially reversible with increased immunosuppression
   c. Implementation: high doses of steroids; if steroids are ineffective, monoclonal antibodies may be administered
4. Chronic rejection
   a. Occurs slowly months to years after transplant
   b. Can be irreversible
   c. Mimics CRF
   d. Implementation: immunosuppressive medications

PRACTICE QUESTIONS

1. The nurse has inserted an indwelling Foley catheter and inflates the balloon. The client immediately complains of pain. Which of the following represents the best plan by the nurse?
   1 Tell the client that the discomfort will pass
   2 Withdraw 1 mL from the balloon of the catheter
   3 Push the catheter farther into the bladder
   4 Deflate the balloon and replace it with another catheter

2. The nurse has an order to obtain a urinalysis from a client with an indwelling urinary catheter. The nurse plans to avoid which of the following, which could contaminate the specimen?
   1 Obtaining the specimen from the urinary drainage bag
   2 Clamping the tubing of the drainage bag
   3 Aspirating a sample from the port on the drainage bag
   4 Wiping the port with an alcohol swab prior to inserting the syringe

3. The nurse is caring for the client who has had a renal biopsy. Which of the following interventions does the nurse avoid in the care of the client after this procedure?
   1 Forcing fluids to at least 3 liters in the first 24 hours
   2 Administering PRN narcotics
   3 Testing serial samples with dipsticks for occult blood
   4 Ambulating the client in the room and hall for short distances

4. The elderly client with cystitis also has an indwelling urinary catheter. The nurse plans to ensure that the nursing assistant does not
   1 Use soap and water to cleanse the perineal area
   2 Keep the drainage bag below the level of the bladder
   3 Use the drainage tubing port to obtain urine samples
   4 Let the drainage tubing rest under the leg

5. The nurse is assisting the client with cystitis with diet selection with an acid ash diet. The nurse encourages the client to eat which of the following foods?
   1 Low-fat milk
   2 Baked haddock
   3 Garden peas
   4 Apples

6. The client with acute pyelonephritis who was started on antibiotic therapy 24 hours ago is still complaining of burning with urination. The nurse checks the physician's orders to see if which of the following medications is prescribed?
   1 Phenazopyridine (Pyridium)
   2 Bethanechol chloride (Urecholine)
   3 Oxybutinin chloride (Ditropan)
   4 Propantheline bromide (Pro-Banthīne)

7. The client who has a history of gout is also diagnosed with urolithiasis. The stones are determined to be of uric acid type. The nurse gives the client instructions in foods to limit, which include
   1 Liver
   2 Apples
   3 Carrots
   4 Milk

8. The nurse is caring for a client who has been diagnosed as having a kidney mass. The client asks the nurse the reason for renal biopsy, when other tests such as CT scan and ultrasound are available. In formulating a response, the nurse incorporates the knowledge that renal biopsy
   1 Helps differentiate between a solid mass and a fluid-filled cyst
   2 Provides an outline of the renal vascular system
   3 Gives specific cytological information about the lesion
   4 Determines if the mass is growing rapidly or slowly

9. The female client is admitted to the emergency department following a fall from a horse. The physician orders insertion of a Foley catheter. The nurse notes blood at the urinary meatus while preparing for the procedure. The nurse should
   1 Use extra povidone-iodine solution in cleansing the meatus
   2 Use a smaller catheter
   3 Administer pain medication before inserting the catheter
   4 Notify the physician

10. The male client has a tentative diagnosis of urethritis. The nurse collects data from the client, knowing that which of the following are manifestations of the disorder?
    1 Hematuria and penile discharge
    2 Hematuria and pyuria
    3 Dysuria and proteinuria
    4 Dysuria and penile discharge

11. The nurse is assisting in planning a teaching session with the female client diagnosed with urethritis due to infection with chlamydia. The nurse plans to include which of the following points in the teaching session?
    1 The most serious complication of this infection is sterility
    2 The infection can be prevented by using spermicide to alter the pH in the perineal area
    3 Medication therapy should be continued for 3 weeks without interruption
    4 Sexual partners during the past 12 months should be notified and treated

12. The male client who is admitted for an unrelated medical problem is diagnosed with urethritis due to chlamydial infection. The nursing assistant assigned to the client asks the nurse what measures are necessary to prevent contraction of the infection during care. The nurse tells the assistant that
    1 Enteric precautions should be instituted for the client
    2 Contact isolation should be initiated because the disease is highly contagious
    3 Universal precautions are quite sufficient because the disease is transmitted sexually
    4 Gloves and mask should be used when in the client's room

13. The client with chlamydial infection has received instructions on self-care and prevention of further infection. The nurse evaluates that the client needs further reinforcement if the client states to
    1 Reduce the chance of reinfection by limiting the number of sexual partners
    2 Use latex condoms to prevent disease transmission
    3 Return to the clinic as requested for follow-up culture in 1 week
    4 Use doxycycline prophylactically to prevent symptoms of *Chlamydia*

14. The nurse is caring for a client with epididymitis. The nurse anticipates which of the following findings on data collection?
    1 Fever, diarrhea, groin pain, and ecchymosis
    2 Fever, nausea and vomiting, and painful scrotal edema
    3 Diarrhea, groin pain, and scrotal edema
    4 Nausea and vomiting, and scrotal edema with ecchymosis

15. The client is in extreme pain from scrotal swelling that is caused by epididymitis. The nurse administers an intramuscular narcotic analgesic in the left arm to relieve the pain. The nurse plans to do which of the following actions next?
    1 Tell the client to do ROM exercises to the left arm to absorb the medication into the bloodstream
    2 Check the name bracelet of the client
    3 Put the side rails up on the bed
    4 Dim the lights in the room

16. The nurse is caring for the client with epididymitis. The nurse avoids using which of the following treatment modalities in the care of the client?
    1 Bed rest
    2 Scrotal elevation
    3 Sitz bath
    4 Use of a heating pad

17. The client has epididymitis as a complication of urinary tract infection. The nurse is giving the client instructions to prevent a recurrence. The nurse evaluates that the client needs further instruction if the client states to
    1 Drink increased amounts of fluids
    2 Continue to take antibiotics until all symptoms are gone
    3 Limit the force of the stream during voiding
    4 Use condoms to eliminate risk from *Chlamydia* and gonorrhea

18. The client with acute prostatitis has difficulty voiding, which is accompanied by pain. The client says to the nurse, "Can't you just put a catheter in so I won't be in this misery when I try to go?" The nurse's response is based on the understanding that catheterization

1 Will prolong the course of the inflammation
2 Could result in obstruction from rebound edema once the catheter is removed
3 Is avoided whenever possible to avoid pushing organisms up into the bladder
4 Could puncture the prostate gland because it is so inflamed

19. The nurse is collecting data from a client who has had benign prostatic hypertrophy (BPH) in the past. To determine if the client is currently experiencing difficulty, the nurse asks the client about the presence of which of the following early symptoms?
    1 Urge incontinence
    2 Nocturia
    3 Decreased force of the urine stream
    4 Urinary retention

20. The client who has a cold is seen in the emergency department with the inability to void. Because the client has a history of BPH, the nurse determines that the client should be questioned about use of which of the following medications?
    1 Diuretics
    2 Antibiotics
    3 Antitussives
    4 Decongestants

21. The client is diagnosed with BPH, and is scheduled for transrectal ultrasound and drawing of a prostate-specific antigen (PSA) level. The client says to the nurse, "I can't remember, can you tell me again why I need these tests to be done?" The nurse responds that the tests
    1 Help to rule out the presence of malignancy
    2 Predict the course of BPH
    3 Pinpoint the likelihood of developing urinary obstruction
    4 Give an indication of whether intermittent self-catheterization is needed

22. The client who has had a prostatectomy has learned perineal exercises to gain control of the urinary sphincter. The nurse evaluates that the client needs further instruction if the client states to perform which of the following as part of these exercises?
    1 Tightening the muscles as if trying to prevent urination
    2 Contracting the abdominal, gluteal, and perineal muscles
    3 Tightening the rectal sphincter while relaxing abdominal muscles
    4 Performing the Valsalva maneuver

23. The client newly diagnosed with chronic renal failure (CRF) has many learning needs about the disease. The nurse prepares a teaching plan for this client to help the client adapt to the disease. The nurse recognizes that which of the following

items pertaining to the client's situation is least likely to interfere with the client's ability to learn?
1 Anxiety
2 Memory deficits
3 Short attention span
4 Presence of family

24. The client with renal failure has a medication order for epoetin alfa (EPO). The nurse administers this medication
1 Subcutaneously
2 Intramuscularly
3 With a full glass of water
4 Diluted in juice to enhance the taste

25. The nurse is working with a client newly diagnosed with chronic renal failure to set up a schedule for hemodialysis. The client states, "This is impossible! How can I even think about leading a normal life again if this is what I'm going to have to do?" The nurse determines that the client is exhibiting
1 Withdrawal
2 Depression
3 Anger
4 Projection

26. The client newly diagnosed with chronic renal failure has recently begun hemodialysis. Knowing that the client is at risk for disequilibrium syndrome, the nurse monitors the client for which of the following?
1 Hypertension, tachycardia, and fever
2 Hypotension, bradycardia, and hypothermia
3 Restlessness, irritability, and generalized weakness
4 Headache, deteriorating level of consciousness, and seizures

27. The client with chronic renal failure has been on dialysis for 3 years. The client is receiving the usual combination of medications for the disease, including aluminum hydroxide as a phosphate-binding agent. The client now presents with mental cloudiness, dementia, and complaints of bone pain. The nurse interprets that these data are compatible with
1 Phosphate overdose
2 Aluminum intoxication
3 Advancing uremia
4 Folic acid deficiency

28. The hemodialysis client with a left arm fistula is at risk for arterial steal syndrome. The nurse monitors this client for which of the following manifestations?
1 Warmth, redness, and pain in the left hand
2 Pallor, diminished pulse, and pain in the left hand

3 Edema and purplish discoloration of the left arm
4 Aching pain, pallor, and edema of the left arm

29. The nurse is reviewing the medical record of a client with a diagnosis of pyelonephritis. Which of the following disorders, if noted on the client's record, does the nurse identify as a risk factor for this disorder?
1 Hypoglycemia
2 Coronary artery disease
3 Diabetes mellitus
4 Orthostatic hypotension

30. The nurse is reviewing the client's record and notes that the physician has documented that the client has a renal disorder. On review of the laboratory results, the nurse most likely expects to note which of the following?
1 Elevated BUN
2 Decreased hemoglobin
3 Decreased RBC count
4 Decreased WBC count

31. A nursing assistant collects a urine specimen from a client and is planning to deliver the specimen to the laboratory after completing morning care to other assigned clients. The licensed practical nurse (LPN) instructs the nursing assistant to place the collected specimen in the refrigerator. The nursing assistant asks the LPN why the urine needs refrigeration. The LPN bases the response on the fact that when urine is allowed to stand unrefrigerated
1 The urine becomes more acidic
2 Bacteria and WBCs decompose
3 The urine clumps
4 The pH decreases

32. The nurse is collecting a 24-hour urine specimen from the client. Which of the following is an inaccurate action when collecting the specimen?
1 Asking the client to void, saving the specimen, and noting the start time
2 Discarding the urine specimen at the start time
3 Placing the specimen on ice or refrigerating it
4 Asking the client to void at the end of the collection and adding this to the collection

33. Which of the following does the nurse include in the plan of care for a client following a renal scan?
1 Place the client on radiation precautions for 18 hours
2 Save all urine in a radiation-safe container for 18 hours
3 Limit contact with the client to 20 minutes per hour
4 No special precautions except to wear gloves if coming in contact with the client's urine

34. The client is scheduled for an intravenous pyelogram (IVP). Prior to the test, the priority nursing action is to
    1 Administer an oral preparation of radiopaque dye
    2 Restrict fluids
    3 Determine a history of allergies
    4 Administer a sedative

35. The nurse instructs the client to obtain a clean-catch urine culture. Which of the following statements, if made by the client, indicates that the client understands the procedure for collecting the specimen?
    1 To empty the bladder into a container so that the full amount of urine can be determined
    2 That a urine specimen will be obtained from a catheter
    3 To cleanse the labia using cleansing towels, void into toilet, and then void into a sterile specimen container
    4 To clean the labia with toilet paper and void into a sterile specimen container

36. Following a renal biopsy, the client complains of pain at the biopsy site, which radiates to the front of the abdomen. The nurse interprets this complaint and further monitors the client for
    1 Bleeding
    2 Infection
    3 Renal colic
    4 A normal expected pain

37. A client is admitted to the hospital and has a diagnosis of early stage of chronic renal failure (CRF). Which of the following does the nurse expect to note on data collection of the client?
    1 Polyuria
    2 Polydypsia
    3 Oliguria
    4 Anuria

38. The nurse is reviewing the medication record of a client diagnosed with CRF. The nurse notes that the client is receiving aluminum hydroxide (Amphojel). The nurse determines that the purpose of this medication is to
    1 Combine with phosphorus and help eliminate phosphates from the body
    2 Prevent ulcers
    3 Promote the elimination of potassium from the body
    4 Prevent constipation

39. The nurse is assisting a client on a low-potassium diet to select food items from the menu. Which of the following food items, if selected by the client, indicates an understanding of this dietary restriction?
    1 Cantaloupe
    2 Spinach
    3 Lima beans
    4 Strawberries

40. The nurse is caring for an 88-year-old woman suspected of having a urinary tract infection (UTI). Which of the following symptoms, if noted in the client, alerts the nurse to the possibility of the presence of a UTI?
    1 Fever
    2 Frequency
    3 Confusion
    4 Urgency

41. The nurse is providing dietary instructions to a client with a diagnosis of acute glomerulonephritis. Which of the following dietary measures is included in the instructions?
    1 Limit fluid intake
    2 Restrict protein intake
    3 Increase the intake of high-fiber foods
    4 Increase the intake of potassium-rich foods

42. The client passes a urinary stone, and laboratory analysis of the stone indicates that it is composed of calcium oxalate. Based on this analysis, which of the following does the nurse include in the dietary instructions?
    1 Increase intake of meat, fish, plums, and cranberries
    2 Avoid citrus fruits and citrus juices
    3 Avoid green, leafy vegetables such as spinach
    4 Increase intake of dairy products

43. The nurse is performing an admission assessment on a client with a diagnosis of bladder cancer. Which of the following symptoms does the nurse most likely expect to note on assessment of this client?
    1 Hematuria
    2 Burning
    3 Urgency
    4 Frequency

44. The client with benign prostatic hypertrophy (BPH) undergoes a transurethral resection (TUR). Postoperatively the client is receiving continuous bladder irrigations. The nurse assesses the client for signs of TUR syndrome. Which of the following data indicates the onset of this syndrome?
    1 Bradycardia and confusion
    2 Tachycardia and diarrhea
    3 Decreased urinary output and bladder spasms
    4 Increased urinary output and anemia

45. The client with prostatitis secondary to kidney infection has received instructions on management of the condition at home and prevention of recurrence. The nurse evaluates that the client understands the instructions if the client verbalizes to
    1 Keep fluid intake to a minimum to decrease the need to void
    2 Exercise as much as possible to stimulate circulation
    3 Stop antibiotic therapy when pain subsides
    4 Use warm sitz baths and analgesics to increase comfort

ANSWERS

1. **4**

RATIONALE: The appropriate procedure if the client complains of pain after insertion is to remove the catheter after deflating the balloon and replace it with another one. This is preferred to option 3, which could make the client more at risk for developing urinary tract infection, since the catheter would be advanced after part of it was resting against the client's external genitalia. Options 1 and 2 are incorrect.

TEST-TAKING STRATEGY: Options 1 and 2 are the least plausible, and should be eliminated first. You would be able to discriminate correctly between options 3 and 4 using principles of aseptic technique.

LEVEL OF COGNITIVE ABILITY: Application
PHASE OF NURSING PROCESS: Planning
CLIENT NEEDS: Physiological Integrity
CONTENT AREA: Adult Health/Renal
REFERENCE
Taylor, C., Lillis, C., & LeMone, P. (1997). *Fundamentals of nursing: The art and science of nursing care* (3rd ed.). Philadelphia: Lippincott-Raven. p. 1237.

2. **1**

RATIONALE: A urine specimen is not taken from the urinary drainage bag. Urine undergoes chemical changes while sitting in the bag, and does not necessarily reflect current client status. In addition, it may become contaminated with bacteria from opening the system.

TEST-TAKING STRATEGY: This question tests a core principle of asepsis. If this question was difficult in any way, take a few moments now to review this key area of nursing practice.

LEVEL OF COGNITIVE ABILITY: Application
PHASE OF NURSING PROCESS: Planning
CLIENT NEEDS: Safe, Effective Care Environment
CONTENT AREA: Adult Health/Renal
REFERENCE
Black, J., & Matassarin-Jacobs, E. (1997). *Medical-surgical nursing: Clinical management for continuity of care* (5th ed.). Philadelphia: W. B. Saunders. pp. 1555–1556.

3. **4**

RATIONALE: Following renal biopsy, the nurse ensures that the client remains in bed for at least 24 hours. Vital signs and puncture site assessments are done frequently during this time. Forcing fluids is done to reduce possible clot formation at the biopsy site. Serial urine samples are hematested with urine dipsticks to evaluate bleeding. Narcotic analgesics are often needed to manage the renal colic pain that some clients feel after this procedure.

TEST-TAKING STRATEGY: Begin to answer this question by recalling that pain and bleeding are potential concerns after this procedure. This allows you to eliminate options 2 and 3. To discriminate between the last two options, you need to recall that forcing fluids will reduce clotting at the site, while ambulation could initiate or enhance bleeding at the biopsy site.

LEVEL OF COGNITIVE ABILITY: Application
PHASE OF NURSING PROCESS: Implementation
CLIENT NEEDS: Physiological Integrity
CONTENT AREA: Adult Health/Renal
REFERENCE
Black, J., & Matassarin-Jacobs, E. (1997). *Medical-surgical nursing: Clinical management for continuity of care* (5th ed.). Philadelphia: W. B. Saunders. p. 1569.

4. **4**

RATIONALE: Proper care of an indwelling catheter is especially important to prevent prolonged infection or reinfection in the client with cystitis. The nurse and all caregivers must use strict aseptic technique when emptying the drainage bag or obtaining urine specimens. The perineal area is cleansed thoroughly using mild soap and water at least twice a day and following a bowel movement. The drainage bag is kept below the level of the bladder to prevent urine from being trapped in the bladder, and for the same reason, the drainage tubing is not placed under the client's leg. The tubing must drain freely at all times.

TEST-TAKING STRATEGY: The wording of the question guides you to look for an incorrect response. Eliminate option 1 first, because this is a basic standard of care for the client with an indwelling catheter. Option 3 is also consistent with principles of asepsis, and is eliminated next. To discriminate between options 2 and 4, recall that option 2 promotes drainage, while option 4 could impede drainage. Thus the answer to the question is option 4, according to the wording of the question.

LEVEL OF COGNITIVE ABILITY: Application
PHASE OF NURSING PROCESS: Implementation
CLIENT NEEDS: Safe, Effective Care Environment
CONTENT AREA: Adult Health/Renal
REFERENCE
Black, J., & Matassarin-Jacobs, E. (1997). *Medical-surgical nursing: Clinical management for continuity of care* (5th ed.). Philadelphia: W. B. Saunders. p. 1573.

5. **2**

RATIONALE: Foods that are allowed on an acid ash diet include meat, fish, shellfish, cheese, eggs, poultry, grains, cranberries, prunes, plums, corn, lentils, and foods with high amounts of chlorine, phosphorus, and sulfur. Foods not included are milk and all milk products; all other vegetables except corn and lentils; all fruits except cranberries, plums, and prunes; and foods containing high amounts of sodium, potassium, calcium, and magnesium.

TEST-TAKING STRATEGY: This question is difficult to answer without specific knowledge of the types of foods that may be included in the acid ash diet. Knowing that most fruits and vegetables are not included on the list may help you to eliminate options 3 and 4. To discriminate between options 1 and 2, it is necessary to know that foods such as meat, fish, cheese, and eggs are included, while milk and milk products are not.

LEVEL OF COGNITIVE ABILITY: Application
PHASE OF NURSING PROCESS: Implementation
CLIENT NEEDS: Health Promotion and Maintenance
CONTENT AREA: Adult Health/Renal
REFERENCE
Black, J., & Matassarin-Jacobs, E. (1997). *Medical-surgical nursing: Clinical management for continuity of care* (5th ed.). Philadelphia: W. B. Saunders. p. 1577.

6. **1**

RATIONALE: The pain experienced with pyelonephritis usually resolves as antibiotic therapy becomes effective. However, clients may be treated for urinary tract pain with phenazopyridine, which is a urinary analgesic. Bethanechol chloride is a cholinergic agent used with neurogenic bladder, or for urinary retention. Oxybutinin and propantheline bromide are antispasmodics that are used to treat bladder spasm.

TEST-TAKING STRATEGY: Specific knowledge of the classifications of these medications is necessary to answer this question correctly. If this question was difficult, take a few moments to review these medications now.
LEVEL OF COGNITIVE ABILITY: Comprehension
PHASE OF NURSING PROCESS: Planning
CLIENT NEEDS: Physiological Integrity
CONTENT AREA: Pharmacology
REFERENCE
Black, J., & Matassarin-Jacobs, E. (1997). *Medical-surgical nursing: Clinical management for continuity of care* (5th ed.). Philadelphia: W. B. Saunders. pp. 1576, 1629.

7. **1**

RATIONALE: Foods containing high amounts of purines should be avoided in the client with uric acid stones. This includes limiting or avoiding organ meats, such as liver, brain, heart, kidney, and sweetbreads. Other foods to avoid include herring, sardines, anchovies, meat extracts, consommés, and gravies. Foods that are low in purines include all fruits, many vegetables, milk, cheese, eggs, refined cereals, sugars and sweets, coffee, tea, chocolate, and carbonated beverages.
TEST-TAKING STRATEGY: To answer this question, begin by examining the options and classifying the types of food sources they represent. Options 2 and 3 represent foods that are grown, whereas options 1 and 4 represent foods that derive from animal sources. Since purines are end products of protein metabolism, eliminate options 2 and 3 first. To discriminate between options 1 and 4, you need to know that organ meats such as liver provide a greater quantity of protein than milk. With this in mind, choose option 1 over option 4.
LEVEL OF COGNITIVE ABILITY: Application
PHASE OF NURSING PROCESS: Implementation
CLIENT NEEDS: Health Promotion and Maintenance
CONTENT AREA: Adult Health/Renal
REFERENCE
Lutz, C., & Przytulski, K. (1997). *Nutrition and diet therapy* (2nd ed.). Philadelphia: F. A. Davis. p. 400.

8. **3**

RATIONALE: Renal biopsy is a definitive test that gives specific information about whether the lesion is benign or malignant. An ultrasound discriminates between a fluid-filled cyst and a solid mass. Renal arteriography outlines the renal vascular system.
TEST-TAKING STRATEGY: Begin to answer this question by eliminating options 1 and 2 first. Basic knowledge of the purposes of biopsy helps you discard these quickly. To discriminate between options 3 and 4, remember that with biopsy the cells are examined under a microscope. This examination then yields specific information about the type of neoplastic cell. While some types of cancer grow more quickly than others, it is not possible to determine this by biopsy. Thus, you would choose option 3 as the better answer.
LEVEL OF COGNITIVE ABILITY: Comprehension
PHASE OF NURSING PROCESS: Planning
CLIENT NEEDS: Physiological Integrity
CONTENT AREA: Adult Health/Renal
REFERENCE
Black, J., & Matassarin-Jacobs, E. (1997). *Medical-surgical nursing: Clinical management for continuity of care* (5th ed.). Philadelphia: W. B. Saunders. p. 1671.

9. **4**

RATIONALE: The presence of blood at the urinary meatus may indicate urethral trauma or disruption. The nurse notifies the physician, knowing that the client should not be catheterized until the cause of the bleeding is determined by diagnostic testing.
TEST-TAKING STRATEGY: This question is straightforward in wording and intent. Basic knowledge of catheter insertion allows you to eliminate each of the incorrect options readily. If this question was difficult, take a few moments now to review this content area briefly.
LEVEL OF COGNITIVE ABILITY: Application
PHASE OF NURSING PROCESS: Implementation
CLIENT NEEDS: Physiological Integrity
CONTENT AREA: Adult Health/Renal
REFERENCE
Black, J., & Matassarin-Jacobs, E. (1997). *Medical-surgical nursing: Clinical management for continuity of care* (5th ed.). Philadelphia: W. B. Saunders. p. 1619.

10. **4**

RATIONALE: Urethritis in the male client often results from chlamydial infection, and is characterized by dysuria, which is accompanied by a clear to mucopurulent discharge. Because this disorder often coexists with gonorrhea, diagnostic tests are done for both, and include culture and rapid assays.
TEST-TAKING STRATEGY: Begin to answer this question by eliminating options 1 and 2. Urethritis is generally accompanied by dysuria in the male client, which is present only in options 3 and 4. Knowing that the problem originates in the urethra, not in the kidney, you can then eliminate the option with proteinuria, which indicates a problem with kidney function. This leaves option 4 as the correct answer. The male client with urethritis has dysuria and discharge from the penis.
LEVEL OF COGNITIVE ABILITY: Comprehension
PHASE OF NURSING PROCESS: Data Collection
CLIENT NEEDS: Physiological Integrity
CONTENT AREA: Adult Health/Renal
REFERENCE
Black, J., & Matassarin-Jacobs, E. (1997). *Medical-surgical nursing: Clinical management for continuity of care* (5th ed.). Philadelphia: W. B. Saunders. p. 2469.

11. **1**

RATIONALE: The most serious complication of chlamydial infection is sterility. The infection can be prevented by the use of latex condoms. It is treated with doxycycline for 7 days, or with azithromycin as a single dose. All sexual partners during the 30 days before diagnosis should be notified, examined, and treated as necessary.
TEST-TAKING STRATEGY: Eliminate option 2 first as a possible answer, using principles of infection control. Knowing that most courses of antibiotic therapy generally extend from 7 to 10 days may help you to eliminate option 3 next. To discriminate accurately between options 1 and 4, it is necessary to know either that sterility is a serious and permanent complication or that partners within the last month should be notified and treated as needed.
LEVEL OF COGNITIVE ABILITY: Application
PHASE OF NURSING PROCESS: Planning
CLIENT NEEDS: Health Promotion and Maintenance
CONTENT AREA: Adult Health/Renal
REFERENCE
Black, J., & Matassarin-Jacobs, E. (1997). *Medical-surgical nursing: Clinical management for continuity of care* (5th ed.). Philadelphia: W. B. Saunders. p. 2470.

12. **3**

RATIONALE: Chlamydial infection is a sexually transmitted disease, and is frequently called non-gonococcal urethritis in the male client. It requires no special precautions. Caregivers cannot acquire the disease during administration of care, and standard universal precautions is the only measure that needs to be used.

TEST-TAKING STRATEGY: This question is straightforward. A basic knowledge of infection control and disease transmission guides you to select option 3 as correct. If this question was difficult for you, take a few moments to review transmission of this disorder and universal precautions.

LEVEL OF COGNITIVE ABILITY: Comprehension
PHASE OF NURSING PROCESS: Implementation
CLIENT NEEDS: Safe, Effective Care Environment
CONTENT AREA: Adult Health/Renal
REFERENCE
Black, J., & Matassarin-Jacobs, E. (1997). *Medical-surgical nursing: Clinical management for continuity of care* (5th ed.). Philadelphia: W. B. Saunders. p. 2470.

13. **4**

RATIONALE: Antibiotics are not taken prophylactically to prevent acquisition of urethritis from *Chlamydia*. The risk of reinfection can be reduced by limiting the number of sexual partners and by the use of condoms. In some instances, follow-up culture is requested in 4 to 7 days to confirm a cure.

TEST-TAKING STRATEGY: The wording of the question guides you to look for an incorrect response. Options 1 and 2 are the most obviously correct and are therefore eliminated as possible answers to the question. Knowing the basic principles of antibiotic therapy allows you to choose option 4, since antibiotics are not used intermittently at will for prophylaxis of this infection.

LEVEL OF COGNITIVE ABILITY: Comprehension
PHASE OF NURSING PROCESS: Evaluation
CLIENT NEEDS: Health Promotion and Maintenance
CONTENT AREA: Adult Health/Renal
REFERENCE
Black, J., & Matassarin-Jacobs, E. (1997). *Medical-surgical nursing: Clinical management for continuity of care* (5th ed.). Philadelphia: W. B. Saunders. p. 2470.

14. **2**

RATIONALE: Typical signs and symptoms of epididymitis include scrotal pain and edema, which are often accompanied by fever, nausea and vomiting, and chills. It is most often caused by infection, although sometimes it can be caused by trauma. It needs to be correctly distinguished from testicular torsion.

TEST-TAKING STRATEGY: Any disorder that ends in "itis" results from inflammation or infection. Therefore, an expected finding is elevated temperature. With this in mind, eliminate options 3 and 4, because they do not contain fever as part of the response. Knowing that ecchymosis results from bleeding, which is not part of this clinical picture, helps you to choose option 2 over option 1 as the answer.

LEVEL OF COGNITIVE ABILITY: Comprehension
PHASE OF NURSING PROCESS: Data Collection
CLIENT NEEDS: Physiological Integrity
CONTENT AREA: Adult Health/Renal

REFERENCE
Black, J., & Matassarin-Jacobs, E. (1997). *Medical-surgical nursing: Clinical management for continuity of care* (5th ed.). Philadelphia: W. B. Saunders. p. 2381.

15. **3**

RATIONALE: The client who receives a narcotic analgesic should immediately have the side rails raised on the bed to prevent injury once the medication has taken effect. Dimming the light in the room is the next most helpful action. The name bracelet should have been checked before administering the medication. It is unnecessary to do range of motion to the site of injection.

TEST-TAKING STRATEGY: Begin to answer this question by eliminating option 2, because this should have been done before administering the medication. Option 1 is not necessary, and may be eliminated next. To discriminate between options 3 and 4, note that the question asks you for the action to be taken next. With this in mind, you would choose option 3 over option 4. Although option 4 is a correct answer, it would be done upon leaving the room. As part of protecting the client's safety after administration of a narcotic analgesic, you would put the side rails up first.

LEVEL OF COGNITIVE ABILITY: Application
PHASE OF NURSING PROCESS: Implementation
CLIENT NEEDS: Safe, Effective Care Environment
CONTENT AREA: Adult Health/Renal
REFERENCE
Black, J., & Matassarin-Jacobs, E. (1997). *Medical-surgical nursing: Clinical management for continuity of care* (5th ed.). Philadelphia: W. B. Saunders. p. 2381.

16. **4**

RATIONALE: Common interventions used in the treatment of epididymitis include bed rest, elevation of the scrotum with a Bellevue bridge, ice packs, sitz baths, analgesics, and antibiotics. A heating pad is not used because direct application of heat could increase blood flow to the area and increase the swelling.

TEST-TAKING STRATEGY: Begin to answer this question by eliminating options 1 and 2, because they are obviously the most helpful in the care of the client. In examining options 3 and 4, note that they both address the application of heat to the client. A sitz bath uses a milder temperature and the heat is moist and soothing. Knowing that direct heat may increase inflammation with tissue that is already at risk would guide you to choose option 4 as the item to avoid.

LEVEL OF COGNITIVE ABILITY: Application
PHASE OF NURSING PROCESS: Implementation
CLIENT NEEDS: Physiological Integrity
CONTENT AREA: Adult Health/Renal
REFERENCE
Black, J., & Matassarin-Jacobs, E. (1997). *Medical-surgical nursing: Clinical management for continuity of care* (5th ed.). Philadelphia: W. B. Saunders. p. 2381.

17. **2**

RATIONALE: The client who experiences epididymitis from urinary tract infection should increase intake of fluids to flush the urinary system. Since organisms can be forced into the vas deferens and epididymis from strain or pressure during voiding, the client should limit the force of the stream. Condom use can help to prevent urethritis and epididymitis from STDs. Antibiotics are always taken until the full course of therapy is completed.

TEST-TAKING STRATEGY: The wording of the question guides you to look for an incorrect response. Since option 1 is consistent with good practices in the prevention of UTI, this option may be eliminated first. To eliminate options 3 and 4, it is necessary to know that the force of stream should be limited to prevent backflow into the epididymis, and that condoms are helpful in preventing this disorder from occurring as a complication of an STD. Remember that antibiotics are not stopped when symptoms subside, but must be taken until the full course of therapy is completed.
LEVEL OF COGNITIVE ABILITY: Comprehension
PHASE OF NURSING PROCESS: Evaluation
CLIENT NEEDS: Health Promotion and Maintenance
CONTENT AREA: Adult Health/Renal
REFERENCE

Black, J., & Matassarin-Jacobs, E. (1997). *Medical-surgical nursing: Clinical management for continuity of care* (5th ed.). Philadelphia: W. B. Saunders. p. 2381.

18. **3**

RATIONALE: Occasionally, the client with acute prostatitis needs urinary catheterization if the client cannot void at all. Otherwise, catheterization is avoided to prevent introducing bacteria into the bladder by pushing them up the urethra. Catheterization does not prolong the course of the inflammation, nor does it cause rebound edema when it is discontinued. There is no reported risk of prostate gland puncture from this procedure, although it may be painful.
TEST-TAKING STRATEGY: Option 4 is the least plausible of all the choices and is eliminated first. Option 1 is also not very plausible and may be eliminated next. In comparing the remaining two responses, knowledge of transmission of infection guides you to choose option 3 over option 2.
LEVEL OF COGNITIVE ABILITY: Comprehension
PHASE OF NURSING PROCESS: Planning
CLIENT NEEDS: Physiological Integrity
CONTENT AREA: Adult Health/Renal
REFERENCE

Black, J., & Matassarin-Jacobs, E. (1997). *Medical-surgical nursing: Clinical management for continuity of care* (5th ed.). Philadelphia: W. B. Saunders. p. 2372.

19. **3**

RATIONALE: Decreased force in the stream of urine is an early sign of BPH. The stream later becomes weak and dribbling. The client may then develop hematuria, frequency, urgency, urge incontinence, and nocturia. If untreated, complete obstruction and urinary retention can occur.
TEST-TAKING STRATEGY: Note that the question asks for an early symptom. If you know that BPH can lead to urinary obstruction, you can then work backward from the most severe symptom to the least, which should also be the earliest. Option 4 is obviously the most severe of symptoms, and therefore is eliminated first. Options 1 and 2 are also more severe than option 3, which guides you to select option 3 as the answer to the question.
LEVEL OF COGNITIVE ABILITY: Comprehension
PHASE OF NURSING PROCESS: Data Collection
CLIENT NEEDS: Physiological Integrity
CONTENT AREA: Adult Health/Renal
REFERENCE

Black, J., & Matassarin-Jacobs, E. (1997). *Medical-surgical nursing: Clinical management for continuity of care* (5th ed.). Philadelphia: W. B. Saunders. p. 2352.

20. **4**

RATIONALE: In the client with BPH, episodes of urinary retention can be triggered by certain medications, such as decongestants, anticholinergics, and antidepressants. The client should be questioned about use of these medications if presenting with urinary retention. Retention can also be precipitated by other factors, such as alcoholic beverages, infection, bed rest, and becoming chilled.
TEST-TAKING STRATEGY: The question is asking you about medications that could exacerbate or contribute to urinary retention in the client with BPH. Diuretics help voiding, and therefore option 1 is readily eliminated. Antibiotics have no effect at all, and thus option 2 is eliminated as well. To discriminate between options 3 and 4, it is necessary to know that medications that contain anticholinergics may cause urinary retention. This guides you to choose option 4 over option 3 as the correct answer. Antitussives have no effect on urinary retention.
LEVEL OF COGNITIVE ABILITY: Comprehension
PHASE OF NURSING PROCESS: Data Collection
CLIENT NEEDS: Physiological Integrity
CONTENT AREA: Adult Health/Renal
REFERENCE

Black, J., & Matassarin-Jacobs, E. (1997). *Medical-surgical nursing: Clinical management for continuity of care* (5th ed.). Philadelphia: W. B. Saunders. p. 2352.

21. **1**

RATIONALE: A transrectal ultrasound and PSA level help to rule out the possibility of prostate cancer. They do not predict the course of BPH or the development of complications such as urinary obstruction. These tests have nothing to do with determining the need for self catheterization.
TEST-TAKING STRATEGY: Begin to answer this question by eliminating options 2 and 3. Diagnostic tests do not predict the course of a disease or the likelihood of developing complications (such as obstruction). Similarly, diagnostic tests will not determine whether self-catheterization is needed. Therefore, this option is eliminated as well. This leaves option 1 as the correct answer. Choose this option also by recalling that biopsy is done to rule out malignancy.
LEVEL OF COGNITIVE ABILITY: Comprehension
PHASE OF NURSING PROCESS: Implementation
CLIENT NEEDS: Physiological Integrity
CONTENT AREA: Adult Health/Renal
REFERENCE

Black, J., & Matassarin-Jacobs, E. (1997). *Medical-surgical nursing: Clinical management for continuity of care* (5th ed.). Philadelphia: W. B. Saunders. p. 2352.

22. **4**

RATIONALE: The Valsalva maneuver is avoided following prostatectomy because it increases the risk of bleeding in the postoperative period. An acceptable exercise is tightening the abdominal, gluteal, and perineal muscles, as if trying to prevent urination. Another acceptable exercise is tightening the rectal sphincter while relaxing the abdominal muscles; this prevents the Valsalva maneuver from occurring.
TEST-TAKING STRATEGY: Notice that the type of movement in the exercises described in options 1, 2, and 3 are all muscle-tightening movements. On the other hand, the Valsalva maneuver in option 4 involves bearing down or a pushing type of movement. Knowing that the answer to the question is not likely to be one that is similar to other

options, choose the Valsalva maneuver (option 4) as the item to avoid.
LEVEL OF COGNITIVE ABILITY: Comprehension
PHASE OF NURSING PROCESS: Evaluation
CLIENT NEEDS: Health Promotion and Maintenance
CONTENT AREA: Adult Health/Renal
REFERENCE

Black, J., & Matassarin-Jacobs, E. (1997). *Medical-surgical nursing: Clinical management for continuity of care* (5th ed.). Philadelphia: W. B. Saunders. p. 2363.

23. **4**

RATIONALE: The client with CRF may have several barriers to learning. Anxiety about the disease and its ramifications may frequently interfere with learning. Physiological effects of the disease process also impair the client's mental functioning. Specifically, the client may exhibit a short attention span and have memory deficits. This usually improves once hemodialysis has begun. The presence of family is helpful, since the family needs to understand the disease and treatment, and may help reinforce information with the client after the formal teaching session is over.
TEST-TAKING STRATEGY: This question asks for the least interfering variable. Knowing that anxiety commonly interferes with learning, you would eliminate option 1 first. Options 2 and 3 are similar in that they reflect neurological impairment. In this case, they are due to physiological effects of the disease on the nervous system. Recall that similar options are not likely to be correct. This leaves option 4 as the correct answer. The presence of family does not automatically interfere with learning; in fact, they may be quite helpful.
LEVEL OF COGNITIVE ABILITY: Comprehension
PHASE OF NURSING PROCESS: Data Collection
CLIENT NEEDS: Psychosocial Integrity
CONTENT AREA: Adult Health/Renal
REFERENCE

Black, J., & Matassarin-Jacobs, E. (1997). *Medical-surgical nursing: Clinical management for continuity of care* (5th ed.). Philadelphia: W. B. Saunders. p. 1657.

24. **1**

RATIONALE: Epoetin alfa is erythropoietin that has been manufactured through the use of recombinant DNA technology. It is used to treat anemia in the client with chronic renal failure. The medication may be administered subcutaneously or intravenously.
TEST-TAKING STRATEGY: Specific knowledge of epoetin alfa is necessary to answer this question. If the medication or its methods of administration are unfamiliar to you, take a few moments to review this medication.
LEVEL OF COGNITIVE ABILITY: Application
PHASE OF NURSING PROCESS: Implementation
CLIENT NEEDS: Physiological Integrity
CONTENT AREA: Pharmacology
REFERENCE

Black, J., & Matassarin-Jacobs, E. (1997). *Medical-surgical nursing: Clinical management for continuity of care* (5th ed.). Philadelphia: W. B. Saunders p. 1654.

25. **3**

RATIONALE: Psychosocial reactions to chronic renal failure and hemodialysis are varied, and may include anger. Other reactions include personality changes, emotional lability, withdrawal, and depression. The individual client's response may vary depending on the client's personality and support systems. The client in this question is exhibiting anger. The client has not projected blame on the nurse, nor does the client's statement reflect withdrawal or depression.
TEST-TAKING STRATEGY: A knowledge of basic communication theory helps you to answer this question. This helps you to eliminate each of the incorrect options systematically.
LEVEL OF COGNITIVE ABILITY: Comprehension
PHASE OF NURSING PROCESS: Data Collection
CLIENT NEEDS: Psychosocial Integrity
CONTENT AREA: Adult Health/Renal
REFERENCE

Black, J., & Matassarin-Jacobs, E. (1997). *Medical-surgical nursing: Clinical management for continuity of care* (5th ed.). Philadelphia: W. B. Saunders pp. 1646–1647.

26. **4**

RATIONALE: Disequilibrium syndrome is characterized by headache, mental confusion, decreasing level of consciousness, nausea, vomiting, twitching, and possible seizure activity. It is caused by rapid removal of solutes from the body during hemodialysis. At the same time, the blood-brain barrier interferes with the efficient removal of wastes from brain tissue. As a result, water goes into cerebral cells because of the osmotic gradient, causing brain swelling and onset of symptoms. It most often occurs in clients who are new to dialysis, and is prevented by dialyzing for shorter times or at reduced blood flow rates.
TEST-TAKING STRATEGY: Familiarity with the causes and symptoms of disequilibrium syndrome is necessary to answer this question correctly. If this question was difficult, take a few moments to review this syndrome.
LEVEL OF COGNITIVE ABILITY: Application
PHASE OF NURSING PROCESS: Data Collection
CLIENT NEEDS: Physiological Integrity
CONTENT AREA: Adult Health/Renal
REFERENCE

Black, J., & Matassarin-Jacobs, E. (1997). *Medical-surgical nursing: Clinical management for continuity of care* (5th ed.). Philadelphia: W. B. Saunders p. 1654.

27. **2**

RATIONALE: Aluminum intoxication may occur when there is accumulation of aluminum, an ingredient in many phosphate-binding antacids. It results in mental cloudiness, dementia, and bone pain from infiltration of the bone with aluminum. This condition was formerly known as dialysis dementia. It may be treated with aluminum chelating agents, which make aluminum available to be dialyzed from the body. It can be prevented by avoiding or limiting the use of phosphate-binding agents that contain aluminum.
TEST-TAKING STRATEGY: To answer this question correctly, it is necessary to understand the potential implications of long-term use of aluminum-containing phosphate-binding agents by the hemodialysis client. If this question was difficult, take a few moments to review this information now.
LEVEL OF COGNITIVE ABILITY: Comprehension
PHASE OF NURSING PROCESS: Data Collection
CLIENT NEEDS: Physiological Integrity
CONTENT AREA: Adult Health/Renal
REFERENCE

Black, J., & Matassarin-Jacobs, E. (1997). *Medical-surgical nursing: Clinical management for continuity of care* (5th ed.). Philadelphia: W. B. Saunders. p. 1654.

28. **2**

RATIONALE: Arterial steal syndrome results from vascular insufficiency after creation of a fistula. The client exhibits pallor and diminished pulse distal to the fistula and complains of pain distal to the fistula that is due to tissue ischemia. Warmth, redness, and pain more likely characterize a problem with infection. The patterns described in options 3 and 4 are incorrect.
TEST-TAKING STRATEGY: Knowledge of arterial steal syndrome and its signs and symptoms is needed to answer this question correctly. If needed, take a few moments now to review this material.
LEVEL OF COGNITIVE ABILITY: Comprehension
PHASE OF NURSING PROCESS: Data Collection
CLIENT NEEDS: Physiological Integrity
CONTENT AREA: Adult Health/Renal
REFERENCE
Luckmann, J. (1997). *Saunders manual of nursing care*. Philadelphia: W. B. Saunders. p. 1195.

29. **3**

RATIONALE: Risk factors associated with pyelonephritis include diabetes mellitus, hypertension, chronic renal calculi, chronic cystitis, structural abnormalities of the urinary tract, presence of urinary stones, and indwelling or frequent urinary catheterization.
TEST-TAKING STRATEGY: Eliminate options 1 and 4 first as least likely risk factors. From the remaining options, remember that diabetes mellitus can cause renal complications. This will assist in directing you to the correct option.
LEVEL OF COGNITIVE ABILITY: Comprehension
PHASE OF NURSING PROCESS: Data Collection
CLIENT NEEDS: Health Promotion and Maintenance
CONTENT AREA: Adult Health/Renal
REFERENCE
Black, J., & Matassarin-Jacobs, E. (1997). *Medical-surgical nursing: Clinical management for continuity of care* (5th ed.). Philadelphia: W. B. Saunders. p. 1628.

30. **1**

RATIONALE: BUN is the most frequently used laboratory test to determine renal function. The BUN starts to rise when the glomerular filtration rate falls below 40%. A decreased hemoglobin and RBC count may be noted if bleeding from the urinary tract occurs or if erythropoietic function by the kidney is impaired. An increased WBC is most likely to be noted in renal disease.
TEST-TAKING STRATEGY: Note the key words "most likely expects to note" in the stem of the question. Eliminate option 4 first. Although options 2 and 3 may be noted in some renal disorders, option 1 is the most likely laboratory finding. Review significant laboratory tests now if you had difficulty with this question.
LEVEL OF COGNITIVE ABILITY: Comprehension
PHASE OF NURSING PROCESS: Data Collection
CLIENT NEEDS: Physiological Integrity
CONTENT AREA: Adult Health/Renal
REFERENCE
Black, J., & Matassarin-Jacobs, E. (1997). *Medical-surgical nursing: Clinical management for continuity of care* (5th ed.). Philadelphia: W. B. Saunders. p. 1562.

31. **2**

RATIONALE: Refrigeration preserves the elements of urine, but the delay in testing can cause crystals to precipitate. If the specimen stands at room temperature, the warmth causes bacteria and WBCs to decompose. When urine is allowed to stand unrefrigerated, the urea breaks down to ammonia and becomes more alkaline. The pH decreases in an acidic condition.
TEST-TAKING STRATEGY: Careful reading will assist you to easily eliminate option 3. Eliminate options 1 and 4 next because they are similar. pH decreases in acidic conditions. This leaves option 2 as the likely option.
LEVEL OF COGNITIVE ABILITY: Comprehension
PHASE OF NURSING PROCESS: Implementation
CLIENT NEEDS: Physiological Integrity
CONTENT AREA: Adult Health/Renal
REFERENCE
McMorrow, M. E., & Malarkey, L. (1998). *Laboratory and diagnostic tests: A pocket guide*. Philadelphia: W. B. Saunders. p. 329.

32. **1**

RATIONALE: Since the 24-hour urine is a timed quantitative determination, it is essential to start the test with an empty bladder. The urine collection should be refrigerated or placed on ice to prevent changes in urine. Fifteen minutes prior to the end of the collection time, the client should be asked to void and this specimen is added to the collection.
TEST-TAKING STRATEGY: Note that options 1 and 2 are addressing the same issue and are different in regards to this procedure. This would lead you to think that one of these options is the correct option. Try to think about the purpose of this timed test and eliminate option 2 because it would make sense that this test should be started when the client has an empty bladder. Review this procedure now if you had difficulty with this question.
LEVEL OF COGNITIVE ABILITY: Application
PHASE OF NURSING PROCESS: Implementation
CLIENT NEEDS: Physiological Integrity
CONTENT AREA: Adult Health/Renal
REFERENCE
McMorrow, M. E., & Malarkey, L. (1998). *Laboratory and diagnostic tests: A pocket guide*. Philadelphia: W. B. Saunders. p. 329.

33. **4**

RATIONALE: There are no specific precautions following a renal scan. If the client is able, urination into a commode is acceptable without risk from the small amount of radioactive material to be excreted. The nurse wears gloves to maintain body secretion precautions.
TEST-TAKING STRATEGY: Knowledge regarding the renal scan is required to answer this question. Knowing that there is generally no danger from the small amount of radioactive material used in this procedure will easily direct you to option 4. Review this procedure now if you had difficulty with this question.
LEVEL OF COGNITIVE ABILITY: Application
PHASE OF NURSING PROCESS: Planning
CLIENT NEEDS: Safe, Effective Care Environment
CONTENT AREA: Adult Health/Renal
REFERENCE
Ignatavicius, D., Workman, M., & Mishler, M. (1999). *Medical-surgical nursing across the health care continuum* (3rd ed.). Philadelphia: W. B. Saunders. p. 1815.

34. **3**

RATIONALE: The iodine-based dye used during the IVP can cause allergic reactions such as itching, hives, rash, tight feeling in the throat, shortness of breath, and broncho-spasm. Assessing for allergies is the priority.

TEST-TAKING STRATEGY: Note the key word "priority" in the stem of the question. Use the nursing process as a guide. Options 1, 2, and 4 address implementation. Option 3 is the only option that addresses data collection.
LEVEL OF COGNITIVE ABILITY: Application
PHASE OF NURSING PROCESS: Implementation
CLIENT NEEDS: Physiological Integrity
CONTENT AREA: Adult Health/Renal
REFERENCE
Chernecky, C., & Berger, B. (1997). *Laboratory tests and diagnostic procedures* (2nd ed.). Philadelphia: W. B. Saunders. p. 643.

35. **3**

RATIONALE: Urine specimens for cultures should be obtained using proper cleansing and voiding techniques to avoid contamination from external sources. The use of paper towels will contaminate the specimen. The procedure described in option 1 would not provide a clean specimen. It is not necessary to obtain the specimen via a catheter.
TEST-TAKING STRATEGY: Note the key words "clean catch." These words should assist in eliminating options 1 and 4 and easily direct you to option 3. If you had difficulty with this question, take time now to review the procedure for this type of urine collection.
LEVEL OF COGNITIVE ABILITY: Comprehension
PHASE OF NURSING PROCESS: Evaluation
CLIENT NEEDS: Safe, Effective Care Environment
CONTENT AREA: Adult Health/Renal
REFERENCE
Leahy, J., & Kizilay, P. (1998). *Foundations of nursing practice: A nursing process approach.* Philadelphia: W. B. Saunders. p. 416.

36. **1**

RATIONALE: If pain originates at the biopsy site and begins to radiate to the flank area and around the front of the abdomen, bleeding should be suspected. Hypotension, a decreasing hematocrit, and gross or microscopic hematuria would also indicate bleeding. Signs of infection would not appear immediately following a biopsy. Pain of this nature is not normal. There are no data to support the presence of renal colic.
TEST-TAKING STRATEGY: You can easily eliminate options 3 and 4. Recalling that signs of infection may not appear immediately following biopsy will assist in directing you to option 1.
LEVEL OF COGNITIVE ABILITY: Comprehension
PHASE OF NURSING PROCESS: Data Collection
CLIENT NEEDS: Physiological Integrity
CONTENT AREA: Adult Health/Renal
REFERENCE
Black, J., & Matassarin-Jacobs, E. (1997). *Medical-surgical nursing: Clinical management for continuity of care* (5th ed.). Philadelphia: W. B. Saunders. p. 1569.

37. **1**

RATIONALE: Polyuria occurs early in CRF and if untreated can cause severe dehydration. Polyuria progresses to anuria, and the client loses all normal functions of the kidney. Oliguria and anuria are not early signs, and polydypsia is unrelated to CRF.
TEST-TAKING STRATEGY: Note the key word "early" in the question. Eliminate options 3 and 4 because they are similar. From the remaining options select option 1 because

this option relates to renal function and is the correct answer to this question. Review the early and the later signs of CRF now if you had difficulty with this question.
LEVEL OF COGNITIVE ABILITY: Comprehension
PHASE OF NURSING PROCESS: Data Collection
CLIENT NEEDS: Physiological Integrity
CONTENT AREA: Adult Health/Renal
REFERENCE
Black, J., & Matassarin-Jacobs, E. (1997). *Medical-surgical nursing: Clinical management for continuity of care* (5th ed.). Philadelphia: W. B. Saunders. p. 1644.

38. **1**

RATIONALE: Amphojel binds with phosphate in the intestines to be excreted in the feces, thus lowering phosphorus levels. It can cause constipation and it does not promote the elimination of potassium. It may be used in the treatment of hyperacidity associated with gastric ulcers, but this is not the purpose of its use in the client with renal failure.
TEST-TAKING STRATEGY: Knowledge regarding the purpose of this medication in CRF is required to answer this question. If you are unfamiliar with this medication, review now.
LEVEL OF COGNITIVE ABILITY: Comprehension
PHASE OF NURSING PROCESS: Planning
CLIENT NEEDS: Physiological Integrity
CONTENT AREA: Adult Health/Renal
REFERENCE
Hodgson, B., & Kizior, R. (2000). *Saunders nursing drug handbook 2000.* Philadelphia: W. B. Saunders. p. 34.

39. **3**

RATIONALE: Cantaloupe (1/4 small), spinach (1/2 cup cooked) and strawberries (1 1/4 cups) are high-potassium foods and average 7 mEq per serving. Lima beans (1/3 cup) average 3 mEq per serving.
TEST-TAKING STRATEGY: Use the process of elimination, remembering that many fruits and green, leafy vegetables are high in potassium. This may assist in directing you to option 3.
LEVEL OF COGNITIVE ABILITY: Comprehension
PHASE OF NURSING PROCESS: Evaluation
CLIENT NEEDS: Health Promotion and Maintenance
CONTENT AREA: Adult Health/Renal
REFERENCE
Black, J., & Matassarin-Jacobs, E. (1997). *Medical-surgical nursing: Clinical management for continuity of care* (5th ed.). Philadelphia: W. B. Saunders. p. 313.

40. **3**

RATIONALE: In an elderly client, the only symptom of a UTI may be something as vague as increasing mental confusion or frequent unexplained falls. Frequency and urgency may commonly occur in an elderly client and fever can be associated with a variety of conditions.
TEST-TAKING STRATEGY: Note the client's age in the question. Eliminate options 2 and 4 because they may commonly occur in an elderly client. Eliminate option 1 next because fever can be associated with a variety of conditions. Review clinical manifestations of UTI that occur in the elderly now if you had difficulty with this question.
LEVEL OF COGNITIVE ABILITY: Comprehension
PHASE OF NURSING PROCESS: Data Collection
CLIENT NEEDS: Physiological Integrity
CONTENT AREA: Adult Health/Renal

REFERENCE
Ignatavicius, D., Workman, M., & Mishler, M. (1999). *Medical-surgical nursing across the health care continuum* (3rd ed.). Philadelphia: W. B. Saunders. p. 1822.

41. 2

RATIONALE: In acute glomerulonephritis it is important to protect the kidneys while they are recovering their function. The diet is generally high-calorie and low-protein. This diet avoids protein catabolism and allows the kidneys to rest.
TEST-TAKING STRATEGY: Knowledge regarding the treatment measures in acute glomerulonephritis is required to answer this question. Recalling that protein increases the workload of the kidneys will assist in directing you to option 2.
LEVEL OF COGNITIVE ABILITY: Application
PHASE OF NURSING PROCESS: Implementation
CLIENT NEEDS: Health Promotion and Maintenance
CONTENT AREA: Adult Health/Renal
REFERENCE
Black, J., & Matassarin-Jacobs, E. (1997). *Medical-surgical nursing: Clinical management for continuity of care* (5th ed.). Philadelphia: W. B. Saunders. p. 1632.

42. 3

RATIONALE: Oxalate is found in dark green foods such as spinach. Other foods that raise urinary oxalate are rhubarb, strawberries, chocolate, wheat bran, nuts, beets, and tea.
TEST-TAKING STRATEGY: Knowledge regarding the foods that raise urinary oxalate will assist in answering this question. Remembering that green, leafy foods are high in oxalate will assist in directing you to option 3. Review these foods now if you had difficulty with this question.
LEVEL OF COGNITIVE ABILITY: Application
PHASE OF NURSING PROCESS: Implementation
CLIENT NEEDS: Health Promotion and Maintenance
CONTENT AREA: Adult Health/Renal
REFERENCE
Ignatavicius, D., Workman, M., & Mishler, M. (1999). *Medical surgical nursing across the health care continuum* (3rd ed.). Philadelphia: W. B. Saunders. p. 1839.

43. 1

RATIONALE: Gross, painless hematuria is most frequently the first manifestation of bladder cancer. As the disease progresses the client may experience dysuria, frequency, and urgency.
TEST-TAKING STRATEGY: The issue of the question relates specifically to bladder cancer. Focusing on this issue should easily direct you to option 1. If you are unfamiliar with the specific manifestations associated with bladder cancer, review now.

LEVEL OF COGNITIVE ABILITY: Comprehension
PHASE OF NURSING PROCESS: Data Collection
CLIENT NEEDS: Physiological Integrity
CONTENT AREA: Adult Health/Renal
REFERENCE
Black, J., & Matassarin-Jacobs, E. (1997). *Medical-surgical nursing: Clinical management for continuity of care* (5th ed.). Philadelphia: W. B. Saunders. p. 1583.

44. 1

RATIONALE: TUR syndrome is caused by increased absorption of nonelectrolyte irrigating fluid used during surgery. The client may show signs of cerebral edema and increased intracranial pressure such as increased blood pressure, bradycardia, confusion, disorientation, muscle twitching, visual disturbances, and nausea and vomiting.
TEST-TAKING STRATEGY: Knowledge regarding TUR syndrome is required to answer this question. If you can recall that increased intracranial pressure is the concern, you can be easily directed to option 1. Review this disorder now if you had difficulty with this question.
LEVEL OF COGNITIVE ABILITY: Comprehension
PHASE OF NURSING PROCESS: Data Collection
CLIENT NEEDS: Physiological Integrity
CONTENT AREA: Adult Health/Renal
REFERENCE
Monahan, F., & Neighbors, M. (1998). *Medical-surgical nursing: Foundations for clinical practice* (2nd ed.). Philadelphia: W. B. Saunders. p. 1712.

45. 4

RATIONALE: Treatment of prostatitis includes medication with antibiotics, analgesics, and stool softeners. The client is also taught to rest, increase fluid intake; and use sitz baths for comfort. Antimicrobial therapy is always continued until the prescription is completely finished.
TEST-TAKING STRATEGY: Eliminate option 3 first because stopping medication therapy before the end of the course is contraindicated. Option 1 is also eliminated, because fluid intake should be increased. To discriminate between the last two options correctly, it is necessary to understand that sitz baths provide comfort, or that rest is helpful in the healing process. Knowledge of either of these concepts helps you to choose option 4 as the correct answer.
LEVEL OF COGNITIVE ABILITY: Comprehension
PHASE OF NURSING PROCESS: Evaluation
CLIENT NEEDS: Health Promotion and Maintenance
CONTENT AREA: Adult Health/Renal
REFERENCE
Black, J., & Matassarin-Jacobs, E. (1997). *Medical-surgical nursing: Clinical management for continuity of care* (5th ed.). Philadelphia: W. B. Saunders. p. 2372.

BIBLIOGRAPHY

Black, J., & Matassarin-Jacobs, E. (1997). *Medical-surgical nursing: Clinical management for continuity of care* (5th ed.). Philadelphia: W. B. Saunders.

Chernecky, C., & Berger, B. (1997). *Laboratory tests and diagnostic procedures* (2nd ed.). Philadelphia: W. B. Saunders.

Cox, H., Hinz, M., Lubno, M., et al. (1997). *Clinical applications of nursing diagnosis: Adult, child, women's, psychiatric, gerontic and home health considerations* (3rd ed.). Philadelphia: F. A. Davis.

Hodgson, B., & Kizior, R. (2000). *Saunders nursing drug handbook 2000*. Philadelphia: W. B. Saunders.

Ignatavicius, D., Workman, M., & Mishler, M. (1999). *Medical-surgical nursing across the health care continuum* (3rd ed.). Philadelphia: W. B. Saunders.

Lehne, R. (1998). *Pharmacology for nursing care* (3rd ed.). Philadelphia: W. B. Saunders.

Leahy, J., & Kizilay, P. (1998). *Foundations of nursing practice: A nursing process approach*. Philadelphia: W. B. Saunders.

Luckmann, J. (1997). *Saunders manual of nursing care*. Philadelphia: W. B. Saunders.

Lutz, C., & Przytulski, K. (1997). *Nutrition and diet therapy* (2nd ed.). Philadelphia: F. A. Davis.

McMorrow, M. E., & Malarkey, L. (1998). *Laboratory and diagnostic tests: A pocket guide*. Philadelphia: W. B. Saunders.

Monahan, F., & Neighbors, M. (1998). *Medical-surgical nursing: Foundations for clinical practice* (2nd ed.). Philadelphia: W. B. Saunders.

O'Toole, M. (1997). *Miller-Keane encyclopedia & dictionary of medicine, nursing, & allied health* (6th ed.). Philadelphia: W. B. Saunders.

Taylor, C., Lillis, C., & LeMone, P. (1997). *Fundamentals of nursing: The art and science of nursing care* (3rd ed.). Philadelphia: Lippincott-Raven.

CHAPTER 51

Renal Medications

....

I. Urinary Tract Antiseptics (Box 51-1)

A. Description
  1. Inhibit the growth of bacteria in the urine
  2. Act as disinfectants within urinary tract
  3. Used to treat urinary tract infections
  4. These medications do not achieve effective antibacterial concentrations in blood or tissues and therefore cannot be used for infections at sites outside the urinary tract

B. Side effects and nursing considerations
  1. Nitrofurantoin (Furadantin, Macrodantin, Macrobid)
    a. Gastrointestinal (GI) effects such as anorexia, nausea, vomiting, and diarrhea
    b. Pulmonary reactions such as dyspnea, chest pain, chills, fever, cough, and alveolar infiltrates
    c. Hematologic effects such as agranulocytosis, leukopenia, thrombocytopenia, and megaloblastic anemia
    d. Peripheral neuropathy such as muscle weakness, tingling sensations, and numbness
    e. Neurological effects such as headache, vertigo, drowsiness, and nystagmus
    f. Produces a harmless brown color to the urine
    g. Pulmonary reactions resolve in 2 to 4 days following cessation of treatment
    h. Administration with milk or meals will minimize GI distress
    i. Contraindicated in clients with renal impairment
    j. Instruct the client in expected side effects and those requiring notifying the physician
  2. Methenamine (Mandelamine, Hiprex, Urex)
    a. Relatively safe and well tolerated
    b. May cause gastric distress
    c. Chronic high-dose therapy can cause bladder irritation
    d. Can cause crystalluria and should not be used in clients with renal impairment
    e. Decomposition of medication generates ammonia; therefore, it should not be used for clients with liver dysfunction
    f. Requires acidic urine with pH of 5.5 or less
    g. Ingestion of large amounts of fluid will reduce antibacterial effects by diluting the medication and raising the urinary pH
    h. Should not be combined with sulfonamides because of the risk of crystalluria and urinary tract injury
    i. Clients taking this medication should not be given alkalinizing agents
  3. Nalidixic acid (NegGram)
    a. GI disturbances such as nausea, vomiting, and abdominal discomfort
    b. Rash
    c. Visual disturbances
    d. Photosensitivity reactions
    e. May produce intracranial hypertension in pediatric clients and should not be administered to children under age 3 months
    f. When used for more than 2 weeks, blood cell counts and liver function tests should be performed
    g. Can intensify the effects of oral anticoagulants
    h. Contraindicated in clients with a history of convulsive disorders
  4. Cinoxacin (Cinobac)

BOX 51-1. Urinary Tract Antiseptics

Nitrofurantoin (Furadantin, Macrodantin, Macrobid)
Methenamine (Mandelamine, Hiprex, Urex)
Nalidixic acid (NegGram)
Cinoxacin (Cinobac)
Norfloxacin (Noroxin)

---

a. Side effects are similar to nalidixic acid
b. Dosage should be reduced in clients with renal impairment; failure to do so could result in accumulation of medication to toxic levels
5. Norfloxacin (Noroxin)
   a. Can cause fatigue, headache, nausea, constipation, rash, and elevated liver function tests
   b. Encourage the client to increase fluids
   c. Advise the client to take medication 1 hour before or 2 hours after meals because food may hamper absorption

II. Sulfonamides (Box 51–2)

A. Description
1. Suppress bacterial growth by inhibiting synthesis of folic acid
2. Active against a broad spectrum of microbes
B. Side effects and nursing considerations
1. Hypersensitivity reactions such as rash, fever, and photosensitivity can occur
2. Stevens-Johnson syndrome, the most severe hypersensitivity response; produces symptoms that include widespread lesions of the skin and mucous membranes, with fever, malaise, and toxemia
3. Can cause hemolytic anemia and agranulocytosis, leukopenia, and thrombocytopenia
4. Should be discontinued if any sort of a rash is observed
5. Instruct the client to take medication on an empty stomach with a full glass of water
6. Clients should be instructed to avoid prolonged exposure to sunlight, wear protective clothing, and apply a sunscreen to exposed skin
7. Adults should maintain a daily urine output of 1200 mL by consuming 8 to 10 glasses of water each day to minimize the risk of renal damage from the medication
8. Can intensify the effects of warfarin (Coumadin), phenytoin (Dilantin), and oral hypoglycemics
9. Administer with caution in clients with renal impairment
10. Contraindicated in infants under age 2 months and in pregnant women or mothers who are breast-feeding
11. Contraindicated if a hypersensitivity exists to sulfonamides, sulfonylureas, thiazide, or loop diuretics

III. Trimethoprim (Proloprim, Trimpex)

A. Description
1. Active against a broad spectrum of microbes
2. Suppresses bacterial synthesis of DNA, RNA, and proteins
B. Side effects and nursing considerations
1. Itching and rash are the most frequent side effects
2. GI reactions such as epigastric distress, nausea and vomiting, glossitis, and stomatitis occur occasionally
3. Megaloblastic anemia, thrombocytopenia, and neutropenia may occur in individuals with preexisting folate deficiency
4. If early signs of bone marrow suppression occur such as sore throat, fever, or pallor, a complete blood count (CBC) should be performed
5. Contraindicated in women who are pregnant or are breast-feeding
6. Contraindicated in clients with folate deficiency

IV. Trimethoprim-Sulfamethoxazole (TMP-SMZ)

A. Description
1. A fixed-dose combination product (TMP-SMZ) that is a powerful broad-spectrum antimicrobial preparation
2. Trade names include Bactrim, Cotrim, and Septra
B. Side effects and nursing considerations
1. Nausea, vomiting, and rash are the most common side effects
2. Can cause megaloblastic anemia in clients who are folate deficient
3. Can cause central nervous system (CNS) effects such as headache, depression, and hallucinations
4. Hyperkalemia can occur
5. Toxicities may occur, such as hypersensitivity reactions, blood dyscrasias, and renal damage
6. Contraindicated during pregnancy and lactation, for infants under age 2 months, in clients with a folate deficiency, and in clients with a history of hypersensitivity to sulfonamides and chemically related medications

V. Cholinergic (Box 51–3)

A. Description
1. Used to treat nonobstructive urinary retention and neurogenic bladder
2. Used to increase bladder tone and function

BOX 51–2. Sulfonamides

Sulfisoxazole (Gantrisin)
Sulfamethoxazole (Gantanol, Urobak)
Sulfadiazine
Sulfacytine (Renoquid)
Sulfamethizole (Thiosulfil Forte)
Trisulfapyrimidines (Triple Sulfa No. 2)

BOX 51–3. Cholinergic

Bethanechol chloride (Duvoid, Urecholine)

B. Side effects
   1. Headache
   2. Hypotension
   3. Flushing and sweating
   4. Increased salivation
   5. Abdominal cramps
   6. Nausea, vomiting, and diarrhea
   7. Urinary urgency
   8. Bronchoconstriction
C. Nursing considerations
   1. Do not administer if the client has urinary obstruction
   2. Never administered by intramuscular (IM) or intravenous (IV) route
   3. Monitor intake and output (I&O)
   4. Monitor for increased bladder tone and function
   5. Administer on an empty stomach to decrease nausea and vomiting
   6. Monitor for cholinergic overdose
   7. Have atropine sulfate (antidote) readily available

VI. Antispasmodics

A. Description
   1. Oxybutynin chloride (Ditropan) relaxes smooth muscles of the urinary tract
   2. Propantheline bromide (Pro-Banthīne) decreases bladder muscle spasms
B. Oxybutynin chloride
   1. Side effects
      a. Leukopenia
      b. Anxiety
      c. Anorexia, nausea, and vomiting
      d. Palpitations
      e. Bradycardia
   2. Nursing considerations
      a. Do not administer in clients with known hypersensitivity, GI or genitourinary (GU) obstruction, glaucoma, severe colitis, or myasthenia gravis
      b. Instruct the client to avoid hazardous activities
C. Propantheline bromide (Pro-Banthīne)
   1. Side effects
      a. Palpitations and tachycardia
      b. Blurred vision
      c. Confusion in elderly clients
      d. Constipation
      e. Dry mouth
      f. Decreased sweating
      g. Urinary hesitancy and urgency
   2. Nursing considerations
      a. Monitor I&O
      b. Provide gum or hard candy for dry mouth

BOX 51–4. Urinary Analgesic

Phenazopyridine HCl (Pyridium)

   c. Do not administer to clients with narrow-angle glaucoma, obstructive uropathy, GI disease, or ulcerative colitis

VII. Urinary Analgesic (Box 51–4)

A. Description
   1. Used for pain from urinary tract irritation or infection
   2. Administered with an antibiotic because it does not treat infection, it treats only pain
B. Side effects
   1. Nausea
   2. Headache
   3. Vertigo
C. Nursing considerations
   1. Instruct the client that urine will turn red or orange
   2. Contraindicated in renal or hepatic disease

VIII. Hematopoietic Growth Factor (Box 51–5)

A. Description
   1. Used to stimulate red blood cell (RBC) production
   2. Reverses anemia associated with **chronic renal failure**
   3. Initial effects can be seen within 1 to 2 weeks, and the hematocrit reaches normal levels (30%–33%) in 2 to 3 months
B. Side effect: major side effect is hypertension
C. Nursing considerations
   1. Monitor hematocrit levels
   2. Monitor vital signs, especially blood pressure for hypertension
   3. The extent of hypertension is directly related to the rate of rise in the hematocrit
   4. Contraindicated in clients with uncontrolled hypertension or hypersensitivity to mammalian cell-derived products or human albumin
   5. Use with caution in clients with cancers of myeloid origin

IX. Preventing Organ Rejection (Box 51–6)

A. Description
   1. Cyclosporine (Sandimmune, Neoral) acts on T lymphocytes to suppress production of

BOX 51–5. Hematopoietic Growth Factor

Epoetin alfa (Epogen, Procrit)

BOX 51–6. Preventing Organ Rejection

IMMUNOSUPPRESSANTS
Cyclosporine (Sandimmune, Neoral)
Tacrolimus (Prograf)

CYTOTOXIC MEDICATIONS
Azathioprine (Imuran)
Mycophenolate mofetil (CellCept)

GLUCOCORTICOID
Prednisone (Deltasone)

ANTIBODIES
Muromonab-CD3 (Orthoclone OKT3)
Lymphocyte immune globulin, antithymocyte globulin (equine) (Atgam)

---

     interleukin-2, gamma interferon, and other cytokines

2. Tacrolimus (Prograf) prevents T cells from producing interleukin-2, gamma interferon, and other cytokines
3. Azathioprine (Imuran) suppresses cell-mediated and humoral immune responses by inhibiting the proliferation of B and T lymphocytes
4. Mycophenolate mofetil (CellCept) causes selective inhibition of B and T lymphocyte proliferation
5. Muromonab-CD3 (Orthoclone OKT3) blocks all T cell functions
6. Therapeutic effect of lymphocyte immune globulin results from a decrease in the number and activity of thymus-derived lymphocytes

B. Cyclosporine (Sandimmune, Neoral)
1. Used to prevent rejection of allogeneic kidney transplant
2. Prednisone (Deltasone) is usually administered concurrently
3. Oral administration is preferred; IV administration is reserved for clients who cannot take the medication orally
4. Blood levels should be measured periodically
5. The most common adverse effects are nephrotoxicity, infection, hypertension, tremor, and hirsutism
6. Clients should be informed about the possibility of renal damage and liver damage and the need for periodic blood urea nitrogen (BUN), creatinine, and liver function tests
7. Clients should be instructed to monitor for early signs of infection and to report these signs immediately
8. Instruct the client to dispense the oral liquid into a glass container using a specially calibrated pipette, mix well, and drink immediately; rinse the container with diluent and drink to ensure ingestion of the complete dose; dry the outside of the pipette and return to its cover for storage
9. Instruct the client to mix the concentrated medication solution with milk, chocolate milk, or orange juice just before administration
10. Assure the client that hirsutism is reversible
11. Grapefruit juice can raise cyclosporine levels, thereby increasing the risk of toxicity
12. Phenytoin, phenobarbital, rifampin, and TMP-SMZ can decrease cyclosporine levels
13. Ketoconazole, erythromycin, and amphotericin B can elevate cyclosporine levels
14. Renal damage can be intensified by the concurrent use of other nephrotoxic medications
15. Contraindicated in the presence of hypersensitivity, pregnancy, and breast-feeding; recent inoculation with live virus vaccines; and recent contact with an active infection such as chickenpox or herpes zoster
16. Is embryotoxic, and women of childbearing age should use a mechanical form of contraception and avoid oral contraceptives

C. Tacrolimus (Prograf)
1. Nephrotoxicity is the major concern
2. Other common reactions include neurotoxicity, GI effects, hypertension, hyperkalemia, and hyperglycemia
3. Increases the risk of infection and lymphomas
4. Concurrent use of glucocorticoids is recommended

D. Azathioprine (Imuran)
1. Used as an adjunct to cyclosporine and glucocorticoids to help suppress transplant rejection
2. Can cause neutropenia and thrombocytopenia from bone marrow suppression
3. Contraindicated in pregnancy and is associated with an increased incidence of neoplasms

E. Mycophenolate mofetil (CellCept)
1. Used in combination with cyclosporine and glucocorticoids
2. Major adverse effects include diarrhea, severe neutropenia, vomiting, and sepsis
3. Associated with an increased risk of infection and malignancies
4. Absorption is decreased by the use of magnesium and aluminum antacids and by cholestyramine (Questran, Prevalite)
5. Contraindicated in pregnancy

F. Muromonab-CD3 (Orthoclone OKT3)
1. Used to prevent acute allograft rejection of kidney transplants
2. Adverse reactions include fever, chills, dyspnea, chest pain, and nausea and vomiting

G. Lymphocyte immune globulin, antithymocyte globulin (equine) (Atgam)

1. Used to prevent rejection of renal transplants
2. Usually administered with glucocorticoids and azathioprine
3. Adverse reactions include chills, fever, leukopenia, and skin reactions

PRACTICE QUESTIONS

1. Cinoxacin (Cinobac) is prescribed for the client with a urinary tract infection. The nurse tells the client to take the medication
   1 1 hour before meals
   2 With meals
   3 At bedtime
   4 In the morning prior to breakfast

2. Laboratory analysis of a urine for culture and sensitivity reveals a gram-negative bacterial infection. Nalidixic acid (NegGram) is prescribed for the client. The nurse questions the prescription if the client has which of the following disorders?
   1 Diabetes mellitus
   2 Seizure disorder
   3 Coronary artery disease
   4 Peptic ulcer disease

3. Norfloxacin (Noroxin) is prescribed for a client with *Pseudomonas* infection of the urinary tract. The nurse tells the client to take the medication
   1 With meals
   2 At bedtime
   3 2 hours after meals
   4 With a snack in the late afternoon

4. Nitrofurantoin (Macrodantin) is prescribed for the client with an acute urinary tract infection. Which of the following food items does the nurse instruct the client to avoid during the administration of this medication?
   1 Orange juice
   2 Cranberry juice
   3 Prune juice
   4 Rhubarb

5. Methenamine mandelate (Mandelamine) is prescribed for the client with a gram-positive urinary tract infection. The nurse questions the prescription if which of the following preexisting disorders is noted in the client's record?
   1 Cirrhosis
   2 Diabetes mellitus
   3 Peripheral vascular disease
   4 Hypothyroidism

6. The client receiving nitrofurantoin (Macrodantin) calls the physician's office complaining of side effects related to the medication. Which of the following side effects indicates the need to stop the treatment with this medication?
   1 Anorexia
   2 Nausea
   3 Cough and chest pain
   4 Diarrhea

7. Nitrofurantoin (Macrodantin) is prescribed for an adult client for treatment of acute urinary tract infection (UTI). Which of the following is the appropriate adult dose?
   1 50 mg three to four times daily
   2 100 mg three times daily
   3 300 mg administered at bedtime
   4 1 g distributed evenly throughout the day

8. Methenamine (Mandelamine) is prescribed for the client with a chronic urinary tract infection. The nurse administers the medication, knowing that the mechanism of action is which of the following?
   1 Inhibits the replication of bacterial DNA
   2 Denatures bacterial proteins
   3 Decreases bladder muscle spasms
   4 Relaxes smooth muscles of the urinary tract

9. Nalidixic acid (NegGram) is prescribed for the client with a urinary tract infection. Reviewing the client's record, the nurse notes that the client is taking warfarin (Coumadin) on a daily basis. Which of the following prescriptions does the nurse anticipate because the client is on this oral anticoagulant?
   1 An increase in the anticoagulation dosage
   2 A reduction in the anticoagulation dosage
   3 The need to discontinue the warfarin during therapy
   4 The need to administer an alternative medication to treat the urinary tract infection

10. Nalidixic acid (NegGram) is prescribed for the adult client with urinary tract infection. The normal adult dosage for this medication is
    1 1 g four times daily for a period of 1 week
    2 500 mg daily administered at bedtime
    3 250 mg administered BID
    4 100 mg administered TID

11. Cinoxacin (Cinobac), a urinary antiseptic, is prescribed for the client. The nurse reviews the client's record, knowing that this medication is contraindicated in which of the following disorders?
    1 Hepatic disease
    2 Renal disease
    3 Diabetes insipidus
    4 Congestive heart failure

12. The nurse is reinforcing discharge instructions to a client receiving sulfisoxazole (Gantrisin). Which of the following is included in the plan of care for instructions?
    1 Restrict fluid intake
    2 Maintain a high fluid intake
    3 Decrease the dosage when symptoms are improving to prevent an allergic response
    4 If the urine turns dark brown, call the physician immediately

13. Sulfamethoxazole (Gantanol) is prescribed for a client with a urinary tract infection. The client is a diabetic and is receiving tolbutamide (Orinase). Based on the administration of these two medications in combination, which of the following does the nurse anticipate might be prescribed?
    1 A decreased dosage of the tolbutamide
    2 An increased dosage of the tolbutamide
    3 A decreased dosage of the sulfamethoxazole
    4 An increased dosage of the sulfamethoxazole

14. Trimethoprim-sulfamethoxazole (Bactrim) is prescribed for the client. The nurse tells the client to report which of the following symptoms if it developed during the course of this medication therapy?
    1 Headache
    2 Nausea
    3 Diarrhea
    4 Sore throat

15. Phenazopyridine (Pyridium) is prescribed for the client for symptomatic relief of pain resulting from a lower urinary tract infection. The nurse tells the client
    1 To take the medication prior to meals
    2 That a reddish orange discoloration of the urine may occur
    3 To discontinue the medication if a headache occurs
    4 To take the medication at bedtime

16. Bethanechol (Urecholine) is prescribed for the client with urinary retention. The nurse reviews the client's record, knowing that which of the following preexisting disorders is a contraindication to the administration of this medication?
    1 Neurogenic atony
    2 Urinary strictures
    3 Gastroesophageal reflux
    4 Gastric atony

17. Bethanechol (Urecholine) is prescribed for the client. The nurse tells the client to take the medication
    1 With meals
    2 2 hours after meals
    3 With a snack in the afternoon
    4 At bedtime with crackers and cheese

18. Bethanechol (Urecholine) is prescribed for the client. The normal adult oral dosage of this medication ranges from
    1 10 to 50 mg three to four times a day
    2 50 to 100 mg three to four times a day
    3 100 mg every 4 hours
    4 100 mg at bedtime

19. The nurse is administering 5 mg of bethanechol (Urecholine) subcutaneously to a client with urinary retention. Which of the following does the nurse prepare to have readily available when administering this medication?
    1 Protamine sulfate
    2 Vitamin K
    3 Atropine sulfate
    4 Mucomyst

20. The nurse administering bethanechol (Urecholine) is monitoring for acute toxicity associated with the medication. Which of the following is not a manifestation associated with overdose?
    1 Salivation
    2 Sweating
    3 Bradycardia
    4 Severe hypertension

21. Bethanechol (Urecholine) is prescribed for the client with urinary retention. An injectable form of bethanechol is available for use. The nurse informs the client of the physician's order, knowing that the medication will be administered
    1 Intravenously
    2 Intramuscularly
    3 Intradermally
    4 Subcutaneously

22. Oxybutynin (Ditropan) is prescribed for the client with neurogenic bladder. The nurse monitors the client, knowing that which of the following indicates a possible toxic effect related to this medication?
    1 Bradycardia
    2 Pallor
    3 Restlessness
    4 Drowsiness

23. Propantheline bromide (Pro-Banthine) is prescribed for the client with bladder spasms. Which of the following disorders, if noted in the client's record, alerts the nurse to question the prescription for this medication?
    1 Glaucoma
    2 Hypothyroidism
    3 Myxedema
    4 Coronary artery disease

24. Following kidney transplant, cyclosporine (Sandimmune) is prescribed for the client. Which of the following laboratory results indicates an adverse effect from the use of this medication?
    1 Decreased white blood cell (WBC) count
    2 Decreased hemoglobin
    3 Elevated BUN
    4 Decreased creatinine

25. The nurse is providing dietary instructions to a client who has been prescribed cyclosporine. Which of the following food items does the nurse instruct the client to avoid?
    1 Orange juice
    2 Grapefruit juice

3 Red meats
4 Green, leafy vegetables

26. Cyclosporine (Sandimmune) is prescribed for the client following a kidney transplant. The nurse is most concerned if it is noted that the client is presently taking which of the following prescribed medications?
    1 Digoxin (Lanoxin)
    2 Propranolol (Inderal)
    3 Phenytoin (Dilantin)
    4 Prednisone (Deltasone)

27. The nurse is caring for a client who will be receiving amphotericin B. The nurse notes that the client is also taking cyclosporine to prevent rejection of a kidney transplant performed 2 years ago. Which of the following prescriptions does the nurse anticipate to be prescribed for this client during the administration of these medications concurrently?
    1 An increased amount of amphotericin B
    2 A decreased amount of amphotericin B
    3 An increased amount of cyclosporine
    4 A decreased amount of cyclosporine

28. The nurse reinforces instructions to the client prescribed to take cyclosporine (Sandimmune) oral solution. Which of the following instructions does the nurse reinforce?
    1 Dilute the medication in a Styrofoam cup prior to administration
    2 Avoid diluting the concentrate for administration
    3 Mix the concentration with chocolate milk
    4 Mix the concentration with grapefruit juice

29. The nurse reinforces instructions regarding the administration of cyclosporine (Sandimmune) to a client. Which of the following statements, if made by the client, indicates the need for further instruction?
    1 "I need to mix the concentrate well and drink it immediately."
    2 "After taking the medication, I need to rinse the container with diluent and drink it to ensure that I have taken the complete dose."
    3 "I will purchase a dropper from the pharmacy to calibrate the amount of medication that I need."
    4 "I will mix the concentrate with orange juice to improve the taste."

30. The nurse is monitoring a client receiving cyclosporine (Sandimmune). Which of the following indicates to the nurse that the client is experiencing an adverse effect from this medication?
    1 Nausea
    2 Alopecia
    3 Tremor
    4 Hypotension

31. Tacrolimus (Prograf) is prescribed for a client for prevention of organ rejection following renal transplant. Which of the following does the nurse expect to be prescribed for this client during the administration of this medication?
    1 Prednisone (Deltasone)
    2 Erythromycin (E-Mycin)
    3 Fluconazole (Diflucan)
    4 Phenytoin (Dilantin)

32. Tacrolimus (Prograf) is prescribed for the client. Which of the following disorders, if noted on the client's record, indicates that the medication needs to be administered with caution?
    1 Diabetes insipidus
    2 Coronary artery disease
    3 Renal insufficiency
    4 Ulcerative colitis

33. The nurse is reviewing the laboratory results documented in the record of a client receiving tacrolimus (Prograf). Which of the following indicates to the nurse that the client is experiencing an adverse effect of the medication?
    1 WBC of 6000/μL
    2 Blood glucose of 200 mg/dL
    3 Potassium level 3.8 mEq/L
    4 Platelet count 300,000 cells/μL

34. Muromonab-CD3 (Orthoclone OKT3) is prescribed for a client to manage allograft rejection following a renal transplant. The nurse administers the medication, knowing that the primary mechanism of action of this medication is that it
    1 Binds to the CD3 site and blocks all T cell functions
    2 Inhibits the proliferation of B lymphocytes
    3 Cross-links DNA, causing cell injury and death
    4 Suppresses B lymphocytes

35. Mycophenolate mofetil (CellCept) is prescribed for a client as prophylaxis of organ rejection following allogeneic renal transplant. Which of the following instructions does the nurse reinforce regarding administration of this medication?
    1 Administer following meals
    2 Open the capsule and mix with food for administration
    3 Contact the physician if a sore throat occurs
    4 Take the medication with a magnesium-type antacid

36. Azathioprine (Imuran) is prescribed for the client to suppress rejection of a renal transplant. The nurse administers the medication, knowing that the mechanism of action of this medication is that it
    1 Inhibits the proliferation of B and T lymphocytes
    2 Cross-links DNA

3 Blocks all T cell functions

4 Decreases the activity of thymus-derived lymphocytes

37. The client with chronic renal failure (CRF) is receiving epoetin alfa (Epogen). The nurse is reviewing the laboratory results and notes that which of the following results indicates a therapeutic effect of the medication?
    1 WBC count of 6000/μL
    2 Hematocrit count of 32%
    3 Platelet count of 400,000 cells/μL
    4 BUN of 15 mg/dL

38. Epoetin alfa (Epogen) has been prescribed for the client with chronic renal failure (CRF). The nurse will prepare to administer this medication by which of the following routes?
    1 PO
    2 IM
    3 Intradermally
    4 Subcutaneously

39. The nurse is monitoring the client receiving epoetin alfa (Epogen) for adverse effects of the medication. The nurse notes that which of the following indicates an adverse effect?
    1 Hypotension
    2 Hypertension
    3 Depression
    4 Bradycardia

40. The nurse is reviewing the laboratory studies of a client receiving epoetin alfa (Epogen). The nurse expects to note a therapeutic effect of this medication
    1 After 1 week of therapy
    2 Immediately
    3 3 days after therapy
    4 2 weeks after therapy

41. The nurse is reinforcing instructions to a client regarding how to administer epoetin alfa (Epogen) by subcutaneous route. The nurse tells the client to
    1 Shake the bottle before use
    2 Keep the vial of medication at room temperature
    3 Use only 1 dose per vial
    4 Use alcohol to clean the top of the vial when reused

42. Aluminum hydroxide (Amphojel) is prescribed for the client with chronic renal failure (CRF). The nurse instructs the client to take this medication
    1 On an empty stomach
    2 At bedtime
    3 With meals
    4 In the morning upon arising

43. A most common side effect associated with the administration of aluminum hydroxide (Amphojel) is
    1 Diarrhea
    2 Constipation
    3 Muscle weakness
    4 Headache

44. The client with hyperphosphatemia is receiving aluminum hydroxide (Amphojel). The usual adult dosage for this medication is
    1 10 mL BID
    2 15 mL TID
    3 30 mL QD
    4 30 mL TID

45. The client with chronic renal failure is receiving ferrous sulfate (Feosol). Which of the following is a common side effect associated with this medication?
    1 Diarrhea
    2 Constipation
    3 Headache
    4 Weakness

ANSWERS

1. **2**

RATIONALE: Cinoxacin is a urinary antiseptic and is administered with meals to decrease GI side effects. Options 1, 3, and 4 are incorrect.
TEST-TAKING STRATEGY: Eliminate options 1, 3, and 4 because they are similar in that they all indicate taking the medication on an empty stomach. If you are unfamiliar with this medication, take time now to review.
LEVEL OF COGNITIVE ABILITY: Application
PHASE OF NURSING PROCESS: Implementation
CLIENT NEEDS: Health Promotion and Maintenance
CONTENT AREA: Pharmacology

REFERENCE
Black, J., & Matassarin-Jacobs, E. (1997). *Medical-surgical nursing: Clinical management for continuity of care* (5th ed.). Philadelphia: W. B. Saunders. p. 1575.

2. **2**

RATIONALE: Nalidixic acid is used for acute and chronic UTIs, especially gram-negative bacterial infections. The medication is contraindicated in clients with a history of convulsions. It is used with caution in clients with liver or renal disorders.
TEST-TAKING STRATEGY: Knowledge regarding the contraindications associated with this medication is required to answer the question. Review this medication now if you had difficulty with this question.

LEVEL OF COGNITIVE ABILITY: Application
PHASE OF NURSING PROCESS: Implementation
CLIENT NEEDS: Safe, Effective Care Environment
CONTENT AREA: Pharmacology
REFERENCE
Black, J., & Matassarin-Jacobs, E. (1997). *Medical-surgical nursing: Clinical management for continuity of care* (5th ed.). Philadelphia: W. B. Saunders. p. 1575.

3. **3**

RATIONALE: Norfloxacin is administered 1 hour before or 2 hours after meals because food may hamper absorption. The normal dosage is 400 mg orally (PO) BID for 7 to 10 days for mild infections and for 10 to 21 days for severe infections.
TEST-TAKING STRATEGY: Eliminate options 1 and 4 first because they are similar. To discriminate between the remaining options, knowledge that this medication is administered more than once daily will direct you to option 3. Review this medication now if you had difficulty with this question.
LEVEL OF COGNITIVE ABILITY: Application
PHASE OF NURSING PROCESS: Implementation
CLIENT NEEDS: Health Promotion and Maintenance
CONTENT AREA: Pharmacology
REFERENCE
Black, J., & Matassarin-Jacobs, E. (1997). *Medical-surgical nursing: Clinical management for continuity of care* (5th ed.). Philadelphia: W. B. Saunders. p. 1575.

4. **4**

RATIONALE: When a client is receiving nitrofurantoin, the urinary pH must be maintained in an acid range. The client needs to be instructed to consume an acid ash diet. Rhubarb will reduce the acidity of the urine, and should be avoided when the client requires an acid ash urine.
TEST-TAKING STRATEGY: Note the key word "avoid" in the stem of the question. Knowledge that this medication requires that the urinary pH be maintained in an acid range will assist in directing you to option 4. Review this medication now if you had difficulty with this question.
LEVEL OF COGNITIVE ABILITY: Application
PHASE OF NURSING PROCESS: Implementation
CLIENT NEEDS: Health Promotion and Maintenance
CONTENT AREA: Pharmacology
REFERENCE
Black, J., & Matassarin-Jacobs, E. (1997). *Medical-surgical nursing: Clinical management for continuity of care* (5th ed.). Philadelphia: W. B. Saunders. p. 1575.

5. **1**

RATIONALE: Methenamine is contraindicated in clients with renal or hepatic disease or clients with severe dehydration. The nurse should question the physician's prescription for this medication in the client with cirrhosis.
TEST-TAKING STRATEGY: Knowledge that this medication is contraindicated in hepatic disease will easily direct you to option 1. If you are unfamiliar with this medication, take time now to review.
LEVEL OF COGNITIVE ABILITY: Application
PHASE OF NURSING PROCESS: Implementation
CLIENT NEEDS: Safe, Effective Care Environment
CONTENT AREA: Pharmacology
REFERENCE
Black, J., & Matassarin-Jacobs, E. (1997). *Medical-surgical nursing: Clinical management for continuity of care* (5th ed.). Philadelphia: W. B. Saunders. p. 1575.

6. **3**

RATIONALE: Gastrointestinal effects are the most frequent adverse reactions to this medication and can be minimized by administering the medication with milk or meals. Pulmonary reactions, manifested as dyspnea, chest pain, chills, fever, cough, and the presence of alveolar infiltrates on x-ray film, would indicate the need to stop the treatment. These symptoms should resolve in 2 to 4 days following discontinuation of this medication.
TEST-TAKING STRATEGY: Eliminate options 1, 2, and 4 because they are GI-related side effects. If you are unfamiliar with this medication, take time now to review this medication.
LEVEL OF COGNITIVE ABILITY: Comprehension
PHASE OF NURSING PROCESS: Data Collection
CLIENT NEEDS: Physiological Integrity
CONTENT AREA: Pharmacology
REFERENCE
Lehne, R. (1998). *Pharmacology for nursing care* (3rd ed.). Philadelphia: W. B. Saunders. p. 903.

7. **1**

RATIONALE: For treatment of acute urinary tract infection (UTI), the adult dosage is 50 mg three to four times a day. For prophylaxis of recurrent UTI, low doses are employed, such as 50 to 100 mg at bedtime for adults.
TEST-TAKING STRATEGY: Knowledge regarding the normal adult dosage of nitrofurantoin is required to answer this question. If you are unfamiliar with this medication, take time now to review.
LEVEL OF COGNITIVE ABILITY: Comprehension
PHASE OF NURSING PROCESS: Planning
CLIENT NEEDS: Physiological Integrity
CONTENT AREA: Pharmacology
REFERENCE
Lehne, R. (1998). *Pharmacology for nursing care* (3rd ed.). Philadelphia: W. B. Saunders. p. 904.

8. **2**

RATIONALE: Methenamine, under acidic conditions, decomposes into ammonia and formaldehyde. The formaldehyde denatures bacterial proteins, causing death. Nalidixic acid is a medication that inhibits the replication of bacterial DNA. Antispasmodics relax smooth muscle of the urinary tract and decrease bladder muscle spasms.
TEST-TAKING STRATEGY: Eliminate options 3 and 4 because they are similar. From the remaining options, it is necessary to know the action of this medication. If you had difficulty with this question, take time now to review this medication.
LEVEL OF COGNITIVE ABILITY: Comprehension
PHASE OF NURSING PROCESS: Implementation
CLIENT NEEDS: Physiological Integrity
CONTENT AREA: Pharmacology
REFERENCE
Lehne, R. (1998). *Pharmacology for nursing care* (3rd ed.). Philadelphia: W. B. Saunders. p. 904.

9. **2**

RATIONALE: Nalidixic acid can intensify the effects of oral anticoagulants. When an oral anticoagulant is combined with nalidixic acid, a reduction in the anticoagulant dosage may be needed.

TEST-TAKING STRATEGY: Option 3 can be eliminated as the least likely choice. Next, eliminate option 1 as the next least likely prescription. From the remaining options, the most likely choice, based on the situation presented, is option 2. Review this medication now if you had difficulty with this question.
LEVEL OF COGNITIVE ABILITY: Comprehension
PHASE OF NURSING PROCESS: Planning
CLIENT NEEDS: Physiological Integrity
CONTENT AREA: Pharmacology
REFERENCE
Lehne, R. (1998). *Pharmacology for nursing care* (3rd ed.). Philadelphia: W. B. Saunders. p. 905.

10. **1**

RATIONALE: Nalidixic acid is dispensed in tablets of 250 mg, 500 mg, and 1 g, and in a suspension of 50 mg/mL for oral use. Adult dosage is 1 g four times a day for 1 week. It should not be administered to children younger than 3 months of age because it may produce intracranial hypertension.
TEST-TAKING STRATEGY: Knowledge regarding the normal adult dosage of nalidixic acid is required to answer this question. If you are unfamiliar with this medication, take time now to review.
LEVEL OF COGNITIVE ABILITY: Comprehension
PHASE OF NURSING PROCESS: Planning
CLIENT NEEDS: Physiological Integrity
CONTENT AREA: Pharmacology
REFERENCE
Lehne, R. (1998). *Pharmacology for nursing care* (3rd ed.). Philadelphia: W. B. Saunders. p. 905.

11. **2**

RATIONALE: Cinoxacin should be administered with caution in clients with renal impairment. The dosage should be reduced, and failure to do so could result in accumulation of cinoxacin to toxic levels. The disorders in options 1, 3, and 4 are not contraindications to this medication.
TEST-TAKING STRATEGY: Knowledge that this medication is to be used with caution in clients with renal impairment will easily direct you to option 2. If you are unfamiliar with this medication. take time now to review.
LEVEL OF COGNITIVE ABILITY: Comprehension
PHASE OF NURSING PROCESS: Implementation
CLIENT NEEDS: Physiological Integrity
CONTENT AREA: Pharmacology
REFERENCE
Lehne, R. (1998). *Pharmacology for nursing care* (3rd ed.). Philadelphia: W. B. Saunders. p. 905.

12. **2**

RATIONALE: Each dose of sulfisoxazole should be administered with a full glass of water, and the client should maintain a high fluid intake. The medication is more soluble in alkaline urine. The client should not be instructed to taper or discontinue the dose. Some forms of sulfisoxazole such as Azo Gantrisin cause the urine to turn dark brown or red. This does not indicate the need to notify the physician.
TEST-TAKING STRATEGY: Use the process of elimination. General principles related to medication administration will assist in eliminating option 3. For the remaining options, recalling that this medication is a sulfonamide will assist in directing you to option 2. Review this medication now if you had difficulty with this question.
LEVEL OF COGNITIVE ABILITY: Application

PHASE OF NURSING PROCESS: Implementation
CLIENT NEEDS: Health Promotion and Maintenance
CONTENT AREA: Pharmacology
REFERENCE
Black, J., & Matassarin-Jacobs, E. (1997). *Medical-surgical nursing: Clinical management for continuity of care* (5th ed.). Philadelphia: W. B. Saunders. p. 1576.

13. **1**

RATIONALE: Sulfonamides can intensify the effects of warfarin (Coumadin), phenytoin, and oral hypoglycemics, such as tolbutamide. When combined with sulfonamides, these medications may require a reduction in dosage.
TEST-TAKING STRATEGY: Options 3 and 4 can be eliminated as the least likely choices. From the remaining options, the most likely choice, based on the situation presented, is option 1. Review medication interactions associated with sulfonamides now if you had difficulty with this question.
LEVEL OF COGNITIVE ABILITY: Comprehension
PHASE OF NURSING PROCESS: Planning
CLIENT NEEDS: Physiological Integrity
CONTENT AREA: Pharmacology
REFERENCE
Lehne, R. (1998). *Pharmacology for nursing care* (3rd ed.). Philadelphia: W. B. Saunders. p. 897.

14. **4**

RATIONALE: Clients taking trimethoprim-sulfamethoxazole should be informed about early signs of blood disorders that can occur from this medication. These signs include sore throat, fever, or pallor, and the client should be instructed to notify the physician if these symptoms occur. The other options do not require physician notification.
TEST-TAKING STRATEGY: Knowledge that this medication can cause blood dyscrasias is required to answer the question. If you are unfamiliar with this medication, take time now to review.
LEVEL OF COGNITIVE ABILITY: Application
PHASE OF NURSING PROCESS: Implementation
CLIENT NEEDS: Health Promotion and Maintenance
CONTENT AREA: Pharmacology
REFERENCE
Lehne, R. (1998). *Pharmacology for nursing care* (3rd ed.). Philadelphia: W. B. Saunders. p. 897.

15. **2**

RATIONALE: The client should be instructed that a reddish orange discoloration of urine may occur. The client should also be instructed that this discoloration can stain fabric. The medication should be taken after meals to reduce the possibility of GI upset. Headache is an occasional side effect of the medication and does not warrant discontinuation of the medication.
TEST-TAKING STRATEGY: Eliminate options 1 and 4 first because they are similar. From the remaining options, eliminate option 3 because the nurse would not advise the client to discontinue this medication. Review this medication now if you had difficulty with this question.
LEVEL OF COGNITIVE ABILITY: Application
PHASE OF NURSING PROCESS: Implementation
CLIENT NEEDS: Health Promotion and Maintenance
CONTENT AREA: Pharmacology
REFERENCE
Hodgson, B., & Kizior, R. (1999). *Saunders nursing drug handbook 1999*. Philadelphia: W. B. Saunders. p. 813.

16. **2**

RATIONALE: Bethanechol can be hazardous to clients with urinary tract obstruction or weakness of the bladder wall. The medication has the ability to contract the bladder and thereby increase pressure within the urinary tract. Elevation of pressure within the urinary tract could rupture the bladder in clients with these conditions.
TEST-TAKING STRATEGY: Knowledge regarding the contraindications associated with this medication is required to answer this question. Noting that the medication is used for urinary retention may assist in directing you to option 2. Review this medication now if you had difficulty with this question.
LEVEL OF COGNITIVE ABILITY: Comprehension
PHASE OF NURSING PROCESS: Implementation
CLIENT NEEDS: Physiological Integrity
CONTENT AREA: Pharmacology
REFERENCE
Lehne, R. (1998). *Pharmacology for nursing care* (3rd ed.). Philadelphia: W. B. Saunders. p. 122.

17. **2**

RATIONALE: Administration of bethanechol with meals can cause nausea and vomiting in the client. To avoid this problem, oral doses should be administered 1 hour before meals or 2 hours after meals.
TEST-TAKING STRATEGY: Note that options 1, 3, and 4 are similar in that they all suggest administering the medication with a food item. Review this medication now if you had difficulty with this question.
LEVEL OF COGNITIVE ABILITY: Application
PHASE OF NURSING PROCESS: Implementation
CLIENT NEEDS: Health Promotion and Maintenance
CONTENT AREA: Pharmacology
REFERENCE
Lehne, R. (1998). *Pharmacology for nursing care* (3rd ed.). Philadelphia: W. B. Saunders. p. 122.

18. **1**

RATIONALE: The normal adult dosage of bethanechol ranges from 10 to 50 mg three to four times daily.
TEST-TAKING STRATEGY: Knowledge regarding the normal dosage of this medication is required to answer this question. Learn this dosage now if you had difficulty with this question.
LEVEL OF COGNITIVE ABILITY: Comprehension
PHASE OF NURSING PROCESS: Planning
CLIENT NEEDS: Physiological Integrity
CONTENT AREA: Pharmacology
REFERENCE
Lehne, R. (1998). *Pharmacology for nursing care* (3rd ed.). Philadelphia: W. B. Saunders. p. 122.

19. **3**

RATIONALE: Cholinergic overdose can occur with bethanechol. The antidote is atropine sulfate administered subcutaneously (SC) or IV, which should be readily available for use should overdose occur. Protamine sulfate is the antidote for heparin. Vitamin K is the antidote for warfarin. Mucomyst is the antidote for acetaminophen overdose.
TEST-TAKING STRATEGY: Knowledge regarding the antidotes for certain medication overdoses is required to answer this question. If you could not answer this question, be sure to learn these antidotes now.

LEVEL OF COGNITIVE ABILITY: Application
PHASE OF NURSING PROCESS: Planning
CLIENT NEEDS: Physiological Integrity
CONTENT AREA: Pharmacology
REFERENCE
Lehne, R. (1998). *Pharmacology for nursing care* (3rd ed.). Philadelphia: W. B. Saunders. p. 127.

20. **4**

RATIONALE: Overdose produces manifestations of excessive muscarinic stimulation such as salivation, sweating, involuntary urination and defecation, bradycardia, and severe hypotension. Treatment includes supportive measures and the administration of atropine sulfate SC or IV.
TEST-TAKING STRATEGY: Knowledge of the signs of cholinergic overdose is required to answer this question. If you are unfamiliar with these signs, learn them now.
LEVEL OF COGNITIVE ABILITY: Comprehension
PHASE OF NURSING PROCESS: Data Collection
CLIENT NEEDS: Physiological Integrity
CONTENT AREA: Pharmacology
REFERENCE
Lehne, R. (1998). *Pharmacology for nursing care* (3rd ed.). Philadelphia: W. B. Saunders. p. 127.

21. **4**

RATIONALE: The injectable form of bethanechol is intended for subcutaneous administration only. Bethanechol must never be injected IM or IV since the resulting high drug levels can cause severe toxicity, such as bloody diarrhea, bradycardia, profound hypotension, and cardiovascular collapse.
TEST-TAKING STRATEGY: Knowledge regarding the route of administration of this medication is required to answer this question. If you did not know the answer to this question, learn this administration route now.
LEVEL OF COGNITIVE ABILITY: Comprehension
PHASE OF NURSING PROCESS: Implementation
CLIENT NEEDS: Physiological Integrity
CONTENT AREA: Pharmacology
REFERENCE
Lehne, R. (1998). *Pharmacology for nursing care* (3rd ed.). Philadelphia: W. B. Saunders. pp. 122–123.

22. **3**

RATIONALE: Overdosage produces CNS excitation, such as nervousness, restlessness, hallucinations, and irritability. Other signs of overdose include either hypotension or hypertension, confusion, tachycardia, flushed or red face, and signs of respiratory depression. Drowsiness is a frequent side effect of the medication, but does not indicate toxicity.
TEST-TAKING STRATEGY: Knowledge regarding the manifestations related to toxicity is required to answer this question. If you are unfamiliar with this medication, take time now to review.
LEVEL OF COGNITIVE ABILITY: Comprehension
PHASE OF NURSING PROCESS: Data Collection
CLIENT NEEDS: Physiological Integrity
CONTENT AREA: Pharmacology
REFERENCE
Hodgson, B., & Kizior, R. (1999). *Saunders nursing drug handbook 1999*. Philadelphia: W. B. Saunders. p. 799.

23. 1

RATIONALE: Propantheline is contraindicated in clients with narrow-angle glaucoma, obstructive uropathy, GI disease, or ulcerative colitis. Options 2, 3, and 4 are not contraindications to the use of this medication.
TEST-TAKING STRATEGY: Eliminate options 2 and 3 because they are similar. From the remaining options, it is necessary to know the contraindications associated with the medication. Review these contraindications now if you had difficulty with this question.
LEVEL OF COGNITIVE ABILITY: Comprehension
PHASE OF NURSING PROCESS: Planning
CLIENT NEEDS: Safe, Effective Care Environment
CONTENT AREA: Pharmacology
REFERENCE
Lehne, R. (1998). *Pharmacology for nursing care* (3rd ed.). Philadelphia: W. B. Saunders. p. 124.

24. 3

RATIONALE: Nephrotoxicity can occur from the use of cyclosporine. Nephrotoxicity is evaluated by monitoring for an elevated BUN and serum creatinine level. Cyclosporine does not depress the bone marrow.
TEST-TAKING STRATEGY: Eliminate options 1 and 2 first because they are unrelated to renal function. Next, eliminate option 4 because the creatinine level would be elevated, not decreased. Option 3 is the only option that indicates an increased level of a renal function test.
LEVEL OF COGNITIVE ABILITY: Comprehension
PHASE OF NURSING PROCESS: Data Collection
CLIENT NEEDS: Physiological Integrity
CONTENT AREA: Pharmacology
REFERENCE
Lehne, R. (1998). *Pharmacology for nursing care* (3rd ed.). Philadelphia: W. B. Saunders. p. 729.

25. 2

RATIONALE: A compound present in grapefruit juice inhibits metabolism of cyclosporine. As a result, consuming grapefruit juice can raise cyclosporine levels by 50% to 100%, thereby greatly increasing the risk of toxicity.
TEST-TAKING STRATEGY: Note the key word "avoid." Knowledge regarding substances that inhibit the metabolism of cyclosporine is required to answer this question. If you had difficulty with this question, review this very important medication now.
LEVEL OF COGNITIVE ABILITY: Application
PHASE OF NURSING PROCESS: Implementation
CLIENT NEEDS: Health Promotion and Maintenance
CONTENT AREA: Pharmacology
REFERENCE
Lehne, R. (1998). *Pharmacology for nursing care* (3rd ed.). Philadelphia: W. B. Saunders. pp. 729–730.

26. 3

RATIONALE: Medications known to lower cyclosporine levels include phenytoin, phenobarbital, rifampin, and trimethoprim-sulfamethoxazole. Cyclosporine levels should be monitored and the dosage adjusted in clients taking these medications.
TEST-TAKING STRATEGY: Knowledge regarding the medications that lower cyclosporine levels is required to

answer this question. If you are unfamiliar with these medications, take time now to review important points related to cyclosporine.
LEVEL OF COGNITIVE ABILITY: Comprehension
PHASE OF NURSING PROCESS: Data Collection
CLIENT NEEDS: Physiological Integrity
CONTENT AREA: Pharmacology
REFERENCE
Lehne, R. (1998). *Pharmacology for nursing care* (3rd ed.). Philadelphia: W. B. Saunders. pp. 729–730.

27. 4

RATIONALE: Amphotericin B as well as erythromycin and ketoconazole can elevate cyclosporine levels. When either of these medications is combined with cyclosporine, the dosage of cyclosporine must be reduced to prevent accumulation to toxic levels.
TEST-TAKING STRATEGY: Knowledge regarding the medications that elevate cyclosporine levels is required to answer this question. If you are unfamiliar with these medications, take time now to review important points related to cyclosporine.
LEVEL OF COGNITIVE ABILITY: Comprehension
PHASE OF NURSING PROCESS: Planning
CLIENT NEEDS: Physiological Integrity
CONTENT AREA: Pharmacology
REFERENCE
Lehne, R. (1998). *Pharmacology for nursing care* (3rd ed.). Philadelphia: W. B. Saunders. pp. 729–730.

28. 3

RATIONALE: To improve palatability, the client should be taught to mix the concentrated medication solution with chocolate milk or orange juice just before administration. Grapefruit juice can raise cyclosporine levels. Instruct the client to dispense the oral liquid into a glass container using a specially calibrated pipette; mix well and drink immediately; rinse the container with diluent and drink it to ensure ingestion of the complete dose; dry the outside of the pipette and return to its cover for storage.
TEST-TAKING STRATEGY: Knowledge regarding the administration of the oral concentrate is required to answer this question. If you are unfamiliar with this procedure, review now.
LEVEL OF COGNITIVE ABILITY: Application
PHASE OF NURSING PROCESS: Implementation
CLIENT NEEDS: Health Promotion and Maintenance
CONTENT AREA: Pharmacology
REFERENCE
Lehne, R. (1998). *Pharmacology for nursing care* (3rd ed.). Philadelphia: W. B. Saunders. p. 734.

29. 3

RATIONALE: The client needs to be instructed to dispense the oral liquid into a glass container using a specially calibrated pipette. The client should not use any other type of dropper to calibrate the amount of prescribed medication. Options 1, 2, and 4 are incorrect options.
TEST-TAKING STRATEGY: Note the key words "indicate the need for further instruction." Knowledge regarding the administration of the oral concentrate is required to answer this question. If you are unfamiliar with this procedure, review now.

LEVEL OF COGNITIVE ABILITY: Comprehension
PHASE OF NURSING PROCESS: Evaluation
CLIENT NEEDS: Health Promotion and Maintenance
CONTENT AREA: Pharmacology
REFERENCE
Lehne, R. (1998). *Pharmacology for nursing care* (3rd ed.). Philadelphia: W. B. Saunders. p. 734.

30. 3

RATIONALE: The most common adverse effects of cyclosporine are nephrotoxicity, infection, hypertension, tremor, and hirsutism. Of these, nephrotoxicity and infection are the most serious.
TEST-TAKING STRATEGY: Knowledge regarding the adverse effects associated with cyclosporine is required to answer this question. If you are unfamiliar with these effects, review now.
LEVEL OF COGNITIVE ABILITY: Comprehension
PHASE OF NURSING PROCESS: Data Collection
CLIENT NEEDS: Physiological Integrity
CONTENT AREA: Pharmacology
REFERENCE
Lehne, R. (1998). *Pharmacology for nursing care* (3rd ed.). Philadelphia: W. B. Saunders. p. 729.

31. 1

RATIONALE: Tacrolimus is an alternative medication to cyclosporine for prevention of organ rejection in clients receiving transplant. The medication is somewhat more effective than cyclosporine but is also more toxic. Concurrent use of glucocorticoids is recommended during administration of this medication.
TEST-TAKING STRATEGY: Knowledge that glucocorticoids are administered concurrently with some medications used to prevent organ rejection will easily direct you to option 1. Review this medication now if you are unfamiliar with it.
LEVEL OF COGNITIVE ABILITY: Comprehension
PHASE OF NURSING PROCESS: Planning
CLIENT NEEDS: Physiological Integrity
CONTENT AREA: Pharmacology
REFERENCE
Lehne, R. (1998). *Pharmacology for nursing care* (3rd ed.). Philadelphia: W. B. Saunders. p. 731.

32. 3

RATIONALE: Tacrolimus is used with caution in immunosuppressed clients and in clients with renal or hepatic function impairment. It is contraindicated in clients with hypersensitivity to this medication or hypersensitivity to cyclosporine.
TEST-TAKING STRATEGY: Many medications affect renal and hepatic function. If you had to select an option and were unsure of the correct answer, select the option that addresses renal or hepatic function. Review the cautions and contraindications associated with the administration of this medication now if you had difficulty with this question.
LEVEL OF COGNITIVE ABILITY: Comprehension
PHASE OF NURSING PROCESS: Data Collection
CLIENT NEEDS: Physiological Integrity
CONTENT AREA: Pharmacology
REFERENCE
Hodgson, B., & Kizior, R. (1999). *Saunders nursing drug handbook 1999.* Philadelphia: W. B. Saunders. p. 960.

33. 2

RATIONALE: Nephrotoxicity is a major concern with this medication. Other common reactions include neurotoxicity evidenced by headache, tremor, and insomnia; GI effects such as diarrhea, nausea, and vomiting; hypertension; hyperkalemia; and hyperglycemia.
TEST-TAKING STRATEGY: Use the process of elimination, noting that options 1, 3, and 4 represent normal values. Option 2 is the only abnormal value reflecting an elevation. Review these normal laboratory values now if you had difficulty with this question.
LEVEL OF COGNITIVE ABILITY: Comprehension
PHASE OF NURSING PROCESS: Data Collection
CLIENT NEEDS: Physiological Integrity
CONTENT AREA: Pharmacology
REFERENCE
Lehne, R. (1998). *Pharmacology for nursing care* (3rd ed.). Philadelphia: W. B. Saunders. p. 731.

34. 1

RATIONALE: Muromonab is a monoclonal antibody. Upon binding to the CD3 site, the antibody blocks all T cell function. Options 2, 3, and 4 are not actions of this medication.
TEST-TAKING STRATEGY: Knowledge regarding the action of this medication is required to answer this question. If you are unfamiliar with this medication, take time now to review.
LEVEL OF COGNITIVE ABILITY: Comprehension
PHASE OF NURSING PROCESS: Implementation
CLIENT NEEDS: Physiological Integrity
CONTENT AREA: Pharmacology
REFERENCE
Lehne, R. (1998). *Pharmacology for nursing care* (3rd ed.). Philadelphia: W. B. Saunders. p. 733.

35. 3

RATIONALE: Mycophenolate mofetil should be administered on an empty stomach. The capsules should not be opened or crushed. The client should contact the physician if unusual bleeding or bruising, sore throat, mouth sores, abdominal pain, or fever occurs. Antacids containing magnesium and aluminum may decrease the absorption of the medication and therefore should not be taken with the medication. The medication is given in combination with corticosteroids and cyclosporine.
TEST-TAKING STRATEGY: Knowledge regarding the teaching points associated with the administration of this medication is required to answer this question. Review this medication now if you had difficulty with it.
LEVEL OF COGNITIVE ABILITY: Application
PHASE OF NURSING PROCESS: Implementation
CLIENT NEEDS: Health Promotion and Maintenance
CONTENT AREA: Pharmacology
REFERENCE
Hodgson, B., & Kizior, R. (1999). *Saunders nursing drug handbook 1999.* Philadelphia: W. B. Saunders. pp. 709–711.

36. 1

RATIONALE: Azathioprine suppresses cell-mediated and humoral immune responses by inhibiting the proliferation of B and T lymphocytes. It is generally used as an adjunct to cyclosporine and glucocorticoids to help suppress transplant rejection.

TEST-TAKING STRATEGY: Knowledge regarding the action of this medication is required to answer this question. If you are unfamiliar with this medication, take time now to review.
LEVEL OF COGNITIVE ABILITY: Comprehension
PHASE OF NURSING PROCESS: Implementation
CLIENT NEEDS: Physiological Integrity
CONTENT AREA: Pharmacology
REFERENCE
Lehne, R. (1998). *Pharmacology for nursing care* (3rd ed.). Philadelphia: W. B. Saunders. p. 732.

37. **2**

RATIONALE: Epoetin alfa is used to reverse anemia associated with CRF. Therapeutic effect is seen when the hematocrit is between 30% and 33%.
TEST-TAKING STRATEGY: Relate the name of the medication, Epogen, to the potential action or effect. The only laboratory test that would reflect the effect of this medication is identified in option 2. Review the therapeutic effect of this medication now if you had difficulty with this question.
LEVEL OF COGNITIVE ABILITY: Analysis
PHASE OF NURSING PROCESS: Evaluation
CLIENT NEEDS: Physiological Integrity
CONTENT AREA: Pharmacology
REFERENCE
Lehne, R. (1998). *Pharmacology for nursing care* (3rd ed.). Philadelphia: W. B. Saunders. p. 567.

38. **4**

RATIONALE: Epoetin alfa is administered parenterally either IV or SC. Administration is by IV bolus for dialysis clients and by IV bolus or SC injection for nondialysis clients. It cannot be given orally because it is a glycoprotein and it would be degraded in the gastrointestinal tract.
TEST-TAKING STRATEGY: Knowledge regarding the administration of this medication is required to answer this question. If you are unfamiliar with this important medication, take time now to review.
LEVEL OF COGNITIVE ABILITY: Application
PHASE OF NURSING PROCESS: Planning
CLIENT NEEDS: Physiological Integrity
CONTENT AREA: Pharmacology
REFERENCE
Lehne, R. (1998). *Pharmacology for nursing care* (3rd ed.). Philadelphia: W. B. Saunders. p. 567.

39. **2**

RATIONALE: Epoetin alfa is generally well tolerated. The most significant adverse effect is hypertension. Occasionally, tachycardia may occur as a side effect. It may also cause an improved sense of well-being.
TEST-TAKING STRATEGY: Knowledge regarding the significant side effect associated with epoetin alfa is required to answer this question. Review this important medication now if you had difficulty with this question.
LEVEL OF COGNITIVE ABILITY: Comprehension
PHASE OF NURSING PROCESS: Data Collection
CLIENT NEEDS: Physiological Integrity
CONTENT AREA: Pharmacology
REFERENCE
Lehne, R. (1998). *Pharmacology for nursing care* (3rd ed.). Philadelphia: W. B. Saunders. p. 567.

40. **4**

RATIONALE: Epoetin alfa stimulates erythropoiesis. It takes 2 to 6 weeks after initiation of therapy before a clinically significant increase in hematocrit is observed. Therefore, this medication is not intended for clients who require immediate correction of severe anemia, and it is not a substitute for emergency transfusions.
TEST-TAKING STRATEGY: Knowledge that the medication stimulates erythropoiesis will assist in directing you to option 4. If you are unfamiliar with this medication and its therapeutic effects, review now.
LEVEL OF COGNITIVE ABILITY: Analysis
PHASE OF NURSING PROCESS: Evaluation
CLIENT NEEDS: Physiological Integrity
CONTENT AREA: Pharmacology
REFERENCE
Kuhn, M. (1998). *Pharmacotherapeutics: A nursing process approach* (4th ed.). Philadelphia: F. A. Davis. p. 567.

41. **3**

RATIONALE: The client should be instructed not to shake the bottle. The medication should be refrigerated at all times. The client should use only 1 dose per vial and not reenter the vial. Unused portions need to be discarded.
TEST-TAKING STRATEGY: Note that options 3 and 4 are identifying opposite actions. This should provide you with the clue that one of these options may be the correct one. If you are not familiar with the teaching points related to this medication, review them now.
LEVEL OF COGNITIVE ABILITY: Application
PHASE OF NURSING PROCESS: Implementation
CLIENT NEEDS: Health Promotion and Maintenance
CONTENT AREA: Pharmacology
REFERENCE
Kuhn, M. (1998). *Pharmacotherapeutics: A nursing process approach* (4th ed.). Philadelphia: F. A. Davis. p. 569.

42. **3**

RATIONALE: The client who is receiving aluminum hydroxide should take the medication with meals. The phosphate-binding effect is best when it is taken with food. If tablets are used, they should be chewed well before swallowing.
TEST-TAKING STRATEGY: Note that options 1, 2, and 4 are similar in that they all suggest administering the medication without a food item. Review this medication now if you had difficulty with this question.
LEVEL OF COGNITIVE ABILITY: Application
PHASE OF NURSING PROCESS: Implementation
CLIENT NEEDS: Health Promotion and Maintenance
CONTENT AREA: Pharmacology
REFERENCE
Kuhn, M. (1998). *Pharmacotherapeutics: A nursing process approach* (4th ed.). Philadelphia: F. A. Davis. p. 574.

43. **2**

RATIONALE: Aluminum-containing antacids are constipating and the client should be instructed to take a stool softener or additional bulk-type laxatives to relieve this uncomfortable side effect. Options 1, 3, and 4 are not side effects of this medication.
TEST-TAKING STRATEGY: Knowledge regarding the purpose and side effects associated with this important med-

ication is required to answer this question. If you are unfamiliar with this medication, take time now to review.
LEVEL OF COGNITIVE ABILITY: Comprehension
PHASE OF NURSING PROCESS: Data Collection
CLIENT NEEDS: Physiological Integrity
CONTENT AREA: Pharmacology
REFERENCE
Kuhn, M. (1998). *Pharmacotherapeutics: A nursing process approach* (4th ed.). Philadelphia: F. A. Davis. p. 574.

44. **4**

RATIONALE: The usual adult dose of aluminum hydroxide is 30 to 60 mL or 1 to 3 capsules before each meal, or three times a day.
TEST-TAKING STRATEGY: Knowledge regarding the usual adult dosage for aluminum hydroxide is required to answer this question. If you are unfamiliar with this important medication, take time now to review.
LEVEL OF COGNITIVE ABILITY: Comprehension
PHASE OF NURSING PROCESS: Planning
CLIENT NEEDS: Physiological Integrity
CONTENT AREA: Pharmacology

REFERENCE
Kuhn, M. (1998). *Pharmacotherapeutics: A nursing process approach* (4th ed.). Philadelphia: F. A. Davis. p. 567.

45. **2**

RATIONALE: Ferrous sulfate is an iron supplement used to treat anemia. Constipation is a frequent and uncomfortable side effect associated with the administration of oral iron supplements. Stool softeners are often prescribed to prevent constipation.
TEST-TAKING STRATEGY: Recalling that oral iron can cause constipation will easily direct you to option 2. If you had difficulty with this question, take time now to review the side effects of ferrous sulfate.
LEVEL OF COGNITIVE ABILITY: Comprehension
PHASE OF NURSING PROCESS: Data Collection
CLIENT NEEDS: Physiological Integrity
CONTENT AREA: Pharmacology
REFERENCE
deWit, S. (1998). *Essentials of medical-surgical nursing* (4th ed.). Philadelphia: W. B. Saunders. p. 484.

BIBLIOGRAPHY

Asperheim, M. K. (1996). *Pharmacology: An introductory text* (8th ed.). Philadelphia: W. B. Saunders.

Black, J., & Matassarin-Jacobs, E. (1997). *Medical-surgical nursing: Clinical management for continuity of care* (5th ed.). Philadelphia: W. B. Saunders.

deWit, S. (1998). *Essentials of medical-surgical nursing* (4th ed.). Philadelphia: W. B. Saunders.

Eckler, J., & Fair, J. (1996). *Pharmacology essentials*. Philadelphia: W. B. Saunders.

Hodgson, B., & Kizior, R. (1999). *Saunders nursing drug handbook 1999*. Philadelphia: W. B. Saunders.

Kuhn, M. (1998). *Pharmacotherapeutics: A nursing process approach* (4th ed.). Philadelphia: F. A. Davis.

Lehne, R. (1998). *Pharmacology for nursing care* (3rd ed.). Philadelphia: W. B. Saunders.

UNIT XV

....

The Adult Client with an Eye/Ear Disorder

PYRAMID TERMS

Astigmatism—Corneal curvature; eye may be hyperopic or myopic.

Cataracts—An opacity of the lens that distorts the image projected onto the retina and can progress to blindness.

Conductive Hearing Loss—When sound waves are blocked to the inner ear fibers because of external ear or middle ear disorders. Disorders can often be corrected with no damage to hearing, or minimal permanent hearing loss.

Cycloplegia—Refers to the paralysis of the ciliary muscles. Cycloplegia causes blurred vision because the shape of the lens can no longer be adjusted to near vision.

Fenestration—Removal of the stapes with a small hole drilled in the footplate; a prosthesis is connected between the incus and footplate. Sounds cause the prosthesis to vibrate in the same manner as did the stapes.

Glaucoma—Increased intraocular pressure as a result of inadequate drainage of aqueous humor from the canal of Schlemm or overproduction of aqueous humor. The condition damages the optic nerve and can result in blindness.

Hyperopia—Farsightedness; objects converge to a point behind the retina. Vision beyond 20 feet is normal but near vision is poor. Correction is done by a convex lens.

Legally Blind—If the best visual acuity with corrective lenses in the better eye is 20/200 or less, or if visual acuity is less than 20 degrees of the visual field in the better eye.

Meniere's Syndrome—A syndrome also called endolymphatic hydrops, which refers to dilation of the endolymphatic system either by overproduction or decreased reabsorption of endolymphatic fluid. It is characterized by tinnitus, unilateral sensorineural hearing loss, and vertigo.

Miosis—Refers to a constricted pupil.

Miotics—Medications that cause contraction of the pupil.

Mydriasis—Refers to a dilated pupil.

Mydriatics—Medications that dilate the pupil.

Myopia—Nearsightedness; rays coming from an object are focused in front of the retina. Near vision is normal but distant vision is defective. A biconcave lens is used for correction.

Otosclerosis—Disease of the labyrinthine capsule of the middle ear that results in a bony overgrowth of tissue surrounding the ossicles. Causes the development of irregular areas of new bone formation and causes fixation of the bones. Stapes fixation leads to a conductive hearing loss.

Presbycusis—Common cause of sensorineural hearing loss associated with aging.

Retinal Detachment—Occurs when the layers of the retina separate due to the accumulation of fluid between them, or when both retinal layers elevate away from choroid as a result of a tumor. Partial separation becomes complete if untreated. When detachment becomes complete, blindness occurs.

Sensorineural Hearing Loss—A pathological process of the inner ear or of the sensory fibers that lead to the cerebral cortex. It is often permanent and measures must be taken to reduce further damage or to attempt to amplify sound as a means of improving hearing to some degree.

◢ PYRAMID TO SUCCESS

Pyramid points focus on nursing interventions for clients with impairment in sight or hearing and on the nursing care related to disorders such as cataracts, glaucoma, and retinal detachment. Pyramid points also focus on emergency interventions for eye and ear disorders and injuries. Review nursing care related to organ donation for the donor and the recipient. Pyramid points also focus on client instructions related to medication administration, sensory perceptual alterations and safety issues, and available support systems.

NURSING PROCESS

DATA COLLECTION
Risk factors related to eye or ear disorders
Visual impairment
Hearing impairment
Signs of infection
Risk for injury
Ability to care for self

PLANNING	IMPLEMENTATION	EVALUATION
The client remains oriented to the environment.	Identify factors that contribute to sensory or perceptual alterations. Orient client to environment. Increase amount of stimuli to achieve appropriate sensory input.	The client interacts appropriately with the environment. The client demonstrates the ability to compensate for sensory deficits by maximizing the use of unimpaired senses.
PLANNING	IMPLEMENTATION	EVALUATION
The client remains free of infection. The client identifies factors that increase the risk of infection.	Monitor vital signs. Monitor for signs of infection. Instruct client regarding signs of infection and methods to avoid infection.	Vital signs remain normal. The client verbalizes the signs of infection. The client verbalizes methods to avoid infection.
PLANNING	IMPLEMENTATION	EVALUATION
The client remains free from injury.	Identify the risk for injury. Initiate safety precautions.	The client remains free of injury.
PLANNING	IMPLEMENTATION	EVALUATION
The client identifies limitations related to self-care.	Discuss limitations in self-care with client. Encourage independence in self-care.	The client participates in self-care to the optimal level.
PLANNING	IMPLEMENTATION	EVALUATION
The client identifies behaviors that reduce fear.	Provide verbal and nonverbal reassurances that may assist in reducing fear. Encourage client to verbalize feelings related to fear.	The client verbalizes comfort and measures that reduce fear.
PLANNING	IMPLEMENTATION	EVALUATION
The client identifies behaviors that may decrease social isolation.	Encourage client to schedule time for social interaction.	The client identifies community resources that assist in decreasing social isolation.
PLANNING	IMPLEMENTATION	EVALUATION
The client identifies the consequences of noncompliant behavior.	Identify probable causes of noncompliant behavior. Involve the client in identifying the importance of compliant behavior.	The client complies with the described plan of care.

◢ CLIENT NEEDS

SAFE, EFFECTIVE CARE ENVIRONMENT

Communication techniques for impaired vision and hearing
Client rights
Informed consent for invasive procedures
Organ donation
Accident prevention related to sensory impairments
Asepsis with procedures and treatments
Standard (universal) precautions

HEALTH PROMOTION AND MAINTENANCE

Aging process
Expected body image changes
The prevention and early detection of health problems and diseases related to the eye and the ear
Home care instructions following procedures related to the eye and ear
Instructions regarding the administration of eye and ear medications
Reinforcement regarding the importance of compliance to the prescribed therapy

PSYCHOSOCIAL INTEGRITY

The ability to cope with feelings of isolation and loss of independence
The threat to vision or hearing loss
Sensory perceptual alterations
Family support systems
Available community resources

PHYSIOLOGICAL INTEGRITY

Care for assistive devices such as glasses, contact lenses, and hearing aids
Self-care limitations
Medications, actions, agents, side effects, and adverse effects
Complications related to procedures
Expected responses to therapy
Cataracts
Glaucoma
Retinal detachment
Initial treatment for eye and ear emergencies
Organ donation
Hearing or visual loss

BIBLIOGRAPHY

deWit, S. (1998). *Essentials of medical-surgical nursing* (4th ed.). Philadelphia: W. B. Saunders.
Hill, S., & Howlett, H. (1997). *Success in practical nursing: Personal and vocational issues* (3rd ed.). Philadelphia: W. B. Saunders.
Leahy, J., & Kizilay, P. (1998). *Foundations of nursing practice: A nursing process approach*. Philadelphia: W. B. Saunders.

Luckmann, J. (1997). *Saunders manual of nursing care*. Philadelphia: W. B. Saunders.
Monahan, F., & Neighbors, M. (1998). *Medical-surgical nursing: Foundations for clinical practice* (2nd ed.). Philadelphia: W. B. Saunders.
National Council of State Boards of Nursing (1998). *National Council detailed test plan for the NCLEX-PN examination*. Chicago: Author.
O'Toole, M. (1997). *Miller-Keane encyclopedia & dictionary of medicine, nursing, & allied health* (6th ed.). Philadelphia: W. B. Saunders.

CHAPTER 52

The Eye and the Ear

I. Anatomy and Physiology of the Eye

A. The Eye
   1. The eye is 1 inch in diameter
   2. It is located in the anterior portion of the orbit
   3. The orbit is the bony structure of the skull that surrounds the eye and offers protection to the eye
B. Layers of the eye
   1. External layer
      a. The fibrous coat that supports the eye
      b. Contains the sclera, which is an opaque white tissue
      c. Contains the cornea, which is a dense transparent layer
   2. Middle layer
      a. The second layer of the eyeball
      b. Is vascular and heavily pigmented
      c. Consists of the choroid, the ciliary body, and the iris
      d. The choroid is the dark brown membrane located between the sclera and the retina
      e. The choroid lines most of the sclera and is attached to the retina, but can easily detach from the sclera
      f. The choroid contains many blood vessels and supplies nutrients to the retina
      g. The ciliary body connects the choroid with the iris and secretes aqueous humor that helps give the eye its shape
      h. The iris is the colored portion of the eye, is located in front of the lens, and has a central circular opening called the pupil
   3. Internal layer
      a. Consists of the retina
      b. The retina is a thin, delicate structure in which the fibers of the optic nerve are distributed
      c. The retina is bordered externally by the choroid and sclera and internally by the vitreous
      d. The retina contains blood vessels and photoreceptors called rods and cones
C. Vitreous body
   1. Contains a gelatinous substance that occupies the vitreous chamber, which is the space between the lens and the retina
   2. It transmits light and gives shape to the posterior eye
D. Vitreous
   1. A gel-like substance that maintains the shape of the eye
   2. Provides additional physical support to the retina
E. Rods and cones
   1. Rods are responsible for peripheral vision and function at reduced levels of illumination
   2. Cones function at bright levels of illumination and are responsible for color vision and central vision
F. Optic disk
   1. A creamy pink to white depressed area in the retina
   2. The optic nerve enters and exits the eyeball at this area
   3. This area is called the blind spot because it contains only nerve fibers, lacks photoreceptor cells, and is insensitive to light
G. Macula lutea
   1. A small, oval, yellowish pink area located lateral and temporal to the optic disk
   2. The central depressed part of the macula is the fovea centralis where most acute vision occurs
H. Aqueous humor
   1. A clear watery fluid that fills the anterior and posterior chambers of the eye
   2. Produced by the ciliary processes; the fluid drains into the canal of Schlemm
   3. The anterior chamber lies between the cornea and the iris
   4. The posterior chamber lies between the iris and lens
I. Canal of Schlemm
   1. A passageway that extends completely around the eye
   2. Permits fluid to drain out of the eye into the systemic circulation so a constant intraocular pressure is maintained

J. Lens
  1. A transparent circular structure behind the iris and in front of vitreous body
  2. Bends rays of light so that the light falls on the retina
K. Pupils
  1. Control the amount of light that enters the eye and reaches the retina
  2. Darkness produces dilation
  3. Light produces constriction
L. Conjunctiva
  1. The thin transparent mucous membrane
  2. Lines the posterior surface of each eyelid and is located over the sclera
M. Lacrimal gland
  1. Produces tears
  2. Tears are drained throughout the punctum into the lacrimal duct and sac
N. Eye muscles
  1. Muscles do not work independently but work in conjunction with the muscle that produces the opposite movement
  2. Rectus muscles: exert their pull when the eye turns temporally
  3. Oblique muscles: exert their pull when the eye turns nasally
O. Nerves
  1. Cranial nerve III: oculomotor
  2. Cranial nerve IV: trochlear
  3. Cranial nerve VI: abducens
  4. Cranial nerve II: optic nerve (nerve of sight)
P. Blood vessels
  1. Ophthalmic artery: major artery supplying the structures in the eye
  2. Ophthalmic veins: venous drainage occurs through the veins

II. Anatomy and Physiology of the Ear

A. Functions
  1. Hearing
  2. Maintenance of balance
B. External ear
  1. Embedded in the temporal bone bilaterally at the level of the eyes
  2. Extends from the auricle through the external canal to the tympanic membrane or eardrum
  3. Includes the mastoid process, which is the body ridge located over the temporal bone
C. Middle ear
  1. Consists of the medial side of the tympanic membrane
  2. Contains three bony ossicles
    a. Malleus
    b. Incus
    c. Stapes
  3. The tympanic membrane is a thick transparent sheet of tissue that provides a barrier between the external and the middle ear
  4. The middle ear is protected from the inner ear

by the round and the oval window membranes
  5. The eustachian tube opens into the middle ear and allows for equalization of pressure on both sides of the tympanic membrane
D. Inner ear
  1. Contains the semicircular canals, the cochlea, and the distal end of the eighth cranial nerve
  2. The semicircular canals contain fluid and hair cells connected to sensory nerve fibers of the vestibular portion of eighth cranial nerve
  3. Maintains sense of balance or equilibrium
  4. Cochlea: spiral-shaped organ of hearing
  5. Organ of Corti: receptor and organ of hearing
  6. Eighth cranial nerve:
    a. Cochlear branch: transmits neuroimpulses from the cochlea to the brain where they are interpreted as sound
    b. Vestibular branch: maintains balance and equilibrium
E. Hearing and equilibrium
  1. The external ear conducts sound waves to the middle ear
  2. The middle ear, also called the tympanic cavity, conducts sound vibrations to the inner ear
  3. The middle ear is filled with air, which is kept at atmospheric pressure by the opening of the eustachian tube
  4. The inner ear contains sensory receptors for sound and for equilibrium
  5. The receptors in the inner ear transmit sound waves and changes in body position to the nerve impulses

III. Assessment of Vision

A. Acuity
  1. Visual acuity tests measure the client's distance and near vision
  2. Snellen chart
    a. A simple tool to record visual acuity
    b. The client stands 20 feet from the chart and covers one eye and uses the other eye to read the line that appears most clearly
    c. If the client is able to do this accurately, the client reads the next lower line
    d. This sequence is repeated until the client is unable to correctly identify more than half of the characters on the line
    e. The procedure is repeated for the other eye
    f. The findings are recorded as a comparison with what the client can read at 20 feet
    g. A result of 20/50 means that the client is able to read at 20 feet from the chart what a healthy eye can read at 50 feet
    h. Clients who wear corrective lenses other than for reading should have their vision tested with the lens in place
B. Confrontational test: performed to examine visual fields or peripheral vision
C. Extraocular muscle function: the client holds the

head still and is asked to move the eyes and to follow a small object through the six cardinal positions of gaze

D. Color vision: the standard tests for color vision involve picking numbers or letters out of a complex and colorful picture such as with the use of an Ishihara chart

E. Pupils
   1. Round and of equal size
   2. Increasing light causes pupillary constriction
   3. Decreasing light causes pupillary dilation
   4. Constriction of both pupils is a normal response to direct light
   5. The client is asked to look straight ahead while the examiner quickly brings a beam of a flashlight in from the side and directs it onto the eye
   6. The constriction of the eye is a direct response to the shining of a flashlight into that eye; constriction of the opposite eye is known as a consensual response

F. Sclera and cornea
   1. Normal sclera color is white
   2. A yellow color to the sclera may indicate jaundice or systemic problems
   3. In a dark-skinned person, the sclera may appear yellow; pigmented dots may be present
   4. The cornea is transparent, smooth, shiny, and bright
   5. Cloudy areas or specks on the cornea may be the result of an accident or eye injury

G. Ophthalmoscopy
   1. An instrument is used to examine the external structures and the interior of the eye
   2. The room is darkened so that the pupil will dilate

IV. Diagnostic Tests for the Eye

A. Fluorescein angiography
   1. Description: detailed imaging and recording of ocular circulation by a series of photographs after the administration of a dye
   2. Implementation preprocedure
      a. Assess the client for allergies and previous reactions to dyes
      b. Obtain an informed consent form
      c. A mydriatic medication, which causes pupil dilation, is instilled in the eye 1 hour before the test
      d. The dye is injected into a vein of the client's arm
      e. Inform the client that the dye may cause the skin to appear yellow for several hours after the test and is gradually eliminated through the urine
      f. The client may experience nausea, vomiting, sneezing, paresthesia of the tongue, or pain at the injection site
      g. If hives appear, oral or intramuscular (IM) antihistamine, such as diphenhydramine (Benadryl), is administered as prescribed

3. Implementation, postprocedure
   a. Encourage rest
   b. Encourage fluids to remove the dye from the client's system
   c. Remind the client that the yellow skin appearance will disappear
   d. Instruct the client that the urine will appear bright green until the dye is excreted
   e. Instruct the client to avoid direct sunlight for a few hours after the test
   f. Instruct the client that the photophobia will continue until pupil dilation returns to normal

B. Computed tomography
   1. Description
      a. A beam of x-ray scans the skull and orbits of the eye
      b. Contrast material is not usually administered
   2. Implementation
      a. No special client preparation or follow-up care is required
      b. Instruct the client that he or she will be positioned in a confined space and need to keep the head still during the procedure

C. Slit lamp
   1. Description
      a. Allows examination of the anterior ocular structures under microscopic magnification
      b. The client leans on a chin rest to stabilize the head while a narrowed beam of light is aimed so it illuminates only a narrow segment of the eye
   2. Implementation
      a. Explain the procedure to the client
      b. Advise the client about the brightness of the light and the need to look forward at a point over the examiner's ear

D. Corneal staining
   1. Description
      a. Instillation of a topical dye into the conjuctival sac to outline irregularities of the corneal surface that are not easily visible
      b. The eye is viewed through a blue filter, and a bright green color indicates areas of a nonintact corneal epithelium
   2. Implementation
      a. If the client wears contact lenses, they must be removed
      b. The client is instructed to blink after the dye has been applied to distribute the dye evenly across the cornea

E. Tonometry
   1. Description
      a. The test is primarily used to assess for an increase in intraocular pressure and potential **glaucoma**
      b. Normal ocular pressure is 10 to 21 mmHg
   2. Implementation
      a. Each eye is anesthetized

b. The client is asked to stare forward at a point above the examiner's ear
c. A flattened cone is brought in contact with the cornea
d. The amount of pressure needed to flatten the cornea is measured
e. The client must be instructed to avoid rubbing the eye following the examination if the eye has been anesthetized and the potential for scratching the cornea exists

V. Assessment of the Ear

A. Otoscopic examination
 1. A speculum is introduced into the external canal to visualize the tympanic membrane
 2. The normal external canal is pink and intact without lesions and with various amounts of cerumen and fine little hairs
 3. The tympanic membrane is transparent, opaque, pearly gray, slightly concave, and is intact and free from lesions
B. Auditory assessment
 1. Sound is transmitted by air conduction and bone conduction
 2. Air conduction takes two to three times longer than bone conduction
 3. Hearing loss is categorized as **conductive**, **sensorineural**, and mixed **conductive** and **sensorineural**
 4. **Conductive hearing loss** is caused by any physical obstruction to the transmission of sound waves
 5. **Sensorineural hearing loss** is a result of a defect in the organ of hearing, in the eighth cranial nerve, or in the brain itself
 6. A mixed **conductive, sensorineural hearing loss** results in profound hearing loss
 7. Tuning fork tests: the Weber and the Rinne tuning fork tests assist in distinguishing **conductive hearing loss** from **sensorineural hearing loss**
C. Vestibular assessment
 1. Test for falling: a significant sway or a fall is a positive Romberg sign
 2. Test for past pointing
  a. The normal test response is that the client can easily return to the point of reference
  b. Clients with vestibular function problems lack a normal sense of position and are unable to return their extended fingers to the point of reference; instead, they deviate either to the right or the left of the reference point
 3. Gaze nystagmus evaluation: any spontaneous nystagmus, a constant and involuntary cyclic movement of the eyeball in any direction, represents problems with the vestibular system
 4. Hallpike's maneuver
  a. Assesses for positional vertigo or induced dizziness

b. A positive test results in nystagmus after 5 to 10 seconds

VI. Diagnostic Tests for the Ear

A. Tomography
 1. Description
  a. Assesses the mastoid, middle ear, and inner ear structures; aids in the diagnosis of **conductive** and **sensorineural hearing loss**
  b. Multiple x-rays of the head are performed; especially helpful in the diagnostic of acoustic tumors
 2. Implementation
  a. All jewelry is removed
  b. Lead eye shields are used to cover the cornea to diminish the radiation dose to the eyes
  c. The client must remain still in a supine position
  d. No follow-up care is required
B. Audiometry
 1. Description
  a. Measures hearing acuity using pure tone audiometry and speech audiometry
  b. Pure tone audiometry is used to identify problems with hearing, speech, music, and other sounds in the environment
  c. In speech audiometry, the client's ability to hear spoken words is measured
  d. After testing, audiogram patterns are depicted on a graph to determine the type and level of the hearing loss
 2. Implementation: instruct the client to identify the sounds as they are heard
C. Caloric test (bithermal test)
 1. Description
  a. Performed to evaluate the client experiencing dizziness
  b. Nystagmus, nausea, vomiting, or ataxia may indicate a pathological condition of the labyrinth system, whereas a decreased response may indicate that the vestibular system is affected
 2. Implementation
  a. Warm water causes a greater response than cold water
  b. Warm-water caloric testing precedes cool-water caloric testing
  c. A 30-second irrigation with 120 to 200 mL of water at 44°C (111.2°F) is used first, followed by irrigation with water at 30°C (86°F)
  d. The client must assume a supine position with the eyes closed and head elevated to 30 degrees
  e. The character and duration of the eye movements are measured
  f. Following the procedure, the client begins taking clear fluids slowly and cautiously because nausea and vomiting may occur

g. Assistance with ambulation may also be necessary following the procedure

VII. Disorders of the Eye

A. Risk factors related to eye disorders (Box 52–1)
B. **Legally blind**
1. Description: if the best visual acuity with corrective lenses in the better eye is 20/200 or less, or if the widest diameter of the visual field in that eye is no greater than 20 degrees
2. Implementation
   a. When speaking to the client who has limited sight or blindness, the nurse uses a normal tone of voice
   b. Orient the client to the environment
   c. Use a focal point and provide further orientation to the environment from that focal point
   d. Allow the client to touch objects in the room
   e. Use the clock placement of foods on the meal tray to orient the client
   f. When ambulating, allow the client to grasp the nurse's arm at the elbow; the arm is kept close to the nurse's body so that the client can detect the direction of movement
   g. Instruct the client to remain one step behind the nurse when ambulating
   h. Instruct the client in the use of the cane used for the blind client, which is differentiated from other canes by its straight shape and white color with red tip
   i. Instruct the client that the cane is held in the dominant hand several inches off the floor
   j. Instruct the client that the cane sweeps the ground where the client's foot will be placed next, to determine the presence of obstacles
   k. Alert the client when you are approaching
   l. Provide radios, TVs, and clocks that give the time orally or provide Braille watches
   m. Promote independence as much as is possible
C. **Cataracts**
1. Description
   a. An opacity of the lens that distorts the image projected onto the retina and which can progress to blindness
   b. Causes include the aging process (senile **cataracts**), inherited (congenital **cataracts**), injury (traumatic **cataracts**),

and as a result of another eye disease (secondary **cataracts**)
   c. Intervention is indicated when visual acuity has been reduced to a level that the client finds to be unacceptable or adversely affecting lifestyle
2. Data collection
   a. Opaque or cloudy white pupil
   b. Gradual loss of vision
   c. Blurred vision
   d. Decreased color perception
   e. Vision that is better in dim light with pupil dilation
3. Implementation
   a. Surgical removal of the lens, one eye at a time
   b. Extracapsular extraction: the lens is lifted out without removing the lens capsule; may be performed by phacoemulsification in which the lens is broken up by ultrasonic vibrations and extracted
   c. Intracapsular extraction: the lens is removed within its capsule through a small incision
   d. A lens implantation may be performed at the time of the surgical procedure
4. Preoperative implementation: administer preoperative eye medications including **mydriatics** and cycloplegics as prescribed
5. Postoperative implementation
   a. Elevate the head of the bed 30 to 45 degrees
   b. Turn the client to the back or nonoperative side
   c. Maintain an eye patch; orient the client to the environment
   d. Position the client's personal belongings to the nonoperative side
   e. Use side rails for safety
   f. Assist with ambulation
6. Client education (Box 52–2)
D. **Glaucoma**
1. Description
   a. Increased intraocular pressure as a result of inadequate drainage of aqueous humor from the canal of Schlemm or overproduction of aqueous humor
   b. The condition damages the optic nerve and can result in blindness
2. Types (Box 52–3)
3. Data collection
   a. Progressive loss of peripheral vision
   b. Elevated intraocular pressure (normal pressure is 10 to 21 mmHg)
   c. Vision worsening in the evening with difficulty adjusting to dark rooms
   d. Blurred vision and progressive loss of central vision
   e. Halos around white lights
   f. Frontal headaches and eye pain
4. Implementation acute **glaucoma**
   a. Treated as a medical emergency and

BOX 52–2. Client Education Following Cataract Surgery

Avoid eye straining

Avoid rubbing or placing pressure on the eyes

Avoid rapid movements, straining, sneezing, coughing, bending, vomiting, and lifting objects over 5 pounds

Instruct the client in measures to prevent constipation

Instruct the client and significant other on dressing changes and prescribed eye drops and medications

Wipe excess drainage or tearing with a sterile wet cotton ball from the inner to the outer canthus

Instruct the client and significant other in the use of an eye shield at bedtime

Instruct the client that if a lens implant is not performed, the eye cannot accommodate and glasses must be worn at all times

Instruct the client that cataract glasses act as magnifying glasses and replace central vision only

Instruct clients that cataract glasses magnify and objects will appear closer; therefore, they need to accommodate, judge distance, and climb stairs carefully

Instruct the client that contact lenses will provide sharp visual acuity but that dexterity is needed to insert them

Advise the client to contact the physician for any decrease in vision, severe eye pain, or increase in eye discharge

---

medications are administered as prescribed to lower intraocular pressure

   b. Prepare the client for peripheral iridectomy, which allows aqueous humor to flow from the posterior to the anterior chamber

5. Implementation chronic **glaucoma**

   a. Instruct the client on the importance of medications (**miotics**) to constrict the pupils, carbonic anhydrase inhibitors and beta blockers to decrease the production of aqueous humor

   b. Instruct the client on the need for lifelong medication use

---

BOX 52–3. Types of Glaucoma

Acute Closed-Angle or *Narrow-Angle Glaucoma*: results from obstruction to outflow of aqueous humor

Chronic Closed-Angle Glaucoma: follows an untreated attack of acute closed-angle glaucoma

Chronic Open-Angle Glaucoma: results from overproduction or obstruction to the outflow of aqueous humor

Acute: a rapid onset of intraocular pressure greater than 50 to 70 mmHg

Chronic: a slow, progressive, gradual onset of intraocular pressure greater than 30 to 50 mmHg

---

   c. Instruct the client to wear a Medic-Alert bracelet

   d. Instruct the client to avoid anticholinergic medications

   e. Instruct the client to report eye pain, halos around the eyes, and changes in vision to the physician

   f. Instruct the client that when maximal medical therapy has failed to halt the progression of visual field loss and optic nerve damage, surgery will be recommended

   g. Prepare the client for trabeculoplasty as prescribed to facilitate aqueous humor drainage

   h. Prepare the client for trabeculectomy as prescribed, which allows drainage of aqueous humor into the conjunctival spaces by the creation of an opening

E. **Retinal detachment**

   1. Description

      a. Occurs when the layers of the retina separate because of the accumulation of fluid between them, or when both retinal layers elevate away from choroid as a result of a tumor

      b. Partial separation becomes complete if untreated

      c. When detachment becomes complete, blindness occurs

   2. Data collection

      a. Flashes of light

      b. Floaters

      c. Increase in blurred vision

      d. Sense of a curtain being drawn over the eyes

      e. Loss of a portion of the visual field

   3. Immediate implementation

      a. Provide bed rest

      b. Cover both eyes with patches to prevent further detachment

      c. Position the client's head as prescribed

      d. Protect the client from injury

      e. Avoid jerky head movements and minimize eye stress

      f. Speak to the client before approaching

      g. Prepare the client for surgical procedures as prescribed

   4. Surgical procedures

      a. Draining fluid from the subretinal space so that the retina can return to the normal position

      b. Sealing retinal breaks by cryosurgery, a cold probe applied to the sclera, to stimulate an inflammatory response leading to adhesions

      c. Diathermy, the use of electrode needle and heat through the sclera, to stimulate an inflammatory response

      d. Laser therapy, to stimulate an inflammatory response, to seal small retinal tears before the detachment occurs

e. Scleral buckling, to hold the choroid and retina together with a splint, until scar tissue forms, closing the tear

f. Insertion of gas or silicone oil to encourage attachment because these agents have a specific gravity less than vitreous or air, and can float against the retina

5. Postoperative implementation

a. Maintain eye patches bilaterally as prescribed

b. Monitor for hemorrhage

c. Prevent nausea and vomiting and monitor for restlessness, which can cause hemorrhage

d. Monitor for sudden, sharp eye pain (notify the physician)

e. Encourage deep breathing but avoid coughing

f. Provide bed rest for 1 to 2 days as prescribed

g. Position the client as prescribed

h. If gas has been inserted, position as prescribed on the abdomen and turn the head so the unaffected eye is down

i. Assist the client with activities of daily living

j. Avoid sudden head movements or anything that increases intraocular pressure

k. Instruct the client to limit reading for 3 to 5 weeks

l. Instruct the client to avoid squinting, straining and constipation, lifting heavy objects, and bending from the waist

m. Instruct the client to wear dark glasses during the day and an eyepatch at night

n. Encourage follow-up care because of the danger of recurrence or occurrence in the other eye

F. Hyphema

1. Description

a. The presence of blood in the anterior chamber that occurs as a result of an injury

b. The condition usually resolves in 5 to 7 days

2. Implementation

a. Encourage rest with client in semi-Fowler's position

b. Avoid sudden eye movements for 3 to 5 days to decrease likelihood of bleeding

c. Administer cycloplegic eye drops as prescribed to place the eye at rest

d. Instruct the client in the use of eye shields or eyepatches as prescribed

e. Instruct the client to restrict reading and watching television

G. Contusions

1. Description

a. Bleeding into the soft tissue as a result of an injury

b. Causes a black eye; the discoloration disappears in approximately 10 days

c. Visual acuity is usually not affected

d. Pain, photophobia, edema, and diplopia may occur

2. Implementation

a. Place ice on the eye immediately

b. Instruct the client to get an eye examination

H. Foreign bodies

1. Description: an object such as dust that enters the eye

2. Implementation

a. Have the client look upward; expose the lower lid, wet a cotton-tipped applicator with sterile normal saline, and gently twist the swab over the particle and remove it

b. If the particle cannot be seen, have the client look downward, place a cotton-tipped applicator horizontally on the outer surface of the upper eyelid, grasp the lashes, and pull the upper lid outward and over the cotton applicator; if the particle is seen, gently twist the swab over it to remove

I. Penetrating objects

1. Description: an injury that occurs to the eye in which an object penetrates the eye

2. Implementation

a. Never remove the object because it may be holding ocular structures in place

b. The object must be removed by the physician

c. Cover the object with a cup

d. Do not allow the client to bend

e. Do not place pressure on the eye

f. The client is to be seen by a physician immediately

J. Chemical burns

1. Description: an eye injury in which a caustic substance enters the eye

2. Implementation

a. Flush the eyes at the site of injury with water for at least 15 to 20 minutes

b. At the scene of the accident, obtain a sample of the chemical involved

c. At the emergency department, the eye is irrigated with gentle solutions such as normal saline or an ophthalmic irrigation solution

d. The solution is directed across the cornea and toward the lateral canthus

e. Prepare the client for visual acuity assessment

f. Apply antibiotic ointment as prescribed

g. Cover the eye with a patch as prescribed

K. Enucleation and exenteration

1. Description

a. Enucleation: removal of the entire eyeball

b. Exenteration: removal of the eyeball and surrounding tissues and bone

c. Performed for the removal of ocular tumors

d. After the eye is removed, a ball implant is inserted to provide a firm base for socket prosthesis and to facilitate the best cosmetic result

e. A prosthesis is fitted approximately 1 month after surgery

2. Preoperative implementation
   a. Provide emotional support to the client
   b. Encourage the client to verbalize feelings related to loss

3. Postoperative implementation
   a. Monitor vital signs
   b. Monitor pressure patch or dressing
   c. Report changes in vital signs or the presence of bright red drainage on the pressure patch or dressing

L. Organ donation
   1. Donor eyes
      a. Obtained from cadavers
      b. Must be enucleated soon after death because of rapid cell death
      c. Must be stored in a preserving solution
      d. Storage, handling, and coordination of donor tissue with surgeons is provided by a network of state eye bank associations across the country

   2. Care to deceased client as a potential eye donor
      a. Raise the head of the bed 30 degrees
      b. Instill antibiotic eye drops as prescribed
      c. Close the eyes and apply a small ice pack to the closed eyes
      d. The family and the physician are contacted to discuss the option of eye donation

   3. Preoperative care to the recipient
      a. Recipient may be told of the tissue availability only several hours to 1 day before the surgery
      b. Assist in alleviating client anxiety
      c. Monitor the eyes for signs of infection
      d. Report the presence of any redness, watery, or purulent drainage or edema around the eye
      e. Instill antibiotic drops into the eye as prescribed to reduce the number of microorganisms present

   4. Postoperative care to the recipient
      a. The eye is covered with a pressure patch and protective shield that is left in place until the next day
      b. Do not remove or change the dressing without a physician's order
      c. Monitor vital signs
      d. Monitor level of consciousness
      e. Assess dressing
      f. Position the client on the nonoperative side to reduce intraocular pressure
      g. Orient the client frequently
      h. Monitor for complications of bleeding,

wound leakage, infection, and graft rejection

   i. Instruct the client how to apply a patch and eye shield
   j. Instruct the client to wear the eye shield at night for 1 month and whenever around small children or pets
   k. Advise the client not to rub the eye

5. Graft rejection
   a. Can occur at any time
   b. Inform the client of the signs of rejection
   c. Signs include redness, swelling, decreased vision, and pain (RSVP)
   d. Treated with topical corticosteroids

VIII. Disorders of the Ear

A. Risk factors related to ear disorders (Box 52–4)
B. **Conductive hearing loss**
   1. Description
      a. When sound waves are blocked to the inner ear fibers because of external ear or middle ear disorders
      b. Disorders can often be corrected with no damage to hearing, or minimal permanent hearing loss
   2. Causes
      a. Any inflammatory process or obstruction of the external or middle ear
      b. Tumors
      c. **Otosclerosis**
      d. A build-up of scar tissue on the ossicles from previous middle ear surgery

C. **Sensorineural hearing loss**
   1. Description
      a. A pathological process of the inner ear or of the sensory fibers that lead to the cerebral cortex
      b. Is often permanent and measures must be taken to reduce further damage or to attempt to amplify sound as a means of improving hearing to some degree
   2. Causes
      a. Damage to the inner ear structures
      b. Damage to cranial nerve VIII
      c. Prolonged exposure to loud noise
      d. Medications
      e. Trauma
      f. Inherited disorders
      g. Metabolic and circulatory disorders
      h. Infections
      i. Surgery
      j. **Meniere's syndrome**

BOX 52–4. Risk Factors of Ear Disorders	
Infection	Medications
Trauma	Tumors
Ototoxicity	Aging process

BOX 52–5. Signs of Hearing Loss

Frequently asking people to repeat statements
Straining to hear
Turning head or leaning forward to favor one ear
Shouting in conversation
Ringing in the ears
Failing to respond when not looking in the direction of the sound
Irritability
Answering questions incorrectly
Raising the volume of the television or radio
Avoiding large groups
Better understanding of speech when in small groups
Withdrawing from social interactions

D. Mixed hearing loss: client has both **sensorineural** and **conductive hearing loss**
E. Signs of hearing loss and facilitating communication (Boxes 52–5 and 52–6)
F. Cochlear implantation
   1. Used for **sensorineural hearing loss**
   2. A small computer converts sound waves into electrical impulses that directly stimulate nerve fibers
   3. Electrodes are placed by the internal ear with a computer device attached to the external ear

---

BOX 52–6. Facilitating Communication

Using written words if the client is able to see, read, and write
Providing plenty of light in the room
Facing the client when speaking
Talking in a room without distracting noises
Moving close to the client and speaking slowly and clearly
Getting the attention of the client before you begin to speak
Keeping hands and other objects away from the mouth when talking to the client
Talking in lower tones, because shouting is not helpful
Rephrasing sentences and repeating information
Validating with the client the understanding of statements made by asking the client to repeat what was said
Reading lips
Encouraging the client to wear glasses when talking to someone to improve vision for lip reading
Sign language, which combines speech with hand movements that signify letters, words, or phrases
Use of telephone amplifiers
Installing flashing lights that are activated by ringing of the telephone or doorbell
Using specially trained dogs that help the client be aware of sound and alert the client of potential dangers

---

G. Hearing aids
   1. Used for the client with **conductive hearing loss**
   2. Can help the client with **sensorineural** loss, although it is not as effective
   3. A difficulty that exists is the amplification of background noise as well as voices
   4. Client education (Box 52–7)
H. **Presbycusis**
   1. Description
      a. Associated with aging
      b. Leads to degeneration or atrophy of the ganglion cells in the cochlea and a loss of elasticity of the basilar membranes
      c. Leads to compromise of the vascular supply to the inner ear with changes in several areas of the ear structure
   2. Data collection
      a. Hearing loss is gradual and bilateral
      b. Clients state they have no problem with hearing, but they cannot understand what the words are
      c. Client thinks that the speaker is mumbling
I. External otitis
   1. Description
      a. Infective inflammatory or allergic responses involving the structure of the external auditory canal or the auricles
      b. An irritating or infective agent comes in contact with the epithelial layer of the external ear that leads to either an allergic response or signs and symptoms of an infection
      c. The skin becomes red, swollen, and tender to touch on movements
      d. The extensive swelling of the canal can lead to **conductive hearing loss** because of obstruction

---

BOX 52–7. Client Education Regarding a Hearing Aid

Encourage the client to start using the hearing aid slowly to develop an adjustment to the device
Adjust the volume to the minimal hearing level to prevent feedback squealing
Teach the client to concentrate on the sounds that are to be heard and to filter out background noise
Instruct the client to clean the ear mold frequently with mild soap and water
Avoid excessive wetting of hearing aid and try to keep the hearing aid dry
Clean the ear cannula of the hearing aid with a toothpick or pipe cleaner
Turn off the hearing aid after removal from the ear and remove the battery when not in use
Keep extra batteries on hand
Keep hearing aid in a safe place
Prevent hair sprays, oils, or other hair and face products from coming in contact with the receiver of the hearing aid

e. It is more common in children, occurs more often in hot, humid environments, and is termed "swimmer's ear"

f. Prevention includes the elimination of irritating or infecting agents

2. Data collection
   a. Pain, itching, redness, and edema
   b. Plugged feeling in the ear
   c. Exudate
   d. Hearing loss

3. Implementation
   a. Apply heat locally for 20 minutes three times a day
   b. Encourage bed rest to assist in reducing pain
   c. Administer antibiotics or steroids as prescribed
   d. Administer analgesics such as aspirin or acetaminophen (Tylenol) for the pain as prescribed
   e. Instruct the client that ears should be kept clean and dry
   f. Instruct the client to use ear plugs for swimming
   g. Instruct the client that cotton-tipped applicators should not be used to dry ears because their use can lead to trauma to the canal
   h. Instruct the client that irritating agents such as hair products or headphones should be discontinued

J. Otitis media
   1. Description: an acute or chronic infective inflammatory or allergic response involving the structure of the middle ear
   2. Chronic otitis media
      a. Surgical treatment is necessary to restore hearing
      b. The type of surgery can vary and include either a simple reconstruction of the tympanic membrane, a myringoplasty, or replacement of the ossicles within the middle ear
      c. A tympanoplasty, a reconstruction of the middle ear, may be attempted to improve **conductive hearing loss**
   3. Data collection
      a. Pain from pressure in the ear
      b. Hearing loss
      c. Tinnitus, dizziness, or vertigo
      d. Fever, headache, and malaise
      e. Nausea and vomiting
      f. Bulging tympanic membrane
      g. Fluid behind the tympanic membrane
   4. Implementation
      a. Provide bed rest to limit head movements and prevent pain
      b. Administer localized heat as prescribed
      c. Administer antibiotics as prescribed
      d. Administer analgesics such as aspirin and acetaminophen (Tylenol) as prescribed
      e. Administer oral and nasal antihistamines

and decongestants to decrease mucus production and decrease levels of fluid in the middle ear

5. Myringotomy
   a. Surgically performed perforation of the tympanic membrane
   b. Allows drainage of middle ear fluids and thus alleviates pain
   c. Client Education (Box 52–8)

6. Needle aspiration: to remove fluid from middle ear

7. Insertion of a grommet: placed through the tympanic membrane to allow continuous drainage of the middle ear

8. Postoperative implementation for middle ear surgery
   a. Inform the client that initial hearing after surgery is diminished because of the packing in the ear canal, and that hearing improvement will occur after the ear canal packing is removed
   b. Keep the dressing clean and dry
   c. Keep the client flat with operative ear up for at least 12 hours as prescribed
   d. Administer antibiotics as prescribed
   e. Instruct clients that they may return to work in approximately 3 weeks postoperatively as prescribed

K. Mastoiditis
   1. Description
      a. May be acute or chronic and results from untreated or inadequately treated chronic or acute otitis media
      b. The pain is not relieved by myringotomy
   2. Data collection
      a. Swelling behind the ear and pain with minimal movement of the head
      b. Cellulitis on the skin or external scalp over the mastoid process

---

BOX 52–8. Client Education Following Myringotomy

Avoid strenuous activities
Avoid rapid head movements, bouncing, or bending
Avoid straining on bowel movement
Avoid drinking through a straw
Avoid traveling by air
Avoid forceful coughing
Avoid contact with persons with colds
Instruct the client that if necessary to blow his or her nose, blow one side at a time with the mouth open
Avoid washing hair, showering, or getting the head wet for 1 week
Instruct the client to keep ears dry for 6 weeks by keeping a ball of cotton coated with petroleum jelly in the ear and to change cotton ball daily
Instruct the client to change ear dressings every 24 hours as prescribed
Instruct the client to report excessive ear drainage to the physician

c. A reddened, dull, thick, immobile tympanic membrane with or without perforation

d. Tender and enlarged postauricular lymph nodes

e. Low-grade fever, malaise, and anorexia

3. Implementation

a. Prepare the client for surgical removal of infected material if necessary

b. Simple or modified radical mastoidectomy with tympanoplasty is the most common treatment

c. Once tissue that is infected is removed, tympanoplasty is performed to reconstruct the ossicles and the tympanic membranes in an attempt to restore normal hearing

4. Postoperative implementation

a. Monitor for dizziness

b. Monitor for signs of meningitis as evidenced by a stiff neck and vomiting

c. Prepare for a wound dressing change 24 hours' postoperatively

d. Monitor the surgical incision for edema, drainage, and redness

e. Position the client flat with the operative side up as prescribed

f. Restrict the client to bed with bedside commode privileges for 24 hours as prescribed

g. Assist the client with getting out of bed to prevent falling or injuries from dizziness

h. With reconstruction of ossicles via graft, precautions are taken to prevent dislodging of graft

L. **Otosclerosis**

1. Description

a. Disease of the labyrinthine capsule of the middle ear that results in a bony overgrowth of tissue surrounding the ossicles

b. Causes the development of irregular areas of new bone formation and causes the fixation of the bones

c. Stapes fixation leads to a **conductive hearing loss**

d. If the disease involves the inner ear, **sensorineural hearing loss** is present

e. It is not uncommon to have bilateral involvement, although hearing loss may be worse in one ear

f. The cause is unknown, although it is thought to have a familial tendency

g. Nonsurgical intervention promotes the improvement of hearing through amplification

h. Surgical intervention involves removal of the bony growth that is causing the hearing loss

i. A partial stapedectomy or complete stapedectomy with prosthesis (**fenestration**) may be surgically performed

2. Data collection

a. Slowly progressing **conductive hearing loss**

b. Bilateral hearing loss

c. A ringing or roaring type of constant tinnitus

d. Loud sounds heard in the ear when chewing

e. Pinkish discoloration (Schwartz's sign) of the tympanic membrane, which indicates vascular changes within the ear

M. **Fenestration**

1. Description

a. Removal of the stapes with a small hole drilled in the footplate; a prosthesis is connected between the incus and footplate

b. Sounds cause the prosthesis to vibrate in the same manner as did the stapes

c. Complications include complete hearing loss, prolonged vertigo, infection, or facial nerve damage

2. Preoperative implementation

a. Instruct the client in measures to prevent middle ear or external ear infections

b. Instruct the client to avoid excessive nose blowing

c. Instruct the client not to clean the ear canal with any foreign object

d. Instruct the client to remove hearing aid 2 weeks before surgery to ensure the integration of local tissue

3. Postoperative implementation

a. Inform the client that hearing is initially worse after the surgical procedure because of swelling and that no noticeable improvement in hearing may occur for as long as 6 weeks

b. Inform the client that the Gelfoam ear packing interferes with hearing but is used to decrease bleeding

c. Assist with ambulating during the first 1 to 2 days after surgery

d. Provide side rails when the client is in bed

e. Administer antibiotics, antivertiginous, and pain medications as prescribed

f. Monitor for facial nerve damage, weakness, changes in tactile sensation, changes in taste sensation, vertigo, nausea, and vomiting

g. Instruct the client to move the head slowly when changing positions to prevent vertigo

h. Instruct the client to avoid persons with upper respiratory tract infections

i. Instruct the client to avoid showering and getting the head and wound wet

j. Instruct the client to refrain from using small objects to clean the external ear canal

k. Instruct the client to avoid rapid, extreme changes in pressure caused by quick head movements, sneezing, nose blowing, straining, and changes in altitude

l. Instruct the client to avoid changes in middle ear pressure because they could dislodge the graft or prosthesis

N. Labyrinthitis
1. Description: Infection of the labyrinth that occurs as a complication of acute or chronic otitis media
2. Data collection
   a. Hearing loss that may be permanent on the affected side
   b. Tinnitus
   c. Spontaneous nystagmus to the affected side
   d. Vertigo
   e. Nausea and vomiting
3. Implementation
   a. Monitor for signs of meningitis, the most common complication, as evidenced by headache, stiff neck, and lethargy
   b. Administer systemic antibiotics as prescribed
   c. Advise the client to stay in bed in a darkened room
   d. Administer antiemetics and antivertiginous medications as prescribed
   e. Instruct the client that the vertigo subsides as the inflammation resolves
   f. Instruct the client that balance problems that persist may require gait training through physical therapy

O. **Meniere's syndrome**
1. Description
   a. A syndrome also called endolymphatic hydrops, which refers to dilation of the endolymphatic system either by overproduction or decreased reabsorption of endolymphatic fluid
   b. Symptoms occur in attacks and last for several days and the client becomes totally incapacitated during the attacks
   c. Initial hearing loss is reversible, but as the frequency of attacks continues, hearing loss becomes permanent
   d. Repeated damage to the cochlea caused by increased fluid pressure leads to permanent hearing loss
2. Data collection
   a. Feelings of fullness in the ear
   b. Tinnitus, as a continuous low-pitched roar or humming sound, is present much of the time, but worsens just before and during severe attacks
   c. Hearing loss is worse during an attack
   d. Vertigo, such as periods of whirling, that might cause the client to fall to the ground
   e. Vertigo that is so intense that even while lying down the client holds the bed or ground in an attempt to prevent the whirling
   f. Nausea and vomiting
   g. Nystagmus
   h. Severe headaches

3. Nonsurgical implementation
   a. Prevent injury during vertigo attacks
   b. Provide bed rest in a quiet environment
   c. Instruct the client to move the head slowly to prevent worsening of the vertigo
   d. Initiate salt and fluid restrictions as prescribed
   e. Instruct the client to stop smoking
   f. Administer nicotinic acid as prescribed for its vasodilatory effect
   g. Administer antihistamines as prescribed, which will reduce the production of histamine and inflammation
   h. Administer antiemetics, tranquilizers, and sedatives as prescribed, to calm the client and allow the client to rest, and to control vertigo, nausea, and vomiting
4. Surgical implementation
   a. Performed when medical therapy is ineffective and the functional level of the client has decreased significantly
   b. Endolymphatic drainage and insertion of a shunt may be performed early in the course of the disease to assist with the drainage of excess fluids
   c. A resection of the vestibular nerve or total removal of the labyrinth or a labyrinthectomy may be performed
5. Postoperative implementation
   a. Monitor packing and dressing of the ear
   b. Speak to the client on the side of the unaffected ear
   c. Monitor neurological status
   d. Maintain side rails
   e. Assist with ambulating
   f. Encourage the use of a bedside commode
   g. Administer antivertiginous and antiemetic medications as prescribed

P. Acoustic neuroma
1. Description
   a. A benign tumor of the vestibular or acoustic nerve
   b. The tumor may cause damage to hearing and to facial movements and sensations
   c. Treatment includes surgical removal of the tumor via craniotomy
   d. Care is taken to preserve the function of facial nerve
   e. The tumor rarely recurs after surgical removal
   f. Postoperative nursing care is similar to postoperative craniotomy care
2. Data collection
   a. Symptoms usually begin with tinnitus and progress to gradual **sensorineural hearing loss**
   b. As the tumor enlarges, damage to adjacent cranial nerves occurs

Q. Trauma
1. Description
   a. The tympanic membrane has a limited

stretching ability and gives way under high pressure

b. Foreign objects placed in the external canal may exert pressure on the tympanic membrane and cause perforation

c. If the object continues through the canal, the bony structure of the stapes, incus, and malleus may be damaged

d. A blunt injury to the basal skull and ear can damage the middle ear structures through fractures extending to the middle ear

e. Excessive nose blowing and rapid changes of pressure that occur with nonpressurized air flights can increase pressure in the middle ear

f. Depending on the damage to the ossicles, hearing loss may or may not return

2. Implementation

a. Tympanic membrane perforations usually heal within 24 hours

b. Surgical reconstruction of the ossicles and tympanic membrane through tympanoplasty or myringoplasty may be performed to improve hearing

R. Cerumen and foreign bodies

1. Description

a. Cerumen or wax is the most common cause of impacted canals

b. Foreign bodies can include vegetables, beads, pencil erasers, or insects

2. Data collection

a. Sensation of fullness in the ear with or without hearing loss

b. Pain, itching, or bleeding

3. Cerumen

a. Irrigation may be performed to remove cerumen

b. Irrigation is contraindicated in clients with a history of tympanic membrane perforation

4. Foreign bodies

a. With a foreign object of vegetable matter, irrigation is used with care because this material expands with hydration

b. Insects are killed before removal, unless they can be coaxed out by flashlight or a humming noise

c. Mineral oil or alcohol may be instilled to suffocate the insect, which is then removed using ear forceps

d. A small ear forceps is used to remove the object; pushing the object farther into the canal and damaging the tympanic membrane is avoided

PRACTICE QUESTIONS

1. The nurse is asked to test the visual acuity of a client using a Snellen chart. The nurse prepares to perform the test, knowing that which of the following identifies the accurate procedure for this visual acuity test?

1 Both eyes are tested together followed by the testing of the right and then the left eye

2 The right eye is tested, followed by the left eye, then both eyes are tested

3 The client is asked to stand 40 feet from the chart and is asked to read the largest line on the chart

4 The client is asked to stand 40 feet from the chart and to read the line that can be read 20 feet away by an individual with unimpaired vision

2. The client's vision is tested with a Snellen chart. The results of the tests are documented as 20/60. The nurse interprets this as

1 The client can read at a distance of 60 feet what a client with normal vision can read at 20 feet

2 The client is legally blind

3 The client's vision is normal

4 The client can only read at a distance of 20 feet what a client with normal vision can read at 60 feet

3. The clinic notes that following several eye examinations, the physician has documented a diagnosis of legal blindness in the client's chart. Which of the following does the nurse expect to note documented as the result of the Snellen chart test?

1 20/20 vision

2 20/40 vision

3 20/60 vision

4 20/200 vision

4. The nurse is preparing the client for eye testing and the examiner is planning to test the eyes using the confrontational method. The nurse tells the client that this test is performed to

1 Examine visual fields or peripheral vision

2 Check for glaucoma

3 Check for color blindness

4 Examine pupil constriction

5. Tonometry is performed on the client with a suspected diagnosis of glaucoma. The nurse reviews the test results as documented in the client's chart and understands that normal intraocular pressure is

1 2 to 7 mmHg

2 10 to 21 mmHg

3 22 to 30 mmHg

4 31 to 35 mmHg

6. The nurse is assisting in developing a plan of care for the client scheduled for cataract surgery. The nurse makes suggestions regarding the plan, knowing that which of the following problems is most specifically associated with this type of surgery?

1. Self-care deficit
2. Alteration in nutrition
3. Sensory perceptual alteration
4. Anxiety

7. The nurse is reviewing the health record of a client diagnosed with glaucoma. The chief clinical manifestation that the nurse expects to note in the early stages of cataract formation is
   1. Eye pain
   2. Floating spots
   3. Blurred vision
   4. Diplopia

8. The nurse is assigned to administer the prescribed eye drops for a client preparing for cataract surgery. Which of the following types of eye drops does the nurse expect to be prescribed?
   1. An osmotic diuretic
   2. A miotic agent
   3. A mydriatic medication
   4. A thiazide diuretic

9. The nurse is assigned to care for a client following a cataract extraction. The nurse plans to position the client
   1. On the operative side
   2. On the nonoperative side
   3. Prone
   4. Supine

10. During the early postoperative stage, the cataract extraction client complains of nausea and severe eye pain over the operative site. What is the initial nursing action in this situation?
    1. Report the client's complaints
    2. Administer the ordered pain medication and antiemetic
    3. Reassure the client that this is normal
    4. Turn the client on the operative side

11. The client is being discharged from the ambulatory care unit following cataract removal. The nurse reinforces instructions regarding home care. Which of the following, if stated by the client, indicates effective teaching?
    1. "I will take aspirin if I have any discomfort."
    2. "I will sleep on the side that I was operated on."
    3. "I will wear my eye shield at night and my glasses during the day."
    4. "I will not lift anything if it weighs more than 10 pounds."

12. The client is diagnosed with glaucoma. Which of the following data gathered by the nurse indicates a risk factor associated with glaucoma?
    1. A history of migraine headaches
    2. Frequent urinary tract infections
    3. Cardiovascular disease
    4. Frequent upper respiratory infections

13. The client with glaucoma asks the nurse if complete vision will return. The most appropriate response is
    1. "Although some vision has been lost and cannot be restored, further loss may be prevented by adhering to the treatment plan."
    2. "Your vision will return as soon as the medication begins to work."
    3. "Your vision will never return to normal."
    4. "Your vision loss is temporary and will return in about 3 to 4 weeks."

14. The nurse is assisting in developing a teaching plan for the client with glaucoma. Which of the following instructions does the nurse suggest to include in the plan of care?
    1. Decrease fluid intake to control the intraocular pressure
    2. Avoid reading the newspaper and watching TV
    3. Decrease the amount of salt in the diet
    4. Eye medications will need to be administered for the rest of your life

15. The nurse is assigned to care for a client with a detached retina. Which of the following assessment signs does the nurse expect to be documented in the client's record?
    1. Pain in the affected eye
    2. Blurred vision
    3. A sense of a curtain falling across the field of vision
    4. A yellow discoloration of the sclera

16. The nurse is assigned to care for a client with a diagnosis of detached retina. Which of the following findings indicates that bleeding has occurred as a result of retinal detachment?
    1. Complaints of a burst of black spots or floaters
    2. A sudden sharp pain in the eye
    3. Total loss of vision
    4. A reddened conjunctiva

17. The client with retinal detachment is admitted to the nursing unit in preparation for a scleral buckling procedure. Which of the following does the nurse anticipate to be prescribed?
    1. Bathroom privileges only
    2. Elevating the head of the bed to 45 degrees
    3. Placing an eye patch over the client's affected eye
    4. Wearing dark glasses to read or watch TV

18. The client arrives in the emergency department following an automobile accident. The client's forehead hit the steering wheel and a hyphema is diagnosed. The nurse prepares to position the client
    1. Flat on bed rest
    2. On bed rest in a semi-Fowler's position
    3. In the lateral position on the affected side
    4. In lateral position on the unaffected side

19. The client sustains a contusion of the eyeball following a traumatic injury with a blunt object. The nurse prepares to initiate which of the following immediately?
    1 Notify the physician
    2 Irrigate the eye with cool water
    3 Apply ice to the affected eye
    4 Accompany the client to the emergency department

20. The client arrives in the emergency department with a penetrating eye injury from wood chips while cutting wood. The nurse checks the eye and notes the piece of wood protruding form the eye. The nurse immediately prepares the client for which of the following?
    1 Removal of the piece of wood using a sterile eye clamp
    2 Application of an eye patch
    3 Visual acuity tests
    4 Irrigation of the eye with sterile saline

21. The client sustains a chemical eye injury from a splash of battery acid. The nurse prepares the client for which of the following immediate measures?
    1 Assessment of visual acuity
    2 Irrigation of the eye with sterile normal saline
    3 Swabbing the eye with antibiotic ointment
    4 Covering the eye with a pressure patch

22. The nurse is caring for a client following enucleation. The nurse notes the presence of bright red drainage on the dressing. Which of the following actions is most appropriate?
    1 Report the findings
    2 Continue to monitor vital signs
    3 Document the finding
    4 Mark the drainage on the dressing and monitor for any increase in bleeding

23. The nurse is preparing to administer ear drops to an adult client. The nurse administers the ear drops, knowing that which of the following is the appropriate procedure?
    1 Pull the pinna up and back
    2 Pull the earlobe down and back
    3 Instruct the client to stand and lean to one side
    4 Tilt the client's head forward and down

24. The nurse is preparing to perform a voice test to check the client's hearing. The nurse performs the procedure, knowing that which of the following describes the accurate procedure?
    1 Stand 4 feet away from the client to ensure that the client can hear at this distance
    2 Quietly whisper a statement and ask the client to repeat it
    3 Whisper a statement with the examiner's back facing the client

    4 Whisper a statement while the client blocks both ears

25. The nurse is assisting the physician with performing a Weber test on a client. The nurse understands that this test checks for
    1 Visual loss
    2 Cataract development
    3 Hearing loss
    4 Nystagmus

26. The nurse is caring for a client who is hearing impaired. Which of the following approaches will facilitate communication?
    1 Speak frequently
    2 Speak loudly
    3 Speak directly into the impaired ear
    4 Speak in a normal tone

27. A client arrives at the emergency department with a foreign body in the left ear that has been determined to be an insect. Which of the following interventions does the nurse anticipate to be prescribed initially?
    1 Irrigation of the ear
    2 Instillation of diluted alcohol
    3 Instillation of antibiotic ear drops
    4 Instillation of corticosteroid ointment

28. The nurse notes that the physician has documented a diagnosis of presbycusis on the client's chart. The nurse understands that this condition is most accurately described as
    1 A sensorineural loss that occurs with aging
    2 A conductive hearing loss that occurs with aging
    3 Tinnitus that occurs with aging
    4 Nystagmus that occurs with aging

29. The nurse is reinforcing discharge instructions for a client who had a fenestration procedure for the treatment of otoselerosis. Which of the following, if stated by the client, indicates that teaching was effective?
    1 "I should drink liquids through a straw for the next 2 to 3 weeks."
    2 "It is OK to take a shower and wash my hair."
    3 "I will take stool softeners as prescribed by my doctor."
    4 "I can resume my tennis lesions starting next week."

30. A client with Meniere's disease is experiencing severe vertigo. The nurse instructs the client to do which of the following to assist in controlling the vertigo?
    1 Increase fluid intake to 3000 mL a day
    2 Avoid sudden head movements
    3 Lie still and watch TV
    4 Increase sodium in the diet

31. The nurse is assigned to care for a client hospitalized with Meniere's disease. The nurse expects that which of the following would most likely be prescribed for the client?
    1 Low-cholesterol diet
    2 Low-sodium diet
    3 Low-carbohydrate diet
    4 Low-fat diet

32. The nurse is caring for a client following craniotomy for removal of an acoustic neuroma. The nurse understands that assessment of which of the following cranial nerves identifies a complication specifically associated with this surgery?
    1 Cranial nerve I, olfactory
    2 Cranial nerve III, oculomotor
    3 Cranial nerve IV, trochlear
    4 Cranial nerve VII, facial nerve

33. The nurse is monitoring a client with a blunt head injury sustained from a motor vehicle accident. Which of the following indicates a basal skull fracture as a result of the injury?
    1 Purulent drainage from the auditory canal
    2 Bloody or clear drainage from the auditory canal
    3 Epistaxis
    4 Periorbital edema

34. The nurse is reviewing the record of a client with mastoiditis. The nurse expects to note which of the following regarding the results of the otoscopic examination?
    1 A pink-colored tympanic membrane
    2 A pearly colored tympanic membrane
    3 A red, dull, thick, and immobile tympanic membrane
    4 A transparent and clear tympanic membrane

35. The client is diagnosed with a disorder involving the inner ear. The nurse caring for the client understands that which of the following is the most common client complaint associated with a disorder involving the inner ear?
    1 Hearing loss
    2 Pruritus
    3 Tinnitus
    4 Burning in the ear

36. The nurse is assigned to care for a client with a diagnosis of Meniere's disease. The nurse plans care, knowing that this condition is a disorder of the
    1 External ear canal
    2 Tympanic membrane
    3 Middle ear
    4 Inner ear

37. The nurse is caring for a client who will be undergoing surgical treatment for Meniere's disease. The nurse plans care understanding that surgical treatment for this disorder is performed to

    1 Provide relief from accumulation of inner ear fluid in the endolymphatic sac
    2 Repair the tympanic membrane
    3 Replace the stapes footplate
    4 Provide relief from accumulation of fluid in the middle ear

38. The nurse is assigned to care for a client with Meniere's disease. The nurse reviews the physician's orders. The nurse plans care, knowing that which of the following is not prescribed for the client?
    1 Increased fluid intake
    2 Low-sodium diet
    3 Vasodilating medications
    4 Mild sedative

39. The nurse is reviewing the health care record of a client with a diagnosis of otosclerosis. The nurse expects to note documentation of which early symptom of this disorder?
    1 Ringing in the ears
    2 Blurred vision
    3 Headache
    4 Vertigo

40. Surgery has been recommended for the client with otosclerosis and the client tells the nurse that surgery is not desired. The client asks the nurse about alternative methods to improve hearing. The most appropriate response is which of the following?
    1 "There are no other methods to improve hearing."
    2 "You need to have surgery since it has been recommended."
    3 "A hearing aid may improve your hearing."
    4 "Your physician is the best. You need to do what the physician suggests."

41. The nurse is caring for a hospitalized client with an acute attack from Meniere's disease. The client verbalizes concern because the client has experienced a hearing loss as a result of the attack. Which of the following responses does the nurse make to the client regarding the hearing loss?
    1 "It will take several weeks before the hearing returns."
    2 "The hearing loss will fluctuate for a period of 1 week."
    3 "The attack leaves a hearing loss in the involved ear."
    4 "The hearing will return to normal."

42. The nurse is reviewing the physician's orders on a client admitted to the hospital with a diagnosis of an acute attack of Meniere's disease. Which of the following orders if noted on the client's chart does the nurse question?
    1 The administration of a sedative
    2 The administration of an antihistamine
    3 The administration of a vasoconstrictor
    4 Bed rest

43. The nurse is reinforcing discharge instructions to the client who was hospitalized for an acute attack of Meniere's disease. Which of the following statements if made by the client indicates a need for further education?
    1 "I need to take the diuretics to decrease the fluid in the ear."
    2 "I need to take the antihistamine as prescribed."
    3 "I need to take a vasodilator."
    4 "It is not necessary to restrict salt in my diet."

44. A client with a diagnosis of otosclerosis is admitted to the ambulatory care unit for stapedectomy. The nurse reinforces instructions with the client regarding home care following the procedure. Which of the following statements if made by the client indicates a need for further education?
    1 "I need to keep water out of the ear canal for at least 3 weeks."
    2 "I need to avoid air travel for at least 6 months."
    3 "I need to notify the physician if I experience any persistent dizziness."
    4 "I need to avoid bending and lifting heavy objects for at least 3 weeks."

45. The nurse is reinforcing discharge instructions with a client who is being discharged following a fenestration procedure for the treatment of otosclerosis. Which of the following is included in the list of instructions prepared for the client?
    1 "It is OK to begin golf lessons."
    2 "It is all right to take a shower daily."
    3 "You need to avoid air travel."
    4 "You need to avoid bending activities for 1 week."

46. A myringotomy is performed on a client in the ambulatory care center. The ambulatory care nurse calls the client 24 hours after the procedure to evaluate the status of the client. The client reports to the nurse that a small amount of brownish drainage has been coming from the ear. Which of the following instructions does the nurse provide to the client?
    1 Contact the physician
    2 Lie on the unaffected side to prevent the drainage

    3 Continue to monitor the drainage because this is normal and may occur for 24 to 48 hours following the surgery
    4 Place a cotton plug in the ear to absorb the drainage

47. The nurse is reinforcing instructions to a client regarding the use of a hearing aid. Which of the following statements if made by the client indicates a need for further education?
    1 "I should keep an extra battery available at all times."
    2 "I should wash the ear mold frequently with mild soap and water."
    3 "I should turn the hearing aid off after removing it from the ear."
    4 "I should not wear the hearing aid during an ear infection."

48. The nurse assesses the client with a blunt head injury sustained from a motor vehicle accident. The nurse notes the presence of bloody drainage from the auditory canal. Which of the following nursing actions is most appropriate?
    1 Document the findings
    2 Place a gauze pad over the ear to absorb the drainage
    3 Report the findings
    4 Continue to monitor the drainage

49. A client with Meniere's disease has been given suggestions for methods to control vertigo. The nurse evaluates that the client understands the information presented if the client states to
    1 Cut down smoking to 10 cigarettes per day
    2 Increase sodium in the diet
    3 Increase fluid intake to 3000 mL a day
    4 Avoid sudden head movements

50. The nurse is trying to communicate with a hearing-impaired client. Which of the following strategies by the nurse is least helpful when talking to this client?
    1 To avoid showing frustration through facial expression
    2 Smiling continuously during conversation
    3 Facing the client directly while speaking
    4 Facing the client so that light falls on own face

ANSWERS

1. **2**

RATIONALE: Visual acuity is tested in one eye at a time, then in both eyes together with the client comfortably seated. Begin with the right eye while the left eye is covered, then test the left eye with the right eye covered, followed by testing both eyes together. Visual acuity is measured with or without corrective lenses and the client stands 20 feet from the chart.

TEST-TAKING STRATEGY: Use the process of elimination. Remember that normal visual acuity as measured by a Snellen chart is 20/20 vision. This should help you eliminate options 3 and 4. It is best to test each eye separately first, then test both eyes together. This most accurately assesses visual acuity. Review this basic procedure now if you had difficulty with this question.

LEVEL OF COGNITIVE ABILITY: Application
PHASE OF NURSING PROCESS: Planning
CLIENT NEEDS: Physiological Integrity
CONTENT AREA: Adult Health/Eye
REFERENCE
deWit, S. (1998). *Essentials of medical-surgical nursing* (4th ed.). Philadelphia: W. B. Saunders. p. 931.

2. **4**

RATIONALE: Vision that is 20/20 is normal, that is, the client is able to read from 20 feet what a person with normal vision can read from 20 feet. A client with a visual acuity of 20/60, can only read at a distance of 20 feet what a person with normal vision can read at 60 feet.

TEST-TAKING STRATEGY: Understanding how to interpret the results of this visual acuity test is necessary to answer this question. If you had difficulty with this question, take time now to review.

LEVEL OF COGNITIVE ABILITY: Comprehension
PHASE OF NURSING PROCESS: Data Collection
CLIENT NEEDS: Physiological Integrity
CONTENT AREA: Adult Health/Eye
REFERENCE
Monahan, F., & Neighbors, M. (1998). *Medical-surgical nursing: Foundations for clinical practice* (2nd ed.). Philadelphia: W. B. Saunders. p. 1940.

3. **4**

RATIONALE: Legal blindness is defined as 20/200 or less with corrected vision (glasses or contact lenses), or less than 20 degrees of visual field in the better eye. Options 1, 2, and 3 are incorrect descriptions.

TEST-TAKING STRATEGY: Knowledge regarding the definition of legal blindness is required to answer this question. If you had difficulty with this question, take time now to review.

LEVEL OF COGNITIVE ABILITY: Comprehension
PHASE OF NURSING PROCESS: Data Collection
CLIENT NEEDS: Physiological Integrity
CONTENT AREA: Adult Health/Eye
REFERENCE
Monahan, F., & Neighbors, M. (1998). *Medical-surgical nursing: Foundations for clinical practice* (2nd ed.). Philadelphia: W. B. Saunders. p. 1958.

4. **1**

RATIONALE: The confrontational method of eye testing is used to examine visual fields or peripheral vision. Tonom-etry is used to check for glaucoma. An Ishihara chart is used to check color vision. A flashlight is used to check pupillary response to light.

TEST-TAKING STRATEGY: Knowledge regarding the procedure for checking peripheral vision by the confrontational method is required to answer this question. Use the process of elimination, and if you had difficulty with this question, take time now to review this visual test.

LEVEL OF COGNITIVE ABILITY: Comprehension
PHASE OF NURSING PROCESS: Implementation
CLIENT NEEDS: Physiological Integrity
CONTENT AREA: Adult Health/Eye
REFERENCE
Monahan, F., & Neighbors, M. (1998). *Medical-surgical nursing: Foundations for clinical practice* (2nd ed.). Philadelphia: W. B. Saunders. p. 1943.

5. **2**

RATIONALE: Tonometry is the method of measuring intraocular fluid pressure using a calibrated instrument that indents or flattens the corneal apex. Pressures between 10 and 21 mmHg are considered within the normal range.

TEST-TAKING STRATEGY: Knowledge regarding the normal intraocular pressure is required to answer this question. If you had difficulty with this question, take time now to learn this normal value.

LEVEL OF COGNITIVE ABILITY: Comprehension
PHASE OF NURSING PROCESS: Data Collection
CLIENT NEEDS: Physiological Integrity
CONTENT AREA: Adult Health/Eye
REFERENCE
deWit, S. (1998). *Essentials of medical-surgical nursing* (4th ed.). Philadelphia: W. B. Saunders. p. 933.

6. **3**

RATIONALE: The most specifically associated problem for the client scheduled for cataract surgery is sensory perceptual alteration (visual) related to lens extraction and replacement. Options 1 and 2 may also be concerns but would occur as a result of a sensory perceptual alteration. Option 4 can occur with any type of surgical procedure.

TEST-TAKING STRATEGY: Use the process of elimination, focusing on the type of surgery. Remember disorders of the eye or ear relate to sensory perceptual alterations.

LEVEL OF COGNITIVE ABILITY: Comprehension
PHASE OF NURSING PROCESS: Planning
CLIENT NEEDS: Psychosocial Integrity
CONTENT AREA: Adult Health/Eye
REFERENCE
deWit, S. (1998). *Essentials of medical-surgical nursing* (4th ed.). Philadelphia: W. B. Saunders. p. 940.

7. **3**

RATIONALE: A gradual painless blurring of central vision is the chief clinical manifestation of a cataract. Early symptoms include slightly blurred vision and a decrease in color perception. Options 1, 2, and 4 are not specifically associated with a cataract.

TEST-TAKING STRATEGY: Note the key word "chief." Recall the pathophysiology related to cataract development. As a cataract develops, the lens of the eye becomes opaque. This description will assist in directing you to the correct option. If you had difficulty with this question, take time now to review the signs associated with cataract development.

LEVEL OF COGNITIVE ABILITY: Comprehension
PHASE OF NURSING PROCESS: Data Collection
CLIENT NEEDS: Physiological Integrity
CONTENT AREA: Adult Health/Eye
REFERENCE
deWit, S. (1998). *Essentials of medical-surgical nursing* (4th ed.). Philadelphia: W. B. Saunders. p. 940.

8. 3

RATIONALE: A mydriatic medication produces mydriasis or dilation of the pupil. Mydriatic medications are used preoperatively in the cataract client. These medications act by dilating the pupils. They also constrict blood vessels. A miotic agent constricts the pupil. An osmotic agent acts to decrease intraocular pressure. A thiazide diuretic promotes the excretion of body fluid. A thiazide diuretic is not likely to be prescribed for a client with a cataract.
TEST-TAKING STRATEGY: Knowledge regarding the actions of the specific medications identified in the options is required to answer this question. Read the question carefully, noting that the client is being prepared for eye surgery. Dilation of the eye is necessary prior to cataract extraction. Review the preparation of a client for cataract surgery now if you had difficulty with this question.
LEVEL OF COGNITIVE ABILITY: Comprehension
PHASE OF NURSING PROCESS: Planning
CLIENT NEEDS: Physiological Integrity
CONTENT AREA: Adult Health/Eye
REFERENCE
deWit, S. (1998). *Essentials of medical-surgical nursing* (4th ed.). Philadelphia: W. B. Saunders. p. 940.

9. 2

RATIONALE: Postoperatively, cataract extraction clients should be positioned on their backs in semi-Fowler's position or on the nonoperative side to prevent edema in the surgical site. Options 1, 3, and 4 are incorrect positions and will cause swelling at the surgical site.
TEST-TAKING STRATEGY: Use the process of elimination. Remember, edema to the surgical site can occur following the trauma of surgery. Think about the principles of gravity and the prevention of the accumulation of fluid around the surgical site. This will assist in directing you to the correct option. If you had difficulty with this question, take time now to review postoperative care of a client following cataract surgery.
LEVEL OF COGNITIVE ABILITY: Application
PHASE OF NURSING PROCESS: Planning
CLIENT NEEDS: Physiological Integrity
CONTENT AREA: Adult Health/Eye
REFERENCE
Monahan, F., & Neighbors, M. (1998). *Medical-surgical nursing: Foundations for clinical practice* (2nd ed.). Philadelphia: W. B. Saunders. p. 1975.

10. 1

RATIONALE: Severe pain or pain accompanied by nausea is an indicator of increased intraocular pressure and should be reported to the physician immediately. Options 2, 3, and 4 are incorrect.
TEST-TAKING STRATEGY: Note the key word "severe." Eliminate option 3 as this is not a normal condition. The client should not be turned to the operative side; therefore, eliminate option 4. Noting the key word in the question should direct you to eliminating option 2. If you had diffi-

culty with this question, take time now to review the postoperative complications of cataract surgery requiring physician notification.
LEVEL OF COGNITIVE ABILITY: Application
PHASE OF NURSING PROCESS: Implementation
CLIENT NEEDS: Physiological Integrity
CONTENT AREA: Adult Health/Eye
REFERENCE
Monahan, F., & Neighbors, M. (1998). *Medical-surgical nursing: Foundations for clinical practice* (2nd ed.). Philadelphia: W. B. Saunders. pp. 1977–1978.

11. 3

RATIONALE: The client is instructed to wear a metal or plastic shield to protect the eye from accidental injury and is instructed not to rub the eye. Glasses may be worn during the day. Aspirin or medications containing aspirin are not to be administered or taken by the client and the client is instructed to take acetaminophen (Tylenol) as needed for pain. The client is instructed not to sleep on the side of the body that was operated on. The client is not to lift more than 5 pounds.
TEST-TAKING STRATEGY: Note the key words "indicates effective teaching." Use the process of elimination and knowledge regarding the postoperative care following this procedure. If you had difficulty with this question, take time now to review these client instructions.
LEVEL OF COGNITIVE ABILITY: Comprehension
PHASE OF NURSING PROCESS: Evaluation
CLIENT NEEDS: Health Promotion and Maintenance
CONTENT AREA: Adult Health/Eye
REFERENCE
Monahan, F., & Neighbors, M. (1998). *Medical-surgical nursing: Foundations for clinical practice* (2nd ed.). Philadelphia: W. B. Saunders. p. 1977.

12. 3

RATIONALE: Hypertension, cardiovascular disease, diabetes, and obesity are associated with the development of glaucoma. Smoking, ingestion of caffeine or large amounts alcohol, illicit drugs, corticosteroids, altered hormone levels, posture, and eye movements may cause varying transient increases in intraocular pressure.
TEST-TAKING STRATEGY: Use knowledge regarding the risk factors associated with glaucoma to answer this question. If you had difficulty with this question, take time now to review the risk factors associated with this disorder.
LEVEL OF COGNITIVE ABILITY: Comprehension
PHASE OF NURSING PROCESS: Data Collection
CLIENT NEEDS: Health Promotion and Maintenance
CONTENT AREA: Adult Health/Eye
REFERENCE
Monahan, F., & Neighbors, M. (1998). *Medical-surgical nursing: Foundations for clinical practice* (2nd ed.). Philadelphia: W. B. Saunders. p. 1978.

13. 1

RATIONALE: Vision loss to glaucoma is irreparable. Reassure the client that although some vision has been lost and cannot be restored, further loss may be prevented by adhering to the treatment plan. Options 2 and 4 are incorrect. Option 3 does not provide reassurance to the client.
TEST-TAKING STRATEGY: Knowledge regarding the effects of glaucoma on vision is required to answer this question. Read the options carefully. Eliminate option 3 as this option does not provide a reassuring response and will

produce anxiety in the client as it is stated. Note that option 1 is more global, addressing the importance of compliance with the treatment plan.
LEVEL OF COGNITIVE ABILITY: Application
PHASE OF NURSING PROCESS: Implementation
CLIENT NEEDS: Psychosocial Integrity
CONTENT AREA: Adult Health/Eye
REFERENCE
Monahan, F., & Neighbors, M. (1998). *Medical-surgical nursing: Foundations for clinical practice* (2nd ed.). Philadelphia: W. B. Saunders. pp. 1979–1980.

14. **4**

RATIONALE: The administration of eye drops is a critical component of the treatment plan for the client with glaucoma. The client needs to be instructed that medications will need to be taken for the rest of his or her life. Limiting fluids and reducing salt will not decrease intraocular pressure. Option 2 is not necessary.
TEST-TAKING STRATEGY: Use the process of elimination. Knowing that medications are an integral component of the treatment plan will assist in directing you to the correct option. Review the treatment associated with the care of the client with glaucoma now if you had difficulty with this question.
LEVEL OF COGNITIVE ABILITY: Application
PHASE OF NURSING PROCESS: Planning
CLIENT NEEDS: Health Promotion and Maintenance
CONTENT AREA: Adult Health/Eye
REFERENCE
Monahan, F., Neighbors, M. (1998). *Medical-surgical nursing: Foundations for clinical practice* (2nd ed.). Philadelphia: W. B. Saunders. p. 1979.

15. **3**

RATIONALE: A characteristic clinical manifestation of retinal detachment described by clients is the feeling that a shadow or curtain is falling across the field of vision. There is no pain associated with detachment of the retina. A retinal detachment is an ophthalmic emergency and even more so if visual acuity is still normal. Options 2 and 4 are not specifically associated with a detached retina.
TEST-TAKING STRATEGY: Knowledge regarding the clinical manifestations associated with retinal detachment is required to answer this question. Retinal detachment can occur suddenly and is an ophthalmic emergency. Review the clinical manifestations associated with this condition now if you had difficulty with this question.
LEVEL OF COGNITIVE ABILITY: Comprehension
PHASE OF NURSING PROCESS: Data Collection
CLIENT NEEDS: Physiological Integrity
CONTENT AREA: Adult Health/Eye
REFERENCE
Monahan, F., & Neighbors, M. (1998). *Medical-surgical nursing: Foundations for clinical practice* (2nd ed.). Philadelphia: W. B. Saunders. p. 1982.

16. **1**

RATIONALE: Complaints of a sudden burst of black spots or floaters indicate that bleeding has occurred as a result of the detachment. Options 2, 3, and 4 are not specifically associated with bleeding as a result of a detached retina.
TEST-TAKING STRATEGY: Knowledge regarding the signs of hemorrhage associated with retinal detachment is required to answer this question. Hemorrhage is a serious complication associated with retinal detachment. Review

the clinical manifestations associated with the complications of a detached retina now if you had difficulty with this question.
LEVEL OF COGNITIVE ABILITY: Comprehension
PHASE OF NURSING PROCESS: Data Collection
CLIENT NEEDS: Physiological Integrity
CONTENT AREA: Adult Health/Eye
REFERENCE
Monahan, F., & Neighbors, M. (1998). *Medical-surgical nursing: Foundations for clinical practice* (2nd ed.). Philadelphia: W. B. Saunders. p. 1983.

17. **3**

RATIONALE: The nurse places an eye patch over the client's affected eye to reduce eye movement. Some clients may need bilateral patching. Depending on the location and size of the retinal break, activity restrictions including watching TV may be needed immediately. These restrictions are necessary to prevent further tearing or detachment and to promote drainage of any subretinal fluid. The nurse positions the client as prescribed by the physician.
TEST-TAKING STRATEGY: Use the process of elimination. Eliminate options that suggest activity such as in options 1 and 4. Remember that the eye needs to be protected and rested. This should direct you to the correct option. If you had difficulty with this question, take time now to review care to the client with retinal detachment.
LEVEL OF COGNITIVE ABILITY: Application
PHASE OF NURSING PROCESS: Planning
CLIENT NEEDS: Physiological Integrity
CONTENT AREA: Adult Health/Eye
REFERENCE
Monahan, F., & Neighbors, M. (1998). *Medical-surgical nursing: Foundations for clinical practice* (2nd ed.). Philadelphia: W. B. Saunders. p. 1984.

18. **2**

RATIONALE: A hyphema is the presence of blood in the anterior chamber. It is produced when a force is sufficient to break the integrity of the blood vessels in the eye. It can be caused by direct injury such as penetrating injury from a BB pellet, or indirectly such as from striking the forehead on a steering wheel during an accident. The client is treated by bed rest in a semi-Fowler's position to assist gravity in keeping the hyphema away from the optical center of the cornea.
TEST-TAKING STRATEGY: Use the process of elimination. Placing the client flat will produce an increase in pressure at the injured site. Note that option 2 is the only option that identifies a position different from the other options. Take time now to review care to the client with hyphema if you had difficulty with this question.
LEVEL OF COGNITIVE ABILITY: Application
PHASE OF NURSING PROCESS: Planning
CLIENT NEEDS: Physiological Integrity
CONTENT AREA: Adult Health/Eye
REFERENCE
Monahan, F., & Neighbors, M. (1998). *Medical-surgical nursing: Foundations for clinical practice* (2nd ed.). Philadelphia: W. B. Saunders. p. 1987.

19. **3**

RATIONALE: Treatment for a contusion begins at the time of injury. Ice is applied immediately. The client should receive a thorough eye examination to rule out the presence of other eye injuries. Eye irrigation is not indicated in a contusion. Options 1 and 4 will delay immediate treatment. Following the application of ice, the physician is notified.

TEST-TAKING STRATEGY: Knowledge regarding the initial treatment following a contusion to the eye is required to answer this question. Use the process of elimination, noting the key word "immediately." Review this content now if you had difficulty with this question.

LEVEL OF COGNITIVE ABILITY: Application
PHASE OF NURSING PROCESS: Planning
CLIENT NEEDS: Physiological Integrity
CONTENT AREA: Adult Health/Eye
REFERENCE
Ignatavicius, D., Workman, M., & Mishler, M. (1999). *Medical-surgical nursing: Across the health care continuum* (3rd ed.). Philadelphia: W. B. Saunders. p. 1188.

20. **3**

RATIONALE: If the laceration is the result of a penetrating injury, an object may be noted protruding from the eye. This object must never be removed except by the ophthalmologist, because it may be holding ocular structures in place. Application of an eye patch or irrigation of the eye may disrupt the foreign body and cause further tearing of the cornea.

TEST-TAKING STRATEGY: Use the process of elimination. Note the key word "penetrating." This should indicate that a laceration has occurred and that interventions are directed at preventing further disruption of the integrity of the eye. The only option that is accurate in the options presented is to prepare for testing visual acuity. Review this content now if you had difficulty with this question.

LEVEL OF COGNITIVE ABILITY: Application
PHASE OF NURSING PROCESS: Planning
CLIENT NEEDS: Physiological Integrity
CONTENT AREA: Adult Health/Eye
REFERENCE
Monahan, F., & Neighbors, M. (1998). *Medical-surgical nursing: Foundations for clinical practice* (2nd ed.). Philadelphia: W. B. Saunders. p. 1987.

21. **2**

RATIONALE: Emergency care following a chemical burn to the eye includes irrigating the eye immediately with sterile normal saline or ocular irrigating solution. The irrigation should be maintained for at least 10 minutes. Following this emergency treatment, visual acuity is assessed. Options 3 and 4 are not immediate measures.

TEST-TAKING STRATEGY: Read the question carefully, noting the type of injury to the eye. The question asks about emergency care; therefore, in this type of injury, it is necessary to irrigate the eye first. Review this content now if you had difficulty with this question.

LEVEL OF COGNITIVE ABILITY: Application
PHASE OF NURSING PROCESS: Planning
CLIENT NEEDS: Physiological Integrity
CONTENT AREA: Adult Health/Eye
REFERENCE
Monahan, F., & Neighbors, M. (1998). *Medical-surgical nursing: Foundations for clinical practice* (2nd ed.). Philadelphia: W. B. Saunders. p. 1989.

22. **1**

RATIONALE: If the nurse notes the presence of bright red drainage on the dressing, it must be reported to the physician, because this can indicate hemorrhage. Options 2, 3, and 4 will delay necessary treatment.

TEST-TAKING STRATEGY: Note the key words "bright red." Bright red drainage indicates active bleeding. The physician needs to be notified if this type of drainage occurs. Review postoperative complications associated with an enucleation now if you had difficulty with this question.

LEVEL OF COGNITIVE ABILITY: Application
PHASE OF NURSING PROCESS: Implementation
CLIENT NEEDS: Physiological Integrity
CONTENT AREA: Adult Health/Eye
REFERENCE
Monahan, F., & Neighbors, M. (1998). *Medical-surgical nursing: Foundations for clinical practice* (2nd ed.). Philadelphia: W. B. Saunders. p. 1955.

23. **1**

RATIONALE: The nurse tilts the client's head slightly away and pulls the pinna up and back. Instructing the client to stand and lean to one side is inappropriate and unsafe.

TEST-TAKING STRATEGY: Use the process of elimination, noting that the question addresses an adult client. Use basic knowledge regarding the administration of ear medications in selecting the correct option. In the adult, the pinna is pulled up and back.

LEVEL OF COGNITIVE ABILITY: Application
PHASE OF NURSING PROCESS: Implementation
CLIENT NEEDS: Physiological Integrity
CONTENT AREA: Adult Health/Ear
REFERENCE
Monahan, F., & Neighbors, M. (1998). *Medical-surgical nursing: Foundations for clinical practice* (2nd ed.). Philadelphia: W. B. Saunders. p. 2000.

24. **2**

RATIONALE: The examiner stands 1 to 2 feet away from the client and asks the client to block one external ear canal. The nurse quietly whispers a statement and asks the client to repeat it. Each ear is tested separately. Options 3 and 4 are not measures that effectively check hearing. Option 1 checks distance hearing.

TEST-TAKING STRATEGY: Knowledge regarding the implementation of this examination is required to answer this question. Eliminate options 3 and 4 because they are not measures that effectively check hearing. Eliminate option 1, because distance hearing is not the issue of the question. Review this simple test now if you had difficulty with this question.

LEVEL OF COGNITIVE ABILITY: Application
PHASE OF NURSING PROCESS: Implementation
CLIENT NEEDS: Physiological Integrity
CONTENT AREA: Adult Health/Ear
REFERENCE
Monahan, F., & Neighbors, M. (1998). *Medical-surgical nursing: Foundations for clinical practice* (2nd ed.). Philadelphia: W. B. Saunders. p. 2001.

25. **3**

RATIONALE: The Weber tuning fork test assesses for conductive or sensorineural hearing loss. Options 1, 2, and 4 are incorrect.

TEST-TAKING STRATEGY: Knowledge regarding the purpose of the Weber tuning fork test is required to answer this question. Recalling that this is a test to determine the type of hearing loss will easily direct you to option 3. Review the purpose of this test now if you had difficulty with this question.

LEVEL OF COGNITIVE ABILITY: Comprehension

PHASE OF NURSING PROCESS: Data Collection
CLIENT NEEDS: Physiological Integrity
CONTENT AREA: Adult Health/Ear
REFERENCE
Monahan, F., & Neighbors, M. (1998). *Medical-surgical nursing: Foundations for clinical practice* (2nd ed.). Philadelphia: W. B. Saunders. p. 2001.

26. **4**

RATIONALE: Speak in a normal tone to the client with impaired hearing and do not shout. Talk directly to the client while facing the client and speak clearly. If the client does not seem to understand what is said, express it differently. Moving closer to the client and toward the better ear may facilitate communication, but avoid talking directly into the impaired ear.
TEST-TAKING STRATEGY: Knowledge regarding effective communication techniques for the hearing impaired is required to answer this question. Use the process of elimination. If you had difficulty with this question, take time now to review these techniques
LEVEL OF COGNITIVE ABILITY: Application
PHASE OF NURSING PROCESS: Implementation
CLIENT NEEDS: Physiological Integrity
CONTENT AREA: Adult Health/Ear
REFERENCE
deWit, S. (1998). *Essentials of medical-surgical nursing* (4th ed.). Philadelphia: W. B. Saunders. p. 957.

27. **2**

RATIONALE: Insects are killed before removal unless they can be coaxed out by a flashlight or a humming noise. Mineral oil or diluted alcohol is instilled into the ear to suffocate the insect, which is then removed by using ear forceps. When the foreign object is vegetable matter, irrigation is not used because this material expands with hydration and the impaction becomes worse. Options 1, 3, and 4 may be prescribed after the initial treatment if necessary and if inflammation or infection is a concern.
TEST-TAKING STRATEGY: Use the process of elimination and knowledge regarding care to the client with a foreign body in the ear to answer this question. If you had difficulty with this question, take time now to review the care required.
LEVEL OF COGNITIVE ABILITY: Comprehension
PHASE OF NURSING PROCESS: Planning
CLIENT NEEDS: Physiological Integrity
CONTENT AREA: Adult Health/Ear
REFERENCE
Ignatavicius, D., Workman, M. & Mishler, M. (1999). *Medical surgical nursing: Across the health care continuum* (3rd ed.). Philadelphia: W. B. Saunders. p. 1370.

28. **1**

RATIONALE: Presbycusis is a type of hearing loss that occurs with aging. It is a gradual sensorineural loss caused by nerve degeneration in the inner ear or auditory nerve. Options 2, 3, and 4 are not accurate descriptions.
TEST-TAKING STRATEGY: Knowledge regarding the description of presbycusis is required to answer this question. If you are unfamiliar with this condition, take time now to review this age-related disorder.
LEVEL OF COGNITIVE ABILITY: Comprehension
PHASE OF NURSING PROCESS: Data Collection
CLIENT NEEDS: Physiological Integrity

CONTENT AREA: Adult Health/Ear
REFERENCE
Monahan, F., & Neighbors, M. (1998). *Medical-surgical nursing: Foundations for clinical practice* (2nd ed.). Philadelphia: W. B. Saunders. p. 1997.

29. **3**

RATIONALE: Following ear surgery, clients need to avoid straining when having a bowel movement. Clients need to be instructed to avoid drinking with a straw for 2 to 3 weeks, avoid air travel, and avoid coughing excessively. Clients need to avoid getting their heads wet, washing their hair, and showering for 1 week. Clients need to avoid rapidly moving the head, bouncing, and bending over for 3 weeks.
TEST-TAKING STRATEGY: Note the key words "teaching was effective." Consider the anatomical area of the client's condition and the surgical procedure in eliminating the incorrect options. If you had difficulty with this question, take time now to review client instructions following ear surgery.
LEVEL OF COGNITIVE ABILITY: Comprehension
PHASE OF NURSING PROCESS: Evaluation
CLIENT NEEDS: Health Promotion and Maintenance
CONTENT AREA: Adult Health/Ear
REFERENCE
Monahan, F., & Neighbors, M. (1998). *Medical-surgical nursing: Foundations for clinical practice* (2nd ed.). Philadelphia: W. B. Saunders. p. 2015.

30. **2**

RATIONALE: The nurse instructs the client to make slow head movements to prevent worsening of the vertigo. Dietary changes such as salt and fluid restrictions that reduce the amount of endolymphatic fluid are sometimes prescribed. Watching TV can increase the vertigo.
TEST-TAKING STRATEGY: Identify the issue of the question. The issue is vertigo. Note the relationship between vertigo and the correct option, avoiding sudden head movements. If you had difficulty with this question, take time now to review measures that will reduce vertigo in the client with Meniere's disease.
LEVEL OF COGNITIVE ABILITY: Application
PHASE OF NURSING PROCESS: Implementation
CLIENT NEEDS: Physiological Integrity
CONTENT AREA: Adult Health/Ear
REFERENCE
Monahan, F., & Neighbors, M. (1998). *Medical-surgical nursing: Foundations for clinical practice* (2nd ed.). Philadelphia: W. B. Saunders. p. 829.

31. **2**

RATIONALE: Dietary changes such as salt and fluid restrictions that reduce the amount of endolymphatic fluid are sometimes prescribed. Options 1, 3, and 4 are not specific dietary prescriptions for this condition.
TEST-TAKING STRATEGY: Knowledge regarding the pathophysiology related to Meniere's disease is required to answer this question. From this point, use of the process of elimination. Review the pathophysiology related to this condition and the treatment now if you had difficulty with this question.
LEVEL OF COGNITIVE ABILITY: Comprehension
PHASE OF NURSING PROCESS: Planning
CLIENT NEEDS: Physiological Integrity
CONTENT AREA: Adult Health/Ear

REFERENCE
Monahan, F., & Neighbors, M. (1998). *Medical-surgical nursing: Foundations for clinical practice* (2nd ed.). Philadelphia: W. B. Saunders. p. 829.

32. **4**

RATIONALE: Treatment for acoustic neuroma is surgical removal via a craniotomy. Extreme care is taken to preserve remaining hearing and preserve the function of the facial verve. Acoustic neuromas rarely occur following surgical removal.
TEST-TAKING STRATEGY: Use knowledge regarding the anatomical location of acoustic neuromas to answer this question. If you had difficulty with this question, take time now to review the complications associated with this surgical procedure.
LEVEL OF COGNITIVE ABILITY: Analysis
PHASE OF NURSING PROCESS: Data Collection
CLIENT NEEDS: Physiological Integrity
CONTENT AREA: Adult Health/Ear
REFERENCE
Monahan, F., & Neighbors, M. (1998). *Medical-surgical nursing: Foundations for clinical practice* (2nd ed.). Philadelphia: W. B. Saunders. p. 828.

33. **2**

RATIONALE: Bloody or clear watery drainage from the auditory canal indicates a cerebrospinal leak following trauma and suggests a basal skull fracture. This warrants immediate attention. Option 1 is indicative of an infectious process. Options 3 and 4 are not specifically associated with a basal skull fracture.
TEST-TAKING STRATEGY: Knowledge regarding the signs associated with a basal skull fracture is required to answer this question. If you had difficulty with this question, take time now to review these signs.
LEVEL OF COGNITIVE ABILITY: Analysis
PHASE OF NURSING PROCESS: Data Collection
CLIENT NEEDS: Physiological Integrity
CONTENT AREA: Adult Health/Ear
REFERENCE
Monahan, F., & Neighbors, M. (1998). *Medical-surgical nursing: Foundations for clinical practice* (2nd ed.). Philadelphia: W. B. Saunders. p. 818.

34. **3**

RATIONALE: Otoscopic examination in a client with mastoiditis reveals a red, dull, thick, and immobile tympanic membrane with or without perforation. Postauricular lymph nodes are tender and enlarged. Clients also have a low-grade fever, malaise, anorexia, swelling behind the ear, and pain with minimal movement of the head. Options 1, 2, and 4 are not findings that are noted in this examination in the client with mastoiditis.
TEST-TAKING STRATEGY: Knowledge regarding the assessment findings associated with mastoiditis is required to answer this question. If you had difficulty with this question, take time now to review the assessment findings associated with this disorder.
LEVEL OF COGNITIVE ABILITY: Comprehension
PHASE OF NURSING PROCESS: Data Collection
CLIENT NEEDS: Physiological Integrity
CONTENT AREA: Adult Health/Ear
REFERENCE
Monahan, F., & Neighbors, M. (1998). *Medical-surgical nursing: Foundations for clinical practice* (2nd ed.). Philadelphia: W. B. Saunders. p. 2012.

35. **3**

RATIONALE: Tinnitus is the most common complaint of clients with otologic disorders, especially disorders involving the inner ear. Symptoms of tinnitus range from mild ringing in the ear, which can go unnoticed during the day, to a loud roaring in the ear, which can interfere with the client's thinking process and attention span. Hearing loss may occur. Options 2 and 4 are not specifically associated with inner ear problems.
TEST-TAKING STRATEGY: Knowledge regarding symptoms associated with inner ear disorders is required to answer this question. Use the process of elimination, recalling the functions of the inner ear to select the correct option. Review inner ear problems and the associated findings now if you had difficulty with this question.
LEVEL OF COGNITIVE ABILITY: Comprehension
PHASE OF NURSING PROCESS: Data Collection
CLIENT NEEDS: Physiological Integrity
CONTENT AREA: Adult Health/Ear
REFERENCE
Monahan, F., & Neighbors, M. (1998). *Medical-surgical nursing: Foundations for clinical practice* (2nd ed.). Philadelphia: W. B. Saunders. p. 2013.

36. **4**

RATIONALE: Meniere's disease is a disorder of the labyrinth of the inner ear. This disorder does not affect the external ear, tympanic membrane, or the middle ear.
TEST-TAKING STRATEGY: Knowledge that a symptom of Meniere's disease is tinnitus will assist in directing you to option 4. If you are unfamiliar with this disorder, take time now to review.
LEVEL OF COGNITIVE ABILITY: Comprehension
PHASE OF NURSING PROCESS: Planning
CLIENT NEEDS: Physiological Integrity
CONTENT AREA: Adult Health/Ear
REFERENCE
O'Toole, M. (1997). *Miller-Keane encyclopedia & dictionary of medicine, nursing, & allied health* (6th ed.). Philadelphia: W. B. Saunders. p. 982.

37. **1**

RATIONALE: Surgical treatment for Meniere's disease involves relief from accumulation of inner ear fluid in the endolymphatic sac. Procedures may be directed toward relief of pressure by the bony structures surrounding the sac or toward opening the sac and diverting the flow of endolymph by means of a shunt to the mastoid bone or to the subarachnoid space. Options 2, 3, and 4 are procedures that are unrelated to Meniere's disease.
TEST-TAKING STRATEGY: Knowledge that Meniere's disease affects the inner ear will assist in directing you to option 1. If you are unfamiliar with this disorder and the surgical procedures, take time now to review.
LEVEL OF COGNITIVE ABILITY: Comprehension
PHASE OF NURSING PROCESS: Planning
CLIENT NEEDS: Physiological Integrity
CONTENT AREA: Adult Health/Ear
REFERENCE
O'Toole, M. (1997). *Miller-Keane encyclopedia & dictionary of medicine, nursing, & allied health* (6th ed.). Philadelphia: W. B. Saunders. p. 982.

38. 1

RATIONALE: A low-sodium diet, elimination or restriction of fluids, and vasodilating medications are used in the treatment of Meniere's disease to assist in reducing the accumulation of inner ear fluid in the endolymphatic sac.
TEST-TAKING STRATEGY: Recalling that in Meniere's disease an accumulation of inner ear fluid occurs will assist in directing you to option 1. If you are unfamiliar with this disease, take time now to review.
LEVEL OF COGNITIVE ABILITY: Comprehension
PHASE OF NURSING PROCESS: Planning
CLIENT NEEDS: Physiological Integrity
CONTENT AREA: Adult Health/Ear
REFERENCE
O'Toole, M. (1997). *Miller-Keane encyclopedia & dictionary of medicine, nursing, & allied health* (6th ed.). Philadelphia: W. B. Saunders. p. 982.

39. 1

RATIONALE: Otosclerosis involves the formation of spongy bone in the capsule of the labyrinth of the ear, often causing the auditory ossicles to become fixed and less able to pass on vibrations when sound enters the ear. An early symptom is ringing in the ears, but the most noticeable symptom is progressive hearing loss. Options 2, 3, and 4 are not associated with this condition.
TEST-TAKING STRATEGY: Note the key word "early." Knowledge that this disorder involves the ear will assist in eliminating options 2 and 3. Focusing on the key word will assist in directing you to option 1. If you had difficulty with this question, take time now to review this disorder.
LEVEL OF COGNITIVE ABILITY: Comprehension
PHASE OF NURSING PROCESS: Data Collection
CLIENT NEEDS: Physiological Integrity
CONTENT AREA: Adult Health/Ear
REFERENCE
O'Toole, M. (1997). *Miller-Keane encyclopedia & dictionary of medicine, nursing, & allied health* (6th ed.). Philadelphia: W. B. Saunders. p. 1167.

40. 3

RATIONALE: Clients with otosclerosis who do not desire surgery may have their hearing loss relieved by the use of a hearing aid. Options 1, 2, and 4 are inappropriate responses.
TEST-TAKING STRATEGY: Use therapeutic communication techniques. Eliminate options 2 and 4 first because they are similar and provide advice to the client. Next eliminate option 1 because it is incorrect and nontherapeutic. Review the surgical treatment for otosclerosis now if you had difficulty with this question.
LEVEL OF COGNITIVE ABILITY: Application
PHASE OF NURSING PROCESS: Implementation
CLIENT NEEDS: Psychosocial Integrity
CONTENT AREA: Adult Health/Ear
REFERENCE
O'Toole, M. (1997). *Miller-Keane encyclopedia & dictionary of medicine, nursing, & allied health* (6th ed.). Philadelphia: W. B. Saunders. p. 1167.

41. 3

RATIONALE: After the acute phase, remission occurs, but symptoms will recur with 2 or 3 acute attacks per year. As this pattern of attacks and remissions develops, fewer symptoms occur during the acute phase. A complete remission eventually occurs with some degree of hearing loss varying from slight to complete. It takes several weeks before all symptoms subside after an attack, leaving a loss of hearing in the involved ear. Options 1, 2, and 4 are incorrect.
TEST-TAKING STRATEGY: Knowledge that a hearing loss occurs to some degree with an acute attack of Meniere's disease is required to answer this question. If you are unfamiliar with the effects of Meniere's disease on hearing, take time now to review.
LEVEL OF COGNITIVE ABILITY: Application
PHASE OF NURSING PROCESS: Implementation
CLIENT NEEDS: Physiological Integrity
CONTENT AREA: Adult Health/Ear
REFERENCE
Beare, P., & Myers, J. (1998). *Adult health nursing* (3rd ed.) St. Louis: Mosby–Year Book. p. 1180.

42. 3

RATIONALE: Medical interventions during the acute phase of Meniere's disease include using atropine or diazepam (Valium) to decrease the autonomic nervous system function. Diphenhydramine (Benadryl) may be prescribed for its antihistamine effects, and a vasodilator will also be prescribed. The client will remain on bed rest during the acute attack, and when allowed to be out of bed, the client will need assistance with walking, sitting, or standing.
TEST-TAKING STRATEGY: Knowledge regarding the pathophysiology associated with Meniere's disease is required to answer this question. Use the process of elimination in considering the correct response. If you are unfamiliar with the treatment measures for this disorder, take time now to review.
LEVEL OF COGNITIVE ABILITY: Comprehension
PHASE OF NURSING PROCESS: Planning
CLIENT NEEDS: Safe, Effective Care Environment
CONTENT AREA: Adult Health/Ear
REFERENCE
Beare, P., & Myers, J. (1998). *Adult health nursing* (3rd ed.) St. Louis: Mosby–Year Book. p. 1180.

43. 4

RATIONALE: Management during remission includes diuretics to decrease the fluid and thereby decrease pressure in the endolymphs. Antihistamines, vasodilators, and diuretics may be prescribed for the client. A low-salt diet is prescribed for the client to reduce fluids. The major goal of treatment is to preserve the client's hearing, and careful medical management helps achieve this in most clients with Meniere's disease.
TEST-TAKING STRATEGY: Knowledge that Meniere's disease occurs as a result of a disturbance in the fluid of the endolymphatic system is required to answer this question. This knowledge and the process of elimination will easily direct you to option 4. If you are unfamiliar with the management of this disorder during remission, take time now to review.
LEVEL OF COGNITIVE ABILITY: Comprehension
PHASE OF NURSING PROCESS: Evaluation
CLIENT NEEDS: Health Promotions and Maintenance
CONTENT AREA: Adult Health/Ear
REFERENCE
Beare, P., & Myers, J. (1998). *Adult health nursing* (3rd ed.) St. Louis: Mosby–Year Book. p. 1180.

44. 2

RATIONALE: Following stapedectomy, the client is instructed to keep water out of the ear canal for at least 3 weeks and to avoid swimming for 6 weeks. The client is also instructed to avoid coughing and sneezing and to avoid bending and lifting heavy objects or other strenuous activities for at least 3 weeks. Air travel is avoided for 4 weeks. If the client develops sudden hearing loss, fever, or severe persistent vertigo or dizziness, the physician should be notified.

TEST-TAKING STRATEGY: Knowledge regarding the discharge instructions following stapedectomy is required to answer this question. Note the key words "indicates a need for further education." Read each option carefully, noting the time frame and the activities described in the options. Eliminate options 1 and 4 first because of the similar time frames. Eliminate option 3 next because of the word "persistent." If you are unfamiliar with the client teaching points following this procedure, take time now to review.

LEVEL OF COGNITIVE ABILITY: Comprehension
PHASE OF NURSING PROCESS: Evaluation
CLIENT NEEDS: Health Promotion and Maintenance
CONTENT AREA: Adult Health/Ear
REFERENCE
Beare, P., & Myers, J. (1998). *Adult health nursing* (3rd ed.) St. Louis: Mosby–Year Book. p. 2017.

45. 3

RATIONALE: Following ear surgery, clients need to avoid straining when having a bowel movement. Clients need to be instructed to avoid drinking with a straw for 2 to 3 weeks, avoid air travel, and avoid coughing excessively. Clients need to avoid getting their heads wet, washing their hair, and showering for 1 week. Clients need to avoid rapidly moving the head, bouncing, and bending over for 3 weeks.

TEST-TAKING STRATEGY: Note that the question asks for the instruction that will be included in the plan of care. Consider the anatomical area of the client's condition and the surgical procedure in eliminating the incorrect options. If you had difficulty with this question, take time now to review client instructions following ear surgery.

LEVEL OF COGNITIVE ABILITY: Application
PHASE OF NURSING PROCESS: Planning
CLIENT NEEDS: Health Promotion and Maintenance
CONTENT AREA: Adult Health/Ear
REFERENCE
Monahan, F., & Neighbors, M. (1998). *Medical-surgical nursing: Foundations for clinical practice* (2nd ed.). Philadelphia: W. B. Saunders. p. 2015.

46. 3

RATIONALE: A small amount of brownish or reddish drainage is normal for 24 to 48 hours following the surgery. Excessive drainage, especially clear fluid, should be reported immediately. Options 1, 2, and 4 are inaccurate instructions.

TEST-TAKING STRATEGY: Knowledge regarding the normal expectations following this procedure is required to answer this question. Read each option carefully and use the process of elimination. If you are unfamiliar with the normal findings following myringotomy, take time now to review.

LEVEL OF COGNITIVE ABILITY: Application
PHASE OF NURSING PROCESS: Implementation
CLIENT NEEDS: Physiological Integrity
CONTENT AREA: Adult Health/Ear
REFERENCE
Monahan, F., & Neighbors, M. (1998). *Medical-surgical nursing: Foundations for clinical practice* (2nd ed.). Philadelphia: W. B. Saunders. p. 2006.

47. 3

RATIONALE: Nurses should have a basic knowledge of the care for a hearing aid to assist the client in its use. The client should be instructed to turn the hearing aid off prior to removing it from the ear to prevent squealing feedback. The hearing aid should be turned off when not in use and the client should always keep an extra battery available. The client should wash the ear mold frequently with mild soap and water and use a pipe cleaner to clean the cannula. The client should not wear the hearing aid during an ear infection.

TEST-TAKING STRATEGY: Use the process of elimination to answer this question. Read each option carefully. Knowledge regarding squealing feedback will assist in directing you to the correct option. If you had difficulty with this question, take time now to review the use of the hearing aid.

LEVEL OF COGNITIVE ABILITY: Comprehension
PHASE OF NURSING PROCESS: Evaluation
CLIENT NEEDS: Health Promotion and Maintenance
CONTENT AREA: Adult Health/Ear
REFERENCE
deWit, S. (1998). *Essentials of medical-surgical nursing* (4th ed.). Philadelphia: W. B. Saunders. p. 963.

48. 3

RATIONALE: Bloody or clear watery drainage from the auditory canal indicates a cerebrospinal leak following trauma and suggests a basal skull fracture. This warrants immediate attention and the physician should be notified. Options 1, 2, and 4 are inappropriate nursing actions.

TEST-TAKING STRATEGY: Use the process of elimination to answer the question. Eliminate options 1 and 4 first because they are similar. Knowledge that the presence of bloody or clear drainage from the auditory canal suggests the presence of a basal skull fracture will easily direct you to option 3. If you had difficulty with this question, take time now to review the complications following a head injury.

LEVEL OF COGNITIVE ABILITY: Application
PHASE OF NURSING PROCESS: Implementation
CLIENT NEEDS: Physiological Integrity
CONTENT AREA: Adult Health/Ear
REFERENCE
O'Toole, M. (1997). *Miller-Keane encyclopedia & dictionary of medicine, nursing, & allied health* (6th ed.). Philadelphia: W. B. Saunders. pp. 328, 751, 1658.

49. 4

RATIONALE: The client should move the head slowly to prevent worsening of the vertigo. Salt and fluid restrictions are sometimes prescribed to reduce the amount of endolymphatic fluid. Clients are advised to stop smoking because of its vasoconstrictive effects.

TEST-TAKING STRATEGY: Identify the issue of the question, which is vertigo. Note the relationship between vertigo and the correct option, avoiding sudden head movements. If you had difficulty with this question, take time now to review measures that will reduce vertigo in the client with Meniere's disease.

LEVEL OF COGNITIVE ABILITY: Comprehension
PHASE OF NURSING PROCESS: Evaluation
CLIENT NEEDS: Health Promotion and Maintenance
CONTENT AREA: Adult Health/Ear

REFERENCE
deWit, S. (1998). *Essentials of medical-surgical nursing* (4th ed.). Philadelphia: W. B. Saunders. p. 962.

50. 2

RATIONALE: Clients who are hearing impaired rely on visual cues to assist them to comprehend the conversation of others. Smiling continuously is the least helpful strategy because the smile distorts the appearance of the mouth if the client is trying to read lips. Facing the client and standing so there is light on the nurse's face are helpful because they assist the client to lip read. Taking care not to show frustration or annoyance with the client's impairment is also helpful to preserve the client's self-esteem.

TEST-TAKING STRATEGY: Note the key words "least helpful." To answer this question carefully, you must be familiar with general communication strategies as well as those that are helpful for the hearing impaired. If this question was difficult, take time to review this material now.
LEVEL OF COGNITIVE ABILITY: Application
PHASE OF NURSING PROCESS: Implementation
CLIENT NEEDS: Psychosocial Integrity
CONTENT AREA: Adult Health/Ear
REFERENCE
deWit, S. (1998). *Essentials of medical-surgical nursing* (4th ed.). Philadelphia: W. B. Saunders. p. 957.

BIBLIOGRAPHY

Beare, P., & Myers, J. (1998). *Adult health nursing* (3rd ed.). St. Louis: Mosby–Year Book. p. 1685.
deWit, S. (1998). *Essentials of medical-surgical nursing* (4th ed.). Philadelphia: W. B. Saunders.
Hodgson, B., & Kizior, R. (2000). *Saunders nursing drug handbook 2000.* Philadelphia: W. B. Saunders.
Ignatavicius, D., Workman, M., & Mishler, M. (1999). *Medical-surgical nursing: Across the health care continuum* (3rd ed.). Philadelphia: W. B. Saunders.
Leahy, J., & Kizilay, P. (1998). *Foundations of nursing practice: A nursing process approach.* Philadelphia: W. B. Saunders.
Luckmann, J. (1997). *Saunders manual of nursing care.* Philadelphia: W. B. Saunders.
Monahan, F., & Neighbors, M. (1998). *Medical-surgical nursing: Foundations for clinical practice* (2nd ed.). Philadelphia: W. B. Saunders.
O'Toole, M. (1997). *Miller-Keane encyclopedia & dictionary of medicine, nursing & allied health* (6th ed.). Philadelphia: W. B. Saunders.

CHAPTER 53

Ophthalmic and Otic Medications

. . . .

I. Ophthalmic Medication Administration
(Box 53–1)

A. Guidelines for the use of eye medications
1. Eye medications are usually in the form of drops or ointments
2. To prevent overflow of medication into the nasal and pharyngeal passages, thus reducing systemic absorption, instruct the client to occlude the nasolacrimal duct with one finger for 1 to 2 minutes after instilling the medication
3. When two or more eye medications are to be administered, wait at least 3 minutes between medications
4. Wash hands carefully before administering eye medications to avoid contaminating the eye or applicator
5. Wash hands after administering eye medications to rinse off any residue
6. Use a separate bottle or tube of medication for each client to avoid accidental cross contamination
7. Place ordered dose of eye medication in the lower conjunctival sac, never directly onto the cornea
8. Avoid touching any part of the eye with the dropper or applicator
9. Administer drops or liquid preparations before ointments
10. Administer glucocorticoid preparations before other medications
11. Monitor the pulse of clients receiving beta blockers
12. If the pulse is below 50 to 60 beats/minute

(bpm) in an adult receiving a beta blocker, withhold the next dose of medication and notify the registered nurse (RN) and/or the physician
13. Instruct the client how to instill medication correctly and supervise instillation until the client can do it safely
14. Instruct the client to read labels carefully to ensure administration of the correct medication and correct strength
15. Remind the client to keep these medications out of the reach of children
16. Instruct the client to avoid driving or operating hazardous equipment if vision is blurred
17. Inform the client that they may be unable to drive home after eye examinations when medications to dilate the pupil (**mydriatics**) or medications to paralyze the ciliary muscle (**cycloplegics**) are used
18. If photophobia occurs, instruct the client to wear sunglasses and avoid bright lights
19. Instruct the client to administer a missed dose as soon as remembered, unless the next dose is scheduled in 1 to 2 hours
20. Inform the client with **glaucoma** that the disorder cannot be cured, only controlled
21. Reinforce the importance of using medications to treat **glaucoma** as prescribed and not to discontinue these medications without consulting the physician
22. Inform the client that medications used to treat **glaucoma** may cause pain and blurred vision, especially when therapy is begun
23. Instruct the client to report the development of any eye irritation
24. Inform the client using eye gel to store the gel at room temperature or in the refrigerator but not to freeze it
25. Instruct the client to discard unused eye gel kept at room temperature after 8 weeks

---

BOX 53–1. Abbreviations

Left eye (OS)	Both eyes (OU)
Right eye (OD)	

26. Inform the client that soft contact lenses may absorb certain eye medications and that preservatives in eye medications may discolor the contact lenses
27. Advise the client wearing contact lenses to question the physician carefully about special precautions to observe
28. In infants, inform the parents that atropine eye drops may contribute to abdominal distention
29. Instruct parents to keep a record of the bowel movements of infants being administered atropine eye drops
30. Auscultate bowel sounds of infants and children receiving atropine eye drops

B. Instillation of eye medications
1. Drops
   a. Wash hands
   b. Put gloves on
   c. Check the name, strength, and expiration date of the medication
   d. Instruct the client to tilt the head backward, open the eyes, and look up
   e. Pull lower lid down against the cheekbone
   f. Hold the bottle like a pencil with the tip downward
   g. Holding the bottle, gently rest the wrist of the hand on the client's cheek
   h. Squeeze the bottle gently to allow the drop to fall into the conjunctival sac
   i. Instruct the client to close eyes gently and not to squeeze eyes shut
   j. Wait 3 to 5 minutes before instilling another drop to promote maximal absorption of the medication
   k. Do not allow the medication bottle to come in contact with the eyeball
2. Ointments
   a. Hold the ointment tube near, but not touching, the eye or eyelashes
   b. Squeeze a thin ribbon of ointment along the lining of the sac from the inner to the outer canthus
   c. Instruct the client to close the eyes gently
   d. Instruct the client that vision may be blurred by the ointment

II. Mydriatic/Cycloplegic and Anticholinergic Medications (Box 53–2)

A. Description
1. **Mydriatics** and **cycloplegics** dilate the pupils **(mydriasis)** and relax the ciliary muscles **(cycloplegia)**, causing blurred vision
2. Anticholinergics block responses of the sphincter muscle in the ciliary body, producing **mydriasis** and **cycloplegia**; are used preoperatively or for eye examinations to produce mydriasis; and are contraindicated in clients with **glaucoma** because of the risk of increased intraocular pressure
3. **Mydriatics** are contraindicated in cardiac

BOX 53–2. Mydriatic/Cycloplegic Eye Medications

Atropine sulfate (Isopto Atropine, Ocu-Tropine)
Scopolamine hydrobromide (Isopto Hyoscine)
Cyclopentolate HCl (Cyclogyl)
Homatropine hydrobromide (Isopto Homatropine)
Tropicamide (Mydriacyl)
Dipivefrin HCl (Propine)
Epinephrine HCl (Epifrin, Glaucon)
Epinephryl borate (Epinal, Eppy/N)
Phenylephrine HCl (AK-Dilate)

---

dysrhythmias and cerebral atherosclerosis and should be used with caution in the elderly and clients with prostatic hypertrophy, diabetes mellitus, or parkinsonism

B. Side effects
1. Tachycardia
2. Photophobia
3. Conjunctivitis
4. Dermatitis

C. Atropine toxicity
1. Dry mouth
2. Blurred vision
3. Photophobia
4. Tachycardia
5. Fever
6. Urinary retention
7. Constipation
8. Headache or brow pain
9. Confusion
10. Worsening of narrow-angle **glaucoma**

D. Systemic reactions of anticholinergics
1. Dry mouth and skin
2. Fever
3. Thirst
4. Confusion
5. Hyperactivity

E. Implementation
1. Monitor for allergic response
2. Assess for risk of injury
3. Monitor for urinary retention and constipation
4. Inform the client that a burning sensation may occur on instillation
5. Instruct the client not to drive or operate machinery for 24 hours after instillation of medication unless otherwise directed by the physician
6. Instruct the client to wear sunglasses until the effects of the medication wear off
7. Instruct the client to notify the physician if blurring of vision, loss of sight, headache or brow pain, difficulty breathing, sweating, or flushing occurs

III. Anti-Infective Eye Medications (Box 53–3)

A. Description: kill or inhibit the growth of bacteria, fungi, and viruses

---

BOX 53–3. Anti-Infective Eye Medications

ANTIBACTERIAL

Chloramphenicol (Chloromycetin, Chloroptic)
Ciprofloxacin HCl (Cipro)
Erythromycin (Ilotycin)
Gentamicin sulfate (Garamycin, Genoptic)
Norfloxacin (Chibroxin)
Tobramycin (Nebcin, Tobrex)
Silver nitrate 1%

ANTIFUNGAL

Natamycin (Natacyn ophthalmic)

ANTIVIRAL

Idoxuridine (Herplex Liquifilm)
Trifluridine (Viroptic)
Vidarabine (Vira-A ophthalmic)

B. Side effects
  1. Superinfection
  2. Global irritation
C. Implementation
  1. Assess for risk of injury
  2. Instruct the client to wash hands thoroughly and frequently
  3. Instruct the client to continue treatment as prescribed
  4. Inform the client that if improvement does not occur to notify the physician

IV. Anti-Inflammatory Eye Medications
(Box 53–4)

A. Description
  1. Control inflammation, thereby reducing vision loss and scarring
  2. Used for uveitis, allergic conditions, and inflammation of the conjunctiva, cornea, and lids
B. Side effects
  1. **Cataracts**
  2. Increased intraocular pressure
  3. Impaired healing
  4. Masking signs and symptoms of infection

BOX 53–4. Anti-Inflammatory Eye Medications

Dexamethasone (Maxidex)
Diclofenac sodium (Voltaren)
Flurbiprofen sodium (Ocufen)
Suprofen (Profenal)
Ketorolac tromethamine (Acular)
Medrysone (HMS, Liquifilm)
Prednisolone acetate (Predforte, Econopred)
Prednisolone sodium phosphate (AK-Pred, Inflamase)
Rimaxolone (Vexol)

BOX 53–5. Topical Anesthetics for the Eye

Proparacaine HCl (Ophthaine, Ophthetic)
Tetracaine hydrochloride (Pontocaine)

C. Implementation
  1. Assess for risk of injury
  2. Instruct the client to wash the hands thoroughly and frequently
  3. Instruct the client to continue treatment as prescribed
  4. Instruct the client that if improvement does not occur to notify the physician
  5. Note that dexamethasone (Maxidex) should not be used for eye abrasions and wounds

V. Topical Anesthetics for the Eye (Box 53–5)

A. Description
  1. Produce corneal anesthesia
  2. Used for anesthesia for eye examinations, surgery, or to remove foreign bodies from the eye
B. Side effects
  1. Temporary stinging or burning of the eye
  2. Temporary loss of corneal reflex
C. Implementation
  1. Assess for risk of injury
  2. Note that the medications should not be given to the client for home use and are not to be self-administered by the client
  3. Note that the blink reflex is temporarily lost and that the corneal epithelium needs to be protected
  4. Provide an eye patch to protect the eye from injury until the corneal reflex returns

VI. Eye Lubricants (Box 53–6)

A. Description
  1. Replace tears or add moisture to the eyes
  2. Moisten contact lenses or an artificial eye
  3. Protect the eyes during surgery or diagnostic procedures
  4. Used for keratitis, during anesthesia, or in a disorder that results in decreased blinking
B. Side effect: burning on instillation
C. Implementation
  1. Inform the client that burning may occur on instillation
  2. Be alert to allergic responses to the preservatives in the lubricants

---

BOX 53–6. Eye Lubricants

Hydroxypropyl methylcellulose (Lacril, Isopto Plain)
Petroleum-based ointment (Artificial Tears, Liquifilm Tears)

BOX 53–7. Miotics

CHOLINERGICS

Acetylcholine chloride (Miochol)
Carbachol (Miostat)
Pilocarpine HCl (Isopto Carpine)
Pilocarpine nitrate (Ocusert Pilo-20, Ocusert Pilo-40)
Echothiophate iodide (Phospholine Iodide)

CHOLINESTERASE MEDICATIONS

Physostigmine salicylate (Isopto Eserine)
Demecarium bromide (Humorsol)
Isoflurophate (Floropryl)

VII. Miotics (Box 53–7)

A. Description
  1. Reduce intraocular pressure by constricting the pupil and contracting the ciliary muscle, thereby increasing the blood flow to the retina and decreasing retinal damage and loss of vision
  2. Open the anterior chamber angle and increase the outflow of aqueous humor
  3. Used to treat **glaucoma**
  4. Used to achieve **miosis** during eye surgery
  5. Contraindicated in clients with **retinal detachment**, adhesions between the iris and lens, or in inflammatory diseases
  6. Use with caution in clients with asthma, hypertension, corneal abrasion, hyperthyroidism, coronary vascular disease, urinary tract obstruction, gastrointestinal (GI) obstruction, ulcer disease, parkinsonism, and bradycardia
B. Side effects
  1. **Myopia**
  2. Headache or eye pain
  3. Decreased vision in poor light
  4. Local irritation
  5. Systemic effects
    a. Flushing and diaphoresis
    b. GI upset and diarrhea
    c. Frequent urination
    d. Increased salivation
    e. Muscle weakness
    f. Respiratory difficulty
  6. Toxicity
    a. Vertigo
    b. Bradycardia
    c. Tremors
    d. Hypotension
    e. Seizures
C. Implementation
  1. Monitor vital signs
  2. Assess for risk of injury
  3. Assess the client for the degree of diminished vision
  4. Monitor for postural hypotension and instruct the client to change positions slowly

  5. Monitor for respiratory difficulty
  6. Maintain oral hygiene because of the increase in salivation
  7. Instruct the client not to stop the medication suddenly
  8. Instruct the client to avoid activities such as driving while vision is impaired
  9. Instruct the client with **glaucoma** to read labels on over-the-counter medications and to avoid atropine-like medications because atropine will increase intraocular pressure
  10. Note that atropine sulfate is the antidote for pilocarpine

VIII. Ocusert System

A. Description
  1. Ocusert is a thin eye wafer impregnated with time-released pilocarpine
  2. It is placed in the upper or lower cul-de-sac of the eye
  3. The pilocarpine is released over 1 week, and the disk is replaced every 7 days
  4. Drawbacks of its use include sudden leakage of pilocarpine, migration of the system over the cornea, and unnoticed loss of the system
B. Implementation
  1. Determine the client's ability to insert the medication disk
  2. Store medication in the refrigerator
  3. Instruct the client to discard damaged or contaminated disks
  4. Inform the client that temporary stinging is expected but to notify the physician if blurred vision or brow pain occurs
  5. Instruct the client to check for the presence of the disk in the conjunctival sac daily at bedtime and upon arising
  6. Since vision may change in the first few hours after the eye system is inserted, instruct the client when replacing the disk to do so at bedtime

IX. Beta-Adrenergic–Blocking Eye Medications (Box 53–8)

A. Description
  1. Reduce intraocular pressure by decreasing sympathetic impulses and decreasing aqueous humor production without affecting **accommodation** or pupil size
  2. Used to treat chronic open-angle **glaucoma**
  3. Contraindicated in clients with asthma

BOX 53–8. Beta-Adrenergic–Blocking Eye Medications

Betaxolol HCl (Betopic)
Levobunolol HCl (Betagan Liquifilm)
Timolol maleate (Timoptic)

BOX 53–9. Carbonic Anhydrase Inhibitors Eye Medications

Acetazolamide (Diamox)
Dichlorophenamide (Daranide)
Dorzolamide (Trusopt)
Methazolamide (Neptazane)

---

because systemic absorption can cause increased airway resistance
4. Use with caution in clients receiving beta blockers
B. Side effects
1. Ocular irritation
2. Visual disturbances
3. Bradycardia
4. Hypotension
5. Bronchospasm
C. Implementation
1. Monitor vital signs, especially blood pressure and pulse before administering medication
2. If the pulse is 60 or below or if the systolic blood pressure is below 90 mmHg, hold the medication and contact the RN and/or the physician
3. Monitor for shortness of breath
4. Assess for risk of injury
5. Instruct the client to notify the physician if shortness of breath occurs
6. Instruct the client not to discontinue the medication abruptly
7. Instruct the client to change positions slowly to avoid orthostatic hypotension
8. Instruct the client to avoid hazardous activities
9. Instruct the client to avoid over-the-counter medications without the physician's approval

X. Carbonic Anhydrase Inhibitors (Box 53–9)

A. Description
1. Interfere with the production of carbonic acid, which leads to decreased aqueous humor formation and decreased intraocular pressure
2. Used for long-term treatment of open-angle **glaucoma**
3. Contraindicated in clients allergic to sulfonamides
B. Side effects
1. Anorexia and GI disturbances
2. Paresthesias in the fingers, toes, and face
3. Polyuria
4. Photosensitivity
5. Lethargy
6. Hypokalemia
7. Renal calculi
C. Implementation
1. Monitor vital signs
2. Monitor visual acuity
3. Assess for risk of injury
4. Monitor I&O and weight

5. Maintain oral hygiene
6. Monitor for signs of hypokalemia
7. Increase fluid intake unless contraindicated
8. Advise the client to avoid prolonged exposure to the sunlight
9. Instruct the client not to discontinue the medication abruptly
10. Instruct the client to avoid hazardous activities while vision is impaired

XI. Osmotic Medications (Box 53–10)

A. Description
1. Lower intraocular pressure
2. Used in emergency treatment of acute closed-angle **glaucoma**
3. Used preoperatively and postoperatively to decrease vitreous humor volume
B. Side effects
1. Headache
2. Nausea, vomiting, and diarrhea
3. Disorientation
4. Electrolyte imbalances
C. Implementation
1. Monitor vital signs
2. Monitor visual acuity
3. Assess for risk for injury
4. Monitor I&O and weight
5. Monitor for signs of electrolyte imbalances
6. Increase fluid intake unless contraindicated
7. Monitor for changes in level of orientation

XII. Otic Medication Administration
(Box 53–11)

A. Administering drops
1. In an adult, pull the auricle up and back to straighten the external canal to instill ear drops
2. Pull the auricle down and back for infants and children younger than 3 years of age
3. Pull the auricle up and back for older children
B. Irrigation of the ear
1. Assist the RN or physician with the procedure
2. Prepare to warm irrigating solution to 100°F because solutions that are not close to the client's body temperature will cause ear injury, nausea, and vertigo
3. If a perforation of the eardrum is suspected, irrigation is not done

XIII. Anti-Infective Ear Medications
(Box 53–12)

A. Description
1. Kill or inhibit growth of bacteria

BOX 53–10. Osmotic Medications for the Eye

Glycerin	Mannitol (Osmitrol)
Isosorbide (Ismotic)	Urea (Ureaphil)

BOX 53-11. Medications That Affect Hearing

ANTIBIOTICS

Amikacin (Amikin)
Chloramphenicol (Chloromycetin, Chloroptic, Ophthoclor)
Erythromycin (E-Mycin, ERYC, Ery-Tab, PCE Dispertabs, Ilotycin)
Gentamicin (Garamycin)
Streptomycin sulfate (Streptomycin)
Tobramycin sulfate (Nebcin)
Vancomycin (Vancocin)

DIURETICS

Acetazolamide (Diamox)
Furosemide (Lasix)
Ethacrynic acid (Edecrin)

OTHERS

Cisplatin (Platinol, Platinol-AQ)
Nitrogen mustard
Quinine (Quinamm)
Quinidine (Cardioquin, Quinaglute, Quinidex)

---

2. Used for otitis media or otitis externa
3. Contraindicated if a prior hypersensitivity exists
B. Side effect: overgrowth of nonsusceptible organisms
C. Implementation
   1. Monitor vital signs
   2. Assess for allergies
   3. Monitor for pain
   4. Instruct the client to report dizziness, fatigue, fever, or sore throat, which may be indicative of a superimposed infection
   5. Instruct the client to complete the entire course of the medication
   6. Instruct the client to keep ear canals dry

BOX 53-12. Anti-Infective Ear Medications

Amoxicillin (Amoxil)
Ampicillin trihydrate (Polycillin)
Cefaclor (Ceclor)
Clindamycin HCl (Cleocin)
Trimethoprim (TMP) and sulfamethoxazole (SMZ) (Bactrim, Cotrim, and Septra)
Erythromycin (Ilotycin, E-Mycin)
Penicillin V potassium (Pen-V)
Loracarbef (Lorabid)
Clarithromycin (Biaxin)
Chloramphenicol (Chloromycetin Otic)
Polymyxin B sulfate (Aerosporin)
Tetracycline HCl (Achromycin)
Acetic acid and aluminum acetate (Otic Domeboro)

BOX 53-13. Antihistamines and Decongestants

Triprolidine and pseudoephedrine (Actifed)
Naphazoline HCl (Allerest, Albalon)
Chlorpheniramine (Chlor-Trimeton, Teldrin)
Brompheniramine (Bromphen, Dimetane)
Terfenadine (Seldane)
Clemastine (Tavist)
Cetirizine (Zyrtec)
Astemizole (Hismanal)

XIV. Antihistamines and Decongestants
(Box 53-13)

A. Description
   1. Produce vasoconstriction
   2. Reduce respiratory tissue edema to open obstructed eustachian tubes
   3. Used for acute otitis media
B. Side effects
   1. Drowsiness
   2. Blurred vision
   3. Dry mucous membranes
C. Implementation
   1. Inform the client that drowsiness, blurred vision, and a dry mouth may occur
   2. Instruct the client to increase fluid intake unless contraindicated and to suck on hard candy to alleviate the dry mouth
   3. Instruct the client to avoid hazardous activities if drowsiness occurs

XV. Local Anesthetics

A. Description
   1. Blocks nerve conduction at or near the application site to control pain
   2. Used for pain associated with ear infections
B. Medication: Benzocaine (Americaine Otic; Tympagesic)
C. Side effects
   1. Allergic reaction
   2. Irritation
D. Implementation
   1. Monitor for effectiveness if used for pain relief
   2. Monitor for irritation or allergic reaction

XVI. Ceruminolytic Medications (Box 53-14)

A. Description: used to loosen and remove impacted wax from the ear canal

---

BOX 53-14. Ceruminolytic Medications

Carbamide peroxide (Debrox)
Boric acid (Ear-Dry)
Trolamine polypeptide oleate-condensate (Cerumenex)

B. Side effects
   1. Irritation
   2. Redness or swelling of the ear canal
C. Implementation
   1. Instruct the client not to use drops more often than prescribed
   2. Keep the container tightly closed and away from moisture
   3. Avoid touching the ear with the dropper
   4. Instruct the client to follow the physician's directions regarding removal of cerumen
   5. Instruct the client to notify the physician if redness, pain, or swelling persists

PRACTICE QUESTIONS

1. In preparation for cataract surgery, the nurse is to administer cyclopentolate HCl (Cyclogyl) eye drops. The nurse administers the medication knowing that the purpose of this medication is to
   1 Provide lubrication to the operative eye
   2 Produce miosis of the operative eye
   3 Dilate the pupil of the operative eye
   4 Constrict the pupil of the operative eye

2. The nurse is reinforcing instructions to the client regarding the administration of the prescribed eye drops. Which of the following statements by the client indicates a need for further education?
   1 "I can tilt my head back, pull down on the lower lid, and place the drop in the lower lid."
   2 "I can lie down, pull down on the lower lid, and place the drop in the lower lid."
   3 "I can lie down, pull up on the upper lid, and place the drop in the lower lid."
   4 "I can lie on my side opposite to the eye in which I am going to place the drop. I will put the drop in the corner of the lid nearest my nose then slowly turn to my other side while blinking."

3. The nurse is preparing to administer ear drops to an infant. The nurse plans to
   1 Pull up and back on the auricle and direct the solution onto the eardrum
   2 Pull down and back on the auricle and direct the solution onto the eardrum
   3 Pull the ear down and back and direct the solution toward the wall of the canal
   4 Pull up and back on the earlobe and direct the solution toward the wall of the canal

4. To minimize the systemic effects that eye drops can produce, the nurse plans to instruct the client to
   1 Eat prior to instilling the drops
   2 Swallow several times after instilling the drops
   3 Blink vigorously to encourage tearing after instilling the drops

4 Occlude the nasolacrimal duct with a finger for several minutes after instilling the drops

5. The client is receiving both epinephrine HCl (Epifrin, Glaucon) and timolol maleate (Timoptic) eye drops. When instructing the client on the administration of the eye drops the nurse plans to tell the client to
   1 Administer the epinephrine HCl first, followed by the timolol maleate
   2 Administer the timolol maleate first, followed by the epinephrine HCl
   3 Administer epinephrine HCl in the morning and the timolol maleate in the evening
   4 Wait 3 minutes between the instillation of each medication

6. The licensed practical nurse (LPN) is assigned to care for a client with glaucoma. The LPN reviews the client's medication record and notifies the registered nurse (RN) if which of the following medications is noted on the client's record?
   1 Carbachol (Miostat)
   2 Pilocarpine HCl (Isopto Carpine)
   3 Pilocarpine nitrate (Ocusert Pilo-20, Ocusert Pilo-40)
   4 Atropine sulfate (Isopto Atropine, Ocutropine)

7. A miotic medication has been prescribed for the client with glaucoma. The client asks the nurse about the purpose of the medication. The nurse tells the client that
   1 "The medication will lower the pressure in your eye and increase the blood flow to the retina."
   2 "The medication will help to dilate the eye to prevent pressure from occurring."
   3 "The medication will relax the muscles of the eye and prevent blurred vision."
   4 "The medication will help to block the responses that are sent to the muscles in the eye."

8. Pilocarpine HCl (Isopto Carpine) is prescribed for the client with glaucoma. Which of the following medications does the nurse plan to have available in the event of systemic toxicity?
   1 Naloxone hydrochloride (Narcan)
   2 Pindolol (Visken)
   3 Atropine sulfate
   4 Mesoridazine besylate (Serentil)

9. Betaxolol HCl (Betopic) eye drops have been prescribed for the client with glaucoma. Which of the following nursing actions is most appropriate related to monitoring for the side effects of this medication?
   1 Monitor temperature
   2 Monitor blood pressure

   3   Monitor urine for sugar and acetone
   4   Monitor peripheral pulses

10. The nurse is assisting the physician with performing an ear irrigation on an assigned client. The nurse plans to

   1   Position the client to turn the head so that the ear to be irrigated in facing upward
   2   Warm the irrigating solution to 100°F
   3   Cool the irrigating solution to 85°F
   4   Position the client with the affected side up following the irrigation

ANSWERS

1. **3**

RATIONALE: Cyclopentolate is a rapidly acting mydriatic and cycloplegic medication. It is effective in 25 to 75 minutes, and accommodation returns in 6 to 24 hours. Cyclopentolate is used for preoperative mydriasis. Options 1, 2, and 4 are not actions of this medication.
TEST-TAKING STRATEGY: Use the process of elimination. Options 2 and 4 are similar because miosis refers to a constricted pupil. Note that the question identifies a client being prepared for eye surgery. The pupil would need to be dilated for the surgical procedure. Review the action and purpose of this medication now if you had difficulty with this question.
LEVEL OF COGNITIVE ABILITY: Comprehension
PHASE OF NURSING PROCESS: Implementation
CLIENT NEEDS: Physiological Integrity
CONTENT AREA: Adult Health/Eye
REFERENCE
Lehne, R. (1998). *Pharmacology for nursing care* (3rd ed.). Philadelphia: W. B. Saunders. p. 1050.

2. **3**

RATIONALE: The client can either lie down or sit with the head tilted back. The lower lid should be pulled downward with the thumb or fingers. The client holds the bottle like a pencil, with the tip downward, and squeezes the bottle gently, allowing one drop to fall into the sac. The client gently closes the eye. An alternative method for clients who blink very easily is to place the client in the supine position with the head turned to one side. The eye to receive the eye drops should be uppermost. With the eye closed, drop the prescribed dose on the inner canthus of the eye. Have the client turn from side to midline and to other side while blinking. The eyedrops will move via gravity and surface tension into the conjunctival sac.
TEST-TAKING STRATEGY: Note the key words "a need for further education." Knowing that the client places drops into the eye by pulling down on the lower lid will direct you to the correct option. Review the procedure for the administration of eye medications now if you had difficulty with this question.
LEVEL OF COGNITIVE ABILITY: Comprehension
PHASE OF NURSING PROCESS: Evaluation
CLIENT NEEDS: Health Promotion and Maintenance
CONTENT AREA: Adult Health/Eye
REFERENCE
Leahy, J., & Kizilay, P. (1998). *Foundations of nursing practice: A nursing process approach.* Philadelphia: W. B. Saunders. p. 487.

3. **3**

RATIONALE: When administering ear drops to an infant, pull the ear down and straight back. In the adult or a child older than 3 years, pull up and back on the auricle to straighten the auditory canal. Administer the medication by aiming it at the wall of the canal rather than directly onto the eardrum.
TEST-TAKING STRATEGY: Eliminate options 1 and 2 because you would not direct ear solution directly onto the eardrum. Remember that in a child younger than 3 years pulling the ear down and straight back is the correct procedure for administering ear medications. Review the procedure for the administration of ear medications now if you had difficulty with this question.
LEVEL OF COGNITIVE ABILITY: Application
PHASE OF NURSING PROCESS: Planning
CLIENT NEEDS: Physiological Integrity
CONTENT AREA: Child Health
REFERENCE
Leahy, J., & Kizilay, P. (1998). *Foundations of nursing practice: A nursing process approach.* Philadelphia: W. B. Saunders. p. 497.

4. **4**

RATIONALE: Applying pressure on the nasolacrimal duct prevents systemic absorption of the medication. Options 1, 2, and 3 will not prevent this occurrence.
TEST-TAKING STRATEGY: Use the process of elimination. Eliminate options 1 and 2 because eating and swallowing are similar and are unrelated to the systemic absorption of an eye medication. Blinking vigorously to produce tearing may result in the loss of the administered medication.
LEVEL OF COGNITIVE ABILITY: Application
PHASE OF NURSING PROCESS: Planning
CLIENT NEEDS: Health Promotion and Maintenance
CONTENT AREA: Adult Health/Eye
REFERENCE
Leahy, J., & Kizilay, P. (1998). *Foundations of nursing practice: A nursing process approach.* Philadelphia: W. B. Saunders. pp. 487, 490.

5. **4**

RATIONALE: When two or more medications are to be administered, the client should wait 3 minutes between instillations. Options 1, 2, and 3 are incorrect.
TEST-TAKING STRATEGY: Knowledge regarding the administration of more than one eye medication is helpful to answer this question. Note that option 4 is different from the other options and provides specific information related to the question. Review the administration of eye medications now if you had difficulty with this question.
LEVEL OF COGNITIVE ABILITY: Application
PHASE OF NURSING PROCESS: Planning
CLIENT NEEDS: Health Promotion and Maintenance
CONTENT AREA: Adult Health/Eye
REFERENCE
Clark, J., Queener, S., & Karb, V. (1997). *Pharmacologic basis of nursing practice* (5th ed.). St. Louis: Mosby–Year Book. p. 835.

6. 4

RATIONALE: Atropine sulfate is a mydriatic and cycloplegic medication and its use is contraindicated in clients with glaucoma. Mydriatic medications dilate the pupil and can cause an increase in intraocular pressure. Options 1, 2, and 3 are miotic agents used in the treatment of glaucoma.
TEST-TAKING STRATEGY: Knowledge regarding the classifications of the medications identified in the options will assist you in answering the question. Remember that my"d"riatics "d"ilate, and these medications are contraindicated in glaucoma.
LEVEL OF COGNITIVE ABILITY: Application
PHASE OF NURSING PROCESS: Implementation
CLIENT NEEDS: Safe, Effective Care Environment
CONTENT AREA: Adult Health/Eye
REFERENCE
Hodgson, B., & Kizior, R. (1999). *Saunders nursing drug handbook 1999.* Philadelphia: W. B. Saunders. p. 83.

7. 1

RATIONALE: Miotics are used to lower the intraocular pressure, thereby increasing blood flow to the retina and decreasing retinal damage and loss of vision. Options 2, 3, and 4 all describe actions related to mydriatic medications, which primarily dilate the pupils and relax the ciliary muscles.
TEST-TAKING STRATEGY: Knowledge regarding the action of miotics is required to answer this question. Note that the client has glaucoma. This should provide you with the clue to direct you to the correct option. Remember, prevention of increased intraocular pressure is the goal in clients with glaucoma.
LEVEL OF COGNITIVE ABILITY: Application
PHASE OF NURSING PROCESS: Implementation
CLIENT NEEDS: Health Promotion and Maintenance
CONTENT AREA: Adult Health/Eye
REFERENCE
Kee, J., & Hayes, E. (1997). *Pharmacology: A nursing process approach* (2nd ed.). Philadelphia: W. B. Saunders. p. 584.

8. 3

RATIONALE: Systemic absorption of pilocarpine HCl can produce toxicity and includes manifestations of vertigo, bradycardia, tremors, hypotension, and seizures. Atropine sulfate must be available in the event of systemic toxicity. Mesoridazine besylate is an antipsychotic medication. Pindolol is a beta-adrenergic blocker. Naloxone hydrochloride is an opioid antagonist used to reverse narcotic-induced respiratory depression.
TEST-TAKING STRATEGY: Knowledge regarding antidotes related to various medications is required to answer this question. Atropine sulfate is the antidote for systemic reactions that occur with pilocarpine. Take time now to review antidotes if you had difficulty with this question.

LEVEL OF COGNITIVE ABILITY: Application
PHASE OF NURSING PROCESS: Planning
CLIENT NEEDS: Physiological Integrity
CONTENT AREA: Adult Health/Eye
REFERENCE
Kee, J., & Hayes, E. (1997). *Pharmacology: A nursing process approach* (2nd ed.). Philadelphia: W. B. Saunders. p. 587.

9. 2

RATIONALE: This medication is an antiglaucoma medication and a beta-adrenergic blocker. Hypotension manifested as dizziness, nausea, diaphoresis, headache, fatigue, constipation, and diarrhea are systemic effects of the medication. The nurse monitors the client's blood pressure. Options 1, 3, and 4 are not related to side effects associated with this medication.
TEST-TAKING STRATEGY: Knowledge regarding the systemic effects related to this medication is required to answer the question. Use the ABCs, airway, breathing, and circulation. Although option 4 is also related to circulation monitoring, the blood pressure is the more global option. Take time now to review the side effects of this medication if you had difficulty with this question.
LEVEL OF COGNITIVE ABILITY: Application
PHASE OF NURSING PROCESS: Implementation
CLIENT NEEDS: Physiological Integrity
CONTENT AREA: Adult Health/Eye
REFERENCE
Hodgson, B., & Kizior, R. (1999). *Saunders nursing drug handbook 1999.* Philadelphia: W. B. Saunders. pp. 109–111.

10. 2

RATIONALE: Irrigation solutions that are not close to the client's body temperature can be uncomfortable and may cause injury, nausea, and vertigo. Position the client so that the ear to be irrigated is facing downward as this allows gravity to assist in the removal of the ear wax and solution. Following the irrigation, the client is to lie on the affected side for a while to finish the drainage of the irrigating solution.
TEST-TAKING STRATEGY: Knowledge regarding the procedure for ear irrigation is necessary to answer the question. Visualizing the procedure will assist in eliminating options 1 and 4. Recalling that the irrigating solution should be close to body temperature will assist in eliminating option 3. Review this procedure now if you had difficulty with this question.
LEVEL OF COGNITIVE ABILITY: Application
PHASE OF NURSING PROCESS: Planning
CLIENT NEEDS: Physiological Integrity
CONTENT AREA: Adult Health/Eye
REFERENCE
Leahy, J., & Kizilay, P. (1998). *Foundations of nursing practice: A nursing process approach.* Philadelphia: W. B. Saunders. p. 490.

BIBLIOGRAPHY

Clark, J., Queener, S., & Karb, V. (1997). *Pharmacologic basis of nursing practice* (5th ed.). St. Louis: Mosby–Year Book.
Hodgson, B., & Kizior, R. (1999). *Saunders nursing drug handbook 1998.* Philadelphia: W. B. Saunders.

Kee, J., & Hayes, E. (1997). *Pharmacology: A nursing process approach* (2nd ed.). Philadelphia: W. B. Saunders.
Leahy, J., & Kizilay, P. (1998). *Foundations of nursing practice: A nursing process approach.* Philadelphia: W. B. Saunders.
Lehne, R. (1998). *Pharmacology for nursing care* (3rd ed.). Philadelphia: W. B. Saunders.

UNIT XVI

....

The Adult Client with a Neurological Disorder

PYRAMID TERMS

Agnosia—The inability to use an object correctly.

Apraxia—The inability to carry out a purposeful activity.

Decerebrate Posturing (Abnormal Extension Response)—Client stiffly extends one or both arms and possibly the legs. Indicates a brain stem lesion.

Decorticate Posturing (Abnormal Flexion Response)—Client flexes one or both arms on the chest and may stiffly extend the legs. Indicates a nonfunctioning cortex.

Flaccid Posturing—Client displays no motor response in any extremity.

Glasgow Coma Scale—A method of assessing a client's neurological condition. A scoring system based on a scale of 1 to 15 points. A score below 8 indicates coma is present. Eye-opening is the most important indicator.

Hemianopia—Blindness in half the visual field.

Homonymous Hemianopia—Blindness in the same visual field of both eyes.

Increased Intracranial Pressure—An increase in intracranial pressure caused by trauma, hemorrhage, growths or tumors, hydrocephalus, edema, or inflammation. Can impede circulation to the brain and absorption of cerebrospinal fluid (CSF), and affect the functioning of nerve cells and lead to brain stem compression and death.

Unconscious Client—A state of depressed cerebral functioning with unresponsiveness to sensory and motor function. Some of the causes include head trauma, cerebral toxins, shock, hemorrhage, tumor, or infections.

PYRAMID TO SUCCESS

Pyramid points related to neurological disorders focus on safety issues, care to the unconscious client, monitoring for increased intracranial pressure, monitoring level of consciousness, positioning clients, implementation during a seizure, the cerebrovascular accident (CVA) client, Parkinson's disease, and care to the client with myasthenia gravis. Altered body image and psychosocial issues that occur as a result of the neurological disorder are also a focus of the Pyramid to Success.

NURSING PROCESS

DATA COLLECTION

Airway
Level of consciousness
Vital signs
Headache
Orientation of person, place, and time
Pupils
Changes in mentation and personality
Speech and/or visual disturbance

Alterations in memory, thinking, and judgment
Sensory and motor function
Response to stimuli, both verbal and tactile
Response to painful stimuli; purposeful, nonpurposeful, posturing, or no response
Nutritional status
Bowel and bladder function
Psychosocial issues

PLANNING	IMPLEMENTATION	EVALUATION
The client will maintain a respiratory rate between 16 and 24 respirations per minute. The client performs coughing and deep-breathing exercises and uses an incentive spirometry.	Monitor respiratory status. Encourage coughing and deep-breathing exercises. Instruct client on the use of an incentive spirometer.	Airway remains patent. Lungs remain clear and free of secretions. The client will not experience respiratory complications.
The client remains oriented. The client will exhibit no further deterioration in neurological status.	Monitor vital signs. Monitor neurological status. Monitor level of consciousness. Monitor sensory and motor abilities. Monitor color, motion, and sensation in affected area. Monitor for adequate and palpable pulses. Monitor for signs of increased intracranial pressure. Report changes in neurological status.	Vital signs and neurological status remain stable. Adequate tissue perfusion is maintained.
The client drinks and eats adequate amounts of fluid, food, and fiber.	Weigh client. Encourage foods and fluids. Monitor I&O. Instruct client regarding the need for adequate fluids and fiber in the diet.	Nutritional status is adequate.
Client remains free of skin breakdown as a result of immobility.	Turn and reposition client. Monitor skin integrity. Instruct client in the importance of turning and repositioning.	The client's skin remains intact.
The client reports reasonable comfort.	Assist client to identify comfort measures. Administer pain measures. Note and document effectiveness of pain measures. Instruct client regarding administration of prescribed medications and measures to reduce pain.	Client remains comfortable and reasonably free of pain.
The client learns to perform activities of daily living as independently as possible. The client verbalizes acceptance of mobility limitations.	Turn and reposition client. Assist client with mobility as necessary. Encourage out-of-bed activities as prescribed. Instruct client in the use of assistive devices.	The client complies with exercise programs and prescribed treatments. Client demonstrates correct use of assistive devices.

PLANNING	IMPLEMENTATION	EVALUATION
The client requests assistance with mobilization activities, as needed. The client participates in care.	Assess client's ability to perform self-care activities. Assist client in care, promoting independence as much as possible.	Client participates in self-care to optimal level. Client performs independent self-care activities to optimal level of functioning.
The client maintains controlled continence.	Monitor bowel sounds. Monitor urinary output. Encourage optimal activity to stimulate bowel elimination. Initiate a bowel or bladder control program as appropriate.	Client remains free of elimination alterations.
The client avoids physical injury. The client achieves optimal level of independence without injury.	Assess client's motor and sensory deficit to determine safety needs. Provide appropriate assistive devices to prevent injury. Keep environment free of obstructions. Document client's safe performance of activities.	Client remains free of injury.
The client participates actively in the decision-making process.	Encourage client to make own decisions. Assist client to recognize own strengths and available support systems.	Client utilizes available support systems.
The client shares grief and loss with a significant person. The client verbalizes feelings about the physical disabilities.	Encourage client to express grief. Encourage client to verbalize grief with significant other. Assist to mobilize support resources.	The client begins to cope with changes caused by the disability. Client verbalizes adjustment or adaptation to the disability.

◆ CLIENT NEEDS

SAFE, EFFECTIVE CARE ENVIRONMENT

Advance directives
Advocacy
Client rights
Confidentiality
Informed consent for invasive procedures
Accident prevention related to neurological deficits
Asepsis with procedures and treatments
Standard (universal) precautions
Consultation and referrals

HEALTH PROMOTION AND MAINTENANCE

Expected body image changes resulting from neurological deficits
Prevention and early detection of health problems associated with neurological deficits
Home care instructions regarding care related to neurological disorder
Reinforcement regarding the importance of prescribed therapy

PSYCHOSOCIAL INTEGRITY

The ability to cope with feelings of isolation and loss of independence

Coping mechanisms
Sensory and perceptual alterations
Grief and loss
Cultural, religious, and spiritual influences
Support systems and utilization of community resources
Body image changes

PHYSIOLOGICAL INTEGRITY

Use of assistive devices for mobility
Promoting normal elimination patterns
Measures to promote comfort
Promoting self-care measures
Pharmacological medications, actions, agents, side effects, and adverse effects
Complications related to procedures
Emergency care
Increased intracranial pressure
Assessing level of consciousness
Positioning clients
Implementation during a seizure
The CVA client
Parkinson's disease
Myasthenia gravis

BIBLIOGRAPHY

deWit, S. (1998). *Essentials of medical-surgical nursing* (4th ed.). Philadelphia: W. B. Saunders.

Hill, S., & Howlett, H. (1997). *Success in practical nursing: Personal and vocational issues* (3rd ed.). Philadelphia: W. B. Saunders.

Leahy, J., & Kizilay, P. (1998). *Foundations of nursing practice: A nursing process approach.* Philadelphia: W. B. Saunders.

Luckmann, J. (1997). *Saunders manual of nursing care.* Philadelphia: W. B. Saunders.

Monahan, F., & Neighbors, M. (1998). *Medical-surgical nursing: Foundations for clinical practice* (2nd ed.). Philadelphia: W. B. Saunders.

National Council of State Boards of Nursing. (1998). *National Council detailed test plan for the NCLEX-PN examination.* Chicago: Author.

O'Toole, M. (1997). *Miller-Keane encyclopedia & dictionary of medicine, nursing, & allied health* (6th ed.). Philadelphia: W. B. Saunders.

CHAPTER 54

Neurological System

. . . .

I. Anatomy and Physiology of the Brain and Spinal Cord

A. Cerebrum
   1. Consists of the right and left hemispheres
   2. Each hemisphere receives sensory information from the opposite side of the body and controls the skeletal muscles of the opposite side
   3. Governs sensory and motor activity
   4. Governs thought and learning
B. Cerebral cortex (Box 54–1)
   1. Outer gray layer
   2. Divided into four lobes
   3. Responsible for the conscious activities of the cerebrum
C. Basal ganglia
   1. Cell bodies in white matter
   2. Assists the cerebral cortex in producing smooth, voluntary movements
D. Diencephalon
   1. Thalamus
      a. Relays sensory impulses to the cortex
      b. Provides a thalamic pain gate
      c. Part of the reticular activating system
   2. Hypothalamus

   a. Regulates autonomic responses of the sympathetic and parasympathetic nervous systems
   b. Regulates stress response, sleep, appetite, body temperature, fluid balance, and emotions
   c. Responsible for the production of hormones secreted by the pituitary gland and hypothalamus
E. Brain stem
   1. Midbrain
      a. Responsible for motor coordination
      b. Visual reflex and auditory relay centers
   2. Pons
      a. Contains respiratory centers
      b. Regulates breathing
   3. Medulla oblongata
      a. Contains all afferent and efferent tracts
      b. Contains cardiac, respiratory, vomiting, and vasomotor centers
      c. Controls heart rate, respiration, blood vessel diameter, sneezing, swallowing, vomiting, and coughing
F. Cerebellum
   1. Coordinates smooth muscle movement
   2. Coordinates posture, equilibrium, and muscle tone
G. The spinal cord
   1. Provides neuron and synapse networks to produce involuntary responses to sensory stimulation
   2. Allows for control of the number of pain impulses that pass through the spinal cord on their way to the brain
   3. Carries sensory information to, and motor information from, the brain
   4. Extends from the first cervical to the second lumbar vertebra
   5. Protected by the meninges, cerebrospinal fluid, and adipose tissue
   6. Horns
      a. Inner column of gray matter contains two anterior and two posterior horns
      b. Posterior horns connect with afferent (sensory) nerve fibers

---

BOX 54–1. Cerebral Cortex

FRONTAL LOBE
Broca's area for speech
Prefontal lobe controls morals, emotions, and judgments

PARIETAL LOBE
Interprets pain, touch, temperature, and pressure

TEMPORAL LOBE
Auditory center
Wenicke's area for sensory and speech

OCCIPITAL LOBE
Visual area

---

c. Anterior horns contain efferent (motor) nerve fibers
7. Nerve tracts
   a. White matter contains the nerve tract
   b. Ascending tracts (sensory pathway)
   c. Descending tract (motor pathway)
H. Meninges
   1. Dura mater is the tough and fibrous membrane
   2. Arachnoid membrane is the delicate membrane and contains subarachnoid fluid
   3. Pia mater is the vascular membrane
   4. Subarachnoid space is formed by the arachnoid membrane and the pia mater
I. Cerebrospinal fluid
   1. Secreted in the ventricles and circulates through the ventricles to the subarachnoid layer of the meninges where it is reabsorbed
   2. Circulates in the subarachnoid space
   3. Normal pressure is 60 to 180 mmH$_2$O
   4. Normal volume is 125 to 150 mL
   5. Acts as a protective cushion
   6. Aids in the exchange of nutrients and wastes
J. Ventricles
   1. Four ventricles
   2. Communicate between the subarachnoid space
   3. Produce and circulate cerebrospinal fluid
K. Blood supply
   1. Right and left internal carotids
   2. Right and left vertebral arteries
   3. These arteries supply the brain via an anastomosis at the base of the brain called the circle of Willis
L. Neurotransmitters
   1. Acetylcholine
   2. Norepinephrine
   3. Dopamine
   4. Serotonin
   5. Amino acids
   6. Polypeptides
M. Neurons
   1. The cell body
   2. Contains the axons and dendrites
   3. Neurons carrying impulses to the central nervous system (CNS) are called sensory neurons
   4. Neurons carrying impulses away from the central nervous system (CNS) are called motor neurons
   5. Synapse is the chemical transmission of impulses from one neuron to another
N. Axons and dendrites
   1. The axon conducts impulses from the cell body
   2. The dendrites receive stimuli from the body and transmit them to the axon
   3. Protected and insulated by Schwann's cells
   4. The Schwann's cell sheath is called the neurolemma
   5. Neurons do not reproduce after the neonatal period

6. If an axon or dendrite is damaged, it will die and be slowly replaced only if the neurolemma is intact and the cell body has not died
O. Spinal nerves
   1. 31 pairs of spinal nerves
   2. Mixed nerve fibers are formed by the joining of the anterior motor and posterior sensory roots
   3. Posterior roots contain afferent (sensory) nerve fibers
   4. Anterior roots contain efferent (motor) nerve fibers
P. Autonomic nervous system
   1. Sympathetic (adrenergic) fibers dilate pupils, increase heart rate and rhythm, contract blood vessels, and relax smooth muscles of the bronchi
   2. Parasympathetic (cholinergic) fibers produce the opposite effect

II. Diagnostic Tests

A. Skull and spinal x-ray
   1. Description
      a. X-rays of the skull reveal the size and shape of the skull bones, suture separation in infants, fractures or bony defects, erosion, or calcification
      b. Spinal x-rays identify fractures, dislocation, compression, curvature, erosion, narrowed spinal cord, and degenerative processes
   2. Implementation preprocedure
      a. Provide nursing support for the confused, combative, or ventilator-dependent client
      b. Maintain immobilization of the neck if a spinal fracture is suspected
      c. Remove metal items from body parts
      d. If the client has thick and heavy hair, this should be documented, as it may affect interpretation of the x-ray film
   3. Implementation postprocedure: maintain immobilization until results are known
B. CT (computed tomography) scan
   1. Description
      a. A type of brain scanning that may require an injection of a dye
      b. Used to detect intracranial bleeding, space-occupying lesions, cerebral edema, infarctions, hydrocephalus, cerebral atrophy, and shifts of brain structures
   2. Implementation preprocedure
      a. Obtain informed consent if a dye is used
      b. Monitor for allergies to iodine, contrast dyes, or shellfish
      c. Instruct clients that they will need to lie still and flat during the test
      d. Instruct clients that they will need to hold their breath when requested
      e. Initiate an IV if prescribed
      f. Remove objects from the head such as wigs, barrettes, earrings, and hairpins

g. Monitor for claustrophobia

h. Inform clients that they may hear mechanical noises as the scanning occurs

i. Inform clients that they may feel a hot, flushed sensation and a metallic taste in the mouth when the dye is injected

j. Note that some clients may be given the dye even if they report an allergy, and are pretreated with an antihistamine and corticosteroids prior to the injection, to reduce the severity of a reaction

3. Implementation postprocedure

a. Provide replacement fluids as diuresis from the dye is expected

b. Monitor for allergic reaction to dye

c. Monitor dye injection site for bleeding or hematoma, and monitor extremity for color, warmth, and the presence of distal pulses

C. Magnetic resonance imaging (MRI)

1. Description

a. A noninvasive procedure that identifies types of tissues and identifies tumors and vascular abnormalities

b. Similar to the CT scan but provides more detailed pictures than the CT scan and does not expose the client to ionizing radiation

2. Implementation preprocedure

a. Remove all metal objects from the client

b. Determine if the client has a pacemaker, implanted defibrillator, or metal implants such as a hip prosthesis or vascular clips because these clients cannot have this test performed

c. Remove IV fluid pumps during the test

d. Provide precautions for the client with pulse oximetry as it can cause a burn during testing if coiled around the body or a body part

e. Provide data collection of the client with claustrophobia

f. Administer medication as prescribed for the client with claustrophobia

g. Determine if the use of a contrast agent is to be used, and follow the prescription related to the administration of food, fluids, and medications

h. Instruct clients that they will need to remain still during the procedure

3. Implementation postprocedure

a. The client may resume normal activities

b. Expect diuresis if a contrast agent is used

D. Lumbar puncture

1. Description

a. Insertion of a spinal needle through L3–L4 interspace into the lumbar subarachnoid space to obtain cerebrospinal fluid (CSF), measure CSF fluid or pressure, or to instill air, dye, or medications

b. Contraindicated in clients with **increased intracranial pressure** because the procedure will cause a rapid decrease in pressure within the CSF around the spinal cord, leading to brain herniation

2. Implementation preprocedure

a. Obtain an informed consent

b. Have the client empty the bladder

3. Implementation during the procedure

a. Position the client in the lateral recumbent position and have the client draw the knees up to the abdomen and chin onto the chest

b. Assist with the collection of specimens (label the specimens in sequence)

c. Maintain strict asepsis

4. Implementation postprocedure

a. Monitor vital signs and neurological signs

b. Position the client flat as prescribed

c. Force fluids

d. Monitor I&O

E. Myelogram

1. Description: injection of dye or air into subarachnoid space to detect abnormalities of the spinal cord and vertebrae

2. Implementation preprocedure

a. Obtain informed consent

b. Provide hydration for at least 12 hours before the test

c. Monitor for allergies to iodine

d. If the client is taking a phenothiazine, hold the medication because this medication lowers the seizure threshold

e. Premedicate for sedation as prescribed

3. Implementation postprocedure

a. Monitor vital signs and neurological assessment frequently as prescribed

b. If a water-based dye is used, elevate the head 15 to 30 degrees for 8 hours as prescribed

c. If an oil-based dye is used, keep the client flat 6 to 8 hours as prescribed

d. If air is used, keep the head lower than the trunk

e. Administer analgesics for headache or backache as prescribed

f. Force fluids

g. Monitor I&O

h. Monitor for bladder distention and voiding

F. Cerebral angiography

1. Description: injection of a contrast through the femoral artery into the carotid arteries to visualize the cerebral arteries and monitor for lesions

2. Implementation preprocedure

a. Obtain informed consent

b. Monitor the client for allergies to iodine and shellfish

c. Encourage hydration for 2 days before the test

d. NPO 4 to 6 hours prior to the test as prescribed

e. Obtain a baseline neurological assessment

f. Mark the peripheral pulses

g. Remove metal items from the hair

h. Administer premedication as prescribed
3. Implementation postprocedure
    a. Monitor neurological status and vital signs frequently until stable
    b. Monitor for swelling in the neck and for difficulty swallowing and notify the physician if these symptoms occur
    c. Maintain bed rest for 12 hours as prescribed
    d. Elevate the head of the bed 15 to 30 degrees only if prescribed
    e. Keep the bed flat if the femoral artery is used
    f. Monitor peripheral pulses
    g. Immobilize the puncture site for 12 hours as prescribed
    h. Apply sandbags and a pressure dressing to the injection site as prescribed
    i. Place ice to the puncture site as prescribed
    j. Force fluids
G. Electroencephalography (EEG)
1. Description: a graphic recording of the electrical activity of the superficial layers of the cerebral cortex
2. Implementation preprocedure
    a. Wash the client's hair
    b. Inform the client that electrodes are attached to the head and that electricity does not enter the head
    c. Withhold stimulants, antidepressants, tranquilizers, and anticonvulsants for 24 to 48 hours prior to the test as prescribed
    d. Allow the client to have breakfast if prescribed
    e. Premedicate for sedation as prescribed
3. Implementation postprocedure
    a. Wash the client's hair
    b. Maintain side rails and safety precautions if the client was sedated
H. Caloric testing (oculovestibular testing)
1. Description: provides information about the function of the vestibular portion of the eighth cranial nerve and aids in the diagnosis of cerebellum and brain stem lesions
2. Procedure
    a. Patency of the external canal is confirmed
    b. Cold or warm water is introduced into the external auditory canal
    c. Stimulation of the auditory canal with warm water produces a horizontal nystagmus toward the side of the irrigated ear when the vestibular eighth cranial nerve is normal
    d. Stimulation of the auditory canal with cold water produces a horizontal nystagmus away from the side of the irrigated ear if the brain stem is intact

III. Neurological Assessment

A. Assessment of risk factors
1. Trauma
2. Hemorrhage
3. Tumors
4. Infection
5. Toxicity
6. Metabolic disorders
7. Hypoxic conditions
8. Deficiency conditions
9. Hypertension
10. Cigarette smoking
11. Stress
B. Assessment of the cranial nerves
1. Cranial nerve I (olfactory) sensory, smell
    a. Have the client close eyes and occlude one nostril with a finger
    b. Ask clients to identify nonirritating odors such as coffee, tea, cloves, soap, chewing gum, and peppermint
    c. Repeat the test on the other nostril
2. Cranial nerve II (optic) sensory, vision
    a. Monitor visual acuity with a Snellen chart or newspaper or ask the client to count how many fingers the examiner is holding up
    b. Check visual fields by confrontation
    c. Have the client sit directly in front of examiner and stare at the examiner's nose
    d. The examiner slowly moves a finger from the periphery toward the center until the client says it can be seen
    e. Check color vision by asking the client to name the color of several nearby objects
3. Cranial nerve III (oculomotor); cranial nerve IV (trochlear); cranial nerve VI (abducens)
    a. The motor functions of these nerves overlap; therefore, they need to be tested together
    b. First, inspect the eyelids for ptosis (drooping), then assess ocular movements and note any eye deviation
    c. Test accommodation and direct and consensual light reflexes
    d. Cranial nerve III (oculomotor) motor: assesses pupillary constriction, upper eyelid elevation, and most eye movement
    e. Cranial nerve IV (trochlear) motor: assesses downward and inward eye movement
    f. Cranial nerve VI (abducens): assesses lateral eye movement
4. Cranial nerve V (trigeminal) sensory and motor
    a. Assesses sensation to the cornea, nasal and oral mucosa, facial skin, and mastication
    b. To test motor function, ask the client to close the jaws tightly then try to separate the clenched jaw
    c. Test the corneal reflex by lightly

touching the client's cornea with a cotton wisp

d. Check sensory function by asking the client to close the eyes, then lightly touch the forehead, cheeks, and chin noting if the touch can be felt equally on both sides

5. Cranial nerve VII (facial) sensory and motor
   a. Test taste perception on the anterior two thirds of the tongue
   b. Have the client show the teeth
   c. Attempt to close the client's eyes against resistance and ask the client to puff out the cheeks
   d. Place sugar, salt, or vinegar on the front of the tongue and have the client identify these substances by their taste

6. Cranial nerve VIII (acoustic) sensory
   a. The ability to hear tests the cochlear portion
   b. The sense of equilibrium tests the vestibular portion
   c. Check the client's ability to hear a watch ticking or a whisper
   d. Observe the client's balance and observe for swaying when walking or standing

7. Cranial nerve IX (glossopharyngeal) sensory and motor
   a. Assesses swallowing ability
   b. Assesses sensation to the pharyngeal soft palate and tonsillar mucosa, and taste perception on the posterior third of the tongue and salivation

8. Cranial nerve X (vagus) sensory and motor
   a. Assesses swallowing and phonation, sensation to the exterior ear's posterior wall, and sensation behind the ear
   b. Assesses sensation to the thoracic and abdominal viscera

9. Cranial nerve IX (glossopharyngeal); cranial nerve X (vagus)
   a. Have the client identify a taste at the back of the tongue
   b. Inspect the soft palate and observe for symmetrical elevation when the client says "aah"
   c. Touch the posterior pharyngeal wall with a tongue depressor to elicit a gag reflex

10. Cranial nerve XI (spinal accessory) motor
    a. Assesses uvula and soft palate movement and sternocleidomastoid and trapezius muscles
    b. Assesses upper portion of trapezius muscle, which governs shoulder movement and neck rotation
    c. Palpate and inspect the sternocleidomastoid muscle as the client pushes the chin against the examiner's hand
    d. Palpate and inspect the trapezius muscle

as the client shrugs shoulders against the examiner's resistance

11. Cranial nerve XII (hypoglossal) motor
    a. Assesses tongue movements involved in swallowing and speech
    b. Observe the tongue for asymmetry, atrophy, deviation to one side, and fasciculations
    c. Ask the client to push the tongue against a tongue depressor, then have the client move the tongue rapidly in and out and from side to side

C. Assessment of level of consciousness
   1. Assesses cerebral function
   2. Monitor client behavior to determine level of consciousness such as confusion, delirium, unconsciousness, stupor, and coma

D. Assessment of vital signs: monitor for blood pressure or pulse changes, which may indicate **increased intracranial pressure (ICP)**

E. Assessment of respirations (Box 54–2)

F. Monitoring of temperature
   1. An elevated temperature increases the brain's metabolic rate
   2. An early rise in temperature indicates a dysfunction of the hypothalamus or brain stem
   3. A slow rise in temperature may indicate infection

G. Assessment of pupils
   1. Size
   2. Equality
   3. Reactions to light described as brisk, slow, or fixed
   4. Unusual eye movements
   5. Unilateral pupil dilation indicates compression of the third cranial nerve

---

BOX 54–2. Types of Respirations

CHEYNE-STOKES

Rhythmical with periods of apnea
Can indicate a metabolic dysfunction or dysfunction in the cerebral hemisphere or basal ganglia

NEUROGENIC HYPERVENTILATION

Regular rapid and deep sustained respirations
Indicates a dysfunction to the low midbrain and middle pons

APNEUSTIC

Irregular respirations with pauses at the end of inspiration and expiration
Indicates a dysfunction to the mid- or caudal pons

ATAXIC

Totally irregular in rhythm and depth
Indicates a dysfunction in the medulla

CLUSTER

Clusters of breaths with irregularly spaced pauses
Indicates a dysfunction in the medulla and pons

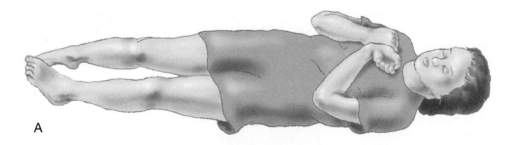

A

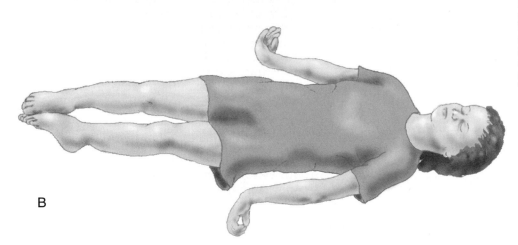

B

FIGURE 54–1. Posturing. *A,* Decorticate posturing. *B,* Decerebrate posturing. (From Ignatavicius, D., Workman, M., & Mishler, M. [1999]. *Medical-surgical nursing: Across the health care continuum* [3rd ed.]. Philadelphia: W. B. Saunders.)

6. Midposition, fixed pupil indicates midbrain injury
7. Pinpoint, fixed indicates pontine damage

H. Assessment of motor function
   1. Muscle tone, including strength and equality
   2. Voluntary and involuntary movements
   3. Purposeful and nonpurposeful movements

I. Monitoring for posturing (Fig. 54–1)
   1. Posturing indicates a deterioration of the condition
   2. Flexor **(decorticate posturing)**
      a. Client flexes one or both arms on the chest and may stiffly extend the legs
      b. Indicates a nonfunctioning cortex
   3. Extensor **(decerebrate posturing)**
      a. Client stiffly extends one or both arms and possibly the legs

   b. Indicates a brain stem lesion
   4. **Flaccid posturing:** client displays no motor response in any extremity

J. Assessment of reflexes (Box 54–3)

K. Assessment of meningeal irritation (Box 54–4)
   1. Nuchal rigidity
   2. Irritability
   3. Fever

L. Assessment of the autonomic system
   1. Sympathetic functions/adrenergic responses
      a. Increased pulse and blood pressure
      b. Dilated pupils
      c. Decreased peristalsis
      d. Increases perspiration
   2. Parasympathetic function/cholinergic responses
      a. Decreased pulse and blood pressure
      b. Constricted pupils
      c. Increased salivation
      d. Increased peristalsis

BOX 54–3. Reflexes

BABINSKI REFLEX

Dorsiflexion of the ankle and great toe with fanning of the other toes
Indicates a disruption of the pyramidal tract

CORNEAL REFLEX

Loss of the blink reflex
Indicates a dysfunction of cranial nerve V

GAG REFLEX

Loss of the gag reflex
Indicates a dysfunction of cranial nerves IX and X

BOX 54–4. Signs of Meningeal Irritation

BRUDZINSKI'S SIGN

Flexion of the head causes flexion of both thighs at the hips, and knee flexion

KERNIG'S SIGN

Flexion of the thigh and knee to right angles and when extended, causes spasm of hamstring and pain

e. Dilated blood vessels

f. Bladder contraction

M. Assessment of sensory function

1. Touch
2. Pressure
3. Pain
4. Bladder control
5. Bowel control

N. **Glasgow Coma Scale** (Box 54–5)

1. A method of assessing a client's neurological condition
2. A scoring system based on a scale of 1 to 15 points
3. A score below 8 indicates coma is present
4. Eye opening is the most important indicator

IV. The Unconscious Client

A. Description

1. A state of depressed cerebral functioning with unresponsiveness to sensory and motor function
2. Some of the causes include head trauma, cerebral toxins, shock, hemorrhage, tumor, or infections

B. Data collection

1. Unarousable
2. Primitive or no response to painful stimuli
3. Altered respirations
4. Decreased cranial nerve and reflex activity

C. Implementation (Box 54–6)

V. Increased Intracranial Pressure (ICP)

A. Description

1. An **increase in intracranial pressure** caused by trauma, hemorrhage, growths or tumors, hydrocephalus, edema, or inflammation

---

BOX 54–5. Glasgow Coma Scale

MOTOR RESPONSE POINTS

Obeys a simple response = 6
Localizes painful stimuli = 5
Normal flexion (withdrawal) = 4
Abnormal flexion (decorticate posturing) = 3
Extensor response (decerebrate posturing) = 2
No motor response to pain = 1

VERBAL RESPONSE POINTS

Oriented = 5
Confused conversation = 4
Inappropriate words = 3
Responds with incomprehensible sounds = 2
No verbal response = 1

EYE-OPENING POINTS

Spontaneous = 4
In response to sound = 3
In response to pain = 2
No response even to painful stimuli = 1

BOX 54–6. Care to the Unconscious Client

Monitor patency of airway and keep an airway and emergency equipment at the bedside
Monitor blood pressure, pulse, and heart sounds
Monitor respiratory and circulatory status
Suction PRN
Monitor neurological status including LOC, pupillary reactions, motor and sensory function
Position client in semi-Fowler's
Change position of client every 2 hours, avoiding injury when turning
Avoid Trendelenburg position
Use side rails at all times
Monitor for edema
Monitor for dehydration
Monitor I&O and daily weight
Maintain NPO status until consciousness returns
Maintain nutrition, fluid, and electrolyte balance
Check gag and swallowing reflex before resuming diet and begin with ice chips and fluids
Monitor intravenous or enteral feedings as prescribed
Monitor bowel sounds
Monitor elimination patterns
Monitor for constipation, impaction, and paralytic ileus
Maintain urinary output to prevent stasis, infection, and calculi formation
Monitor the status of skin integrity
Initiate measures to prevent skin breakdown
Provide frequent mouth care
Remove dentures and contact lenses
Monitor eyes for corneal reflex and irritation and instill artificial tears or cover with eyepatches
Monitor drainage from the ears or nose for the presence of cerebrospinal fluid
Assume that the unconscious client can hear
Avoid restraints
Do not leave the client unattended if unstable
Initiate seizure precautions if necessary
Provide range of motion exercises to prevent contractures
Use a footboard or high-top sneakers to prevent foot drop
Use splints to prevent wrist deformities
Initiate physical therapy as appropriate

2. Can impede circulation to the brain, impede the absorption of CSF, affect the functioning of nerve cells, and lead to brain stem compression and death

B. Data collection

1. Monitor level of consciousness (LOC), which is the most sensitive and earliest indication of **increasing intracranial pressure**
2. Declining LOC from restlessness to confusion and coma
3. Headache
4. Abnormal respirations
5. Rise in blood pressure with widening pulse pressure
6. Slowing of pulse
7. Elevated temperature

8. Vomiting
9. Pupil changes
10. Changes in motor function from weakness to hemiplegia, a positive Babinski reflex, posturing such as decorticate, decerebrate, and seizures
11. Late signs of **increased ICP** include increased systolic blood pressure, widened pulse pressure, and slowed heart rate

C. Implementation
1. Elevate the head of the bed 30 to 40 degrees as prescribed
2. Avoid Trendelenburg position
3. Prevent flexion of the neck and hips
4. Monitor respiratory status and prevent hypoxia
5. Avoid the administration of morphine to prevent the occurrence of hypoxia
6. Maintain mechanical ventilation as prescribed maintaining the $PaCO_2$ at 30 to 35 mmHg, which will result in vasoconstriction of the cerebral blood vessels, decreased blood flow, and, thus, decreased **ICP**
7. Maintain body temperature
8. Prevent shivering, which can raise **intracranial pressure**
9. Decrease environmental stimuli
10. Monitor electrolyte levels and acid-base balance
11. Monitor I&O
12. Limit fluid intake to 1200 mL/day
13. Instruct the client to avoid straining activities such as coughing and sneezing
14. Instruct the client to avoid the Valsalva maneuver

D. Surgical intervention (Box 54–7)

VI. Hyperthermia

A. Description
1. A temperature of 106°F, which increases the cerebral metabolism and increases the risk of hypoxia
2. The causes include infection, heat stroke, exposure to high environmental temperatures, and dysfunction of the thermoregulatory center

B. Data collection
1. Temperature of 106°F

BOX 54–7. Surgical Intervention for ICP

VENTRICULOPERITONEAL SHUNT
Description:
Shunts CSF from the ventricles into the peritoneum
Implementation postprocedure:
Position client supine and turn from back to unoperative side
Monitor for signs of increasing intracranial pressure due to shunt failure
Monitor for signs of infection

BOX 54–8. Medications to Prevent Shivering

CHLORPROMAZINE HYDROCHLORIDE (THORAZINE)
Depresses thermoregulation in the hypothalamus and reduces peripheral vasoconstriction, muscle tone, and shivering

MEPERIDINE HYDROCHLORIDE (DEMEROL)
Relaxes the smooth muscle and reduces shivering

---

2. Shivering
3. Nausea and vomiting

C. Implementation
1. Maintain a patent airway
2. Initiate seizure precautions
3. Monitor I&O and monitor skin and mucous membranes for signs of dehydration
4. Monitor lung sounds
5. Monitor for irregularities
6. Monitor peripheral pulses for systemic blood flow
7. Induce normothermia with fluids, cool baths, fans, or hypothermia blanket

D. Inducing normothermia
1. Prevent shivering, which will increase cerebrospinal fluid pressure and oxygen consumption
2. Monitor neurological changes
3. Monitor for infection and respiratory complications because hypothermia may mask signs of infection
4. Monitor for cardiac irregularities
5. Monitor I&O
6. Administer medications as prescribed to prevent shivering
7. Prevent trauma to the skin and tissues
8. Apply lotion to the skin frequently
9. Inspect for frostbite

E. Medications to prevent shivering (Box 54–8)

VII. Head Injury

A. Description
1. A trauma to the skull resulting in mild to extensive damage to the brain
2. Immediate complications include cerebral bleeding, hematomas, uncontrolled **increased ICP,** infections, and seizures
3. Changes in personality or behavior, cranial nerve deficits, and any other residual deficits depend on the area of the brain damage and the extent of the damage

B. Types of head injuries (Box 54–9)
1. Open
   a. Scalp lacerations
   b. Fractures in the skull
   c. Interruption of the dura mater
2. Closed
   a. Concussions

BOX 54-9. Types of Head Injuries

CONCUSSION

A jarring of the brain within the skull with temporary loss of consciousness

CONTUSION

A bruising type injury to brain
It may occur with subdural or extradural collections of blood

SKULL FRACTURES

Linear
Depressed
Compound
Comminuted

EPIDURAL HEMATOMA

The most serious type of hematoma; forms rapidly and results from an arterial bleed
Forms between the dura and the skull from a tear in the meningeal artery
A surgical emergency

SUBDURAL HEMATOMA

Forms slowly and results from a venous bleed
It occurs under the dura, due to tears in the veins crossing the subdural space

SUBARACHNOID HEMORRHAGE

Bleeding directly into the brain, ventricles, or the subarachnoid space

INTRACEREBRAL HEMORRHAGE

Multiple hemorrhages around a contused area

---

        b. Contusions
        c. Fractures
C. Hematoma
    1. Description: can occur as a result of a subarachnoid hemorrhage or an intracerebral hemorrhage
    2. Data collection
        a. Assessment findings will be dependent on the injury
        b. Clinical manifestations usually result from **increased intracranial pressure**
        c. Changing neurological signs in the client
        d. Level of consciousness (LOC)
        e. Airway and breathing pattern
        f. Vital signs for signs of **increasing ICP**
        g. Headache, nausea, and vomiting
        h. Visual disturbances, pupillary changes, papilledema, and extraocular eye movements
        i. Nuchal rigidity
        j. CSF drainage from the ears or nose
        k. Weakness and paralysis
        l. Posturing
        m. Decreased sensation or absence of feeling
        n. Reflex activity
        o. Seizure activity
    3. Implementation
        a. Monitor respiratory status and maintain a patent airway as increased CO_2 levels increase cerebral edema
        b. Monitor neurological status and vital signs including temperature
        c. Monitor for **increased intracranial pressure (ICP)**
        d. Maintain head elevation to reduce venous pressure
        e. Prevent neck flexion
        f. Initiate normothermia measures for increased temperature
        g. Monitor cranial nerve function, reflexes, and motor and sensory function
        h. Initiate seizure precautions
        i. Monitor for pain and restlessness
        j. Avoid morphine sulfate as it is a respiratory depressant and may **increase intracranial pressure (ICP)**
        k. Monitor for drainage from the nose or ears because this fluid may be cerebrospinal fluid (CSF)
        l. Do not attempt to clean the nose, suction, or allow the client to blow the nose if drainage occurs
        m. Do not clean the ear if drainage is noted but apply a loose, dry, sterile dressing
        n. Check drainage for presence of cerebrospinal fluid (CSF)
        o. Notify the physician if drainage from ears or nose is noted
        p. Instruct the client to avoid coughing because this **increases intracranial pressure (ICP)**
        q. Monitor for signs of infection
        r. Prevent complications of immobility
D. Craniotomy
    1. Description
        a. A surgical procedure that involves an incision through the cranium to remove accumulated blood or a tumor
        b. Complications of the procedure include **increased intracranial pressure** from cerebral edema, hemorrhage, or obstruction of the normal flow of cerebrospinal fluid
        c. Additional complications include hematomas, hypovolemic shock, hydrocephalus, respiratory and neurogenic complications, pulmonary edema, and wound infections
        d. Complications related to fluid and electrolyte imbalances include diabetes insipidus and inappropriate secretion antidiuretic hormone syndrome
    2. Implementation preoperatively
        a. Explain procedure to the client and family
        b. Ensure that informed consent has been obtained
        c. Prepare to shave client's head as prescribed and cover head with appropriate covering
        d. Stabilize the client prior to surgery
    3. Implementation postoperatively (Box 54–10)
    4. Postoperative positioning (Box 54–11)

BOX 54–10. Nursing Care Following Craniotomy

Monitor vital signs and neurologic status every 30 minutes to 1 hour

Monitor for increased intracranial pressure

Monitor for decreased level of consciousness, motor weakness or paralysis, aphasia, visual changes, and personality changes

Check physician's orders regarding client positioning

Avoid extreme hip or neck flexion and maintain head in midline neutral position

Provide a quiet environment

Monitor head dressing frequently for signs of drainage

Mark the area of drainage once each nursing shift for baseline comparison

Monitor the Hemovac or Jackson-Pratt drain, which may be in place for 24 hours

Maintain suction on the Hemovac or drain

Measure drainage from the Hemovac or drain every 8 hours and record the amount and color

Notify physician if drainage is greater than the normal 30–50 mL per shift

Notify physician immediately of excessive amounts of drainage or a saturated head dressing

Record strict measurement of hourly I&O

Maintain fluid restriction to 1500 mL/day as prescribed

Monitor electrolyte values

Monitor for cardiac irregularities that may occur as a result of fluid and electrolyte imbalance

Apply ice packs or cool compresses as prescribed for periorbital edema and ecchymosis of one or both eyes, which is not an unusual occurrence

Provide range of motion exercises every 8 hours

Place antiembolism stockings on the client as prescribed

Administer anticonvulsants, antacids, corticosteroids, and antibiotics as prescribed

Administer analgesics as codeine and acetaminophen (Tylenol) as prescribed for pain

BOX 54–11. Client Positioning Following Craniotomy

Positions prescribed following craniotomy vary with the type of surgery and the specific postoperative physician's orders

Always check physician's orders regarding client positioning

Incorrect positioning may cause serious and possibly fatal complications

REMOVAL OF A BONE FLAP FOR DECOMPRESSION

To facilitate brain expansion, the client should be turned from the back to the unoperative side, but not to the side operated on

POSTERIOR FOSSA SURGERY

To protect the operative site from pressure and minimize tension on the suture line, position client on the side, with a pillow under the head for support, and not on the back

INFRATENTORIAL SURGERY

Involves surgery below the brain's tentorium

The physician may order a flat position without head elevation or may order the head of the bed to be elevated at 30 to 45 degrees

Do not elevate the head of the bed in the acute phase of care following surgery without a physician's order

SUPRATENTORIAL SURGERY

Involves surgery above the brain's tentorium

The physician may order the head of the bed to be elevated at 30 degrees to promote venous outflow through the jugular veins

Do not lower the head of the bed in the acute phase of care following surgery without a physician's order

VIII. Spinal Cord Injury

A. Description (Box 54–12)
1. Trauma to the spinal cord causing partial or complete disruption of the nerve tracts and neurons
2. The injury can range from a concussion to a contusion, laceration, or compression of the cord
3. Spinal cord edema develops, and necrosis of the spinal cord can develop due to compromised capillary circulation and venous return
4. Loss of motor function, sensation, reflex activity, and bowel and bladder control may result
5. The most common causes include motor vehicle accidents, falls, sporting and industrial accidents, and gunshot or stab wounds
6. Complications related to the injury include respiratory failure, autonomic dysreflexia, spinal shock, further cord damage, and death
B. Most frequently involved vertebrae
1. Cervical 5, 6, and 7
2. Thoracic 12
3. Lumbar 1
C. Transection of the cord
1. Complete transection of the cord
   a. The spinal cord is completely severed with total loss of sensation, movement, and reflex activity below the level of injury
   b. If the cord has not suffered irreparable

BOX 54–12. Effects of the Spinal Cord Injury

QUADRIPLEGIA

Injury occurring from C1 through C8

Paralysis involving all four extremities

PARAPLEGIA

Injury occurring from T1 through L4

Paralysis involving only the lower extremities

damage, early treatment is needed to prevent partial damage from developing into total and permanent damage

2. Partial transection of the cord
   a. The spinal cord is partially damaged or severed
   b. The symptoms depend on the extent and location of the damage

D. Types of injuries
   1. Anterior cord syndrome
      a. Damage to the anterior portion of the gray and white matter of the spinal cord
      b. Motor function, pain, and temperature sensation are lost below the level of injury; however, the sensations of touch, position, and vibration remain intact
   2. Posterior cord injury
      a. Damage to the posterior portion of the gray and white matter of the spinal cord
      b. Motor function remains intact but the client experiences a loss of vibratory sense, crude touch, and position sensation
   3. Central cord syndrome
      a. Occurs from a lesion in the central portion of the spinal cord
      b. Loss of motor function is more pronounced in the upper extremities and varying degrees and patterns of sensation remain intact
   4. Brown-Séquard Syndrome
      a. Results from penetrating injuries that cause hemisection of the spinal cord or injuries that affect half of the cord
      b. Motor function, proprioception, vibration and deep touch sensations are lost on the same side of the body (ipsilateral) as the lesion
      c. On the opposite side of the body (contralateral) from the injury, the sensations of pain, temperature, and light touch are affected

E. Assessment of spinal cord injuries
   1. Depends on the level of the cord injury
   2. The level of spinal cord injury is the lowest spinal cord segment with intact motor and sensory function
   3. Respiratory status
   4. Motor and sensory changes below the level of injury
   5. Total sensory loss and motor paralysis below the level of injury
   6. Loss of reflexes below the level of injury
   7. Loss of bladder and bowel control
   8. Urinary retention and bladder distention
   9. Presence of sweat, which does not occur on paralyzed areas

F. Cervical injuries
   1. C2–3 injury is usually fatal
   2. C4 is the major innervation to the diaphragm by the phrenic nerve
   3. Involvement above C4 causes respiratory difficulty and paralysis of all four extremities

4. Client may have movement in the shoulder if the injury is at C5 or below

G. Thoracic level injuries
   1. Loss of movement of the chest, trunk, bowel, bladder, and legs depending on the level of injury
   2. Leg paralysis (paraplegia)
   3. Autonomic dysreflexia with lesions above T6 and in cervical lesions
   4. Visceral distention from a distended bladder or impacted rectum may cause reactions such as sweating, bradycardia, hypertension, nasal stuffiness, "gooseflesh"

H. Lumbar and sacral level injuries
   1. Loss of movement and sensation of the lower extremities
   2. S2 and S3 center on micturation; therefore, below this level the bladder will contract but not empty (neurogenic bladder)
   3. Injury above S2 in males allows them to have an erection, but they are unable to ejaculate due to sympathetic nerve damage
   4. Injury between S2 and S4 damages the sympathetic and parasympathetic responses, preventing erection or ejaculation

I. Emergency implementation
   1. Emergency management is critical because improper handling can cause further damage and loss of neurological function
   2. Maintain a patent airway
   3. Always suspect spinal cord injury until this injury is ruled out
   4. Immobilize the client on a spinal backboard with the head in a neutral position to prevent an incomplete injury from becoming complete
   5. Prevent head flexion, rotation, or extension
   6. During immobilization, maintain traction and alignment on the head by placing hands on either side of the head by the ears
   7. Maintain an extended position
   8. Log roll the client
   9. No part of the body should be twisted or turned nor should the client be allowed to assume a sitting position
   10. In the emergency department, a client who has sustained a severe cervical injury should be placed immediately in skeletal traction via skull tongs or halo vest to immobilize the cervical spine and reduce the fracture and dislocation

J. Implementation during hospitalization
   1. Respiratory system
      a. Monitor respiratory status because paralysis of the intercostal and abdominal muscles occurs with C4 injuries
      b. Monitor arterial blood gases and maintain mechanical ventilation if prescribed to prevent respiratory arrest, especially with cervical injuries
      c. Encourage deep breathing and the use of an incentive spirometer

d. Monitor for signs of infection, particularly pneumonia
2. Cardiovascular system
   a. Monitor for cardiac dysrhythmias
   b. Monitor for signs of hemorrhage or bleeding around the fracture site
   c. Monitor for signs of shock such as hypotension, tachycardia, and a weak and thready pulse
   d. Monitor lower extremities for deep vein thrombosis
   e. Measure circumference of the calf and thigh
   f. Apply thigh-high antiembolism stockings as prescribed
   g. Remove antiembolism stockings daily to assess the skin
   h. Monitor for orthostatic hypotension when repositioning the client
3. Neuromuscular system
   a. Monitor neurological status
   b. Monitor motor and sensory status to determine the level of injury
   c. Monitor motor ability by testing the client's ability to squeeze the hands, spread the fingers, move the toes, turn the feet
   d. Monitor sensation by pinching skin, or pricking with a pin, starting at the shoulders and working down the extremities
   e. Monitor for signs of autonomic dysreflexia and spinal shock
   f. Immobilize the client to promote healing and prevent further injury
   g. Monitor pain
   h. Initiate measures to reduce pain
   i. Administer analgesics as prescribed
   j. Monitor for complications of immobility
   k. Prepare the client for decompression laminectomy, spinal fusion, or insertion of steel rods if prescribed
   l. Collaborate with the physical therapist and occupational therapist to determine appropriate exercise techniques, to assess the need for hand and wrist splints, and to develop an appropriate plan to prevent foot drop
4. Gastrointestinal system
   a. Monitor the abdomen for distention and hemorrhage
   b. Monitor bowel sounds and monitor for paralytic ileus
   c. Prevent bowel retention
   d. Initiate a bowel control program as appropriate
   e. Maintain adequate nutrition and a high-fiber diet
5. Renal system
   a. Prevent bladder retention
   b. Initiate a bladder control program as appropriate
   c. Maintain fluid and electrolyte balance
   d. Maintain adequate fluid intake of 2000 mL daily
   e. Monitor for urinary tract infection and calculi
6. Integumentary system
   a. Monitor skin integrity
   b. Turn client every 2 hours
7. Psychosocial integrity
   a. Monitor psychosocial status
   b. Encourage the client to express feelings of anger and depression
   c. Discuss sexual concerns of the client
   d. Promote self-care, setting realistic goals based on the client's potential functional level
   e. Encourage contact with appropriate community resources

K. Spinal shock
1. Description
   a. Also known as neurogenic shock
   b. A sudden depression of reflex activity in the spinal cord below the level of injury (areflexia)
   c. Occurs within the first hour of injury and lasts days to months
   d. The muscles become completely paralyzed and flaccid and reflexes are absent
   e. Spinal shock ends when the reflexes are regained
2. Data collection
   a. Flaccid paralysis
   b. Hypotension
   c. Bradycardia
   d. Loss of reflex activity below the level of injury
   e. Paralytic ileus
3. Implementation
   a. Monitor for signs of spinal shock following spinal cord injury
   b. Monitor for hypotension and bradycardia
   c. Monitor for reflex activity
   d. Monitor bowel sounds
   e. Monitor for bowel and bladder retention
   f. Provide supportive measures as prescribed based on the presence of symptoms
   g. Monitor for the return of reflexes

L. Autonomic dysreflexia
1. Description
   a. Also known as hyperreflexia
   b. Commonly caused by visceral distention from a distended bladder or impacted rectum
   c. A neurological emergency and must be treated immediately to prevent a hypertensive stroke
   d. It generally occurs after the period of spinal shock is resolved
   e. Occurs with lesions above T6 and in cervical lesions
2. Data collection
   a. Hypertension
   b. Bradycardia

c. Flushing of the face and neck
d. Severe, throbbing headache
e. Nasal stuffiness
f. Piloerection (gooseflesh)
g. Sweating
h. Nausea
i. Restlessness
j. Dilated pupils and blurred vision

3. Implementation
   a. Notify the physician if signs of autonomic dysreflexia occur
   b. Monitor for potential cause and remove the stimulus
   c. Monitor vital signs, particularly blood pressure every 15 minutes
   d. Raise the head of the bed to high Fowler's
   e. Loosen tight clothing
   f. Monitor for bladder distention and prepare for urinary catheterization
   g. If a urinary catheter is present, check for kinks in the tubing and for drainage
   h. Monitor for a fecal impaction and disimpact immediately
   i. Administer antihypertensives as prescribed

M. Cervical traction for cervical injuries (Fig. 54–2)
   1. Description
      a. Skeletal traction used to stabilize fractures or dislocations of the cervical or upper thoracic spine
      b. Two types of equipment used for cervical traction are skull tongs and halo traction
   2. Skull tongs
      a. Skull tongs are inserted into the outer aspect of the client's skull and traction is applied
      b. Weights are attached to the tongs and the client is used as countertraction
      c. Monitor neurological status of the client
      d. Determine the amount of weight prescribed to be added to the traction

e. Ensure that weights hang securely and freely at all times
f. Ensure the ropes for the traction remain within the pulley
g. Maintain body alignment and maintain care of the client on Roto-Rest bed, Stryker, or Foster frame as prescribed
h. Turn the client every 2 hours
i. Monitor insertion site of the tongs for infection
j. Provide sterile pin site care as prescribed

3. Halo traction
   a. Consists of a headpiece with four pins, two anterior and two posterior, inserted into the client's skull, then a halo jacket or cast is applied
   b. Once the fracture is stable, the headpiece can be attached to a body jacket called a halo vest
   c. Monitor the client's neurological status for changes in movement or decreased strength
   d. Never move or turn the client by holding or pulling on the halo device
   e. Monitor for tightness of the jacket by ensuring that one finger can be placed under the jacket
   f. Monitor skin integrity to ensure that the jacket or cast is not causing pressure
   g. Provide sterile pin site care as prescribed

4. Client education for halo vest (Box 54–13)

N. Implementation for thoracic and lumbar/sacral injuries
   1. Bed rest
   2. Immobilization with a fiberglass or plastic body cast
   3. Use of a brace or corset when the client is out of bed

O. Surgical implementation for thoracic and lumbar/sacral injuries

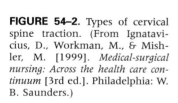

FIGURE 54–2. Types of cervical spine traction. (From Ignatavicius, D., Workman, M., & Mishler, M. [1999]. *Medical-surgical nursing: Across the health care continuum* [3rd ed.]. Philadelphia: W. B. Saunders.)

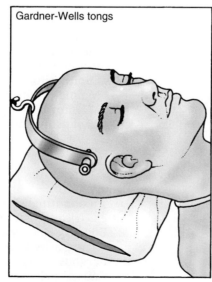

Gardner-Wells tongs

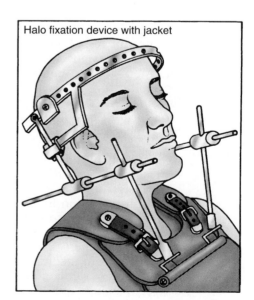

Halo fixation device with jacket

BOX 54–13. Client Education for a Halo Vest

Notify physician if halo vest or ring bolts loosen

Use fleece or foam inserts to relieve pressure points

Keep vest lining dry

Clean the pin site daily

Notify the physician if redness, swelling, drainage, open areas, pain, tenderness, or a clicking sound occurs from the pin site

A sponge bath or tub bath is allowed; showers are prohibited

Inspect the skin under the vest daily for breakdown using a flashlight

Do not use any products other than shampoo on the hair

When shampooing the hair, cover the vest with plastic

When getting out of bed, roll onto the side and push on the mattress with arms

Never use the metal frame for turning or lifting

Use a rolled towel or pillowcase between the back of the neck and the bed, or next to the cheek when lying on the side, and raise the head of the bed to increase sleep comfort

Adapt clothing to fit over the halo

Eat foods high in protein and calcium to promote bone healing

Have the correct size wrench available at all times for an emergency

If cardiopulmonary resuscitation is required, the anterior portion of the vest will be loosened and the posterior portion well remain in place to provide stability

---

1. Decompressive laminectomy
   a. Removal of one or more laminae
   b. Allows for cord expansion from edema
   c. Performed if conventional methods fail to prevent neurological deterioration
2. Spinal fusion and Harrington rod insertion
   a. Used for thoracic spinal injuries
   b. Insertion of a metal or steel rod to stabilize thoracic spine
3. Implementation postoperatively
   a. Monitor for respiratory impairment
   b. Monitor vital signs, motor function, sensation, and circulatory status in lower extremities
   c. Encourage breathing exercises
   d. Monitor for signs of fluid and electrolyte imbalance
   e. Observe for complications of immobility
   f. Keep the client flat
   g. Provide cast care if the client is in a full body cast
   h. Turn and reposition frequently by log rolling side to back to side using turning sheets and pillows between the legs to maintain alignment
   i. Administer pain medication as prescribed
   j. Maintain NPO status until the client is actively passing flatus

k. Monitor bowel sounds
l. Provide the use of a fracture bed pan
m. Monitor I&O
n. Provide a diet high in protein, iron, and thiamine and low in calcium

P. Medications
1. Dexamethasone (Decadron)
   a. Used for its anti-inflammatory and edema-reducing effects
   b. May interfere with healing
2. Dextran
   a. A plasma expander
   b. Used to increase capillary blood flow within the spinal cord and to prevent or treat hypotension
3. Dantrolene (Dantrium)/baclofen (Lioresal)
   a. Used for clients with upper motor neuron injuries
   b. Controls muscle spasticity

IX. Cerebral Aneurysm

A. Description
1. Dilation of the walls of a weakened cerebral artery
2. Can lead to rupture
B. Data collection
1. Pain
2. Diplopia
3. Blurred vision
4. Tinnitus
5. Nausea
6. Hemiparesis
7. Nuchal rigidity
8. Irritability
9. Seizures
C. Implementation
1. Maintain a patent airway (suction only with a physician's order)
2. Administer oxygen as prescribed
3. Monitor vital signs and for hypertension or dysrhythmias
4. Avoid rectal temperatures
5. Maintain bed rest in semi-Fowler's position or side-lying position
6. Maintain a darkened room without stimulation
7. Limit visitors
8. Maintain fluid restrictions
9. Monitor I&O
10. Avoid stimulants in the diet

X. Seizures

A. Description
1. An abnormal sudden, excessive discharge of electrical activity within the brain
2. Epilepsy is a disorder characterized by chronic seizure activity and indicates brain or central nervous system (CNS) irritation
3. Causes include genetic factors, trauma,

tumors, circulatory or metabolic disorders, toxicity, or infections
    4. Status epilepticus involves a rapid succession of epileptic spasms without intervals of consciousness; it is a potential complication that can occur with any type of seizure, and brain damage may result
B. Types of seizures (Table 54–1)
    1. Generalized seizures
        a. Tonic-clonic (grand mal)
        b. Absence (petit mal)
        c. Myoclonic
        d. Atonic or akinetic (drop attacks)
    2. Partial seizures
        a. Simple partial
        b. Complex partial
C. Data collection
    1. Seizure history
    2. Type of seizure
    3. Occurrences before, during, and after the seizure
    4. Prodromal signs such as mood changes, irritability, and insomnia
    5. Aura, a sensation that warns the client of the impending seizure
    6. Loss of motor activity or bowel and bladder function or loss of consciousness during the seizure
    7. Occurrences during the postictal state such as headache, loss of consciousness, sleepiness, impaired speech, or thinking
D. Implementation
    1. Note the time and duration of the seizure
    2. Monitor behavior at the onset of the seizure, if the client experienced an aura, if a change in facial expression occurred, or if a sound or cry occurred from the client

3. If the client is standing, place the client on the floor and protect the head and body
4. Maintain a patent airway (do not force the jaws open)
5. Administer oxygen
6. Prepare to suction
7. Turn the client's head to the side
8. Prevent injury during the seizure
9. Remain with the client
10. Do not restrain the client
11. Loosen restrictive clothing
12. Note the type, character, and progression of the movements during the seizure
13. Monitor for incontinence
14. Medications such as IV diazepam (Valium), phenytoin (Dilantin), and phenobarbital sodium (Luminal) are administered to stop the seizure
15. Document the characteristics of the seizure
16. Monitor behavior following seizure such as the state of consciousness, motor ability, and speech ability
17. Instruct the client on the importance of lifelong medication and the need for follow-up medication blood levels
18. Instruct the client to avoid alcohol, excessive stress, and fatigue
19. Encourage the client to contact available community resources such as the Epilepsy Foundation

XI. Cerebral Vascular Accident (CVA)

A. Description
    1. A sudden focal neurological deficit due to cerebral vascular disease

Table 54–1. Types of Seizures

Generalized Seizures	*Partial Seizures*
Tonic-Clonic (Grand Mal)	*Simple Partial*
May begin with an aura The tonic phase involves the stiffening or rigidity of the muscles of the arms and legs and usually lasts 10–20 seconds followed by loss of consciousness The clonic phase consists of hyperventilation and jerking of the extremities and usually lasts about 30 seconds Full recovery from the seizure may take several hours	Produces sensory symptoms accompanied by motor symptoms that are localized or confined to a specific area. The client remains conscious and may report an aura.
Absence (Petit Mal)	*Complex Partial*
Brief seizure lasting seconds; the individual may or may not lose consciousness No loss or change in muscle tone occurs Seizures may occur several times during a day The victim appears to be day dreaming These type of seizures are more common in children	A psychomotor seizure The area of the brain most involved is the temporal lobe Characterized by periods of altered behavior that the client is not aware of The client loses consciousness for a few seconds
Myoclonic	
A seizure that presents as a brief generalized jerking or stiffening of extremities The victim may fall to ground from the seizure	
Atonic or Akinetic (Drop Attacks)	
A sudden momentary loss of muscle tone The victim may fall to ground as a result of the seizure	

2. A syndrome in which the cerebral circulation is interrupted causing neurological deficits
3. Cerebral anoxia lasting longer than 10 minutes causes cerebral infarction with irreversible change
4. Surrounding cerebral edema and congestion cause further dysfunction
5. Diagnosis is determined by CT scan, EEG, and cerebral arteriography
6. The permanent disability cannot be determined until the cerebral edema subsides
7. The order in which function may return is facial, swallowing, lower limb, speech, and arms

B. Causes
   1. Thrombosis
   2. Embolism
   3. Hemorrhage from rupture of a vessel
   4. Transient ischemia attack (TIA)
C. Risk factors
   1. Atherosclerosis
   2. Hypertension
   3. Anticoagulation therapy
   4. Diabetes
   5. Stress
   6. Obesity
   7. Oral contraceptives
D. Data collection (Table 54–2; Box 54–14)
   1. Airway patency
   2. Slow bounding pulse
   3. Cheyne-Stokes respirations
   4. Hypertension
   5. Headache, nausea, and vomiting
   6. Dizziness and vertigo
   7. Facial drooping
   8. Nuchal rigidity

Table 54–2. Left and Right Hemisphere Lesions

Findings depend on area of brain affected
Lesions in the cerebral hemisphere result in manifestations on the contralateral side, which is the side of the body opposite the cerebral accident.

Left Hemisphere Lesion	Right Hemisphere Lesion
Aphasia both expressive and receptive	Disoriented to time, place, and person
Agraphia—difficulty writing	Cannot recognize faces
Alexia—reading problems	Spatial—perceptual deficits
No memory deficit	Neglect of left side
Deficits in the right visual field such as reading problems and inability to discriminate words and letters	Client unaware of paralyzed side
	Loss of depth perception
	Impulsive
No hearing deficit	Unaware of neurologic deficits
Behavior slow, cautious, and disorganized	Confabulates
	Euphoric; impaired sense of humor
Anxious when attempting a new task	Constantly smiles
Depression	Denies illness
Sense of guilt	Poor judgment
Quick anger and frustration	Overestimates ability
Feelings of worthlessness	Loss of ability to hear tonal variations
Worries over the future	

BOX 54–14. Assessment Findings in a CVA

AGNOSIA
Inability to use an object correctly

APRAXIA
Inability to carry out a purposeful activity

HEMIANOPIA
Blindness in half of the visual field

HOMONYMOUS HEMIANOPIA
Blindness in the same visual field of both eyes
Note: With visual problems, client must turn head to scan complete range of vision

---

9. Diplopia and nystagmus
10. Papilledema
11. Blindness
12. Ataxia
13. Dysarthria
14. Dysphagia
15. Speech changes
16. Decreased sensation to pressure, heat, and cold
17. Bowel and bladder dysfunctions
18. Emotional changes
19. Paralysis

E. Aphasia
   1. Expressive
      a. Damage in Broca's area of the frontal brain
      b. Client understands what is said, but is unable to verbally communicate
   2. Receptive
      a. Injury involving Wernicke's area in the temporoparietal area
      b. Client is unable to understand the spoken and often the written word
   3. Global or mixed: language dysfunction in both the areas of expression and reception
   4. Implementation for aphasia
      a. Provide repetitive directions
      b. Break tasks down to one step at a time
      c. Repeat names of objects frequently used
      d. Use a picture board or communication board

F. Implementation during the acute phase of CVA
   1. Maintain a patent airway and administer oxygen as prescribed
   2. Monitor vital signs
   3. Maintain a blood pressure of 150/100 to maintain cerebral perfusion after a CVA
   4. Suction but never suction nasally and for no longer than 10 seconds to prevent **increasing ICP**
   5. Monitor for **increasing ICP** because the client is at most risk during first 72 hours
   6. Position the client on the side with the head of the bed elevated 15 to 30 degrees as prescribed
   7. Monitor LOC, pupillary response, motor and

sensory response, cranial nerve function, and reflexes

8. Maintain a quiet environment and provide minimal handling of the client to prevent further bleeding
9. Administer IVs as prescribed
10. Insert a Foley catheter as prescribed
11. Maintain fluid and electrolyte balance
12. Prepare to administer anticoagulants, antiplatelets, diuretics, antihypertensives, and anticonvulsants as prescribed
13. Establish a form of communication system

G. Implementation in the postacute phase of CVA
   1. Continue with implementation from the acute phase
   2. Position the client 2 hours on the unaffected side, 20 minutes on the affected side
   3. Position the client in the prone position if necessary, for 30 minutes three times daily
   4. Provide skin, mouth, and eye care
   5. Perform passive range of motion exercises to prevent contractures
   6. Place antiembolism stockings on the client
   7. Measure thighs and calves for increase in size and monitor for positive Homans' sign
   8. Monitor for gag reflex and the ability to swallow
   9. Provide sips of fluids and slowly advance the diet to foods that are easy to chew and swallow
   10. Provide soft and semisoft foods and fluids rather than thin liquids because clients are better able to tolerate these types of food
   11. When eating, position the client sitting in a chair, or sitting up in bed with the head and neck positioned slightly forward and flexed
   12. Place food in the back of the mouth on the unaffected side to prevent trapping of food in the affected cheek

H. Implementation in the chronic phase of CVA
   1. Provide eye care for visual deficits
   2. Approach the client from the nonaffected side
   3. Place the client's personal objects within the visual field
   4. Instruct the client with visual problems to turn the head from side to side
   5. Place a patch over affected eye if the client has diplopia
   6. Increase mobility as tolerated
   7. Encourage fluids and high-fiber diet
   8. Administer stool softeners as prescribed
   9. Encourage the client to express feelings
   10. Encourage independence in activities of daily living
   11. Monitor the need for assistive devices such as a cane, walker, splints, or braces
   12. Teach transfer technique from bed to chair, and chair to bed
   13. Provide gait training
   14. Initiate physical and occupational therapy
   15. Refer to speech and language pathologist

XII. Multiple Sclerosis (MS)

A. Description
   1. A chronic, progressive, noncontagious, degenerative disease of the central nervous system (CNS) characterized by demyelinization of the neurons
   2. It usually occurs between the ages of 20 and 40 and consists of periods of remissions and exacerbations
   3. The causes are unknown but thought to be due to autoimmune response or viral infection
   4. Precipitating factors include pregnancy, fatigue, stress, infection, and trauma
   5. EEG findings are abnormal
   6. A lumbar puncture indicates increased gamma globulin but the serum globulin level is normal

B. Data collection
   1. Fatigue and weakness
   2. Ataxia and vertigo
   3. Tremors and spasticity of the lower extremities
   4. Paresthesias
   5. Blurred vision and diplopia
   6. Nystagmus
   7. Dysphasia
   8. Decreased perception to pain, touch, and temperature
   9. Bladder and bowel disturbances including urgency, frequency, retention, and incontinence
   10. Abnormal reflexes including hyperreflexia, absent reflexes, and positive Babinski reflex
   11. Emotion changes such as apathy, euphoria, irritability, and depression
   12. Memory changes and confusion

C. Implementation (Box 54–15)
   1. Provide bed rest during exacerbation
   2. Protect the client from injury by providing safety measures
   3. Place an eye patch on the eye for diplopia
   4. Monitor for potential complications such as urinary tract infections, calculi, decubiti ulcers, respiratory tract infections, and contractures
   5. Promote regular elimination by bladder and bowel training
   6. Encourage independence
   7. Assist the client to establish a regular exercise and rest program
   8. Monitor the need for and provide assistive devices
   9. Initiate physical and speech therapy
   10. Instruct the client to avoid fatigue, stress, infection, overheating, and chilling
   11. Instruct the client to balance moderate activity with rest periods
   12. Instruct the client to increase fluids and eat a balanced diet including low-fat, high-fiber, and high-potassium foods
   13. Instruct clients in safety measures related to

BOX 54–15. Medications Used with Multiple Sclerosis

STEROIDS

Used to reduce edema and the inflammatory response

Used to decrease the length of time the client's symptoms are exacerbated and improve the degree of recovery

IMMUNOSUPPRESSIVES

Used for the treatment of chronic progressive MS to stabilize the disease process

BACLOFEN (LIORESAL), DANTROLENE (DANTRIUM), or DIAZEPAM (VALIUM)

Used to lessen muscle spasticity

CARBAMAZEPINE (TEGRETOL)

Used to treat paresthesias

PROPRANOLOL (INDERAL) and CLONAZEPAM (CLONOPIN)

Used to treat cerebellar ataxia

BETHANECHOL (URECHOLINE)

Used to prevent urinary retention

OXYBUTYNIN CHLORIDE (DITROPAN)

Used to increase bladder capacity

---

sensory loss such as regulating the temperature of bathwater and avoiding heating pads

14. Instruct clients in safety measures related to motor loss such as avoiding the use of scatter rugs and using assistive devices such as a walker or cane

15. Instruct client in the self-administration of prescribed medications

16. Provide information about National Multiple Sclerosis Society

◆ XIII. Myasthenia Gravis

A. Description
   1. A neuromuscular disease characterized by marked weakness and abnormal fatigue of the voluntary muscles
   2. A defect in the transmission of nerve impulses at the myoneural junction occurs
   3. Causes include insufficient secretion of acetylcholine, excessive secretion of cholinesterase, or unresponsiveness of the muscle fibers to acetylcholine

B. Data collection
   1. Weakness and fatigue
   2. Difficulty chewing
   3. Dysphagia
   4. Ptosis
   5. Diplopia
   6. Weak, hoarse voice
   7. Difficulty breathing
   8. Diminished breath sounds

9. Respiratory paralysis and failure

C. Implementation
   1. Monitor respiratory status and the ability to cough and deep breathe adequately
   2. Monitor for respiratory failure
   3. Maintain suctioning and emergency equipment at bedside
   4. Monitor vital signs
   5. Monitor speech and swallowing abilities to prevent aspiration
   6. Encourage the client to sit up when eating
   7. Monitor muscle status
   8. Instruct the client to conserve strength
   9. Plan short activities that coincide with times of maximal muscle strength
   10. Monitor for myasthenic and cholinergic crisis
   11. Administer anticholinesterase medications as prescribed
   12. Instruct the client to avoid stress, infection, fatigue, and over-the-counter drugs
   13. Instruct clients to wear a Medic-Alert bracelet
   14. Inform the client about services from the Myasthenia Gravis Foundation

D. Anticholinesterase medications
   1. Action: increase levels of acetylcholine at myoneural junction
   2. Medications
      a. Neostigmine (Prostigmin)
      b. Pyridostigmine (Mestinon)
      c. Physostigmine (Antilirium)
      d. Edrophonium (Tensilon)
   3. Side effects
      a. Sweating
      b. Salivation
      c. Nausea
      d. Diarrhea and abdominal cramps
      e. Bradycardia
      f. Hypotension
   4. Implementation
      a. Administer medications on time
      b. Administer medication 30 minutes before meals with milk and crackers to reduce GI upset
      c. Monitor and record muscle strength
      d. Note that excessive doses lead to cholinergic crisis
      e. Have the antidote (atropine) available

E. Myasthenic crisis
   1. Description
      a. Acute exacerbation of disease
      b. Caused by a rapid, unrecognized progression of the disease, an inadequate amount of medication, infection, fatigue, or stress
   2. Data collection
      a. Weakness
      b. Dyspnea
      c. Dysphagia
      d. Restlessness
      e. Difficulty speaking
   3. Implementation
      a. Monitor for signs of myasthenic crisis

b. Increase anticholinesterase medication

F. Cholinergic crisis

1. Description
   a. Depolarization of the motor end plates
   b. Caused by overmedication with anticholinesterase
2. Data collection
   a. Restlessness
   b. Weakness
   c. Dysphagia
   d. Dyspnea
   e. Nausea, vomiting, and diarrhea
   f. Fasciculations
   g. Sweating
   h. Salivation
   i. Increased bronchial secretions
3. Implementation
   a. Hold anticholinesterase medication
   b. Prepare to administer the antidote, atropine, if prescribed

G. Tensilon (edrophonium) test

1. Description: test done to diagnose myasthenia gravis and to differentiate between myasthenic crisis and cholinergic crisis
2. To diagnose myasthenia gravis
   a. Tensilon injection is given to the client
   b. Positive for myasthenia: client shows improvement in muscle strength after the administration of Tensilon
   c. Negative for myasthenia: the client shows no improvement in muscle strength, and strength may even deteriorate after injection of Tensilon
3. To differentiate crisis
   a. Myasthenic crisis: Tensilon is administered, and if strength improves, the client needs more medication
   b. Cholinergic crisis: Tensilon is administered, and if weakness is more severe, an overdose of medication has occurred; administer atropine, the antidote, as prescribed

XIV. Parkinson's Disease

A. Description

1. A degenerative disease caused by the depletion of dopamine that interferes with the inhibition of excitatory impulses
2. It results in a dysfunction of the extrapyramidal system
3. It is a slow, progressive disease that results in a crippling disability
4. The debilitation can result in falls, self-care deficits, depression, and failure of body systems
5. Mental deterioration occurs late in the disease

B. Data collection

1. Bradykinesia, abnormal slowness of movement, and sluggishness of physical and mental responses
2. Aching shoulders and arms

3. Monotonous speech
4. Handwriting that becomes progressively smaller
5. Tremors in hands and fingers at rest (pill rolling)
6. Tremors increasing when fatigued and decreasing with purposeful activity or sleep
7. Rigidity with jerky interrupted movements
8. Restlessness and pacing
9. Blank facial expression
10. Drooling
11. Difficulty swallowing and speaking
12. Loss of coordination and balance
13. Shuffling steps, stooped position and propulsive gait

C. Implementation (Box 54–16)

1. Monitor neurological status
2. Monitor ability to swallow and chew
3. Provide high-calorie, high-protein, high-fiber, soft diet with small, frequent feedings
4. Increase fluids to 2000 mL/day
5. Promote independence along with safety measures
6. Avoid rushing clients with activities
7. Assist with ambulation
8. Provide assistive devices
9. Instruct the client to wear low-heeled shoes
10. Encourage the client to lift the feet when walking and to avoid prolonged sitting
11. Provide a firm mattress and position the client prone, without a pillow, to facilitate proper posture
12. Instruct the proper posture by teaching the client to hold hands behind the back to keep the spine and neck erect
13. Monitor for constipation
14. Promote physical therapy and rehabilitation
15. Administer anticholinergic medications as prescribed to treat tremors and rigidity and to inhibit the action of acetylcholine
16. Administer antiparkinsonian medications to increase the level of dopamine in the central nervous system (CNS)
17. Instruct the client to avoid foods high in vitamin B_6 because they block the effects of antiparkinsonian drugs
18. Instruct the client to avoid MAO inhibitors because they will precipitate hypertensive crisis

---

BOX 54–16. Medications to Treat Parkinson's

Amantadine hydrochloride (Symadine, Symmetrel)
Ethopropazine hydrochloride (Parsidol)
Levodopa (Dopar, Larodopa)
Carbidopa and levodopa (Sinemet)
Trihexphenidyl hydrochloride (Artane)
Procyclidine hydrochloride (Kemadrin)
Benztropine mesylate (Cogentin)
Bromocriptine (Parlodel)

XV. Trigeminal Neuralgia

A. Description
   1. A sensory disorder of the fifth cranial nerve
   2. Results in severe, recurrent, sharp facial pain along the trigeminal nerve
B. Data collection
   1. Pain on the lips, gums, nose, or across the cheeks
   2. Situations that stimulate symptoms such as cold, washing the face, chewing, and food or fluids of extreme temperatures
C. Implementation (Box 54–17)
   1. Identify then instruct the client to avoid situations that cause pain
   2. Instruct the client to avoid hot or cold foods and fluids
   3. Provide small feedings of liquid and soft foods
   4. Instruct clients to chew food on the unaffected side
   5. Administer medications as prescribed
D. Surgical implementation
   1. An alcohol injection along the affected portion of the nerve to produce anesthesia of the nerve may provide relief of pain for up to 16 months
   2. Retrogasserian rhizotomy or total severance of the sensory root of the trigeminal nerve
   3. Jannetta procedure, that surgically relocates the artery that is compressing the trigeminal nerve
   4. Electrocoagulation or percutaneous radiofrequency rhizotomy to create a heat lesion

XVI. Bell's Palsy (Facial Paralysis)

A. Description
   1. A lower motor neuron lesion of the seventh cranial nerve that may occur as a result of trauma, hemorrhage, meningitis, or a tumor
   2. It results in paralysis of one side of the face
   3. Recovery usually occurs in a few weeks without residual effects
B. Data collection
   1. Inability to raise the eyebrows, frown, smile, close the eyelids, or puff out the cheeks
   2. Upward movement of the eye when attempting to close the eyelid
   3. Loss of taste
C. Implementation
   1. Encourage active facial exercises to prevent the loss of muscle tone

---

BOX 54–17. Medications to Treat Trigeminal Neuralgia

Carbamazepine (Tegretol)
Phenytoin (Dilantin)
Baclofen (Lioresal)

---

   2. Provide a face sling to prevent stretching of weak muscles
   3. Protect the eyes from dryness and to prevent injury
   4. Promote good oral care
   5. Instruct the client to chew on the unaffected side
   6. Administer analgesics and steroids as prescribed

XVII. Guillain-Barré Syndrome

A. Description
   1. An acute infectious neuronitis of the cranial and peripheral nerves
   2. The immune system overreacts to the infection and destroys the myelin sheath
   3. It is usually preceded by a mild upper respiratory infection or gastroenteritis
   4. The recovery is a slow process and can take years
   5. The major concern is difficulty breathing
B. Data collection
   1. Paresthesias
   2. Weakness of lower extremities
   3. Gradual progressive weakness of upper extremities and facial muscles
   4. Can progress to respiratory failure
   5. Cardiac dysrhythmias
   6. Cerebrospinal fluid reveals an elevated protein level
   7. EEG is abnormal
C. Implementation
   1. Care is directed toward the treatment of symptoms
   2. Monitor respiratory status
   3. Provide respiratory treatments
   4. Prepare to initiate respiratory support
   5. Monitor cardiac status
   6. Monitor for complications of immobility
   7. Provide client and family support

XVIII. Amyotrophic Lateral Sclerosis

A. Description
   1. Also known as Lou Gehrig's disease
   2. A progressive degenerative disease involving the motor system
   3. The sensory and autonomic systems are not involved and mental status changes do not result from the disease
   4. The cause of the disease may be related to an excess of glutamate, a chemical responsible for relaying messages between the motor neurons
   5. As the disease progresses, muscle weakness and atrophy develop until a flaccid quadriplegia develops
   6. Eventually the respiratory muscles become affected, leading to respiratory compromise, pneumonia, and death
   7. There is no known cure and the treatment is symptomatic

B. Data collection
   1. Fatigue
   2. Fatigue while talking
   3. Muscle weakness
   4. Muscle atrophy
   5. Tongue atrophy
   6. Dysphagia
   7. Weakness of the hands and arms
   8. Fasciculations of the face
   9. Nasal quality of speech
   10. Dysarthria

C. Implementation
   1. Care is directed toward the treatment of symptoms
   2. Monitor respiratory status
   3. Provide respiratory treatments
   4. Prepare to initiate respiratory support
   5. Monitor for complications of immobility
   6. Provide client and family support

XIX. Encephalitis

A. Description
   1. An inflammation of the brain parenchyma and often the meninges
   2. Affects the cerebrum, the brain stem, and/or the cerebellum
   3. Most often caused by a viral agent, although bacteria, fungi, or parasites may also be involved
   4. Viral encephalitis is almost always preceded by a viral infection

B. Transmission
   1. Arboviruses can be transmitted to humans through the bite of an infected mosquito or tick
   2. Echovirus, coxsackievirus, poliovirus, herpes zoster, and viruses that cause mumps and chickenpox are common enteroviruses associated with encephalitis
   3. Herpes simplex type 1 virus can cause viral encephalitis
   4. Amebic meningoencephalitis can enter the nasal mucosa of people swimming in warm freshwater ponds and lakes

C. Data collection
   1. Presence of cold sores, lesions, or ulcerations of the oral cavity
   2. History of insect bites and swimming in fresh water
   3. Exposure to infectious diseases
   4. Travel to areas where disease is prevalent
   5. Fever
   6. Nausea and vomiting
   7. Stiff neck
   8. Changes in LOC and mental status
   9. Symptoms of **increased ICP**
   10. Motor dysfunction and focal neurological deficits

D. Implementation
   1. Monitor vital and neurological signs
   2. Monitor LOC using the **Glasgow Coma Scale**
   3. Monitor mental status changes and personality and behavior changes
   4. Monitor for signs of **increased intracranial pressure**
   5. Monitor for presence of nuchal rigidity and a positive Kernig's or **Brudzinski's sign** indicating meningeal irritation
   6. Assist the client to turn, cough, and deep breathe frequently
   7. Elevate the head of the bed 30 to 45 degrees
   8. Monitor for muscle and neurological deficits
   9. Administer acyclovir (Zovirax) as prescribed
   10. Initiate rehabilitation as needed for motor dysfunction or neurological deficits

XX. Meningitis

A. Description
   1. Inflammation of the arachnoid and pia mater of the brain and spinal cord
   2. Caused by bacterial and viral organisms, although fungal and protozoal meningitis also occurs
   3. Predisposing factors include skull fractures, brain or spinal surgery, sinus or upper respiratory infections, the use of nasal sprays, and individuals with compromised immune systems
   4. CSF fluid is analyzed to determine the diagnosis and the type of meningitis

B. Transmission
   1. Direct contact including droplet spread
   2. Occurs in areas of high population density, crowded living areas, and prisons

C. Data collection
   1. Mild lethargy
   2. Memory changes
   3. Short attention span
   4. Bewilderment
   5. Personality and behavior changes
   6. Severe headache
   7. Generalized muscle aches and pains
   8. Nausea and vomiting
   9. Fever and chills
   10. Tachycardia
   11. Deterioration in level of consciousness
   12. Red macular rash with meningococcal meningitis
   13. Abdominal and chest pain with viral meningitis
   14. Photophobia
   15. Signs of meningeal irritation as nuchal rigidity and a positive Kernig's and Brudzinski's sign

D. Implementation
   1. Monitor vital signs and neurological signs
   2. Monitor for signs of **increasing ICP**
   3. Initiate seizure precautions
   4. Monitor for seizure activity
   5. Monitor or signs of meningeal irritation

6. Perform cranial nerve assessment
7. Monitor vascular status
8. Maintain isolation precautions as necessary with bacterial meningitis
9. Maintain urine and stool precautions with viral meningitis
10. Maintain respiratory isolation for the client with pneumococcal meningitis
11. Elevate the head of the bed 30 degrees and avoid neck flexion and extreme hip flexion
12. Prevent stimulation and restrict visitors
13. Administer analgesics as prescribed
14. Administer antibiotics as prescribed

PRACTICE QUESTIONS

1. The client has an impairment of cranial nerve II. Specific to this impairment, the nurse plans to do which of the following to ensure client safety?
   1 Provide a clear path for ambulation without obstacles
   2 Test the temperature of the shower water
   3 Speak loudly to the client
   4 Check the temperature of the food on the dietary tray

2. The client has a cerebellar lesion. The nurse evaluates that the client is adapting successfully to this problem if the client demonstrates proper use of which of the following items?
   1 Adaptive eating utensils
   2 Walker
   3 Raised toilet seat
   4 Slider board

3. The nurse is planning care for the client who displays confusion secondary to a neurological problem. Which of the following approaches by the nurse is least helpful in assisting this client?
   1 Giving simple, clear directions
   2 Providing a stable environment
   3 Providing sensory cues
   4 Encouraging multiple visitors at one time

4. The client with a neurological impairment experiences urinary incontinence. Which of the following nursing actions is most helpful in assisting the client adapt to this alteration?
   1 Establishing a toileting schedule
   2 Inserting a Foley catheter
   3 Using adult diapers
   4 Padding the bed with an absorbent cotton pad

5. The nurse has obtained a personal and family history for the client with a neurological disorder. Which of the following factors in the client's history does not give the client added risk for neurological problems?
   1 Previous back injury
   2 Allergy to pollen
   3 History of hypertension
   4 History of headaches

6. The client with right leg hemiplegia has a nursing diagnosis of Impaired Physical Mobility. The nurse evaluates that the family needs reinforcement of teaching if the nurse observes which of the following being done by the family?
   1 Encouraging the client to stand unassisted on the leg
   2 Active range of motion (ROM) to the affected leg
   3 Passive ROM to the affected leg
   4 Application of a premolded splint

7. The nurse is preparing the client who is scheduled to have a cerebral angiogram. The nurse checks the client for
   1 Allergy to salmon
   2 Allergy to iodine or shellfish
   3 Claustrophobia
   4 Excessive weight

8. The client admitted with a neurological problem indicates to the nurse that magnetic resonance imaging (MRI) may be done. The nurse interprets that the client may be ineligible for this diagnostic procedure based on the client's history of
   1 Hypertension
   2 Chronic obstructive pulmonary disorder
   3 Heart failure
   4 Prosthetic valve replacement

9. The client is having a lumbar puncture (LP) performed. The nurse plans to position the client in which of the following positions for the procedure?
   1 Side-lying, with legs pulled up and head bent down onto the chest
   2 Side-lying, with a pillow under the hip
   3 Prone, in slight Trendelenburg
   4 Prone, with a pillow under the abdomen

10. The client is somewhat nervous about having magnetic resonance imaging (MRI). Which of the following statements by the nurse provides the most reassurance to the client about the procedure?
    1 "It is necessary to remove any metal or metal containing objects before having the MRI done, to avoid the metal being drawn into the magnetic field."
    2 "The MRI machine is a long, hollow narrow tube, and may make you feel somewhat claustrophobic."
    3 "Even though you are alone in the scanner, you will be in voice communication with the technologist during the procedure."
    4 "You will be able to eat before the procedure unless you get nauseated easily. If so, you should eat lightly."

11. The client has just undergone computed tomography (CT) scanning with a contrast medium.

The nurse evaluates that the client understands postprocedure care if the client verbalizes to
1 Eat lightly for the remainder of the day
2 Rest quietly for the remainder of the day
3 Hold medications for at least 4 hours
4 Force fluids for the day

12. The nurse is admitting the client to the short stay unit following a myelogram. A water-based contrast agent was used. The nurse plans which of the following activity restrictions for the client?
1 Bed rest for 6 to 8 hours, with the head of the bed elevated 15 to 30 degrees
2 Bed rest for 2 to 4 hours, with the head of the bed elevated 15 to 30 degrees
3 Bed rest for 6 to 8 hours, with the head of the bed flat
4 Bed rest for 2 to 4 hours, with the head of the bed flat

13. The nurse is administering mouth care to an unconscious client. The nurse should avoid doing which of the following?
1 Positioning the client on the side
2 Using products with lemon or alcohol
3 Cleansing the mucous membranes with toothettes
4 Brushing the teeth with a small toothbrush

14. The nurse is trying to help the family of an unconscious client cope with the situation. Which of the following interventions does the nurse plan to incorporate into the care routine for the client?
1 Discouraging the family from touching the client
2 Explaining equipment and procedures on an ongoing basis
3 Ensuring adherence to visiting hours to ensure client's rest
4 Encouraging the family not to "give in" to their feelings of grief

15. The nurse is suctioning the unconscious client with a tracheostomy. The nurse avoids which of the following actions?
1 Keeping a supply of suction catheters at the bedside
2 Auscultating breath sounds to determine need for suctioning
3 Hyperoxygenating the client before, during, and after suctioning
4 Making sure not to suction for longer than 30 seconds

16. The nurse has applied a hypothermia blanket to a client with a fever. The nurse inspects the skin frequently to detect which complication of hypothermia blanket use?
1 Skin breakdown
2 Frostbite

3 Arterial insufficiency
4 Venous insufficiency

17. The nurse is caring for an unconscious client who is experiencing persistent hyperthermia with no signs and symptoms of infection. The nurse interprets that there may be damage to the client's thermoregulatory center in the
1 Cerebrum
2 Cerebellum
3 Hippocampus
4 Hypothalamus

18. The client seeking treatment for an episode of hyperthermia is being discharged to home. The nurse evaluates that the client needs clarification of discharge instructions if the client states to
1 Stay in a cool environment when possible
2 Increase fluid intake for the next 24 hours
3 Monitor voiding for adequacy of urine output
4 Resume a full activity level immediately

19. The nurse is caring for the client with an increased intracranial pressure (ICP). The nurse monitors for which of the following trends in vital signs if the intracranial pressure is rising?
1 Increasing temperature, increasing pulse, increasing respirations, decreasing BP
2 Increasing temperature, decreasing pulse, decreasing respirations, increasing BP
3 Decreasing temperature, decreasing pulse, increasing respirations, decreasing BP
4 Decreasing temperature, increasing pulse, decreasing respirations, increasing BP

20. The nurse is positioning the client with increased intracranial pressure (ICP). Which of the following positions does the nurse avoid?
1 Head turned to the side
2 Head midline
3 Neck in neutral position
4 Head of bed elevated 30 to 45 degrees

21. The client recovering from head injury is arousable and participating in care. The nurse would evaluate that the client understands measures to prevent elevations in intracranial pressure if the nurse observes the client doing which of the following activities?
1 Exhaling during repositioning
2 Isometric exercises
3 Blowing the nose
4 Coughing vigorously

22. The family of an unconscious client with increased intracranial pressure is talking at the client's bedside. They are discussing the client's condition, and wondering if the client will ever recover. The nurse intervenes, based on the understanding that
1 The family needs immediate crisis intervention

2 The family could benefit from a conference with the physician

3 It is possible the client can hear the family

4 The client might have wanted a visit from the hospital chaplain

23. The nurse is providing care to the client with increased intracranial pressure (ICP). Which of the following approaches may not be beneficial in controlling the client's ICP from an environmental viewpoint?

1 Maintaining a calm atmosphere

2 Reducing environmental noise

3 Clustering nursing activities to be done all at one time

4 Allowing the client uninterrupted time for sleep

24. The client has clear fluid leaking from the nose following basilar skull fracture. The nurse determines that this is cerebrospinal fluid (CSF) if it

1 Clumps together on the dressing and has a pH of 7

2 Separates into concentric rings and tests positive for glucose

3 Is grossly bloody in appearance and has a pH of 6

4 Is clear in appearance and tests negative for glucose

25. The client is admitted for observation after an auto accident with probable minor head injury. The nurse plans on leaving the cervical collar in place until

1 The physician makes rounds

2 The family comes to visit

3 The result of spinal x-rays are known

4 The nurse needs to do physical care

26. The client was seen and treated in the emergency department for a concussion. The nurse evaluates that the family needs reinforcement of the discharge instructions if they verbalize to call the physician for which of the following client signs and symptoms?

1 Difficulty speaking

2 Difficulty awakening

3 Vomiting

4 Minor headache

27. The nurse is caring for a client who has undergone craniotomy with a supratentorial incision. The nurse uses which of the following postoperative positions?

1 Head of the bed flat; head and neck midline

2 Head of the bed flat; head turned to the non-operative side

3 Head of the bed elevated 30 to 45 degrees; head and neck midline

4 Head of the bed elevated 30 to 45 degrees; head turned to the operative side

28. The nurse is preparing to give the postcraniotomy client medication for incisional pain. The family asks the nurse why the client is receiving codeine sulfate and not "something stronger." In formulating a response, the nurse incorporates the understanding that codeine

1 Is one of the strongest narcotic analgesics available

2 Cannot lead to physical or psychological dependence

3 Does not cause gastrointestinal upset or constipation as other narcotics do

4 Does not alter respirations or mask neurological signs as other narcotics do

29. The nurse is assisting in preparing home care instructions for the postcraniotomy client. Which of the following items does the nurse not include in the instructions?

1 Tub bath or shower is permitted, but keep the scalp dry until sutures are removed

2 Use a check-off system for anticonvulsant medications to avoid missing doses

3 The client after craniotomy will not hear sounds clearly unless they are loud

4 If the client is prone to seizures or gets dizzy spells, someone should be with the client while walking

30. The nurse notes documentation of a nursing diagnosis of Body Image Disturbance for the client after craniotomy. The nurse evaluates that the client has not met the outcome criteria by discharge if the client

1 Wears a turban to cover the incision

2 States an intention to purchase a hairpiece until the hair has grown back

3 Verbalizes that periorbital bruising will disappear over time

4 Indicates that facial puffiness will be a permanent problem

31. The client with a cervical spine injury has Crutchfield tongs applied in the emergency department. The nurse avoids which of the following when planning care for this client?

1 Use of a Roto-Rest bed

2 Assessment of the integrity of the weights and pulleys

3 Comparing the amount of ordered traction with the amount in use

4 Removing the weights to reposition the client

32. The client with spinal cord injury becomes angry and belligerent whenever the nurse tries to administer care. The nurse should

1 Advise the client that rehabilitation progresses more quickly with cooperation

2 Acknowledge the client's anger and continue to encourage participation in care

3 Leave the client alone until ready to participate

4 Ask the family to deliver the care

33. The nurse has completed reinforcing discharge instructions for the client with application of a halo vest. The nurse evaluates that the client needs further clarification of the instructions if the client states to
   1 Use caution since the vest alters balance
   2 Wash the skin daily under the lamb's-wool liner of the vest
   3 Use a straw for drinking
   4 Drive only during the daytime

34. The client with spinal cord injury expresses little interest in food, and is very particular about the choice of meals that are actually eaten. The nurse interprets that
   1 Meal choices represent an area of client control, and should be encouraged as much as is nutritionally reasonable
   2 Anorexia is a sign of clinical depression, and a referral to a psychologist is needed
   3 The client has compulsive habits, which should be ignored as long as they are not harmful
   4 The client probably has a naturally slow metabolism, and the decreased nutritional intake won't matter

35. The client with paraplegia has a Risk for Injury related to spasticity of leg muscles. Which of the following items does the nurse not include in a plan to minimize the risk of injury to the client?
   1 Removing potentially harmful objects near the spastic limbs
   2 Performing range of motion to the affected limbs
   3 Use of padded restraints to immobilize the limb
   4 Use of PRN orders for muscle relaxants such as baclofen (Lioresal)

36. The nurse is teaching the paraplegic client measures to promote skin integrity. Which of the following instructions is least helpful to the client?
   1 Shifting weight every 2 hours while in a wheelchair
   2 Using a mirror to inspect for redness and breakdown twice a week
   3 Checking the bottom sheet for wetness and wrinkles
   4 Using a pressure relief pad while in a wheelchair

37. The client who is paraplegic after spinal cord injury has been taught muscle strengthening exercises for the upper body. The nurse evaluates that the client will obtain the least muscle-strengthening benefit from which of the following activities?
   1 Doing push-ups in a prone position
   2 Extending the arms while holding weights

38. The nurse is caring for the client who has suffered spinal cord injury. The nurse further monitors the client for signs of autonomic dysreflexia and suspects this complication if which of the following is noted?
   1 Severe, throbbing headache
   2 Pallor of the face and neck
   3 Sudden tachycardia
   4 Severe and sudden hypotension

39. The family of a spinal cord–injured client rushes to the nursing station saying that the client needs immediate help. Upon entering the room, the nurse notes that the client is diaphoretic with a flushed face and neck, and complains of severe headache. The pulse is 40 and BP is 230/100 mmHg. The nurse acts quickly, knowing the client is experiencing
   1 Spinal shock
   2 Malignant hypertension
   3 Pulmonary embolism
   4 Autonomic dysreflexia

40. The client with spinal cord injury is prone to experiencing autonomic dysreflexia. The nurse avoids which of the following measures to minimize the risk of recurrence?
   1 Strict adherence to a bowel retraining program
   2 Limiting bladder catheterization to once every 12 hours
   3 Keeping the linen wrinkle-free under the client
   4 Avoiding unnecessary pressure on the lower limbs

41. The client with spinal cord injury suddenly experiences an episode of autonomic dysreflexia. After checking vital signs, the nurse immediately
   1 Lowers the head of the bed and administers an antihypertensive agent
   2 Removes the noxious stimulus and administers an antihypertensive agent
   3 Lowers the head of the bed and removes the noxious stimulus
   4 Raises the head of the bed and removes the noxious stimulus

42. The nurse is planning care for the client in spinal shock. Which of the following actions is least helpful in minimizing the effects of vasodilatation below the level of the injury?
   1 Monitoring vital signs before and during position changes
   2 Using vasopressor medications as prescribed
   3 Moving the client quickly as one unit
   4 Applying TEDS or compression stockings

43. The nurse is caring for a client with an intracranial aneurysm who was previously alert. Which

3 Doing active range of motion to finger joints
4 Squeezing rubber balls

of the following findings is not an early indication that the level of consciousness (LOC) is deteriorating?
1 Slight slurring of speech
2 Ptosis of the left eyelid
3 Mild drowsiness
4 Less frequent spontaneous speech

44. The nurse is planning to put aneurysm precautions in place for the client with a cerebral aneurysm. Which of the following items is not included as part of the precautions?
1 Avoidance of pushing or straining, such as with defecation
2 Maintaining the head of bed at 15 degrees
3 Limiting cigarettes to three per day
4 Provision of physical aspects of care by the nurse

45. The nurse is monitoring the client who is experiencing seizure activity. The nurse does not need to determine information about which of the following items as part of routine monitoring of seizures?
1 Duration of the seizure
2 What the client ate in the 2 hours preceding seizure activity
3 Seizure progression and type of movements
4 Changes in pupil size or eye deviation

46. The nurse is planning to institute seizure precautions for a client who is being admitted from the emergency department. Which of the following measures does the nurse avoid in planning for the client's safety?
1 Placing an airway, oxygen, and suction equipment at the bedside
2 Padding the side rails of the bed
3 Putting a padded tongue blade at the head of the bed
4 Having IV equipment ready for insertion of IV access

47. The nurse is caring for the client who begins to experience seizure activity while in bed. Which of the following actions by the nurse is contraindicated?
1 Loosening restrictive clothing
2 Removing the pillow and raising padded side rails
3 Restraining the client's limbs
4 Positioning the client to the side if possible, with the head flexed forward

48. The nurse has given medication instructions to the client receiving phenytoin (Dilantin). The nurse evaluates that the client has adequate understanding if the client states
1 The medication dose may be self-adjusted depending on side effects
2 Alcohol is not contraindicated while taking this medication
3 Good oral hygiene is needed, including brushing and flossing
4 The morning dose of the medication should be taken before a serum drug level is drawn

49. The nurse is planning care for the client with hemiparesis of the right arm and leg. The nurse incorporates in the care plan to place objects
1 Within the client's reach, on the right side
2 Within the client's reach, on the left side
3 Just out of the client's reach, on the right side
4 Just out of the client's reach, on the left side

50. The client with CVA has residual dysphagia. When a diet order is initiated, the nurse avoids doing which of the following?
1 Giving the client thin liquids
2 Thickening liquids to the consistency of oatmeal
3 Placing food on the unaffected side of the mouth
4 Allowing plenty of time for chewing and swallowing

51. The nurse has instructed the family of a CVA client who has homonymous hemianopia about measures to help the client overcome the deficit. The nurse evaluates that the family understands the measures to use if they state to
1 Place objects in the client's impaired field of vision
2 Approach the client from the impaired field of vision
3 Remind the client to turn the head to scan the lost visual field
4 Discourage the client from wearing eyeglasses

52. The nurse is trying to communicate with a CVA client with aphasia. Which of the following actions by the nurse is least helpful to the client?
1 Speaking to the client at a slower rate
2 Completing the sentences that the client cannot finish
3 Looking directly at the client during attempts at speech
4 Allowing plenty of time for the client to respond

53. The client with diplopia has been taught to use an eyepatch to promote better vision and prevent injury. The nurse evaluates that the client has correct understanding of the use of the patch if the client states to
1 Use the patch only when vision is especially troublesome
2 Wear the patch for 1 hour at a time
3 Wear the patch continuously, alternating eyes each day
4 Wear the patch continuously, alternating eyes each week

54. A client receives a dose of edrophonium (Tensilon) intravenously. The client shows improve-

ment in muscle strength for a period of time following the injection. The nurse interprets that this finding is compatible with
1 Multiple sclerosis
2 Amyotrophic lateral sclerosis
3 Myasthenia gravis
4 Muscular dystrophy

55. The client with myasthenia gravis is having difficulty speaking. The speech is dysarthritic and has a nasal tone. The nurse plans to avoid using which of the following communication strategies when working with this client?
1 Repeating what the client said to verify the message
2 Encouraging the client to speak quickly
3 Using a communication board when necessary
4 Asking yes and no questions when able

56. The client has experienced an episode of myasthenic crisis. The nurse identifies whether the client has precipitating factors such as
1 Too little exercise
2 Increased intake of fatty foods
3 Omitted doses of medication
4 Excess medication

57. The nurse is teaching the client with myasthenia gravis about prevention of myasthenic and cholinergic crises. The nurse tells the client that this is most effectively done by
1 Doing all chores early in the day while less fatigued
2 Taking medications on time to maintain therapeutic blood levels
3 Doing muscle-strengthening exercises
4 Eating large, well-balanced meals

58. The nurse has instructed the client with myasthenia gravis about ways to manage own health at home. The nurse evaluates that the client needs more information if the client makes which of the following statements?
1 "I should take my medications an hour before mealtime."
2 "I've made arrangements to get a portable resuscitation bag and home suction equipment."
3 "Going to the beach will be a nice, relaxing form of activity."
4 "Here's the Medic-Alert bracelet I obtained."

59. The client with Parkinson's disease is embarrassed about the symptoms of the disorder, and is bored and lonely. The nurse plans which of the following approaches as most therapeutic in assisting the client to cope with the disease?
1 Plan only a few activities for the client during the day
2 Assist the client with ADLs as much as possible

3 Encourage and praise perseverance in exercising and performing ADLs
4 Cluster activities at the end of the day when the client is most bored

60. The client with Parkinson's disease is experiencing a parkinsonian crisis. The nurse immediately places the client
1 In a quiet, dim room with respiratory and cardiac support available
2 In a high Fowler's position, with a nasogastric tube at the bedside
3 In a room near the nursing station, which is near the code cart
4 In a bed with padded side rails, with limb restraints nearby

61. The nurse has given instructions to the client with Parkinson's disease about maintaining mobility. The nurse evaluates that the client understands the directions if the client states to
1 Exercise in the evening to combat fatigue
2 Rock back and forth to start movement with bradykinesia
3 Sit in soft, deep chairs
4 Buy clothes with many buttons to maintain finger dexterity

62. The nurse has given suggestions to the client with trigeminal neuralgia about strategies to minimize episodes of pain. The nurse evaluates that the client needs reinforcement of information if the client makes which of the following statements?
1 "I will wash my face with cotton pads."
2 "I'll have to start chewing on the unaffected side."
3 "I should rinse my mouth sometimes if tooth brushing is painful."
4 "I'll try to eat my food either very warm or very cold."

63. The nurse has given the client with Bell's palsy instructions on preserving muscle tone in the face and preventing denervation. The nurse evaluates the client needs additional information if the client states to
1 Expose the face to cold and drafts
2 Massage the face with a gentle upward motion
3 Wrinkle the forehead, blow out the cheeks, and whistle
4 Use a device for electrical stimulation of the face

64. The nurse is admitting a client with Guillain-Barré syndrome to the nursing unit. The client has an ascending paralysis to the level of the waist. Knowing the complications of the disorder, the nurse takes which of the following items into the client's room?
1 Nebulizer and pulse oximeter
2 Flashlight and incentive spirometer

3 ECG monitoring electrodes and intubation tray

4 Blood pressure cuff and flashlight

65. The client is admitted with an exacerbation of multiple sclerosis (MS). The nurse is assessing the client for possible precipitating risk factors. Which of the following factors, if stated by the client, does the nurse note as being unrelated to the exacerbation?

1 A stressful week at work

2 Ingestion of more fruits and vegetables

3 A recent bout of the flu

4 Inability to sleep well

ANSWERS

1. **1**

RATIONALE: Cranial nerve II is the optic nerve, which governs vision. The nurse can provide safety for the visually impaired client by clearing the path of obstacles when ambulating. Testing the shower water temperature is useful if there is impairment of peripheral nerves. Speaking loudly may help overcome deficit of cranial nerve VIII (vestibulocochlear). Cranial nerves VII (facial) and IX (glossopharyngeal) control taste from the anterior two-thirds and posterior one-third of the tongue, respectively.

TEST-TAKING STRATEGY: Knowledge of the cranial nerves is needed to answer this question accurately. Review them briefly if you had difficulty with this question.

LEVEL OF COGNITIVE ABILITY: Application

PHASE OF NURSING PROCESS: Planning

CLIENT NEEDS: Safe, Effective Care Environment

CONTENT AREA: Adult Health/Neurological

REFERENCE

Black, J., & Matassarin-Jacobs, E. (1997). *Medical-surgical nursing: Clinical management for continuity of care* (5th ed.). Philadelphia: W. B. Saunders. pp. 712–713, 719.

2. **2**

RATIONALE: The cerebellum is responsible for balance and coordination. A walker provides stability for the client during ambulation. Adaptive eating utensils may be beneficial when the client has partial paralysis of the hand. A raised toilet seat is useful when the client does not have the mobility or ability to flex the hips. A slider board is used in transferring a client from a bed to stretcher or wheelchair.

TEST-TAKING STRATEGY: To answer this question correctly, you must know that the cerebellum controls balance and coordination. This immediately helps you eliminate options 3 and 4. To help you choose between options 1 and 2, adaptive eating utensils are used when there is loss of fine-motor coordination, such as with cerebrovascular accident. The walker would help the client maintain balance.

LEVEL OF COGNITIVE ABILITY: Comprehension

PHASE OF NURSING PROCESS: Evaluation

CLIENT NEEDS: Health Promotion and Maintenance

CONTENT AREA: Adult Health/Neurological

REFERENCE

Black, J., & Matassarin-Jacobs, E. (1997). *Medical-surgical nursing: Clinical management for continuity of care* (5th ed.). Philadelphia: W. B. Saunders. p. 712.

3. **4**

RATIONALE: Clients with cognitive impairment from neurological dysfunction respond best to a stable environment, which is limited in the amounts and type of sensory input. The nurse can provide sensory cues and give clear, simple directions in a positive manner. Confusion and agitation can be minimized by reducing environmental stimuli (such as television or multiple visitors) and keeping familiar personal articles (such as family pictures) at the bedside.

TEST-TAKING STRATEGY: This question asks for the least helpful action, which makes you look for an incorrect response. The client who is confused can handle limited amounts of information at one time, which makes option 4 the correct answer to this question.

LEVEL OF COGNITIVE ABILITY: Application

PHASE OF NURSING PROCESS: Planning

CLIENT NEEDS: Psychosocial Integrity

CONTENT AREA: Adult Health/Neurological

REFERENCE

deWit, S. (1998). *Essentials of medical-surgical nursing* (4th ed.). Philadelphia: W. B. Saunders. p. 281.

4. **1**

RATIONALE: A bladder retraining program, such as use of a toileting schedule, may be helpful to clients experiencing urinary incontinence. A Foley catheter should be used only when necessary due to risk of infection. Use of diapers or pads is the least acceptable alternative because the risk of skin breakdown is great.

TEST-TAKING STRATEGY: This question can be answered most easily by looking at it from a client safety viewpoint. Since Foley catheters carry risk of infection, and the use of diapers or pads carries the risk of skin breakdown, the only acceptable answer is the toileting schedule.

LEVEL OF COGNITIVE ABILITY: Application

PHASE OF NURSING PROCESS: Implementation

CLIENT NEEDS: Physiological Integrity

CONTENT AREA: Adult Health/Neurological

REFERENCE

deWit, S. (1998). *Essentials of medical-surgical nursing* (4th ed.). Philadelphia: W. B. Saunders. p. 346.

5. **2**

RATIONALE: Previous neurological problems such as headaches or back injuries place the client more at risk for development of a neurological disorder. Chronic diseases such as hypertension and diabetes mellitus also place the client at greater risk. Assessment of allergies is a routine part of the health history, regardless of the nature of the client's problem.

TEST-TAKING STRATEGY: This question is fairly straightforward. Each of the incorrect responses for the question has an actual or potential neurological association. Allergies indicate a disturbance of the immune system. Review the risks associated with neurological problems now if you had difficulty with this question.

LEVEL OF COGNITIVE ABILITY: Comprehension
PHASE OF NURSING PROCESS: Data Collection
CLIENT NEEDS: Physiological Integrity
CONTENT AREA: Adult Health/Neurological
REFERENCE
deWit, S. (1998). *Essentials of medical-surgical nursing* (4th ed.). Philadelphia: W. B. Saunders. pp. 326–327.

6. **1**

RATIONALE: The question is worded to elicit an unsafe action on the part of the family. Depending on the client's functional ability, either passive or active ROM is indicated to keep the joint moving freely. Application of a premolded splint also keeps the limb aligned and in good position. The client should not attempt to stand unsupported on a weak or paralyzed limb. The inability to bear weight will cause the client to fall.
TEST-TAKING STRATEGY: This question tests fundamental concepts of impaired mobility and corrective actions. If you had any difficulty with this question, you may want to review these concepts now.
LEVEL OF COGNITIVE ABILITY: Comprehension
PHASE OF NURSING PROCESS: Evaluation
CLIENT NEEDS: Health Promotion and Maintenance
CONTENT AREA: Adult Health/Neurological
REFERENCE
deWit, S. (1998). *Essentials of medical-surgical nursing* (4th ed.). Philadelphia: W. B. Saunders. p. 341.

7. **2**

RATIONALE: The client undergoing cerebral angiography is assessed for possible allergy to the contrast dye, which can be determined by questioning the client about allergies to iodine or shellfish. Salmon is irrelevant to the question. Claustrophobia and excessive weight are areas of concern with magnetic resonance imaging.
TEST-TAKING STRATEGY: This concept is fundamental for angiography of any group of blood vessels. Memorize this now if you have not already. It is likely you could encounter this type of question in some form.
LEVEL OF COGNITIVE ABILITY: Application
PHASE OF NURSING PROCESS: Data Collection
CLIENT NEEDS: Physiological Integrity
CONTENT AREA: Adult Health/Neurological
REFERENCE
deWit, S. (1998). *Essentials of medical-surgical nursing* (4th ed.). Philadelphia: W. B. Saunders. p. 332.

8. **4**

RATIONALE: The client having an MRI has all metallic objects removed, because of the magnetic field generated by the device. A careful history is done to determine if any metal objects are inside the client, such as orthopedic hardware, pacemakers, artificial heart valves, aneurysm clips, or intrauterine devices. These may heat up, become dislodged, or malfunction during this procedure. The client may be ineligible if there is significant risk.
TEST-TAKING STRATEGY: You will note that each of the incorrect options is a medical disorder. The correct answer is the name of a surgical procedure in which an artificial valve (sometimes metal) is implanted. An important concept with regard to MRI is the avoidance of any metal objects in the vicinity of the machine. Review the contraindications related to this procedure now if you had difficulty with this question.

LEVEL OF COGNITIVE ABILITY: Comprehension
PHASE OF NURSING PROCESS: Data Collection
CLIENT NEEDS: Physiological Integrity
CONTENT AREA: Adult Health/Neurological
REFERENCE
deWit, S. (1998). *Essentials of medical-surgical nursing* (4th ed.). Philadelphia: W. B. Saunders. p. 671.

9. **1**

RATIONALE: The client undergoing LP is positioned lying on the side, with the legs pulled up to the abdomen, and with the head bent down onto the chest. This position helps to open the spaces between the vertebrae.
TEST-TAKING STRATEGY: Knowing that an LP is the introduction of a needle into the subarachnoid space, it is reasonable that the position of the client must facilitate this. The correct answer is the only position that flexes the vertebrae for easier needle insertion. Review positioning procedures for an LP now if you had difficulty with this question.
LEVEL OF COGNITIVE ABILITY: Application
PHASE OF NURSING PROCESS: Planning
CLIENT NEEDS: Physiological Integrity
CONTENT AREA: Adult Health/Neurological
REFERENCE
Black, J., & Matassarin-Jacobs, E. (1997). *Medical-surgical nursing: Clinical management for continuity of care* (5th ed.). Philadelphia: W. B. Saunders. p. 733.

10. **3**

RATIONALE: The MRI scanner is a hollow tube that gives some clients a feeling of claustrophobia. Metal objects must be removed before the procedure so they are not drawn in to the magnetic field. The client may eat and take all prescribed medications before the procedure. If a contrast medium is used, the client may wish to eat lightly if the client has a tendency to get nauseated easily. The client lies supine on a padded table, which moves into the imager. The client must lie still during the procedure. The imager makes tapping noises while scanning. The client is alone in the imager, but the nurse can reassure the client that the technician is in voice communication with the client at all times.
TEST-TAKING STRATEGY: The statements in each of the options is correct. However, the question asks which of them will give the most reassurance to the client. While all statements are factually true, the correct option is the only one that provides a measure of reassurance to the client. Review MRI now if you had difficulty with this question.
LEVEL OF COGNITIVE ABILITY: Application
PHASE OF NURSING PROCESS: Implementation
CLIENT NEEDS: Psychosocial Integrity
CONTENT AREA: Adult Health/Neurological
REFERENCE
Black, J., & Matassarin-Jacobs, E. (1997). *Medical-surgical nursing: Clinical management for continuity of care* (5th ed.). Philadelphia: W. B. Saunders. p. 732.

11. **4**

RATIONALE: After CT scanning, the client may resume all usual activities. The client should be encouraged to take in extra fluids to replace those lost with diuresis from the contrast dye.
TEST-TAKING STRATEGY: Looking at the available choices, option 3 makes the least sense and should be eliminated first. Knowing that there is no special aftercare

lets you eliminate options 1 and 2 next. Review the procedure related to CT scanning now if you had difficulty with this question.
LEVEL OF COGNITIVE ABILITY: Comprehension
PHASE OF NURSING PROCESS: Evaluation
CLIENT NEEDS: Health Promotion and Maintenance
CONTENT AREA: Adult Health/Neurological
REFERENCE
Black, J., & Matassarin-Jacobs, E. (1997). *Medical-surgical nursing: Clinical management for continuity of care* (5th ed.). Philadelphia: W. B. Saunders. p. 731.

12. **1**

RATIONALE: Following a myelogram, the client is placed on bed rest for 6 to 8 hours. When a water-based contrast medium is used, the client is positioned with the head of bed elevated 15 to 30 degrees. With the use of an oil-based medium, the head of the bed is positioned flat (even though the contrast is aspirated out after the procedure).
TEST-TAKING STRATEGY: This question is asking for knowledge of two separate items; e.g., length of bed rest and head position. With a myelogram procedure, if you reason that the longer the bed rest, the less likelihood of complications, then you can narrow your choices to options 1 and 3. If you can remember that "oil rises, so keep the head low," you will be able to choose correctly. Review postprocedure care following a myelogram now if you had difficulty with this question.
LEVEL OF COGNITIVE ABILITY: Application
PHASE OF NURSING PROCESS: Planning
CLIENT NEEDS: Physiological Integrity
CONTENT AREA: Adult Health/Neurological
REFERENCE
Black, J., & Matassarin-Jacobs, E. (1997). *Medical-surgical nursing: Clinical management for continuity of care* (5th ed.). Philadelphia: W. B. Saunders. pp. 735–736.

13. **2**

RATIONALE: The unconscious client is positioned on the side during mouth care to prevent aspiration. The teeth are brushed at least twice daily using a small toothbrush. The gums, tongue, roof of the mouth, and oral mucous membranes are cleaned with toothettes to avoid encrustation and infection. The lips are coated with water-soluble lubricant to prevent drying, cracking, and encrustation. The use of products with lemon or alcohol should be avoided because they have a drying effect.
TEST-TAKING STRATEGY: The question asks what the nurse should avoid. Standard mouth care procedures include use of toothbrush and toothettes, so these may eliminated first. Knowing that the unconscious client is at risk of aspiration tells you that option 1 is correct also. This leaves option 2 as incorrect, because repeated use of these products could dry and crack the oral mucous membranes.
LEVEL OF COGNITIVE ABILITY: Application
PHASE OF NURSING PROCESS: Implementation
CLIENT NEEDS: Physiological Integrity
CONTENT AREA: Adult Health/Neurological
REFERENCE
Black, J., & Matassarin-Jacobs, E. (1997). *Medical-surgical nursing: Clinical management for continuity of care* (5th ed.). Philadelphia: W. B. Saunders. p. 758.

14. **2**

RATIONALE: Families often need assistance to cope with the sudden severe illness of a loved one. The nurse can help the family of an unconscious client by assisting them to work through their feelings of grief. The nurse should explain all equipment, treatments and procedures, and supplement or reinforce information given by the physician. Family should be encouraged to touch and speak to the client, and to become involved in the client's care to the extent they are comfortable. The nurse should allow the family to stay with the client to the extent possible, and should encourage them to eat and sleep adequately to maintain their strength.
TEST-TAKING STRATEGY: The options seem to revolve around two themes: the adjustment of the family to the situation and the involvement or interaction with the client and care. Each of the incorrect options either inhibits the family's coping or distances the family from the client or the client's care. Avoid selecting these types of options.
LEVEL OF COGNITIVE ABILITY: Application
PHASE OF NURSING PROCESS: Planning
CLIENT NEEDS: Psychosocial Integrity
CONTENT AREA: Adult Health/Neurological
REFERENCE
Black, J., & Matassarin-Jacobs, E. (1997). *Medical-surgical nursing: Clinical management for continuity of care* (5th ed.). Philadelphia: W. B. Saunders. p. 762.

15. **4**

RATIONALE: Suction equipment should be kept at the bedside of an unconscious client, regardless of whether an artificial airway is used. The nurse auscultates breath sounds every 2 to 4 hours, or more frequently if there is need. The client should be hyperoxygenated before, during, and after suctioning to minimize cerebral hypoxia. The client should not be suctioned for longer than 10 seconds at one time, to prevent cerebral hypoxia and a rise in intracranial pressure.
TEST-TAKING STRATEGY: The question is worded to make you seek an incorrect nursing action. Each of the first three options is standard suctioning procedure. The only option that is different, and dangerous, is option 4. If you had difficulty with this question, review suctioning procedures now.
LEVEL OF COGNITIVE ABILITY: Application
PHASE OF NURSING PROCESS: Implementation
CLIENT NEEDS: Physiological Integrity
CONTENT AREA: Adult Health/Neurological
REFERENCE
deWit, S. (1998). *Essentials of medical-surgical nursing* (4th ed.). Philadelphia: W. B. Saunders. p. 422.

16. **1**

RATIONALE: When a hypothermia blanket is used, the skin is inspected frequently for pressure points, which over time could lead to skin breakdown.
TEST-TAKING STRATEGY: Options 3 and 4 may be eliminated first because they are other health problems. The temperature of the blanket is not cold enough to produce frostbite. This leaves skin breakdown as the correct answer. Review the complications associated with the use of a hypothermia blanket now if you had difficulty with this question.
LEVEL OF COGNITIVE ABILITY: Application
PHASE OF NURSING PROCESS: Data Collection
CLIENT NEEDS: Physiological Integrity
CONTENT AREA: Adult Health/Neurological

REFERENCE
Black, J., & Matassarin-Jacobs, E. (1997). *Medical-surgical nursing: Clinical management for continuity of care* (5th ed.). Philadelphia: W. B. Saunders. p. 800.

17. **4**

RATIONALE: Hypothalamic damage causes hyperthermia, which may also be called "central fever." It is characterized by a persistent high fever with no diurnal variation. There is also an absence of sweating.
TEST-TAKING STRATEGY: Knowledge of the location of the brain's thermoregulatory center is needed to answer this question. Eliminate options 1 and 2 first because they are responsible for higher mental functions and balance, respectively. Relate hyperthermia with hypothalamus.
LEVEL OF COGNITIVE ABILITY: Comprehension
PHASE OF NURSING PROCESS: Data Collection
CLIENT NEEDS: Physiological Integrity
CONTENT AREA: Adult Health/Neurological
REFERENCE
Monahan, F., & Neighbors, M. (1998). *Medical-surgical nursing: Foundations for clinical practice* (2nd ed.). Philadelphia: W. B. Saunders. p. 720.

18. **4**

RATIONALE: Discharge instructions for the client hospitalized for hyperthermia include prevention of heat related disorders, increased fluid intake for 24 hours, self-monitoring of voiding, and the importance of staying in a cool environment and resting.
TEST-TAKING STRATEGY: This question is worded to elicit the least appropriate activity upon discharge. Options 2 and 3 relate to maintaining and monitoring fluid balance, and are therefore eliminated. A cool environment is appropriate, so this is eliminated also. Resumption of full activity is not helpful; rather, rest periods are indicated, so this is the correct option.
LEVEL OF COGNITIVE ABILITY: Comprehension
PHASE OF NURSING PROCESS: Evaluation
CLIENT NEEDS: Health Promotion and Maintenance
CONTENT AREA: Adult Health/Neurological
REFERENCE
Luckmann, J. (1997). *Saunders manual of nursing care.* Philadelphia: W. B. Saunders. p. 1735.

19. **2**

RATIONALE: A change in vital signs may be a late sign of increased ICP. Trends include increasing temperature and blood pressure, and decreasing pulse and respirations. Respiratory irregularities may also arise.
TEST-TAKING STRATEGY: This question looks complex, but can be logically answered. If you remember that temperature rises, then you are able to eliminate options 3 and 4. If you know that the client becomes bradycardic, or know that the BP rises, you are able to make the correct choice. Review the signs of increased intracranial pressure now if you had difficulty with this question.
LEVEL OF COGNITIVE ABILITY: Application
PHASE OF NURSING PROCESS: Data Collection
CLIENT NEEDS: Physiological Integrity
CONTENT AREA: Adult Health/Neurological
REFERENCE
Monahan, F., & Neighbors, M. (1998). *Medical-surgical nursing: Foundations for clinical practice* (2nd ed.). Philadelphia: W. B. Saunders. p. 730.

20. **1**

RATIONALE: The head of the client with increased ICP should be positioned so the head is in a neutral, midline position. The nurse should avoid flexing or extending the neck, or turning the neck side to side. The head of the bed should be raised 30 to 45 degrees. Use of proper positions promotes venous drainage from the cranium to keep intracranial pressure down.
TEST-TAKING STRATEGY: This question is asking which position will be detrimental to the client with increased ICP. This would be one that interferes either with arterial circulation to the brain, or with venous drainage from the brain. The only position that meets one of these criteria is option 1. Review client positioning with ICP now if you had difficulty with this question.
LEVEL OF COGNITIVE ABILITY: Application
PHASE OF NURSING PROCESS: Implementation
CLIENT NEEDS: Physiological Integrity
CONTENT AREA: Adult Health/Neurological
REFERENCE
Monahan, F., & Neighbors, M. (1998). *Medical-surgical nursing: Foundations for clinical practice* (2nd ed.). Philadelphia: W. B. Saunders. p. 732.

21. **1**

RATIONALE: Activities that increase intrathoracic and intra-abdominal pressures cause indirect elevation of the ICP. Some of these activities include isometric exercises, Valsalva maneuver, coughing, sneezing, and blowing the nose. Exhaling during activities such as repositioning or pulling up in bed opens the glottis, which prevents intrathoracic pressure from rising.
TEST-TAKING STRATEGY: Evaluate each of the options in terms of the tension it puts on the body. Doing so will help you eliminate each of the incorrect options systematically. Review the measures that will reduce or prevent increased intracranial pressure if you had difficulty with this question.
LEVEL OF COGNITIVE ABILITY: Comprehension
PHASE OF NURSING PROCESS: Evaluation
CLIENT NEEDS: Health Promotion and Maintenance
CONTENT AREA: Adult Health/Neurological
REFERENCE
Monahan, F., & Neighbors, M. (1998). *Medical-surgical nursing: Foundations for clinical practice* (2nd ed.). Philadelphia: W. B. Saunders. p. 730.

22. **3**

RATIONALE: Some clients who have awakened from an unconscious state have reported they remember hearing specific voices and conversations. Family and staff should assume the client's sense of hearing is still intact, and act accordingly. Research has also demonstrated that positive outcomes are associated with coma stimulation, that is, speaking to and touching the client.
TEST-TAKING STRATEGY: The nurse would not infer that the client wants a visit from the chaplain based on the family speaking over the client at the bedside, so that can be eliminated first. The family demonstrates no evidence of crisis, and they seem to be well informed. This eliminates options 1 and 2. Option 3 is the only correct choice.
LEVEL OF COGNITIVE ABILITY: Comprehension
PHASE OF NURSING PROCESS: Implementation
CLIENT NEEDS: Psychosocial Integrity
CONTENT AREA: Adult Health/Neurological

REFERENCE
Black, J., & Matassarin-Jacobs, E. (1997). *Medical-surgical nursing: Clinical management for continuity of care* (5th ed.). Philadelphia: W. B. Saunders. p. 762.

23. 3

RATIONALE: Nursing interventions should be spaced out over the shift to minimize the risk of a sustained rise in ICP. If possible, activities known to raise the ICP should be avoided where possible. Other interventions to control the ICP include maintaining a calm, quiet environment, and avoiding emotional stress and interruption of sleep.
TEST-TAKING STRATEGY: This question tests the concept that stimulation raises the ICP. If you know this, you will be able to eliminate each of the incorrect options as you read them. Review nursing care to the client with increased intracranial pressure now if you had difficulty with this question.
LEVEL OF COGNITIVE ABILITY: Application
PHASE OF NURSING PROCESS: Implementation
CLIENT NEEDS: Physiological Integrity
CONTENT AREA: Adult Health/Neurological
REFERENCE
Monahan, F., & Neighbors, M. (1998). *Medical-surgical nursing: Foundations for clinical practice* (2nd ed.). Philadelphia: W. B. Saunders. p. 730.

24. 2

RATIONALE: Leakage of CSF from the ears or nose may accompany basilar skull fracture. It can be distinguished from other body fluids because the drainage will separate into bloody and yellow concentric rings on dressing material, called Halo's sign. It also tests positive for glucose.
TEST-TAKING STRATEGY: The key to answering this question lies in knowing that CSF contains glucose, while other secretions, such as mucus, do not. Knowing that CSF separates into rings will also help you with this particular question. Review testing for CSF fluid now if you had difficulty with this question.
LEVEL OF COGNITIVE ABILITY: Comprehension
PHASE OF NURSING PROCESS: Data Collection
CLIENT NEEDS: Physiological Integrity
CONTENT AREA: Adult Health/Neurological
REFERENCE
Monahan, F., & Neighbors, M. (1998). *Medical-surgical nursing: Foundations for clinical practice* (2nd ed.). Philadelphia: W. B. Saunders. p. 754.

25. 3

RATIONALE: There is a significant association between cervical spine injury and head injury. For this reason, the nurse leaves any form of spinal immobilization in place until lateral cervical spine x-rays rule out fracture or other damage.
TEST-TAKING STRATEGY: This question is rather straightforward. The reason for spinal immobilization is to protect the spine from movement, which could cause further damage if the cervical spine is injured. If x-ray results are negative, there is no reason to leave the collar in place. Take a few moments to review emergency care if this question was difficult. In this scenario, the results of the x-ray are the key to further intervention.
LEVEL OF COGNITIVE ABILITY: Application
PHASE OF NURSING PROCESS: Planning
CLIENT NEEDS: Physiological Integrity
CONTENT AREA: Adult Health/Neurological

REFERENCE
Black, J., & Matassarin-Jacobs, E. (1997). *Medical surgical nursing: Clinical management for continuity of care* (5th ed.). Philadelphia: W. B. Saunders. pp. 824–825.

26. 4

RATIONALE: A concussion after head injury is a temporary loss of consciousness (from a few seconds to a few minutes) without evidence of structural damage. After concussion, the family is taught to monitor the client and to call the physician or return the client to the emergency department for signs and symptoms, including confusion, difficulty awakening or speaking, one-sided weakness, vomiting, or severe headache. Minor headache is expected.
TEST-TAKING STRATEGY: To answer this question, you need to be familiar with neurological signs and symptoms of increased intracranial pressure (ICP). Vomiting and neurologic deficits (in this case, speaking), indicate increased intracranial pressure. Decreasing LOC (difficulty arousing) is an early sign of increasing ICP. For these reasons, eliminate each of these options and choose the minor headache, which is expected.
LEVEL OF COGNITIVE ABILITY: Comprehension
PHASE OF NURSING PROCESS: Evaluation
CLIENT NEEDS: Health Promotion and Maintenance
CONTENT AREA: Adult Health/Neurological
REFERENCE
Monahan, F., & Neighbors, M. (1998). *Medical-surgical nursing: Foundations for clinical practice* (2nd ed.). Philadelphia: W. B. Saunders. p. 730.

27. 3

RATIONALE: Following supratentorial surgery, the head is kept at a 30- to 45-degree angle. The head and neck should not be angled either anteriorly or laterally, but rather should be kept in a neutral (midline) position. This will promote venous return through the jugular veins, which will help prevent a rise in intracranial pressure.
TEST-TAKING STRATEGY: This question tests knowledge of differences in positioning the craniotomy client with an infratentorial versus supratentorial incision. If you know that with supra- "keep the head up," and with infra- "keep the head down," you can eliminate options 1 and 2. Knowing how to position the head for optimal venous drainage helps you to select option 3 over option 4. Review client positioning following craniotomy now if you had difficulty with this question.
LEVEL OF COGNITIVE ABILITY: Application
PHASE OF NURSING PROCESS: Implementation
CLIENT NEEDS: Physiological Integrity
CONTENT AREA: Adult Health/Neurological
REFERENCE
Black, J., & Matassarin-Jacobs, E. (1997). *Medical-surgical nursing: Clinical management for continuity of care* (5th ed.). Philadelphia: W. B. Saunders. p. 853.

28. 4

RATIONALE: Codeine is the narcotic analgesic of choice for clients after craniotomy. It is often combined with a nonnarcotic analgesic such as acetaminophen for added effect. It does not alter the respiratory rate or mask neurological signs as other narcotics do. Side effects of codeine include gastrointestinal upset and constipation. The drug can lead to physical and psychological dependence with chronic use.

TEST-TAKING STRATEGY: This question tests your knowledge of codeine as a narcotic analgesic. General knowledge about narcotic analgesics as a class helps you to eliminate options 2 and 3. Since codeine is not the strongest narcotic available, you eliminate option 1 next. This leaves the correct option, which is codeine's advantage of not masking neurological signs.
LEVEL OF COGNITIVE ABILITY: Comprehension
PHASE OF NURSING PROCESS: Implementation
CLIENT NEEDS: Physiological Integrity
CONTENT AREA: Pharmacology
REFERENCE
Black, J., & Matassarin-Jacobs, E. (1997). *Medical-surgical nursing: Clinical management for continuity of care* (5th ed.). Philadelphia: W. B. Saunders. p. 855.

29. **3**

RATIONALE: Seizures are a potential complication that can occur for up to 1 year after surgery. For this reason, the client must diligently take anticonvulsant medications. The client and family are encouraged to keep track of doses administered. The family should learn seizure precautions, and accompany the client while ambulating if dizziness or seizures tend to occur. The suture line is kept dry until sutures are removed to prevent infection. The postcraniotomy client is typically sensitive to loud noises, and can find them irritating (loud television). Awareness control of environmental noise by others is helpful to this client.
TEST-TAKING STRATEGY: Begin to answer this question by eliminating option 1 first, since it is a general teaching point appropriate after many types of surgery. If you know that seizures are a potential postoperative risk up to a year after surgery, this eliminates options 2 and 4 as well. This leaves option 3 as the correct answer. Many clients after craniotomy have sensitivity to or are irritated by loud noises.
LEVEL OF COGNITIVE ABILITY: Application
PHASE OF NURSING PROCESS: Planning
CLIENT NEEDS: Health Promotion and Maintenance
CONTENT AREA: Adult Health/Neurological
REFERENCE
Monahan, F., & Neighbors, M. (1998). *Medical-surgical nursing: Foundations for clinical practice* (2nd ed.). Philadelphia: W. B. Saunders. p. 758.

30. **4**

RATIONALE: After craniotomy, clients may experience difficulty with altered personal appearance. The nurse can help by listening to client concerns, and by clarifying any misconceptions about facial edema, periorbital bruising, and hair loss (which are temporary). The nurse can encourage the client to participate in self-grooming and use personal articles of clothing. Finally, the nurse can suggest the use of a turban, followed by a hairpiece, to help the client adapt to the temporary change in appearance.
TEST-TAKING STRATEGY: The wording of this question makes you look for an incorrect statement or a maladaptive response. Options 1 and 2 both indicate adaptive responses, and are therefore eliminated. Knowing that facial edema and bruising are temporary helps you to choose option 4 over option 3.
LEVEL OF COGNITIVE ABILITY: Comprehension
PHASE OF NURSING PROCESS: Evaluation
CLIENT NEEDS: Psychosocial Integrity
CONTENT AREA: Adult Health/Neurological

REFERENCE
Monahan, F., & Neighbors, M. (1998). *Medical-surgical nursing: Foundations for clinical practice* (2nd ed.). Philadelphia: W. B. Saunders. p. 758.

31. **4**

RATIONALE: Crutchfield tongs are applied after drilling holes in the client's skull under local anesthesia. Weights are attached to the tongs, which exert pulling pressure on the longitudinal axis of the cervical spine. Serial x-rays of the cervical spine are taken, with weights being gradually added until x-ray reveals that the vertebral column is realigned. After that, weights may be gradually reduced to a point that maintains alignment. The client with Crutchfield tongs is placed on a Stryker frame or Roto-Rest bed. The nurse ensures that weights hang freely, and the amount of weight matches the current order. The nurse also inspects the integrity and position of the ropes and pulleys. The nurse does not remove the weights to administer care.
TEST-TAKING STRATEGY: The question asks for an action that is to be avoided, so the correct answer is an item that would be contraindicated. Knowing the basics of traction is sufficient to answer this question. Since options 2 and 3 are correct, and option 4 is not, then option 4 must be the answer to the question as stated. Review nursing care related to the client with cervical tongs now if you had difficulty with this question.
LEVEL OF COGNITIVE ABILITY: Application
PHASE OF NURSING PROCESS: Planning
CLIENT NEEDS: Physiological Integrity
CONTENT AREA: Adult Health/Neurological
REFERENCE
Monahan, F., & Neighbors, M. (1998). *Medical-surgical nursing: Foundations for clinical practice* (2nd ed.). Philadelphia: W. B. Saunders. p. 861.

32. **2**

RATIONALE: Adjusting to paralysis is difficult both physically and psychosocially for the client and family. The nurse recognizes that the client goes through the grieving process in adjusting to the loss, and may move back and forth among the stages of grief. The nurse acknowledges the client's feelings while continuing to meet the client's physical needs and encouraging independence.
TEST-TAKING STRATEGY: This question can be answered easily by examining the impact or outcome of each of the options. The nurse cannot leave the client alone until the client is ready (option 3), so this can be eliminated first. The family is also in crisis and needs the nurse's support (option 4), and should not be relied upon for care. Option 1 represents a factual, but noncaring approach to the client, which is also not therapeutic. This leaves option 2 as the best choice of the available responses. Also, option 2 acknowledges the client's feelings.
LEVEL OF COGNITIVE ABILITY: Application
PHASE OF NURSING PROCESS: Implementation
CLIENT NEEDS: Psychosocial Integrity
CONTENT AREA: Adult Health/Neurological
REFERENCE
Black, J., & Matassarin-Jacobs, E. (1997). *Medical-surgical nursing: Clinical management for continuity of care* (5th ed.). Philadelphia: W. B. Saunders. p. 910.

33. **4**

RATIONALE: The halo device alters balance and can cause fatigue due to its weight. The client should cleanse the skin daily under the vest to protect the skin from ulceration, and use powder or lotions sparingly or not at all. The wool liner should be changed if odor becomes a problem. The client should have food cut into small pieces to facilitate chewing and use straws for drinking. Pin care is done as instructed. The client may not drive because the device impairs the range of vision.

TEST-TAKING STRATEGY: To answer this question successfully, it is necessary to know that a halo brace or vest is used to allow mobility for the client who needs continuous cervical traction. It maintains the head and spine in a neutral position. With this in mind, it may be fairly easy to choose option 4 as the correct answer to the question as stated. The inability to turn the head without turning the torso makes driving contraindicated. Review client education points related to a halo vest now if you had difficulty with this question.

LEVEL OF COGNITIVE ABILITY: Comprehension
PHASE OF NURSING PROCESS: Evaluation
CLIENT NEEDS: Health Promotion and Maintenance
CONTENT AREA: Adult Health/Neurological
REFERENCE
Monahan, F., & Neighbors, M. (1998). *Medical-surgical nursing: Foundations for clinical practice* (2nd ed.). Philadelphia: W. B. Saunders. p. 824.

34. 1

RATIONALE: Depression is frequently seen in the client with spinal cord injury, and may be exhibited as a loss of appetite. The client should be allowed to choose the types of food eaten, and when they are eaten as much as is feasible, since it is one of the few areas of control that the client has left.

TEST-TAKING STRATEGY: The nurse does not make the diagnosis of clinical depression, which makes option 2 an unreasonable choice. For the same reason, the option related to compulsive habits should be eliminated. There is no evidence in the question to demonstrate that the client has a slow metabolic rate, so this is eliminated next. The option that is left is the correct choice, that is, leaving the client as much control as possible.

LEVEL OF COGNITIVE ABILITY: Comprehension
PHASE OF NURSING PROCESS: Data Collection
CLIENT NEEDS: Psychosocial Integrity
CONTENT AREA: Adult Health/Neurological
REFERENCE
Black, J., & Matassarin-Jacobs, E. (1997). *Medical-surgical nursing: Clinical management for continuity of care* (5th ed.). Philadelphia: W. B. Saunders. p. 898.

35. 3

RATIONALE: Range of motion exercises are beneficial in stretching muscles, which may diminish spasticity. Removing potentially harmful objects is a good safety measure. Use of muscle relaxants is also indicated if the spasms cause discomfort to the client or pose a risk to the client's safety. Use of limb restraints will not alleviate spasticity and could harm the client.

TEST-TAKING STRATEGY: The wording of the question guides you to look for a response that is potentially harmful to the client. Each of the incorrect options can be eliminated systematically, if you evaluate the options by looking for those interventions that would pose a risk to the client. Restraints should be avoided.

LEVEL OF COGNITIVE ABILITY: Application
PHASE OF NURSING PROCESS: Planning

CLIENT NEEDS: Safe, Effective Care Environment
CONTENT AREA: Adult Health/Neurological
REFERENCE
Black, J., & Matassarin-Jacobs, E. (1997). *Medical-surgical nursing: Clinical management for continuity of care* (5th ed.). Philadelphia: W. B. Saunders. pp. 900–901.

36. 2

RATIONALE: To prevent pressure ulcers from developing, the paraplegic client should shift weight in the wheelchair every 2 hours, and use a pressure relief pad. While in bed, the bottom sheet should be free of wrinkles and wetness. The client should use a mirror to inspect the skin twice a day (morning and evening) to assess for redness, edema, and breakdown. General additional measures include a nutritious diet and meticulous skin care.

TEST-TAKING STRATEGY: This question asks for the "least helpful" measure. Each of the responses appears reasonable on first inspection. With a closer look, however, you will notice that the time frame for inspecting the skin is much too infrequent, making this the correct response to the question as stated. Prioritization is required to answer this question.

LEVEL OF COGNITIVE ABILITY: Application
PHASE OF NURSING PROCESS: Implementation
CLIENT NEEDS: Health Promotion and Maintenance
CONTENT AREA: Adult Health/Neurological
REFERENCE
deWit, S. (1998). *Essentials of medical-surgical nursing* (4th ed.). Philadelphia: W. B. Saunders. p. 266.

37. 3

RATIONALE: Range of motion to the finger joints prevents contractures, but does not actively strengthen muscle groups needed for self-mobilization with paraplegia. Other activities that are more effective include push-ups from a prone position, sit-ups from a sitting position, extending the arms while holding weights, and squeezing rubber balls or crumpling newspaper.

TEST-TAKING STRATEGY: This question can be answered by thinking about the energy expenditure of the muscle groups involved in the activities listed in each option. The one that will involve the least energy expenditure (and therefore the least amount of muscle development) is the range of motion exercises, which makes it the correct answer to this question as stated.

LEVEL OF COGNITIVE ABILITY: Comprehension
PHASE OF NURSING PROCESS: Evaluation
CLIENT NEEDS: Health Promotion and Maintenance
CONTENT AREA: Adult Health/Neurological
REFERENCE
Monahan, F., & Neighbors, M. (1998). *Medical-surgical nursing: Foundations for clinical practice* (2nd ed.). Philadelphia: W. B. Saunders. p. 739.

38. 1

RATIONALE: The client with spinal cord injury is at risk for autonomic dysreflexia with an injury above the level of T7. It is characterized by severe, throbbing headache, flushing of the face and neck, bradycardia, and sudden severe hypertension. Other signs include nasal stuffiness, blurred vision, nausea, and sweating. It is a life-threatening syndrome triggered by a noxious stimulus below the level of the injury.

TEST-TAKING STRATEGY: To answer this question correctly, it is necessary to know what causes autonomic dysreflexia. It results from the sudden exaggerated response of the sympathetic nervous system to a noxious stimulus. A massive sympathetic nervous system response causes severe hypertension. This would account for the throbbing headache (the correct answer), and cause flushing of the face and neck. Baroreceptors sense the sudden hypertension, causing a reflex bradycardia. The pulse and BP changes with autonomic dysreflexia are actually the opposite of what would occur with hypovolemic shock. Review the signs of autonomic dysreflexia now if you had difficulty with this question.
LEVEL OF COGNITIVE ABILITY: Comprehension
PHASE OF NURSING PROCESS: Data Collection
CLIENT NEEDS: Physiological Integrity
CONTENT AREA: Adult Health/Neurological
REFERENCE
Black, J., & Matassarin-Jacobs, E. (1997). *Medical-surgical nursing: Clinical management for continuity of care* (5th ed.). Philadelphia: W.B. Saunders. pp. 894–895.

39. **4**

RATIONALE: The client with spinal cord injury is at risk for autonomic dysreflexia with an injury above the level of T7. It is characterized by severe, throbbing headache, flushing of the face and neck, bradycardia, and sudden severe hypertension. Other signs include nasal stuffiness, blurred vision, nausea, and sweating. It is a life-threatening syndrome triggered by a noxious stimulus below the level of the injury.
TEST-TAKING STRATEGY: Begin to answer this question by eliminating options 1 and 3. The client in spinal shock is hypotensive (not hypertensive), and the client's clinical picture does not match pulmonary embolism. (It may be useful to know also that autonomic dysreflexia does not occur until spinal shock resolves.) The word "hypertension" may have caught your eye in option 2, but knowing that malignant hypertension occurs with anesthesia causes you to eliminate this option as well.
LEVEL OF COGNITIVE ABILITY: Comprehension
PHASE OF NURSING PROCESS: Data Collection
CLIENT NEEDS: Physiological Integrity
CONTENT AREA: Adult Health/Neurological
REFERENCE
Black, J., & Matassarin-Jacobs, E. (1997). *Medical-surgical nursing: Clinical management for continuity of care* (5th ed.). Philadelphia: W. B. Saunders. pp. 894–895.

40. **2**

RATIONALE: The most frequent cause of autonomic dysreflexia is a distended bladder. Straight catheterization should be done every 4 to 6 hours, and Foley catheters should be checked frequently to prevent kinks in the tubing. Constipation and fecal impaction are other causes, so maintaining bowel regularity is important. Other causes include stimulation of the skin from tactile, thermal, or painful stimuli. The nurse administers care to minimize risk in these areas.
TEST-TAKING STRATEGY: The easiest way to answer questions of this nature is to remember that autonomic dysreflexia is caused by noxious stimuli to the bowel, bladder, or skin. With this in mind, you can easily eliminate each of the incorrect options for this question. Review the measures to minimize the risk of autonomic dysreflexia now if you had difficulty with this question.

LEVEL OF COGNITIVE ABILITY: Application
PHASE OF NURSING PROCESS: Implementation
CLIENT NEEDS: Physiological Integrity
CONTENT AREA: Adult Health/Neurological
REFERENCE
Monahan, F., & Neighbors, M. (1998). *Medical-surgical nursing: Foundations for clinical practice* (2nd ed.). Philadelphia: W. B. Saunders. p. 823.

41. **4**

RATIONALE: Key nursing actions are to sit the client up in bed, remove the noxious stimulus, and bring the blood pressure under control with antihypertensive medication per protocol. The nurse can also clearly label the client's chart identifying the risk for autonomic dysreflexia. Client and family should be taught to recognize, and later manage, the signs and symptoms of this syndrome.
TEST-TAKING STRATEGY: Note the word "immediately" in the stem. This is a clue that the first item in each option must be the first action. If you know to raise the head of the client's bed first (to try to minimize cerebral hypertension), then this eliminates each of the incorrect responses. Review immediate nursing interventions for the client experiencing autonomic dysreflexia if you had difficulty with this question.
LEVEL OF COGNITIVE ABILITY: Application
PHASE OF NURSING PROCESS: Implementation
CLIENT NEEDS: Physiological Integrity
CONTENT AREA: Adult Health/Neurological
REFERENCE
Monahan, F., & Neighbors, M. (1998). *Medical-surgical nursing: Foundations for clinical practice* (2nd ed.). Philadelphia: W. B. Saunders. p. 825.

42. **3**

RATIONALE: Reflex vasodilatation below the level of spinal cord injury places the client at risk of orthostatic hypotension, which may be profound. Measures to minimize this include measuring vital signs before and during position changes, use of a tilt table in early mobilization, and changing the client's position slowly. Venous pooling can be reduced by using TEDS or pneumatic boots. Vasopressor medications are used per protocol.
TEST-TAKING STRATEGY: Reflex vasodilatation below the level of the injury causes hypotension. The question asks which is the least helpful in minimizing the hypotensive effect. Venous compression (option 4) is helpful, and so is eliminated as the correct answer. Options 1 and 2 are helpful, and are eliminated next. Knowing that quick position changes and movement aggravate hypotension helps you be sure that you have selected the correct option.
LEVEL OF COGNITIVE ABILITY: Application
PHASE OF NURSING PROCESS: Planning
CLIENT NEEDS: Physiological Integrity
CONTENT AREA: Adult Health/Neurological
REFERENCE
Monahan, F., & Neighbors, M. (1998). *Medical-surgical nursing: Foundations for clinical practice* (2nd ed.). Philadelphia: W. B. Saunders. p. 824.

43. **2**

RATIONALE: Ptosis of the eyelid is due to pressure on and dysfunction of cranial nerve III. Once this occurs, this is ongoing and does not relate to LOC. Early changes in LOC relate to alertness and verbal responsiveness. Less frequent speech, slight slurring of speech, and mild drowsiness are early signs of decreasing LOC.

TEST-TAKING STRATEGY: The question asks for which assessment is not an early sign of LOC deterioration. Thus, the answer is either a later sign or one that is unrelated. If you know that LOC includes orientation, awareness, and verbal responsiveness, then you would eliminate each of the incorrect options systematically. Review the early signs of decreasing LOC now if you had difficulty with this question.

LEVEL OF COGNITIVE ABILITY: Comprehension
PHASE OF NURSING PROCESS: Data Collection
CLIENT NEEDS: Physiological Integrity
CONTENT AREA: Adult Health/Neurological
REFERENCE
Monahan, F., & Neighbors, M. (1998). *Medical-surgical nursing: Foundations for clinical practice* (2nd ed.). Philadelphia: W. B. Saunders. p. 815.

44. 3

RATIONALE: Aneurysm precautions include placing the client on bed rest in a quiet setting. Lights are kept dim to minimize environmental stimulation. Any activity that increases BP or impedes venous return from the brain is prohibited, such as pushing, pulling, sneezing, coughing, or straining. The nurse provides all physical care to minimize increases in BP. For the same reason, visitors, radio, television, and reading materials are prohibited or limited. Stimulants such as caffeine and nicotine are prohibited; decaffeinated coffee or tea may be used.

TEST-TAKING STRATEGY: To answer this question you must understand that a global principle in aneurysm precautions is to limit the amount of stimulation (in any form) that the client receives, and to prevent increased intracranial pressure (ICP). Options 1 and 2 are effective in promoting venous drainage from the brain (to keep ICP down), and are part of the precautions. Option 4 limits the amount of stimulation and exertion by the client, and is also part of the precautions. Nicotine must be completely eliminated, which makes this the answer to the question. Review aneurysm precautions now if you had difficulty with this question.

LEVEL OF COGNITIVE ABILITY: Application
PHASE OF NURSING PROCESS: Planning
CLIENT NEEDS: Physiological Integrity
CONTENT AREA: Adult Health/Neurological
REFERENCE
Monahan, F., & Neighbors, M. (1998). *Medical-surgical nursing: Foundations for clinical practice* (2nd ed.). Philadelphia: W. B. Saunders. p. 372.

45. 2

RATIONALE: Typically, seizure assessment includes the time the seizure began, part(s) of the body affected, the type of movements and progression of the seizure, changes in pupil size, eye deviation or nystagmus, client condition during the seizure, and postictal status.

TEST-TAKING STRATEGY: The response about the client's intake prior to the seizure suggests worry about vomiting and subsequent aspiration. The nurse is concerned about aspiration, not from vomiting, but from inhalation of the client's own saliva. Since all other options are standard assessments, this is the answer to the question. Review nursing assessment during a seizure, if you had difficulty answering this question.

LEVEL OF COGNITIVE ABILITY: Application

PHASE OF NURSING PROCESS: Data Collection
CLIENT NEEDS: Physiological Integrity
CONTENT AREA: Adult Health/Neurological
REFERENCE
Monahan, F., & Neighbors, M. (1998). *Medical-surgical nursing: Foundations for clinical practice* (2nd ed.). Philadelphia: W. B. Saunders. p. 799.

46. 3

RATIONALE: Seizure precautions may vary somewhat from agency to agency, but they generally have some commonalities. Usually an airway, oxygen, and suctioning equipment are kept available at the bedside. The side rails of the bed are padded, and the bed is kept in the lowest position. The client has an IV in place to have a readily accessible route if anticonvulsant medications must be administered. The use of padded tongue blades is highly controversial, and they should not be kept at the bedside. Forcing a tongue blade into the mouth during a seizure will more likely harm the client who bites down during seizure activity. Risks include blocking the airway from improper placement, chipping the client's teeth, and subsequent risk of aspirating tooth fragments. If the client has an aura before the seizure, it may give the nurse enough time to place an oral airway before seizure activity begins.

TEST-TAKING STRATEGY: This question must be evaluated from the perspective of causing possible harm. No harm can come to the client from any of the options except for the tongue blade. Review seizure precautions now if you had difficulty with this question.

LEVEL OF COGNITIVE ABILITY: Application
PHASE OF NURSING PROCESS: Planning
CLIENT NEEDS: Safe, Effective Care Environment
CONTENT AREA: Adult Health/Neurological
REFERENCE
Monahan, F., & Neighbors, M. (1998). *Medical-surgical nursing: Foundations for clinical practice* (2nd ed.). Philadelphia: W. B. Saunders. p. 798.

47. 3

RATIONALE: Nursing actions during a seizure include providing for privacy, loosening restrictive clothing, removing the pillow and raising the side rails in bed, and placing the client on one side with the head flexed forward, if possible, to allow the tongue to fall forward and facilitate drainage. The limbs are never restrained, because the strong muscle contractions could cause the client harm. If the client is not in bed when seizure activity begins, the nurse lowers the client to the floor if possible, protects the head with a pad against injury, and moves furniture that may injure the client. Other aspects of care are as described for the client who is in bed.

TEST-TAKING STRATEGY: This question must be evaluated from the perspective of causing possible harm. No harm can come to the client from any of the options except for restraining the limbs. Avoid restraints. Review care to a client during a seizure now if you had difficulty with this question.

LEVEL OF COGNITIVE ABILITY: Application
PHASE OF NURSING PROCESS: Implementation
CLIENT NEEDS: Physiological Integrity
CONTENT AREA: Adult Health/Neurological
REFERENCE
Monahan, F., & Neighbors, M. (1998). *Medical-surgical nursing: Foundations for clinical practice* (2nd ed.). Philadelphia: W. B. Saunders. pp. 798–799.

48. 3

RATIONALE: Typical anticonvulsant medication instructions include taking the dose daily to keep the blood level of the medication constant; having a serum drug level drawn before taking the morning dose; avoiding abruptly stopping the medication; avoiding alcohol; checking with the physician before taking OTC medications; avoiding activities where alertness and coordination are required until medication effects are known; providing good oral hygiene and getting regular dental care; and carrying a Medic-Alert bracelet or tag.

TEST-TAKING STRATEGY: Options 1 and 2 can be eliminated fairly easily after reading this question, since they are the least likely choices for being correct. Of the two remaining options, medications are not generally taken just prior to drawing therapeutic serum levels, because the results would be artificially high. This leaves oral hygiene as the correct option, due to the risk of gingival hyperplasia. Review client education related to phenytoin (Dilantin) now if you had difficulty with this question.

LEVEL OF COGNITIVE ABILITY: Comprehension
PHASE OF NURSING PROCESS: Evaluation
CLIENT NEEDS: Health Promotion and Maintenance
CONTENT AREA: Adult Health/Neurological
REFERENCE
Monahan, F., & Neighbors, M. (1998). *Medical-surgical nursing: Foundations for clinical practice* (2nd ed.). Philadelphia: W. B. Saunders. p. 796.

49. 2

RATIONALE: Hemiparesis is a weakness of the face, arm, and leg on one side. The client with one-sided hemiparesis benefits from having objects placed on the unaffected side and within reach. Other helpful activities with hemiparesis include ROM exercises to the affected side, and muscle-strengthening exercises to the unaffected side.

TEST-TAKING STRATEGY: Begin to answer this question by eliminating options 3 and 4 as potentially hazardous to the client. This question tests your ability to distinguish between hemiparesis and unilateral neglect. The client with hemiparesis has weakness on one side, and therefore objects should be place on the stronger side. With unilateral neglect, objects are placed on the affected side to train the client to attend to that part of the environment. Knowing this, pick option 2 over option 1. Review care to the client with hemiparesis now if you had difficulty with this question.

LEVEL OF COGNITIVE ABILITY: Application
PHASE OF NURSING PROCESS: Planning
CLIENT NEEDS: Safe, Effective Care Environment
CONTENT AREA: Adult Health/Neurological
REFERENCE
Monahan, F., & Neighbors, M. (1998). *Medical-surgical nursing: Foundations for clinical practice* (2nd ed.). Philadelphia: W. B. Saunders. p. 807.

50. 1

RATIONALE: Before the client with dysphagia is started on a diet, the gag and swallow reflexes must have returned. The client is assisted with meals as needed, and is given ample time to chew and swallow. Food is placed on the unaffected side of the mouth. Liquids are thickened to avoid aspiration.

TEST-TAKING STRATEGY: This question asks you to identify an incorrect item. Option 4 is generally a good action for all clients. Option 3 is correct because the client has better sensation and motion on the unaffected side of the mouth. This narrows your options to two opposing concepts, thin versus thick liquids. Thickened liquids are easier for the client with impaired facial motion and swallowing ability to manage. Knowing this enables you to choose option 1 as the action to avoid. Review care to the client with residual dysphagia now if you had difficulty with this question.

LEVEL OF COGNITIVE ABILITY: Application
PHASE OF NURSING PROCESS: Implementation
CLIENT NEEDS: Physiological Integrity
CONTENT AREA: Adult Health/Neurological
REFERENCE
Black, J., & Matassarin-Jacobs, E. (1997). *Medical-surgical nursing: Clinical management for continuity of care* (5th ed.). Philadelphia: W. B. Saunders. p. 796.

51. 3

RATIONALE: Homonymous hemianopia is loss of one half of the visual field. The client with homonymous hemianopia should have objects placed in the intact field of vision, and the nurse should also approach the client from the intact side. The nurse instructs the client to scan the environment to overcome the visual deficit, and does client teaching from within the intact field of vision. The nurse encourages the use of personal eyeglasses, if they are available.

TEST-TAKING STRATEGY: To answer this question accurately, you must be able to distinguish between homonymous hemianopia and unilateral neglect. Clients are approached differently with these two deficits. The similarity is that the client must be taught to scan the environment, which is also the answer to this question. Review the concept of homonymous hemianopia if you are unfamiliar with it.

LEVEL OF COGNITIVE ABILITY: Comprehension
PHASE OF NURSING PROCESS: Evaluation
CLIENT NEEDS: Health Promotion and Maintenance
CONTENT AREA: Adult Health/Neurological
REFERENCE
Monahan, F., & Neighbors, M. (1998). *Medical-surgical nursing: Foundations for clinical practice* (2nd ed.). Philadelphia: W. B. Saunders. p. 1940.

52. 2

RATIONALE: Clients with aphasia after CVA often fatigue easily and have a short attention span. General guidelines when trying to communicate with the aphasic client include speaking more slowly and allowing adequate response time, listening to and watching attempts to communicate, and trying to put the client at ease with a caring and understanding manner. Avoid shouting (the client is not deaf), appearing rushed for a response, and letting family members give all the responses for the client.

TEST-TAKING STRATEGY: This question tests a fundamental concept in communicating with the aphasic client. If this question was difficult, take a few moments now to review these communication strategies.

LEVEL OF COGNITIVE ABILITY: Application
PHASE OF NURSING PROCESS: Implementation
CLIENT NEEDS: Psychosocial Integrity
CONTENT AREA: Adult Health/Neurological
REFERENCE
Black, J., & Matassarin-Jacobs, E. (1997). *Medical-surgical nursing: Clinical management for continuity of care* (5th ed.). Philadelphia: W. B. Saunders. p. 805.

53. 3

RATIONALE: Placing an eyepatch over one eye in the client with diplopia removes the second image and restores more normal vision. The patch is alternated on a daily basis to maintain the strength of the extraocular muscles of the eyes.

TEST-TAKING STRATEGY: Knowing that an eyepatch will help diplopia only while it is worn, you can first eliminate options 1 and 2 as not helpful. If you know that the extraocular muscles weaken with eyepatch use, select option 3 over 4, because these are small muscles that would lose strength fairly rapidly.

LEVEL OF COGNITIVE ABILITY: Comprehension
PHASE OF NURSING PROCESS: Evaluation
CLIENT NEEDS: Physiological Integrity
CONTENT AREA: Adult Health/Neurological
REFERENCE

Black, J., & Matassarin-Jacobs, E. (1997). *Medical-surgical nursing: Clinical management for continuity of care* (5th ed.). Philadelphia: W. B. Saunders. p. 803.

54. 3

RATIONALE: Myasthenia gravis can often be diagnosed based on clinical signs and symptoms. The diagnosis can be confirmed by injecting the client with a dose of Tensilon. This drug inhibits the breakdown of an enzyme in the neuromuscular junction, so more acetylcholine binds onto receptors. If the muscle is strengthened for 3 to 5 minutes after this injection, it confirms a diagnosis of myasthenia gravis. Another drug, neostigmine may also be used because the effect last for 1 to 2 hours, giving a better analysis. For either drug, atropine should be available as the antidote.

TEST-TAKING STRATEGY: Knowledge of the purpose and expected findings of the Tensilon test is required to answer this question. If this is unfamiliar, take time now to review. You are likely to see questions related to the Tensilon test.

LEVEL OF COGNITIVE ABILITY: Comprehension
PHASE OF NURSING PROCESS: Data Collection
CLIENT NEEDS: Physiological Integrity
CONTENT AREA: Pharmacology
REFERENCE

Black, J., & Matassarin-Jacobs, E. (1997). *Medical-surgical nursing: Clinical management for continuity of care* (5th ed.). Philadelphia: W. B. Saunders. pp. 884–885.

55. 2

RATIONALE: The client has speech that is nasal in tone and dysarthritic due to cranial nerve involvement of the muscles governing speech. The nurse listens attentively and verbally, verifies what the client has said, asks questions requiring a yes or no response, and develops alternative communication methods (letter board, picture board, pen and paper, flash cards). Encouraging the client to speak quickly is unsuccessful and counterproductive.

TEST-TAKING STRATEGY: There are some techniques that are useful in communicating with clients with speech impairment, regardless of the specific cause of the difficulty. Options 3 and 4 are classic examples of alternative communication methods that are useful, so you would eliminate them items to avoid. Since option 1 is also helpful, this leaves option 2 as the correct answer to the question as stated. Speaking quickly is difficult for a client with a speech impairment.

LEVEL OF COGNITIVE ABILITY: Application

PHASE OF NURSING PROCESS: Planning
CLIENT NEEDS: Psychosocial Integrity
CONTENT AREA: Adult Health/Neurological
REFERENCE

Monahan, F., & Neighbors, M. (1998). *Medical-surgical nursing: Foundations for clinical practice* (2nd ed.). Philadelphia: W. B. Saunders. p. 782.

56. 3

RATIONALE: Myasthenic crisis is often caused by undermedication, and responds to administration of cholinergic medications such as neostigmine and pyridostigmine. Cholinergic crisis (the opposite problem) is caused by excess medication and responds to withholding of medications. Too little exercise and fatty food intake are incorrect. Overexertion and overeating could possibly trigger myasthenic crisis.

TEST-TAKING STRATEGY: To answer this question most easily, it is necessary to know that undermedication is a common cause of myasthenic crisis. Take a few moments to review the causes if you are unfamiliar with them.

LEVEL OF COGNITIVE ABILITY: Comprehension
PHASE OF NURSING PROCESS: Data Collection
CLIENT NEEDS: Physiological Integrity
CONTENT AREA: Adult Health/Neurological
REFERENCE

Black, J., & Matassarin-Jacobs, E. (1997). *Medical-surgical nursing: Clinical management for continuity of care* (5th ed.). Philadelphia: W. B. Saunders. p. 885.

57. 2

RATIONALE: Clients with myasthenia gravis are taught to space out activities over the day to conserve energy and restore muscle strength. It is very important to take medications correctly to maintain blood levels that are not too low or too high. Muscle-strengthening exercises are not helpful and can fatigue the client. Overeating is a cause of exacerbation of symptoms, as well as exposure to heat, crowds, erratic sleep habits, and emotional stress.

TEST-TAKING STRATEGY: If you know that common causes of myasthenic and cholinergic crises are undermedication and overmedication, respectively, you should be able to easily eliminate each of the incorrect options to this question. No other option prevents both of those complications. It is extremely important that these clients take medications on time to maintain therapeutic blood levels. Review measures to prevent myasthenic and cholinergic crises now if you are unfamiliar with them.

LEVEL OF COGNITIVE ABILITY: Application
PHASE OF NURSING PROCESS: Implementation
CLIENT NEEDS: Health Promotion and Maintenance
CONTENT AREA: Adult Health/Neurological
REFERENCE

Monahan, F., & Neighbors, M. (1998). *Medical-surgical nursing: Foundations for clinical practice* (2nd ed.). Philadelphia: W. B. Saunders. p. 782.

58. 3

RATIONALE: Most ongoing treatment for myasthenia gravis in done in outpatient settings, and the client needs to be aware of the lifestyle changes needed to maintain independence. Taking medications an hour before mealtime gives greater muscle strength for chewing, and is indicated. The client should have portable suction equipment and a portable resuscitation bag available in case of respiratory distress. The client should carry medical identification about the condition. The client should avoid activities that could worsen the symptoms, including stress, infection, heat, surgery, or alcohol.

TEST-TAKING STRATEGY: Options 2 and 4 are very reasonable courses of action, and so they are eliminated as possible answers to this question as stated. To discriminate between the remaining two options, you would need to know that premedication an hour before meals gives strength to the muscles (for chewing and swallowing), and that heat and infection (crowds at the beach) trigger myasthenic crisis. Review client education points with myasthenia gravis.

LEVEL OF COGNITIVE ABILITY: Comprehension
PHASE OF NURSING PROCESS: Evaluation
CLIENT NEEDS: Health Promotion and Maintenance
CONTENT AREA: Adult Health/Neurological
REFERENCE

Monahan, F., & Neighbors, M. (1998). *Medical-surgical nursing: Foundations for clinical practice* (2nd ed.). Philadelphia: W. B. Saunders. p. 784.

59. 3

RATIONALE: The client with Parkinson's disease tends to become withdrawn and depressed, and should become an active participant in own care to prevent this. There should be planned activities throughout the day to inhibit daytime sleeping and boredom. The nurse gives the client encouragement and praises the client for perseverance. Exercise helps prevent progression of the disease and self-care improves self-esteem.

TEST-TAKING STRATEGY: Options 1 and 4 are the least plausible of all available answers, and so they may be eliminated first. Option 2 is well intentioned, but is not therapeutic in helping the client to cope with the disease. Option 3 is the best choice.

LEVEL OF COGNITIVE ABILITY: Application
PHASE OF NURSING PROCESS: Planning
CLIENT NEEDS: Psychosocial Integrity
CONTENT AREA: Adult Health/Neurological
REFERENCE

Monahan, F., & Neighbors, M. (1998). *Medical-surgical nursing: Foundations for clinical practice* (2nd ed.). Philadelphia: W. B. Saunders. p. 788.

60. 1

RATIONALE: Parkinsonian crisis can occur with emotional trauma or sudden withdrawal of medications. The client exhibits severe tremors, rigidity, and bradykinesia. The client also displays anxiety, is diaphoretic, and has tachycardia and hyperpnea. The client should be placed in a quiet, dim room and respiratory, and cardiac support should be available.

TEST-TAKING STRATEGY: Option 4 is not indicated and is eliminated first. Option 3 is not an immediate concern and is also discarded. Of the remaining two, there is nothing about parkinsonian crisis that warrants placement of an NG tube. This leaves the correct option, which is to put the client in a dim, quiet room and provide for support of cardiac and respiratory symptoms. Review nursing care for parkinsonian crisis now if you had difficulty with this question.

LEVEL OF COGNITIVE ABILITY: Application
PHASE OF NURSING PROCESS: Implementation
CLIENT NEEDS: Physiological Integrity
CONTENT AREA: Adult Health/Neurological

REFERENCE

Black, J., & Matassarin-Jacobs, E. (1997). *Medical-surgical nursing: Clinical management for continuity of care* (5th ed.). Philadelphia: W. B. Saunders. p. 879.

61. 2

RATIONALE: The client with Parkinson's disease should exercise in the morning when energy levels are highest. The client should avoid sitting in soft, deep chairs, because they are difficult to get up from. The client can rock back and forth to initiate movement. The client should buy clothes with Velcro fasteners and slide locking buckles to support the ability to dress self.

TEST-TAKING STRATEGY: Option 1 is not useful to clients with fatigue from any disorder, so this option may be eliminated first. Knowing that the client with Parkinson's has difficulty with movement and dexterity helps you eliminate options 3 and 4 next. Thus you are left with the correct answer, which is avoiding sitting in deep, soft chairs. Review client teaching points with Parkinson's disease now if you had difficulty with this question.

LEVEL OF COGNITIVE ABILITY: Comprehension
PHASE OF NURSING PROCESS: Evaluation
CLIENT NEEDS: Health Promotion and Maintenance
CONTENT AREA: Adult Health/Neurological
REFERENCE

Black, J., & Matassarin-Jacobs, E. (1997). *Medical-surgical nursing: Clinical management for continuity of care* (5th ed.). Philadelphia: W. B. Saunders. p. 881.

62. 4

RATIONALE: Facial pain can be minimized by using cotton pads to wash the face, and using room temperature water. The client should chew on the unaffected side of the mouth, eat a soft diet, and take in foods and beverages at room temperature. If tooth brushing triggers pain, sometimes an oral rinse after meals is helpful instead.

TEST-TAKING STRATEGY: To answer this question most easily, you should know that the pain of trigeminal neuralgia is triggered by mechanical or thermal stimuli. This will help you eliminate each of the incorrect options systematically. Very hot or cold foods are likely to trigger the pain, not relieve it. Review client education points now if you had difficulty with this question.

LEVEL OF COGNITIVE ABILITY: Comprehension
PHASE OF NURSING PROCESS: Evaluation
CLIENT NEEDS: Health Promotion and Maintenance
CONTENT AREA: Adult Health/Neurological
REFERENCE

Monahan, F., & Neighbors, M. (1998). *Medical-surgical nursing: Foundations for clinical practice* (2nd ed.). Philadelphia: W. B. Saunders. p. 829.

63. 1

RATIONALE: Prevention of muscle atrophy with Bell's palsy is accomplished with the use of facial massage, facial exercises, and electrical stimulation of the nerves. Exposure to cold or drafts is avoided. Local application of heat to the face may improve blood flow and provide comfort.

TEST-TAKING STRATEGY: Evaluate each of the options with regard to their effect on preserving muscle tone in the face. Options 2, 3, and 4 are plausible choices. Option 1 is unrelated to muscle tone and is also contraindicated in clients with this condition. Because of this, option 1 is the answer to this question as stated.

LEVEL OF COGNITIVE ABILITY: Comprehension
PHASE OF NURSING PROCESS: Evaluation
CLIENT NEEDS: Health Promotion and Maintenance
CONTENT AREA: Adult Health/Neurological
REFERENCE
Monahan, F., & Neighbors, M. (1998). *Medical-surgical nursing: Foundations for clinical practice* (2nd ed.). Philadelphia: W. B. Saunders. p. 829.

64. **3**

RATIONALE: The client with Guillain-Barré syndrome is at risk for respiratory failure because of ascending paralysis. An intubation tray should be available for use. Another complication of this syndrome is cardiac dysrhythmias, which necessitates the use of ECG monitoring. Because the client is immobilized, the nurse should routinely assess for deep-vein thrombosis and pulmonary embolism.
TEST-TAKING STRATEGY: With an ascending paralysis, the client is at risk for involvement of respiratory muscles and subsequent respiratory failure. This knowledge makes you look for an option that coincides with this line of thought. Option 3 is the only option that includes an intubation tray, which would be needed if the client status deteriorated to needing intubation and mechanical ventilation. This option most directly addresses airway.
LEVEL OF COGNITIVE ABILITY: Application
PHASE OF NURSING PROCESS: Implementation

CLIENT NEEDS: Physiological Integrity
CONTENT AREA: Adult Health/Neurological
REFERENCE
Monahan, F., & Neighbors, M. (1998). *Medical-surgical nursing: Foundations for clinical practice* (2nd ed.). Philadelphia: W. B. Saunders. p. 773.

65. **2**

RATIONALE: The onset or exacerbation of MS is preceded by a number of different factors. These include emotional stress, fatigue, infection, physical injury, and pregnancy. There are no known methods of primary prevention. Intake of fruit and vegetables is an unrelated item.
TEST-TAKING STRATEGY: If you examine each of the options, all but the fruit and vegetables option involves physiological or psychological stress. Since this is the option that is different than the others, it is a likely choice for being the correct answer. Review the precipitating risk factors associated with MS now if you had difficulty with this question.
LEVEL OF COGNITIVE ABILITY: Application
PHASE OF NURSING PROCESS: Data Collection
CLIENT NEEDS: Physiological Integrity
CONTENT AREA: Adult Health/Neurological
REFERENCE
Black, J., & Matassarin-Jacobs, E. (1997). *Medical-surgical nursing: Clinical management for continuity of care* (5th ed.). Philadelphia: W. B. Saunders. p. 873.

BIBLIOGRAPHY

Black, J., & Matassarin-Jacobs, E. (1997). *Medical-surgical nursing: Clinical management for continuity of care* (5th ed.). Philadelphia: W. B. Saunders.

Chernecky, C., & Berger, B. (1997). *Laboratory tests and diagnostic procedures* (2nd ed.). Philadelphia: W. B. Saunders.

Deglin, J., & Vallerand, A. (1999). *Davis's drug guide for nurses* (6th ed.). Philadelphia: F. A. Davis.

deWit, S. (1998). *Essentials of medical-surgical nursing* (4th ed.). Philadelphia: W. B. Saunders.

Hodgson, B., & Kizior, R. (2000). *Saunders nursing drug handbook 2000*. Philadelphia: W. B. Saunders.

Ignatavicius, D., Workman, M., & Mishler, M. (1999). *Medical-surgical nursing across the health care continuum* (3rd ed.). Philadelphia: W. B. Saunders.

Jaffee, M., & McVan, B. (1997). *Davis's laboratory and diagnostic test handbook*. Philadelphia: F. A. Davis.

Lehne, R. (1998). *Pharmacology for nursing care* (3rd ed.). Philadelphia: W. B. Saunders.

Luckmann, J. (1997). *Saunders manual of nursing care*. Philadelphia: W. B. Saunders.

Monahan, F., & Neighbors, M. (1998). *Medical-surgical nursing: Foundations for clinical practice* (2nd ed.). Philadelphia: W. B. Saunders.

O'Toole, M. (1997). *Miller-Keane encyclopedia & dictionary of medicine, nursing, & allied health* (6th ed.). Philadelphia: W. B. Saunders.

CHAPTER 55

Neurological Medications

. . . .

I. Skeletal Muscle Relaxants

A. Description
  1. Acts directly on the neuromuscular junction or indirectly on the central nervous system (CNS)
  2. Centrally acting muscle relaxants depress neuron activity in the spinal cord or brain
  3. Peripherally acting muscle relaxants act directly on the skeletal muscles
  4. Used to prevent or relieve muscle spasms, to treat spasticity associated with spinal cord disease or lesions, for painful musculoskeletal conditions, and for chronic debilitating disorders, such as multiple sclerosis, cerebrovascular accident (CVA), or cerebral palsy
  5. Contraindicated in severe liver or renal disease and in severe heart disease
  6. Should not be taken with CNS depressants, such as barbiturates, narcotics, and alcohol; sedatives; hypnotics; or tricylic antidepressants
  7. Chronic high-dose therapy can cause physical dependence; withdrawal should be done slowly
B. Medications (Box 55–1)
C. Side effects and implementation: refer to chapter 57 for information regarding the side effects and implementation measures for the client taking a skeletal muscle relaxant

II. Antimyasthenic Medications

A. Description
  1. Relieve muscle weakness associated with myasthenia gravis by blocking acetylcholine breakdown at the neuromuscular junction
  2. Used to treat or diagnose myasthenia gravis or to distinguish cholinergic crisis from myasthenic crisis
  3. Neostigmine bromide (Prostigmin), pyridostigmine bromide (Mestinon),

ambenonium (Mytelase) are used to control myasthenic symptoms
  4. Edrophonium chloride (Tensilon) is used to diagnose myasthenia gravis and to distinguish cholinergic crisis from myasthenic crisis
B. Medications (Box 55–2)
C. Side effects: cholinergic crisis (Box 55–3)
D. Implementation
  1. Check neuromuscular status, including reflexes, muscle strength, and gait
  2. Monitor clients for signs and symptoms of medication overdose (cholinergic crisis) and underdose (myasthenic crisis)
  3. Instruct the client to take medications on time to prevent weakness, because weakness can impair the client's ability to breathe and swallow
  4. Instruct the client to take medication before meals for best absorption
  5. Instruct clients to wear a MedicAlert bracelet
  6. Note that antimyasthenic therapy is lifelong therapy
  7. Evaluate for medication effectiveness, which is based on the improvement of neuromuscular symptoms or strength without cholinergic signs and symptoms
  8. When edrophonium (Tensilon) is being

BOX 55–1. Skeletal Muscle Relaxants

Baclofen (Lioresal)
Carisoprodol (Soma)
Cyclobenzaprine hydrochloride (Flexeril)
Dantrolene (Dantrium)
Diazepam (Valium)
Methocarbamol (Robaxin)
Orphenadrine (Norflex)
Chlorzoxazone (Paraflex, Parafon Forte)
Chlorphenesin carbamate (Maolate)
Meprobamate (Equanil, Miltown)

BOX 55-2. Antimyasthenic Medications

Edrophonium chloride (Tensilon)
Neostigmine bromide (Prostigmin)
Pyridostigmine bromide (Mestinon)
Ambenonium (Mytelase)

administered, have emergency resuscitation equipment on hand and atropine available for cholinergic crisis

E. **Tensilon Test**
1. Tensilon is injected IV by the physician
2. The **Tensilon test** can cause ventricular fibrillation and cardiac arrest
3. Atropine is the antidote for overdose
4. To diagnose:
   a. If ptosis is immediately corrected after administration of the medication, the diagnosis is most likely myasthenia gravis
   b. Most myasthenic clients will show a marked improvement in muscle tone within 30 to 60 seconds after injection, and the muscle improvement lasts 4 to 5 minutes
5. To determine cholinergic crisis (overdose with anticholinesterase) or myasthenic crisis (undermedication):
   a. In cholinergic crisis, muscle tone does not improve after the administration of Tensilon, and muscle twitching may be noted around the eyes and face
   b. A Tensilon injection makes the client in cholinergic crisis temporarily worse (negative Tensilon test)
   c. A Tensilon injection temporarily improves the condition when the client is in myasthenic crisis (positive Tensilon test)

III. Antiparkinsonian Medications

A. Description
1. Stores the balance of the neurotransmitters acetylcholine and dopamine in the CNS, decreasing the signs and symptoms of Parkinson's disease
2. These medications include the dopaminergics,

which stimulate the dopamine receptors, and the anticholinergics, which block the cholinergic receptors
3. Used for drug-induced parkinsonism, in which neuroleptic agents block dopamine receptors in the CNS, leading to functional loss of dopamine activity
4. Used for Parkinson's disease, in which dopamine-containing neurons in the basal ganglia are destroyed or deficient, which causes loss of fine motor control
B. Dopaminergic medications
1. Description
   a. Stimulate the dopamine receptors
   b. Increase the amount of dopamine available in the CNS or enhance neurotransmission of dopamine
   c. Contraindicated in cardiac, renal, or mental health disorders
   d. Levodopa taken with monoamine oxidase inhibitor (MAOI) antidepressant can cause a hypertensive crisis
2. Medications (Box 55-4)
3. Side effects
   a. Dyskinesia
   b. Involuntary body movements
   c. Tachycardia
   d. Nausea and vomiting
   e. Urinary retention
   f. Constipation
   g. Dizziness
   h. Orthostatic hypotension
   i. Confusion
   j. Mood changes
   k. Hallucinations
4. Implementation
   a. Monitor vital signs
   b. Monitor for risk for injury
   c. Instruct the client to take medication with food if nausea and vomiting occur
   d. Monitor for signs and symptoms of parkinsonism, such as rigidity, tremors, akinesia, and bradykinesia; a stooped forward posture; shuffling gait; and masked facies
   e. Monitor for signs of dyskinesia
   f. Instruct clients on carbidopa-levodopa (Sinemet) to eat low-protein foods, because high-protein diets interfere with medication transport to the CNS
   g. Instruct the client to change positions slowly to minimize orthostatic hypotension

BOX 55-3. Signs of Cholinergic Crisis

GI disturbances
Nausea
Vomiting
Diarrhea
Abdominal cramps
Increased salivation and tearing
Miosis
Hypertension
Sweating
Increased bronchial secretion

BOX 55-4. Dopaminergic Medications

Amantadine (Symmetrel)
Bromocriptine (Parlodel)
Carbidopa
Levodopa; carbidopa (Sinemet)
Pergolide (Permax)
Selegiline hydrochloride (Eldepryl)

h. Instruct clients not to discontinue the medication abruptly
i. Instruct clients to report side effects and symptoms of dyskinesia
j. Instruct the client to avoid alcohol
k. Monitor clients for improvement in signs and symptoms of parkinsonism without the development of severe side effects from the medications
l. Inform the client that urine or perspiration may be discolored and that this is harmless, but it may stain clothing
m. Advise the diabetic client that glucose testing should not be done through urine testing because the results will not be reliable
n. When administering levodopa, instruct the client to avoid excessive vitamin B_6 intake to prevent medication reactions

IV. Anticholinergic-Blocking Medications

A. Description
1. Block the cholinergic receptors in the CNS, thereby suppressing acetylcholine activity
2. Reduce the rigidity and some of the tremors, but have a minimal effect on the bradykinesia
3. Contraindicated in clients with glaucoma
4. Clients with chronic obstructive lung diseases can develop dry, thick mucous secretions
B. Medications (Box 55–5)
C. Side effects
1. Blurred vision
2. Dry mouth, dry secretions
3. Increased pulse rate
4. Constipation
5. Urinary retention
6. Restlessness and confusion
7. Photophobia
D. Implementation
1. Obtain a medication history
2. Monitor vital signs
3. Monitor for risk of injury
4. Monitor for signs and symptoms of parkinsonism, such as rigidity, tremors, akinesia, and bradykinesia; a stooped forward posture; shuffling gait; and masked facies
5. Monitor client for improvement in signs and symptoms

BOX 55–5. Anticholinergic-Blocking Medications

Benztropine mesylate (Cogentin)
Trihexyphenidyl hydrochloride (Artane)
Biperiden hydrochloride (Akineton)
Ethopropazine hydrochloride (Parsidol)
Orphenadrine hydrochloride (Disipal)
Orphenadrine citrate (Banflex, Norflex)
Procyclidine hydrochloride (Kemadrin)

---

6. Assess client's bowel and urinary function and monitor for urinary retention and constipation
7. Monitor for involuntary movements
8. Encourage the client to avoid alcohol, smoking, caffeine, and aspirin to decrease gastric acidity
9. Instruct the client to consult with a physician before taking any nonprescription medications
10. Instruct clients to minimize dry mouth by increasing fluid intake and by using ice chips, hard candy, or gum
11. Instruct clients to prevent constipation by increasing fluid and fiber in the diet
12. Instruct the client to use sunglasses in direct sun because of possible photophobia
13. Instruct clients to have routine eye examinations to assess for intraocular pressure

V. Anticonvulsant Medications

A. Description
1. Used to depress abnormal neuronal discharges and prevent the spread of seizures
2. Use with caution in clients on anticoagulants, aspirin, sulfonamides, cimetidine (Tagamet), and antipsychotics
3. Absorption is decreased with the use of antacids, calcium preparations, and antineoplastic medications
B. Implementation for clients on anticonvulsants
1. Initiate seizure precautions
2. Monitor urinary output
3. Monitor liver and renal function tests
4. Monitor for signs of medication toxicity, which would include CNS depression, ataxia, nausea, vomiting, drowsiness, dizziness, restlessness, and visual disturbances
5. Instruct clients to take anticonvulsants with food to decrease GI irritation but to avoid milk and antacids, which impair the absorption of anticonvulsants
6. Instruct the client taking liquid medication to shake it well before ingesting
7. Instruct clients not to discontinue medication
8. Instruct clients not to consume alcohol
9. Instruct clients to use caution when driving or performing activities that require alertness
10. Instruct clients to wear a Medic-Alert bracelet
11. Encourage clients to follow up with periodic blood studies related to determining toxicity
12. Instruct the client to avoid over-the-counter medications
13. Instruct the diabetic client to monitor serum glucose levels closely
14. Inform clients that urine may be a harmless pink-red or red-brown color
15. Instruct clients to maintain good oral hygiene and to use a soft toothbrush

---

BOX 55–6. Hydantoins
Phenytoin (Dilantin) Mephenytoin (Mesantoin) Ethotoin (Peganone)

16. Instruct the client in the need for preventive dental check-ups
17. Instruct the client to report symptoms of sore throat, bruising, and nosebleeds, which may indicate a blood dyscrasia
18. Instruct clients to inform the physician if adverse reactions, such as gingivitis, nystagmus, slurred speech, rash, or dizziness occurs
19. If a seizure occurs, assess seizure activity including location and duration
20. Protect clients from hazards in the environment during a seizure

C. Hydantoins (Box 55–6)
1. Used to treat seizures
2. Phenytoin (Dilantin) is also used to treat dysrhythmias
3. Side effects
  a. Gingival hyperplasia
  b. Reddened gums that bleed easily
  c. Slurred speech
  d. Confusion
  e. Depression
  f. Nausea, vomiting, and constipation
  g. Headaches
  h. Blood dyscrasias
  i. Decreased platelet count
  j. Decreased white blood cell count
  k. Elevated blood glucose
  l. Alopecia
  m. Hirsutism
4. Implementation
  a. Oral tube feedings may interfere with the absorption of oral phenytoin (Dilantin) and diminish the medication's effectiveness; therefore, feedings should be scheduled as far as possible from the phenytoin (Dilantin) administration
  b. Monitor therapeutic serum levels to assess for toxicity
  c. Monitor for signs of toxicity
  d. When IV phenytoin is administered, it is diluted in normal saline because dextrose causes the medication to precipitate
  e. Instruct clients about the importance of

BOX 55–7. Barbiturates
Phenobarbital (Luminal) Primidone (Mysoline) Amobarbital (Amytal) Mephobarbital (Mebaral)

BOX 55–8. Benzodiazepines
Clonazepam (Klonopin) Clorazepate (Tranxene) Diazepam (Valium) Lorazepam (Ativan)

good oral hygiene and regular dental exams
  f. Instruct clients to consult with a physician before taking other medications to ensure compatibility with anticonvulsants
D. Barbiturates (Box 55–7)
1. Used for grand mal seizures and acute episodes of seizures due to status epilepticus
2. May also be used as adjuncts to anesthesia
3. Side effects
  a. Drowsiness
  b. Dizziness
  c. Hypotension
  d. Respiratory depression
  e. Tolerance to the medication
E. Benzodiazepines (Box 55–8)
1. To treat absence (petite mal) seizures
2. Diazepam (Valium) is used to treat status epilepticus, anxiety, and skeletal muscle spasms
3. Clorazepate (Tranxene) is used as adjunctive therapy for partial seizures
4. Side effects
  a. Ataxia
  b. Respiratory and cardiac depression
  c. Medication tolerance
  d. Drug dependency
F. Succinimides (Box 55–9)
1. Used to treat absence (petite mal) seizures
2. Side effects
  a. Anorexia, nausea, vomiting
  b. Blood dyscrasias
G. Oxazolidinediones (Box 55–10)
1. Used for absence (petite mal) seizures
2. Side effects
  a. Sedation
  b. Photophobia
H. Iminostilbenes
1. Used in treating seizure disorders that have not responded to other anticonvulsants
2. Used to treat trigeminal neuralgia
3. Medication: carbamazepine (Tegretol)
4. Side effects
  a. Drowsiness
  b. Dizziness

BOX 55–9. Succinimides
Ethosuximide (Zarontin) Methsuximide (Celontin) Phensuximide (Milontin)

BOX 55–10. Oxazolidinediones

Paramethadione (Paradione)
Trimethadione (Tridione)

   c. Nausea, vomiting
   d. Constipation or diarrhea
   e. Visual abnormalities
   f. Dry mouth
   g. Headache
   h. Water retention
   i. Increased sweating
 I. Valproates (Box 55–11)
   1. Used to treat grand mal, petit mal, myoclonic, and psychomotor seizures
   2. Side effects
     a. Nausea and vomiting
     b. Abdominal cramps
     c. Diarrhea or constipation
     d. Hepatotoxicity

VI. Central Nervous System Stimulants

A. Description
   1. Amphetamines and caffeine stimulate the cerebral cortex of the brain
   2. Analeptics and caffeine act on the brain stem and medulla to stimulate respirations
   3. Anorexiants act on the cerebral cortex and hypothalamus to suppress appetite
   4. Used to treat narcolepsy and attention deficit hyperactivity disorders
   5. Used to treat respiratory depression after anesthesia
   6. Used as adjunctive therapy for obesity
B. Amphetamines
   1. Medications (Box 55–12)
   2. Side effects
     a. Sleeplessness
     b. Tremors
     c. Irritability and restlessness
     d. Heart palpitations and tachycardia
     e. Hypertension
     f. Dry mouth
     g. Anorexia and weight loss
     h. Diarrhea or constipation
     i. Impotence
     j. Dependence and tolerance
C. Anorexiants
   1. Medications (Box 55–13)
   2. Side effects
     a. Nervousness, irritability, and restlessness
     b. Insomnia

BOX 55–11. Valproates

Valproic acid (Depakene)
Divalproex sodium (Depakote)

BOX 55–12. Amphetamines

Amphetamine sulfate
Dextroamphetamine sulfate (Dexedrine)
Methamphetamine hydrochloride (Desoxyn)
Methylphenidate hydrochloride (Ritalin)
Pemoline (Cylert)

   c. Heart palpitations
   d. Hypertension
D. Analeptics
   1. Medications
     a. Caffeine (Tirend, Vivarin)
     b. Theophylline, also a bronchodilator, may be used for newborns with apnea to stimulate respirations
   2. Side effects
     a. Nervousness and restlessness
     b. Tremors and twitching
     c. Palpitations
     d. Insomnia
     e. Diuresis
     f. GI irritation
     g. Tinnitus
E. CNS stimulant for migraines
   1. Sumatriptan succinate (Imitrex)
   2. Promotes vasoconstriction of the carotid arteries
F. Respiratory stimulant
   1. Doxapram hydrochloride (Dopram)
   2. Used to treat sedative hypnotic overdose to correct respiratory depression
G. Implementation for CNS stimulants
   1. Monitor vital signs
   2. Assess mental status
   3. Assess height, weight, and growth of children
   4. Monitor complete blood count (CBC), white blood count (WBC), and platelet counts before and during therapy
   5. Monitor for side effects
   6. Monitor sleep patterns

BOX 55–13. Anorexiants

Diethylpropion hydrochloride (Tenuate, Tepanil, Dospan)
Fenfluramine hydrochloride (Pondimin)
Mazindol (Sanorex, Mazanor)
Phendimetrazine tartrate (Adipost, Trimcaps, Prelu-2)
Phenmetrazine hydrochloride (Preludin)
Phentermine hydrochloride (Fastin, Ionamin, Adipex-P)
Benzphetamine hydrochloride (Didrex)
Dextroamphetamine sulfate (Dexedrine)
Phenylpropanolamine hydrochloride (Acutrim, Control, Dexatrim, Prolamine)

7. Monitor for withdrawal symptoms, such as nausea, vomiting, weakness, and headache
8. Instruct the client to take medication before meals
9. Instruct the client to avoid foods and beverages containing caffeine to prevent additional stimulation
10. Instruct clients to read labels on over-the-counter products because many contain caffeine
11. Instruct clients to avoid alcohol
12. Instruct clients not to discontinue medication abruptly
13. Instruct the client to take the last daily dose of CNS stimulant at least 6 hours before bedtime to prevent insomnia
14. Monitor for drug dependence and abuse with amphetamines
15. If a child is taking a CNS stimulant, instruct the parents to notify the school nurse
16. Monitor for calming effects of CNS stimulants within 3 to 4 weeks on children with attention deficit hyperactivity disorder
17. Monitor growth in children on long-term therapy with methylphenidate hydrochloride (Ritalin)

VII. Nonnarcotic Analgesics

A. Nonsteroidal anti-inflammatory drugs (NSAIDs)
  1. Description
     a. NSAIDs are aspirin and aspirin-like medications that inhibit the synthesis of prostaglandins
     b. They act as an analgesic to relieve pain, as an antipyretic to reduce body temperature, and as an anticoagulant to inhibit platelet aggregation
     c. Used to relieve inflammation and pain and in the treatment of rheumatoid arthritis, bursitis, tendinitis, osteoarthritis, and acute gout
     d. Contraindicated in hypersensitivity or liver or renal disease
     e. Aspirin should not be taken by children with flu symptoms because of the risk of Reye's syndrome
     f. Aspirin should not be taken if the client is on an anticoagulant
     g. Aspirin and an NSAID should not be taken together because aspirin decreases the blood level and the effectiveness of the NSAID
     h. NSAIDs can increase the effects of warfarin (Coumadin), sulfonamides, cephalosporins, and phenytoin (Dilantin)
     i. Hypoglycemia may result if ibuprofen (Motrin) is taken with insulin or an oral hypoglycemic medication
     j. A high risk of toxicity exists if ibuprofen (Motrin) is taken concurrently with calcium blockers

---

BOX 55–14. Nonsteroidal Anti-Inflammatory Medications (NSAIDs)

Aspirin (ASA, Bayer, Ecotrin)
Diflunisal (Dolobid)
Indomethacin (Indocin)
Sulindac (Clinoril)
Tolmetin (Tolectin)
Phenylbutazone (Butazolidin)
Fenoprofen calcium (Nalfon)
Flurbiprofen sodium (Ansaid, Ocufen)
Ibuprofen (Motrin, Advil, Nuprin, Medipren)
Ketoprofen (Orudis)
Naproxen (Naprosyn)
Oxaprozin (Daypro)
Meclofenamate (Meclomen)
Mefenamic acid (Ponstel)
Piroxicam (Feldene)
Diclofenac sodium (Voltaren)
Etodolac (Lodine)
Ketorolac tromethamine (Toradol)

---

2. Medications (Box 55–14)
3. Side effects (Table 55–1)
4. Implementation
   a. Assess client for allergies
   b. Obtain a medication history on the client
   c. Ask client about a history of gastric upset or bleeding or liver disease
   d. Check the client for GI upset during medication administration
   e. Monitor for signs of bleeding, such as tarry stools, bleeding gums, petechiae, ecchymosis, and purpura
   f. Monitor for edema
   g. Monitor serum salicylate (aspirin) level when client is taking high doses
   h. Instruct the client to take medication with water, milk, or food
   i. Enteric-coated form or buffered form of aspirin can be taken to decrease gastric distress; instruct clients that enteric-coated tablets cannot be crushed or broken
   j. Advise clients to inform other health care professionals that they are taking high doses of aspirin
   k. Note that aspirin should be discontinued 3 to 7 days prior to surgery to reduce the risk of bleeding

Table 55–1. Side Effects of Aspirin and NSAIDs

Aspirin	*NSAIDs*
Drowsiness	Hypotension
Tinnitus	Sodium and water retention
Headaches	Gastric irritation
Flushing	Blood dyscrasias
Dizziness	Dizziness
GI symptoms	Tinnitus
Visual changes	Pruritus

l. Instruct clients to avoid alcoholic beverages

B. Acetaminophen (Tylenol)
1. Description
   a. Inhibits prostaglandin synthesis
   b. Used to decrease pain and fever
   c. Contraindicated in hepatic or renal disease, alcoholism, and hypersensitivity
2. Side effects
   a. Anorexia, nausea, and vomiting
   b. Rash
   c. Hypoglycemia
   d. Oliguria
   e. Hepatotoxicity
3. Implementation
   a. Monitor vital signs
   b. Assess the client for history of liver dysfunction
   c. Monitor for hepatic damage, which includes nausea, vomiting, diarrhea, and abdominal pain
   d. Monitor liver enzyme tests
   e. Instruct the client that self-medication should not be used longer than 10 days for an adult and 5 days for a child
   f. Note that the antidote is acetylcysteine (Mucomyst)
   g. Evaluate for the effectiveness of the medication

VIII. Narcotic Analgesics

A. Description
1. Suppress pain impulses but can suppress respiration and coughing by acting on the respiratory and cough center in the medulla of the brain stem
2. Can produce euphoria and sedation
3. Can cause physical dependence
B. Medications (Box 55–15)
1. Codeine sulfate
   a. Effective cough suppressant at low doses
   b. Can cause constipation
2. Hydromorphone hydrochloride (Dilaudid)
   a. Can decrease respirations
   b. Can cause constipation
3. Meperidine (Demerol)
   a. Can decrease blood pressure and cause dizziness
   b. Can increase intracranial pressure in head injuries
4. Morphine sulfate
   a. Can cause respiratory depression, orthostatic hypotension, and constipation
   b. May cause nausea and vomiting because of increased vestibular sensitivity
5. Oxycodone with aspirin (Percodan)
   a. Should not be taken by clients allergic to aspirin
   b. Can cause gastric irritation and should be taken with food or plenty of liquids
6. Propoxyphene napsylate (Darvon-N) and propoxyphene hydrochloride (Darvon)

BOX 55–15. Narcotic Analgesics

Codeine sulfate
Hydromorphone hydrochloride (Dilaudid)
Meperidine (Demerol)
Morphine sulfate
Oxycodone hydrochloride with acetaminophen (Percocet)
Oxycodone with aspirin (Percodan)
Propoxyphene napsylate (Darvon-N)
Propoxyphene hydrochloride (Darvon)
Buprenorphine hydrochloride (Buprenex)
Butorphanol tartrate (Stadol)
Dezocine (Dalgan)
Nalbuphine hydrochloride (Nubain)
Methadone hydrochloride (Dolophine)
Pentazocine (Talwin)
Pentazocine hydrochloride (Talwin Compound)
Hydrocodone (Hycodan)
Levorphanol tartrate (Levo-Dromoran)
Fentanyl (Duragesic, Sublimaze)
Sufentanil citrate (Sufenta)
Oxycodone hydrochloride (Roxicodone)
Oxymorphone hydrochloride (Numorphan)

---

   a. Darvon compound contains aspirin and should not be taken in clients allergic to aspirin
   b. Darvocet-N contains acetaminophen
7. Nalbuphine hydrochloride (Nubain): preferable for treating the pain of a myocardial infarction (MI) because it reduces the oxygen needs of the heart without reducing blood pressure
8. Methadone hydrochloride (Dolophine)
   a. Dilute doses of oral concentrate with at least 90 mL of water
   b. Dilute dispersible tablets in at least 120 mL of water, orange juice, or acidic fruit beverage
   c. Used as a replacement medication for opiate dependence or to facilitate withdrawal
9. Pentazocine (Talwin) and pentazocine hydrochloride (Talwin Compound)
   a. Increase blood pressure and cardiac workload
   b. Cause dysphoria rather than euphoria
10. Hydrocodone (Hycodan): frequently used for cough suppression

C. Implementation
1. Monitor vital signs
2. Assess client thoroughly before administering pain medication
3. Initiate nursing measures such as massage, distraction, deep breathing and relaxation exercises, and the application of heat or cold as prescribed; provide care and comfort prior to administering the narcotic analgesic
4. Administer medications 30 to 60 minutes before painful activities
5. Monitor respiratory rate and if the rate is less

than 12 breaths per minute in an adult, hold medication unless ventilatory support is provided
6. Monitor pulse, and if bradycardia develops, withhold the dose and notify the physician
7. Monitor blood pressure for hypotension
8. Encourage activities such as turning, deep breathing, and incentive spirometry to prevent atelectasis and pneumonia
9. Monitor level of consciousness (LOC)
10. Initiate safety precautions such as side rails, a nightlight, and supervised ambulation; discourage smoking
11. Monitor I&O and for urinary retention
12. Instruct the client to take oral doses with milk or a snack to reduce gastric irritation
13. Instruct the client to avoid alcohol
14. Instruct clients to avoid activities that require alertness

D. Morphine sulfate
1. Description
    a. Used for acute pain due to MI or cancer, for dyspnea due to pulmonary edema, and as a preoperative medication
    b. Contraindicated in severe respiratory disorders, head injury or **increased intracranial pressure,** severe renal disease, or seizure activity
    c. Used with caution in clients with shock or blood loss
2. Side effects
    a. Respiratory depression
    b. Orthostatic hypotension
    c. Urinary retention
    d. Nausea, vomiting, and constipation
    e. Cough suppression
    f. Reduction in pupillary size
3. Implementation
    a. Note that the antidote for morphine overdose is naloxone (Narcan)
    b. Monitor vital signs
    c. Note rate and depth of respirations; respirations of less than 10 per minute can indicate respiratory distress
    d. Monitor urinary output, which should be at least 600 mL/day
    e. Monitor bowel sounds for decreased peristalsis because constipation can occur
    f. Monitor for pupil changes because pinpoint pupils can indicate morphine overdose
    g. Avoid alcohol or CNS depressants because they can cause respiratory depression
    h. Instruct clients to report dizziness or difficulty breathing
    i. Assess risk for injury; assist the client with activities and ambulation

E. Meperidine (Demerol)
1. Description
    a. Used for acute pain and as a preoperative medication
    b. Contraindicated in head injuries and

increased intracranial pressure, respiratory disorders, hypotension, shock, severe hepatic and renal disease, and in clients taking MAOI
    c. Should not be taken with alcohol or sedative hypnotics because it may increase the CNS depression
2. Side effects
    a. Hypotension
    b. Respiratory depression
    c. Tachycardia
    d. Drowsiness
    e. Urinary retention and/or constipation
    f. Nausea and vomiting
    g. Headache and dizziness
    h. Blurred vision
    i. Tinnitus
    j. Tremors
3. Implementation
    a. Monitor vital signs
    b. Monitor for respiratory dysfunction and hypotension
    c. Have naloxone (Narcan) available for overdose
    d. Monitor for urinary retention
    e. Monitor bowel sounds and for constipation
    f. Monitor mental status
    g. Initiate safety precautions
    h. Instruct the client not to consume alcohol

IX. Narcotic Antagonist

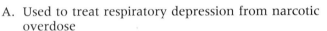

A. Used to treat respiratory depression from narcotic overdose
B. Medication: naloxone hydrochloride (Narcan)
C. Implementation
1. Monitor blood pressure, pulse, and respiratory rate every 5 minutes initially, tapering to every 15 minutes, then every 30 minutes until stable
2. Assist with placing the client on a cardiac monitor
3. Monitor I&O
4. Auscultate bowel sounds
5. Have resuscitation equipment available
6. Do not leave the client unattended
7. Monitor the client closely for several hours because when the effects of the antagonist wear off, the client may again display signs of narcotic overdose

X. Osmotic Diuretics (Box 55–16)

A. Description
1. Increase osmotic pressure of the glomerular

BOX 55–16. Osmotic Diuretics
Mannitol (Osmitrol)
Urea (Ureaphil)

BOX 55–17. Corticosteroids

Betamethasone (Celestone)
Cortisone acetate (Cortone)
Dexamethasone (Decadron)
Hydrocortisone (Cortef, Hydrocortone)
Methylprednisolone (Depo-Medrol, Medrol, Solu-
  Medrol)
Prednisolone (Delta-Cortef, Hydeltrasol)
Prednisone (Deltasone)

filtrate inhibiting reabsorption of water and
electrolytes
2. Used for oliguria and to prevent renal failure
3. Used to decrease intracranial pressure
4. Used to decrease intraocular pressure in
   narrow-angle glaucoma
5. Mannitol is used with chemotherapy to
   induce diuresis
B. Side effects
1. Fluid and electrolyte imbalances
2. Pulmonary edema from the rapid shifts of
   fluid
3. Nausea and vomiting
4. Tachycardia from the rapid fluid loss
5. Hyponatremia and dehydration
C. Implementation
1. Monitor vital signs
2. Monitor weight and urine output
3. Monitor electrolyte levels
4. Monitor for signs of pulmonary edema
5. Monitor for signs of dehydration
6. Monitor neurological status and for signs of
   decreasing intracranial pressure if appropriate
7. Change the client's position slowly to prevent
   orthostatic hypotension

◆ **XI. Corticosteroids** (Box 55–17)

A. Description
1. Inhibit accumulation of inflammatory cells at
   inflammation sites
2. Prevent and suppress cell and tissue immune
   reactions
3. Used to treat cerebral edema
4. Side effects can occur primarily if the
   medication is prescribed long term
◆ B. Side effects and implementation: refer to Chapter
43 for information regarding the side effects and
implementation measures for the client taking a
corticosteroid

PRACTICE QUESTIONS

1. The nurse is caring for a client diagnosed with
Bell's palsy. The client has been taking acetaminophen (Tylenol) and a Tylenol overdose is suspected. The nurse anticipates that the antidote to
be prepared is

  1 Auranofin (Ridaura)
  2 Fludarabine (Fludara)
  3 Acetylcysteine (Mucomyst)
  4 Pentostatin (Nipent)

2. The client with trigeminal neuralgia tells the
nurse that acetaminophen (Tylenol) is taken on
a frequent daily basis for relief of generalized
discomfort. Which of the following indicates toxicity associated with the medication?
  1 Platelet count of 400,000 cells/μl
  2 A direct bilirubin level of 2 mg/dL
  3 Prothrombin time of 12 seconds
  4 Sodium of 140 mEq/L

3. The nurse is assisting in preparing to administer
acetylcysteine (Mucomyst) to the client with an
overdose of acetaminophen (Tylenol). Which of
the following are appropriate actions when administering this antidote?
  1 Mixing the medication in a flavored ice drink
and allowing the client to drink the medication through a straw
  2 Administering the medication by IM, mixed
in 10 mL of normal saline
  3 Administering the medication by IM in the
gluteal muscle
  4 Administering the medication subcutaneously
in the deltoid muscle

4. The client is receiving baclofen (Lioresal) for
muscle spasms due to a spinal cord injury. The
nurse monitors the client knowing that which of
the following indicates a side effect related to this
medication?
  1 Photosensitivity
  2 Slurred speech
  3 Hypertension
  4 Muscle pain

5. The client is suspected of having myasthenia gravis. The physician administers edrophonium
(Tensilon) by IV to determine the diagnosis. The
nurse understands that which of the following
indicates the diagnosis of myasthenia gravis following administration of this medication?
  1 An increase in muscle strength
  2 A decrease in muscle strength
  3 Joint pain
  4 Feelings of faintness, dizziness, hypotension,
and signs of flushing in the client

6. The client with myasthenia gravis is suspected of
having cholinergic crisis. Which of the following
symptoms indicates that this crisis exists?
  1 Hypotension
  2 Hypertension
  3 Mouth sores
  4 Ataxia

7. The client with myasthenia gravis is receiving pyridostigmine (Mestinon). The nurse monitors for signs and symptoms of cholinergic crisis due to overdose of the medication. The nurse checks the medication supply to ensure that which medication is available for administration if a cholinergic crisis occurs?
   1 Vitamin K
   2 Protamine sulfate
   3 Acetylcysteine (Mucomyst)
   4 Atropine sulfate

8. The client with myasthenia gravis becomes increasingly weaker. The physician prepares to identify whether the client is reacting to an overdose of the medication (cholinergic crisis) or an increasing severity of the disease (myasthenic crisis). An injection of edrophonium (Tensilon) is administered. Which of the following indicates that the client is in cholinergic crisis?
   1 An improvement of the weakness
   2 A temporary worsening of the condition
   3 No change in the condition
   4 Complaints of muscle spasms

9. The client with myasthenia gravis verbalizes complaints of feeling much weaker than normal. The physician plans to implement a diagnostic test to determine if the client is experiencing a myasthenic crisis. The physician administers edrophonium (Tensilon). Which of the following indicates that the client is experiencing a myasthenic crisis?
   1 Increasing weakness
   2 No change in the condition
   3 A temporary improvement in the condition
   4 An increase in muscle spasms

10. Levodopa (Carbidopa) is prescribed for the client with Parkinson's disease. The nurse monitors the client for adverse reactions to the medication. Which of the following indicates that the client is experiencing an adverse reaction?
    1 Pruritus
    2 Hypertension
    3 Tachycardia
    4 Impaired voluntary movements

11. Phenytoin (Dilantin), 100 mg PO three times daily, has been prescribed for the client for seizure control. The nurse reinforces intructions regarding the medication to the client. Which of the following statements, if made by the client, indicates effective teaching?
    1 "It's OK to break the capsules to make it easier for me to swallow them."
    2 "I will use a soft toothbrush to brush my teeth."
    3 "If I forget to take my medication, I can wait until the next dose and eliminate that dose."
    4 "If my throat becomes sore, it's a normal effect of the medication and it's nothing to be concerned about."

12. The client is taking phenytoin (Dilantin) for seizure control. A serum drug level is drawn. Which of the following indicates a therapeutic serum drug range?
    1 5 to 10 μg/mL
    2 10 to 20 μg/mL
    3 20 to 30 μg/mL
    4 30 to 40 μg/mL

13. A nonsteroidal anti-inflammatory drug (NSAID) is prescribed for the client. To promote the best absorption of the medication, the nurse instructs the client to take the medication
    1 60 minutes before meals
    2 After meals
    3 With 8 oz of milk
    4 With an antacid

14. The nurse is caring for a client who is taking phenytoin (Dilantin) for control of seizures. During data collection, the nurse notes that the client is taking birth control pills. Which of the following information should the nurse provide to the client?
    1 The increased risk of thrombophlebitis exists while taking phenytoin (Dilantin) and birth control pills together
    2 The potential decreased effectiveness of the birth control pills exists while taking phenytoin (Dilantin)
    3 The client may stop the medication if it is causing severe gastrointestinal effects
    4 Pregnancy should be avoided while taking phenytoin (Dilantin)

15. A client with trigeminal neuralgia is being treated with carbamazepine (Tegretol). Which of the following laboratory results indicates that the client is experiencing an adverse reaction to the medication?
    1 White blood cell count of 3000/μl
    2 Blood urea nitrogen (BUN) 15 mg/dL
    3 Sodium 140 mEq/L
    4 Uric acid 5.0 ng/dL

16. A client with multiple sclerosis is receiving diazepam (Valium), a centrally acting skeletal muscle relaxant. Which of the following indicates that the client is experiencing a side effect related to this medication?
    1 Headache
    2 Increased salivation
    3 Urinary retention
    4 Drowsiness

17. The nurse is caring for a client receiving morphine sulfate SC for pain. Since morphine has

been prescribed for this client, which of the following nursing actions is included in the plan of care?
1 Monitor the client's temperature
2 Force fluids
3 Maintain the client in a supine position
4 Encourage the client to cough and deep breathe

18. Meperidine (Demerol) is prescribed for the client with pain. Which of the following does the nurse monitor as a side effect of this medication?
1 Hypertension
2 Bradycardia
3 Diarrhea
4 Urinary retention

19. The nurse is caring for a client with severe back pain. Codeine sulfate has been prescribed for the client. Which of the following does the nurse include in the plan of care while the client is taking this medication?
1 Monitor for hypertension
2 Restrict fluid intake
3 Monitor bowel activity
4 Monitor peripheral pulses

20. Dantrolene (Dantrium) is prescribed for a client with spinal cord injury for discomfort due to spasticity. The nurse tells the client about the importance of follow-up and the need for which of the following blood studies?
1 Sedimentation rate
2 White blood cell count
3 Liver function
4 Creatinine

21. The client with epilepsy is taking the prescribed dose of phenytoin (Dilantin) to control seizures. A phenytoin blood level is drawn and the results reveal a level of 35 µg/mL. Which of the following symptoms is expected as a result of this laboratory finding?
1 No symptoms because this is a normal therapeutic level
2 Slurred speech
3 Tachycardia
4 Nystagmus

22. The physician initiates levodopa therapy for the client with Parkinson's disease. A few days after the client starts the medication, the client complains of nausea and vomiting. The nurse's best instruction to the client is that
1 This is an expected side effect of the drug
2 Taking the medication with food will help to prevent the nausea
3 Taking an antiemetic is the best measure to prevent the nausea
4 The nausea and vomiting will decrease when the dose of levodopa is stabilized

23. Mannitol (Osmitrol) is being administered to a client with increased intracranial pressure following a head injury. The nurse assisting in caring for the client knows that which of the following indicates the therapeutic action of this medication?
1 Induces diuresis by raising the osmotic pressure of glomerular filtrate, thereby inhibiting tubular reabsorption of water and solutes
2 Prevents diuresis by promoting the reabsorption of sodium and water in the loop of Henle
3 Prevents the filtration of sodium and water through the kidneys
4 Prevents the filtration of sodium and potassium through the kidneys

24. Carbamazepine (Tegretol) is prescribed for a client with a diagnosis of psychomotor seizures. The nurse reviews the client's health history, knowing that this medication is contraindicated if which of the following disorders is present?
1 Liver disease
2 Headaches
3 Hypothyroidism
4 Diabetes mellitus

25. The client is admitted to the hospital with complaints of back spasms. The client states, "I have been taking two or three aspirin every 4 hours for the last week and it hasn't helped my back." Aspirin intoxication is suspected. Which of the following symptoms indicates aspirin intoxication?
1 Diarrhea
2 Constipation
3 Tinnitus
4 Photosensitivity

ANSWERS

1. 3

RATIONALE: The antidote for acetaminophen is acetylcysteine. Auranofin is a gold preparation used in rheumatoid arthritis. Fludarabine and pentostatin are antineoplastic agents.

TEST-TAKING STRATEGY: Knowledge regarding the antidote for acetaminophen and the drug classifications noted in the options, will assist you in answering this question. It is important to know the antidote for various medications. If you had difficulty with this question, take time now to review antidotes.

LEVEL OF COGNITIVE ABILITY: Comprehension
PHASE OF NURSING PROCESS: Planning
CLIENT NEEDS: Physiological Integrity
CONTENT AREA: Pharmacology
REFERENCE

Hodgson, B., & Kizior, R. (1999). *Saunders nursing drug handbook 1999.* Philadelphia: W. B. Saunders. p. 10.

2. 2

RATIONALE: In adults, overdose of acetaminophen causes liver damage. Option 2 is an indicator of liver function, and is the only option that indicates an abnormal laboratory value. The normal direct bilirubin is 0 to 0.4 mg/dL. The normal platelet count is 150,000 to 400,000 cells/μl. The normal prothrombin time is 10 to 13 seconds. The normal sodium is 135 to 145 mEq/l.

TEST-TAKING STRATEGY: Knowledge that acetaminophen causes liver damage and knowledge of the normal laboratory results will be helpful in answering this question. Reviewing the laboratory values in the options will direct you to option 2, the abnormal value. Also, of all of the options, the bilirubin is the most directly related laboratory value to liver function.

LEVEL OF COGNITIVE ABILITY: Comprehension
PHASE OF NURSING PROCESS: Data Collection
CLIENT NEEDS: Physiological Integrity
CONTENT AREA: Pharmacology
REFERENCE

Hodgson, B., & Kizior, R. (1999). *Saunders nursing drug handbook 1999.* Philadelphia: W. B. Saunders. p. 8.

3. 1

RATIONALE: Because acetylcysteine has a pervasive flavor of rotten eggs, it must be disguised in a flavored ice drink, and is preferably drunk through a straw to minimize contact with the mouth. It is not administered by IM or SC route.

TEST-TAKING STRATEGY: Knowing that the medication is a solution that is also used for nebulization treatments will assist you in selecting the option that indicates an oral route. Note that options 2, 3, and 4 indicate parenteral administration and option 1, the correct option, indicates oral administration.

LEVEL OF COGNITIVE ABILITY: Application
PHASE OF NURSING PROCESS: Implementation
CLIENT NEEDS: Physiological Integrity
CONTENT AREA: Pharmacology
REFERENCE

Hodgson, B., & Kizior, R. (1999). *Saunders nursing drug handbook 1999.* Philadelphia: W. B. Saunders. p. 11.

4. 2

RATIONALE: Side effects of baclofen include drowsiness, dizziness, weakness, and nausea. Occasional side effects include headache, paresthesia of the hands and feet, constipation or diarrhea, anorexia, hypotension, confusion, and nasal congestion. Paradoxical CNS excitement and restlessness can occur along with slurred speech, tremor, dry mouth, nocturia, and impotence.

TEST-TAKING STRATEGY: Knowledge regarding the medication is required to answer the question. Option 2 is the option that is most closely associated with a neurological disorder. If you had difficulty with this question, take time now to review the side effects related to baclofen.

LEVEL OF COGNITIVE ABILITY: Application
PHASE OF NURSING PROCESS: Data Collection
CLIENT NEEDS: Physiological Integrity
CONTENT AREA: Pharmacology
REFERENCE

Hodgson, B., & Kizior, R. (1999). *Saunders nursing drug handbook 1999.* Philadelphia: W. B. Saunders. pp. 95–96.

5. 1

RATIONALE: Edrophonium (Tensilon) is a short-acting acetylcholinesterase inhibitor used as a diagnostic agent. When a new client with suspected myasthenia gravis is given the medication intravenously, an increase in muscle strength should be seen in 1 to 3 minutes. If no response occurs, another dose of edrophonium is given over the next 2 minutes, and muscle strength is again tested. If no increase in muscle strength occurs with this higher dose, the muscle weakness is not caused by myasthenia gravis. Clients receiving injections of this medication commonly demonstrate a drop in blood pressure, feel faint and dizzy, and are flushed.

TEST-TAKING STRATEGY: Knowledge regarding this medication as a diagnostic tool for myasthenia gravis is required to answer this question. Take time now to review this medication as a diagnostic tool for suspected myasthenia gravis.

LEVEL OF COGNITIVE ABILITY: Comprehension
PHASE OF NURSING PROCESS: Data Collection
CLIENT NEEDS: Physiological Integrity
CONTENT AREA: Pharmacology
REFERENCE

Hodgson, B., & Kizior, R. (1999). *Saunders nursing drug handbook 1999.* Philadelphia: W. B. Saunders. p. 1135.

6. 2

RATIONALE: Cholinergic crisis occurs with an overdose of medication. Indications of cholinergic crisis include GI disturbances, nausea, vomiting, diarrhea, abdominal cramps, increased salivation and tearing, miosis, hypertension, sweating, and increased bronchial secretions.

TEST-TAKING STRATEGY: Knowledge regarding both cholinergic and myasthenic crisis is required to answer this question. Take time now to review both cholinergic and myasthenic crisis if you had difficulty with this question.

LEVEL OF COGNITIVE ABILITY: Comprehension
PHASE OF NURSING PROCESS: Data Collection
CLIENT NEEDS: Physiological Integrity
CONTENT AREA: Pharmacology
REFERENCE

deWit, S. (1998). *Essentials of medical-surgical nursing* (4th ed.). Philadelphia: W. B. Saunders. p. 383.

7. 4

RATIONALE: The antidote for cholinergic crisis is atropine sulfate. Vitamin K is the antidote for warfarin. Protamine sulfate is the antidote for heparin, and acetylcysteine is the antidote for acetaminophen.
TEST-TAKING STRATEGY: Knowledge regarding antidotes for the various medications is required to answer this question. Review antidotes now if you had difficulty with this question.
LEVEL OF COGNITIVE ABILITY: Comprehension
PHASE OF NURSING PROCESS: Planning
CLIENT NEEDS: Physiological Integrity
CONTENT AREA: Pharmacology
REFERENCE
Hodgson, B., & Kizior, R. (1999). *Saunders nursing drug handbook 1999.* Philadelphia: W. B. Saunders. p. 1097.

8. 2

RATIONALE: An edrophonium injection makes the client in cholinergic crisis temporarily worse. This in known as a negative Tensilon test.
TEST-TAKING STRATEGY: Knowledge regarding the use of this medication as a diagnostic tool to differentiate between cholinergic and myasthenic crisis is required to answer this question. Take time now to review this diagnostic test and the differences between cholinergic and myasthenic crisis.
LEVEL OF COGNITIVE ABILITY: Analysis
PHASE OF NURSING PROCESS: Data Collection
CLIENT NEEDS: Physiological Integrity
CONTENT AREA: Pharmacology
REFERENCE
Monahan, F., & Neighbors, M. (1998). *Medical-surgical nursing: Foundations for clinical practice* (2nd ed.). Philadelphia: W. B. Saunders. p. 783.

9. 3

RATIONALE: Edrophonium is administered to determine whether the client is reacting to an overdose of a medication (cholinergic crisis) or an increasing severity of the disease (myasthenic crisis). When the edrophonium injection is given and the condition improves temporarily, the client in myasthenic crisis. This is known as a positive Tensilon test.
TEST-TAKING STRATEGY: Knowledge regarding the use of this medication as a diagnostic tool to differentiate between cholinergic and myasthenic crisis is required to answer this question. Take time now to review this diagnostic test and the differences between cholinergic and myasthenic crisis.
LEVEL OF COGNITIVE ABILITY: Analysis
PHASE OF NURSING PROCESS: Data Collection
CLIENT NEEDS: Physiological Integrity
CONTENT AREA: Pharmacology
REFERENCE
Monahan, F., & Neighbors, M. (1998). *Medical-surgical nursing: Foundations for clinical practice* (2nd ed.). Philadelphia: W. B. Saunders. p. 783.

10. 4

RATIONALE: Dyskinesia and impaired voluntary movement may occur with high levodopa dosages. Nausea, anorexia, dizziness, orthostatic hypotension, bradycardia, and akinesia (the temporary muscle weakness that lasts 1 min-

ute to 1 hour, also known as "on-off phenomenon") are frequent side effects of the medication.
TEST-TAKING STRATEGY: Knowledge regarding the adverse effects of levodopa is required to answer this question. Options 2 and 3 are cardiac-related options, so these options can be eliminated first. Note that the question asks for an adverse reaction; therefore, select option 4 over option 1 as the correct answer. Review the adverse effects of levodopa now if you had difficulty with this question.
LEVEL OF COGNITIVE ABILITY: Comprehension
PHASE OF NURSING PROCESS: Data Collection
CLIENT NEEDS: Physiological Integrity
CONTENT AREA: Pharmacology
REFERENCE
Lehne, R. (1998). *Pharmacology for nursing care* (3rd ed.). Philadelphia: W. B. Saunders. p. 194.

11. 2

RATIONALE: Phenytoin is an anticonvulsant. Gingival hyperplasia, bleeding, swelling, and tenderness of the gums can occur with the use of this medication. The client needs to be taught good oral hygiene, gum massage, and the need for regular dentist visits. The client should not skip medication doses because this could precipitate a seizure. Capsules should not be chewed or broken; they must be swallowed. The client needs to be instructed to report a sore throat, fever, glandular swelling, or any skin reaction—this indicates hematological toxicity.
TEST-TAKING STRATEGY: Note the key words "indicates effective teaching." Eliminate option 3 because the client needs to be encouraged to take medications on time. Also, eliminate option 4 because the client needs to report these symptoms to the physician. Remember, phenytoin capsules should not be broken. Take time now to review the side effects related to phenytoin if you had difficulty with this question.
LEVEL OF COGNITIVE ABILITY: Comprehension
PHASE OF NURSING PROCESS: Evaluation
CLIENT NEEDS: Health Promotion and Maintenance
CONTENT AREA: Pharmacology
REFERENCE
Hodgson, B., & Kizior, R. (1999). *Saunders nursing drug handbook 1999.* Philadelphia: W. B. Saunders. p. 823.

12. 2

RATIONALE: The therapeutic serum drug level range for phenytoin (Dilantin) is 10 to 20 µg/mL.
TEST-TAKING STRATEGY: Knowledge regarding the therapeutic serum range of this medication is required to answer the question. A helpful hint may be to remember that the theophylline therapeutic range and the acetaminophen therapeutic is the same as the phenytoin therapeutic range. Remembering this may assist you when answering questions related to any of these three medications.
LEVEL OF COGNITIVE ABILITY: Analysis
PHASE OF NURSING PROCESS: Data Collection
CLIENT NEEDS: Physiological Integrity
CONTENT AREA: Pharmacology
REFERENCE
Hodgson, B., & Kizior, R. (1999). *Saunders nursing drug handbook 1999.* Philadelphia: W. B. Saunders. p. 824.

13. 1

RATIONALE: NSAIDs should be given 30 to 60 minutes before or 2 hours after meals to promote the best absorption. Administering the medication with meals, milk, or an antacid will slow the absorption of the medication.

TEST-TAKING STRATEGY: Note the similarity between options 2, 3, and 4. Each of these options indicates administering the medication with a food, fluid, or an antacid. Also, note the key words "best absorption." Review this medication now if you had difficulty with this question.

LEVEL OF COGNITIVE ABILITY: Application
PHASE OF NURSING PROCESS: Implementation
CLIENT NEEDS: Health Promotion and Maintenance
CONTENT AREA: Pharmacology
REFERENCE
Eckler, J., & Fair, J. (1996). *Pharmacology essentials*. Philadelphia: W. B. Saunders. p. 179.

14. **2**

RATIONALE: Phenytoin enhances the rate of estrogen metabolism, which can decrease the effectiveness of some birth control pills. Options 1, 3, are 4 are not accurate.

TEST-TAKING STRATEGY: Knowledge regarding medication interactions while taking phenytoin is required to answer the question. Option 1 would cause anxiety in the client. A client should not be instructed to stop anticonvulsant medication. Pregnancy does not need to be "avoided." Review drug interactions related to phenytoin now, if you had difficulty with this question.

LEVEL OF COGNITIVE ABILITY: Application
PHASE OF NURSING PROCESS: Implementation
CLIENT NEEDS: Health Promotion and Maintenance
CONTENT AREA: Pharmacology
REFERENCE
Lehne, R. (1998). *Pharmacology for nursing care* (3rd ed.). Philadelphia: W. B. Saunders. p. 209.

15. **1**

RATIONALE: Adverse effects of carbamazepine appears as blood dyscrasias, including aplastic anemia, agranulocytosis, thrombocytopenia, leukopenia, cardiovascular disturbances, thrombophlebitis, dysrhythmias, and dermatological effects.

TEST-TAKING STRATEGY: Knowledge regarding the adverse effects related to this medication is required to answer the question. If you are familiar with normal laboratory values, you will note that the only option that indicates an abnormal value is option 1. Review the signs of adverse reactions related to this medication now if you had difficulty with this question.

LEVEL OF COGNITIVE ABILITY: Analysis
PHASE OF NURSING PROCESS: Data Collection
CLIENT NEEDS: Physiological Integrity
CONTENT AREA: Pharmacology
REFERENCE
Hodgson, B., & Kizior, R. (1999). *Saunders nursing drug handbook 1999*. Philadelphia: W. B. Saunders. p. 145.

16. **4**

RATIONALE: Incoordination and drowsiness are common side effects resulting from this medication. Options 1, 2, and 3 are incorrect.

TEST-TAKING STRATEGY: Note that the question addresses a centrally acting skeletal muscle relaxant. This may assist you in the process of elimination and direct you to the correct option of drowsiness. If you had difficulty with this question, take time now to review the side effects associated with diazepam.

LEVEL OF COGNITIVE ABILITY: Comprehension
PHASE OF NURSING PROCESS: Data Collection

CLIENT NEEDS: Physiological Integrity
CONTENT AREA: Pharmacology
REFERENCE
Hodgson, B., & Kizior, R. (1999). *Saunders nursing drug handbook 1999*. Philadelphia: W. B. Saunders. p. 308.

17. **4**

RATIONALE: Morphine suppresses the cough reflex. Clients need to be encouraged to cough and deep breathe to prevent pneumonia. Options 1, 2, and 3 are not specifically associated with this medication.

TEST-TAKING STRATEGY: Knowledge that morphine suppresses the cough reflex and the respiratory reflex should lead you to the correct option. Additionally, use your ABCs when selecting the correct option.

LEVEL OF COGNITIVE ABILITY: Application
PHASE OF NURSING PROCESS: Planning
CLIENT NEEDS: Physiological Integrity
CONTENT AREA: Pharmacology
REFERENCE
Hodgson, B., & Kizior, R. (1999). *Saunders nursing drug handbook 1999*. Philadelphia: W. B. Saunders. p. 706.

18. **4**

RATIONALE: Side effects of this medication include respiratory depression, orthostatic hypotension, tachycardia, drowsiness and mental clouding, constipation, and urinary retention.

TEST-TAKING STRATEGY: Knowledge regarding side effects associated with narcotic analgesics will assist you in answering the question. If you had difficulty with this question, take time now to review the medication.

LEVEL OF COGNITIVE ABILITY: Comprehension
PHASE OF NURSING PROCESS: Data Collection
CLIENT NEEDS: Physiological Integrity
CONTENT AREA: Pharmacology
REFERENCE
Hodgson, B., & Kizior, R. (1999). *Saunders nursing drug handbook 1999*. Philadelphia: W. B. Saunders. p. 638.

19. **3**

RATIONALE: While the client is taking codeine sulfate, the nurse monitors vital signs for hypotension. The nurse also increases fluid intake, palpates the bladder for urinary retention, auscultates bowel sounds, and monitors the pattern of daily bowel activity and stool consistency. The nurse should monitor respiratory status and initiate breathing and coughing exercises. Additionally, the nurse monitors the efectiveness of the pain medication.

TEST-TAKING STRATEGY: Use the process of elimination, recalling that codeine can cause constipation. If you had difficulty with this question, take time now to review nursing measures related to the administration of codeine sulfate.

LEVEL OF COGNITIVE ABILITY: Application
PHASE OF NURSING PROCESS: Planning
CLIENT NEEDS: Physiological Integrity
CONTENT AREA: Pharmacology
REFERENCE
Hodgson, B., & Kizior, R. (1999). *Saunders nursing drug handbook 1999*. Philadelphia: W. B. Saunders. p. 251.

20. **3**

RATIONALE: Dantrolene can cause liver damage and the nurse should monitor the liver function studies. Baseline

liver function studies are done before therapy starts, and regular liver function studies are performed throughout therapy. Dantrolene is discontinued if no relief of spasticity is achieved in 6 weeks.
TEST-TAKING STRATEGY: Knowledge that this medication is hepatotoxic will direct you to the correct option. If you had difficulty with this question, take time now to review.
LEVEL OF COGNITIVE ABILITY: Comprehension
PHASE OF NURSING PROCESS: Implementation
CLIENT NEEDS: Physiological Integrity
CONTENT AREA: Pharmacology
REFERENCE
Hodgson, B., & Kizior, R. (1999). *Saunders nursing drug handbook 1999*. Philadelphia: W. B. Saunders. p. 284.

21. **2**

RATIONALE: The therapeutic phenytoin level is 10 to 20 μg/mL. At greater than 20 μg/mL, involuntary movements of the eyeballs (nystagmus) appears. At greater than 30 μg/mL, ataxia and slurred speech arise.
TEST-TAKING STRATEGY: Knowledge regarding the therapeutic phenytoin level is required to answer this question. Take time now to review therapeutic levels and associated signs, if you had difficulty with this question.
LEVEL OF COGNITIVE ABILITY: Analysis
PHASE OF NURSING PROCESS: Data Collection
CLIENT NEEDS: Physiological Integrity
CONTENT AREA: Pharmacology
REFERENCE
Hodgson, B., & Kizior, R. (1999). *Saunders nursing drug handbook 1999*. Philadelphia: W. B. Saunders. p. 823.

22. **2**

RATIONALE: The best instruction by the nurse is that food will prevent the nausea. Antiemetics from the phenothiazine class should not be used since they block the therapeutic action of dopamine. The other options are incorrect.
TEST TAKING STRATEGY: Note the key word "best" and focus on the issue of the question. It is best to use nonpharmacological approaches first to alleviate the nausea. Additionally, the nurse cannot prescribe medications. Review this medication now if you had difficulty with this question.
LEVEL OF COGNITIVE ABILITY: Application
PHASE OF NURSING PROCESS: Implementation
CLIENT NEEDS: Physiological Integrity
CONTENT AREA: Pharmacology
REFERENCE
Lehne, R. (1998). *Pharmacology for nursing care* (3rd ed.). Philadelphia: W. B. Saunders. p. 203.

23. **1**

RATIONALE: Mannitol is an osmotic diuretic that induces diuresis by raising the osmotic pressure of glomerular filtrate, thereby inhibiting tubular reabsorption of water and solutes. It is used to reduce intracranial pressure in the client with head trauma.
TEST-TAKING STRATEGY: Read the question carefully, noting that it presents a client with increased intracranial pressure. The only option that suggests an action that will produce diuresis and thus reduce intracranial pressure is option 1. If you had difficulty with this question, take time now to review the action of mannitol.
LEVEL OF COGNITIVE ABILITY: Analysis
PHASE OF NURSING PROCESS: Evaluation
CLIENT NEEDS: Physiological Integrity
CONTENT AREA: Pharmacology
REFERENCE
Hodgson, B., & Kizior, R. (1999). *Saunders nursing drug handbook 1999*. Philadelphia: W. B. Saunders. p. 620.

24. **1**

RATIONALE: Carbamazepine is contraindicated in liver disease, and liver function tests are routinely prescribed for baseline purposes and are monitored during therapy. It is also contraindicated if the client has a history of blood dyscrasias.
TEST-TAKING STRATEGY: Knowledge regarding the contraindications associated with carbamazepine is required to answer this question. Review this medication now if you are unfamiliar with it.
LEVEL OF COGNITIVE ABILITY: Comprehension
PHASE OF NURSING PROCESS: Data Collection
CLIENT NEEDS: Physiological Integrity
CONTENT AREA: Pharmacology
REFERENCE
Eckler, J., & Fair, J. (1996). *Pharmacology essentials*. Philadelphia: W. B. Saunders. p. 244.

25. **3**

RATIONALE: Mild intoxication with acetylsalicylic acid (aspirin) is called salicylism and is commonly experienced when the daily dosage is more than 4 g. Tinnitus (ringing in the ears) is the most frequent effect noted with intoxication. Hyperventilation may occur because aspirin stimulates the respiratory center. Fever may result because aspirin interferes with the metabolic pathways coupling oxygen consumption and heat production. Options 1, 2, and 4 are incorrect.
TEST-TAKING STRATEGY: Focus on the issue of the question, aspirin intoxication. Options 1 and 2 relate to GI symptoms. Option 3, the correct answer, is the indicator of toxicity. If you had difficulty with this question, take time now to review aspirin intoxication.
LEVEL OF COGNITIVE ABILITY: Comprehension
PHASE OF NURSING PROCESS: Data Collection
CLIENT NEEDS: Physiological Integrity
CONTENT AREA: Pharmacology
REFERENCE
Hodgson, B., & Kizior, R. (1999). *Saunders nursing drug handbook 1999*. Philadelphia: W. B. Saunders. p. 76.

BIBLIOGRAPHY

Eckler, J., & Fair, J. (1996). *Pharmacology essentials*. Philadelphia: W. B. Saunders.
Hodgson, B., & Kizior, R. (1999). *Saunders snursing drug handbook 1999*. Philadelphia: W. B. Saunders.

Lehne, R. (1998). *Pharmacology for nursing care* (3rd ed.). Philadelphia: W. B. Saunders.
Luckmann, J. (1997). *Saunders manual of nursing care*. Philadelphia: W. B. Saunders.
Monahan, F., & Neighbors, M. (1998). *Medical-surgical nursing: Foundations for clinical practice* (2nd ed.). Philadelphia: W. B. Saunders.

UNIT XVII

....

The Adult Client with a Musculoskeletal Disorder

PYRAMID TERMS

Casts—Made of plaster or fiberglass to provide immobilization of bone and joints after a fracture or injury.

Compartment Syndrome—Increased pressure within one or more compartments causing massive compromise of circulation to an area and causing irreversible neuromuscular damage within 4 to 6 hours of its onset if not treated.

External Fixation—Stabilization of a fracture by the use of an external frame, with multiple pins applied through the bone.

Fat Embolism—An embolism that can occur 24 to 48 hours following a fracture or within the first 72 hours.

Internal Fixation—Stabilization of a fracture that involves the application of screws, plates, pins, or nails to hold the fragments in alignment.

Reduction—The procedure that restores the bone to proper alignment.

Traction—Force applied in two directions to reduce and immobilize a fracture.

PYRAMID TO SUCCESS

The Pyramid to Success focuses on the emergency care to a client who sustains a fracture or other musculoskeletal injury, monitoring for complications related to fractures, and interventions if complications occur. Nursing care related to casts and traction is emphasized. Skill related to instructing the client in the use of an assistive device such as a cane, walker, or crutches is a pyramid point. Pyramid points also include postoperative care following hip surgery or amputation, and care to the client with rheumatoid arthritis or osteoporosis. Focus on the points related to the psychosocial effects as a result of the musculoskeletal disorder, such as unexpected body image changes, and the appropriate and available support services needed for the client.

NURSING PROCESS

DATA COLLECTION

Fatigue and weakness
Fever
Weight loss
Inability to perform activities
Limited range of motion
Loss of movement
Asymmetry of limbs or deformed appearance
Tenderness, pain, stiffness, and swelling
Numbness or tingling of extremities
Muscle atrophy
Problems with balance or gait

PLANNING	IMPLEMENTATION	EVALUATION
Client reports the presence of pain. Client uses nonpharmacological measures to reduce pain.	Monitor for pain. Assist client to identify comfort measures to reduce pain. Provide comfort measures. Instruct client in nonpharmacological measures to reduce pain. Administer pain medication as appropriate. Instruct client regarding administration of prescribed medications. Document the effectiveness of pain-reduction techniques.	Client remains comfortable and free of pain.
PLANNING	IMPLEMENTATION	EVALUATION
Client performs coughing and deep-breathing exercises. Client tolerates ambulation activities as prescribed.	Monitor respiratory status for complications related to immobility. Encourage coughing and deep breathing. Turn and reposition client. Perform range of motion exercises as prescribed. Encourage out-of-bed activities as prescribed.	Lungs remain clear and free of secretions.
PLANNING	IMPLEMENTATION	EVALUATION
Client reports adequate sensation in affected area.	Monitor color, motion, and sensation in affected area. Monitor for adequate and palpable pulses.	Palpable pulses are noted. Adequate tissue perfusion in affected area is maintained.
PLANNING	IMPLEMENTATION	EVALUATION
Client remains free of infection.	Monitor temperature. Monitor wound status. Monitor for signs of infection.	Temperature remains within normal limits. Wound remains free of infection.
PLANNING	IMPLEMENTATION	EVALUATION
Client identifies factors that may cause injury. Client avoids situations that may cause physical injury.	Assess clients motor and sensory deficit to determine safety needs. Provide assistive devices as appropriate to prevent injury. Instruct client in the use of assistive devices. Keep environment free of obstructions. Document client's safe performance of activities.	Client demonstrates correct use of assistive devices. Client achieves optimal level of ambulation without injury.
PLANNING	IMPLEMENTATION	EVALUATION
Client remains free of skin breakdown as a result of immobility. Client's surgical wound demonstrates signs of the healing process.	Monitor skin integrity. Turn and reposition client. Monitor surgical wound for signs of healing. Encourage ambulation and out-of-bed activity.	Surgical wound heals. Client's skin remains intact.

PLANNING	IMPLEMENTATION	EVALUATION
Client requests assistance with mobilization activities. Client identifies mobility limitations and restrictions.	Monitor mobility limitations. Assist client with mobility. Provide assistive devices as appropriate for ambulation. Instruct client in the use of assistive devices. Encourage verbalization regarding mobility limitations and restrictions.	Client accepts mobility limitations. Client uses assistive devices appropriately.
PLANNING	IMPLEMENTATION	EVALUATION
Client verbalizes the need for assistance. Client participates in self-care to optimal level.	Assess the need for assistance with self-care. Assist client with self-care needs as necessary. Assist client in care, promoting independence as much as possible.	Client performs independent self-care activities to optimal level of functioning.
PLANNING	IMPLEMENTATION	EVALUATION
Client verbalizes the presence of optimal elimination patterns.	Monitor intake and output (I&O). Monitor bowel sounds. Assess dietary habits. Encourage optimal activity to stimulate bowel elimination. Instruct client regarding the need for adequate fluids and fiber in the diet.	Client remains free of elimination alterations related to immobility.
PLANNING	IMPLEMENTATION	EVALUATION
Client shares grief and loss with a significant person. Client actively participates in the decision-making process.	Encourage client to express grief and loss. Assist client to recognize own strengths and available support systems.	Client uses available support systems.

◆ CLIENT NEEDS

SAFE, EFFECTIVE CARE ENVIRONMENT

Client rights
Confidentiality regarding disorder and plan of care
Informed consent for diagnostic treatments and surgical procedures
Physical therapy and occupational therapy referrals
Dietary consultation
Asepsis related to wounds
Standard precautions
Preventing injury from accidents

HEALTH PROMOTION AND MAINTENANCE

The aging process and disease prevention
Health promotion related to diet and activity
Techniques related to data collection of the musculoskeletal system
Home care instructions regarding care related to musculoskeletal disorder
Reinforcement regarding the importance of prescribed therapy

PSYCHOSOCIAL INTEGRITY

Grief and loss related to mobility limitations and restrictions
The ability to cope with feelings of isolation and loss of independence
Sensory and perceptual alterations
Cultural, religious, and spiritual influences
Situational role changes as a result of musculoskeletal disorder

Unexpected body image changes as a result of injury or disease
Available support systems and use of community resources

PHYSIOLOGICAL INTEGRITY

Use of assistive devices for mobility such as canes, walkers, and crutches
Promoting normal elimination patterns
Measures to promote comfort
Promoting self-care measures
Pharmacological medications, actions, agents, side effects, and adverse effects
Complications related to procedures or injuries
Emergency care for a fracture or other injury
Complications of a fracture
Care related to casts and traction
Postoperative interventions
Rheumatoid arthritis
Osteoporosis

BIBLIOGRAPHY

deWit, S. (1998). *Essentials of medical-surgical nursing* (4th ed.). Philadelphia: W. B. Saunders.

Hill, S. & Howlett, H. (1997). *Success in practical nursing: Personal and vocational issues* (3rd ed.). Philadelphia: W. B. Saunders.

Leahy, J., & Kizilay, P. (1998). *Foundations of nursing practice: A nursing process approach.* Philadelphia: W. B. Saunders.

Luckmann, J. (1997). *Saunders manual of nursing care.* Philadelphia: W. B. Saunders.

Monahan, F., & Neighbors, M. (1998). *Medical-surgical nursing: Foundations for clinical practice* (2nd ed.). Philadelphia: W. B. Saunders.

National Council of State Boards of Nursing (1998). *National Council detailed test plan for the NCLEX-PN examination.* Chicago: Author.

O'Toole, M. (1997). *Miller-Keane encyclopedia & dictionary of medicine, nursing, & allied health* (6th ed.). Philadelphia: W. B. Saunders.

CHAPTER 56

Musculoskeletal System

· ·

I. Anatomy and Physiology

A. Skeleton
1. Axial portion
   a. Cranium
   b. Vertebrae
   c. Ribs
2. Appendicular portion
   a. Limbs
   b. Shoulders
   c. Hips
B. Types of bones (Box 56–1)
1. Spongy bone
   a. Located in the ends of long bones and the center of flat and irregular bones
   b. Can withstand forces applied in many directions
2. Dense (compact) bones
   a. Covers spongy bone
   b. Cylinder around a central marrow cavity
   c. Can withstand force predominantly in one direction
3. Characteristics of the bones
   a. Support and protect structures of the body
   b. Provide attachments for muscles, tendons, and ligaments
   c. Contain tissue in the central cavities, which aids in formation of blood cells
   d. Assists in regulating calcium and phosphate concentrations
4. Bone growth
   a. The length of bone growth is a result of the ossification of the epiphyseal cartilage at the ends of bones, and bone growth stops between the ages of 18 and 25 years
   b. The width of bone growth is a result of the activity of osteoblasts and occurs throughout life but does slow down with the aging process
   c. Bone absorption around the bone marrow continues throughout life; therefore, bones become weaker with aging
C. Types of joints (Table 56–1)
1. Characteristics of the joints
   a. Allow the movement between bones
   b. Formed where two bones join
   c. Surfaces are covered with cartilage
   d. Enclosed in a capsule
   e. Contain a cavity filled with synovial fluid
   f. Ligaments hold the bone and joint in the correct position
   g. Articulation is the meeting point of two or more joints
2. Synovial fluid
   a. Found in joint capsule
   b. Formed by synovial membrane, which lines joint capsule
   c. Lubricates the cartilage
   d. Cushion for shocks
D. Muscles
1. Characteristics of muscles
   a. Made up of bundles of muscle fibers

BOX 56–1. Types of Bones

Long	Flat
Short	Irregular

Table 56–1. Types of Joints

Type	Description
Synarthrosis	Fibrous or fixed joints
	No movement associated with these joints
Amphiarthrosis	Cartilaginous joints
	Slightly movable joints
Diarthrosis	Synovial joints
	Ball-and-socket joints
Condyloid	Freely movable joints
	Synovial joints allow frictionless, painless movement

b. Provide the force to move bones
c. Assist in maintaining posture
d. Assist with heat production

2. The process of contraction and relaxation
   a. Muscle contraction and relaxation require large amounts of adenosine triphosphate (ATP)
   b. Contraction also requires calcium, which functions as a catalyst
   c. Acetylcholine released by the motor end plate of the motor neuron initiates an action potential
   d. Acetylcholine is then destroyed by acetylcholinesterase
   e. Calcium is required to contract muscle fibers and acts as a catalyst for the enzyme needed for the sliding together action of actin and myosin
   f. Following contraction, ATP transports calcium out in order to allow actin and myosin to slide apart and allow the muscle to relax

3. Skeletal muscles
   a. Are attached to two bones and cross at least one joint
   b. The point of origin is the point of attachment on the bone closest to the trunk
   c. The point of insertion is the point of attachment on the bone farthest from the trunk
   d. Skeletal muscles act in groups
   e. Prime movers contract to produce movement
   f. Antagonists relax
   g. Synergists contract to stabilize
   h. Nerves activate and control the muscles

II. Risk Factors Associated with Musculoskeletal Disorders (Box 56–2)

III. Diagnostic Tests

A. X-rays
   1. Description: a commonly used procedure to diagnose disorders of the musculoskeletal system
   2. Implementation
      a. Handle injured area carefully
      b. Administer analgesics as prescribed prior to the procedure, particularly if the client is in pain
      c. Remove any radiopaque objects such as jewelry
      d. Shield the client's testes, ovaries, or pregnant abdomen
      e. The client must lie still during an x-ray
      f. Inform clients that exposure to radiation is minimal and not dangerous
      g. Health care provider is to wear a lead apron if staying in the room with the client

---

BOX 56–2. Risk Factors Associated with Musculoskeletal Disorders

Trauma and injury
Falls
Autoimmune disorders
Infection
Degenerative conditions such as rheumatoid arthritis
Obesity
Calcium deficiency
Postmenopausal states
Metabolic disorders such as diabetes mellitus
Neoplastic disorders
Hyperuricemia
Medications such as corticosteroids

B. Arthrocentesis
   1. Description
      a. Involves aspirating synovial fluid, blood, or pus via a needle inserted into a joint cavity
      b. Medication may be instilled into the joint if necessary to alleviate inflammation
   2. Implementation
      a. Obtain a consent form
      b. Apply a compress bandage postprocedure as prescribed
      c. Instruct the client to rest the joint for 8 to 24 hours' postprocedure
      d. Instruct the client to notify the physician if a fever or swelling of the joint occurs

C. Arthrogram
   1. Description
      a. A radiographic examination of the soft tissues of the joint structures used to diagnose trauma to the joint capsule or ligaments
      b. A local anesthesia is used for the procedure. A contrast medium or air is injected into the joint cavity and the joint is moved through range of motion as a series of x-rays is taken
   2. Implementation
      a. Inform the client to fast from food and fluids for 8 hours prior to the procedure
      b. Assess for client allergies to iodine or seafood prior to the procedure
      c. Obtain a consent form
      d. Inform the client of the need to remain as still as possible except when asked to reposition
      e. Minimize the use of the joint for 12 hours following the procedure
      f. Instruct the client that the joint may be edematous and tender for 1 to 2 days after the procedure and may be treated with ice packs and analgesics as prescribed
      g. Inform the client that if edema and tenderness last longer than 2 days to notify the physician
      h. If knee arthrography was performed, an

Ace wrap over the knee may be prescribed for 3 to 4 days
   i. If air was used for injection, crepitus may be felt in the joint for up to 2 days

D. Arthroscopy
1. Description
   a. Provides an endoscopic examination of various joints
   b. Articular cartilage abnormalities can be assessed, loose bodies can be removed, and the cartilage trimmed
   c. A biopsy may be performed during the procedure
2. Implementation
   a. Instruct the client to fast for 8 to 12 hours prior to the procedure
   b. Obtain a consent form
   c. Administer pain medication as prescribed postprocedure
   d. An elastic wrap should be worn for 2 to 4 days as prescribed
   e. Instruct the client that walking without weight bearing is usually permitted after sensation returns but to limit activity for 1 to 4 days as prescribed
   f. Instruct the client to elevate the extremity as often as possible for 2 days and to place ice on the site to minimize swelling
   g. Reinforce instructions regarding the use of crutches, which may be used for 5 to 7 days postprocedure when walking
   h. Advise the client to notify the physician if fever, increased knee pain, or if edema continues for more than 3 days

E. Bone scan
1. Description
   a. Radioisotopc is injected IV and will collect in areas that indicate abnormal bone metabolism and some fractures if they exist
   b. The isotope is excreted in urine and feces within 48 hours and is not harmful to others
2. Implementation
   a. Hold fluids for 4 hours prior to the procedure
   b. Obtain a consent form
   c. Remove all jewelry and metal objects
   d. Following the injection of the radioisotope, the client must drink 32 ounces of water (if not contraindicated) to promote renal filtering of excess isotope
   e. From 1 to 3 hours after injection, have the client void; then the scanning procedure is performed
   f. Inform the client of the need to lie supine during the procedure and that the procedure is not painful
   g. No special precautions are required after the procedure because a minimal amount of radioactivity exists in the isotope
   h. Monitor the injection site for redness and swelling

   i. Encourage oral fluid intake following the procedure

F. Bone or muscle biopsy
1. Description: may be done during surgery or through aspiration, or punch or needle biopsy
2. Implementation
   a. Obtain a consent form
   b. Monitor for bleeding, swelling, and hematoma or severe pain
   c. Elevate the site for 24 hours following the procedure to reduce edema
   d. Apply ice packs as prescribed to prevent the development of a hematoma
   e. Monitor for signs of infection following the procedure
   f. Inform the client that mild to moderate discomfort is normal following the procedure

G. Electromyography (EMG)
1. Description
   a. Measures electrical potential associated with skeletal muscle contractions
   b. Needles are inserted into the muscle and recordings of muscular electrical activity are traced on recording paper through an oscilloscope
2. Implementation
   a. Obtain a consent form
   b. Instruct the client that the needle insertion is uncomfortable
   c. Instruct the client not to take any stimulants or sedatives 24 hours prior to the procedure
   d. Inform the client that slight bruising may occur at needle insertion sites

H. Myelogram
1. Description: injection of dye or air into subarachnoid space to detect abnormalities of the spinal cord and vertebrae
2. Implementation preprocedure
   a. Obtain a consent
   b. Provide hydration for at least 12 hours before the test
   c. Assess for allergies to iodine
   d. Premedicate for sedation as prescribed
3. Implementation postprocedure
   a. Perform vital signs and neurological assessment frequently as prescribed
   b. If a water-based dye is used, elevate the head 15 to 30 degrees for 8 hours as prescribed
   c. If an oil-based dye is used, keep the client flat 6 to 8 hours as prescribed
   d. If air is used, keep the head lower than the trunk
   e. Force fluids and monitor I&O

IV. Fractures

A. Description: a break in the continuity of the bone caused by trauma, twisting as a result of muscle spasm or indirect loss of leverage, or bone

---

BOX 56–3. Types of Fractures

Closed or simple: skin over the fractured area remains intact
Greenstick: one side of the bone is broken and the other is bent; most commonly seen in children
Transverse: the bone is fractured straight across
Oblique: the break extends in an oblique direction
Spiral: the break partially encircles bone
Comminuted: the bone is splintered or crushed, with three or more fragments
Complete: the bone is completely separated by a break into two parts
Incomplete: a partial break in the bone
Open-Compound: the bone is exposed to air through a break in the skin, and soft tissue injury and infection are common
Impacted: a part of fractured bone is driven into another bone
Depressed: bone fragments are driven inward
Compression: a fractured bone compressed by another bone
Pathological: a fracture due to weakening of the bone structure by pathological processes such as neoplasia or osteomalocia; also called spontaneous fracture

---

decalcification and disease that results in osteopenia
B. Types of fractures (Box 56–3)
C. Data collection in a fracture of an extremity
  1. Pain or tenderness over the involved area
  2. Loss of function
  3. Obvious deformity
  4. Crepitation
  5. Erythema, edema, and ecchymosis
  6. Muscle spasm and impaired sensation
D. Initial care of a fractured extremity (Box 56–4)
  1. Immobilize affected extremity
  2. If a compound fracture exists, splint the extremity and cover the wound with a sterile dressing
E. **Reduction:** restoring the bone to proper alignment
  1. Closed **reduction**
    a. Performed by manual manipulation
    b. May be performed under local or general anesthesia
    c. A **cast** may be applied following **reduction**
  2. Open **reduction**
    a. Involves a surgical intervention
    b. May be treated with **internal fixation** devices

BOX 56–4. Interventions for a Fracture

Reduction	Traction
Fixation	Casts

---

  c. The client may be placed in **traction** or a **cast** following the procedure
F. Fixation
  1. Internal **fixation** (Fig. 56–1)
    a. Follows open **reduction**
    b. Involves the application of screws, plates, pins, or nails to hold the fragments in alignment
    c. May involve the removal of damaged bone and replacement with a prosthesis
    d. Provides immediate bone strength
    e. Risk of infection is associated with the procedure
  2. External **fixation**
    a. An external frame is used, with multiple pins applied through the bone
    b. Provides more freedom of movement than with **traction**
G. **Traction** (Fig. 56–2)
  1. Description
    a. The exertion of a pulling force applied in two directions to reduce and immobilize a fracture
    b. Provides proper bone alignment and reduces muscle spasms
  2. Implementation
    a. Maintain proper body alignment
    b. Ensure that the weights hang freely and do not touch the floor
    c. Do not remove or lift weights without a physician's order
    d. Ensure that pulleys are not obstructed and that ropes in pulleys move freely
    e. Place knots in ropes to prevent slipping
    f. Check ropes for fraying
H. Skeletal **traction** (Fig. 56–3)
  1. Description: mechanically applied to bone using pins, wires, or tongs
  2. Implementation
    a. Monitor color, motion, and sensation (CMS) of the affected extremity
    b. Monitor the insertion sites for redness, swelling, or drainage
    c. Provide insertion site care as prescribed
  3. Cervical tongs and halo fixation device (refer to Chapter 54 regarding care to the client with these devices)
I. Skin **traction** (Box 56–5)
  1. Description: **traction** applied by the use of elastic bandages or adhesive
  2. Cervical skin **traction**
    a. Relieves muscle spasms and compression in upper extremities and the neck

---

BOX 56–5. Types of Skin Traction

Cervical traction	Russell's traction
Buck's traction	Pelvic traction
Bryant's traction	

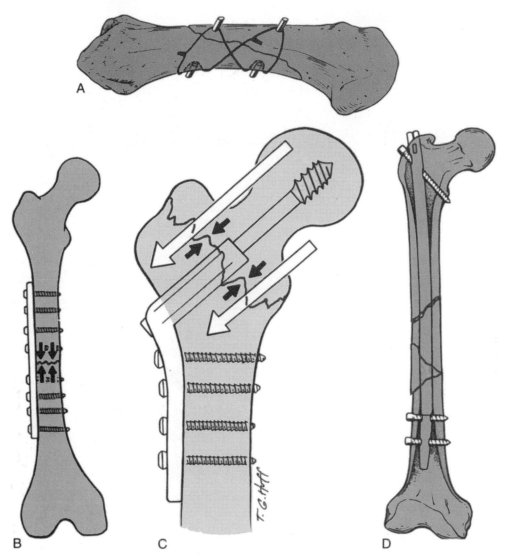

FIGURE 56–1. Examples of internal fixation. *A,* Tension band wiring technique using Kirschner wires for fracture of a phalanx. *B,* Compression plate to the lateral aspect of the femur. *C,* Sliding hip screw. *D,* Static locked intramedullary and fixed to both proximal and distal fragments of the femur. (From Browner, B. D., Jupiter, J. B., Levine, A. M., & Trafton, P. G. [1992]. *Skeletal trauma: Fractures, Dislocations, Ligamentous Injuries.* [2nd ed.]. Philadelphia: W. B. Saunders. pp. 253, 254, 942, 1551.)

b. Uses a head halter and a chin pad to attach the **traction**
c. Use powder to protect the ears from friction rub
d. Position the client with the head of the bed elevated 30 to 40 degrees and attach the weights to a pulley system over the head of the bed
3. Buck's skin traction
  a. Used to alleviate muscle spasms; immobilizes a lower limb by maintaining a straight pull on the limb with the use of weights
  b. A boot appliance is applied to attach to the **traction**
  c. Weight is attached to a pulley; allow weights to hang freely over the edge of the bed

d. Not more than 8 to 10 pounds of weight should be applied
e. Elevate the foot of the bed to provide the **traction**
4. Bryant's and Russell's skin **traction** (refer to Chapter 34 regarding information related to these types of traction)
5. Pelvic skin **traction**
  a. Used to relieve low back, hip, or leg pain and to reduce muscle spasm

---

BOX 56–6. Balanced Suspension

Thomas splint with Pearson attachment
Steinmann pin
Kirschner wires

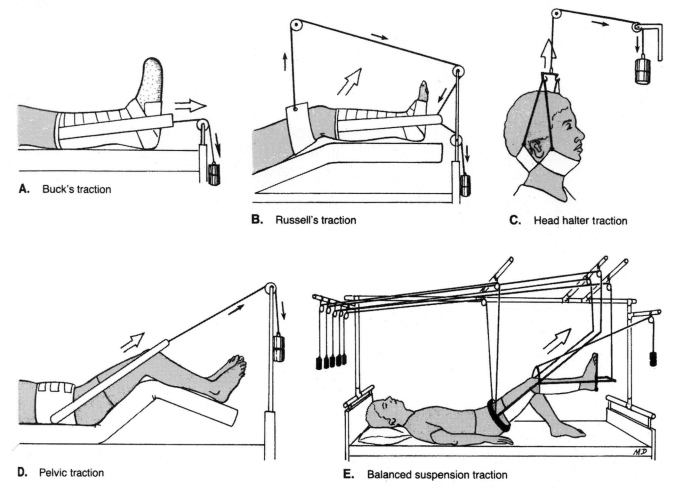

A. Buck's traction

B. Russell's traction

C. Head halter traction

D. Pelvic traction

E. Balanced suspension traction

FIGURE 56–2. Examples of common types of traction. (From Black, J. M., & Matassarin-Jacobs, E. [1993]. *Luckmann and Sorensen's medical-surgical nursing: A psychophysiologic approach.* [4th ed.]. Philadelphia: W. B. Saunders. p. 1885.)

   b. Apply the **traction** snugly over the pelvis and iliac crest and attach to weights
   c. Use measures as prescribed to prevent the client from slipping down in bed
J. Balanced suspension (Box 56–6)
  1. Description
    a. Used with skin or skeletal **traction**

   b. Used to approximate fractures of the femur, tibia, or fibula
   c. Produced by a counterforce other than the client
  2. Implementation
    a. Position the client in low Fowler's, either on the side or back

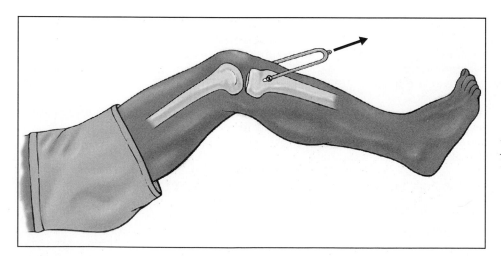

FIGURE 56–3. Skeletal traction. (From Monahan, F., & Neighbors, M. [1998]. *Medical-surgical nursing: Foundations for clinical practice.* [2nd ed.]. Philadelphia: W. B. Saunders. p. 861.)

b. Maintain a 20-degree angle from the thigh to the bed
c. Protect the skin from breakdown
d. Provide pin care if pins are used with the skeletal **traction**
e. Clean pin site with sterile normal saline and hydrogen peroxide or Betadine as prescribed or per agency procedure

K. Dunlop's traction
 1. Description: horizontal traction to align fractures of the humerus; vertical traction maintains the forearm in proper alignment
 2. Implementation: nursing care is similar to Buck's traction

L. Casts
 1. Description: made of plaster or fiberglass to provide immobilization of bone and joints after a fracture or injury
 2. Implementation
  a. Keep the **cast** and extremity elevated
  b. Allow a wet **cast** 24 to 48 hours to dry (synthetic casts dry in 20 minutes)
  c. Handle a wet **cast** with the palms of the hands until dry
  d. Turn the extremity unless contraindicated so that all sides of the wet **cast** will dry
  e. Heat can be used to dry the **cast**
  f. The **cast** will change from a dull to a shiny substance when dry
  g. Examine the skin and **cast** for pressure areas
  h. Monitor the extremity for circulatory impairment such as pain, swelling, discoloration, tingling, numbness, coolness, or diminished pulse
  i. Notify the physician immediately if circulatory compromise occurs
  j. Prepare for bivalving or cutting the **cast** if circulatory impairment occurs (Fig. 56–4)

k. Petal the **cast**; maintain smooth edges around the **cast** to prevent crumbling of the **cast** material
l. Monitor the client's temperature
m. Monitor for the presence of a foul odor, which may indicate infection
n. Monitor drainage by circling the area of drainage on the **cast**
o. Monitor for warmth on the **cast**
p. Monitor for wet spots, which may indicate a need for drying, or the presence of drainage under the **cast**
q. If an open draining area exists on the affected extremity, a cut-out portion of the **cast** or a window will be made by the physician
r. Instruct the client not to stick objects inside the **cast**
s. Teach the client to keep the **cast** clean and dry
t. Instruct the client on isometric exercises to prevent muscle atrophy

V. Crutch Walking

A. Description
 1. An accurate measurement of the client for crutches is important because an incorrect measurement could damage the brachial plexus
 2. The distance between the axilla and arm pieces on the crutches should be two fingerwidths in the axilla space
 3. The elbows should be slightly flexed 20 to 30 degrees when walking
 4. When ambulating with the client, stand on the affected side
 5. Instruct the client never to rest the axilla on the axillary bars
 6. Instruct the client to look up and outward when ambulating
 7. Instruct the client to stop ambulation if numbness or tingling in the hands or arms occurs

B. Crutch gaits (Table 56–2)

C. Assisting the client with crutches to sit and stand
 1. Place the unaffected leg against the front of the chair
 2. Move the crutches to the affected side and grasp the chair's arm with the hand on the unaffected side
 3. Flex the knee of the unaffected leg to lower self into the chair while placing the affected leg straight out in front
 4. Reverse steps to move from a sitting to a standing position

D. Going up and down stairs
 1. Up the stairs
  a. The client moves the unaffected leg up first
  b. The client moves the affected leg and the crutches up

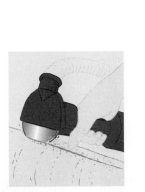
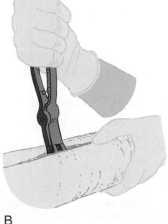

FIGURE 56–4. *A,* Cast saw with its blade. *B,* Cast spreader. (From Black, J., & Matassarin-Jacobs, E. [1997]. *Medical-surgical nursing: A nursing process approach.* [5th ed.]. Philadelphia: W. B. Saunders. p. 2152.)

Table 56–2. Crutch Gaits

Gait	Description	Pattern
Four-point gait	Sequence 1. Advance left crutch. 2. Advance right foot. 3. Advance right crutch. 4. Advance left foot. Advantages: most stable crutch gait. Requirements: partial weight bearing on both legs.	
Three-point gait	Sequence 1. Advance both crutches forward with the affected leg and shift weight to crutches. 2. Advance unaffected leg and shift weight onto it. Advantages: allows the affected leg to be partially or completely free of weight bearing. Requirements: full weight bearing on one leg, balance, and upper-body strength.	
Two-point gait	Sequence 1. Advance left crutch and right foot. 2. Advance right crutch and left foot. Advantages: Faster version of the four-point gait, more normal walking pattern (arms and legs moving in opposition). Requirements: Partial weight bearing on both legs, balance.	

2. Down stairs
   a. The client moves the crutches and the affected leg down
   b. The client moves unaffected leg down

VI. Canes and Walkers

A. Description: made of a lightweight material with a rubber tip at the bottom
B. Implementation
   1. Stand at the affected side of the client when ambulating
   2. The handle should be at the level of the client's greater trochanter
   3. The client's elbow should be flexed at a 25- to 30-degree angle
   4. Instruct the client to hold the cane close to the body
   5. Instruct the client to hold the cane in the hand on the unaffected side so that the cane and weaker leg can work together with each step
   6. Instruct the client to move the cane at the same time as the affected leg
   7. Instruct the client to inspect the rubber tips regularly for worn places
C. Hemicanes or quadripod canes
   1. Used for clients who have the use of only one upper extremity
   2. Hemicanes provide more security than a quadripod cane; however, both types provide more security than a single-tipped cane
   3. Position the cane at the client's unaffected side with the straight nonangled side adjacent to the body
   4. Position the cane 6 inches from client's side with the handgrips level with the greater trochanter
D. Walker
   1. Stand adjacent to the client on the affected side
   2. Instruct the client to put all four points of the walker flat on the floor before putting weight on the hand pieces
   3. Instruct the client to move the walker forward and to walk into it

VII. Complications of Fractures (Box 56–7)

A. Fat embolism
   1. Description
      a. An embolism originating in the bone marrow that occurs after a fracture

BOX 56–7. Complications of Fractures

Compartment syndrome	Avascular necrosis
Fat emboli	Pulmonary emboli
Infection	

b. Clients with long bone fractures are at the greatest risk for development of **fat embolism**

c. Usually occurs within 48 hours following the injury

2. Data collection
   a. Restlessness
   b. Mental status changes
   c. Tachycardia, tachypnea, and hypotension
   d. Dyspnea
   e. Petechial rash over the upper chest and neck

3. Implementation: notify the physician immediately

B. **Compartment syndrome**

1. Description
   a. Increased pressure within one or more compartments causing massive compromise of circulation to an area
   b. Leads to decreased perfusion and tissue anoxia
   c. Within 4 to 6 hours after the onset of **compartment syndrome,** neuromuscular damage is irreversible

2. Data collection
   a. Increased pain and swelling
   b. Pain with passive motion
   c. Inability to move joints
   d. Loss of sensation (paresthesia)
   e. Pulselessness

3. Implementation: notify the physician immediately

C. Infection

1. Description: can be caused by the interruption of the integrity of the skin

2. Data collection
   a. Fever
   b. Pain
   c. Erythema in the area surrounding the fracture
   d. Tachycardia
   e. Elevated WBC count

3. Implementation: notify the physician

D. Avascular necrosis

1. Description: an interruption in the blood supply to the bony tissue, which results in the death of the bone

2. Data collection
   a. Pain
   b. Decreased sensation

3. Implementation
   a. Notify the physician if pain or decreased sensation occurs
   b. Prepare the client for removal of necrotic tissue because it serves as a focus for infection

E. Pulmonary embolism

1. Description: caused by immobility precipitated by a fracture

2. Data collection
   a. Restlessness and apprehension
   b. Dyspnea

c. Diaphoresis

3. Implementation
   a. Notify the physician if signs of emboli are present
   b. Anticoagulant therapy may be prescribed

VIII. Fractured Hip

A. Types

1. Intracapsular
   a. Bone is broken inside the joint
   b. Skin **traction** is applied preoperatively to immobilize and prevent pain
   c. Treatment includes a total hip replacement or **internal fixation** with replacement of the femoral head with a prosthesis (Fig. 56–5)
   d. Avoid hip flexion to prevent displacement

2. Extracapsular
   a. Fracture can occur at the greater trochanter or can be an intertrochanteric fracture
   b. Trochanteric fracture is outside the joint
   c. Preoperative treatment includes balanced suspension **traction**
   d. Avoid hip flexion to prevent displacement
   e. Surgical treatment includes **internal fixation** with nail plate, screws, or wires

B. Implementation postoperatively

1. Maintain leg and hip in proper alignment
2. Prevent flexion or external or internal rotation
3. Turn the client from the back to the unaffected side
4. Do not position to the affected side unless prescribed by the physician
5. Maintain leg abduction to prevent internal or external rotation
6. Use a trochanter roll to prevent external rotation
7. Ensure that hip flexion angle does not exceed 60 to 80 degrees

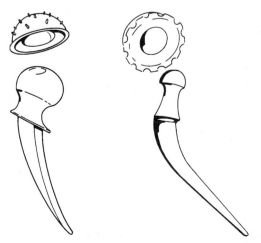

FIGURE 56–5. Hip prostheses. (From deWit, S. [1998]. *Essentials of medical-surgical nursing.* [4th ed.]. Philadelphia: W. B. Saunders. p. 695.)

8. Elevate the head of the bed 30 to 45 degrees for meals only
9. Ambulate as prescribed by the physician
10. Avoid weight bearing on affected leg as prescribed; instruct the client on the use of a walker to avoid weight bearing
11. Keep the operative leg extended, supported, and elevated when getting the client out of bed
12. Avoid hip flexion greater than 90 degrees and avoid low chairs when out of bed
13. Monitor the wound for infection or hemorrhage
14. Monitor circulation and sensation of the affected side
15. Maintain the Hemovac if in place; maintain compression to facilitate drainage and monitor and record Hemovac output
16. Hemovac drainage should continuously decrease in amount, and by 48 hours' postoperatively drainage should be approximately 30 mL in an 8-hour period
17. Maintain the use of antiembolism stockings and encourage the client to flex and extend the feet and ankles
18. Provide continuous passive motion (CPM) the first day postoperatively with increasing degrees of flexion up to 90 degrees as prescribed
19. Instruct the client to avoid crossing the legs and bending-over activities
20. Physical therapy will begin postoperatively as prescribed by the physician

IX. Total Knee Replacement

A. Description: implantation of a device to substitute for the femoral condyles and the tibial joint surfaces
B. Implementation postoperatively
   1. Monitor the incision for drainage and infection
   2. Maintain the Hemovac if in place
   3. Begin CPM 24 to 48 hours as prescribed to exercise the knee and provide moderate flexion and extension
   4. Administer analgesics before CPM to decrease pain
   5. The leg should not be dangled to prevent dislocation
   6. Maintain Ace wrap or antiembolism stockings if prescribed
   7. Out of bed 2 to 3 days postoperatively as prescribed
   8. Avoid weight bearing and instruct the client in crutch walking

X. Herniation: Intervertebral Disk

A. Description: nucleus of the disk protrudes into the annulus, causing nerve compression
B. Cervical disk

1. Occurs at C5 to C6 and C6 to C7 interspaces
2. Diagnosis is determined by cervical myelography
3. Causes pain and stiffness in the neck, top of the shoulders, scapula, upper extremities, and head
4. Produces paresthesia and numbness of the upper extremities
5. Implementation
   a. Provide bed rest to relieve pressure, and reduce inflammation and edema
   b. Provide immobilization as prescribed via cervical collar, **traction,** or brace
   c. Apply hot, moist compresses as prescribed to increase the blood flow and relax spasms
   d. Instruct the client to avoid flexing, extending, or rotating the neck
   e. Instruct the client that while sleeping to avoid the prone position and keep the head in a neutral position using a feather pillow
   f. Instruct the client to avoid long automobile rides
   g. Instruct the client in the use of analgesics, sedatives, anti-inflammatory agents, and steroids as prescribed
   h. Prepare the client for corticosteroid injection into the epidural space if prescribed
   i. Assist the client with the application of a cervical collar or cervical traction as prescribed
6. Cervical collar
   a. Used for cervical disk herniation
   b. Holds the head in a neutral or slightly flexed position
   c. Client may have to wear a cervical collar 24 hours a day
   d. Inspect the skin under the collar for irritation
   e. When pain subsides, the client is taught cervical isometric exercises to strengthen the muscles
C. Lumbar disk
   1. Occurs at L4 to L5 or L5 to S1 interspaces
   2. Diagnosis is determined by lumbar myelography
   3. Postural deformity occurs
   4. Produces muscle weakness, sensory loss, and alteration of the tendon reflexes
   5. The client experiences low back pain and muscle spasms with radiation of the pain into one hip and down the leg (sciatica)
   6. Pain is aggravated by bending, lifting, straining, sneezing, and coughing and is relieved by bed rest
   7. Implementation
      a. Bed rest on a firm mattress in semi-Fowler's with moderate hip and knee flexion
      b. Apply moist heat and massage as prescribed

c. Instruct the client to sleep on the side with knees and hips in a position of flexion with a pillow between the legs

d. Apply pelvic **traction** as prescribed to relieve muscle spasms

e. Begin ambulation gradually as the inflammation and edema subside

f. Instruct the client in the use of muscle relaxants, anti-inflammatory medications, and steroids as prescribed

g. Instruct the client in the use of a corset or brace as prescribed

h. Instruct the client regarding correct posture while sitting, standing, walking and working

i. Instruct the client to lift objects by bending the knees and keeping the back straight, avoiding lifting anything above the elbows

j. Instruct the client regarding a weight-control program as prescribed

k. Instruct the client in an exercise program as prescribed to strengthen abdominal and back muscles

D. Disk surgery (Box 56–8)

1. Implementation preoperatively
   a. Reassure the client that surgery will not weaken the back
   b. Instruct the client regarding coughing and deep-breathing exercises
   c. Instruct the client about log rolling and range of motion exercises

2. Implementation postoperative: cervical disk
   a. Monitor for respiratory difficulty
   b. Encourage coughing and deep breathing
   c. Monitor for hoarseness and the inability to cough effectively because this may indicate laryngeal nerve damage
   d. Use throat sprays or lozenges for a sore throat and do not use those that may numb the throat, to avoid choking
   e. Monitor the wound for drainage
   f. Provide a soft diet if the client complains of dysphagia
   g. Monitor for sudden return of radicular pain, which may indicate that the cervical spine has become unstable

3. Implementation postoperative: lumbar disk
   a. Monitor for wound hemorrhage
   b. Monitor sensation and motor ability of lower extremities as well as color, temperature, and sensation of toes

---

BOX 56–8. Types of Disk Surgery

Diskectomy: removal of herniated disk tissue and related matter
Laminectomy: removal of the lamina
Laminotomy: division of the lamina of a vertebra
Diskectomy with fusion: fusion of vertebrae with bone graft
Chemolysis: injections to dissolve affected disk

---

c. Monitor for urinary retention, paralytic ileus, and constipation

d. Initiate measures to prevent constipation such as high-fiber diet, increased fluids, and stool softeners as prescribed

e. When turning and repositioning the client, place the bed in a flat position and a pillow between the legs; turn the client as a unit (log roll) without twisting the client's back

f. When positioning the client, a pillow is placed under the head with the knees slightly flexed

g. Avoid extreme knee flexion when the client is lying on the side

h. To assist the client out of bed, raise the head of the bed while the client lies on the side; the client's head and shoulders are supported by the first nurse as the client pushes to a sitting position, while the second nurse eases the client's legs over the side of the bed

i. Instruct the client to avoid sitting because it places a strain on surgical site

j. Administer narcotics and sedatives as prescribed to relieve pain and anxiety

k. Encourage early ambulation

l. Assist the client with the use of a back brace or corset if prescribed

XI. Amputation (Fig. 56–6)

A. Description: the surgical removal of a limb or part of a limb

B. Implementation postoperatively

1. Monitor vital signs

2. Monitor for infection and hemorrhage

3. Mark bleeding and drainage on the dressing if it occurs

4. Keep a tourniquet at the bedside

5. Monitor for pulmonary emboli

6. Observe and prevent contractures

7. Monitor for signs of necrosis and neuroma

8. Evaluate for phantom limb pain, explain the sensation to the client, and medicate the client as prescribed

9. During the first 24 hours, elevate the foot of the bed to reduce edema, then keep the bed flat to prevent hip flexion contractures as prescribed

10. Do not elevate the stump itself because elevation can cause flexion contracture of the hip joint

11. After 24 and 48 hours' postoperatively, position the client prone as prescribed to stretch the muscles and prevent flexion contractures of the hip

12. In the prone position, place a pillow under the abdomen and stump and keep the legs close together to prevent abduction

13. Maintain application of an Ace wrap or elastic stump shrinker as prescribed to provide stump shrinkage

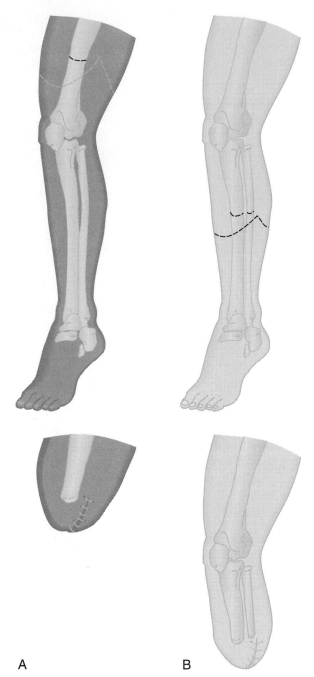

FIGURE 56–6. Above and below the knee amputation. (From Black, J., & Matassarin-Jacobs, E. [1997]. *Medical-surgical nursing: A nursing process approach.* [5th ed.]. Philadelphia: W. B. Saunders. p. 1420.)

14. Remove and rewrap the Ace bandage or elastic stump shrinker three to four times daily as prescribed
15. Wash the stump with mild soap or water and apply lanolin to the skin if dry
16. Massage skin toward the suture line to increase circulation
17. Prepare for a **cast** application if prescribed to prepare the stump for prosthesis
18. Encourage the client to look at the stump
19. Encourage verbalization regarding loss of

body part and assist the client to identify coping mechanisms to deal with loss

C. Implementation of below-the-knee amputation
   1. Prevent edema
   2. Do not allow stump to hang over the edge of the bed
   3. Do not allow the client to sit for long periods
D. Implementation of above-the-knee amputation
   1. Prevent internal or external rotation of the limb
   2. Place a sandbag or rolled towel along the outside of the thigh to prevent rotation
E. Rehabilitation
   1. Instruct the client in crutch walking
   2. Prepare the stump for prosthesis
   3. Prepare the client for the fitting of the stump for prosthesis
   4. Instruct the client in exercises to maintain range of motion
   5. Provide psychosocial support to the client

XII. Rheumatoid Arthritis (RA)

A. Description
   1. Chronic systemic inflammatory disease; the cause is unknown
   2. Leads to destruction of connective tissue and synovial membrane within joints
   3. Weakens and leads to dislocation of the joint and permanent deformity
   4. Formation of pannus occurs at the junction of synovial tissue and articular cartilage projecting into the joint cavity and causing necrosis
   5. Exacerbations are increased by physical or emotional stress
   6. Risk factors include exposure to infectious agents; fatigue and emotional stress can exacerbate the condition
   7. Vasculitis can cause malfunction and eventual failure of an organ or system
B. Data collection
   1. Inflammation, tenderness, and stiffness of the joints
   2. Moderate to severe pain and morning stiffness lasting longer than 30 minutes
   3. Joint deformities, muscle atrophy, and decreased range of motion
   4. Spongy, soft feeling in joints
   5. Low-grade temperature, fatigue, and weakness
   6. Anorexia, weight loss, and anemia
   7. Elevated sedimentation rate and positive rheumatoid factor
   8. X-ray showing joint deterioration
   9. Synovial tissue biopsy presents inflammation
C. Rheumatoid (RA) factor
   1. A blood test used to diagnose rheumatoid arthritis
   2. Values
      a. Nonreactive: 0 to 39 IU/mL

b. Weakly reactive: 40 to 79 IU/mL
c. Reactive: greater than 80 IU/mL

D. Pain
  1. Salicylates
    a. Monitor for side effects including tinnitus, GI upset, or prolonged bleeding time
    b. Administer with meals or a snack
    c. Monitor for abnormal bleeding or bruising
  2. Nonsteroidal anti-inflammatory drugs (NSAIDs)
    a. Administer in combination with salicylates as prescribed if pain and inflammation are not decreased within 6 to 12 weeks following salicylate therapy
    b. Monitor for side effects such as GI upset, CNS manifestations, skin rash, hypertension, fluid retention, and changes in renal function
  3. Corticosteroids: administer as prescribed during exacerbations or severe involvement when commonly used agents are ineffective
  4. Antineoplastic medications: administer as prescribed in clients with life-threatening RA
  5. Gold salts: administer as prescribed in combination with salicylates and NSAIDs to induce remission and decrease pain and inflammation

E. Physical mobility
  1. Preserve joint function
  2. Provide ROM exercises to maintain joint motion and muscle strengthening
  3. Balance rest and activity
  4. Splint during acute inflammation to prevent deformity
  5. Prevent flexion contractures
  6. Apply heat or cold therapy as prescribed to joints
  7. Apply paraffin baths and massage as prescribed
  8. Encourage consistency with exercise program
  9. Instruct the client to stop exercise if pain increases
  10. Exercise only to the point of pain
  11. Avoid weight bearing on inflamed joints

F. Self-care (Box 56–9)
  1. Assess the need for assistive devices such as higher toilet seats, chairs, and wheelchairs to facilitate mobility
  2. Collaborate with occupational therapy to obtain assistive adaptive devices
  3. Instruct the client in alternative strategies for providing activities of daily living

G. Fatigue
  1. Identify factors that may contribute to fatigue
  2. Monitor for signs of anemia
  3. Administer iron, folic acid, and vitamin supplements as prescribed
  4. Monitor for drug-related blood loss by testing the stool for occult blood
  5. Instruct the client in measures to conserve

BOX 56–9. Client Education for RA and DJD

Assist the client to identify and correct hazards in the home

Instruct the client in the correct use of assistive adaptive devices

Instruct in energy conservation measures

Review prescribed exercise program

Instruct the client to sit in a chair with a high, straight back

Instruct the client to use a small pillow only when lying down

Instruct the client in measures to protect joints such as turning doorknobs counterclockwise and using two hands instead of one to hold objects

Instruct the client regarding the prescribed medications

Stress the importance of follow-up visits with the physician

---

energy such as pacing activities and obtaining assistance when possible

H. Body image disturbance
  1. Assess the client's reaction to body change
  2. Encourage the client to verbalize feelings
  3. Assist the client with self-care activities and grooming
  4. Encourage the client to wear street clothes
  5. Provide patience and understanding and be aware that the client may be manipulative and demanding

I. Surgical implementation
  1. Synovectomy: surgical removal of the synovia to help maintain joint function
  2. Arthrodesis: bony fusion of a joint to regain some mobility
  3. Joint replacement (arthroplasty): surgical replacement of diseased joints with artificial joints to restore motion to a joint and function to the muscles, ligaments, and other soft tissue structures that control a joint

XIII. Osteoarthritis (Degenerative Joint Disease, DJD)

A. Description
  1. Progressive degeneration of the joints caused by wear and tear
  2. Causes the formation of bony build-up and the loss of articular cartilage in peripheral and axial joints
  3. Affects the weight-bearing joints and joints that receive the greatest stress such as the knees, toes, and lower spine
  4. The cause is unknown but may be caused by trauma, fractures, infections, or obesity

B. Data collection
  1. Joint pain that occurs early in the disease process diminishes after rest and intensifies after activity
  2. As the disease progresses, pain occurs with slight motion or even at rest

3. Symptoms are aggravated by temperature change and humidity
4. Crepitus
5. Joint enlargement
6. Presence of Heberden's nodes or Bouchard's nodes
7. Limited ROM
8. Difficulty getting up after prolonged sitting
9. Skeletal muscle atrophy
10. Inability to perform activities of daily living
11. Compression of the spine as manifested by radiating pain, stiffness, and muscle spasms in one or both extremities

C. Pain
1. Administer NSAIDs, salicylates, and muscle relaxants as prescribed
2. Prepare the client for corticosteroid injections into joints as prescribed
3. Place the affected joint in a functional position
4. Immobilize the affected joint with a splint or brace
5. Avoid large pillows under the head or knees
6. Provide a bed or foot cradle
7. Position the client prone twice a day
8. Instruct the client on the importance of moist heat, hot packs or compresses, and paraffin dips as prescribed
9. Apply cold applications as prescribed when the joint is acutely inflamed
10. Encourage adequate rest recommending 10 hours of sleep at night and a 1- to 2-hour nap in the afternoon

D. Nutrition
1. Encourage a well-balanced diet
2. Encourage weight loss if necessary

E. Physical mobility
1. Reinforce the exercise program and the importance of participating in the program
2. Instruct the client that exercises should be active rather than passive and to exercise only to the point of pain
3. Instruct the client to stop exercise if pain is increased with exercising
4. Instruct the client to decrease the number of repetitions in an exercise when the inflammation is severe

F. Surgical management
1. Osteotomy: the bone is cut to correct the joint deformity and promote realignment
2. Total joint replacement (TJR)
   a. Performed when all measures of pain relief have failed
   b. Hips and knees are most commonly replaced
   c. Contraindicated in the presence of infection, advanced osteoporosis, and severe inflammation

◆ **XIV. Osteoporosis**

A. Description
1. An age-related metabolic disease

2. Bone demineralization results in the loss of bone mass, leading to fragile and porous bones and subsequent fractures
3. Greater bone resorption than bone formation occurs
4. Occurs most commonly in the wrist, hip, and vertebral column
5. Can occur postmenopausal or as a result of a metabolic disorder or calcium deficiency

B. Data collection
1. Back pain after lifting, bending, or stooping
2. Back pain that increases with palpation
3. Pelvic or hip pain, especially with weight bearing
4. Problems with balance
5. Decline in height from vertebrae compression
6. Kyphosis of the dorsal spine
7. Constipation, abdominal distention, and respiratory impairment as a result of movement restriction and spinal deformity
8. Pathological fractures
9. Appearance of thin porous bone on x-ray

C. Implementation
1. Assess risk for injury
2. Provide a safe and hazard-free environment and assist the client to identify hazards in the home environment
3. Use side rails to prevent falls
4. Move the client gently when turning and repositioning
5. Encourage ambulation; assist with ambulation if the client is unsteady
6. Instruct in the use of assistive devices such as a cane or walker
7. Provide ROM exercises
8. Instruct in the use of good body mechanics
9. Instruct the client in exercises to strengthen abdominal and back muscles in order to improve posture and provide support for the spine
10. Instruct the client to avoid activities that can cause vertebral compression
11. Apply a back brace as prescribed during an acute phase to immobilize the spine and provide spinal column support
12. Encourage the use of a firm mattress
13. Provide a diet high in protein, calcium, vitamins C and D, and iron
14. Encourage adequate fluid intake to prevent renal calculi
15. Instruct the client to avoid alcohol and coffee
16. Administer estrogen or androgens to decrease the rate of bone resorption as prescribed
17. Administer calcium and vitamin D as prescribed for bone metabolism
18. Administer calcitonin as prescribed to inhibit bone loss
19. Administer analgesics, muscle relaxants, and anti-inflammatory medications as prescribed

XV. Gout

A. Description
   1. A systemic disease in which urate crystals deposit in joints and other body tissues
   2. Leads to abnormal amounts of uric acid in the body
   3. Primary gout results from a disorder of purine metabolism
   4. Secondary gout involves excessive uric acid in the blood that is caused by another disease
B. Phases
   1. Asymptomatic
      a. No symptoms
      b. Serum uric acid is elevated
   2. Acute: excruciating pain and inflammation of one or more small joints, especially the great toe
   3. Intermittent: asymptomatic period between acute attacks
   4. Chronic
      a. Results from repeated episodes of acute gout
      b. Results in deposits of urate crystals under the skin and within the major organs, especially the renal system
C. Data collection
   1. Excruciating pain in the involved joints
   2. Swelling and inflammation of joints
   3. Tophi (hard, fairly large and irregular shaped deposits in the skin) that may break open and discharge a yellow gritty substance
   4. Low-grade fever
   5. Malaise and headache
   6. Pruritus
   7. Presence of renal stones
   8. Elevated uric acid levels
D. Implementation
   1. Provide a low-purine diet as prescribed
   2. Instruct the client to avoid foods such as organ meats, wines, aged cheese
   3. Encourage a high fluid intake of 2000 mL to prevent stone formation
   4. Encourage weight-reduction diet if required
   5. Instruct the client to avoid alcohol and fat-starvation diets because they may precipitate a gout attack
   6. Increase urinary pH (above 6) by eating alkaline-ash foods such as citrus fruits and juices, milk, and other dairy products
   7. Provide bed rest during acute attacks
   8. Monitor joint ROM ability and appearance of joints
   9. Position the joint in a mild flexion position during an acute attack
   10. Elevate the affected extremity
   11. Protect the affected joint from excessive movement or direct contact with sheets
   12. Provide heat or cold for local treatments to the affected joint as prescribed
   13. Administer NSAIDs and anti-gout medications as prescribed

PRACTICE QUESTIONS

1. The client is complaining of knee pain. The knee is swollen, reddened, and warm to the touch. The nurse interprets that the client's signs and symptoms are not compatible with
   1 Inflammation
   2 Degenerative disease
   3 Infection
   4 Recent injury

2. The client is treated in the physician's office after a fall, which sprained the ankle. X-ray has ruled out fracture. Before sending the client home, the nurse plans to teach the client about which of the following items to be avoided in the next 24 hours?
   1 Application of a heating pad
   2 Application of an Ace wrap
   3 Resting the foot
   4 Elevating the ankle on a pillow while sitting or lying down

3. The nurse is collecting physical data of the musculoskeletal system on an assigned client. The nurse documents the presence of which of the following as a normal finding?
   1 Fasciculations
   2 Atrophy on the client's dominant side
   3 Hypertrophy on the client's dominant side
   4 Atrophy on the client's nondominant side

4. The nurse has given dietary instructions to a client to minimize the risk of osteoporosis. The nurse evaluates that the client understands the recommended changes if the client verbalizes to increase intake of which of these foods?
   1 Potatoes
   2 Cheese
   3 Fish
   4 Chicken

5. The nurse is providing care to the client following a bone biopsy. Which of the following actions by the nurse is not needed in the care of this client?
   1 Monitoring site for swelling, bleeding, and hematoma
   2 Administering intramuscular (IM) narcotic analgesics
   3 Elevating the limb for 24 hours
   4 Monitoring vitals signs every 4 hours

6. The nurse has reinforced instructions to the client returning home after arthroscopy of the knee. The nurse evaluates that the client understands the instructions if the client states to
   1 Stay off the leg entirely for the rest of the day
   2 Resume strenuous exercise the following day
   3 Refrain from eating food for the remainder of the day
   4 Report fever or site inflammation to the physician

7. The nurse is caring for the client who is going to have an arthrogram using a contrast medium. Which of the following data collected by the nurse is of highest priority?
   1 Allergy to iodine or shellfish
   2 Ability of the client to remain still during the procedure
   3 Whether the client has any remaining questions about the procedure
   4 Whether the client wishes to void before the procedure

8. The client with a bone infection is to have indium imaging done. The client asks the nurse to explain how the procedure is done. The nurse responds that
   1 Indium is injected into the bloodstream and collects in normal bone, but not in infected areas
   2 Indium is injected into the bloodstream and highlights the vascular supply to the bone
   3 A sample of the client's leukocytes is tagged with indium, and will subsequently accumulate in infected bone
   4 A sample of the client's RBCs is tagged with indium, and will highlight normal bone

9. The client with a possible rib fracture has never had a chest x-ray. The nurse plans to tell the client which of the following items about the procedure?
   1 The x-rays stimulate a small amount of pain
   2 It is necessary to remove jewelry and any other metal objects
   3 The client will be asked to breathe in and out during the x-ray
   4 The x-ray technologist will stand next to the client during the x-ray

10. The nurse is teaching the client who is to have a gallium scan about the procedure. The nurse includes which of the following items as part of the instructions?
    1 The gallium will be injected intravenously 2 to 3 hours before the procedure
    2 The procedure takes about 15 minutes to perform
    3 The client must stand erect during the filming
    4 The client should remain on bed rest for the remainder of the day after the scan

11. The client has had a bone scan done. The nurse evaluates that the client understands the elements of follow-up care if the client states to
    1 Report any feelings of nausea or flushing
    2 Ambulate at least three times before the end of the day
    3 Eat only small meals for the remainder of the day
    4 Drink plenty of water for a day or two following the procedure

12. The client seeks treatment in the emergency department for a lower leg injury. There is visible deformity to the lower aspect of the leg, and the injured leg appears shorter than the other. The area is painful, swollen, and becoming ecchymotic. The nurse interprets that this client has experienced a
    1 Contusion
    2 Fracture
    3 Sprain
    4 Strain

13. The nurse is one of several people who witness a vehicle hit a pedestrian at fairly low speed on a small street. The individual is dazed and tries to get up. The leg appears fractured. The nurse
    1 Stays with the person and encourages the person to remain still
    2 Assists the person to get up and walk to the sidewalk
    3 Leaves the person for a few moments to call an ambulance
    4 Tries to manually reduce the fracture

14. The nurse witnesses a client sustain a fall and suspects the leg may be fractured. Which of the following actions is the highest priority?
    1 Take a set of vital signs
    2 Call the radiology department
    3 Reassure the client that everything will be fine
    4 Immobilize the leg before moving the client

15. The nurse in the emergency department is caring for a client with a fractured arm. The nurse evaluates that which of the following items is not necessary before reduction of the fracture in the casting room?
    1 Explanation of the procedure to the client
    2 Administration of an analgesic
    3 Anesthesia consent
    4 Consent for the procedure

16. The nurse plans to reduce the anxiety of a client who is going to have a plaster cast applied by teaching the client about the procedure. The nurse does not include which of the following items in the discussion?
    1 A stockinette will be placed over the leg area to be casted
    2 The cast edges may be trimmed with a cast knife
    3 The cast will give off heat as it dries
    4 The client may bear weight on the cast in one-half hour

17. The nurse is planning to teach the client with a left arm cast about measures to keep the left shoulder from becoming stiff and "frozen." Which of the following suggestions does the nurse include in the teaching plan?

1 Lift the left arm up over the head
2 Lift the right arm up over the head
3 Make a fist with the hand of the casted arm
4 Use a sling on the left arm

18. The client has a fiberglass (nonplaster) cast applied to the lower leg. The client asks the nurse when the client will be able to walk on the cast. The nurse replies that the client will be able to bear weight on the cast
   1 Within 20 to 30 minutes of application
   2 In approximately 8 hours
   3 In 24 hours
   4 In 48 hours

19. The nurse has reinforced instructions with the client with a nonplaster (fiberglass) leg cast on cast care at home. The nurse evaluates that the client needs further instructions if the client makes which of the following statements?
   1 "I should avoid walking on wet, slippery floors."
   2 "It's OK to wipe dirt off the top of the cast with a damp cloth."
   3 "I'm not supposed to scratch the skin underneath the cast."
   4 "If the cast gets wet, I can dry it with a hair dryer turned to the warmest setting."

20. The client with a hip fracture asks the nurse why Buck's extension traction is being applied before surgery. The nurse's response is based on the understanding that Buck's extension traction primarily
   1 Provides rigid immobilization of the fracture site
   2 Provides comfort by reducing muscle spasms and provides fracture immobilization
   3 Lengthens the fractured leg to prevent severing of blood vessels
   4 Allows bone healing to begin before surgery

21. The client in skeletal leg traction with an overbed frame is not allowed to turn from side to side. Which of the following actions by the nurse is most useful in trying to provide good skin care to the client?
   1 Ask the client to lift up by digging into the mattress with the unaffected leg
   2 Push down on the mattress of the bed while administering care
   3 Have another nurse tilt the client anyway
   4 Ask the client to pull up on a trapeze to lift the hips off the bed

22. The nurse is evaluating the pin sites of a client in skeletal traction. The nurse is least concerned with which of the following findings?
   1 Purulent drainage
   2 Serous drainage
   3 Pain at a pin site
   4 Inflammation

23. The client has Buck's extension traction applied to the right leg. The nurse plans which of the following interventions to prevent complications of the device?
   1 Massage the skin of the right leg with lotion every 8 hours
   2 Give pin care once a shift
   3 Inspect the skin on the right leg at least once every 8 hours
   4 Release the weights on the right leg for range of motion exercises daily

24. The nurse is caring for the client who had skeletal traction applied to the left leg. The client is complaining of severe left leg pain. Which of the following actions should the nurse take first?
   1 Medicate the client with an analgesic
   2 Provide pin care
   3 Call the physician immediately
   4 Check the client's alignment in bed

25. The nurse has reinforced instructions regarding specific leg exercises for the client immobilized in right skeletal lower leg traction. The nurse evaluates that the client needs further instruction if the nurse observes the client
   1 Pulling up on the trapeze
   2 Flexing and extending the feet
   3 Performing active ROM to the right ankle and knee
   4 Doing quadriceps- and gluteal-setting exercises

26. The nurse is assessing the casted extremity of a client. The nurse checks for which of the following signs and symptoms indicative of infection?
   1 Coolness and pallor of the extremity
   2 Presence of a "hot spot" on the cast
   3 Diminished distal pulse
   4 Dependent edema

27. The client has sustained a closed fracture and has just had a cast applied to the affected arm. The client is complaining of intense pain. The nurse has elevated the limb, applied an ice bag, and administered an analgesic, which was ineffective in relieving the pain. The nurse interprets that this pain may be due to
   1 Impaired tissue perfusion
   2 The newness of the fracture
   3 The anxiety of the client
   4 Infection under the cast

28. The nurse is assigned to care for a client with multiple trauma admitted to the hospital. The client has a leg fracture and a plaster cast has been applied. In positioning the casted leg, the nurse should
   1 Keep the leg level
   2 Keep the leg level for 3 hours, and elevate it for 1 hour

3 Elevate the leg on pillows continuously for 24 to 48 hours

4 Elevate the leg for 3 hours, and put it flat for 1 hour

29. The client is complaining of skin irritation from the edges of a cast applied the previous day. The nurse plans on which of the following actions?
1 Massaging the skin at the rim of the cast
2 Applying lotion to the skin at the rim of the cast
3 Using a rough file to smooth the cast edges
4 Petaling the cast edges with adhesive tape

30. The client is being discharged to home after application of a plaster leg cast. The nurse evaluates that the client understands proper care of the cast if the client states to
1 Avoid getting the cast wet
2 Use the fingertips to lift and move the leg
3 Cover the casted leg with warm blankets
4 Use a padded coat hanger end to scratch under the cast

31. The client being measured for crutches asks the nurse why the crutches cannot rest up underneath the arm for extra support. The nurse's response is based on the understanding that this could result in
1 Impaired range of motion while the client ambulates
2 Skin breakdown in the area of the axilla
3 Injury to the brachial plexus nerves
4 A fall and further injury

32. The nurse is planning to reinforce instructions to the client about how to stand on crutches. The nurse plans to incorporate into written instructions to place the crutches
1 8 inches to the front and side of the client's toes
2 3 inches to the front and side of the client's toes
3 20 inches to the front and side of the client's toes
4 15 inches to the front and side of the client's toes

33. The nurse is giving the client with a left leg cast crutch walking instructions using the three-point gait. The client is allowed touch-down of the affected leg. The nurse tells the client to advance the
1 Left leg and right crutch, then right leg and left crutch
2 Crutches and then both legs simultaneously
3 Crutches and the right leg, then advance the left leg
4 Crutches and the left leg, then advance the right leg

34. The nurse has given the client instructions regarding crutch safety. The nurse evaluates that the client needs reinforcement of information if the client states
1 The need to have spare crutches and tips available
2 That crutch tips will not slip even when wet
3 Not to use someone else's crutches
4 That crutch tips should be inspected periodically for wear

35. The client has slight weakness in the right leg. Based on this information, the nurse determines that the client would benefit most from the use of a
1 Walker
2 Wooden crutch
3 Lofstrand crutch
4 Straight-leg cane

36. A client who has experienced a CVA has partial hemiplegia of the left leg. The straight-leg cane formerly used by the client is not quite sufficient now. The nurse interprets that the client could benefit from the somewhat greater support and stability provided by a
1 Quad cane
2 Wooden crutch
3 Lofstrand crutch
4 Wheelchair

37. The client with right-sided weakness needs to learn how to use a cane. The nurse plans to teach the client to position the cane by holding it with the
1 Left hand, and placing the cane in front of the left foot
2 Right hand, and placing the cane in front of the right foot
3 Left hand, and 6 inches lateral to the left foot
4 Right hand, and 6 inches lateral to the right foot

38. The client who is learning to use a cane is afraid it will slip with ambulation and cause a fall. The nurse provides the client with the greatest reassurance by telling the client that
1 Canes prevent falls, not cause them
2 The cane has a flared tip with concentric rings to give stability
3 The physical therapist will determine if the cane is inadequate
4 The cane would help to break a fall, even if the client does slip

39. The nurse is evaluating the client's use of a cane for left-sided weakness. The nurse intervenes and corrects the client if the nurse observes that the client
1 Holds the cane on the right side
2 Keeps the cane 6 inches out to the side of the right foot
3 Moves the cane when the right leg is moved
4 Leans on the cane when the right leg swings through

40. The nurse is caring for the client who develops compartment syndrome from a severely fractured arm. The client asks the nurse how this can happen. The nurse's response is based on the understanding that
    1 An injured artery causes impaired arterial perfusion through the compartment
    2 The fascia expands with injury, causing pressure on underlying nerves and muscles
    3 A bone fragment has injured the nerve supply in the area
    4 Bleeding and swelling cause increased pressure in an area that cannot expand

41. The nurse is caring for a client with fresh application of a plaster leg cast. The nurse plans to prevent the development of compartment syndrome by
    1 Elevating the limb and applying ice to the affected leg
    2 Elevating the limb and covering the limb with bath blankets
    3 Placing the leg in a slightly dependent position and applying ice
    4 Keeping the leg horizontal and applying ice to the affected leg

42. The nurse is monitoring a confused elderly client admitted with a hip fracture. Which of the following data obtained by the nurse does not place the client at more risk for altered thought processes?
    1 Stress induced by the fracture
    2 Hearing aid available and in working order
    3 Unfamiliar hospital setting
    4 Eyeglasses left at home

43. The nurse is caring for an elderly client who had a hip pinned after being fractured. In planning nursing care, which of the following does the nurse avoid to minimize the chance for further injury?
    1 Side rails in the "up" position
    2 Use of nightlight in hospital room and bathroom
    3 Call bell placed within reach
    4 Delays in responding to call light

44. The nurse is repositioning the client who has returned to the nursing unit following internal fixation of a fractured right hip. The nurse should use a
    1 Pillow to keep the right leg abducted during turning
    2 Pillow to keep the right leg adducted during turning
    3 Trochanter roll to prevent external rotation while turning
    4 Trochanter roll to prevent abduction while turning

45. The client who has had a right total knee replacement asks the nurse how long the right leg must be kept in the continuous passive motion (CPM) machine. The nurse's response is based on the understanding that the device should be used
    1 For 30 minutes out of every hour
    2 Every other hour for 60 minutes
    3 For 3 hours at a time, followed by 1 hour of rest
    4 For the length of time prescribed by the physician

46. The nurse has an order to get the client out of bed to a chair on the first postoperative day after total knee replacement. The nurse plans to do which of the following to protect the knee joint?
    1 Apply a knee immobilizer before getting the client up, and elevate the client's surgical leg while sitting
    2 Apply an Ace wrap around the dressing and put ice on the knee while sitting
    3 Lift the client to the bedside chair, leaving the CPM machine in place
    4 Obtain a walker to minimize weight bearing by the client on the affected leg

47. The client with diabetes mellitus has had a right below-the-knee amputation. The nurse is especially vigilant in monitoring for which of the following signs and symptoms due to the history of diabetes?
    1 Edema of the stump
    2 Hemorrhage
    3 Separation of wound edges
    4 Slight redness of incision

48. A client is admitted to the nursing unit after a left below-the-knee amputation following a crush injury to the foot and lower leg. The client tells the nurse, "I think I'm going crazy. I can feel my left foot itching." The nurse interprets the client's statement to be
    1 A normal response, and indicates the presence of phantom limb sensation
    2 A normal response, and indicates the presence of phantom limb pain
    3 An abnormal response, and indicates the client needs more psychological support
    4 An abnormal response, and indicates the client is in denial about the limb loss

49. The client is complaining of low back pain with radiation down the left posterior thigh. The nurse continues to collect data from the client to see if the pain is worsened or aggravated by
    1 Bed rest
    2 Application of heat
    3 Bending or lifting
    4 Ibuprofen (Motrin)

50. The client has just undergone spinal fusion after experiencing a herniated lumbar disk. The nurse avoids which of the following to maintain client safety after this procedure?
    1. Log rolling technique for repositioning
    2. Pillows under the length of the legs
    3. Head of the bed flat
    4. Overhead trapeze

51. The nurse has reinforced instructions with a client with herniated lumbar disk about proper body mechanics and other items pertinent to low back care. The nurse evaluates that the client needs further instruction if the client verbalizes to
    1. Get out of bed by sitting straight up and swinging the legs over the side of the bed
    2. Increase fiber and fluids in the diet
    3. Strengthen the back muscles by swimming or walking
    4. Bend at the knees to pick up objects

52. The client who has had spinal fusion and insertion of hardware is extremely concerned with the perceived lengthy rehabilitation period. The client expresses concerns about finances and ability to return to prior employment. The nurse understands that the client's needs could best be addressed by referral to the
    1. Surgeon
    2. Clinical nurse specialist
    3. Social worker
    4. Physical therapist

53. The nurse is planning to reinforce instructions to the client for proper use of thoracolumbarsacral orthosis (TLSO) after spinal fusion with instrumentation. The nurse plans to include which of the following teaching points in discussion with the client?
    1. Areas of skin redness at the edges of the brace indicates a good, snug fit
    2. The device is applied before getting out of bed in the morning
    3. The brace should be applied directly next to the skin
    4. The Velcro closures should be fairly loose to avoid constriction

54. The client is being transferred to the nursing unit from the postanesthesia care unit following spinal fusion with Harrington rod insertion. The nurse prepares to transfer the client from the stretcher to the bed by using
    1. A bath blanket and the assistance of three people
    2. A bath blanket and the assistance of four people
    3. A slider board and the assistance of two people
    4. A slider board and the assistance of four people

55. The client is being discharged to home following spinal fusion with insertion of Harrington rods. The nurse suggests a consultation with the continuing care nurse regarding the need for follow-up modification of the home environment if the client stated that
    1. The bedroom and bath are on the second floor of the home
    2. The bathroom has hand railings in the shower
    3. The family has rented a commode for use by the client
    4. There are three steps to get up to the front door

56. The client with a left arm fracture exhibits loss of sensation in the left fingers, pallor, poor capillary refill, and diminished left radial pulse. The nurse takes which of the following actions?
    1. Administers an analgesic
    2. Checks the circulation again in 30 minutes
    3. Provides range of motion to the fingers of the left hand
    4. Contacts the physician

57. The client is complaining of pain underneath a cast in the area of a bony prominence. The nurse interprets that this client may need to have
    1. The cast replaced with an air splint
    2. Extra padding put over this area of the cast
    3. The cast bivalved
    4. A window cut in the cast

58. The client is fearful about having an arm cast removed. Which of the following actions by the nurse is the most helpful?
    1. Telling the client that the saw makes a frightening noise
    2. Reassuring the client that no one has had an arm lacerated yet
    3. Stating that the hot cutting blades cause burns only very rarely
    4. Showing the client the cast cutter and explaining how it works

59. The client has just had a cast removed, and the underlying skin is yellow-brown and crusted. The nurse gives the client instructions for skin care. The nurse evaluates that the client has misunderstood the directions if the client states to
    1. Soak the skin and wash it gently
    2. Scrub the skin vigorously with soap and water
    3. Apply an emollient lotion to enhance softening
    4. Use a sunscreen on the skin if exposed for a period of time

60. The client has skeletal traction applied to the right leg, and has an overhead trapeze available for use. The nurse monitors which of the following as a high-risk area for pressure and breakdown?

1 Scapulae
2 Back of the head
3 Right heel
4 Left heel

61. The client has been placed in Buck's extension traction. The nurse provides countertraction to reduce shear and friction by
    1 Slightly elevating the head of the bed
    2 Slightly elevating the foot of the bed
    3 Providing an overhead trapeze
    4 Using a footboard

62. The nurse is obtaining a health history from a client and is assessing for risk factors associated with osteoporosis. Which of the following findings is not an associated risk factor?
    1 High-calcium diet consumption
    2 Postmenopausal age
    3 Long-term use of corticosteroids
    4 Family history of osteoporosis

63. The nurse is providing instructions to a client with osteoporosis regarding appropriate food items to include in the diet. Which of the following food items provides the least amount calcium?
    1 Plain yogurt
    2 Seafood
    3 Sardines
    4 Pork

64. The nurse is caring for a client who is having an acute attack of gout. Which of the following is not a component of the plan of care for this client?
    1 Restricting fluids
    2 A low-purine diet
    3 Bed rest
    4 The administration of NSAIDs

65. The nurse is collecting data on a client with a diagnosis of rheumatoid arthritis (RA). Which of the following does the nurse not expect to note in the client?
    1 Complaints of pain that occurs following exercise
    2 Complaints of pain that is more severe upon arising in the morning
    3 Swollen, shiny joints
    4 Skin nodules near bony prominences

ANSWERS

1. **2**

RATIONALE: Redness and heat are associated with musculoskeletal inflammation, infection, or a recent injury. Degenerative disease is accompanied by pain, but there is no redness. Swelling may or may not occur.
TEST-TAKING STRATEGY: Use the process of elimination, recalling the signs of inflammation. This will easily direct you to option 2.
LEVEL OF COGNITIVE ABILITY: Comprehension
PHASE OF NURSING PROCESS: Data Collection
CLIENT NEEDS: Physiological Integrity
CONTENT AREA: Adult Health/Musculoskeletal
REFERENCE
deWit, S. (1998). *Essentials of medical-surgical nursing* (4th ed.). Philadelphia: W. B. Saunders. p. 145.

2. **1**

RATIONALE: Soft-tissue injuries such as sprains are treated by RICE (rest, ice, compression, elevation) for the first 24 hours after the injury. Ice is applied intermittently for 20 to 30 minutes at a time. Heat is not used in the first 24 hours because it could increase venous congestion, which would increase edema and pain.
TEST-TAKING STRATEGY: Note the key word "avoided." It is likely that sprains should be rested and elevated, so these options are eliminated. Use of an Ace wrap is also helpful in reducing the pain and swelling, so this cannot be the answer either. By the process of elimination, heat must be the item to avoid in the first 24 hours.
LEVEL OF COGNITIVE ABILITY: Application
PHASE OF NURSING PROCESS: Planning

CLIENT NEEDS: Physiological Integrity
CONTENT AREA: Adult Health/Musculoskeletal
REFERENCE
deWit, S. (1998). *Essentials of medical-surgical nursing* (4th ed.). Philadelphia: W. B. Saunders. p. 681.

3. **3**

RATIONALE: Hypertrophy, or increased muscle size, on the client's dominant side of up to 1 cm, is considered normal. Atrophy on either side is considered an abnormal finding. Fasciculations are fine muscle twitches that are not normally present.
TEST-TAKING STRATEGY: Use the process of elimination noting the key word "normal." Options 2 and 4 are eliminated first because atrophy is not a normal finding. Knowing that fasciculations are not normal helps you to select option 3 over option 1.
LEVEL OF COGNITIVE ABILITY: Comprehension
PHASE OF NURSING PROCESS: Data Collection
CLIENT NEEDS: Physiological Integrity
CONTENT AREA: Adult Health/Musculoskeletal
REFERENCE
Black, J., & Matassarin-Jacobs, E. (1997). *Medical-surgical nursing: Clinical management for continuity of care* (5th ed.). Philadelphia: W. B. Saunders. p. 2086.

4. **2**

RATIONALE: The major dietary source of calcium is from dairy foods, including milk, yogurt, and a variety of cheeses. Calcium may also be added to certain products, such as orange juice, which is then advertised as being "fortified" with calcium. Calcium supplements are available and recommended for those with typically low calcium intake.

TEST-TAKING STRATEGY: To answer this question, you need to know that calcium is required for the client with osteoporosis and the foods high in calcium. Review this content now, if you had difficulty with this question.
LEVEL OF COGNITIVE ABILITY: Comprehension
PHASE OF NURSING PROCESS: Evaluation
CLIENT NEEDS: Health Promotion and Maintenance
CONTENT AREA: Adult Health/Musculoskeletal
REFERENCE
deWit, S. (1998). *Essentials of medical-surgical nursing* (4th ed.). Philadelphia: W. B. Saunders. pp. 701–702.

5. **2**

RATIONALE: Nursing care after bone biopsy includes monitoring the site for swelling, bleeding, and hematoma formation. The biopsy site is elevated for 24 hours to reduce edema. The vital signs are monitored every 4 hours for 24 hours. The client usually requires mild analgesic; more severe pain usually indicates that complications are arising.
TEST-TAKING STRATEGY: Note the key word "not." One way to approach this question is to look at the method of anesthesia used for this procedure. If you know that this procedure is done under local anesthesia, it makes sense that monitoring vital signs every 4 hours is probably sufficient (option 4). The nurse routinely monitors for complications (option 1). This narrows the choices to site elevation or narcotic analgesics. Of these two, site elevation makes sense to reduce edema, while narcotic administration by the IM route seems excessive for a local procedure. Thus, option 2 is the answer to the question as stated.
LEVEL OF COGNITIVE ABILITY: Application
PHASE OF NURSING PROCESS: Implementation
CLIENT NEEDS: Physiological Integrity
CONTENT AREA: Adult Health/Musculoskeletal
REFERENCE
deWit, S. (1998). *Essential of medical-surgical nursing* (4th ed.). Philadelphia: W. B. Saunders. p. 672.

6. **4**

RATIONALE: After arthroscopy, the client can usually walk carefully on the leg once sensation has returned. The client is instructed to avoid strenuous exercise for at least a few days. The client may resume the usual diet. Signs and symptoms of infection should be reported to the physician.
TEST-TAKING STRATEGY: Note the key words "understand the instructions." Option 2 and 3 are the least plausible and may be eliminated first. To differentiate between the last two, you need to know that the client can walk on the affected leg once sensation has returned. The client is always taught signs and symptoms of infection to report to the physician.
LEVEL OF COGNITIVE ABILITY: Comprehension
PHASE OF NURSING PROCESS: Evaluation
CLIENT NEEDS: Health Promotion and Maintenance
CONTENT AREA: Adult Health/Musculoskeletal
REFERENCE
deWit, S. (1998). *Essential of medical-surgical nursing* (4th ed.). Philadelphia: W. B. Saunders. p. 671.

7. **1**

RATIONALE: Because of the risk of allergy to contrast dye, the nurse places highest priority on identifying whether the client has an allergy to iodine or shellfish. The nurse also reinforces information about the test, tells the client about the need to remain still during the procedure,

and encourages the client to void before the procedure for comfort.
TEST-TAKING STRATEGY: Note the key words "highest priority." This tells you that more than one or all of the options are correct (in fact, they all are). While options 2, 3, and 4 all compete for your priority, only option 1 (allergy to iodine or shellfish) takes obvious first preference. The consequence of possible anaphylactic shock (physiological risk) makes this the correct option.
LEVEL OF COGNITIVE ABILITY: Comprehension
PHASE OF NURSING PROCESS: Data Collection
CLIENT NEEDS: Physiological Integrity
CONTENT AREA: Adult Health/Musculoskeletal
REFERENCE
Monahan, F., & Neighbors, M. (1998). *Medical-surgical nursing: Foundations for clinical practice* (2nd ed.). Philadelphia: W. B. Saunders. p. 850.

8. **3**

RATIONALE: A sample of the client's blood is collected, and the leukocytes are tagged with indium. The leukocytes are then reinjected into the client. They accumulate in infected areas of bone, and can be detected with scanning. No special preparation or aftercare is necessary.
TEST-TAKING STRATEGY: This question is difficult if you are not familiar with the procedure. Look at the information. The client has a bone infection. With any type of infection, leukocytes migrate to the area (and bone is not a highly vascular area). This might suggest option 3 to you as the correct choice in answering this question.
LEVEL OF COGNITIVE ABILITY: Comprehension
PHASE OF NURSING PROCESS: Implementation
CLIENT NEEDS: Physiological Integrity
CONTENT AREA: Adult Health/Musculoskeletal
REFERENCE
Black, J., & Matassarin-Jacobs, E. (1997). *Medical-surgical nursing: Clinical management for continuity of care* (5th ed.). Philadelphia: W. B. Saunders. pp. 2094–2095.

9. **2**

RATIONALE: An x-ray is a photographic image of a part of the body on a special film, which is used to diagnose a wide variety of conditions. The x-ray itself is painless; any discomfort arises from repositioning a painful part for filming. The nurse may want to premedicate a client who is at risk for pain. Any radiopaque objects such as jewelry or other metal must be removed. The client is asked to breathe in deeply, and then hold the breath while the chest x-ray is taken. To minimize risk of radiation exposure, the x-ray technologist stands in a separate area protected by a lead wall. The client also wears a lead shield over the gonads.
TEST-TAKING STRATEGY: Use the process of elimination. Options 1 and 4 are obviously incorrect and are eliminated first. Of the two remaining options, eliminate option 3 because the client needs to be still during the x-ray.
LEVEL OF COGNITIVE ABILITY: Application
PHASE OF NURSING PROCESS: Planning
CLIENT NEEDS: Safe, Effective Care Environment
CONTENT AREA: Adult Health/Musculoskeletal
REFERENCE
Monahan, F., & Neighbors, M. (1998). *Medical-surgical nursing: Foundations for clinical practice* (2nd ed.). Philadelphia: W. B. Saunders. p. 1514.

10. **1**

RATIONALE: A gallium scan is similar to a bone scan, but with injection of gallium isotope instead of technetium

Tc^{99m}. Gallium is injected 2 to 3 hours before the procedure. The procedure takes 30 to 60 minutes to perform. The client must lie still during the procedure. There is no special aftercare.

TEST-TAKING STRATEGY: Use the process of elimination. If you know that a gallium scan is similar to a bone scan, then you could begin by eliminating options 3 and 4. The time frame in option 2 is rather brief, which allows you to choose option 1 as the correct option. Review this test now if you had difficulty with this question.

LEVEL OF COGNITIVE ABILITY: Application
PHASE OF NURSING PROCESS: Implementation
CLIENT NEEDS: Physiological Integrity
CONTENT AREA: Adult Health/Musculoskeletal
REFERENCE
Monahan, F., & Neighbors, M. (1998). *Medical-surgical nursing: Foundations for clinical practice* (2nd ed.). Philadelphia: W. B. Saunders. p. 850.

11. 4

RATIONALE: There are no special restrictions following a bone scan. The client is encouraged to drink large amounts of water for 24 to 48 hours to flush the radioisotope from the system. There are no hazards to the client or staff from the minimal amount of radioactivity of the isotope.

TEST-TAKING STRATEGY: Use the process of elimination. There is no purpose for option 2 or 3, which allows you to eliminate them first. Nausea and flushing could accompany dye injection during a procedure, but this procedure uses radioisotopes, and the question relates to care after the procedure. Thus, this one is eliminated also. The only option left is pushing fluids, which will hasten elimination of the isotope from the client's system.

LEVEL OF COGNITIVE ABILITY: Comprehension
PHASE OF NURSING PROCESS: Evaluation
CLIENT NEEDS: Health Promotion and Maintenance
CONTENT AREA: Adult Health/Musculoskeletal
REFERENCE
deWit, S. (1998). *Essentials of medical-surgical nursing* (4th ed.). Philadelphia: W. B. Saunders. p. 671.

12. 2

RATIONALE: Typical signs and symptoms of fracture include pain, loss of function in the area, deformity, shortening of the extremity, crepitus, swelling, and ecchymosis. Not all fractures lead to the development of every sign. A contusion results from a blow to soft tissue, and causes pain, swelling, and ecchymosis. A sprain is an injury to a ligament caused by a wrenching or twisting motion. Symptoms include pain, swelling, and inability to use the joint or bear weight normally. A strain results from a pulling force on the muscle. Symptoms include soreness and pain with muscle use.

TEST-TAKING STRATEGY: Within the list of signs and symptoms in the question, note the one that states one leg is shorter than another. Only a fractured bone (which shortens with displacement) could cause this sign. This makes it easy to eliminate each of the other incorrect options. Review the signs of a fracture now if you had difficulty with this question.

LEVEL OF COGNITIVE ABILITY: Comprehension
PHASE OF NURSING PROCESS: Data Collection
CLIENT NEEDS: Physiological Integrity
CONTENT AREA: Adult Health/Musculoskeletal

REFERENCE
deWit, S. (1998). *Essentials of medical-surgical nursing* (4th ed.). Philadelphia: W. B. Saunders. p. 682.

13. 1

RATIONALE: With a suspected fracture, the client is not moved unless it is dangerous to remain in that spot. The nurse should remain with the client, and have someone else call for emergency help. A fracture is not reduced at the scene. Before moving the client, the site of fracture is immobilized to prevent further injury.

TEST-TAKING STRATEGY: Use the process of elimination. Options 2 and 4 are the worst choices and should be eliminated first. Either of these options could result in further injury to the client. Of the two remaining options, the most prudent action is for the nurse to remain with the client and have someone else call for emergency assistance. Review immediate care to the client with a fracture now if you had difficulty with this question.

LEVEL OF COGNITIVE ABILITY: Application
PHASE OF NURSING PROCESS: Implementation
CLIENT NEEDS: Physiological Integrity
CONTENT AREA: Adult Health/Musculoskeletal
REFERENCE
deWit, S. (1998). *Essentials of medical-surgical nursing* (4th ed.). Philadelphia: W. B. Saunders. p. 682.

14. 4

RATIONALE: When a fracture is suspected, it is imperative that the area is splinted before the client is moved. Emergency help should be called for if the client is not hospitalized; a physician is called for the hospitalized client. The nurse should remain with the client and provide realistic reassurance. The nurse does not prescribe radiology tests.

TEST-TAKING STRATEGY: Note the key words "highest priority." Eliminate option 2 because the nurse does not order x-rays. Option 3 is eliminated next because the nurse never tells a client that "everything will be fine." Of the last two choices, immobilizing the limb is imperative for the client's safety, which makes it a better choice than taking vital signs. Review care to the client when a fracture is suspected now if you had difficulty with this question.

LEVEL OF COGNITIVE ABILITY: Application
PHASE OF NURSING PROCESS: Implementation
CLIENT NEEDS: Physiological Integrity
CONTENT AREA: Adult Health/Musculoskeletal
REFERENCE
deWit, S. (1998). *Essentials of medical-surgical nursing* (4th ed.). Philadelphia: W. B. Saunders. p. 683.

15. 3

RATIONALE: Before a fracture is reduced, the client is informed about the procedure, and consent is obtained. An analgesic is given as prescribed, because the procedure is painful. Administration of anesthesia may or may not be done, depending on severity. Closed reductions may be done in the emergency room without anesthesia. If anesthesia is used, the procedure is done in the operating room.

TEST-TAKING STRATEGY: Note the key words "not necessary" and "casting room." Options 1 and 4 are obviously needed, so these options are eliminated first. The question specifically states that the procedure is going to be done in the cast room, which helps you to choose option 3 (anesthesia consent) as the unnecessary item. Review the procedure for reduction of a fracture now if you had difficulty with this question.

LEVEL OF COGNITIVE ABILITY: Comprehension
PHASE OF NURSING PROCESS: Evaluation
CLIENT NEEDS: Physiological Integrity
CONTENT AREA: Adult Health/Musculoskeletal
REFERENCE
Monahan, F., & Neighbors, M. (1998). *Medical-surgical nursing: Foundations for clinical practice* (2nd ed.). Philadelphia: W. B. Saunders. p. 918.

16. **4**

RATIONALE: The procedure for casting involves washing and drying the skin and placing a stockinette material over the area to be casted. A roll of padding is then applied smoothly and evenly. The plaster is rolled onto the padding, and the edges are trimmed or smoothed as needed. A plaster cast gives off heat as it dries. A plaster cast can tolerate weight bearing once it is dry, which varies from 24 to 72 hours depending on the nature and thickness of the cast.
TEST-TAKING STRATEGY: Note the key word "not." Familiarity with the different types of casting materials and their differences helps you to answer this question. Options 1, 2, and 3 are all true for plaster casts. Option 4 is true for nonplaster casts.
LEVEL OF COGNITIVE ABILITY: Application
PHASE OF NURSING PROCESS: Planning
CLIENT NEEDS: Physiological Integrity
CONTENT AREA: Adult Health/Musculoskeletal
REFERENCE
deWit, S. (1998). *Essentials of medical-surgical nursing* (4th ed.). Philadelphia: W. B. Saunders. p. 686.

17. **1**

RATIONALE: Immobility and the weight of a casted arm may cause the shoulder above an arm fracture to become stiff. The shoulder of a casted arm should be lifted over the head periodically as a preventive measure. The use of slings further immobilizes the shoulder and may be contraindicated. Making fists with the left hand provides isometric exercise to maintain muscle strength. Range of motion of the affected fingers is also a useful general measure. Lifting the right arm is of no particular value.
TEST-TAKING STRATEGY: Use the process of elimination. Visualize each of the movements and think about the muscle groups that are moved with each. Options 2 and 4 provide for no movement of the left arm and are eliminated first. Making a fist with the hand on the casted arm provides good isometric exercise to the muscles surrounding the fracture, but again, does nothing for the shoulder. The only viable option is raising the arm over the head, which provides some range of motion for the shoulder joint.
LEVEL OF COGNITIVE ABILITY: Application
PHASE OF NURSING PROCESS: Planning
CLIENT NEEDS: Health Promotion and Maintenance
CONTENT AREA: Adult Health/Musculoskeletal
REFERENCE
deWit, S. (1998). *Essentials of medical-surgical nursing* (4th ed.). Philadelphia: W. B. Saunders. pp. 689–690.

18. **1**

RATIONALE: A fiberglass cast is made of water-activated polyurethane materials, which are dry to the touch within minutes and reach full rigid strength in about 20 minutes. Because of this, the client can bear weight on the cast within 20 to 30 minutes.
TEST-TAKING STRATEGY: Familiarity with nonplaster casts is needed to answer this question precisely. Options 3 and 4 should be eliminated first, because these time frames are similar to the drying times for plaster casts. Knowing that the nonplaster type of cast is lighter and dries extremely quickly may help you to choose the 20- to 30-minute time frame as correct.
LEVEL OF COGNITIVE ABILITY: Application
PHASE OF NURSING PROCESS: Implementation
CLIENT NEEDS: Health Promotion and Maintenance
CONTENT AREA: Adult Health/Musculoskeletal
REFERENCE
deWit, S. (1998). *Essentials of medical-surgical nursing* (4th ed.). Philadelphia: W. B. Saunders. p. 687.

19. **4**

RATIONALE: Client instructions should include to avoid walking on wet, slippery floors to prevent falls. Surface soil on a cast may be removed with a damp cloth. If the cast gets wet, it can be dried with a hair dryer set to a cool setting to prevent skin breakdown. If the skin under the cast itches, cool air from a hair dryer may be used to relieve it. The client should never scratch under a cast due to risk of skin breakdown and ulcer formation.
TEST-TAKING STRATEGY: Note the key words "needs further instructions." Options 1 and 3 are certainly true, and are therefore eliminated. Knowledge of nonplaster cast material is needed to discriminate between the last two. A fiberglass cast may be wiped with a damp cloth, because it is water resistant. It may be helpful to remember never to use a hair dryer on a cast, or on the skin under any cast, with the dryer set at the warmest setting; only cool settings are used, to prevent burns.
LEVEL OF COGNITIVE ABILITY: Comprehension
PHASE OF NURSING PROCESS: Evaluation
CLIENT NEEDS: Health Promotion and Maintenance
CONTENT AREA: Adult Health/Musculoskeletal
REFERENCE
Monahan, F., & Neighbors, M. (1998). *Medical-surgical nursing: Foundations for clinical practice* (2nd ed.). Philadelphia: W. B. Saunders. p. 857.

20. **2**

RATIONALE: Buck's extension traction is a type of skin traction often applied after hip fracture before the fracture is reduced in surgery. It reduces muscle spasms and helps to immobilize the fracture. It does not lengthen the leg for the purpose of preventing blood vessel severance. It also does not allow for bony healing to begin.
TEST-TAKING STRATEGY: Use the process of elimination. Options 3 and 4 are the least plausible of all the choices, and should be eliminated first. To discriminate between the last two, note the words "rigid immobilization" in option 1. Since skin traction uses lighter weights than skeletal traction, this type of traction cannot be said to provide rigid immobilization. Review this type of traction now if you had difficulty with this question.
LEVEL OF COGNITIVE ABILITY: Comprehension
PHASE OF NURSING PROCESS: Planning
CLIENT NEEDS: Physiological Integrity
CONTENT AREA: Adult Health/Musculoskeletal
REFERENCE
deWit, S. (1998). *Essentials of medical-surgical nursing* (4th ed.). Philadelphia: W. B. Saunders. p. 689.

21. **4**

RATIONALE: If the client in skeletal traction may not turn from side to side, the nurse should have the client pull up on a trapeze and try to lift the hips off the bed for skin care, bed pan use, and linen changes. If the client is unable to pull up on a trapeze, the nurse can push down on the mattress with one hand while administering care with the other.

TEST-TAKING STRATEGY: Use the process of elimination. Option 3 is contraindicated because it ignores a medical order. Option 1 is not feasible as stated. The client cannot lift up from the bed using one foot only. Options 2 and 4 are both acceptable alternatives. Since the question asks which would be "most useful," the answer is option 4. Providing care to the client who can lift the hips off the bed using a trapeze is easier and more efficient than providing care to one who cannot.

LEVEL OF COGNITIVE ABILITY: Application
PHASE OF NURSING PROCESS: Implementation
CLIENT NEEDS: Physiological Integrity
CONTENT AREA: Adult Health/Musculoskeletal
REFERENCE
Monahan, F., & Neighbors, M. (1998). *Medical-surgical nursing: Foundations for clinical practice* (2nd ed.). Philadelphia: W. B. Saunders. pp. 862–863.

22. **2**

RATIONALE: A small amount of serous oozing is expected at pin insertion sites. Signs of infection such as inflammation, purulent drainage, and pain at the pin site are not expected findings, and should be reported.

TEST-TAKING STRATEGY: Options 1 and 4 seem to indicate an infectious problem, and are eliminated. Note the key words "least concerned with." To discriminate between options 2 and 3, look at them carefully. The complaint of pain is at "a pin site" only. It gives no indication that the pain is related to the fracture or muscle spasm. Since serous drainage is an expected finding, choose this over the complaint of pain as the answer to the question.

LEVEL OF COGNITIVE ABILITY: Comprehension
PHASE OF NURSING PROCESS: Evaluation
CLIENT NEEDS: Physiological Integrity
CONTENT AREA: Adult Health/Musculoskeletal
REFERENCE
Monahan, F., & Neighbors, M. (1998). *Medical-surgical nursing: Foundations for clinical practice* (2nd ed.). Philadelphia: W. B. Saunders. p. 863.

23. **3**

RATIONALE: Buck's extension traction is a type of skin traction. The nurse inspects the skin of the limb in traction at least once every 8 hours for irritation or inflammation. Massaging the skin with lotion is not indicated. The nurse never releases the weights of traction unless specifically ordered by the physician. There are no pins to care for with skin traction.

TEST-TAKING STRATEGY: A baseline knowledge of Buck's extension traction allows you to eliminate options 2 and 4 easily. There are no pins, and the nurse never removes weights without a specific order to do so. Since the apparatus would have to be removed to apply lotion, which is unnecessary, the answer is to inspect the skin. Review care to the client with Buck's extension traction now if you had difficulty with this question.

LEVEL OF COGNITIVE ABILITY: Application
PHASE OF NURSING PROCESS: Planning
CLIENT NEEDS: Physiological Integrity
CONTENT AREA: Adult Health/Musculoskeletal

REFERENCE
Monahan, F., & Neighbors, M. (1998). *Medical-surgical nursing: Foundations for clinical practice* (2nd ed.). Philadelphia: W. B. Saunders. p. 869.

24. **4**

RATIONALE: A client who complains of severe pain may need realignment, or may have traction weights ordered that are too heavy. The nurse realigns the client, and if ineffective, then calls the physician. Severe leg pain, once traction has been established, indicates a problem. Medicating the client should be done after trying to determine and treat the cause. Providing pin care is unrelated to the problem as described.

TEST-TAKING STRATEGY: Note the key word "first." Use the steps of the nursing process. Option 4 is the only option that addresses data collection.

LEVEL OF COGNITIVE ABILITY: Application
PHASE OF NURSING PROCESS: Implementation
CLIENT NEEDS: Physiological Integrity
CONTENT AREA: Adult Health/Musculoskeletal
REFERENCE
deWit, S. (1998). *Essentials of medical-surgical nursing* (4th ed.). Philadelphia: W. B. Saunders. p. 690.

25. **3**

RATIONALE: Exercise is indicated within therapeutic limits for the client in skeletal traction to maintain muscle strength and range of motion. The client may pull up on the trapeze, perform active ROM with uninvolved joints, and do isometric muscle setting exercises (such as quadriceps- and gluteal-setting exercises). The client may also flex and extend the feet.

TEST-TAKING STRATEGY: Note the key words "needs further instruction." Options 1 and 4 are most easily identified as correct actions, and are therefore eliminated as possible answers to this question. To discriminate between options 2 and 3, imagine the lines of pull on the fracture site with the movements described. While flexing and extending the feet does not disrupt the line of pull from the traction, performing active ROM to the affected knee and ankle does.

LEVEL OF COGNITIVE ABILITY: Comprehension
PHASE OF NURSING PROCESS: Evaluation
CLIENT NEEDS: Physiological Integrity
CONTENT AREA: Adult Health/Musculoskeletal
REFERENCE
Monahan, F., & Neighbors, M. (1998). *Medical-surgical nursing: Foundations for clinical practice* (2nd ed.). Philadelphia: W. B. Saunders. p. 863.

26. **2**

RATIONALE: Signs and symptoms of infection under a casted area include odor or purulent drainage from the cast, or the presence of "hot spots," which are areas of the cast that are warmer than others. The physician should be notified if any of these occur. Signs of impaired circulation in the distal limb include coolness and pallor of the skin, diminished arterial pulse, and edema.

TEST-TAKING STRATEGY: Begin to answer this question by thinking of what you would expect to find with infection: redness, swelling, heat, and purulent drainage. With these in mind, options 1 and 3 can be eliminated easily. To discriminate between options 2 and 4, "dependent edema" is not necessarily indicative of infection. Swelling would be

continuous. The "hot spot" on the cast could signify infection underneath that area.
LEVEL OF COGNITIVE ABILITY: Application
PHASE OF NURSING PROCESS: Data Collection
CLIENT NEEDS: Physiological Integrity
CONTENT AREA: Adult Health/Musculoskeletal
REFERENCE
Monahan, F., & Neighbors, M. (1998). *Medical-surgical nursing: Foundations for clinical practice* (2nd ed.). Philadelphia: W. B. Saunders. p. 856.

27. 1

RATIONALE: Most pain associated with fractures can be minimized with rest, elevation, application of cold, and administration of analgesics. Pain that is not relieved from these measures should be reported to the physician, as it may be due to impaired tissue perfusion, tissue breakdown, or necrosis. Since this is a new closed fracture and cast, infection would not have had time to set in.
TEST-TAKING STRATEGY: Use the process of elimination. Options 2 and 3 are the least plausible given the description in the question and are eliminated first. Since the fracture and cast are so new, it is extremely unlikely that infection could have possibly set in. The most likely option is impaired tissue perfusion, since pain from ischemia is not relieved by comfort measures and analgesics.
LEVEL OF COGNITIVE ABILITY: Comprehension
PHASE OF NURSING PROCESS: Data Collection
CLIENT NEEDS: Physiological Integrity
CONTENT AREA: Adult Health/Musculoskeletal
REFERENCE
Monahan, F., & Neighbors, M. (1998). *Medical-surgical nursing: Foundations for clinical practice* (2nd ed.). Philadelphia: W. B. Saunders. p. 858.

28. 3

RATIONALE: A casted extremity is elevated continuously for the first 24 to 48 hours to minimize swelling and to promote venous drainage.
TEST-TAKING STRATEGY: Use the process of elimination. Recall that edema sets in after fracture, and can be augmented by casting. For this reason, options 1 and 2 are the least helpful, and can be eliminated first. There is no useful purpose for the timing in option 4. Review care to the client with a cast if you had difficulty with this question.
LEVEL OF COGNITIVE ABILITY: Application
PHASE OF NURSING PROCESS: Implementation
CLIENT NEEDS: Physiological Integrity
CONTENT AREA: Adult Health/Musculoskeletal
REFERENCE
deWit, S. (1998). *Essentials of medical-surgical nursing* (4th ed.). Philadelphia: W. B. Saunders. p. 687.

29. 4

RATIONALE: The edges of the cast can be petaled with tape to minimize skin irritation. If a client has a cast applied and returns home, the client can be taught to do the same.
TEST-TAKING STRATEGY: Use the process of elimination. Options 1 and 2 are similar, and neither helps to get rid of the cause of the irritation, so they are eliminated first. Imagine the use of a "rough file"; it would create plaster chips and dust that could go underneath the cast. Review cast petaling now if you had difficulty with this question.
LEVEL OF COGNITIVE ABILITY: Application
PHASE OF NURSING PROCESS: Planning

CLIENT NEEDS: Physiological Integrity
CONTENT AREA: Adult Health/Musculoskeletal
REFERENCE
deWit, S. (1998). *Essentials of medical-surgical nursing* (4th ed.). Philadelphia: W. B. Saunders. pp. 687–688.

30. 1

RATIONALE: A plaster cast must remain dry to keep its strength. The cast should be handled using the palms of the hands, not the fingertips, until fully dry. Air should circulate freely around the cast to help it dry; the cast also gives off heat as it dries. The client should never scratch under the cast; a cool hair dryer may be used to eliminate an itch.
TEST-TAKING STRATEGY: Knowledge of cast care is needed to answer this question. Knowing that a wet cast can be dented with the fingertips, causing pressure underneath, helps you to discard option 2 first. Knowing that the cast needs to dry makes you eliminate option 3 next. Option 4 is dangerous to skin integrity and is immediately eliminated. Plaster casts, once they have dried after application, should not become wet.
LEVEL OF COGNITIVE ABILITY: Comprehension
PHASE OF NURSING PROCESS: Evaluation
CLIENT NEEDS: Health Promotion and Maintenance
CONTENT AREA: Adult Health/Musculoskeletal
REFERENCE
deWit, S. (1998). *Essentials of medical-surgical nursing* (4th ed.). Philadelphia: W. B. Saunders. p. 687.

31. 3

RATIONALE: Crutches are measured so that the tops are three to four fingerbreadths or 1 to 2 inches from the axilla. This ensures that the client's axilla are not resting on the crutch, or bearing the weight of the crutch. This could result in injury to the nerves of the brachial plexus.
TEST-TAKING STRATEGY: Use the process of elimination, recalling the anatomy of the arm and axillary area. Review measures for crutch walking now if you had difficulty with this question.
LEVEL OF COGNITIVE ABILITY: Comprehension
PHASE OF NURSING PROCESS: Planning
CLIENT NEEDS: Physiological Integrity
CONTENT AREA: Adult Health/Musculoskeletal
REFERENCE
Monahan, F., & Neighbors, M. (1998). *Medical-surgical nursing: Foundations for clinical practice* (2nd ed.). Philadelphia: W. B. Saunders. p. 880.

32. 1

RATIONALE: The classic tripod position is taught to the client before giving instructions on gait. The crutches are placed anywhere from 6 to 10 inches in front and to the side of the client, depending on the client's body size. This provides a wide enough base of support to the client and improves balance.
TEST-TAKING STRATEGY: Use the process of elimination. Three inches and 20 inches seem excessively short and long, respectively. These two options should be eliminated first. Of the two remaining, 8 inches seems more in keeping with the normal length of a stride than 15 inches for someone wearing a cast, and it is the answer to the question. Review crutch walking now if you had difficulty with this question.
LEVEL OF COGNITIVE ABILITY: Application
PHASE OF NURSING PROCESS: Planning

CLIENT NEEDS: Health Promotion and Maintenance
CONTENT AREA: Adult Health/Musculoskeletal
REFERENCE
Potter, P., & Perry, A. (1997). *Fundamentals of nursing: Concepts, process, and practice* (4th ed.). St. Louis: Mosby–Year Book. p. 936.

33. **4**

RATIONALE: A three-point gait requires good balance and arm strength. The crutches are advanced with the affected leg, and then the unaffected leg is moved forward. Option 1 describes a two-point gait. Option 2 describes a swing-to gait. Option 3 describes the three-point gait used for a right leg problem.
TEST-TAKING STRATEGY: Option 1 does not provide the support needed for the casted extremity described in the question and should be eliminated. Option 2 is not necessary if the client is allowed to let the extremity touch the floor. Of the two remaining, option 4 is the option that provides support to the left leg. Review crutch walking now if you had difficulty with this question.
LEVEL OF COGNITIVE ABILITY: Application
PHASE OF NURSING PROCESS: Implementation
CLIENT NEEDS: Health Promotion and Maintenance
CONTENT AREA: Adult Health/Musculoskeletal
REFERENCE
deWit, S. (1998). *Essentials of medical-surgical nursing* (4th ed.). Philadelphia: W. B. Saunders. p. 680.

34. **2**

RATIONALE: Crutch tips should remain dry. Water could cause slipping by decreasing the surface friction of the rubber tip on the floor. If crutch tips get wet, the client should dry them with a cloth or paper towel. The client should use only crutches measured for the client. The tips should be inspected for wear, and spare crutches and tips should be available if needed.
TEST-TAKING STRATEGY: Note the key words "needs reinforcement." Use the process of elimination. Option 3 is certainly a correct statement, and is therefore eliminated. Options 1 and 4 are also true. Remember, crutch tips can slip when they get wet, posing a possible threat to the unsuspecting client.
LEVEL OF COGNITIVE ABILITY: Comprehension
PHASE OF NURSING PROCESS: Evaluation
CLIENT NEEDS: Health Promotion and Maintenance
CONTENT AREA: Adult Health/Musculoskeletal
REFERENCE
Potter, P., & Perry, A. (1997). *Fundamentals of nursing: Concepts, process, and practice* (4th ed.). St. Louis: Mosby–Year Book. p. 936.

35. **4**

RATIONALE: A straight-leg cane is useful for the client with slight weakness in one leg. A walker is beneficial to the client with greater or bilateral weakness, or is at risk for falls. Wooden crutches are often used by clients with a leg cast. Lofstrand crutches aid clients who need crutches, but have limited arm strength.
TEST-TAKING STRATEGY: Use the process of elimination. Giving a walker to a client with a slight leg weakness is excessive, and is eliminated first. Since there is no evidence in the situation of the question that the client has weight-bearing difficulty, crutches are not indicated either. This leaves the straight leg cane as the correct choice.
LEVEL OF COGNITIVE ABILITY: Comprehension
PHASE OF NURSING PROCESS: Planning

CLIENT NEEDS: Physiological Integrity
CONTENT AREA: Adult Health/Musculoskeletal
REFERENCE
Potter, P., & Perry, A. (1997). *Fundamentals of nursing: Concepts, process, and practice* (4th ed.). St. Louis: Mosby–Year Book. p. 935.

36. **1**

RATIONALE: A quad-cane may be used by the client requiring greater support and stability than is provided by a straight leg cane. The quad-cane provides a four point base of support and is indicated for use by clients with partial or complete hemiplegia. Neither crutches nor a wheelchair are indicated for use with a client such as described in the question.
TEST-TAKING STRATEGY: Use the process of elimination. Giving a wheelchair to a client with partial hemiplegia is excessive, and is eliminated first. Wooden crutches are not indicated, as there is no restriction in weight bearing. A Lofstrand crutch is useful for clients with bilateral weakness. This leaves the quad cane as the correct choice.
LEVEL OF COGNITIVE ABILITY: Comprehension
PHASE OF NURSING PROCESS: Planning
CLIENT NEEDS: Physiological Integrity
CONTENT AREA: Adult Health/Musculoskeletal
REFERENCE
Potter, P., & Perry, A. (1997). *Fundamentals of nursing: Concepts, process, and practice* (4th ed.). St. Louis: Mosby–Year Book. p. 935.

37. **3**

RATIONALE: The client is taught to hold the cane on the opposite side of the weakness. This is because with normal walking the opposite arm and leg move together (called reciprocal motion). The cane is placed 6 inches lateral to the fifth toe.
TEST-TAKING STRATEGY: Knowing that the cane is held at the client's side, not in front, helps you to eliminate options 1 and 2 first. Knowing that the preferred method is to have the cane positioned on the stronger side helps you to choose option 3 over option 4. Remember these important points.
LEVEL OF COGNITIVE ABILITY: Application
PHASE OF NURSING PROCESS: Planning
CLIENT NEEDS: Health Promotion and Maintenance
CONTENT AREA: Adult Health/Musculoskeletal
REFERENCE
Potter, P., & Perry, A. (1997). *Fundamentals of nursing: Concepts, process, and practice* (4th ed.). St. Louis: Mosby–Year Book. p. 935.

38. **2**

RATIONALE: A cane should have a slightly flared tip with flexible concentric rings. This tip acts as a shock absorber and provides optimal stability. Options 1, 3, and 4 are not appropriate.
TEST-TAKING STRATEGY: Options 1 and 4 are the least plausible of all the choices, and may be eliminated first. Neither of these statements provides any reassurance for the client. Option 3 also provides no information to relieve the client's anxiety. Option 2 is the best answer. It is a true statement and addresses in a factual way the client's concerns about safety.
LEVEL OF COGNITIVE ABILITY: Application
PHASE OF NURSING PROCESS: Implementation
CLIENT NEEDS: Psychosocial Integrity
CONTENT AREA: Adult Health/Musculoskeletal

REFERENCE
Monahan, F., & Neighbors, M. (1998). *Medical-surgical nursing: Foundations for clinical practice* (2nd ed.). Philadelphia: W. B. Saunders. p. 880.

39. 3

RATIONALE: The cane is held on the stronger side to minimize stress on the affected extremity and provide a wide base of support. The cane is held 6 inches lateral to the fifth great toe. The cane is moved forward with the affected leg. The client leans on the cane for added support while the stronger side swings through.

TEST-TAKING STRATEGY: The wording of this question guides you to look for an incorrect action. Knowing that the cane is held on the stronger side helps you eliminate options 1 and 2 first. To discriminate between the two remaining choices, recall that the client moves the cane with the weaker leg and leans on it for support when the stronger leg swings through. Review client instructions for cane walking now if you had difficulty with this question.

LEVEL OF COGNITIVE ABILITY: Comprehension
PHASE OF NURSING PROCESS: Evaluation
CLIENT NEEDS: Health Promotion and Maintenance
CONTENT AREA: Adult Health/Musculoskeletal

REFERENCE
Monahan, F., & Neighbors, M. (1998). *Medical-surgical nursing: Foundations for clinical practice* (2nd ed.). Philadelphia: W. B Saunders. p. 880.

40. 4

RATIONALE: Compartment syndrome is caused by bleeding and swelling within a compartment that is lined by fascia, which does not expand. The bleeding and swelling place pressure on the nerves, muscles, and blood vessels in the compartment, triggering the symptoms.

TEST-TAKING STRATEGY: A basic understanding of the concept of a compartment is needed to answer this question. Option 1 should be eliminated first because it is not due to an arterial injury. Knowing that the fascia itself cannot expand eliminates option 2. To discriminate between the last two, it is necessary to know that bleeding and swelling cause the symptoms, not a nerve injury.

LEVEL OF COGNITIVE ABILITY: Comprehension
PHASE OF NURSING PROCESS: Planning
CLIENT NEEDS: Physiological Integrity
CONTENT AREA: Adult Health/Musculoskeletal

REFERENCE
Monahan, F., & Neighbors, M. (1998). *Medical-surgical nursing: Foundations for clinical practice* (2nd ed.). Philadelphia: W. B. Saunders. p. 932.

41. 1

RATIONALE: Compartment syndrome is prevented by controlling edema. This is achieved most optimally with the use of elevation and application of ice.

TEST-TAKING STRATEGY: Knowing that edema is controlled or prevented with limb elevation helps you to eliminate options 3 and 4 as possible answers. To discriminate between the last two options, look at the effects of ice versus bath blankets. Ice will further control edema whereas bath blankets will produce heat and prevent air circulation needed for the cast to dry. Review measures to prevent compartment syndrome now if you had difficulty with this question.

LEVEL OF COGNITIVE ABILITY: Application
PHASE OF NURSING PROCESS: Planning

CLIENT NEEDS: Physiological Integrity
CONTENT AREA: Adult Health/Musculoskeletal

REFERENCE
Monahan, F., & Neighbors, M. (1998). *Medical-surgical nursing: Foundations for clinical practice* (2nd ed.). Philadelphia: W. B. Saunders. p. 933.

42. 2

RATIONALE: Confusion in the elderly client with hip fracture could result from the unfamiliar hospital setting, stress due to the fracture, concurrent systemic diseases, cerebral ischemia, or side effects of medications. Use of eyeglasses and hearing aids enhance the client's interaction with the environment, and can reduce disorientation.

TEST-TAKING STRATEGY: Note the key word "not." Stress from the fracture (option 1) and unfamiliar setting (option 3) are not likely to help the client's functional level, and are eliminated as possible options. Eyeglasses and hearing aids are both useful adjuncts in communicating with a client. Since the eyeglasses were left at home, they are of no use at the current time. The working hearing aid is the answer to the question.

LEVEL OF COGNITIVE ABILITY: Comprehension
PHASE OF NURSING PROCESS: Data Collection
CLIENT NEEDS: Psychosocial Integrity
CONTENT AREA: Adult Health/Musculoskeletal

REFERENCE
Leahy, J., & Kizilay, P. (1998). *Foundations of nursing practice: A nursing process approach.* Philadelphia: W. B. Saunders. p. 1056.

43. 4

RATIONALE: Safe nursing actions intended to prevent injury to the client include keeping side rails up, the bed in the low position, and providing a call bell that is within the client's reach. Responding promptly to the client's use of the call light minimizes the chance that the client will try to get up alone, which could result in a fall.

TEST-TAKING STRATEGY: Note the key word "avoid." Since options 1 and 3 (side rails up and call bell in reach) are standard nursing actions, they are eliminated as possible options. Use of a nightlight helps prevent falls, which is also helpful. This leaves the delay in answering the call light as the correct option. Delays will give the client reason to try to get up unattended, and risk another fall and possible injury.

LEVEL OF COGNITIVE ABILITY: Application
PHASE OF NURSING PROCESS: Planning
CLIENT NEEDS: Safe, Effective Care Environment
CONTENT AREA: Adult Health/Musculoskeletal

REFERENCE
deWit, S. (1998). *Essentials of medical-surgical nursing* (4th ed.). Philadelphia: W. B. Saunders. p. 279.

44. 1

RATIONALE: Following internal fixation of a hip fracture, the client is turned to the affected side or the unaffected side as prescribed by the surgeon. Before moving the client, the nurse places a pillow between the client's legs to keep the affected leg in abduction. The client is then repositioned while proper alignment and abduction are maintained.

TEST-TAKING STRATEGY: A trochanter roll is useful in preventing external rotation, but it is used once the client has been repositioned. It is not used while turning the client. Thus, options 3 and 4 may be readily eliminated. To discriminate between options 1 and 2, use of a pillow would

keep the legs abducted, not adducted. Thus, option 1 is the answer to the question.
LEVEL OF COGNITIVE ABILITY: Application
PHASE OF NURSING PROCESS: Implementation
CLIENT NEEDS: Physiological Integrity
CONTENT AREA: Adult Health/Musculoskeletal
REFERENCE
Monahan, F., & Neighbors, M. (1998). *Medical-surgical nursing: Foundations for clinical practice* (2nd ed.). Philadelphia: W. B. Saunders. p. 866.

45. **4**

RATIONALE: The client who has received a total knee replacement often has the leg put into a CPM machine while in the postanesthesia care unit. The device increases circulation and movement of the knee joint. It should be used as prescribed by the physician.
TEST-TAKING STRATEGY: Knowledge of the purpose and effects of a CPM machine is needed to answer this question correctly. If this question was difficult, take a few moments now to review these concepts.
LEVEL OF COGNITIVE ABILITY: Comprehension
PHASE OF NURSING PROCESS: Planning
CLIENT NEEDS: Physiological Integrity
CONTENT AREA: Adult Health/Musculoskeletal
REFERENCE
Monahan, F., & Neighbors, M. (1998). *Medical-surgical nursing: Foundations for clinical practice* (2nd ed.). Philadelphia: W. B. Saunders. pp. 868, 914.

46. **1**

RATIONALE: The nurse assists the client to get out of bed on the first postoperative day after putting a knee immobilizer on the affected joint for stability. The surgeon orders the weight-bearing limits on the affected leg. The leg is elevated while the client is sitting in the chair to minimize edema.
TEST-TAKING STRATEGY: Use the process of elimination. A compression dressing should already be in place on the wound, so option 2 should be eliminated first. Since the CPM machine is used only while the client is in bed, option 3 is incorrect and is eliminated also. To discriminate between the last two options, knowing that ambulation is not started until the second postoperative day would help you choose correctly. The knee immobilizer should be a natural choice when answering a question about protecting a knee joint.
LEVEL OF COGNITIVE ABILITY: Application
PHASE OF NURSING PROCESS: Planning
CLIENT NEEDS: Physiological Integrity
CONTENT AREA: Adult Health/Musculoskeletal
REFERENCE
Monahan, F., & Neighbors, M. (1998). *Medical-surgical nursing: Foundations for clinical practice* (2nd ed.). Philadelphia: W. B. Saunders. p. 868.

47. **3**

RATIONALE: Clients with diabetes mellitus are more prone to wound infection and delayed wound healing due to the disease. Postoperative stump edema and hemorrhage are complications in the immediate postoperative period that apply to any client with an amputation. Slight redness of the incision is considered normal, as long it is dry and intact.

TEST-TAKING STRATEGY: The question guides you to look for complications that are primarily due to the coexisting condition of diabetes mellitus. Knowing that diabetes increases the client's chances of developing infection and delayed wound healing helps you to eliminate options 1 and 2 first. Choose option 3 over option 4 because separation of wound edges is a more serious problem than a slight redness to the incision line, which is considered normal.
LEVEL OF COGNITIVE ABILITY: Comprehension
PHASE OF NURSING PROCESS: Data Collection
CLIENT NEEDS: Physiological Integrity
CONTENT AREA: Adult Health/Musculoskeletal
REFERENCE
Monahan, F., & Neighbors, M. (1998). *Medical-surgical nursing: Foundations for clinical practice* (2nd ed.). Philadelphia: W. B. Saunders. p. 868.

48. **1**

RATIONALE: Phantom limb sensations are felt in the area of the amputated limb. These can include itching, warmth, and cold. The sensations are due to intact peripheral nerves in the area amputated. Whenever possible, clients should be prepared for these sensations. The client may also feel painful sensations in the amputated limb, called phantom limb pain. The origin of the pain is less well understood, but the client should be prepared for this, too, whenever possible.
TEST-TAKING STRATEGY: Use the process of elimination. By knowing that sensation and pain may be felt in the residual limb helps you to eliminate options 3 and 4 first, because the sensations are not abnormal responses. Select option 1 over option 2 because the client has described an itching sensation, but has not complained of pain in the residual limb.
LEVEL OF COGNITIVE ABILITY: Comprehension
PHASE OF NURSING PROCESS: Data Collection
CLIENT NEEDS: Psychosocial Integrity
CONTENT AREA: Adult Health/Musculoskeletal
REFERENCE
Monahan, F., & Neighbors, M. (1998). *Medical-surgical nursing: Foundations for clinical practice* (2nd ed.). Philadelphia: W. B. Saunders. p. 877.

49. **3**

RATIONALE: Low back pain with radiation into one leg (sciatica) is consistent with herniated lumbar disk. The nurse continues to collect data from the client to see if the pain is aggravated by events that increase intraspinal pressure such as bending, lifting, sneezing, coughing, or when lifting the leg straight up while supine (straight-leg-raising test). Options 1, 2, and 4 assist in alleviating pain.
TEST-TAKING STRATEGY: To answer this question, recall the basic causes of back pain and the factors that alleviate or aggravate it. With this knowledge, recall that bed rest, heat (or sometimes ice), and nonsteroidal anti-inflammatory agents usually relieve back pain, whereas bending, lifting, and straining aggravate it. If this question was difficult, review these concepts now.
LEVEL OF COGNITIVE ABILITY: Comprehension
PHASE OF NURSING PROCESS: Data Collection
CLIENT NEEDS: Physiological Integrity
CONTENT AREA: Adult Health/Musculoskeletal
REFERENCE
deWit, S. (1998). *Essentials of medical-surgical nursing* (4th ed.). Philadelphia: W. B. Saunders. p. 377.

50. 4

RATIONALE: Following spinal fusion, the head of bed is generally kept in a flat position. The client is log rolled from side to side as ordered. Pillows may be placed under the entire length of the legs by surgeon preference to relieve tension on the lower back. The use of an overhead trapeze is contraindicated because its use could promote twisting of the spine after surgery.
TEST-TAKING STRATEGY: Note the key word "avoids." After spinal surgery, the nurse uses positioning techniques and aids that will keep the spine in good alignment. Thus, options 1 and 3 are obviously indicated, and are therefore eliminated as items to avoid as this question asks. To discriminate between the last two items, using pillows under the length of the legs promotes slight flexion of the spine while avoiding pressure on the popliteal space (which predisposes to thrombophlebitis). Using an overbed trapeze could allow the client to twist the spine, which is directly contraindicated. Review postoperative care following spinal fusion now if you had difficulty with this question.
LEVEL OF COGNITIVE ABILITY: Application
PHASE OF NURSING PROCESS: Implementation
CLIENT NEEDS: Physiological Integrity
CONTENT AREA: Adult Health/Musculoskeletal
REFERENCE
Monahan, F., & Neighbors, M. (1998). *Medical-surgical nursing: Foundations for clinical practice* (2nd ed.). Philadelphia: W. B. Saunders. p. 764.

51. 1

RATIONALE: Clients are taught to get out of bed by sliding near to the edge of the mattress. The client then rolls onto one side and pushes up from the bed using one or both arms. The back is kept straight and the legs are swung over the side. Increasing fluids and dietary fiber helps prevent straining at stool, thereby preventing increases in intraspinal pressure. Walking and swimming are excellent exercises for strengthening lower back muscles. Proper body mechanics includes bending at the knees, not the waist, to lift objects.
TEST-TAKING STRATEGY: Note the key words "needs further instruction." Options 3 and 4 are examples of classic interventions that are indicated, and so they are eliminated first. Clients with low back pain should avoid events that increase intraspinal pressure. Option 2 prevents increases in intraspinal pressure. Option 1 causes an increase in intraspinal pressure if you think of the body mechanics involved in getting out of bed this way. Review the principles of proper body mechanics now if you had difficulty with this question.
LEVEL OF COGNITIVE ABILITY: Comprehension
PHASE OF NURSING PROCESS: Evaluation
CLIENT NEEDS: Health Promotion and Maintenance
CONTENT AREA: Adult Health/Musculoskeletal
REFERENCE
Monahan, F., & Neighbors, M. (1998). *Medical-surgical nursing: Foundations for clinical practice* (2nd ed.). Philadelphia: W. B. Saunders. p. 794.

52. 3

RATIONALE: Following spinal surgery, concerns about finances and employment are best handled by referral to a social worker. This individual will provide information about resources available to the client.
TEST-TAKING STRATEGY: An understanding of the roles of the various members of the health care team helps you to answer this question. The physical therapist has the best knowledge of techniques for increasing mobility and endurance. An occupational therapist has knowledge of techniques for ADLs and items related to occupation, but this is not one of the options. The clinical nurse specialist and physician do not have information related to financial resources. Review health care professional roles now if you had difficulty with this question.
LEVEL OF COGNITIVE ABILITY: Comprehension
PHASE OF NURSING PROCESS: Planning
CLIENT NEEDS: Safe, Effective Care Environment
CONTENT AREA: Adult Health/Musculoskeletal
REFERENCE
Monahan, F., & Neighbors, M. (1998). *Medical-surgical nursing: Foundations for clinical practice* (2nd ed.). Philadelphia: W. B. Saunders. p. 765.

53. 2

RATIONALE: A back brace or thoracolumbarsacral orthosis is individually fitted to the client. The brace should not irritate the skin with proper fitting. The brace is applied in the morning before getting out of bed. The closures should be secure, but not overly loose or tight. A layer of clothing is worn between the orthosis and the skin.
TEST-TAKING STRATEGY: Skin irritation is not likely to be a good sign, and should be eliminated first. Loose connections are also not likely to indicate proper fit, so option 4 should be eliminated next. Of the two remaining, do not choose option 3 because the orthosis is likely to become soiled with perspiration of cause skin irritation. Review care to the client with a brace now if you had difficulty with this question.
LEVEL OF COGNITIVE ABILITY: Application
PHASE OF NURSING PROCESS: Planning
CLIENT NEEDS: Physiological Integrity
CONTENT AREA: Adult Health/Musculoskeletal
REFERENCE
Luckmann, J. (1997). *Saunders manual of nursing care.* Philadelphia: W. B. Saunders. pp. 1565, 1567, 1611.

54. 4

RATIONALE: Following spinal fusion, with or without instrumentation, the client is transferred from stretcher to bed using a slider board and the assistance of four people. This permits optimal stabilization and support of the spine, while allowing the client to be moved smoothly and gently.
TEST-TAKING STRATEGY: Use the process of elimination. This question can be answered by analyzing the level of comfort and stability provided to the client's spine with the amounts of assistance given in each option. Using this approach, you can systematically eliminate each of the incorrect options.
LEVEL OF COGNITIVE ABILITY: Application
PHASE OF NURSING PROCESS: Implementation
CLIENT NEEDS: Safe, Effective Care Environment
CONTENT AREA: Adult Health/Musculoskeletal
REFERENCE
Monahan, F., & Neighbors, M. (1998). *Medical-surgical nursing: Foundations for clinical practice* (2nd ed.). Philadelphia: W. B. Saunders. p. 763.

55. 1

RATIONALE: Stair climbing may be restricted or limited for several weeks following spinal fusion with instrumentation. The nurse ensures that resources are in place prior to discharge so that the client may sleep and perform all ADLs on a single living level.

TEST-TAKING STRATEGY: Use the process of elimination. Options 2 and 3 are obviously useful to the client, and can therefore be eliminated. To discriminate between options 1 and 4 (both of which involve stairs), option 4 is the least problematic, while option 1 poses a significant problem to the client who is restricted from stair climbing.

LEVEL OF COGNITIVE ABILITY: Comprehension
PHASE OF NURSING PROCESS: Evaluation
CLIENT NEEDS: Safe, Effective Care Environment
CONTENT AREA: Adult Health/Musculoskeletal
REFERENCE

Monahan, F., & Neighbors, M. (1998). *Medical-surgical nursing: Foundations for clinical practice* (2nd ed.). Philadelphia: W. B. Saunders. p. 764.

56. **4**

RATIONALE: The client with pallor, slow capillary refill, weakened or lost pulse, and absence of sensation or motion to the distal limb may have arterial damage from a lacerated, contused, thrombosed, or severed artery. These signs can occur with constriction from a tight cast as well. Regardless of the cause, the nurse notifies the physician immediately. Emergency intervention is needed, which could include removal of the constricting bandage, fracture reduction, or surgery to repair the area.

TEST-TAKING STRATEGY: Knowing that these signs indicate insufficient arterial circulation, you know that this can lead to irreversible ischemia and damage. Because of this, eliminate options 1 and 3 first as not being helpful. Rechecking the circulation in 30 minutes loses valuable time for action to restore the impaired circulation, and is a poor choice. The physician should be notified immediately.

LEVEL OF COGNITIVE ABILITY: Application
PHASE OF NURSING PROCESS: Implementation
CLIENT NEEDS: Physiological Integrity
CONTENT AREA: Adult Health/Musculoskeletal
REFERENCE

deWit, S. (1998). *Essentials of medical-surgical nursing* (4th ed.). Philadelphia: W. B. Saunders. p. 691.

57. **4**

RATIONALE: A window may be cut in a dried cast to relieve pressure, monitor pulses, relieve discomfort, or to remove drains. Bivalving the cast involves splitting the cast along both sides to allow space for swelling, facilitate taking x-rays, or to make a half-cast for use as an intermittent splint. Padding is not placed on top of a cast. The use of an air splint is not indicated.

TEST-TAKING STRATEGY: Note the key words "bony prominence." Wherever there is a bony prominence, there is a risk of pressure and skin breakdown. If the pressure area is under a cast, the cast must be removed in that area to relieve the pressure. Therefore, options 1 and 3 can be readily eliminated. Since extra padding over the area of the cast does no good either, that option can be eliminated next. This leaves putting a window in the cast as the correct answer. This will relieve the pressure in that one area without disrupting the cast.

LEVEL OF COGNITIVE ABILITY: Comprehension
PHASE OF NURSING PROCESS: Planning

CLIENT NEEDS: Physiological Integrity
CONTENT AREA: Adult Health/Musculoskeletal
REFERENCE

deWit, S. (1998). *Essentials of medical-surgical nursing* (4th ed.). Philadelphia: W. B. Saunders. p. 687.

58. **4**

RATIONALE: Clients may be fearful of having a cast removed due to misconceptions about the cast-cutting blade. The nurse should show the cast cutter to the client before it is used, and explain that the client may feel heat, vibration, and pressure. The cast cutter resembles a small electric saw with a circular blade. The nurse should reassure the client that the blade does not cut like a saw, but instead cuts the cast by vibrating side to side.

TEST-TAKING STRATEGY: Note the key words "most helpful." Option 2 gives no information although it may be well intentioned, and is eliminated first. Options 1 and 3 give accurate information, but are not reassuring. Option 4 gives the client the most reassurance because it best prepares the client for what will occur when the cast is removed.

LEVEL OF COGNITIVE ABILITY: Application
PHASE OF NURSING PROCESS: Implementation
CLIENT NEEDS: Psychosocial Integrity
CONTENT AREA: Adult Health/Musculoskeletal
REFERENCE

Monahan, F., & Neighbors, M. (1998). *Medical-surgical nursing: Foundations for clinical practice* (2nd ed.). Philadelphia: W. B. Saunders. p. 853.

59. **2**

RATIONALE: The skin under a casted area may be discolored and crusted with dead skin layers. The client should gently soak and wash the skin for the first few days. The skin should be patted dry, and a lubricating lotion should be applied. Clients often want to scrub the dead skin away, which irritates the skin. The client should avoid overexposing the skin to the sunlight.

TEST-TAKING STRATEGY: Note the key words "misunderstood." Option 3 is obviously helpful, and therefore cannot be the answer to the question as stated. Option 4 is good advice if the skin has been covered, and is eliminated next. Options 1 and 2 seem to oppose each other, making it likely that one of them is correct. Since vigorous scrubbing is more likely to be irritating than providing gentle soaking, it is the most likely choice as the answer to the question.

LEVEL OF COGNITIVE ABILITY: Comprehension
PHASE OF NURSING PROCESS: Evaluation
CLIENT NEEDS: Health Promotion and Maintenance
CONTENT AREA: Adult Health/Musculoskeletal
REFERENCE

Monahan, F., & Neighbors, M. (1998). *Medical-surgical nursing: Foundations for clinical practice* (2nd ed.). Philadelphia: W. B. Saunders. p. 858.

60. **4**

RATIONALE: Common areas that are under pressure and are at risk for breakdown include the elbows (if they are used for repositioning instead of a trapeze) and the heel of the good leg (which is used as a brace when pushing up in bed). Other pressure points caused by the traction include the ischial tuberosity, popliteal space, and Achilles tendon.

TEST-TAKING STRATEGY: Note the key words "high-risk area." Thus, you would compare each of the options in terms of their relative risk, and choose the one that is greatest. The right heel is eliminated first because it is off the bed in the traction set-up. The overhead trapeze diminishes the likelihood that the scapulae and back of the head would be immobile. This leaves the left heel as the answer to the question. This makes sense, given that the client would use the unaffected heel to push into the mattress during repositioning. With repeated use, this could cause the left heel to become reddened and break down.
LEVEL OF COGNITIVE ABILITY: Comprehension
PHASE OF NURSING PROCESS: Data Collection
CLIENT NEEDS: Physiological Integrity
CONTENT AREA: Adult Health/Musculoskeletal
REFERENCE
Monahan, F., & Neighbors, M. (1998). *Medical-surgical nursing: Foundations for clinical practice* (2nd ed.). Philadelphia: W. B. Saunders. p. 862.

61. 2

RATIONALE: The part of the bed under an area in traction is usually elevated to aid in countertraction. For the client in Buck's extension traction (which is applied to a leg), the foot of the bed is elevated.
TEST-TAKING STRATEGY: To answer this question accurately, you need to understand the principles of traction and countertraction, and be familiar with Buck's extension traction. Option 3 is not used for the purpose of countertraction and is eliminated first. Knowing that Buck's extension traction is applied to the leg helps you eliminate option 1. Of the two remaining choices, option 4 places undue pressure on the client's unaffected foot. Furthermore, a footboard is not used for the purpose of providing countertraction. Option 2 provides a force that opposes the traction force effectively without harming the client.
LEVEL OF COGNITIVE ABILITY: Application
PHASE OF NURSING PROCESS: Implementation
CLIENT NEEDS: Physiological Integrity
CONTENT AREA: Adult Health/Musculoskeletal
REFERENCE
Monahan, F., & Neighbors, M. (1998). *Medical-surgical nursing: Foundations for clinical practice* (2nd ed.). Philadelphia: W. B. Saunders. pp. 861–862.

62. 1

RATIONALE: Risk factors associated with osteoporosis include a diet that is deficient in calcium. Options 2, 3, and 4 include risk factors associated with osteoporesis. Additional risk factors include being sedentary, cigarette smoking, excessive alcohol consumption, chronic illness, and long-term use of anticonvulsants and furosemide.
TEST-TAKING STRATEGY: Knowledge regarding the risk factors associated with osteoporosis is required to answer this question. Review these risk factors now if you are not familiar with them.
LEVEL OF COGNITIVE ABILITY: Comprehension
PHASE OF NURSING PROCESS: Data Collection
CLIENT NEEDS: Health Promotion and Maintenance
CONTENT AREA: Adult Health/Musculoskeletal
REFERENCE
deWit, S. (1998). *Essentials of medical-surgical nursing* (4th ed.). Philadelphia: W. B. Saunders. p. 701.

63. 4

RATIONALE: Foods high in calcium include plain yogurt, dairy products, seafood, sardines, green vegetables, calcium-fortified orange juice, and cereal. Of the items listed in the options, option 4 contains the least amount of calcium.
TEST-TAKING STRATEGY: Note the key word "least." By the process of elimination, you should easily be directed to option 4. Review foods high in calcium now if you had difficulty with this question.
LEVEL OF COGNITIVE ABILITY: Comprehension
PHASE OF NURSING PROCESS: Implementation
CLIENT NEEDS: Health Promotion and Maintenance
CONTENT AREA: Adult Health/Musculoskeletal
REFERENCE
deWit, S. (1998). *Essentials of medical-surgical nursing* (4th ed.). Philadelphia: W. B. Saunders. p. 701.

64. 1

RATIONALE: Ample fluid intake is encouraged to promote excretion of uric acid. The client is placed on bed rest until the pain subsides. A diet low in purine is normally prescribed, which includes a decrease in red and organ meats. NSAIDs are used to reduce pain and inflammation.
TEST-TAKING STRATEGY: Note the key word "not." Also note the key word "acute." This will assist in eliminating options 3 and 4. Knowledge that a low-purine diet may be recommended for the client with gout will easily direct you to option 1. Review care to the client with gout now if you had difficulty with this question.
LEVEL OF COGNITIVE ABILITY: Application
PHASE OF NURSING PROCESS: Planning
CLIENT NEEDS: Health Promotion and Maintenance
CONTENT AREA: Adult Health/Musculoskeletal
REFERENCE
deWit, S. (1998). *Essentials of medical-surgical nursing* (4th ed.). Philadelphia: W. B. Saunders. p. 701.

65. 1

RATIONALE: Rheumatoid arthritis is characterized by chronic joint pain of varying intensity that is more severe upon rising in the morning. The nurse notes that joint involvement is symmetrical and the joints are swollen, shiny, reddened, and painful. Rheumatoid nodules, which are painless subcutaneous movable skin nodules near bony prominences, may occur anywhere on the body.
TEST-TAKING STRATEGY: Note that key word "not." Note that options 1 and 2 are similar in that both address the component of pain and its occurrence. This should lead you to suspect that one of these options is correct. Review the characteristics associated with RA now if you had difficulty with this question.
LEVEL OF COGNITIVE ABILITY: Comprehension
PHASE OF NURSING PROCESS: Data Collection
CLIENT NEEDS: Physiological Integrity
CONTENT AREA: Adult Health/Musculoskeletal
REFERENCE
Monahan, F., & Neighbors, M. (1998). *Medical-surgical nursing: Foundations for clinical practice* (2nd ed.). Philadelphia: W. B. Saunders. p. 891.

BIBLIOGRAPHY

Black, J., & Matassarin-Jacobs, E. (1997). *Medical surgical nursing: Clinical management for continuity of care* (5th ed.). Philadelphia: W. B. Saunders.

Chernecky, C., & Berger, B. (1997). *Laboratory tests and diagnostic procedures* (2nd ed.). Philadelphia: W. B. Saunders.

Deglin, J., & Vallerand, A. (1999). *Davis's drug guide for nurses* (6th ed.). Philadelphia: F. A. Davis.

deWit, S. (1998). *Essentials of medical-surgical nursing* (4th ed.). Philadelphia: W. B. Saunders.

Hodgson, B., & Kizior, R. (2000). *Saunders nursing drug handbook 2000*. Philadelphia: W. B. Saunders.

Leahy, J., & Kizilay, P. (1998). *Foundations of nursing practice: A nursing process approach*. Philadelphia: W. B. Saunders.

Lehne, R. (1998). *Pharmacology for nursing care* (3rd ed.). Philadelphia: W. B. Saunders.

Luckmann, J. (1997). *Saunders manual of nursing care*. Philadelphia: W. B. Saunders.

Monahan, F., & Neighbors, M. (1998). *Medical-surgical nursing: Foundations for clinical practice* (2nd ed.). Philadelphia: W. B. Saunders.

O'Toole, M. (1997). *Miller-Keane encyclopedia & dictionary of medicine, nursing, & allied health* (6th ed.). Philadelphia: W. B. Saunders.

Potter, P., & Perry, A. (1997). *Fundamentals of nursing: Concepts, process, and practice* (4th ed.). St. Louis: Mosby–Year Book.

CHAPTER 57

Musculoskeletal Medications

I. Skeletal Muscle Relaxants (Box 57–1)

A. Description
1. Act directly on the neuromuscular junction or indirectly on the central nervous system (CNS)
2. Centrally acting muscle relaxants depress neuron activity in the spinal cord or brain
3. Peripheral-acting muscle relaxants act directly on the skeletal muscles
4. Used to prevent or relieve muscle spasms, to treat spasticity associated with spinal cord disease or lesions, for painful musculoskeletal conditions, and for chronic debilitating disorders such as multiple sclerosis, cerebrovascular accident (CVA), or cerebral palsy
5. Contraindicated in severe liver, renal, or heart disease
6. Should not be taken with CNS depressants such as barbiturates, narcotics, and alcohol; sedatives; hypnotics; or tricyclic antidepressants

B. Side effects
1. Dizziness and hypotension
2. Drowsiness
3. Dry mouth

BOX 57–1. Skeletal Muscle Relaxants

Baclofen (Lioresal)
Carisoprodol (Soma)
Cyclobenzaprine hydrochloride (Flexeril)
Dantrolene (Dantrium)
Diazepam (Valium)
Methocarbamol (Robaxin)
Orphenadrine (Norflex)
Chlorzoxazone (Paraflex, Parafon Forte)
Chlorphenesin carbamate (Maolate)
Meprobamate (Equanil, Miltown)

---

4. Gastrointestinal (GI) upset
5. Photosensitivity
6. Liver toxicity

C. Implementation
1. Obtain a medication history
2. Monitor vital signs
3. Monitor for CNS side effects
4. Monitor for risk of injury
5. Monitor involved joints and muscles for pain and mobility
6. Monitor liver function tests because hepatotoxicity can occur
7. Monitor renal function
8. Instruct the client to take medication with food to decrease GI upset
9. Instruct the client to report side effects
10. Instruct the client to avoid alcohol and CNS depressants
11. Instruct the client to avoid activities requiring alertness

D. Nursing considerations
1. Baclofen (Lioresal)
   a. Causes CNS effects such as drowsiness, dizziness, weakness, and fatigue
   b. Frequently causes nausea, constipation, and urinary retention
   c. Can be administered by the physician by intrathecal infusion by using an implantable pump
2. Dantrolene (Dantrium)
   a. Acts directly on skeletal muscles to relieve spasticity
   b. Liver damage is the most serious adverse effect
   c. Liver function tests should be monitored prior to the initiation of treatment and during treatment
   d. Can cause GI bleeding, urinary frequency, impotence, photosensitivity, and rash
   e. Instruct the client to wear protective clothing when in the sun

f. Instruct the client to notify the physician if rash, bloody or tarry stool, or yellow discoloration of skin or eyes occurs

3. Cyclobenzaprine hydrochloride (Flexeril)
   a. Contraindicated in clients who have received monoamine oxidase (MAO) inhibitors within 14 days of initiation of cyclobenzaprine therapy, and in clients with cardiac disorders
   b. Used with caution in clients with a history of urinary retention, angle-closure glaucoma, and increased intraocular pressure
   c. Should be used only for short term (2 to 3 weeks of therapy)

4. Methocarbamol (Robaxin)
   a. Parenteral form is contraindicated in clients with renal impairment
   b. Parenteral form can cause anaphylaxis and seizures
   c. Parenteral form can cause hypotension and bradycardia
   d. May cause urine to turn brown, black, or green
   e. Inform the client to notify the physician if blurred vision, nasal congestion, urticaria, or rash occurs

5. Chlorzoxazone (Paraflex, Parafon Forte)
   a. Monitor for hypersensitivity reactions, such as urticaria, redness or itching, and possibly angioedema
   b. May cause malaise and urine discoloration

6. Carisoprodol (Soma)
   a. Advise the client to take medication with food to prevent GI upset
   b. Instruct the client to report to the physician rash or hypersensitivity

II. Antigout Medications (Box 57–2)

A. Description
   1. Decrease inflammation
   2. Reduce uric acid production and increase uric acid excretion
   3. To prevent or relieve gout
   4. Used cautiously in clients with GI, renal, cardiac, and hepatic disease
   5. Allopurinol (Zyloprim) can increase the effect of warfarin and oral hypoglycemic agents

B. Side effects
   1. Headaches
   2. Nausea, vomiting, and diarrhea

BOX 57–2. Antigout Medications

Allopurinol (Zyloprim)
Colchicine
Probenecid (Benemid)
Sulfinpyrazone (Anturane)

---

3. Blood dyscrasias such as bone marrow depression
4. Flushed skin and skin rash
5. Uric acid kidney stones
6. Sore gums
7. Metallic taste

C. Implementation
   1. Monitor serum uric acid levels
   2. Monitor intake and output (I&O)
   3. Maintain a fluid intake of at least 2000 to 3000 mL a day to avoid kidney stones
   4. Monitor complete blood count (CBC) and renal and liver function studies
   5. Instruct the client to avoid alcohol and caffeine because these products can increase uric acid levels
   6. Instruct the client not to take large doses of vitamin C while taking allopurinol (Zyloprim) because kidney stones may occur
   7. Encourage the client to comply with therapy to prevent elevated uric acid levels, which can trigger a gout attack
   8. Instruct the client to avoid foods high in purine such as wine and other forms of alcohol, organ meats, sardines, salmon, and gravy
   9. Instruct the client to take medication with food
   10. Instruct the client to report side effects to the physician
   11. Advise the client to have a yearly eye exam because visual changes can occur from prolonged use of allopurinol (Zyloprim)
   12. Caution the client not to take aspirin with these medications because this could trigger a gout attack
   13. Concurrent use of aspirin causes elevated uric acid levels; clients should be instructed to take acetaminophen (Tylenol)

III. Antiarthritic Medications

A. Nonsteroidal anti-inflammatory drugs (NSAIDs) (Box 57–3)
   1. Description
      a. NSAIDs are aspirin and aspirin-like medications that inhibit the synthesis of prostaglandins
      b. They act as an analgesic to relieve pain, as an antipyretic to reduce body temperature, and as an anticoagulant to inhibit platelet aggregation
      c. Used to relieve inflammation and pain and in the treatment of rheumatoid arthritis, bursitis, tendinitis, osteoarthritis, and acute gout
      d. Contraindicated in hypersensitivity or liver or renal disease
      e. Aspirin should not be taken by children with flu symptoms because of the risk of Reye's syndrome
      f. Aspirin should not be taken if the client is on an anticoagulant

BOX 57-3. Nonsteroidal Anti-Inflammatory Medications (NSAIDs)

Aspirin (acetylsalicylic acid [ASA]; Bayer, Ecotrin)
Diflunisal (Dolobid)
Indomethacin (Indocin)
Sulindac (Clinoril)
Tolmetin (Tolectin)
Phenylbutazone (Butazolidin)
Fenoprofen calcium (Nalfon)
Flurbiprofen sodium (Ansaid, Ocufen)
Ibuprofen (Motrin, Advil, Nuprin, Medipren)
Ketoprofen (Orudis)
Naproxen (Naprosyn)
Oxaprozin (Daypro)
Meclofenamate (Meclomen)
Mefenamic acid (Ponstel)
Piroxicam (Feldene)
Diclofenac sodium (Voltaren)
Etodolac (Lodine)
Ketorolac tromethamine (Toradol)

g. Aspirin and an NSAID should not be taken together because aspirin decreases the blood level and the effectiveness of the NSAID
h. NSAIDs can increase the effects of warfarin, sulfonamides, cephalosporins, and phenytoin (Dilantin)
i. Hypoglycemia may result if ibuprofen (Motrin) is taken with insulin or an oral hypoglycemic medication
j. A high risk of toxicity exists if ibuprofen (Motrin) is taken concurrently with calcium blockers
2. Side effects (Table 57-1)
3. Implementation
a. Assess the client for allergies
b. Obtain a medication history
c. Assess for history of gastric upset or bleeding, or liver disease
d. Monitor the client for GI upset during medication administration
e. Monitor for edema
f. Monitor serum salicylate (aspirin) level when the client is taking high doses
g. Monitor for signs of bleeding such as tarry stools, bleeding gums, petechiae, ecchymosis, and purpura

Table 57-1. Side Effects

Aspirin	*NSAIDs*
Drowsiness	Hypotension
Tinnitus	Sodium and water retention
Pruritus	Gastric irritation
Headaches	Blood dyscrasias
Flushing	Dizziness
Dizziness	Tinnitus
GI symptoms	Pruritus
Visual changes	

BOX 57-4. Gold Therapy Medications

Auranofin (Ridaura)
Aurothioglucose (Solganal)
Gold sodium thiomalate (Myochrysine)

h. Instruct the client to take medication with water, milk, or food
i. Enteric-coated form or buffered form of aspirin can be taken to decrease gastric distress
j. Instruct clients that enteric-coated tablets cannot be crushed or broken
k. Advise clients to inform other health care professionals if they are taking high doses of aspirin
l. Note that aspirin should be discontinued 3 to 7 days prior to surgery to reduce the risk of bleeding
m. Instruct the client to avoid alcoholic beverages
B. Gold therapy (Box 57-4)
1. Description
a. Referred to as chrysotherapy or heavy-metal therapy
b. Depresses migration of leukocytes and suppresses prostaglandin activity
c. Reduces inflammation by decreasing enzyme release and altering the immune response
d. Primarily used for palliative relief of symptoms in rheumatoid arthritis
e. Contraindications are listed in Box 57-5
2. Side effects
a. Dizziness
b. Rash and urticaria
c. Erythema and dermatitis
d. Alopecia
e. Stomatitis
f. Diarrhea
g. Hepatitis
h. Metallic taste in the mouth
i. Blood dyscrasias such as bone marrow suppression
j. Photosensitivity reactions
k. Gold toxicity

BOX 57-5. Contraindications to Gold Therapy

Eczema
Urticaria
Colitis
Hemorrhagic conditions
Systemic lupus erythematosus
Renal or hepatic dysfunction
Uncontrolled diabetes mellitus
Congestive heart failure
Recent radiation therapy

3. Implementation
   a. Obtain the client's health history
   b. Monitor for blood dyscrasias before and during therapy
   c. Monitor for proteinuria and hematuria before and during therapy
   d. When giving gold injection, monitor the client for 30 minutes for possible allergic reaction
   e. Instruct the client to maintain good oral hygiene
   f. Instruct the client to use sunscreen and protective clothing to prevent photosensitivity reactions
   g. Teach the client about the signs and symptoms of gold toxicity, which include pruritus, skin rash, metallic taste, stomatitis, and diarrhea
   h. If toxicity occurs, dimercaprol (BAL in oil) may be prescribed to enhance gold excretion

PRACTICE QUESTIONS

1. Allopurinol (Zyloprim) has been prescribed for the client. The client asks the nurse about the action of the medication. The nurse responds, knowing that it
   1 Is used for the lysis of thrombi obstructing coronary arteries
   2 Prevents calcium ion entry across cell membranes of the cardiac smooth muscle
   3 Decreases sympathetic outflow from the CNS
   4 Decreases uric acid production and reduces uric acid concentrations in both the serum and urine

2. The nurse is caring for a client who is taking allopurinol (Zyloprim). Which of the following medications, if prescribed for the client, does the nurse question?
   1 Mebendazole (Vermox)
   2 Ergonovine maleate (Ergotrate)
   3 Warfarin sodium (Coumadin)
   4 Pentazocine (Talwin)

3. The nurse prepares to reinforce instructions to a client who is taking allopurinol (Zyloprim). The nurse plans to include which of the following in the instructions?
   1 Inform the client that the effect of the medication will occur immediately
   2 Instruct the client to drink 3000 mL of fluid per day
   3 Instruct the client to take the medication on an empty stomach
   4 Inform the client that if swelling of the lips occurs this is a normal, expected response

4. The nurse is caring for a client with unstable angina. The client is taking acetylsalicylic acid (aspirin) on a daily basis to reduce the risk of myocardial infarction (MI). Which of the following medication doses does the nurse expect the client to be taking?
   1 3 g daily
   2 300 to 325 mg daily
   3 1.3 g daily
   4 650 to 700 mg daily

5. Colchicine is prescribed for a client with a diagnosis of gout. The nurse reviews the client's medical history in the health record, knowing that the medication is contraindicated in which of the following disorders?
   1 Renal failure
   2 Hypothyroidism
   3 Diabetes mellitus
   4 Myexdema

6. The nurse is caring for a client who is taking probenecid (Benemid). The client has been instructed to restrict the diet to low-purine foods. Which of the following foods does the nurse instruct the client to avoid?
   1 Potatoes
   2 Ice cream
   3 Spinach
   4 Scallops

7. The physician prescribes auranofin (Ridaura) for the client with rheumatoid arthritis. Which of the following indicates to the nurse that the client is experiencing toxicity related to the medication?
   1 Constipation
   2 Complaints of a metallic taste in the mouth
   3 Ringing in the ears
   4 Joint pain

8. A film-coated form of diflunisal (Dolobid) has been prescribed for a client to treat chronic rheumatoid arthritis. The client calls the clinic nurse because of difficulty swallowing the tablets. Which of the following instructions does the nurse give the client?
   1 Crush the tablets and mix them with food
   2 Open the tablets and mix the contents with food
   3 Swallow the tablets with large amounts of water or milk
   4 Notify the physician for a medication change

9. The physician instructs an elderly client with rheumatoid arthritis to take ibuprofen (Motrin). The nurse reinforces the instructions, knowing that the normal adult dose for this client is which of the following?
   1 100 mg PO BID
   2 200 mg PO BID
   3 300 mg PO TID
   4 1000 mg PO QID

10. Baclofen (Lioresal) is prescribed for the client with multiple sclerosis. The nurse assists in planning care, knowing that the primary therapeutic effect of this medication is which of the following?
    1. Increased muscle tone
    2. Decreased muscle spasms
    3. Decreased local pain and tenderness
    4. Increased range of motion

11. The nurse is monitoring a client receiving baclofen (Lioresal) for side effects related to the medication. Which of the following indicates that the client is experiencing a side effect?
    1. Drowsiness
    2. Diarrhea
    3. Polyuria
    4. Muscular excitability

12. The nurse is reinforcing discharge instructions to a client receiving baclofen (Lioresal). Which of the following does the nurse plan to include in the instructions?
    1. Restrict fluid intake
    2. Avoid the use of alcohol
    3. Stop the medication if diarrhea occurs
    4. Notify the physician if fatigue occurs

13. The adult client with muscle spasms is taking an oral maintenance dose of baclofen (Lioresal). The nurse reviews the medication record, expecting that which of the following doses will be prescribed?
    1. 15 mg QID
    2. 25 mg QID
    3. 30 mg QID
    4. 40 mg QID

14. A client with acute muscle spasms has been taking baclofen (Lioresal). The client calls the clinic nurse because of continuous feelings of weakness and fatigue and asks the nurse about discontinuing the medication. Which of the following responses to the client is most appropriate?
    1. "It is best that you taper the dose if you intend to stop the medication."
    2. "Weakness and fatigue commonly occur and will diminish with continued medication use."
    3. "It is all right to stop the medication if you think that you can tolerate the muscle spasms."
    4. "You should never stop the medication."

15. Dantrolene sodium (Dantrium) is prescribed for the client experiencing flexor spasms. The client asks the nurse about the action of the medication. The nurse responds, knowing that the therapeutic action of this medication is which of the following?
    1. Acts within the spinal cord to suppress hyperactive reflexes

    2. Acts on the CNS to suppress spasms
    3. Acts directly on the skeletal muscle to relieve spasticity
    4. Depresses spinal reflexes

16. The nurse is reviewing the laboratory studies on a client receiving dantrolene sodium (Dantrium). Which of the following laboratory tests would identify an adverse effect associated with the administration of this medication?
    1. Blood urea nitrogen (BUN)
    2. Creatinine
    3. Liver function tests
    4. Hematologic function tests

17. The nurse is reviewing the record of a client who has been prescribed baclofen (Lioresal). Which of the following disorders, if noted in the client's history, alerts the nurse to contact the physician?
    1. Coronary artery disease
    2. Diabetes mellitus
    3. Seizure disorders
    4. Hyperthyroidism

18. Cyclobenzaprine hydrochloride (Flexeril) is prescribed for the client for muscle spasms. The nurse is reviewing the client's record. Which of the following disorders, if noted in the client's record, indicates a need to contact the physician regarding the administration of this medication?
    1. Glaucoma
    2. Hyperthyroidism
    3. Emphysema
    4. Diabetes mellitus

19. The client is to receive a prescription for methocarbamol (Robaxin). The nurse reinforces instructions to the client regarding the medication. Which of the following client statements indicates a need for further education?
    1. "My urine may turn brown or green."
    2. "If my vision becomes blurred I don't need to be concerned about it."
    3. "I might get some nasal congestion from this medication."
    4. "This medication is prescribed to help relieve my muscle spasms."

20. The nurse is reviewing the physician's orders for an adult client who has been admitted to the hospital following a back injury. Carisoprodol (Soma) is prescribed for the client to relieve the muscle spasms. The physician has prescribed 350 mg to be administered QID. When preparing to give this medication, the nurse determines that this dosage is
    1. The normal adult dosage
    2. A lower than normal dosage
    3. A higher than normal dosage
    4. A dosage requiring further clarification

ANSWERS

1. **4**

RATIONALE: Allopurinol is an antigout medication. It decreases uric acid production by inhibiting the enzyme xanthine oxidase, and reduces uric acid concentrations in both serum and urine.
TEST-TAKING STRATEGY: Knowledge regarding this medication is required to answer the question. Use the process of elimination. Note that options 1 and 2 are similar in that they both address a cardiac situation. This leaves options 3 and 4. Knowledge that this medication is in the antigout classification will assist in directing you to the correct option. If you had difficulty with this question, take time now to review the action of allopurinol.
LEVEL OF COGNITIVE ABILITY: Comprehension
PHASE OF NURSING PROCESS: Implementation
CLIENT NEEDS: Physiological Integrity
CONTENT AREA: Pharmacology
REFERENCE
Hodgson, B., & Kizior, R. (2000). *Saunders nursing drug handbook 2000.* Philadelphia: W. B. Saunders. p. 24.

2. **3**

RATIONALE: Allopurinol is an antigout medication that may increase the effect of oral anticoagulants. Warfarin sodium is an anticoagulant, and if this medication is prescribed for the client, the nurse questions the order. Ergonovine is an antimigraine medication. Pentazocine is an opioid analgesic. Mebendazole is an anhelmintic.
TEST-TAKING STRATEGY: Knowledge regarding the medication interactions related to allopurinol is required to answer this question. If you had difficulty with this question, take time now to review the interactions associated with this medication.
LEVEL OF COGNITIVE ABILITY: Application
PHASE OF NURSING PROCESS: Implementation
CLIENT NEEDS: Safe, Effective Care Environment
CONTENT AREA: Pharmacology
REFERENCE
Hodgson, B., & Kizior, R. (2000). *Saunders nursing drug handbook 2000.* Philadelphia: W. B. Saunders. p. 25.

3. **2**

RATIONALE: Clients taking allopurinol are encouraged to drink 3000 mL of fluid a day. A full therapeutic effect may take 1 or more weeks. Allopurinol is to be given with milk or immediately following meals. If clients develop a rash, irritation of the eyes, or swelling of the lips or mouth, they should contact the physician because this may indicate hypersensitivity.
TEST-TAKING STRATEGY: Knowledge regarding client instructions related to this medication will assist in answering the question. Option 4 can be easily eliminated because it indicates a hypersensitivity, which is not a normal expected response. From this point, use the process of elimination and nursing knowledge. If you had difficulty with this question, take time now to review client instructions related to allopurinol.
LEVEL OF COGNITIVE ABILITY: Comprehension
PHASE OF NURSING PROCESS: Planning
CLIENT NEEDS: Health Promotion and Maintenance
CONTENT AREA: Pharmacology

REFERENCE
Hodgson, B., & Kizior, R. (2000). *Saunders nursing drug handbook 2000.* Philadelphia: W. B. Saunders. p. 25.

4. **2**

RATIONALE: Aspirin may be used to reduce the risk of recurrent TIA or stroke, or reduce the risk of MI in clients with unstable angina or with a history of a previous MI. The normal dose for clients being treated with aspirin to decrease thrombosis and MI is 300 to 325 mg daily. Clients being treated to prevent TIAs are usually prescribed 1.3 g daily in 2 to 4 divided doses. Clients with rheumatoid arthritis are treated with 3.2 to 6.0 g daily in divided doses.
TEST-TAKING STRATEGY: Knowledge regarding the use of aspirin as prophylaxis is required to answer this question. Read the question carefully. Note the key words "reduce the risk of MI." This should indicate to you that the client is receiving the medication as a preventive measure, directing you to the lowest dose of medication in the options. If you had difficulty with this question, take time now to review aspirin dosages.
LEVEL OF COGNITIVE ABILITY: Comprehension
PHASE OF NURSING PROCESS: Planning
CLIENT NEEDS: Physiological Integrity
CONTENT AREA: Pharmacology
REFERENCE
Hodgson, B., & Kizior, R. (2000). *Saunders nursing drug handbook 2000.* Philadelphia: W. B. Saunders. p. 76.

5. **1**

RATIONALE: Colchicine is contraindicated in severe GI, renal, hepatic or cardiac disorders, and in clients with blood dyscrasias. Clients with impaired renal function may exhibit myopathy and neuropathy manifested as generalized weakness. This medication should be used with caution in clients with impaired hepatic function, the elderly, and the debilitated.
TEST-TAKING STRATEGY: Use the process of elimination. Note that options 2, 3, and 4 are all endocrine-related disorders. Option 1, the correct option, is different from the others. Review this medication now if you had difficulty with this question.
LEVEL OF COGNITIVE ABILITY: Comprehension
PHASE OF NURSING PROCESS: Data Collection
CLIENT NEEDS: Physiological Integrity
CONTENT AREA: Pharmacology
REFERENCE
Hodgson, B., & Kizior, R. (2000). *Saunders nursing drug handbook 2000.* Philadelphia: W. B. Saunders. p. 252.

6. **4**

RATIONALE: Probenecid is a medication used for clients with gout to inhibit the reabsorption of uric acid by the kidney and promote excretion of uric acid in the urine. Uric acid is produced when purine is catabolized. Clients are instructed to modify their diets and limit excessive purine intake. High-purine foods to avoid or limit include organ meats, roe, sardines, scallops, anchovies, broth, mincemeat, herring, shrimp, mackerel, gravy, and yeast.
TEST-TAKING STRATEGY: Note the key word "avoid." Use the process of elimination. Options 1 and 3 are high-nutrient foods, so eliminate these options first. From this point, use knowledge regarding the purpose of the medication, the treatment for gout, and food sources high in purine to select the correct option. If you had difficulty with

this question, take time now to review foods that are high in purine.
LEVEL OF COGNITIVE ABILITY: Application
PHASE OF NURSING PROCESS: Implementation
CLIENT NEEDS: Health Promotion and Maintenance
CONTENT AREA: Pharmacology
REFERENCE
Hodgson, B., & Kizior, R. (2000). *Saunders nursing drug handbook 2000*. Philadelphia: W. B. Saunders. p. 859.

7. **2**

RATIONALE: Auranofin is the one gold preparation that is given orally rather than by injection. Gastrointestinal reactions including diarrhea, abdominal pain, nausea, and loss of appetite are common early in therapy, but usually subside in the first 3 months. Early symptoms of toxic reactions include a rash, purple blotches, pruritus, mouth lesions, and a metallic taste in the mouth.
TEST-TAKING STRATEGY: Knowledge that auranofin is a gold preparation will assist you in answering the question. Use the process of elimination. Option 4, joint pain, can be eliminated because the medication is administered to reduce the joint pain. Note that the question is asking for a toxic effect; therefore, from the options remaining, you should be directed to the correct option, metallic taste. Remember, gold is a metal. If you had difficulty with this question, take time now to review toxicity related to gold compounds.
LEVEL OF COGNITIVE ABILITY: Comprehension
PHASE OF NURSING PROCESS: Data Collection
CLIENT NEEDS: Physiological Integrity
CONTENT AREA: Pharmacology
REFERENCE
Deglin, J., & Vallerand, A. (1999). *Davis's drug guide for nurses* (6th ed.). Philadelphia: F. A. Davis. p. 451.

8. **3**

RATIONALE: Diflunisal may be given with water, milk, or meals. The tablets should not be crushed or broken open.
TEST-TAKING STRATEGY: Eliminate option 4 first as the least likely option. Next, noting the words "film-coated" will assist in eliminating options 1 and 2. Additionally, these options are similar in that they both suggest breaking the tablets. If you had difficulty with this question, review the procedure for administration now.
LEVEL OF COGNITIVE ABILITY: Application
PHASE OF NURSING PROCESS: Implementation
CLIENT NEEDS: Health Promotion and Maintenance
CONTENT AREA: Pharmacology
REFERENCE
Hodgson, B., & Kizior, R. (2000). *Saunders nursing drug handbook 2000*. Philadelphia: W. B. Saunders. p. 322.

9. **3**

RATIONALE: For acute or chronic rheumatoid arthritis or osteoarthritis, the normal PO adult dose for an elderly client is 300 to 800 mg three to four times daily.
TEST-TAKING STRATEGY: This may be a difficult question. Noting the word "elderly" in the question will assist in eliminating option 4. From the remaining options it is necessary to be familiar with normal dosages. Review the normal dosage for this medication now if you had difficulty with this question.
LEVEL OF COGNITIVE ABILITY: Analysis

PHASE OF NURSING PROCESS: Implementation
CLIENT NEEDS: Physiological Integrity
CONTENT AREA: Pharmacology
REFERENCE
Hodgson, B., & Kizior, R. (2000). *Saunders nursing drug handbook 2000*. Philadelphia: W. B. Saunders. p. 512.

10. **2**

RATIONALE: Baclofen is a skeletal muscle relaxant and acts at the spinal cord level to decrease the frequency and amplitude of muscle spasms in clients with spinal cord injuries or diseases and in clients with multiple sclerosis.
TEST-TAKING STRATEGY: Knowledge that this medication is a skeletal muscle relaxant is required to answer this question. If you knew the action of this medication, you would easily be directed to option 2. Review this medication now if you had difficulty with this question.
LEVEL OF COGNITIVE ABILITY: Comprehension
PHASE OF NURSING PROCESS: Planning
CLIENT NEEDS: Physiological Integrity
CONTENT AREA: Pharmacology
REFERENCE
Lehne, R. (1998). *Pharmacology for nursing care* (3rd ed.). Philadelphia: W. B. Saunders. pp. 222–223.

11. **1**

RATIONALE: Baclofen is a CNS depressant and frequently causes drowsiness, dizziness, weakness, and fatigue. It can also cause nausea, constipation, and urinary retention. Clients should be warned about the possible reactions.
TEST-TAKING STRATEGY: Knowledge that baclofen is a CNS depressant used to treat muscle spasticity will easily direct you to option 1. If you had difficulty with this question, review the side effects of this medication now.
LEVEL OF COGNITIVE ABILITY: Comprehension
PHASE OF NURSING PROCESS: Data Collection
CLIENT NEEDS: Physiological Integrity
CONTENT AREA: Pharmacology
REFERENCE
Lehne, R. (1998). *Pharmacology for nursing care* (3rd ed.). Philadelphia: W. B. Saunders. pp. 222–223.

12. **2**

RATIONALE: Baclofen is a CNS depressant. The client should be cautioned against the use of alcohol and other CNS depressants because baclofen potentiates the depressant activity of these agents. Constipation rather than diarrhea is an adverse effect of baclofen. It is not necessary to restrict fluids, but the client should be warned that urinary retention can occur. Fatigue is related to a CNS effect that is most intense during the early phase of therapy and diminishes with continued medication use. It is not necessary that the client notify the physician.
TEST-TAKING STRATEGY: Knowledge that baclofen is a CNS depressant will easily direct you to option 2. If you were unsure of the correct option, use general principles related to medication administration. Alcohol should be avoided with the use of many medications.
LEVEL OF COGNITIVE ABILITY: Application
PHASE OF NURSING PROCESS: Planning
CLIENT NEEDS: Health Promotion and Maintenance
CONTENT AREA: Pharmacology
REFERENCE
Lehne, R. (1998). *Pharmacology for nursing care* (3rd ed.). Philadelphia: W. B. Saunders. pp. 222–223.

13. **1**

RATIONALE: Baclofen is dispensed in tablets of 10 and 20 mg for oral use. Dosages are low initially and then gradually increased. Maintenance doses range from 15 to 20 mg administered three to four times a day.
TEST-TAKING STRATEGY: Knowledge regarding the normal adult maintenance dosage is required to answer this question. This may be a difficult question, and if you are unfamiliar with this maintenance dosage, learn it now.
LEVEL OF COGNITIVE ABILITY: Analysis
PHASE OF NURSING PROCESS: Planning
CLIENT NEEDS: Physiological Integrity
CONTENT AREA: Pharmacology
REFERENCE

Lehne, R. (1998). *Pharmacology for nursing care* (3rd ed.). Philadelphia: W. B. Saunders. pp. 222–223.

14. **2**

RATIONALE: The client should be instructed that symptoms such as drowsiness, weakness, and fatigue are more intense in the early phase of therapy and diminish with continued medication use. The client should be instructed never to abruptly withdraw or stop the medication because abrupt withdrawal can cause hallucinations, paranoid ideation, and seizures. It is best for the nurse to inform the client that these symptoms will subside and to encourage the client to continue the use of the medication.
TEST-TAKING STRATEGY: Note the key words "most appropriate." Eliminate option 4 first because it is a rather extreme nursing response. Next, eliminate options 1 and 3 because these responses do not represent the scope of nursing practice.
LEVEL OF COGNITIVE ABILITY: Application
PHASE OF NURSING PROCESS: Implementation
CLIENT NEEDS: Health Promotion and Maintenance
CONTENT AREA: Pharmacology
REFERENCE

Lehne, R. (1998). *Pharmacology for nursing care* (3rd ed.). Philadelphia: W. B. Saunders. p. 225.

15. **3**

RATIONALE: Dantrolene sodium acts directly on skeletal muscle to relieve muscle spasticity. The primary action is the suppression of calcium release from the sarcoplasmic reticulum. This in turn decreases the ability of the skeletal muscle to contract.
TEST-TAKING STRATEGY: Options 1, 2, and 4 are all similar in that they address the CNS (spinal cord, CNS, spinal) and the depression of reflexes. Therefore, eliminate these options. Review this medication now if you had difficulty with this question.
LEVEL OF COGNITIVE ABILITY: Comprehension
PHASE OF NURSING PROCESS: Implementation
CLIENT NEEDS: Physiological Integrity
CONTENT AREA: Pharmacology
REFERENCE

Lehne, R. (1998). *Pharmacology for nursing care* (3rd ed.). Philadelphia: W. B. Saunders. p. 223.

16. **3**

RATIONALE: Dose-related liver damage is the most serious adverse effect of dantrolene. To reduce the risk of liver damage, tests of liver function should be performed prior to treatment and throughout the treatment interval. It is administered in the lowest effective dosage for the shortest time necessary.
TEST-TAKING STRATEGY: Eliminate options 1 and 2 because these tests both assess kidney function. From the remaining options, it is necessary to recall that this medication affects liver function. Review this medication now if you had difficulty with this question.
LEVEL OF COGNITIVE ABILITY: Analysis
PHASE OF NURSING PROCESS: Data Collection
CLIENT NEEDS: Physiological Integrity
CONTENT AREA: Pharmacology
REFERENCE

Lehne, R. (1998). *Pharmacology for nursing care* (3rd ed.). Philadelphia: W. B. Saunders. p. 223.

17. **3**

RATIONALE: Clients with seizure disorders may have a lowered seizure threshold when baclofen is administered. Concurrent therapy may require an increase in the anticonvulsive medication.
TEST-TAKING STRATEGY: Knowledge regarding the contraindications and the cautions associated with the administration of baclofen is required to answer this question. If you are unfamiliar with these contraindications and cautions, review them now.
LEVEL OF COGNITIVE ABILITY: Analysis
PHASE OF NURSING PROCESS: Data Collection
CLIENT NEEDS: Safe, Effective Care Environment
CONTENT AREA: Pharmacology
REFERENCE

Kuhn, M. (1998). *Pharmacotherapeutics: A nursing process approach* (4th ed.). Philadelphia: F. A. Davis. p. 317.

18. **1**

RATIONALE: Because this medication has anticholinergic effects, it should be used with caution with clients with a history of urinary retention, angle-closure glaucoma, and increased intraocular pressure. Cyclobenzaprine should be used only for short-term 2- to 3-week therapy.
TEST-TAKING STRATEGY: Knowledge that this medication has anticholinergic effects will easily assist in directing you to option 1. If you are unfamiliar with this medication and the contraindications associated with its administration, review now.
LEVEL OF COGNITIVE ABILITY: Analysis
PHASE OF NURSING PROCESS: Data Collection
CLIENT NEEDS: Safe, Effective Care Environment
CONTENT AREA: Pharmacology
REFERENCE

Kuhn, M. (1998). *Pharmacotherapeutics: A nursing process approach* (4th ed.). Philadelphia: F. A. Davis. p. 317.

19. **2**

RATIONALE: The client needs to be told that the urine may turn brown, black, or green. Other adverse effects include blurred vision, nasal congestion, urticaria, and rash. The client needs to be instructed that if these adverse effects occur, the physician needs to be notified.
TEST-TAKING STRATEGY: Note the key words "need for further education." This may assist you in the process of elimination and direct you to option 2. If you had difficulty with this question, take time now to review.

LEVEL OF COGNITIVE ABILITY: Comprehension
PHASE OF NURSING PROCESS: Evaluation
CLIENT NEEDS: Health Promotion and Maintenance
CONTENT AREA: Pharmacology
REFERENCE
Kuhn, M. (1998). *Pharmacotherapeutics: A nursing process approach* (4th ed.). Philadelphia: F. A. Davis. p. 317.

20. **1**

RATIONALE: The normal adult dosage for carisoprodol is 350 mg PO three to four times daily.

TEST-TAKING STRATEGY: This question may be difficult if you are not familiar with the normal medication dosage. Review this medication now if you had difficulty with this question.
LEVEL OF COGNITIVE ABILITY: Analysis
PHASE OF NURSING PROCESS: Planning
CLIENT NEEDS: Physiological Integrity
CONTENT AREA: Pharmacology
REFERENCE
Deglin, J., & Vallerand, A. (1999). *Davis's drug guide for nurses* (6th ed.). Philadelphia: F. A. Davis. p. 158.

BIBLIOGRAPHY

Deglin, J., & Vallerand, A. (1999). *Davis's drug guide for nurses* (6th ed.). Philadelphia: F. A. Davis.

Hodgson, B., & Kizior, R. (2000). *Saunders nursing drug handbook 2000.* Philadelphia: W. B. Saunders.

Kuhn, M. (1998). *Pharmacotherapeutics: A nursing process approach* (4th ed.). Philadelphia: F. A. Davis.

Lehne, R. (1998). *Pharmacology for nursing care* (3rd ed.). Philadelphia: W. B. Saunders.

Luckmann, J. (1997). *Saunders manual of nursing care.* Philadelphia: W. B. Saunders.

Monahan, F., & Neighbors, M. (1998). *Medical-surgical nursing: Foundations for clinical practice* (2nd ed.). Philadelphia: W. B. Saunders.

O'Toole, M. (1997). *Miller-Keane encyclopedia & dictionary of medicine, nursing, & allied health* (6th ed.). Philadelphia: W. B. Saunders.

UNIT XVIII

....

The Adult Client with an Immune Disorder

PYRAMID TERMS

Acquired Immunity—Received passively from the mother's antibodies, animal serum, or from the production of antibodies in response to a disease. Immunization produces active acquired immunity.

Allergy—An abnormal, individual response to certain substances that normally do not trigger such an exaggerated reaction.

Cellular Response—A delayed response; also called delayed hypersensitivity. Active against slowly developing bacterial infections.

Humoral Response—An immediate response that provides protection against acute, rapidly developing bacterial and viral infections.

Immune Deficiency—The absence or inadequate production of immune bodies.

Natural Immunity—Also called innate immunity. Is present at birth.

PYRAMID TO SUCCESS

Pyramid points focus on the effects of and complications associated with an immune deficiency. Specific focus is on the nursing care related to the disorder, the impact of the treatment or disorder, and client adaptation. Acquired immunodeficiency syndrome is a pyramid focus, along with protecting the client from infection, and preventing the transmission of infection to other individuals. Psychosocial issues relate to social isolation and the body image disturbances that can occur as a result of the immune disorder.

NURSING PROCESS

DATA COLLECTION

Risk factors
Infections
Medication history
Family history
Nutritional status
Drug or alcohol abuse
Occupational or environmental risks

PLANNING	IMPLEMENTATION	EVALUATION
The client will not develop an infection.	Monitor temperature and for signs of infection. Monitor any lesions for drainage. Initiate body and fluid precautions as required.	Temperature remains within normal limits.
The client requests medication for discomfort. The client verbalizes relief of pain from comfort measures and medication.	Rate the client's pain on a scale of 0 to 10. Provide comfort measures and pain medications as required. Monitor and document the effects of pain control measures and pain medications. Describe pain management regimen to client and family.	The client verbalizes ability to cope with pain and measures for pain relief. The client obtains effective relief of pain.
The client verbalizes body image changes.	Encourage client to verbalize the effects of physical and emotional changes. Actively listen to client and family and acknowledge the reality of concerns about treatments, progress, and prognosis.	The client describes actual changes in body function.
The client identifies behaviors that will reduce social isolation.	Identify with the client factors that might contribute to feelings of social isolation. Reinforce efforts by the client, family, and friends to maintain interactions and relationships.	The client identifies resources and support systems that will assist in decreasing social isolation.
The client identifies personal strengths that may promote effective coping.	Assist client to identify personal strengths. Encourage client to express concerns related to problem solving.	The client utilizes support systems. The client verbalizes a plan for accepting the personal health care situation.
The client verbalizes fears related to prognosis.	Encourage and assist the client and family to express fears. Assist to mobilize support services for client and family.	The client demonstrates behaviors that reduce fear.

CLIENT NEEDS

SAFE, EFFECTIVE CARE ENVIRONMENT

Advance directives
Advocacy related to client's decisions
Client rights
Confidentiality regarding diagnosis
Informed consent for treatments and procedures
Consultations and referrals
Handling hazardous and infectious materials
Asepsis
Standard (universal) and protective precautions

HEALTH PROMOTION AND MAINTENANCE

Expected body image changes
Prevention of disease related to infection
Health screening measures
Health promotion programs
Client lifestyle choices

PSYCHOSOCIAL INTEGRITY

Ability to cope, adapt, and/or problem solve during illness or stressful events
Grief and loss related to death and the dying process

Religious, spiritual, and cultural preferences

Assisting the client and family to cope

Assisting in mobilizing appropriate support and resource systems

Promoting a positive environment to maintain optimal quality of life

PHYSIOLOGICAL INTEGRITY

Providing basic care and comfort

Promoting nutrition

Managing pain

Diagnostic tests and laboratory values

Monitoring for the expected and unexpected responses to treatments

Protecting the client from the infection

BIBLIOGRAPHY

deWit, S. (1998). *Essentials of medical-surgical nursing* (4th ed.). Philadelphia: W. B. Saunders.

Hill, S., & Howlett, H. (1997). *Success in practical nursing: Personal and vocational issues* (3rd ed.). Philadelphia: W. B. Saunders.

Ignatavicius, D., Workman, M., & Mishler, M. (1999). *Medical-surgical nursing: Across the health care continuum* (3rd ed.). Philadelphia: W. B. Saunders.

Leahy, J., & Kizilay, P. (1998). *Foundations of nursing practice: A nursing process approach.* Philadelphia: W. B. Saunders.

Luckmann, J. (1997). *Saunders manual of nursing care.* Philadelphia: W. B. Saunders.

Monahan, F., & Neighbors, M. (1998). *Medical-surgical nursing: Foundations for clinical practice* (2nd ed.). Philadelphia: W. B. Saunders.

National Council of State Boards of Nursing (1998). *National Council detailed test plan for the NCLEX-PN examination.* Chicago: Author.

O'Toole, M. (1997). *Miller-Keane encyclopedia & dictionary of medicine, nursing, & allied health* (6th ed.). Philadelphia: W. B. Saunders.

CHAPTER 58

Immune Disorders

. . . .

I. Functions of the Immune System

A. Provides protection against invasion from outside the body, such as microorganisms
B. Protects the body from internal threats
C. Maintains the internal environment by removing dead or damaged cells

II. Immune Response

A. T lymphocytes and B lymphocytes
   1. Migrate to lymphoid tissue where they wait to form either sensitized lymphocytes for cellular immunity or antibodies for humoral immunity
   2. Some B lymphocytes lie dormant until a specific antigen enters the body at which time they greatly increase in number and are available for defense
   3. T lymphocytes are responsible for rejection of transplanted tissue
   4. Both T and B lymphocytes are necessary for normal immune response
B. **Humoral Response**
   1. An immediate response
   2. Provides protection against acute, rapidly developing bacterial and viral infections
C. **Cellular Response**
   1. A delayed response; also called delayed hypersensitivity
   2. Active against slowly developing bacterial infections
   3. Also involved in autoimmune response, some allergic reactions, and rejection of foreign cells

III. Immunity

A. **Natural immunity**
   1. Also called innate
   2. Present at birth
B. **Acquired immunity**
   1. Received passively from the mother's antibodies, animal serum, or from the production of antibodies in response to a disease

2. Immunization produces active **acquired immunity**

IV. Immunizations (refer to Chapter 36 regarding immunizations)

V. Laboratory Studies

A. Antinuclear antibody (ANA)
   1. A blood test used in the differential diagnosis of rheumatic diseases, and to detect antinucleoprotein factors and patterns associated with certain autoimmune diseases
   2. Positive at a titer of 1:20 or 1:40 depending on the laboratory
   3. A positive result does not necessarily confirm a disease
B. Anti-dsDNA antibody test
   1. A blood test done specifically to identify or differentiate DNA antibodies found in systemic lupus erythematosus (SLE) or other rheumatic diseases
   2. Supports a diagnosis, monitors disease activity and response to therapy, and establishes a prognosis for SLE
   3. Values
      a. Negative: less than 70 units by ELISA
      b. Borderline: 70 to 200 units
      c. Positive: greater than 200 units
C. Refer to Chapter 10 for testing related to acquired immunodeficiency syndrome (AIDS)

VI. Immune Deficiency

A. Description
   1. Absence or inadequate production of immune bodies
   2. Can be congenital (primary) or acquired (secondary)
   3. Treatment depends on the inadequacy of immune bodies and its primary cause
B. Data collection
   1. Factors that decrease immune function
   2. Frequent infections

3. Nutritional status
4. Medication history such as corticosteroids
5. History of alcohol or drug abuse

C. Implementation
1. Protect from infection
2. Promote balanced, adequate nutrition
3. Use strict aseptic technique for all procedures
4. Provide psychosocial care regarding lifestyle changes and role changes
5. Instruct the client in measures to prevent infection

VII. Hypersensitivity and Allergy

A. Description
1. An **allergy** is an abnormal, individual response to certain substances that normally do not trigger such an exaggerated reaction
2. In all types of allergies, a reaction occurs only on second and subsequent contacts with the allergen
3. Skin testing may be done to determine the allergen

B. Data collection
1. History of exposure to allergens
2. Itching, tearing, and burning of eyes
3. Itching and burning of the skin
4. Rashes
5. Nose twitching and nasal stuffiness

C. Implementation
1. Identification of the specific allergen
2. Managing the symptoms with the use of antihistamines, anti-inflammatory agents, or cortisone
3. Salves, wet compresses, and soothing baths for local reactions
4. Desensitization programs

VIII. Anaphylaxis

A. Description
1. A serious and dramatic allergic reaction with the release of histamine from the damaged cells
2. Can cause shock and death if not treated immediately

B. Data collection
1. Identification of allergies
2. Difficulty breathing
3. Difficulty swallowing
4. Complaints of a swollen tongue
5. Facial edema and swelling of the lips
6. Skin redness
7. Presence of a rash
8. Skin redness

C. Implementation
1. Establish a patent airway
2. Prepare for the administration of epinephrine (Adrenalin), diphenhydramine hydrochloride (Benadryl), or corticosteroids
3. Provide measures to control shock
4. Provide emotional support

5. Instruct the client to wear a Medic-Alert bracelet
6. Instruct the client in the use of prescribed medication for immediate treatment of a reaction

IX. Autoimmune Disease

A. Description
1. The body is unable to recognize its own cells as a part of itself
2. Can affect collagenous tissue

B. Systemic lupus erythematosus (SLE)
1. Description
   a. A chronic progressive systemic inflammatory disease that can cause major organs and systems to fail
   b. Connective tissue and fibrin deposits in blood vessels on collagen fibers and on organs
   c. Leads to necrosis and/or inflammation in blood vessels, lymph nodes, GI tract, and pleura
   d. There is no cure for the disease
2. Causes
   a. The cause is unknown and it is thought to be due to a defect in the immunological mechanisms or from genetic origin
   b. Precipitating factors include medications, stress, genetic factors, sunlight or ultraviolet light, and pregnancy
3. Data collection
   a. Precipitating factors such as sunlight, stress, and medications
   b. Dry scaly raised rash on the face or upper body
   c. Fever
   d. Weakness, malaise, and fatigue
   e. Anorexia
   f. Weight loss
   g. Photosensitivity
   h. Joint pain
   i. Erythema of the palms
   j. Butterfly erythema of the face
   k. Anemia
   l. Positive antinuclear antibodies (ANA) and lupus erythematosus (LE) prep
   m. Elevated sedimentation rate
4. Implementation
   a. Monitor skin integrity and provide frequent oral care
   b. Instruct the client to clean skin with a mild soap, avoiding harsh and perfumed substances
   c. Assist with the use of ointments and creams for the rash as prescribed
   d. Identify factors contributing to fatigue
   e. Administer iron, folic acid, or vitamin supplements as prescribed if anemia occurs
   f. Provide a high-vitamin and high-iron diet
   g. Provide a high-protein diet if there is no evidence of kidney disease

h. Instruct in measures to conserve energy such as pacing activities and balancing rest with exercise

i. Administer topical or systemic corticosteroids, salicylates and NSAIDs as prescribed for pain and inflammation

j. Administer hydroxychloroquine (Plaquenil) as prescribed to decrease the inflammatory response

k. Instruct the client to avoid exposure to sunlight and ultraviolet light

l. Monitor for proteinuria and red cell casts in the urine

m. Monitor for bruising, bleeding, and injury

n. Assist with plasmapheresis as prescribed to remove autoantibodies and immune complexes from the blood before organ damage occurs

o. Monitor for signs of organ involvement such as pleuritis, nephritis, pericarditis, neuritis, anemia, and peritonitis

p. Note that lupus nephritis occurs early in the disease process

q. Provide supportive therapy as major organs become affected

r. Provide emotional support and encourage the client to verbalize feelings

s. Provide information regarding support groups and encourage use of community resources

C. Scleroderma (progressive systemic sclerosis)

1. Description

a. A chronic connective tissue disease, similar to SLE, characterized by inflammation, fibrosis, and sclerosis

b. Affects the connective tissue throughout the body

c. Causes fibrotic changes involving the skin, synovial membranes, esophagus, heart, lungs, kidneys, and GI tract

d. Treatment is directed toward forcing the disease into remission and slowing its progress.

2. Data collection

a. Pain

b. Stiffness and muscle weakness

c. Pitting edema of the hands and fingers, which progresses to the rest of the body

d. Taut and shiny skin that is free from wrinkles

e. Skin tissue is tight, hard and thick, and loses its elasticity

f. Masklike hard skin that adheres to underlying structures

g. Dysphagia

h. Decreased range of motion

i. Joint contractures

j. Inability to perform activities of daily living

3. Implementation

a. Encourage activity as tolerated

b. Maintain a constant room temperature

c. Provide small frequent meals eliminating foods that stimulate gastric secretions such as spicy foods, caffeine, and alcohol

d. Advise client to sit up for 1 to 2 hours after meals if esophageal involvement exists

e. Provide supportive therapy as major organs become affected

f. Administer corticosteroids as prescribed for inflammation

g. Provide emotional support and encourage the use of resources as necessary

D. Polyarteritis nodosa

1. Description

a. A collagen disease that causes inflammation of the arteries and thickening and impairment of the circulation

b. Treatment is similar to that for systemic lupus erythematosus

c. Affects middle-aged men and involves every body system

d. The cause is unknown and the prognosis is poor

e. Renal disorders and cardiac involvement are the most frequent causes of death

2. Data collection

a. Malaise and weakness

b. Low-grade fever

c. Severe abdominal pain

d. Bloody diarrhea

e. Weight loss

f. Elevated sedimentation rate

3. Implementation

a. Provide supportive care as required

b. Provide a well-balanced diet

c. Administer corticosteroids and analgesics to control pain and inflammation

d. Provide emotional support and encourage the client to verbalize feelings

e. Initiate support services for the client

E. Pemphigus

1. Description

a. A rare disease that occurs predominantly between middle and old age

b. The cause is unknown and the disorder is potentially fatal

c. Initial lesions occur on the oral mucosa and then progress to a generalized distribution

d. Treatment is aimed at suppressing the immune response that causes blister formation

2. Data collection

a. Lesions appear as fragile, flaccid bullae

b. Partial-thickness wounds that bleed, weep, and form crusts when bullae are disrupted

c. Debilitation, malaise, and pain

d. Chewing and swallowing difficulties

e. Nikolsky's sign: separation of the epidermis caused by rubbing the skin

f. Leukocytosis, eosinophilia, and foul-smelling discharge from the skin

3. Implementation
   a. Provide supportive care
   b. Provide oral hygiene and increase fluid intake
   c. Soothe oral lesions
   d. Assist with oatmeal or potassium permanganate baths as prescribed for relief of symptoms
   e. Administer topical or systemic antibiotics as prescribed for secondary infections
   f. Administer corticosteroids and cytotoxic agents as prescribed to bring about remission

X. Acquired Immunodeficiency Syndrome (AIDS)

A. Description
   1. An infectious disease characterized by severe deficits in cellular function
   2. Manifested clinically by opportunistic infection and/or unusual neoplasms
   3. Etiology: human immunodeficiency virus (HIV)
   4. The disease has a long incubation period, sometimes up to 10 years or more
   5. Manifestations may not appear until late in the infection
B. AIDS-related complex (ARC)
   1. Similar to AIDS
   2. Two or more symptoms or two or more laboratory findings characteristic of immunodeficiency
   3. The client is not as ill as the AIDS client
   4. May lead to AIDS
C. High-risk groups
   1. Male homosexuals or bisexuals
   2. Intravenous drug abusers
   3. Persons receiving blood transfusions (hemophiliacs, surgical clients)
   4. Those individuals with frequent exposure to blood and body fluids
   5. Heterosexual contact with high-risk individuals
   6. Babies born to infected mothers
D. Data collection
   1. Malaise and weight loss
   2. Lymphadenopathy of at least 3 months
   3. Leukopenia
   4. Diarrhea
   5. Fatigue
   6. Night sweats
   7. Presence of opportunistic infections
   8. *Pneumocystis carinii* pneumonia (major source of mortality)
   9. Kaposi's sarcoma: purplish red lesions of internal organs and skin
   10. Candidiasis
   11. Fungal infections
   12. Cytomegalovirus (CMV)
E. Implementation
   1. Provide respiratory support

2. Administer respiratory treatments as prescribed
3. Administer oxygen as prescribed
4. Maintain fluid and electrolyte balance
5. Monitor for signs of infection
6. Prevent the spread of infection
7. Initiate standard (universal) precautions
8. Provide comfort as necessary
9. Provide meticulous skin care
10. Provide adequate nutritional support as prescribed
11. Refer to Chapters 22 and 36 for additional information on AIDS

PRACTICE QUESTIONS

1. A client is suspected of having systemic lupus erythematous (SLE). The nurse monitors the client knowing that which of the following is a characteristic sign of SLE?
   1 Rash on the face across the bridge of the nose and on the cheeks
   2 Fatigue
   3 Fever
   4 Elevated red blood cell count

2. The nurse is caring for a client with systemic lupus erythematous (SLE). Which of the following is not a component of the teaching plan for the client to manage fatigue?
   1 Avoid long periods of rest
   2 To sit whenever possible
   3 To take a hot bath in the evening
   4 To engage in moderate low-impact exercise when not fatigued

3. The client has requested and undergone testing for human immunodeficiency virus (HIV). The client now asks what will be done next, since the results of two enzyme-linked immunosorbent assay (ELISA) tests have been positive. The nurse's response is based on the understanding that
   1 The client will probably have a bone marrow biopsy done
   2 A Western blot will be done to confirm these findings
   3 A CD4 cell count will be done to measure T-helper lymphocytes
   4 The client will be definitively diagnosed as HIV positive at this point

4. The nurse is caring for the client with acquired immunodeficiency syndrome (AIDS). The nurse detects early infection with *Pneumocystis carinii* by monitoring the client for which of the following clinical manifestations?
   1 Dyspnea on exertion
   2 Dyspnea at rest
   3 Fever
   4 Cough

5. The client with acquired immunodeficiency syndrome (AIDS) has a concurrent diagnosis of histoplasmosis. The nurse notes during data collection that the client has enlarged lymph nodes. The nurse interprets that
   1 The client has disseminated histoplasmosis
   2 This is a side effect of the medications given to treat AIDS
   3 This indicates that the histoplasmosis is resolving
   4 The client probably has yet another infection that is developing

6. The nurse is caring for the client with acquired immunodeficiency syndrome (AIDS) who is experiencing night fever and night sweats. Which of the following nursing interventions is the least helpful in managing this symptom?
   1 Keep a change of bed linens nearby in case they are needed
   2 Administer an antipyretic after the client spikes the fever
   3 Make sure the pillow has a plastic cover
   4 Keep liquids at the bedside

7. The client exposed to human immunodeficiency virus (HIV) approximately 3 months ago has seroconverted to HIV-positive status. The nurse anticipates that the client will experience which of the following at this time?
   1 Oral lesions
   2 Purplish skin lesions
   3 Chronic cough
   4 No signs and symptoms

8. The client with acquired immunodeficiency syndrome (AIDS) has raised, dark purplish lesions on the trunk of the body. The nurse anticipates that which of the following procedures will be done to confirm whether these lesions are due to Kaposi's sarcoma?
   1 Enzyme-linked immunosorbent assay (ELISA)
   2 Western blot
   3 Skin biopsy
   4 Lung biopsy

9. The nurse participating in a health fair is setting up a booth on prevention of human immunodeficiency virus (HIV) transmission. A poster is planned that will list sexual behaviors in one of two columns, rated "safe" and "not safe." Which of the following behaviors does the nurse place in the "not safe" column?
   1 Use of latex condoms
   2 Use of "natural skin" condoms
   3 Abstinence
   4 Mutual monogamy

10. The client with acquired immunodeficiency syndrome (AIDS) is experiencing nausea and vomiting. The nurse makes which of the following dietary alterations for this client to enhance nutritional intake?
    1 Avoid dairy products and red meat
    2 Plan large, nutritious meals
    3 Add spices to food for added flavor
    4 Serve foods while they are very warm

11. The client with acquired immunodeficiency syndrome (AIDS) has diarrhea from lactose intolerance and a respiratory infection from *Pneumocystis carinii*. In evaluating the documented plan of care for the nursing diagnosis Impaired Gas Exchange, which of the following is not considered by the nurse to be a positive outcome criterion for this client?
    1 No complaints of shortness of breath
    2 Expectorates secretions easily
    3 Has clear breath sounds
    4 Limits fluid intake

12. A client with pemphigus vulgaris is being seen in the clinic on a regular basis. The nurse plans care based on which of the following descriptions of this condition?
    1 The presence of skin vesicles found along the nerve caused by a virus
    2 An autoimmune disorder that causes blistering in the epidermis
    3 The presence of red raised papules and large plaques covered by silvery scales
    4 The presence of tiny red vesicles

13. The nurse is providing dietary instructions to the client with systemic lupus erythematosus (SLE). Which of the following dietary items does the nurse instruct the client to avoid?
    1 Cantaloupe
    2 Broccoli
    3 Turkey
    4 Steak

14. The client is brought to the emergency department and is experiencing an anaphylaxis reaction from eating shellfish. The nurse prepares for which of the following initial actions?
    1 Administration of epinephrine (Adrenalin)
    2 Administration of a corticosteroid
    3 Maintaining a patent airway
    4 Instructing the client on the importance of obtaining a Medic-Alert bracelet

15. The nurse is assisting in planning care for a client with a diagnosis of immune deficiency. The nurse incorporates which of the following as a priority in the plan of care?
    1 Emotional support to decrease fear
    2 Protecting the client from infection
    3 Encouraging discussion about lifestyle changes
    4 Identifying factors that decreased the immune function

16. A client calls the nurse in the emergency department and tells the nurse that he/she was just stung by a bumblebee while gardening. The client is afraid of a severe reaction because the client's neighbor experienced such a reaction the previous week. The most appropriate nursing action is to
    1 Ask the client if he/she ever received a bee sting in the past
    2 Tell the client to call an ambulance for transport to the emergency department
    3 Advise the client to soak the site in hydrogen peroxide
    4 Tell the client not to worry about the sting unless difficult breathing occurs

17. The nurse is assisting in administering immunizations at a health care clinic. The nurse understands that an immunization will provide
    1 Natural immunity from disease
    2 Acquired immunity from disease
    3 Innate immunity from disease
    4 Protection from all diseases

18. The nurse is assigned to care for a client with systemic lupus erythematosus (SLE). The nurse plans care knowing that this disorder is
    1 A local rash that occurs as a result of allergy
    2 An inflammatory disease of collagen contained in connective tissue
    3 A disease caused by a tick bite
    4 A disease caused by the continuous release of histamine in the body

19. The nurse is assigned to care for a client admitted to the hospital with a diagnosis of systemic lupus erythematosus (SLE). The nurse reviews the physician's orders expecting to note that which of the following medications is prescribed?
    1 Antibiotic
    2 Narcotic analgesic
    3 Antidiarrheal
    4 Corticosteroid

20. The nurse administers an injection to a client with a diagnosis of acquired immunodeficiency syndrome (AIDS). After administering the medication, the nurse disposes the used needle by
    1 Placing it in a puncture-resistant container
    2 Laying the needle and syringe on the bedside table and carefully recapping the needle
    3 Asking the client to recap the needle
    4 Recapping the needle before placing it in a puncture-resistant container

ANSWERS

1. **1**

RATIONALE: Skin lesions or rash on the face across the bridge of the nose and on the cheeks is a characteristic sign of SLE. Fever and fatigue may potentially occur before and during exacerbation. Anemia is most likely to occur in SLE.
TEST-TAKING STRATEGY: Note the key words "characteristic sign." Knowledge regarding the manifestations associated with SLE will easily direct you to option 1. If you are unfamiliar with this important disorder, review now.
LEVEL OF COGNITIVE ABILITY: Comprehension
PHASE OF NURSING PROCESS: Data Collection
CLIENT NEEDS: Physiological Integrity
CONTENT AREA: Fundamental Skills
REFERENCE
Monahan, F., & Neighbors, M. (1998). *Medical-surgical nursing: Foundations for clinical practice* (2nd ed.). Philadelphia: W. B. Saunders. p. 1491.

2. **3**

RATIONALE: To help reduce fatigue in the client with SLE, the nurse should instruct the client to sit whenever possible, to avoid hot baths, to schedule moderate low-impact exercises when not fatigued, and to maintain a balanced diet. The client is instructed not to rest for long periods because it promotes joint stiffness.
TEST-TAKING STRATEGY: Note the key words "not" and "manage fatigue." By the process of elimination, you should easily be directed to option 3 as being the action that would exacerbate fatigue. If you had difficulty with this question, take time now to review measures to prevent fatigue.
LEVEL OF COGNITIVE ABILITY: Application
PHASE OF NURSING PROCESS: Implementation
CLIENT NEEDS: Health Promotion and Maintenance
CONTENT AREA: Fundamental Skills
REFERENCE
Monahan, F., & Neighbors, M. (198). *Medical-surgical nursing: Foundations for clinical practice* (2nd ed.). Philadelphia: W. B. Saunders. p. 1493.

3. **2**

RATIONALE: If the results of two ELISA tests are positive, the Western blot is done to confirm the findings. If the result of the Western blot is positive, then the client is considered to be positive for HIV, and infected with the HIV virus.
TEST-TAKING STRATEGY: Knowledge of the procedural steps in diagnosing HIV is needed to answer this question. Review these now if they are unfamiliar to you. This is a subject of great concern to clients, and you want to have the appropriate information to share. The increasing incidence of HIV as a major health problem also makes it a reasonably popular area for testing.
LEVEL OF COGNITIVE ABILITY: Comprehension
PHASE OF NURSING PROCESS: Planning
CLIENT NEEDS: Physiological Integrity
CONTENT AREA: Fundamental Skills
REFERENCE
deWit, S. (1998). *Essentials of medical-surgical nursing* (4th ed.). Philadelphia: W. B. Saunders. p. 186.

4. **4**

RATIONALE: The client with *Pneumocystis carinii* infection usually has a cough as the first symptom, which begins as nonproductive, then progresses to productive. Later signs include fever, dyspnea on exertion, and finally dyspnea at rest.
TEST-TAKING STRATEGY: The key word in the stem of this question is "early." While all of these symptoms may appear at some point in the client with *P. carinii*, knowing that the cough appears first helps to you eliminate each of the other options. Review the early signs of *P. carinii* infection now, if you had difficulty with this question.
LEVEL OF COGNITIVE ABILITY: Comprehension
PHASE OF NURSING PROCESS: Data Collection
CLIENT NEEDS: Physiological Integrity
CONTENT AREA: Fundamental Skills
REFERENCE
Black, J., & Matassarin-Jacobs, E. (1997). *Medical-surgical nursing: Clinical management for continuity of care* (5th ed.). Philadelphia: W. B. Saunders. p. 629.

5. **1**

RATIONALE: Histoplasmosis usually starts as a respiratory infection in the client with AIDS. It then becomes a disseminated infection, with enlargement of lymph nodes, spleen, and liver. Options 2, 3, and 4 are incorrect.
TEST-TAKING STRATEGY: Knowing that lymph nodes may enlarge with generalized infection helps you to narrow the plausible choices to options 1 and 4. Since the stem contains no information that indicates that option 4 is true, option 1 is the correct choice by elimination. Review disseminated infections in the client with AIDS now if you had difficulty with this question.
LEVEL OF COGNITIVE ABILITY: Comprehension
PHASE OF NURSING PROCESS: Data Collection
CLIENT NEEDS: Physiological Integrity
CONTENT AREA: Fundamental Skills
REFERENCE
Ignatavicius, D., Workman, M., & Mishler, M. (1999). *Medical-surgical nursing: Across the health care continuum* (3rd ed.). Philadelphia: W. B. Saunders. p. 446.

6. **2**

RATIONALE: For clients with AIDS who experience night fever and night sweats, it is useful to offer the client an antipyretic of choice prior to going to sleep. It is also helpful to keep a change of bed linens and nightclothes nearby for use. The pillow should have a plastic cover, and a towel may be placed over the pillowcase if there is profuse diaphoresis. The client should have liquids at the bedside to drink.
TEST-TAKING STRATEGY: The wording of the question guides you to look for a response that is not the best or most correct action. Options 1 and 3 are helpful from an environmental viewpoint, so they are eliminated first as answers to this question. Knowing that liquids will help prevent dehydration causes you to eliminate this option next. This leaves option 2 as the answer. Since night fever and sweats occur serially, it is most helpful to give the antipyretic before sleep as a prophylactic measure.
LEVEL OF COGNITIVE ABILITY: Application
PHASE OF NURSING PROCESS: Implementation
CLIENT NEEDS: Physiological Integrity
CONTENT AREA: Fundamental Skills

REFERENCE
Black, J., & Matassarin-Jacobs, E. (1997). *Medical-surgical nursing: Clinical management for continuity of care* (5th ed.). Philadelphia: W. B. Saunders. p. 632.

7. **4**

RATIONALE: The client in stage 1 (seroconversion) acute HIV infection has laboratory documentation of HIV-positive status, but is asymptomatic. Following introduction of the infection and seroconversion in stage 1, the client may remain asymptomatic for a period of 6 months to 11 years or more (stage 2: chronic asymptomatic status). The client's T4 cell count is normal during these two stages. The client will begin to show symptoms in stage 3: symptomatic stage, when the T4 cell count drops below 500/mm.[3] At this time, the client experiences opportunistic infections, including oral (thrush) and skin lesions (Kaposi's sarcoma). The client may also experience signs of respiratory infection in stage 3.
TEST-TAKING STRATEGY: The wording of the question tells you that there are clearly three incorrect options, while only one is correct. Use knowledge of concepts related to seroconversion to help you eliminate each of the incorrect options.
LEVEL OF COGNITIVE ABILITY: Comprehension
PHASE OF NURSING PROCESS: Data Collection
CLIENT NEEDS: Physiological Integrity
CONTENT AREA: Fundamental Skills
REFERENCE
deWit, S. (1998). *Essentials of medical-surgical nursing* (4th ed.). Philadelphia: W. B. Saunders. p. 184.

8. **3**

RATIONALE: The skin biopsy is the procedure of choice to diagnose Kaposi's sarcoma, which frequently complicates the clinical picture of the client with AIDS. Lung biopsy would confirm *Pneumocystis carinii* infection. The ELISA and Western blot are tests to diagnose HIV status.
TEST-TAKING STRATEGY: Begin to answer this question by eliminating options 1 and 2, which are used to diagnose whether the client is HIV positive. Knowledge of the meaning of Kaposi's sarcoma, or attention to the words "lesions" and "trunk" will help you to choose correctly between the remaining two options. Review the diagnostic testing to confirm Kaposi's sarcoma now if you had difficulty with this question.
LEVEL OF COGNITIVE ABILITY: Comprehension
PHASE OF NURSING PROCESS: Data Collection
CLIENT NEEDS: Physiological Integrity
CONTENT AREA: Fundamental Skills
REFERENCE
deWit, S. (1998). *Essentials of medical-surgical nursing* (4th ed.). Philadelphia: W. B. Saunders. p. 190.

9. **2**

RATIONALE: Abstinence is the safest way to avoid HIV infection. The next most reliable method is participation in a mutually monogamous relationship. The use of latex condoms is considered safe, because the latex prevents the transmission of the HIV virus as long as the condom is used properly and remains in place. The use of natural skin condoms is not considered safe because the pores in the condom are large enough for the virus to pass through.
TEST-TAKING STRATEGY: Use knowledge of transmission of sexually transmitted diseases and universal precautions to answer this question. The wording of the question

tells you that there is one option that is dissimilar from the others, which in this case is the correct answer to the question. Review these preventive measures now if you had difficulty with this question.
LEVEL OF COGNITIVE ABILITY: Application
PHASE OF NURSING PROCESS: Planning
CLIENT NEEDS: Health Promotion and Maintenance
CONTENT AREA: Fundamental Skills
REFERENCE
deWit, S. (1998). *Essentials of medical-surgical nursing* (4th ed.). Philadelphia: W. B. Saunders. p. 185.

10. **1**

RATIONALE: The AIDS client with nausea and vomiting should avoid fatty products such as diary products and red meat. Meals should be small and frequent to lessen the chance of vomiting. Spices and odorous foods should be avoided, since they aggravate nausea. Foods are best tolerated either cold or at room temperature.
TEST-TAKING STRATEGY: Use knowledge of the effects of AIDS on the GI tract and general principles for treating nausea and vomiting to answer this question. Doing so will guide you to eliminate each of the incorrect options systematically. Review nutritional support for the client with AIDS now if you had difficulty with this question.
LEVEL OF COGNITIVE ABILITY: Application
PHASE OF NURSING PROCESS: Implementation
CLIENT NEEDS: Physiological Integrity
CONTENT AREA: Fundamental Skills
REFERENCE
Luckmann, J. (1997). *Saunders manual of nursing care.* Philadelphia: W. B. Saunders. p. 1939.

11. **4**

RATIONALE: The status of the client with a diagnosis of Impaired Gas Exchange would be evaluated against the standard outcome criteria for this nursing diagnosis. These would include that the client states that breathing is easier, coughs up secretions effectively, and has clear breath sounds. The client should not limit fluid intake because fluids are needed to decrease the viscosity of secretions for expectoration. The client with diarrhea should also not limit fluid intake because of the risk of dehydration.
TEST-TAKING STRATEGY: Note that the stem of the question contains the key word "not." This tells you that the answer to the question is an incorrect goal for the client. Use knowledge related to airway management and fluid balance and the process of elimination to choose correctly.
LEVEL OF COGNITIVE ABILITY: Analysis
PHASE OF NURSING PROCESS: Evaluation
CLIENT NEEDS: Physiological Integrity
CONTENT AREA: Fundamental Skills
REFERENCE
Luckmann, J. (1997). *Saunders manual of nursing care.* Philadelphia: W. B. Saunders. p. 1495.

12. **2**

RATIONALE: Pemphigus vulgaris is an autoimmune disease that causes blistering in the epidermis. The clients have large flaccid blisters (bullae). Because the blisters are in the epidermis, they have a very tiny covering of skin and break easily, leaving large denuded areas of skin. On initial examination, clients may have crusting areas instead of intact blisters. Option 1 describes herpes zoster. Option 3 describes psoriasis, and option 4 describes eczema.

TEST-TAKING STRATEGY: Knowledge that pemphigus vulgaris is an autoimmune disorder will easily direct you to option 2. If you had difficulty with this question, take time now to review the characteristics of this disorder.
LEVEL OF COGNITIVE ABILITY: Application
PHASE OF NURSING PROCESS: Planning
CLIENT NEEDS: Physiological Integrity
CONTENT AREA: Fundamental Skills
REFERENCE
Beare, P., & Myers, J. (1998). *Adult health nursing* (3rd ed.). St. Louis: Mosby–Year Book. p. 1767.

13. **4**

RATIONALE: The client with SLE is at risk for cardiovascular disorders, such as coronary artery disease and hypertension. The client is advised of lifestyle changes to reduce these risks, which include smoking cessation, prevention of obesity, and hyperlipidemia. The client is advised to reduce salt, fat, and cholesterol intake.
TEST-TAKING STRATEGY: Note the key word "avoid" in the question. Knowledge regarding the risks associated with SLE will assist you in answering this question. Use knowledge regarding basic nutritional components of food items to help direct you to option 4. If you had difficulty with this question, take time now to review therapeutic management of SLE.
LEVEL OF COGNITIVE ABILITY: Application
PHASE OF NURSING PROCESS: Implementation
CLIENT NEEDS: Physiological Integrity
CONTENT AREA: Fundamental Skills
REFERENCE
Black, J., & Matassarin-Jacobs, E. (1997). *Medical-surgical nursing: Clinical management for continuity of care* (5th ed.). Philadelphia: W. B. Saunders. p. 676.

14. **3**

RATIONALE: The initial action is to maintain a patent airway. The client would then receive epinephrine. Corticosteroids may also be prescribed. The client will need to be instructed about wearing a Medic-Alert bracelet, but this is not the initial action.
TEST-TAKING STRATEGY: Use the ABCs, airway, breathing, and circulation, to answer the question. Airway is always the priority.
LEVEL OF COGNITIVE ABILITY: Application
PHASE OF NURSING PROCESS: Planning
CLIENT NEEDS: Physiological Integrity
CONTENT AREA: Fundamental Skills
REFERENCE
deWit, S. (1998). *Essentials of medical-surgical nursing* (4th ed.). Philadelphia: W. B. Saunders. p. 181.

15. **2**

RATIONALE: The client with immune deficiency has inadequate, or the absence of, immune bodies and is at risk for infection. The priority nursing intervention is to protect the client from infection. Options 1, 3, and 4 may be components of care but are not the priority.
TEST-TAKING STRATEGY: Use Maslow's hierarchy of needs theory to answer the question. Remember that physiological needs are the priority. This will easily direct you to option 2. Review the care of a client with immune deficiency now, if you had difficulty with this question.
LEVEL OF COGNITIVE ABILITY: Application
PHASE OF NURSING PROCESS: Planning

CLIENT NEEDS: Physiological Integrity
CONTENT AREA: Fundamental Skills
REFERENCE
deWit, S. (1998). *Essentials of medical-surgical nursing* (4th ed.). Philadelphia: W. B. Saunders. p. 180.

16. 1

RATIONALE: In all types of allergies, a reaction occurs only on second and subsequent contacts with the allergen. The most appropriate action therefore is to ask the client if he or she ever received a bee sting. Option 2 is unnecessary. Option 3 is not appropriate advice. The client should not be told "not to worry."
TEST-TAKING STRATEGY: Use the steps of the nursing process to answer the question. Option 1 is the only option that addresses data collection. Review information related to allergic reactions now if you had difficulty with this question.
LEVEL OF COGNITIVE ABILITY: Application
PHASE OF NURSING PROCESS: Implementation
CLIENT NEEDS: Physiological Integrity
CONTENT AREA: Fundamental Skills
REFERENCE
deWit, S. (1998). *Essentials of medical-surgical nursing* (4th ed.). Philadelphia: W. B. Saunders. p. 181.

17. 2

RATIONALE: Acquired immunity can occur by receiving an immunization that causes antibodies to a specific pathogen to form. Natural (innate) immunity is present at birth. There is not an immunization that protects the client from all diseases.
TEST-TAKING STRATEGY: Use the process of elimination and knowledge regarding immunity to disease to answer the question. Eliminate option 4 first because of the absolute word "all." Next eliminate options 1 and 3 because they are similar. Review natural and acquired immunity now if you had difficulty with this question.
LEVEL OF COGNITIVE ABILITY: Comprehension
PHASE OF NURSING PROCESS: Implementation
CLIENT NEEDS: Physiological Integrity
CONTENT AREA: Fundamental Skills
REFERENCE
deWit, S. (1998). *Essentials of medical-surgical nursing* (4th ed.). Philadelphia: W. B. Saunders. p. 167.

18. 2

RATIONALE: SLE is an inflammatory disease of collagen contained in connective tissue. Options 1, 3, and 4 are not associated with this disease.
TEST-TAKING STRATEGY: Knowledge regarding the characteristics of SLE is required to answer this question. If you are unfamiliar with disorder, take time now to review.
LEVEL OF COGNITIVE ABILITY: Comprehension
PHASE OF NURSING PROCESS: Planning
CLIENT NEEDS: Physiological Integrity
CONTENT AREA: Fundamental Skills
REFERENCE
deWit, S. (1998). *Essentials of medical-surgical nursing* (4th ed.). Philadelphia: W. B. Saunders. p. 181.

19. 4

RATIONALE: Treatment of SLE is based on the systems involved and symptoms. Treatment normally consists of anti-inflammatories, corticosteroids, and immunosuppressants. Options 1, 2, and 3 are not a standard component of medication therapy.
TEST-TAKING STRATEGY: Knowledge regarding the treatment for SLE is required to answer the question. If you are unfamiliar with the treatments normally prescribed in this disease, take time now to review.
LEVEL OF COGNITIVE ABILITY: Comprehension
PHASE OF NURSING PROCESS: Planning
CLIENT NEEDS: Physiological Integrity
CONTENT AREA: Fundamental Skills
REFERENCE
deWit, S. (1998). *Essentials of medical-surgical nursing* (4th ed.). Philadelphia: W. B. Saunders. p. 181.

20. 1

RATIONALE: The correct procedure for needle disposal is to dispose of uncapped needles and sharps in a hard-wall, puncture-resistant container immediately after use. Needles are not recapped.
TEST-TAKING STRATEGY: Use the process of elimination and principles related to the safe disposal of needles and syringes to answer the question. Note that options 2, 3, and 4 are similar in that they all address recapping the needle. Review these principles now if you had difficulty with this question.
LEVEL OF COGNITIVE ABILITY: Application
PHASE OF NURSING PROCESS: Implementation
CLIENT NEEDS: Safe, Effective Care Environment
CONTENT AREA: Fundamental Skills
REFERENCE
deWit, S. (1998). *Essentials of medical-surgical nursing* (4th ed.). Philadelphia: W. B. Saunders. p. 196.

BIBLIOGRAPHY

Beare, P., & Myers, J. (1998). *Adult health nursing* (3rd ed.). St. Louis, MO: Mosby–Year Book.

Black, J., & Matassarin-Jacobs, E. (1997). *Medical-surgical nursing: Clinical management for continuity of care* (5th ed.). Philadelphia: W. B. Saunders.

deWit, S. (1998). *Essentials of medical-surgical nursing* (4th ed.). Philadelphia: W. B. Saunders.

Ignatavicius, D., Workman, M., & Mishler, M. (1999). *Medical-surgical nursing: Across the health care continuum* (3rd ed.). Philadelphia: W. B. Saunders.

Luckmann, J. (1997). *Saunders manual of nursing care.* Philadelphia: W. B. Saunders.

Monahan, F., & Neighbors, M. (1998). *Medical-surgical nursing: Foundations for clinical practice* (2nd ed.). Philadelphia: W. B. Saunders.

CHAPTER 59

Immunologic Medications

I. Anti-Inflammatory Medications

A. Sulfasalazine (Azulfidine)
1. Anti-inflammatory
2. Used to treat toxoplasmosis or nocardiasis
3. Administered orally
4. Can cause renal toxicity
5. Suppresses bone marrow function
6. Increases photosensitivity
7. Monitor urine output and complete blood count (CBC)
8. Monitor client for sore throat, pallor, purpura, jaundice, and weakness
9. Encourage fluids
10. Advise the client to avoid the sun

II. Anti-Infective Medications

A. Pentamidine isethionate (Pentam-300)
1. Anti-infective
2. Used to treat *Pneumocystis carinii* pneumonia
3. Administered by IM or IV route
4. Can cause nephrotoxicity
5. Monitor blood pressure and heart rate (may cause hypotension)
6. Monitor for hypoglycemia
7. Is hepatotoxic and immunosuppressive
8. Monitor liver function tests and complete blood count

B. Metronidazole (Flagyl)
1. Anti-infective
2. Used to treat cryptosporidiosis and giardiasis
3. Administered orally or by IV route
4. Administer with food or milk
5. Monitor for dry mouth, dizziness, or fungal infection
6. Instruct the client to avoid alcohol during treatment

III. Antifungal Medications

A. Ketoconazole (Nizoral)
1. Antifungal
2. Used in the treatment of candidiasis, coccidioidomycosis, or histoplasmosis
3. Administered orally
4. Administer with food or milk
5. Instruct the client to avoid antacids for 2 hours after taking the medication because gastric acid is needed to activate the medication
6. Is hepatotoxic
7. Monitor hepatic function
8. Instruct the client to avoid sun because the medication increases photosensitivity
9. Instruct the client to avoid alcohol during treatment

B. Fluconazole (Diflucan)
1. Antifungal
2. Used to treat candidiasis
3. Administered orally
4. Is hepatotoxic
5. Monitor for abdominal pain, fever, and diarrhea
6. Monitor hepatic function

C. Amphotericin B (Fungizone)
1. Antifungal
2. Used to treat candidiasis and other fungal infections
3. Administered by the IV route
4. Is nephrotoxic
5. Can cause thrombophlebitis
6. Suppresses bone marrow function
7. Monitor renal function
8. Monitor infusion site
9. Monitor CBC

IV. Antivirals

A. Ganciclovir (Cytovene)
1. Antiviral
2. Used to treat cytomegalovirus retinitis
3. Administered orally or by the intravenous route

4. Suppresses bone marrow function
5. Monitor neutrophil and platelet count
6. Administer with food

B. Acyclovir (Zovirax)
1. Antiviral
2. Used to treat herpes simplex, herpes zoster, or varicella zoster
3. May be administered orally or by the IV route
4. Is nephrotoxic
5. Monitor renal function
6. Encourage fluids
7. Is irritating to a blood vessel when administered by the IV route

C. Foscarnet (Foscavir)
1. Antiviral
2. Used in the treatment of cytomegalovirus retinitis in HIV-infected clients
3. Administered by the IV route
4. Is nephrotoxic
5. Monitor renal function

D. Zidovudine (Retrovir, AZT)
1. Antiretroviral (nucleoside reverse transcriptase inhibitor)
2. Indicated for clients with HIV seropositivity
3. Administered orally
4. Suppresses bone marrow function
5. Is hepatotoxic and nephrotoxic
6. Monitor CBC, and hepatic and renal function
7. Monitor for dizziness because the medication crosses the blood-brain barrier
8. Instruct the client that the medication must be administered around the clock

E. Didanosine (Videx)
1. Antiretroviral (nucleoside reverse transcriptase inhibitor)
2. Indicated for clients with HIV seropositivity
3. Administered orally
4. Administer on an empty stomach to enhance absorption
5. Instruct the client to chew tablet or crush
6. Monitor for dizziness, neuropathy, and pancreatitis

F. Lamivudine (Epivir)
1. Antiretroviral (nucleoside reverse transcriptase inhibitor)
2. Indicated for clients with HIV seropositivity
3. Used as a prophylaxis for occupational exposure
4. Administered orally
5. Can cause severe pancreatitis
6. Instruct the client to avoid fatty foods

G. Saquinavir mesylate (Invirase)
1. Antiretroviral (protease inhibitor)
2. Used in combination with other antiretroviral medications in the management of HIV infection
3. Administered orally
4. Administered with meals
5. Is best absorbed if the client consumes high-calorie, high-fat meals
6. It can cause photosensitivity and the client is instructed to avoid sun exposure

H. Ritonavir (Norvir)
1. Antiretroviral (protease inhibitor)
2. Used in combination with other antiretroviral medications in the management of HIV infection
3. Administered orally
4. Administered 1 hour before or 2 hours after meals because it is best absorbed in a fasting state
5. Can increase triglyceride levels
6. Monitor triglyceride levels

I. Stavudine (d4T, Zerit)
1. Antiretroviral (protease inhibitor)
2. Used in the management of HIV infection in clients who do not respond to or who cannot tolerate conventional therapy
3. Administered orally
4. Can cause peripheral neuropathy
5. Monitor the client's gait
6. Ask the client about paresthesias

J. Zalcitabine (ddC)
1. Antiretroviral (nucleoside reverse transcriptase inhibitor)
2. Used in the management of HIV infection with other antiretrovirals such as AZT because of the synergistic effect
3. It has also been used as a single agent in clients who are intolerant of, or who progress on, other regimens
4. Administered orally (with AZT)
5. Can cause serious liver damage
6. Monitor liver function studies

V. Antitubercular Medications

A. Rifampin (Rifadin)
B. Ethambutol (Myambutol)
C. Pyrazinamide
D. Isonazid (INH)
E. Refer to Chapter 47 regarding information related to these medications

VI. Dapsone (DDS)

A. Antifungal, anti-infective, antiprotozoal
B. Used for the treatment of toxoplasmosis
C. Administered orally
D. Suppresses bone marrow activity
E. Can cause anemia, peripheral motor weakness, and liver damage
F. Monitor the CBC
G. Monitor for fever, sore throat, purpura, or jaundice

VII. Pyrimethamine (Daraprim)

A. Antimalarial and antiprotozoal
B. Used in the treatment of toxoplasmosis or *Pneumocyctis carinii* pneumonia
C. Administered orally
D. Supresses bone marrow function
E. Monitor CBC and platelet count
F. Administer with food or milk

PRACTICE QUESTIONS

1. Dapsone (DDS) is prescribed for a client with acquired immunodeficiency syndrome (AIDS) for the treatment of toxoplasmosis. The nurse reinforces medication instructions and tells the client to
   1 Discontinue the medication if nausea and vomiting develop
   2 Plan to take the medication every 6 hours around the clock
   3 Contact the physician if fever or a sore throat occurs
   4 Report to the clinic weekly for the injections

2. Pyrimethamine (Daraprim) has been added to the medication regimen for the client with acquired immunodeficiency syndrome (AIDS). On review of the client's record, the nurse notes this new prescription and plans care knowing that this has been prescribed for the treatment of
   1 Toxoplasmosis
   2 Cardiac irregularities
   3 Kaposi's sarcoma
   4 Nausea and vomiting

3. Saquinavir mesylate (Invirase) is prescribed for the client who is human immunodeficiency virus (HIV) seropositive. The nurse reinforces medication instructions and tells the client to
   1 Take the medication on an empty stomach
   2 Eat low-calorie foods
   3 Eat foods that are low in fat
   4 Avoid sun exposure

4. The client who is human immunodeficiency virus (HIV) seropositive has been taking Ritonavir (Norvir). The client returns to the clinic for follow-up laboratory tests. The nurse reviews the client's record and expects to note a physician's order for which of the following laboratory tests?
   1 Platelet count
   2 Triglyceride level
   3 Prothrombin time (PT)
   4 International normalized ratio (INR)

5. The client who is human immunodeficiency virus (HIV) seropositive has been taking Stavudine (d4T, Zerit). The nurse monitors which of the following most closely while the client is taking this medication?
   1 Appetite
   2 Gait
   3 Gastrointestinal function
   4 Level of consciousness (LOC)

6. The client who is human immunodeficiency virus (HIV) seropositive has been taking zalcitabine (ddC) as a component of treatment. The nurse plans to monitor which of the following most closely while the client is taking this medication?
   1 Liver function studies
   2 Platelet count
   3 Red blood cell count
   4 Glucose level

7. The nurse is assigned to care for a client with cytomegalovirus retinitis and acquired immunodeficiency syndrome (AIDS) who is receiving foscavir (Foscarnet). The nurse checks the latest results of which of the following laboratory studies while the client is taking this medication?
   1 Serum albumin
   2 Serum creatinine
   3 CD4 cell count
   4 Lymphocyte count

8. The client with acquired immunodeficiency syndrome (AIDS) and *Pneumocystis carinii* infection has been receiving pentamidine (Pentam-300). The client develops a fever of 101°F. The nurse does further monitoring of the client, knowing that this sign most likely indicates
   1 The dose of the medication is too low
   2 The client is experiencing toxic effects of the medication
   3 The client has developed inadequacy of thermoregulation
   4 This is a result of another infection, caused by leukopenic effects of the medication

9. The client with acquired immunodeficiency syndrome (AIDS) has been started on therapy with zidovudine (AZT, Retrovir). The nurse carefully monitors which of the following laboratory results during treatment with this medication?
   1 Complete blood count (CBC)
   2 Blood urea nitrogen (BUN)
   3 Blood culture
   4 Blood glucose level

10. The nurse is reviewing the results of serum laboratory studies drawn on a client with acquired immunodeficiency syndrome (AIDS) who is receiving didanosine (Videx). The nurse interprets that the client may very well have the medication discontinued by the physician because of which of the following significantly elevated results?
    1 Serum cholesterol
    2 Serum amylase
    3 Blood glucose
    4 Serum protein

ANSWERS

1. **3**

RATIONALE: Dapsone may be prescribed for the treatment of toxoplasmosis. The medication is taken orally on a daily basis. The medication suppresses bone marrow activity and the CBC is monitored closely. If the client develops fever, sore throat, purpura, or jaundice, the physician is notified. Medications are available to treat nausea and vomiting and the client should not discontinue the dapsone if these symptoms occur but should contact the physician.
TEST-TAKING STRATEGY: Use the process of elimination. Eliminate option 1 first because the nurse would not tell the client to discontinue the medication. Next eliminate options 2 and 4, knowing that the medication is administered orally on a daily basis. Review this medication now if you had difficulty with this question.
LEVEL OF COGNITIVE ABILITY: Application
PHASE OF NURSING PROCESS: Implementation
CLIENT NEEDS: Health Promotion and Maintenance
CONTENT AREA: Pharmacology
REFERENCE
Deglin, J., & Vallerand, A. (1999). *Davis's drug guide for nurses* (6th ed.). Philadelphia: F. A. Davis. p. 1132.

2. **1**

RATIONALE: Pyrimethamine is an antimalarial and an antiprotozoal medication. It is used in the treatment of toxoplasmosis or *Pneumocystis carinii* pneumonia. It is not used to treat nausea, vomiting, cardiac irregularities, or Kaposi's sarcoma.
TEST-TAKING STRATEGY: Knowledge regarding the action and use of pyrimethamine is required to answer this question. If you know that this medication is an antimalarial and an antiprotozoal medication, then you would easily be directed to option 1. Review this medication now if you had difficulty with this medication.
LEVEL OF COGNITIVE ABILITY: Comprehension
PHASE OF NURSING PROCESS: Planning
CLIENT NEEDS: Physiological Integrity
CONTENT AREA: Pharmacology
REFERENCE
Deglin, J., & Vallerand, A. (1999). *Davis's drug guide for nurses* (6th ed.). Philadelphia: F. A. Davis. p. 877.

3. **4**

RATIONALE: Saquinavir is an antiretroviral (protease inhibitor) used in combination with other antiretroviral medications in the management of HIV infection. It is administered with meals and is best absorbed if the client consumes high-calorie, high-fat meals. It can cause photosensitivity, so the client is instructed to avoid sun exposure.
TEST-TAKING STRATEGY: Knowledge regarding this medication is required to answer this question. Options 2 and 3 can be eliminated first, knowing that these dietary measures would not likely be prescribed. For the remaining options, it is necessary to know that this medication can cause photosensitivity. Review this medication now if you had difficulty with this question.
LEVEL OF COGNITIVE ABILITY: Application
PHASE OF NURSING PROCESS: Implementation
CLIENT NEEDS: Health Promotion and Maintenance
CONTENT AREA: Pharmacology
REFERENCE
Ignatavicius, D., Workman, M., & Mishler, M. (1999). *Medical-surgical nursing: Across the health care continuum* (3rd ed.). Philadelphia: W. B. Saunders. p. 453.

4. **2**

RATIONALE: Ritonavir is an antiretroviral (protease inhibitor) used in combination with other antiretroviral medications in the management of HIV infection. It can increase the triglyceride levels and therefore the client's triglyceride level should be monitored. The platelet count, PT, and INR are not laboratory tests that would specifically be monitored in the client on this medication.
TEST-TAKING STRATEGY: Knowledge regarding the side effects of ritonavir is required to answer this question. If you are unfamiliar with this medication, take time now to review.
LEVEL OF COGNITIVE ABILITY: Comprehension
PHASE OF NURSING PROCESS: Planning
CLIENT NEEDS: Physiological Integrity
CONTENT AREA: Pharmacology
REFERENCE
Ignatavicius, D., Workman, M., & Mishler, M. (1999). *Medical-surgical nursing: Across the health care continuum* (3rd ed.). Philadelphia: W. B. Saunders. p. 453.

5. **2**

RATIONALE: Stavudine is an antiretroviral (protease inhibitor) used in the management of HIV infection in clients who do not respond to or who cannot tolerate conventional therapy. The medication can cause peripheral neuropathy and the nurse should closely monitor the client's gait and ask the client about paresthesias.
TEST-TAKING STRATEGY: Knowledge regarding the specific side effects of this medication is required to answer this question. If you are not familiar with this medication and the important data collection measures, take time now to review.
LEVEL OF COGNITIVE ABILITY: Application
PHASE OF NURSING PROCESS: Data Collection
CLIENT NEEDS: Physiological Integrity
CONTENT AREA: Pharmacology
REFERENCE
Ignatavicius, D., Workman, M., & Mishler, M. (1999). *Medical-surgical nursing: Across the health care continuum* (3rd ed.). Philadelphia: W. B. Saunders. p. 453.

6. **1**

RATIONALE: Zalcitabine is an antiretroviral (nucleoside reverse transcriptase inhibitor) used in the management of HIV infection with other antiretrovirals. It can cause serious liver damage, and liver function studies should be monitored closely. Options 2, 3, and 4 are not specifically associated with the use of this medication.
TEST-TAKING STRATEGY: Knowledge regarding the side effects of zalcitabine is required to answer this question. If you are unfamiliar with this medication, take time now to review.
LEVEL OF COGNITIVE ABILITY: Application
PHASE OF NURSING PROCESS: Data Collection
CLIENT NEEDS: Physiological Integrity
CONTENT AREA: Pharmacology
REFERENCE
Ignatavicius, D., Workman, M., & Mishler, M. (1999). *Medical-surgical nursing: Across the health care continuum* (3rd ed.). Philadelphia: W. B. Saunders. p. 453.

7. **2**

RATIONALE: Foscavir is very toxic to the kidneys. Serum creatinine is monitored prior to therapy, two to three times per week during induction therapy, and at least weekly during maintenance therapy. It also may cause decreased levels of calcium, magnesium, phosphorus, and potassium in the bloodstream. Thus, these levels are also measured with the same frequency.

TEST-TAKING STRATEGY: It is necessary to know the toxicities and important side effects of this medication to discriminate among the various options correctly. If needed, take a few moments to review this medication now.

LEVEL OF COGNITIVE ABILITY: Application
PHASE OF NURSING PROCESS: Data Collection
CLIENT NEEDS: Physiological Integrity
CONTENT AREA: Pharmacology
REFERENCE

Deglin, J., & Vallerand, A. (1999). *Davis's drug guide for nurses* (6th ed.). Philadelphia: F. A. Davis. p. 411.

8. **4**

RATIONALE: Frequent side effects of this medication include leukopenia, thrombocytopenia, and anemia. The client should be routinely monitored for signs and symptoms of infection. The client should also have ongoing monitoring of a number of parameters due to the nature and side effects of the medication, including blood glucose, BUN, serum creatinine, CBC, liver function studies, and serum calcium and magnesium levels.

TEST-TAKING STRATEGY: Options 2 and 3 are the least plausible given the information in the question, and are eliminated first. To discriminate between the last two, you need to know that the medication has leukopenic side effects to choose correctly. Review this medication now if you had difficulty with this question.

LEVEL OF COGNITIVE ABILITY: Comprehension
PHASE OF NURSING PROCESS: Data Collection
CLIENT NEEDS: Physiological Integrity
CONTENT AREA: Pharmacology
REFERENCE

Deglin, J., & Vallerand, A. (1999). *Davis's drug guide for nurses* (6th ed.). Philadelphia: F. A. Davis. p. 300.

9. **1**

RATIONALE: A common side effect of this medication therapy is agranulocytopenia and anemia. The nurse carefully monitors CBC results for these changes. With early HIV infection or in the client who is asymptomatic, CBC levels are monitored monthly for 3 months, then every 3 months thereafter. In clients with advanced disease, they are monitored every 2 weeks for the first 2 months, and then once a month if the medication is tolerated well.

TEST-TAKING STRATEGY: It is necessary to know the toxicities and important side effects of this medication to discriminate among the various options correctly. If needed, take a few moments to review this medication now.

LEVEL OF COGNITIVE ABILITY: Application
PHASE OF NURSING PROCESS: Implementation
CLIENT NEEDS: Physiological Integrity
CONTENT AREA: Pharmacology
REFERENCE

Deglin, J., & Vallerand, A. (1999). *Davis's drug guide for nurses* (6th ed.). Philadelphia: F. A. Davis. p. 1051.

10. **2**

RATIONALE: A serum amylase level that is increased 1.5 to 2 times normal may signify pancreatitis in the AIDS client, which is potentially fatal. The medication may have to be discontinued. The medication is also hepatotoxic, and can result in liver failure.

TEST-TAKING STRATEGY: It is necessary to know the toxicities and important side effects of this medication to discriminate among the various options correctly. If needed, take a few moments to review this medication now.

LEVEL OF COGNITIVE ABILITY: Comprehension
PHASE OF NURSING PROCESS: Planning
CLIENT NEEDS: Physiological Integrity
CONTENT AREA: Pharmacology
REFERENCE

Deglin, J., & Vallerand, A. (1999). *Davis's drug guide for nurses* (6th ed.). Philadelphia: F. A. Davis. p. 270.

BIBLIOGRAPHY

Deglin, J., & Vallerand, A. (1999). *Davis's drug guide for nurses* (6th ed.). Philadelphia: F. A. Davis.

deWit, S. (1998). *Essentials of medical-surgical nursing* (4th ed.). Philadelphia: W. B. Saunders.

Ignatavicius, D., Workman, M., & Mishler, M. (1999). *Medical-surgical nursing: Across the health care continuum* (3rd ed.). Philadelphia: W. B. Saunders.

Luckmann, J. (1997). *Saunders manual of nursing care*. Philadelphia: W. B. Saunders.

Monahan, F., & Neighbors, M. (1998). *Medical-surgical nursing: Foundations for clinical practice* (2nd ed.). Philadelphia: W. B. Saunders.

UNIT XIX

....

The Client with a Mental Health Disorder

PYRAMID TERMS

Abuse—An act of misuse, deceit, or exploitation. The wrong or improper use or action toward another individual that results in injury, damage, maltreatment, or corruption.

Addiction—Also known as drug dependence. Incorporates the concepts of loss of control with respect to the use of a drug, taking the drug despite related problems and complications, and a tendency to relapse.

Coping Mechanisms—Methods of adjusting to environmental stress without altering one's own goals or purposes. Can include both conscious and unconscious mechanisms.

Crisis—A temporary state of disequilibrium in which an individual's usual coping mechanisms or problem-solving methods fail. It can result in personality growth or personality disorganization.

Defense Mechanisms—Unconscious intrapsychic processes used to fight off anxiety by preventing the conscious awareness of threatening feelings. These mechanisms can be used in a healthy or unhealthy manner.

Milieu—The physical and social environment in which an individual lives. Milieu therapy focuses on positive physical and social environmental manipulation in order to produce positive change.

Restraints—Physical restraints include any manual method or mechanical device, material, or equipment that inhibits free movement. Chemical restraints include the administration of medications for the specific purpose of inhibiting a specific behavior or movement.

Seclusion—Placing a client alone in a specially designed room for protection and close supervision. It is the last measure in a process to maximize safety to the client and others.

Suicide—The ultimate act of self-destruction in which an individual purposefully ends his or her own life.

Suicide Attempt—Any willfull, self-inflicted, or life-threatening attempt by an individual that has not led to death.

◆ PYRAMID TO SUCCESS

The Pyramid to Success focuses on the therapeutic nurse-client relationship, client rights, and the ethical and legal issues related to the care of the client with a mental health disorder. Pyramid points focus on the use of restraints, seclusion, and electroconvulsive therapy (ECT). Focus on care to the client with an addiction, such as an eating disorder, or drug or alcohol disorder. Additional focus areas include anxiety, depression, suicide, abuse and violence, post-traumatic stress disorders, obsessive-compulsive disorders, schizophrenia, and bipolar disorders. Pyramid points address the use of medications prescribed for the client with a mental health disorder, particularly lithium carbonate (Eskalith) and the benzodiazepines.

NURSING PROCESS

DATA COLLECTION

Physical, social, emotional, intellectual, spiritual, and cultural aspects
Presenting problem, current lifestyle, and life experiences
Physical appearance, such as dress, posture, gait, motor activity level, attitude, behavioral mannerism, and speech
Affect and emotional state
Sensorium, such as attention and alertness, orientation, and memory
Intelligence, insight, and awareness of illness
Personal strengths
Coping mechanisms
Support systems

PLANNING	IMPLEMENTATION	EVALUATION
Client verbalizes willingness to consume adequate nutritional intake.	Assess likes and dislikes of client. Select food items with client as appropriate to meet client's physical and psychosocial needs. Monitor weight. Monitor and document food intake.	Client eats prescribed foods. Client maintains weight.
Client initiates and follows through with personal hygiene measures.	Schedule time to perform personal hygiene and assist client as necessary. Monitor client for maintenance of personal hygiene. Monitor dress and appearance for appropriateness.	Client participates in personal hygiene measures.
Client identifies techniques to induce sleep.	Monitor sleep patterns. Monitor frequency and length of time client is awake at night. Teach relaxation skills and exercises. Decrease intake of caffeine and other stimulants. Discourage daytime napping. Adhere to relaxing bedtime ritual.	Client uses sleep and relaxation techniques. Client sleeps through the night.
Client identifies symptoms that are indicators of anxiety. Client uses anxiety-reducing techniques. Client demonstrates ability to continue with necessary activities.	Monitor and document level of anxiety. Encourage client to verbalize thoughts and feelings to externalize anxiety. Assist client to identify events that have precipitated anxiety in the past. Explore techniques that have and have not reduced anxiety in the past. Assist client to focus on the present situation as a means of identifying coping mechanisms to reduce anxiety. Encourage client to express feelings. Reduce excessive stimulation by providing a quiet environment, limited contact with others, and limiting use of caffeine and other stimulants. Provide appropriate diversion to reduce anxiety. Provide positive reinforcement when client is able to continue with activities of daily living and activities necessary to progress to optimal wellness.	Client verbalizes reduction in anxiety. Client demonstrates ability to focus appropriately.

PLANNING	IMPLEMENTATION	EVALUATION
The client verbalizes anger. The client demonstrates ability to control anger. The client identifies effective ways to express anger in a nondestructive manner.	Identify behaviors that are cues of impending violence against self or others. Identify situations that provoke violence. Encourage client to verbalize anger. Set limits on client's behavior. Explore with client alternative ways of expressing anger. Encourage the use of positive coping mechanisms. Assess and document client's potential for suicide. Initiate suicide precautions as necessary. Follow agency policies and procedures regarding the use of restraints or seclusion.	Client does not harm self or others.
Client will state feelings in a given situation. Client will directly ask for what he or she wants or needs.	Define the nurse-client relationship. Develop a therapeutic relationship. Discuss behavioral expectations and consequences. Acknowledge and reward open communication.	The client is direct in communicating feelings and needs.
The client accepts positive feedback from others. The client identifies things that enhance self-concept. The client practices new behaviors.	Encourage and accept expression of thoughts and feelings. Provide opportunities to problem solve. Encourage client to practice new behaviors in role-playing situations. Provide praise and recognition.	The client will maintain a positive self-concept.
The client will distinguish verbal thoughts from the need to act out on thoughts. The client will seek out nursing staff and request time away from others to deescalate feelings.	Reduce environmental stimulation. Assist client to express thoughts and feelings. Monitor for aggressive or potential self-destructive behaviors. Encourage client to verbalize the need for an environment necessary to deescalate feelings.	The client maintains safety of self and others.
The client will share perceptions of reality with others. The client will list pros and cons of actions before making decisions.	Use a calm, nonthreatening, direct approach. Present reality in a matter of fact, tone, and manner. Orient client to person, place, time, and situation. Encourage reality-oriented conversation and activities.	The client validates reality.
The client will allow contact with others. The client will interact with others.	Promote trust and a therapeutic nurse-client relationship. Assist client to set daily goals. Be realistic about client's tolerance for activity with others.	The client maintains contact with others.
Client/family identifies coping patterns. Client/family participates in decision-making processes.	Assess interaction between client and family. Monitor for potential disruptive behaviors. Promote a trusting relationship with client and family. Encourage client and family to verbalize feelings. Assist client and family to identify personal strengths. Encourage family to participate in client's care. Provide positive reinforcement for effective use of coping mechanisms. Encourage family to express concerns related to home care. Explore available community resources with the family.	Client/family uses appropriate coping mechanisms. Client and family acknowledges change in family roles.

PLANNING	IMPLEMENTATION	EVALUATION
The client follows rules regarding acceptable behavior.	Teach client about personal boundaries. Discuss role expectations with the client. Provide choices whenever possible.	The client accepts limits and takes responsibility for own feelings.
PLANNING	IMPLEMENTATION	EVALUATION
The client takes medications at prescribed times.	Instruct client regarding importance of medication regimen. Assist with initiating referral to community resources and other support services as appropriate.	The client complies with therapeutic regimen.

◆ CLIENT NEEDS

SAFE, EFFECTIVE CARE ENVIRONMENT

Client advocacy
Client rights
Confidentiality
Informed consent related to treatments, such as restraints, seclusion, and electroconvulsive therapy (ECT)
Legal responsibilities related to reporting incidence of violence and abuse
Psychiatric consultations and referrals
Providing safety to client and others
Use of restraints and seclusion

HEALTH PROMOTION AND MAINTENANCE

Health promotion programs related to addictions
Individual lifestyle choices

PSYCHOSOCIAL INTEGRITY

Therapeutic nurse-client relationship
Coping mechanisms

Grief and loss
Religious and spiritual influences on health
Stress management
Support systems
Behavior management
Chemical dependency
Abuse and neglect
Domestic violence
Crisis intervention
Therapeutic environment

PHYSIOLOGICAL INTEGRITY

Personal hygiene measures
Nutrition
Rest and sleep
Elimination
Medication administration
Expected effects of medications
Potential complications related to medications and ECT
Abusive and self-destructive behavior
Alterations in body systems related to addictions

BIBLIOGRAPHY

deWit, S. (1998). *Essentials of medical-surgical nursing* (4th ed.). Philadelphia: W. B. Saunders.

Hill, S., & Howlett, H. (1997). *Success in practical nursing: Personal and vocational issues* (3rd ed.). Philadelphia: W. B. Saunders.

Leahy, J., & Kizilay, P. (1998). *Foundations of nursing practice: A nursing process approach.* Philadelphia: W. B. Saunders.

National Council of State Boards of Nursing (1998). *National Council detailed test plan for the NCLEX-PN examination.* Chicago: Author.

O'Toole, M. (1997). *Miller-Keane encyclopedia & dictionary of medicine, nursing, & allied health* (6th ed.). Philadelphia: W. B. Saunders.

Thompson, J., McFarland, G., Hirsch, J., & Tucker, S. (1997). *Mosby's clinical nursing.* St. Louis: Mosby–Year Book.

Varcarolis, E. (1998). *Foundations of psychiatric mental health nursing* (3rd ed.). Philadelphia: W. B. Saunders.

CHAPTER 60

Foundations of Psychiatric Mental Health Nursing

I. Mental Health

A. A lifelong process of successful adaptation to a changing internal and external environment
B. The individual is in contact with reality and the environment and possesses the ability to love, work, and resolve conflicts

II. Psychiatric/Mental Health Illness

A. Description
   1. Loss of the ability to respond to the environment in ways that are expected by society
   2. Characterized by thought or behavior patterns that cause the individual distress or impaired functioning
B. Personality characteristics
   1. Is unaccepting of self and dislikes self
   2. Has an unrealistic perception of strengths and weaknesses
   3. Thoughts and perceptions may not be reality based
   4. Is unable to find meaning and purpose in life
   5. Lacks direction, has difficulty in meeting own needs, and depends on others
C. Adaptations to stress
   1. Feels out of control with self and with the environment
   2. Has ineffective **coping mechanisms**
D. Interpersonal relationships
   1. Is unable to love and care for others
   2. Is unable to feel loved by others or accept feelings from others

III. Coping and Defense Mechanisms

A. **Coping mechanisms**
   1. Coping involves any effort to decrease the stress response

2. **Coping mechanisms** are usually conscious decisions, can be either constructive or destructive in nature, task-oriented, related to direct problem solving, or can be a defense-oriented response to protect oneself
   3. Destructive **coping mechanisms** often cause a mental health disorder because the problem that causes the disorder is avoided
   4. Neurotic or psychotic behaviors can typically result when **coping mechanisms** become destructive
B. **Defense mechanisms** (Box 60–1)
   1. Usually an unconscious mechanism used to defend against anxiety and stress
   2. Used to release anxiety and to relieve emotional conflict caused by uncomfortable situations that threaten self-esteem
C. Implementation
   1. Identify the client's use of the **defense mechanism**
   2. Determine if the use of the **defense mechanism** characterizes unhealthy adjustment
   3. Avoid criticizing the behavior and the use of **defense mechanisms**
   4. Assist the client to identify the source of the anxiety
   5. Assist the client to explore methods to reduce the anxiety

IV. The Nurse-Client Relationship

A. Principles
   1. Value the client as an individual
   2. Be aware of the client in a holistic manner, including physical needs
   3. Maintain appropriate limits
   4. Remember that empathy is therapeutic and sympathy is nontherapeutic

BOX 60–1. Common Defense Mechanisms

DENIAL

Disowning consciously intolerable thoughts and impulses

DISPLACEMENT

Feelings toward one person are directed to another who is less threatening, therefore satisfying an impulse with a substitute object

IDENTIFICATION

The unconscious attempt to change oneself to resemble an admired person

PROJECTION

Transferring one's internal feelings, thoughts, and unacceptable ideas and traits to someone else

RATIONALIZATION

An attempt to make unacceptable feelings and behavior acceptable by justifying the behavior

REACTION FORMATION

Developing conscious attitudes and behaviors and acting-out behaviors opposite to what one really feels

REGRESSION

Returning to an earlier developmental stage to express an impulse in order to deal with reality

REPRESSION

An unconscious process in which the client blocks undesirable and unacceptable thoughts from conscious expression

SUBLIMATION

Replacement of an unacceptable need, attitude, or emotion with one more socially acceptable

---

5. Maintain honest and open communication
6. Encourage expression of the client's feelings
7. Assist the client to develop resources
B. Phases of the therapeutic relationship
   1. Orientation/initiation phase
      a. Establish boundaries and trust with the client
      b. Identify the expectations of the relationship
      c. Identify anxiety in the client
      d. Review goals with the client
   2. Working/continuation phase
      a. Promote an attitude of acceptance
      b. Continue to identify and evaluate problems
      c. Assist the client to express feelings
      d. Promote insight and the use of constructive **coping mechanisms**
      e. Increase the client's independence
   3. Termination/separation phase
      a. Prepare the client for this phase on initial contact

b. Encourage the client to discuss feelings about this phase
c. Identify and deal with termination and separation issues
d. Evaluate client progress and achievement of goals
e. Encourage the use of support systems
f. Do not promise the client that you will continue the relationship

V. Therapeutic Communication Process

A. Principles
   1. Communication includes both verbal and nonverbal expression
   2. Successful communication includes appropriateness, efficiency, flexibility, and feedback
   3. Anxiety in either the nurse or the client blocks communication
B. Therapeutic communication techniques and blocks to communication (Table 60–1)

VI. Diagnostic and Statistical Manual of Mental Disorders of the American Psychiatric Association (DSM-IV)

A. A classification system used to determine a medical diagnosis
B. Knowledge of the criteria for a particular medical diagnosis will assist the registered nurse in making a clinical decision about a nursing diagnosis

VII. Types of Mental Health Admissions and Discharges (Box 60–2)

A. Voluntary admission
   1. Sought by the client or the client's guardian through a written application to the facility

Table 60–1. Therapeutic Communication Techniques and Blocks to Communication

Therapeutic Techniques	Blocks to Communication
Listening	Giving advice
Being silent	Changing the subject
Respecting the client	Giving approval or disapproval
Providing recognition and acknowledgment	Challenging the client
Providing feedback	Making stereotypical comments
Offering to assist	Making value judgments
Focusing and refocusing	Providing false reassurance
Clarifying and validating	Placing the client's feelings on hold
Reflecting	Asking the client "Why?"
Making observations	Being defensive
Giving information	
Presenting reality	
Summarizing	
Using open-ended questions	
Providing nonverbal encouragement	
Giving neutral responses	
Encouraging the client to make a plan of action	

BOX 60–2. Client Rights

Right to accessible health care
Right to a coordination and continuity of health care
Right to courteous and individualized health care
Right to information about the qualifications, names, and titles of personnel delivering care
Right to refuse observation by those not directly involved in care
Right to privacy and confidentiality
Right to informed consent
Right to treatment
Right to refuse treatment
Right to treatment in the least restrictive setting
Right not to be subjected to unnecessary restraints
Right to habeas corpus; may request a hearing at any time to be released from the hospital
Right to information about diagnosis, prognosis, and treatment
Right to information on the charges of service
Right to communicate with people outside the hospital through correspondence, telephone, and personal visits
Right to keep clothing and personal effects
Right to be employed
Right to religious freedom
Right to execute wills
Right to retain licenses, privileges, or permits established by the law, such as a driver's or professional license

2. Voluntary clients have the right to demand an obtained release
3. If the client is a minor, the release may be dependent on the consent of a parent or guardian

B. Informal admission
 1. A form of voluntary admission
 2. Informal admission permits a client to make a verbal application for the admission similar to that made for the hospital admission for medical treatment

C. Involuntary admission
 1. Involuntary admission is made without the client's consent
 2. Involuntary admission may be necessary when a person is a danger to self or others or is in need of psychiatric treatment or physical care

D. Commitment procedures
 1. A specified number of physicians must certify that the client's mental health justifies detention and treatment
 2. May be emergency, observational or temporary, or indeterminate or extended

E. Emergency involuntary admission
 1. Most states provide for emergency involuntary admission or civil commitment for a specified period (1 to 10 days on average) to prevent dangerous behavior that is likely to cause harm to self or others
 2. Police officers, physicians, and mental health

professionals may be designated to authorize the detention of mentally ill persons who are dangerous to themselves or others

F. Observational or temporary involuntary admission
 1. The primary purpose is observation, diagnosis, and treatment of persons who suffer from mental illness or pose a danger to themselves or others
 2. The length of time is specified by statute, is of longer duration than emergency admission, and varies markedly from state to state

G. Indeterminate, or extended, involuntary hospital admission
 1. Provides extended care and treatment of the mentally ill
 2. Those who undergo extended involuntary admission are committed solely through judicial or administrative action or medical certification
 3. This type of involuntary admission generally lasts 60 to 180 days, but it may be for an indeterminate length of time

H. Release from the hospital
 1. Description
  a. Depends on the client's admission status
  b. Clients who sought informal or voluntary admission have the right to demand and receive release
 2. Discharge
  a. Follow-up care is critical for these clients
  b. Discharge planning is important for the continued well-being of the psychiatric client
  c. After care, case managers are needed to facilitate the client's adaptation back into the community and to provide early referral if the treatment plan is not followed

VIII. Milieu Therapy

A. Description
 1. **Milieu** is the physical and social environment in which an individual lives
 2. Staffed by persons trained to provide support and understanding and to give individual attention
 3. All members contribute to the planning and functioning of the setting

B. Focus
 1. Group and social interaction
 2. Use of community meetings, activity groups, social skills groups, and physical exercise programs

IX. Behavioral Therapy and Behavioral Modification

A. Behavioral therapy
 1. An approach to bring about behavioral change

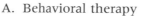

2. It includes a group of diversified approaches for dealing with maladaptive behavior
3. The belief that most behaviors are learned
4. Maladaptive behavior is a way of dealing with stress, and the therapy is an approach to bring about a change in the behavior

B. Self-control therapy
   1. A basic theme is that the talking to self can direct and control actions more effectively
   2. Useful to deal with stress

C. Desensitization
   1. The reduction of intense reactions to a stimulus by repeated exposure to the stimulus in a weaker and milder form
   2. Gradually over a period of time, exposure is increased until the fear of the object or situation has ceased

D. Aversion therapy
   1. Negative reinforcement is a technique to change behavior
   2. Uses negative reinforcement to alter or eliminate an unwanted or negative behavior

E. Modeling: the therapist provides a role model for specified identified behaviors and the client learns through imitation

F. Operant conditioning: includes rewarding a client for desired behaviors and is the basis for behavioral modification

X. Groups and Group Therapy

A. Stages of group development
   1. Initial stage
      a. Involves superficial rather than open and trusting communication
      b. Members are becoming acquainted with each other and are searching for similarity between themselves and other group members
      c. Members may be unclear about the purpose or goals of the group
      d. A certain amount of structuring of group norms, roles, and responsibilities takes place
   2. Working stage
      a. During this stage the real work of the group is accomplished
      b. Members are familiar with each other, the group leader, and the group roles, and they feel free to approach their problems and to attempt to solve their problems
      c. Conflict and cooperation surface during the group's work
   3. Termination stage
      a. The group evaluates the experience and explores members' feelings about it and the impending separation
      b. Provides an opportunity for members who have difficulty with termination to learn to deal more realistically and comfortably with this normal part of human experience

XI. Community Support Groups

A. Promote identification, clarification, understanding, role modeling, feelings of togetherness, and group cohesion
B. Prevent the individual member from feeling lonely and isolated
C. Members are better able to deal with the problems that they brought to the group
D. The outcome is rewarding and the members develop new or more effective patterns of behavior
E. Some groups evolve into educational models that enhance communication, self-image, body image, problem solving, decision making, and growth processes

XII. Family Therapy

A. Specific intervention mode based on the premise that the members, with the presenting symptoms, signal the presence of pain in the whole family
B. The therapist works to assist the family to identify and express their thoughts and feelings, define family roles and rules, try new, more productive styles of relating, and restore strength to the family

PRACTICE QUESTIONS

1. The nurse assists in planning care for a client scheduled to be discharged from a mental health clinic. The nurse knows that unresolved feelings related to loss may be weakened during which phase of the therapeutic nurse-client relationship?
   1 Orientation phase
   2 Working phase
   3 Termination phase
   4 Trusting phase

2. A client with depression who attempted suicide says to the nurse, "I should have died. I've always been a failure. Nothing ever goes right for me." The most therapeutic response by the nurse is
   1 "I don't see you as a failure."
   2 "Feeling like this is all part of being ill."
   3 "You've been feeling like a failure for a while?"
   4 "You have everything to live for."

3. A client states to the nurse, "I haven't slept at all the last couple of nights." Which of the following responses by the nurse illustrates the most therapeutic communication technique for this client?
   1 "Go on..."
   2 "Sleeping?"
   3 "The last couple of nights?"
   4 "You're having difficulty sleeping?"

4. While the male nurse is gathering psychosocial data from a female client, the client states, "I

don't want to discuss this—it's private and personal." Which of the following statements, if made by the male nurse, indicates that the nurse is therapeutic?

1 "This often happens to me. Perhaps you would find it easier to speak to a nurse who is female?"

2 "I am a nurse and as such I'll have you know that all information is kept confidential."

3 "I know that some of these questions are difficult for you, but as a nurse, I must legally respect your confidentiality."

4 "This is difficult for you to speak about, but I am trying to perform a complete data collection and I am no different from a female nurse, if that's your problem."

5. The nurse is caring for a Native American client who says, "I don't want you to touch me. I'll take care of myself!" Which of the following responses is the most therapeutic communication by the nurse?

1 "I will respect your feelings. I'll just leave this cup for you to collect your urine in. After breakfast, I will take more blood from you."

2 "If you didn't want our care, why did you come here?"

3 "Why are you being so difficult? I only want to help you."

4 "Sounds like you're feeling pretty troubled by all of us. Let's work together so you can do everything for yourself as you request."

6. The nurse is assigned to care for a client who is experiencing Altered Thought Processes. The nurse is told that the client believes that the food is being poisoned. Which type of communication technique does the nurse plan to use to encourage the client to discuss feelings?

1 Using open-ended questions and silence

2 Offering opinions about the necessity of adequate nutrition

3 Telling the client about the importance of eating

4 Focusing on self-disclosure regarding food preferences

7. The nurse is assigned to care for a client admitted to the hospital after sustaining an injury from a house fire. The client attempted to save a neighbor involved in the fire but in spite of the client's efforts, the neighbor died. Which of the following actions does the nurse engage in with the client during the working phase of the nurse-client relationship?

1 Identifying the client's potential for self-harm

2 Identifying the client's ability to function

3 Inquiring about the client's perception of the neighbor's death

4 Inquiring about the client's feelings that may block coping

8. A client who has just been sexually assaulted is very quiet and calm. The nurse identifies this behavior as indicative of which defense mechanism?

1 Denial

2 Projection

3 Rationalization

4 Intellectualization

9. The nurse is assisting with the data collection on a client admitted to the psychiatric unit. The nurse reviews the data obtained and identifies which of the following as a potential concern?

1 The presence of bruises on the client's body

2 The client's report of not eating or sleeping

3 The client's report of suicidal thoughts

4 The significant other disapproving of the treatment

10. Laboratory work is prescribed on a client who has been experiencing delusions. When the laboratory technician approaches the client to obtain a specimen of the client's blood, the client begins to shout, "You're all vampires. Let me out of here!" The nurse who is present at the time makes which of the following most appropriate responses?

1 "The technician is not going to hurt you but is going to help you!"

2 "What makes you think that the technician is a vampire?"

3 "The technician will leave and come back later for your blood."

4 "It must be fearful to think others want to hurt you."

11. An inebriated client is brought to the emergency department by the local police. The client is told that the physician will be in to see the client in about 30 minutes. The client becomes very loud and offensive and wants to be seen by the physician immediately. The nurse assisting to care for the client would plan for which of the following most appropriate nursing interventions?

1 Attempt to talk with the client to de-escalate behavior

2 Watch the behavior escalate before intervening

3 Inform the client that he or she will be asked to leave if the behavior continues

4 Offer to take the client to an examination room until he or she can be treated

12. A client is admitted to a psychiatric unit for treatment of psychotic behavior. The client is at the locked exit door and is shouting, "Let me out. There's nothing wrong with me. I don't belong here." The nurse identifies this behavior as

1 Projection

2 Denial

3 Regression

4 Rationalization

13. The client says to the nurse, "I'm going to die, and I wish my family would stop hoping for a cure! I get so angry when they carry on like this! After all, I'm the one who's dying." The most therapeutic response by the nurse is
    1 "You're feeling angry that your family continues to hope for you to be cured?"
    2 "I think we should talk more about your anger with your family."
    3 "Well, it sounds like you're being pretty pessimistic. After all, years ago people died of pneumonia."
    4. "Have you shared your feelings with your family?"

14. The nurse employed in a psychiatric unit is assigned to care for a client admitted to the unit 2 days ago. On review of the client's record, the nurse notes that the admission was an informal voluntary admission. Based on this type of admission, the nurse expects which of the following?
    1 The client will be very resistant to treatment measures
    2 The client's family will be very resistant to treatment measures
    3 The client will be angry and will refuse care
    4 The client will participate in the treatment plan

15. A licensed practical nurse (LPN) enters a client's room, and the client is demanding release from the hospital. The LPN reviews the client's record and notes that the client was admitted 2 days ago for treatment of anxiety disorder, and that the admission was voluntary. The LPN reports the findings to the registered nurse (RN) and expects that the RN will take which of the following actions?
    1 Tell the client that discharge is not possible at this time
    2 Call the client's family
    3 Contact the physician
    4 Persuade the client to stay a few more days

16. A client is admitted to the psychiatric nursing unit. When collecting data from the client, the nurse notes that the client is admitted by involuntary status. Based on this type of admission, the nurse most likely expects that the client
    1 Presents a harm to self
    2 Requested the admission
    3 Consented to the admission
    4 Provided written application to the facility for admission

17. The nurse is caring for a client who is scheduled for electroconvulsive therapy (ECT). The nurse notes that an informed consent has not been obtained for the procedure. On review of the record, the nurse notes that the admission was an involuntary hospitalization. Based on this information, the nurse determines that

    1 An informed consent does not need to be obtained
    2 An informed consent should be obtained from the family
    3 An informed consent needs to be obtained from the client
    4 The physician will obtain the informed consent

18. Following a group therapy session, a client approaches the licensed practical nurse (LPN) and verbalizes a need for seclusion because of uncontrollable feelings. The LPN reports the findings to the registered nurse (RN) and expects that the RN will take which of the following actions?
    1 Inform the client that seclusion has not been prescribed
    2 Obtain an informed consent
    3 Call the client's family
    4 Place the client in seclusion immediately

19. The nurse is providing care to a client admitted to the hospital with a diagnosis of anxiety disorder. The nurse is talking with the client. The client says to the nurse, "I have a secret that I want to tell you. You won't tell anyone about it, will you?" The most appropriate nursing response is which of the following?
    1 "No, I won't tell anyone."
    2 "I cannot promise to keep a secret."
    3 "If you tell me the secret, I will tell it to your doctor."
    4 "If you tell me the secret, I will need to document it in your record."

20. A nurse is greeted by a neighbor in a local grocery store. The neighbor says to the nurse, "How is Carol doing? She is my best friend and is seen at your clinic every week." The most appropriate nursing response is which of the following?
    1 "I'm not supposed to discuss this, but since you are my neighbor, I can tell you that she is doing great!"
    2 "I'm not supposed to discuss this, but since you are my neighbor, I can tell you that she really has some problems!"
    3 "If you want to know about Carol, you need to ask her yourself."
    4 "I cannot discuss any client situation with you."

21. The client was involuntarily admitted to the psychiatric unit because of episodes of extremely violent behavior. The client is demanding to be discharged from the hospital. The licensed practical nurse (LPN) reports the information to the registered nurse (RN) and the RN does not allow the client to leave. The LPN understands that which of the following represents the legal ramifications associated with the RN's behavior?
    1 The RN will be charged with imprisonment
    2 The RN will be charged with assault

3 The RN will be charged with slander
4 No charge will be made against the RN because the RN's actions are reasonable

22. The nurse is preparing the client for the termination phase of the nurse-client relationship. Which of the following nursing tasks does the nurse most appropriately plan for this phase?
1 Identify expected outcomes
2 Plan short-term goals
3 Assist in making appropriate referrals
4 Assist in developing realistic solutions

23. During the termination phase of the nurse-client relationship, the clinic nurse observes that the client continuously demonstrates bursts of anger. The most appropriate interpretation of the behavior is that the client
1 Requires further treatment and is not ready to be discharged
2 Is displaying typical behaviors that can occur during termination
3 Needs to be admitted to the hospital
4 Needs to be referred to the psychiatrist as soon as possible

24. An 18-year-old woman is admitted to an inpatient unit with the diagnosis of anorexia nervosa. A behavioral approach is used as part of her treatment plan. The nurse understands that the purpose of this approach is to
1 Help the client identify and examine dysfunctional thoughts and beliefs
2 Emphasize social interaction with clients who withdraw
3 Provide a supportive environment
4 Examine conflicts and past issues

25. Milieu therapy is prescribed for a client. The nurse understands that this type of therapy can best be described as which of the following?
1 A form of behavior modification therapy
2 A cognitive approach to changing behavior
3 A living, learning, or working environment
4 A behavioral approach to changing behavior

26. Disulfiram (Antabuse) is prescribed for a client with a problem related to alcohol. The nurse

understands that this medication works on the principle of which of the following therapies?
1 Desensitization
2 Self-control therapy
3 Milieu therapy
4 Aversion therapy

27. A client with an eating disorder is attending group meetings with Overeaters Anonymous. Which of the following is not a characteristic of this form of self-help group?
1 People who have a similar problem are able to help others
2 It is designed to serve people who have a common problem
3 The members provide support to each other
4 The leader is a nurse or psychiatrist

28. The client is attending a Gamblers Anonymous meeting for the first time. The model used by this group is the 12-step program developed by Alcoholics Anonymous. The nurse understands that the first step in the 12-step program is which of the following?
1 Stating that the gambling will be stopped
2 Discontinuing relationships with friends who are gamblers
3 Substituting gambling for other activities
4 Admitting to having a problem

29. The nurse is assisting in conducting a group therapy session and a client with a manic disorder is monopolizing the group. The most appropriate nursing action is which of the following?
1 Suggest that the client stop talking and try listening to others
2 Ask the client to leave
3 Tell the client to stop monopolizing the group
4 Refer the client to another group

30. The nurse is assisting in monitoring a group therapy session. During this session, the members are identifying tasks and boundaries. The nurse understands that these activities are characteristic of which stage of group development?
1 Forming
2 Storming
3 Norming
4 Performing

ANSWERS

1. **3**

RATIONALE: Termination often weakens unresolved feelings in the nurse and client. Since this represents a loss for both, unresolved issues that have a loss component may be reawakened during the termination process.
TEST-TAKING STRATEGY: Note the key words "unresolved" and "weakened" in the question. Considering the

phases of the therapeutic nurse-client relationship will easily direct you to option 3. Review these phases now if you had difficulty with this question.
LEVEL OF COGNITIVE ABILITY: Comprehension
PHASE OF NURSING PROCESS: Planning
CLIENT NEEDS: Psychosocial Integrity
CONTENT AREA: Mental Health
REFERENCE
Leahy, J., & Kizilay, P. (1998). *Foundations of nursing practice: A nursing process approach.* Philadelphia: W. B. Saunders. p. 220.

2. 3

RATIONALE: Responding to the feelings expressed by a client is an effective therapeutic communication technique. The correct option is an example of the use of restating. Options 1, 2, and 4 block communication because they minimize the client's experience and do not facilitate exploration of the client's expressed feelings.
TEST-TAKING STRATEGY: Knowledge of the techniques that facilitate therapeutic communication will direct you to the correct option. Select an option that directly addresses client feelings and concerns. Option 3 is the only option that is stated in the form of a question and is open-ended, thus encouraging the verbalization of feelings.
LEVEL OF COGNITIVE ABILITY: Application
PHASE OF NURSING PROCESS: Implementation
CLIENT NEEDS: Psychosocial Integrity
CONTENT AREA: Mental Health
REFERENCE
Leahy, J., & Kizilay, P. (1998). *Foundations of nursing practice: A nursing process approach.* Philadelphia: W. B. Saunders. p. 227.

3. 4

RATIONALE: The most therapeutic nursing communication technique is restatement. Although it is a technique that has a prompting component to it, it repeats the client's major theme, which assists the nurse to obtain a more specific perception of the problem from the client.
TEST-TAKING STRATEGY: Use therapeutic communication techniques. Option 4 will provide the perception of the problem from the client's perspective. Option 1 allows the client to direct the discussion when it needs to be more focused at this point. Option 2 uses reflection that simply repeats the client's last words to prompt further discussion (which is too open-ended). Option 3 focuses on the number of nights rather than the specific problem of sleep.
LEVEL OF COGNITIVE ABILITY: Application
PHASE OF NURSING PROCESS: Implementation
CLIENT NEEDS: Psychosocial Integrity
CONTENT AREA: Mental Health
REFERENCE
Leahy, J., & Kizilay, P. (1998). *Foundations of nursing practice: A nursing process approach.* Philadelphia: W. B. Saunders. pp. 224–229.

4. 3

RATIONALE: When reading the question, you cannot tell whether or not the client is responding to the nurse's gender or is simply uncomfortable sharing personal information. The most therapeutic response for the male nurse is not to bring what may be his own gender issues into the response at this time. Options 1, 2, and 4 are nontherapeutic responses.
TEST-TAKING STRATEGY: Use therapeutic communication techniques. Option 1 is not therapeutic because the response clearly ignores the fact that this is not about the nurse, but is about the client and the client's discomfort. In option 2, the nurse becomes pompous and somewhat angry, which is not therapeutic. In option 4, the nurse begins correctly with an empathic stance but becomes involved in a gender defense and is somewhat defensive.
LEVEL OF COGNITIVE ABILITY: Comprehension
PHASE OF NURSING PROCESS: Evaluation
CLIENT NEEDS: Psychosocial Integrity
CONTENT AREA: Mental Health

REFERENCE
Leahy, J., & Kizilay, P. (1998). *Foundations of nursing practice: A nursing process approach.* Philadelphia: W. B. Saunders. pp. 224–229.

5. 4

RATIONALE: The most therapeutic response is the one that reflects the client's feelings and offers the client control of care. In this way the nurse avoids engaging in a regressive struggle with the client. Native Americans view touch very differently from other Americans.
TEST-TAKING STRATEGY: Use knowledge regarding cultural issues related to Native Americans to answer the question. In option 1, the nurse uses avoidance and information giving. Option 2 is an aggressive and nontherapeutic communication technique. Option 3 is social and nontherapeutic because it labels the client's behavior and is likely to provoke anger from the client.
LEVEL OF COGNITIVE ABILITY: Comprehension
PHASE OF NURSING PROCESS: Implementation
CLIENT NEEDS: Psychosocial Integrity
CONTENT AREA: Mental Health
REFERENCE
Leahy, J., & Kizilay, P. (1998). *Foundations of nursing practice: A nursing process approach.* Philadelphia: W. B. Saunders. pp. 224–229.

6. 1

RATIONALE: Open-ended questions and silence are strategies used to encourage clients to discuss their problem. Options 2 and 3 do not encourage the client to express feelings. The nurse should not offer opinions and should encourage the client to identify the reasons for the behavior. Option 4 is not a client-centered intervention.
TEST-TAKING STRATEGY: Use the process of elimination. Eliminate options 2 and 3 first because they do not support client expression of feelings. Eliminate option 4 next because it is not a client-centered response. Focusing on the client's feelings will easily direct you to option 1.
LEVEL OF COGNITIVE ABILITY: Application
PHASE OF NURSING PROCESS: Planning
CLIENT NEEDS: Psychosocial Integrity
CONTENT AREA: Mental Health
REFERENCE
Leahy, J., & Kizilay, P. (1998). *Foundations of nursing practice: A nursing process approach.* Philadelphia: W. B. Saunders. pp. 225–226.

7. 4

RATIONALE: The client must first deal with feelings and negative responses before being able to work through the meaning of the crisis. Option 4 pertains directly to the client's feelings. Options 1, 2, and 3 do not directly address the client's feelings.
TEST-TAKING STRATEGY: Focus on the issue of the question. Use the process of elimination and focus on the feelings of the client. Review the phases of the nurse-client relationship now if you had difficulty with this question.
LEVEL OF COGNITIVE ABILITY: Application
PHASE OF NURSING PROCESS: Implementation
CLIENT NEEDS: Psychosocial Integrity
CONTENT AREA: Mental Health
REFERENCE
Leahy, J., & Kizilay, P. (1998). *Foundations of nursing practice: A nursing process approach.* Philadelphia: W. B. Saunders. p. 227.

8. 1

RATIONALE: Denial is a response by victims of sexual abuse. It is described as an adaptive and protective reaction. Projection is blaming or "scapegoating." Rationalization is justifying the unacceptable attributes about him or herself. Intellectualization is the excessive use of abstract thinking or generalizations to decrease painful thinking.
TEST-TAKING STRATEGY: Knowledge regarding defense mechanisms is required to answer the question. The key words are "calm" and "quiet." These behaviors are indicative of denial in a sexually abused victim. If you had difficulty with this question, take time now to review content related to the sexually abused victim and defense mechanisms.
LEVEL OF COGNITIVE ABILITY: Comprehension
PHASE OF NURSING PROCESS: Evaluation
CLIENT NEEDS: Psychosocial Integrity
CONTENT AREA: Mental Health
REFERENCE
Varcarolis, E. (1998). *Foundations of psychiatric mental health nursing* (3rd ed.). Philadelphia: W. B. Saunders. p. 421.

9. 3

RATIONALE: The client's thoughts are extremely important when verbalized. Suicidal thoughts are the highest priority. Options 1, 2, and 4 will all affect the treatment of the client but are not of greatest importance at this time.
TEST-TAKING STRATEGY: The client is the focus of the question; therefore, eliminate option 4. Use priorities when selecting from the remaining options. Eliminate option 2 as the least concern among the remaining options. Select option 3 because it directly addresses the client's thoughts.
LEVEL OF COGNITIVE ABILITY: Comprehension
PHASE OF THE NURSING PROCESS: Data Collection
CLIENT NEEDS: Psychosocial Integrity
CONTENT AREA: Mental Health
REFERENCE
deWit, S. (1998). *Essentials of medical-surgical nursing* (4th ed.). Philadelphia: W. B. Saunders. p. 1003.

10. 4

RATIONALE: This response helps the client to focus on the emotion underlying the delusion, but does not argue with it. If the nurse attempts to change the client's mind, the delusion may in fact be even more strongly held.
TEST-TAKING STRATEGY: Knowledge regarding the dynamics of delusions and how delusions meet the client's underlying needs is helpful to answer the question. Option 4 is the only option that recognizes the client's need. Additionally, option 4 focuses on the client's feelings.
LEVEL OF COGNITIVE ABILITY: Application
PHASE OF NURSING PROCESS: Implementation
CLIENT NEEDS: Psychosocial Integrity
CONTENT AREA: Mental Health
REFERENCE
Leahy, J., & Kizilay, P. (1998). *Foundations of nursing practice: A nursing process approach*. Philadelphia: W. B. Saunders. p. 227.

11. 4

RATIONALE: Safety of the client, other clients, and staff is of prime concern. When dealing with an impaired individual, trying to talk may be out of the question. Waiting to intervene could cause the client to become even more agitated and a threat to others. Option 3 would only further aggravate an already agitated individual. Option 4 is in effect an isolation technique that allows for separation from others and provides a less stimulating environment where the client can maintain dignity.
TEST-TAKING STRATEGY: Focus on the issue of the question and use the process of elimination. Noting that the client is inebriated will assist in directing you to option 4, which most directly addresses the situation and the behavior and feelings of the client.
LEVEL OF COGNITIVE ABILITY: Application
PHASE OF NURSING PROCESS: Planning
CLIENT NEEDS: Psychosocial Integrity
CONTENT AREA: Mental Health
REFERENCE
deWit, S. (1998). *Essentials of medical-surgical nursing* (4th ed.). Philadelphia: W. B. Saunders. pp. 1011–1013.

12. 2

RATIONALE: Denial is refusal to admit to a painful reality, which is treated as if it does not exist. In projection, a person unconsciously rejects emotionally unacceptable features and attributes them to other people, objects, or situations. In regression, the client returns to an earlier, more comforting, although less mature way of behaving. Rationalization is justifying illogical or unreasonable ideas, actions, or feelings by developing acceptable explanations that satisfy the teller as well as the listener.
TEST-TAKING STRATEGY: Note the key words "There's nothing wrong with me." Select the response that recognizes the client's attempt to avoid looking at the reality of the situation. If you had difficulty with this question, take time now to review defense mechanisms.
LEVEL OF COGNITIVE ABILITY: Comprehension
PHASE OF NURSING PROCESS: Data Collection
CLIENT NEEDS: Psychosocial Integrity
CONTENT AREA: Mental Health
REFERENCE
Varcarolis, E. (1998). *Foundations of psychiatric mental health nursing* (3rd ed.). Philadelphia: W. B. Saunders. p. 340.

13. 1

RATIONALE: Reflection is the therapeutic communication technique that redirects the client's feelings back in order to validate what the client is saying. Options 2, 3, and 4 are nontherapeutic at this time.
TEST-TAKING STRATEGY: Use therapeutic communication techniques. In option 2 the nurse attempts to use focusing, but the attempt to discuss central issues seems premature. In option 3 the nurse makes a judgment and is nontherapeutic in the one-on-one relationship. In option 4 the nurse is attempting to assess the client's ability to openly discuss feelings with family members. Although this may be appropriate, the timing is somewhat premature and closes off facilitation of the client's feelings.
LEVEL OF COGNITIVE ABILITY: Application
PHASE OF NURSING PROCESS: Implementation
CLIENT NEEDS: Psychosocial Integrity
CONTENT AREA: Mental Health
REFERENCE
Leahy, J., & Kizilay, P. (1998). *Foundations of nursing practice: A nursing process approach*. Philadelphia: W. B. Saunders. pp. 224–226.

14. **4**

RATIONALE: Generally, voluntary admission is sought by the client or client's guardian through a written application to the facility. If the client seeks voluntary admission, the most likely expectation is that the client will participate in the treatment program.

TEST-TAKING STRATEGY: Note the key words "informal voluntary admission." This will easily direct you to option 4. Additionally, note that options 1, 2, and 3 are similar. Review the various types of hospital admission processes now if you had difficulty with this question.

LEVEL OF COGNITIVE ABILITY: Comprehension
PHASE OF NURSING PROCESS: Planning
CLIENT NEEDS: Psychosocial Integrity
CONTENT AREA: Mental Health
REFERENCE

Varcarolis, E. (1998). *Foundations of psychiatric mental health nursing* (3rd ed.). Philadelphia: W. B. Saunders. p. 99.

15. **3**

RATIONALE: Generally, voluntary admission is sought by the client or client's guardian through a written application to the facility. Voluntary clients have the right to demand and obtain release. The best nursing action is to contact the physician.

TEST-TAKING STRATEGY: Noting the type of hospital admission will assist in eliminating option 1. It is inappropriate to "persuade" a client to stay in the hospital. Option 2 should be eliminated based simply on the issue of client rights and the issue of confidentiality. Review the various types of hospital admission and discharge processes now if you had difficulty with this question.

LEVEL OF COGNITIVE ABILITY: Comprehension
PHASE OF NURSING PROCESS: Implementation
CLIENT NEEDS: Safe, Effective Care Environment
CONTENT AREA: Mental Health
REFERENCE

Varcarolis, E. (1998). *Foundations of psychiatric mental health nursing* (3rd ed.). Philadelphia: W. B. Saunders. p. 99.

16. **1**

RATIONALE: Involuntary admission is made without the client's consent. Involuntary admission is necessary when a person is a danger to self or others or is in need of psychiatric treatment or physical care. A specified number of physicians must certify that a person's mental health justifies detention and treatment. Options 2, 3, and 4 describe the process of voluntary admission.

TEST-TAKING STRATEGY: Note the key words "involuntary status." This should easily direct you to option 1. Note that options 2, 3, and 4 are all similar. Review the process of involuntary admission now if you had difficulty with this question.

LEVEL OF COGNITIVE ABILITY: Comprehension
PHASE OF NURSING PROCESS: Data Collection
CLIENT NEEDS: Psychosocial Integrity
CONTENT AREA: Mental Health
REFERENCE

Varcarolis, E. (1998). *Foundations of psychiatric mental health nursing* (3rd ed.). Philadelphia: W. B. Saunders. p. 99.

17. **3**

RATIONALE: Clients who are involuntarily admitted do not lose their right to informed consent. The informed consent needs to be obtained from the client.

TEST-TAKING STRATEGY: Knowledge regarding the hospital admission processes and client's rights is necessary to answer this question. If you had difficulty with this question, focus on the issue of client rights to direct you to option 3. Review client rights now if you had difficulty with this question.

LEVEL OF COGNITIVE ABILITY: Comprehension
PHASE OF NURSING PROCESS: Planning
CLIENT NEEDS: Safe, Effective Care Environment
CONTENT AREA: Mental Health
REFERENCE

Varcarolis, E. (1998). *Foundations of psychiatric mental health nursing* (3rd ed.). Philadelphia: W. B. Saunders. p. 100.

18. **2**

RATIONALE: A client may request to be secluded or restrained. Federal laws require the consent of the client, unless an emergency situation exists in which an immediate risk to the client or others can be documented. The use of seclusion and restraint is permitted only on the written order of a physician, which must be reviewed and renewed every 24 hours, and which also must specify the type of restraint to be used.

TEST-TAKING STRATEGY: Knowledge regarding the legal issues surrounding the use of seclusion and restraints and knowledge regarding the issue of client's rights will easily direct you to option 2. There is no reason to call the family at this time; therefore, eliminate option 3. Knowing that a physician's written order is necessary will assist in eliminating option 4. Option 1 is not the best choice because this information, if given to a client experiencing uncontrollable feelings, may cause escalation of the feelings.

LEVEL OF COGNITIVE ABILITY: Comprehension
PHASE OF NURSING PROCESS: Planning
CLIENT NEEDS: Safe, Effective Care Environment
CONTENT AREA: Mental Health
REFERENCE

Varcarolis, E. (1998). *Foundations of psychiatric mental health nursing* (3rd ed.). Philadelphia: W. B. Saunders. pp. 100, 321.

19. **2**

RATIONALE: The nurse should never promise to keep a secret. Secrets are appropriate in a social relationship but not in a therapeutic one. The nurse needs to be honest with the client and tell the client that a promise cannot be made to keep the secret.

TEST-TAKING STRATEGY: Use the process of elimination. Option 1 can be easily eliminated because it is inappropriate. Also, options 3 and 4 are not only inappropriate, but are to an extent threatening and may even block further communication.

LEVEL OF COGNITIVE ABILITY: Application
PHASE OF NURSING PROCESS: Implementation
CLIENT NEEDS: Psychosocial Integrity
CONTENT AREA: Mental Health
REFERENCE

Varcarolis, E. (1998). *Foundations of psychiatric mental health nursing* (3rd ed.). Philadelphia: W. B. Saunders. p. 200.

20. **4**

RATIONALE: A nurse is required to maintain confidentiality regarding clients and their care. Confidentiality is basic to the therapeutic relationship and is a client's right. Option 3 is correct in a sense; however, it is a rather blunt statement. Both options 1 and 2 identify statements that do not maintain client confidentiality.

TEST-TAKING STRATEGY: Focus on the issue of the question, maintaining confidentiality. This should easily assist you in eliminating options 1 and 2. From the remaining options, select option 4 over option 3 because it is more direct and correct. Option 3 is a rather blunt and somewhat rude statement. Review confidentiality issues now if you had difficulty with this question.
LEVEL OF COGNITIVE ABILITY: Application
PHASE OF NURSING PROCESS: Implementation
CLIENT NEEDS: Safe, Effective Care Environment
CONTENT AREA: Mental Health
REFERENCE
deWit, S. (1998). *Essentials of medical-surgical nursing* (4th ed.). Philadelphia: W. B. Saunders. p. 1066.

21. 4

RATIONALE: False imprisonment is an act with the intent to confine a person to a specific area. A nurse can be charged with false imprisonment if the nurse prohibits a client from leaving the hospital if the client was voluntarily admitted and if there are no agency or legal policies for detaining the client. On the other hand, if the client was involuntarily admitted or had agreed to an evaluation before discharge, the nurse's actions are reasonable.
TEST-TAKING STRATEGY: Noting the key words "involuntarily admitted" will easily direct you to eliminate option 1 and direct you to option 4. Options 2 and 3 are unrelated to the issue of the question and can be easily eliminated. Review the issues related to false imprisonment and hospital admissions now if you had difficulty with this question.
LEVEL OF COGNITIVE ABILITY: Comprehension
PHASE OF NURSING PROCESS: Evaluation
CLIENT NEEDS: Safe, Effective Care Environment
CONTENT AREA: Mental Health
REFERENCE
Varcarolis, E. (1998). *Foundations of psychiatric mental health nursing* (3rd ed.). Philadelphia: W. B. Saunders. p. 106.

22. 3

RATIONALE: Tasks of the termination phase include evaluating client performance, evaluating achievement of expected outcomes, evaluating future needs, making appropriate referrals, and dealing with the common behaviors associated with termination. Options 1, 2, and 4 identify the tasks of the working phase of the relationship.
TEST-TAKING STRATEGY: Noting the key words "termination phase" should easily direct you to option 3. If you are unfamiliar with the appropriate tasks of the phases of the nurse-client relationship, take time now to review.
LEVEL OF COGNITIVE ABILITY: Application
PHASE OF NURSING PROCESS: Planning
CLIENT NEEDS: Psychosocial Integrity
CONTENT AREA: Mental Health
REFERENCE
Leahy, J., & Kizilay, P. (1998). *Foundations of nursing practice: A nursing process approach.* Philadelphia: W. B. Saunders. p. 220.

23. 2

RATIONALE: In the termination phase of a relationship, it is normal for a client to demonstrate a number of regressive behaviors. Typical behaviors include return of symptoms, anger, withdrawal, and minimizing the relationship. The anger that the client is experiencing is a normal behavior during the termination phase and does not necessarily indicate the need for hospitalization or treatment.

TEST-TAKING STRATEGY: Note the key words "termination phase." This alone may assist in directing you to option 2. Additionally, note the similarity between options 1, 3, and 4. These options address the need for further supervised treatment. If you are unfamiliar with the client behaviors associated with the termination phase, take time now to review.
LEVEL OF COGNITIVE ABILITY: Comprehension
PHASE OF NURSING PROCESS: Evaluation
CLIENT NEEDS: Psychosocial Integrity
CONTENT AREA: Mental Health
REFERENCE
Leahy, J., & Kizilay, P. (1998). *Foundations of nursing practice: A nursing process approach.* Philadelphia: W. B. Saunders. p. 220.

24. 1

RATIONALE: Behavioral therapy is used to help clients identify and examine dysfunctional thoughts as well as identify and examine values and beliefs that maintain these thoughts. Options 2, 3, and 4 are incorrect.
TEST-TAKING STRATEGY: Note the key word "behavioral." Focusing on this key word should direct you to option 1. If you are unfamiliar with this type of therapy and its purpose, take time now to review.
LEVEL OF COGNITIVE ABILITY: Comprehension
PHASE OF NURSING PROCESS: Planning
CLIENT NEEDS: Psychosocial Integrity
CONTENT AREA: Mental Health
REFERENCE
Varcarolis, E. (1998). *Foundations of psychiatric mental health nursing* (3rd ed.). Philadelphia: W. B. Saunders. p. 812.

25. 3

RATIONALE: Milieu therapy, or "therapeutic community," has as its locus a living, learning, or working environment. Although milieu therapy may include behavioral approaches, its primary locus is described in option 3.
TEST-TAKING STRATEGY: Knowledge regarding the components of milieu therapy is required to answer this question. Note that options 1, 2, and 4 are similar and that option 3 identifies a global description.
LEVEL OF COGNITIVE ABILITY: Comprehension
PHASE OF NURSING PROCESS: Planning
CLIENT NEEDS: Psychosocial Integrity
CONTENT AREA: Mental Health
REFERENCE
Varcarolis, E. (1998). *Foundations of psychiatric mental health nursing* (3rd ed.). Philadelphia: W. B. Saunders. p. 58.

26. 4

RATIONALE: Aversion therapy, also known as aversion conditioning or negative reinforcement, is a technique used to change behavior. In this therapy, a stimulus (alcohol) attractive to the client is paired with an unpleasant event in hopes of instituting the stimulus with negative properties.
TEST-TAKING STRATEGY: Knowledge that aversion therapy is a form of negative reinforcement will easily direct you to the correct option. If you had difficulty with this question, take time now to review this form of therapy.
LEVEL OF COGNITIVE ABILITY: Comprehension
PHASE OF NURSING PROCESS: Planning
CLIENT NEEDS: Psychosocial Integrity
CONTENT AREA: Mental Health

REFERENCE
Varcarolis, E. (1998). *Foundations of psychiatric mental health nursing* (3rd ed.). Philadelphia: W. B. Saunders. p. 58.

27. **4**

RATIONALE: The sponsor of a self-help group is an experienced member of the group. A nurse or psychiatrist may be asked by the group to serve as a resource but would not be the leader of the group. Options 1, 2, and 3 are characteristics of a self-help group.
TEST-TAKING STRATEGY: Note the key word "not" in the stem of the question. Note that options 1, 2, and 3 are all similar. This should easily direct you to option 4. Review the characteristics of a self-help group now if you had difficulty with this question.
LEVEL OF COGNITIVE ABILITY: Comprehension
PHASE OF NURSING PROCESS: Planning
CLIENT NEEDS: Psychosocial Integrity
CONTENT AREA: Mental Health
REFERENCE
Varcarolis, E. (1998). *Foundations of psychiatric mental health nursing* (3rd ed.). Philadelphia: W. B. Saunders. p. 258.

28. **4**

RATIONALE: The first step in the 12-step program is to admit that a problem exists. Options 1 and 2 are unrealistic as a first step in the process to recovery. Although option 3 may be a strategy, it is not the first step.
TEST-TAKING STRATEGY: Note the key words "first step" in the question. This will easily assist in directing you to option 4. If you are unfamiliar with the 12-step program, take time now to review.
LEVEL OF COGNITIVE ABILITY: Comprehension
PHASE OF NURSING PROCESS: Data Collection
CLIENT NEEDS: Psychosocial Integrity
CONTENT AREA: Mental Health
REFERENCE
Varcarolis, E. (1998). *Foundations of psychiatric mental health nursing* (3rd ed.). Philadelphia: W. B. Saunders. p. 258.

29. **1**

RATIONALE: If a client is monopolizing the group it is important that the nurse be direct and decisive. The best action is to suggest that the client stop talking and try listening to others. Although option 3 may be a direct response, option 1 is the most therapeutic direct statement. Options 2 and 4 are inappropriate.
TEST-TAKING STRATEGY: Eliminate options 2 and 4 first because they are similar. Use therapeutic communication techniques to assist in directing you to option 1. If you had difficulty with this question, take time now to review therapeutic communication techniques.
LEVEL OF COGNITIVE ABILITY: Application
PHASE OF NURSING PROCESS: Implementation
CLIENT NEEDS: Psychosocial Integrity
CONTENT AREA: Mental Health
REFERENCE
Varcarolis, E. (1998). *Foundations of psychiatric mental health nursing* (3rd ed.). Philadelphia: W. B. Saunders. p. 262.

30. **1**

RATIONALE: In the forming or initial stage, the members are identifying tasks and boundaries. Storming involves responding emotionally to tasks. In the norming stage, members express intimate personal opinions and feelings about personal tasks. In the performing stage, members direct group energy toward the completion of tasks.
TEST-TAKING STRATEGY: Note the key word "identifying" in the question. This key word should assist in directing you to option 1. If you had difficulty with this question, take time now to review the stages of group development.
LEVEL OF COGNITIVE ABILITY: Comprehension
PHASE OF NURSING PROCESS: Data Collection
CLIENT NEEDS: Psychosocial Integrity
CONTENT AREA: Mental Health
REFERENCE
Varcarolis, E. (1998). *Foundations of psychiatric mental health nursing* (3rd ed.). Philadelphia: W. B. Saunders. p. 264.

BIBLIOGRAPHY

Brent, N. (1997). *Nurses and the law.* Philadelphia: W. B. Saunders.
deWit, S. (1998). *Essentials of medical-surgical nursing* (4th ed.). Philadelphia: W. B. Saunders.

Leahy, J., & Kizilay, P. (1998). *Foundations of nursing practice: A nursing process approach.* Philadelphia: W. B. Saunders.
O'Toole, M. (1997). *Miller-Keane encyclopedia & dictionary of medicine, nursing, & allied health* (6th ed.). Philadelphia: W. B. Saunders.
Varcarolis, E. (1998). *Foundations of psychiatric mental health nursing* (3rd ed.). Philadelphia: W. B. Saunders.

CHAPTER 61

Mental Health Disorders

I. Anxiety

A. Description
   1. A subjective, individual experience
   2. A normal response to stress
   3. A feeling of apprehension, uneasiness, uncertainty, or dread
   4. Occurs as a result of threats that may be misperceived or misinterpreted
   5. May precede new experiences
   6. Occurs as a result of a threat to identity or self-esteem
   7. May result when values are threatened

B. Types of anxiety
   1. Normal: a healthy type of anxiety
   2. Acute: precipitated by imminent loss or change that threatens the sense of security
   3. Chronic: anxiety that the individual has lived with for a long time

C. Levels of anxiety
   1. Mild
      a. Associated with the tension of everyday life
      b. The individual is alert
      c. The perceptual field is increased
      d. Can be motivating, produce growth and creativity, and increase learning
   2. Moderate
      a. The focus is on immediate concerns
      b. Narrows the perceptual field
      c. Selective inattentiveness occurs
      d. Learning and problem solving still take place
   3. Severe
      a. Feeling that something bad is about to happen
      b. A significant reduction in perceptual field occurs
      c. Focus is on specific details or scattered details
      d. All behavior is directed at relieving the anxiety
      e. Learning and problem solving are not possible
      f. The individual needs direction to focus
   4. Panic
      a. Associated with dread and terror and a sense of impending doom
      b. The personality is disorganized
      c. The individual is unable to communicate or function effectively
      d. Increased motor activity occurs
      e. Loss of rational thoughts with distorted perception
      f. Inability to concentrate
      g. If prolonged, panic can lead to exhaustion and death

D. Implementation
   1. Recognize the anxiety
   2. Establish trust
   3. Protect the client
   4. Do not attack **coping mechanisms**
   5. Do not force the client into situations that provoke anxiety
   6. Decrease stimulation in the environment
   7. Modify the environment by setting limits or limiting the interaction with others
   8. Provide creative outlets
   9. Provide activities that limit the amount of time for destructive behavior
   10. Promote relaxation techniques
   11. Administer antianxiety medications as prescribed

E. Implementation: mild to moderate levels
   1. Help the client identify the anxiety
   2. Encourage the client to talk about feelings and concerns
   3. Help the client identify thoughts and feelings that occur prior to the onset of anxiety
   4. Encourage problem solving
   5. Encourage gross motor exercise

F. Implementation: severe to panic levels
   1. Reduce the anxiety quickly

2. Use a calm manner
3. Always remain with the client
4. Minimize environmental stimuli
5. Provide clear, simple statements
6. Use a low-pitched voice
7. Attend to the physical needs of the client
8. Provide gross motor activity
9. Administer antianxiety medications as prescribed

II. Generalized Anxiety Disorder

A. Description
   1. An unrealistic anxiety in which the cause can usually be identified
   2. Physical symptoms occur
B. Data collection
   1. Chronic muscular tension
   2. Restlessness
   3. Episodes of trembling and shakiness
   4. Chronic fatigue
   5. Dizziness
   6. Inability to relax
   7. Inability to concentrate
   8. Sleep problems
   9. Inability to recognize the connection between anxiety and physical symptoms
   10. The client is focused on the physical discomfort
C. Panic disorder
   1. Description
      a. The cause usually cannot be identified
      b. It produces a sudden onset with feelings of intense apprehension and dread
      c. Severe recurrent, intermittent anxiety attacks, lasting 5 to 30 minutes
   2. Data collection
      a. Choking sensation
      b. Labored breathing
      c. Pounding heart
      d. Chest pain
      e. Dizziness
      f. Nausea
      g. Blurred vision
      h. Numbness or tingling of extremities
      i. A sense of unreality and helplessness
      j. A fear of being trapped and going crazy
      k. A fear of dying
   3. Implementation
      a. Attend to physical symptoms
      b. Assist the client to identify the thoughts that arouse the anxiety and identify the basis for these thoughts
      c. Assist the client to change unrealistic thoughts to more realistic thoughts
      d. Utilize cognitive restructuring
      e. Administer antianxiety medications as prescribed

III. Post-Traumatic Stress Disorder

A. Description: after experiencing a psychologically traumatic event, outside the range of usual experience, the individual reexperiences the event via recurrent and intrusive dreams or flashbacks
B. Stressors
   1. A natural disaster
   2. Combat
   3. Victim of rape
   4. Accidents
   5. Victim of crime or violence
   6. Victim of sexual, physical, and emotional **abuse**
   7. Reexperiencing the event as flashbacks
C. Data collection
   1. Emotional numbness
   2. Detachment
   3. Depression
   4. Anxiety
   5. Sleep disturbances and nightmares
   6. Hypervigilance
   7. Guilt about surviving
   8. Poor concentration and avoidance of activities that trigger the memory of the event
D. Implementation
   1. Desensitization through gradual exposure to the event or situations similar to the event
   2. Instructing the client in relaxation techniques
   3. Providing individual therapy addressing loss of control issues or anger
   4. Using support groups
   5. Using hypnotherapy

IV. Phobias

A. Description
   1. An irrational fear of an object or situation that persists although the person may recognize it as unreasonable
   2. Is associated with panic level anxiety and the anxiety is severe if the object, situation, or activity cannot be avoided
   3. **Defense mechanisms** commonly used include repression and displacement
B. Types
   1. Agoraphobia
      a. Fear of being alone in open or public places where escape might be difficult
      b. The individual may not leave home
      c. The individual experiences fear or a sense of helplessness or embarrassment if the attack occurs
      d. The individual avoids situations that may trigger the attack
   2. Social phobia
      a. Fear of situations in which one might be embarrassed or criticized and the fear of making a fool of oneself
      b. Can include the fear of eating in public, public speaking, or performing
   3. Specific phobia: a fear of a single object, activity, or situation such as snakes, closed spaces, and flying

C. Implementation
   1. Stay with the client when the anxiety is high to promote safety and security
   2. Identify the basis of the anxiety
   3. Allow the client to verbalize feelings about the anxiety-producing object or situation because frequently talking about the feared object is the first step in the desensitization process
   4. Desensitization by gradually introducing the individual to the feared object or situation in small doses
   5. Teach relaxation techniques such as breathing exercises, muscle-relaxation exercises, and visualization of pleasant situations
   6. Do not force contact with the phobic object or situation

V. Obsessive-Compulsive Disorder

A. Obsessions: preoccupation with persistent intrusive thoughts and ideas
B. Compulsions
   1. Repeated performance of rituals or purposeless behaviors designed to prevent some event, divert unacceptable thoughts, and decrease anxiety
   2. Obsessions and compulsions often occur together and can disrupt normal activities
   3. Anxiety occurs if obsessions or compulsions are resisted, and from being powerless to resist the thoughts or rituals
   4. Obsessive thoughts can involve issues of violence, aggression, sexual behavior, orderliness, or religion
   5. Intrusive thoughts uncontrollably interrupt conscious thoughts and the ability to function
C. Behavior patterns
   1. Decrease the anxiety
   2. Are associated with the obsessive thoughts
   3. Neutralize the thought
   4. During stressful times, the ritualistic behavior increases
   5. **Defense mechanisms** include repression, displacement, and undoing
D. Implementation
   1. Identify the situations that precipitate the behavior
   2. Do not interrupt the compulsive behaviors
   3. Allow time for the client to perform rituals
   4. Provide for client safety related to the behaviors
   5. Implement a schedule for the client that distracts from the behaviors
   6. Set limits on rituals that may interfere with the client's physical well-being to protect from physical harm
   7. Encourage the client to verbalize concerns
   8. Gradually assist the client to decrease the frequency of compulsive behaviors by establishing a written contract

BOX 61–1. Types of Somatoform Disorders
Somatization disorder Hypochondriasis Conversion disorder

VI. Somatoform Disorders

A. Description
   1. Characterized by persistent worry or complaints regarding physical illness when there are no supporting physical findings
   2. The client focuses on the physical signs and symptoms and is unable to control them
   3. The physical signs and symptoms increase with psychosocial stressors
   4. The anxiety is redirected into a somatic concern.
B. Somatization disorder (Box 61–1)
   1. Description
      a. Occurs over a period of years and usually presents before age 30
      b. The client has multiple physical complaints involving multiple systems
      c. The emotional stress can result from anxiety, fear, depression, worry, or repressed anger
      d. The client may unconsciously use somatization for secondary gains such as increased attention and decreased responsibilities
   2. Data collection
      a. Physical complaints of abdominal pain, denial of emotional problems, signs of anxiety, fear, and low self-esteem
      b. Psychosexual symptoms
      c. Secondary gain
C. Hypochondriasis
   1. Description
      a. The preoccupation with fears of having a serious disease
      b. No evidence of physical illness exists
      c. Causes a significant impaired social and occupational functioning
   2. Data collection
      a. Preoccupation with physical functioning
      b. Frequent somatic complaints
      c. Difficulty expressing feelings
      d. Extensive use of home remedies or nonprescription medications
      e. Repeatedly visiting the doctor
      f. Secondary gain
      g. Fatigue and insomnia
      h. Anxiety
D. Conversion disorder
   1. Description
      a. A physical symptom or a deficit suggesting loss or altered body function related to psychological conflict or a neurological disorder

b. An expression of a psychologic conflict or need
c. The most common conversion symptoms are blindness, deafness, paralysis, and the inability to talk
d. There is no organic cause
e. Symptoms are not intentionally produced by the client
f. Symptoms are directly related to conflict and decrease anxiety

2. Data collection
   a. "La Belle Indifference"—unconcerned with symptoms
   b. Physical limitation or disability
   c. Feelings of guilt, anxiety, or frustration
   d. Low self-esteem and feelings of inadequacy
   e. Unexpressed anger or conflict
   f. Secondary gain

3. Implementation
   a. Obtain a nursing history and assess for physical problems
   b. Do not reinforce the sick role
   c. Discourage verbalization about physical symptoms by not responding with positive reinforcement
   d. Explore with the client the needs being met by symptoms
   e. Assist the client to identify alternative ways of meeting needs
   f. Assist the client to relate feelings and conflicts to physical symptoms
   g. Allow a specific time period to discuss physical complaints because the client will feel less threatened if this behavior is limited rather than stopped completely
   h. Assure the client that physical illness has been ruled out
   i. Explore the source of anxiety and stimulate verbalization of anxiety
   j. Encourage the use of relaxation techniques as the anxiety increases
   k. Convey your understanding that symptoms are real to the client
   l. Implement pain-reduction measures as required
   m. Report and assess any new physical complaint
   n. Encourage diversional activities to decrease the client's focus on self
   o. Provide positive feedback for accomplishments to increase self-esteem
   p. Assist clients in recognizing their feelings and emotions
   q. Contract with the client to engage in relationships with others to redirect interest
   r. Administer antianxiety medications as prescribed

VII. Dissociative Disorder

A. Description
   1. A disruption in integrative functions of memory, consciousness, or identity
   2. Associated with exposure to a traumatic event

B. Dissociative identity disorder (multiple personality)
   1. Description
      a. Two or more fully developed distinct and unique personalities within the person
      b. Personalities may take full control of the client, one at a time
      c. The personalities may or may not be aware of each other
   2. Data collection
      a. The inability to recall important information too extensive to be explained by ordinary forgetfulness
      b. Transition from one personality to the other is related to stress and is sudden
      c. Dissociation is used as a method of distancing and defending self from anxiety and traumatizing experiences

C. Dissociative amnesia
   1. Description
      a. Inability to recall important personal information because it is anxiety provoking
      b. Memory impairment may be impartial or almost complete
   2. Data collection
      a. Localized—the client blocks out all memories about a specific period
      b. Selective—the client recalls some but not all memories about a specific period
      c. Generalized—loss of all memory about past life

D. Dissociative fugue
   1. Description
      a. The assumption of a new identity in a new environment
      b. The disorder may occur suddenly
   2. Data collection
      a. May drift from place to place
      b. Develops few social relationships
      c. When the fugue lifts the client returns home and is unable to recall the fugue state

E. Depersonalization disorder
   1. Description: an altered self-perception in which one's own reality is temporarily lost or changed
   2. Data collection
      a. Feelings of detachment
      b. Intact reality testing

F. Implementation
   1. Develop a trusting relationship with the client
   2. Encourage verbal expression of painful experiences, anxieties, and concerns
   3. Explore methods of coping
   4. Identify sources of conflict
   5. Focus on the clients' strengths and skills
   6. Orient the client
   7. Provide nondemanding simple routines
   8. Allow the client to progress at own pace
   9. Use stress-reduction techniques
   10. Use individual, group, and/or family psychotherapy to integrate dissociated aspects of personality or memory and to expand self-awareness

◆ VIII. Bipolar Disorder

A. Description
   1. Characterized by episodes of mania and depression with periods of normal mood and activity in between
   2. The treatment medication of choice is lithium carbonate (Eskalith), which can be toxic and therefore requires the regular monitoring of serum lithium levels
B. Data collection (Box 61–2)
◆ C. Implementation for mania
   1. Remove hazardous objects from the environment
   2. Monitor the client's sleep patterns
   3. Assess the client closely for fatigue
   4. Provide frequent rest periods
   5. Use comfort measures to promote sleep
   6. Provide a private room if possible
   7. Administer hypnotic or sedative medication as prescribed
   8. Encourage the client to ventilate feelings
   9. Use calm, slow interactions
   10. Help the client focus on one topic during the conversation

---

BOX 61–2. Bipolar Disorders

MANIA

Inappropriate affect
Restlessness
Flight of ideas
Inability to eat or sleep because of involvement in more important things
Extroverted personality
Delusional self-confidence
Initiation of activity
High and unstable affect
Becomes angry quickly
Pressure of speech
Grandiose and persecutory delusions
Inappropriate dress
Urgent motor activity
Significant decrease in appetite
Inability to sleep yet still active
Sexually promiscuous
Distracted by environmental stimuli
Unlimited energy

DEPRESSION

Decreased emotion and physical activity
Inability to make quick decisions
Introverted personality
Lack of initiative
Lack of self-confidence
Internalizing hostility
Loss of interest in appearance
Lack of energy
Easily fatigued
Withdrawn from groups
Lack of sexual interest

---

   11. Ignore or distract the client from grandiose thinking
   12. Present reality to the client
   13. Don't argue with the client
   14. Limit group activities and assess the client's tolerance level
   15. Provide high-calorie finger foods and fluids
   16. Supervise the client's choice of clothing
   17. Reduce environmental stimuli
   18. Set limits on inappropriate behaviors
   19. Provide physical activities and outlets for tension
   20. Avoid competitive games
   21. Provide gross motor activities such as walking
   22. Provide simple and direct explanations for routine procedures
   23. Provide structured activities or one-to-one activities with the nurse
   24. Supervise administration of medication

IX. Schizophrenia

A. Description
   1. A group of mental disorders characterized by psychotic features, inability to trust others, disordered thought processes, and disrupted interpersonal relationships
   2. Schizophrenia causes disturbances in affect, mood, behavior, and thought processes
B. Data collection
   1. Physical characteristics
      a. Disheveled appearance
      b. Body image distortions
      c. Preoccupied with somatic complaints
      d. Neglects eating, sleeping, and elimination
   2. Motor activity (Box 61–3)
      a. Catatonic, posturing—holding bizarre postures for long periods
      b. Catatonic excitement—moving excitedly with no environmental stimuli
      c. May be totally immobilized
      d. Unable to respond to commands, or responds only to commands
      e. Waxy flexibility
      f. Movements may be repetitive or stereotyped
      g. Motor activity may be increased as evidenced by agitation, pacing, inability to sleep, loss of appetite and weight, and impulsiveness
      h. May be unable to initiate activity, known as volition or anergia
   3. Emotional characteristics
      a. Mistrust
      b. Views the world as threatening and unsafe
      c. Feelings not easily interpreted
      d. Ambivalence manifested as compulsive rituals, negativism, and overcompliance

BOX 61–3. Abnormal Motor Behaviors

DESCRIPTION

Abnormal motor behavior or activity, displayed by the mentally ill client, occurring as a result of a psychiatric disorder

TYPES OF ABNORMAL MOTOR BEHAVIORS

Akathisia
Displaying motor restlessness and muscular quivering; the client is unable to sit or lie quietly

Echolalia
Repeating the speech of another person

Echopraxia
Repeating the movements of another person

Parkinson-like Symptoms
Making masklike faces, drooling, and having shuffling gait, tremors, and muscular rigidity

Waxy Flexibility
Having one's arms or legs placed in a certain position and holding that same position for hours

Dyskinesia
Impairment of the power of voluntary movements

---

    e. May display feelings of helplessness, anxiety, anger, guilt and depression, and decreased self-esteem

4. Compulsive rituals: attempts to solve conflicting feelings by constant, repetitive activity, which may be stereotyped or seem meaningless
5. Overcompliance: attempts to deny responsibility for any action by doing only what another exactly instructs
6. Affective disturbances
    a. Flat affect or inappropriate affect
    b. Altered thought processes
7. Thought processes
    a. Impaired reality testing
    b. Fragmentation of thoughts
    c. Blocking
    d. Loose associations
    e. Autistic thinking
    f. Perceives environment in a totally self-centered way
    g. Neologisms
    h. Magical thinking
    i. Unable to conceptualize meaning in words or thoughts
    j. Unable to organize facts logically
    k. Delusions
8. Types of delusions (Box 61–4)
    a. Loss of reference in which the client believes that certain events, situations, or interactions are directly related to self
    b. Delusions of persecution in which clients believe that they are being harassed, threatened, or persecuted by some powerful force
    c. Delusions of grandeur in which the client attaches special significance to self in relation to others or the universe and has an exaggerated sense of self that has no basis in reality
    d. Somatic delusions in which clients believe that their bodies are changing or responding in an unusual way that has no basis in reality
9. Perceptual distortions (Box 61–5)
    a. Illusions that may be brief experiences with a misinterpretation or exaggeration of reality
    b. Hallucinations such as perceiving objects, sensations, or images with no basis in reality (Box 61–6)
10. Language and communication disturbances (Box 61–7)
    a. Related to disorders in the thought process
    b. Unable to organize language
    c. Difficulty communicating clearly
    d. Inappropriate responses to a situation
    e. A single word or phrase may represent the whole meaning of the conversation and clients may feel they have communicated adequately
    f. May develop private language
C. Types of schizophrenia
  1. Paranoid schizophrenia
    a. Suspiciousness
    b. Hostility
    c. Delusions
    d. Auditory hallucinations
    e. Anxiety and anger
    f. Aloofness
    g. Persecutory themes
    h. Violence
  2. Disorganized schizophrenia
    a. Extreme social withdrawal

BOX 61–4. Delusions

DESCRIPTION

A false belief held to be true even when there is evidence to the contrary

TYPES

PERSECUTION

The thought that one is being singled out for harm by others

GRANDEUR

The false belief that one is a very powerful and important person

JEALOUSY

The false belief that one's partner or mate is going out with other people

BOX 61–5. Abnormal Thought Processes

DESCRIPTION

Abnormal thought processes, displayed by the mentally ill client, occurring as a result of a psychiatric disorder

NEOLOGISMS

Words that an individual makes up that only have meaning for the individual; is often part of a delusional system

LOOSENESS OF ASSOCIATION

The individual's thinking is haphazard, illogical, and confused and connections in thought are interrupted; seen mostly in schizophrenic disorders

FLIGHT OF IDEAS

A constant flow of speech in which the individual jumps from one topic to another in rapid succession; there is a connection between topics although it is sometimes difficult to identify; is seen in manic states

BLOCKING

A sudden cessation of a thought in the middle of a sentence; the client is unable to continue the train of thought; often sudden new thoughts come up unrelated to the topic

CIRCUMSTANTIALITY

Before getting to the point or answering a question, the individual gets caught up in countless details and explanations

CONFABULATION

Filling a memory gap with detailed fantasy believed by the teller; the purpose of confabulation is to maintain self-esteem; seen in organic conditions such as Korsakoff's psychosis

WORD SALAD

A mixture of words and phrases that have no meaning

BOX 61–6. Preoccupation in Thought Content

HALLUCINATIONS

Description

A sense perception for which no external stimuli exists

Can have an organic or functional etiology

TYPES

Visual

Seeing things that are not there

Auditory

Hearing voices when none are present

Olfactory

Smelling smells that do not exist

Tactile

Feeling touch sensations in the absence of stimuli

Gustatory

Experiencing taste in the absence of stimuli

---

    b. Delusions and hallucinations
    c. Disorganized speech
    d. Disorganized or catatonic behavior
    e. Flat affect
    f. Social withdrawal
  5. Residual schizophrenia
    a. Diagnosed as schizophrenic in the past
    b. May last for many years
    c. The client exhibits marked social isolation and withdrawal and impaired role functioning
D. Implementation (Box 61–8)
E. Implementation: active hallucinations
  1. Monitor for hallucination cues
  2. Intervene with a one-to-one contact

BOX 61–7. Language and Communication Disturbance

Neologism—a new word devised that has special meaning only to the client

Echolalia—repetition of words or phrases heard from another person

Verbigeration—purposeless repetition of words or phrases

Metonymic speech—mental confusion exhibited by the use of a word that is not the precise term intended but is of similar meaning

Clang association—repetition of words or phrases that are similar in sound but in no other way

Word salad—form of speech in which words or phrases are connected meaninglessly

Stilted language—an inappropriate and overly formal communication pattern usually written and seems artificial and intellectual

Pressured speech—speaks as if the words are being forced out quickly

Mutism—absence of verbal speech

---

    b. Disorganized speech or behavior
    c. Flat or inappropriate affect
    d. Silliness unrelated to speech
    e. Stereotyped behaviors
    f. Grimacing mannerisms
    g. Inability to perform activities of daily living
3. Catatonic schizophrenia
    a. Marked psychomotor disturbances
    b. Immobility
    c. Stupor
    d. Waxy flexibility
    e. Excessive purposeless motor activity
    f. Echolalia
    g. Automatic obedience
    h. Stereotyped or repetitive behavior
4. Undifferentiated schizophrenia
    a. Does not meet criteria for paranoid, disorganized, or catatonic schizophrenia

BOX 61–8. Implementation for Schizophrenia

Assess client's physical needs
Set limits on client's behavior when it interferes with others and becomes disruptive
Maintain a safe environment
Initiate one-to-one interactions and progress to small groups as tolerated
Spend time with client even if client is unable to respond
Monitor for altered thought processes
Maintain ego boundaries and avoid touching the client
Limit time of interaction with client
Avoid an overly warm approach
A neutral approach is less threatening
Do not make promises to client that cannot be kept
Establish daily routines
Assist client to improve grooming and accept responsibility for personal care
Sit with client in silence if necessary
Provide short, brief, and frequent contact with client
Tell client when you are leaving
Tell client when you don't understand
Do not "go along" with the client's delusions or hallucinations
Provide simple concrete activities such as puzzles or word games
Reorient the client as necessary
Assist client to establish what is real and unreal
Stay with the client if the client is frightened
Speak to the client in a simple, direct, and concise manner
Reassure the client that the environment is safe
Remove the client from group situations if the client's behavior is too bizarre, disturbing, or dangerous to others
Set realistic goals
Initially do not offer choices to the client and gradually assist the client in making own decisions
Assess physical needs
Use containers for food especially with the paranoid schizophrenic
Provide a radio or tape player at night for insomnia
Explain in detail everything you are doing
Set limits on the client's behavior if client is unable to do so
Decrease excessive stimuli in the environment
Monitor for suicide risk
Assist the client to use alternative means to express feelings through music or art therapy or writing

3. Decrease stimuli or move the client to another area
4. Avoid conveying to the client that you are also experiencing the hallucination
5. Respond verbally to anything real that the client talks about
6. Avoid touching the client
7. Encourage the client's expression of feelings
8. During hallucination, attempt to engage the client's attention through a concrete activity
9. Accept behavior and do not joke about or judge the client's behavior

10. Provide easy activities and a structured environment with routine activities of daily living
11. Monitor for signs of increasing fear, anxiety, or agitation
12. Provide **seclusion** as necessary
13. Administer medications as prescribed

F. Implementation delusions
   1. Interact on the basis of reality
   2. Encourage the client to express feelings
   3. Do not dispute with the client or try to convince the client that delusions are false
   4. Begin with activities on a one-to-one basis
   5. Alter hospital routines as necessary such as using canned or packaged food, food in containers, or food from home
   6. Recognize accomplishments and provide positive feedback for successes

X. Paranoid Disorders

A. Description
   1. The client demonstrates suspiciousness and mistrust of others
   2. The client is often viewed by others as hostile, stubborn, and defensive
   3. Concrete, pervasive, delusional system characterized by persecutory and grandiose beliefs
B. Behaviors
   1. Suspicious and mistrustful
   2. Emotionally distant
   3. Distorts reality
   4. Poor insight
   5. Hypervigilance
   6. Low self-esteem
   7. Highly sensitive, difficulty in admitting own error, and takes pride in being correct
   8. Hypercritical and intolerant of others
   9. Hostile, aggressive, and quarrelsome
   10. Evasive
   11. Concrete thinking
C. Delusions
   1. Serves purpose in establishing identity and self-esteem
   2. Grandiose and persecutory delusions
   3. Process of delusion includes denial, projection, and rationalization
   4. As trust in others increases, the need for delusions decreases
D. Types
   1. Paranoid personality
      a. Suspicious
      b. Nonpsychotic
      c. No hallucinations or delusions
      d. No symptoms of schizophrenia
   2. Paranoid state
      a. Onset abrupt in response to stress and subsides when stress decreases
      b. No hallucinations but experiences paranoid delusions

    c. May be sensitive and suspicious before development of delusions
    d. Psychotic state
    e. No symptoms of schizophrenia
  3. Paranoia
    a. Client appears normal except for delusional system
    b. Single highly organized delusional system
    c. Not bizarre
    d. No hallucinations
    e. Reserved and sensitive before onset
    f. Psychotic state
    g. No symptoms of schizophrenia
  4. Paranoid schizophrenia
    a. Prior to onset the client becomes cold, withdrawn, distrustful, resentful, argumentative, sarcastic, and defiant
    b. Bizarre, numerous, and changeable delusions
    c. Delusions become less logical as the client becomes more disorganized
    d. Persecutory hallucinations
    e. Psychotic state
    f. All symptoms of schizophrenia present
E. Implementation (Box 61–9)

XI. Personality Disorders

A. Description
  1. Includes various inflexible maladaptive behavior patterns or traits that may impair functioning and relationships
  2. Individuals usually remain in touch with reality and typically have a lack of insight into their behavior
  3. Stress exacerbates manifestations of personality disorder
  4. In severe cases personality disorder may deteriorate to a psychotic state
B. Characteristics
  1. Poor impulse control
    a. Acting out to manage internal pain
    b. Forms of acting out include physical and verbal attacks, manipulation, substance **abuse,** promiscuous sexual behaviors, and **suicide attempts**
  2. Mood characteristics
    a. Experience abandonment and depression
    b. Moods include rage, guilt, fear, and emptiness
  3. Impaired judgment
    a. Have difficulty with problem solving
    b. Unable to perceive consequences of behavior
  4. Impaired reality testing: distort reality and often project their own feelings onto others
  5. Impaired object relations: rigid and inflexible and have difficulty in intimate relationships
  6. Impaired self-perception: distorted self-perception and experience self-hate or self-idealization

---

BOX 61–9. Implementation for Paranoid Disorders

Assess for suicide risk
Diminish suspicious behavior
Establish trusting relationship
Promote increased self-esteem
Remain calm, nonthreatening, and nonjudgmental
Provide continuity of care
Respond honestly to the client
Follow through on commitments made to the client
Acknowledge client's feelings but tell client that you do not share their interpretation of an event
Provide a daily schedule of activities
Assist client to identify diversionary activities
Gradually introduce client to groups
Refocus conversation to reality-based topics
Use role playing to help the client identify thoughts and feelings
Provide positive reinforcement for successes
Do not argue with delusions
Use concrete, specific words
Do not be secretive with the client
Do not whisper in client's presence
Assure clients they will be safe
Involve the client in noncompetitive tasks
Provide the client the opportunity to complete small tasks
Monitor eating, drinking, sleeping, and elimination patterns
Limit physical contact
Monitor for agitation and decrease stimuli as needed

---

  7. Impaired thought processes
    a. Concrete or diffuse thinking
    b. Difficulty concentrating
    c. Impaired memory
  8. Impaired stimulus barrier
    a. Unable to regulate incoming sensory stimuli
    b. Increased excitability
    c. Excessive response to noise and light
    d. Poor attention span
    e. Agitated
    f. Insomnia
C. Schizoid personality disorder
  1. Description: characterized by an inability to form warm, close social relationships
  2. Data collection
    a. Social detachment and lack of close relationships
    b. Interest in solitary activities
    c. Aloof and indifferent
    d. Restricted expression of emotions
    e. Lack of interest in others
D. Schizotypal personality disorder
  1. Description: exhibit abnormal or highly unusual thoughts, perceptions, and speech and behavior patterns
  2. Data collection
    a. Suspicious
    b. Paranoia
    c. Magical thinking

     d. Odd thinking and speech

     e. Relationship deficits

E. Paranoid personality disorder

  1. Description: characterized by suspiciousness and mistrust of others

  2. Data collection

     a. Suspicious and distrusting

     b. Argumentative

     c. Hostile, aloof

     d. Rigid, critical, and controlling of others

     e. Grandiosity

F. Histrionic personality disorder

  1. Description

     a. Characterized by overly dramatic and intensely expressive behavior

     b. The client is lively and dramatic and enjoys being the center of attention

     c. Interpersonal relations may be poor

  2. Data collection

     a. Attention seeking

     b. Needs to be the center of attention

     c. Sexually seductive or provocative

     d. Self-dramatizing and theatrical

     e. Overly concerned with appearance

     f. Has romantic fantasies and controls partners

     g. Bores easily

     h. Displays dependency

G. Narcissistic personality disorder

  1. Description

     a. Characterized by an increased sense of self-importance

     b. The client is preoccupied with fantasies and unlimited success and has a constant need for attention and admiration

  2. Data collection

     a. Grandiosity

     b. Requires admiration and inflated accomplishments

     c. Overestimates abilities and underestimates contributions of others

     d. Lacks empathy and sensitivity to the needs of others

H. Avoidant personality disorder

  1. Description: characterized by social withdrawal and extreme sensitivity to potential rejection

  2. Data collection

     a. Feelings of inadequacy

     b. Hypersensitive to reactions of others and reacts poorly to criticism

     c. Social inhibition

     d. Lack of support system

I. Dependent personality disorder

  1. Description

     a. The individual lacks self-confidence and the ability to function independently

     b. Passively allows others to make decisions and assume responsibility for major areas in their life

  2. Data collection

     a. Difficulty making decisions

     b. Lacks autonomy

     c. Cannot tolerate being alone and must always have a close relationship

     d. Needs others to assume responsibility and make decisions

J. Obsessive-compulsive personality disorder

  1. Description: the client has difficulty expressing warm and tender emotions and reflects perfectionism, stubbornness, the need to control others, and a devotion to work

  2. Data collection

     a. Orderliness and perfectionism

     b. Overly conscientious

     c. Inflexible and preoccupied with details and rules

     d. Devoted to work and lacks leisure activities and friendships

     e. Miserly and stubborn

     f. Hoards worthless objects

K. Antisocial personality disorder

  1. Description

     a. A pattern of irresponsible and antisocial behavior

     b. Characterized by selfishness, inability to maintain lasting relationships, poor sexual adjustment, failure to except social norms, irritability, and aggressiveness

  2. Data collection

     a. Perceives the world as hostile

     b. Superficial charm and hostility

     c. No shame or guilt

     d. Self-centered

     e. Unreliable

     f. Easily bored

     g. Poor work history

     h. Unable to tolerate frustration

     i. Views others as objects to be manipulated

     j. Poor judgment

     k. Impulsive

L. Borderline personality disorder

  1. Description

     a. Characterized by instability in interpersonal relationships, mood, and self-image

     b. Behavior may be impulsive and unpredictable

  2. Data collection

     a. Unclear identity

     b. Unstable and intense

     c. Extreme shifts in mood

     d. Easily angered

     e. Easily bored

     f. Argumentative

     g. Depression

     h. Self-destructive behavior

     i. Manipulation

     j. Unable to tolerate anxiety

     k. Chronic feelings of emptiness and fear of being alone

     l. Splitting

M. Passive-aggressive personality disorder

  1. Description

     a. Characterized by passively expressing

covert aggression rather than dealing with it directly

b. The behavior can interfere with both social and work activities

2. Data collection
   a. Procrastination
   b. Stubbornness
   c. Intentional inefficiency
   d. Forgetfulness
   e. Dependency

N. Implementation
   1. Maintain safety against self-destructive behaviors
   2. Allow the client to make choices and be as independent as possible
   3. Encourage the client to discuss feelings rather than act them out
   4. Provide consistency in response to the client's acting-out behaviors
   5. Discuss expectations and responsibilities with the client
   6. Discuss the consequences that will follow certain behaviors
   7. Inform the client that harm to self, others, and property is unacceptable
   8. Identify splitting behavior
   9. Assist the client to deal directly with anger
   10. Develop a written contract with the client
   11. Encourage the client to keep a journal recording daily feelings
   12. Encourage the client to participate in group activities and praise nonmanipulative behavior
   13. Set and maintain limits to decrease manipulative behavior
   14. Remove the client from group situations in which attention-seeking behaviors occur
   15. Provide realistic praise for positive behaviors in social situations

XII. Electroconvulsive Therapy (ECT)

A. Description
   1. An effective treatment for depression that consists of inducing a grand mal seizure by passing an electrical current through electrodes that are attached to the temples
   2. The administration of a muscle relaxant minimizes seizure activity, preventing damage to long bones and cervical vertebrae
   3. The usual course is 6 to 12 treatments given two to three times per week
   4. Maintenance ECT once a month may help to decrease prolapse rate for clients with recurrent depression
   5. ECT is not a permanent cure
   6. Not necessarily effective in clients with dysrhythmic depression or those with depression and personality disorders, those with drug dependence, or those with depression secondary to situational or social difficulties

7. Risk clients include clients with recent MI, CVA, or cerebral vascular malformation, or clients with intracranial mass lesions

B. Uses
   1. Clients with major depressive and bipolar depressive disorders especially when psychotic symptoms are present such as delusions of guilt, somatic delusions, and delusions of infidelity
   2. Clients who have depression with marked psychomotor retardation and stupor
   3. Manic clients whose conditions are resistant to lithium and antipsychotic medications and in clients who are rapid cyclers (a client with a bipolar disorder who has many episodes of mood swings close together)
   4. Clients with schizophrenia, especially catatonia; those with schizoaffective syndromes; and psychotic clients

C. Indications for use
   1. When antidepressant medications have no effect
   2. When there is a need for rapid definitive response when a client is suicidal or homicidal
   3. The client is in extreme agitation or stupor
   4. The risks of other treatments outweigh the risk of ECT
   5. The client has a history of poor medication response, a history of good ECT response, or both
   6. The client prefers it

D. Preprocedure
   1. Explain the procedure to the client
   2. Encourage the client to discuss feelings, including myths regarding ECT
   3. Teach the client and family what to expect
   4. Informed consent must be obtained when voluntary clients are being treated
   5. For involuntary clients, when informed consent cannot be obtained, permission may be obtained from the next of kin, although in some states the permission for ECT must be court ordered
   6. NPO after midnight or at least 4 hours prior to treatment
   7. Baseline vital signs are taken
   8. The client is requested to void
   9. Hairpins, contact lenses, and dentures are removed
   10. Administer preoperative medication if prescribed; glycopyrrolate (Robinul) or atropine may be prescribed to prevent aspiration and to minimize bradydysrhythmias in response to electrical stimulants

E. During the procedure
   1. Place a blood pressure cuff on one of the client's arms
   2. An IV line is inserted and EEG and ECG electrodes are attached
   3. A pulse oximeter is placed onto the client's finger

4. Blood pressure is monitored throughout treatment
5. Medications administered may include short-acting anesthetics such as methohexital sodium (Brevital), thiopental (Pentothal), and a muscle relaxant such as succinylcholine (Anectine)
6. 100% oxygen by mask via positive pressure is administered throughout the procedure
7. An airway or bite block is placed to prevent biting the tongue
8. Electrical stimulus is given and the seizure should last 30 to 60 seconds

F. Postprocedure
1. Client will go to a properly staffed recovery room with the blood pressure cuff and oximeter in place, where oxygen, suction, and other emergency equipment is available
2. Once the client is awake, talk to the client and take vital signs
3. The client may be confused; provide frequent orientation (brief, distinct, and simple) and reassurance
4. The client returns to the nursing unit when a 90% oxygen saturation level is present, vital signs are stable, and mental status is satisfactory
5. Assess the gag reflex prior to giving the client fluids, food, or medication

G. Potential side effects
1. Major side effects with bilateral treatment are confusion, disorientation, and short-term memory loss
2. The client may be confused and disorientated upon awakening
3. Memory deficits may occur but memory usually recovers completely, although some clients have memory loss lasting up to 6 months

XIII. Cognitive Impairment Disorders

A. Dementia and Alzheimer's disease (refer to Chapter 65 for information regarding dementia and Alzheimer's disease)
B. Autistic disorder
1. A rare developmental disorder that includes characteristics such as lack of social response and interaction
2. Withdrawal from social contact
3. Impaired communication
4. Bizarre mannerism
5. If the child can talk, the child uses speech not for communication but to repeat words or phrases meaninglessly
6. The child may develop an unusual attachment to a significant object and display frequent rocking, spinning, twirling, or other bizarre behaviors
C. Attention deficit hyperactivity disorder (ADHD)
1. Known as hyperactivity

2. The child cannot sustain concentration to complete a task
3. The child has little impulse control and exhibits continual frequently disruptive activity
4. The child has a short attention span and difficulty with organizing and completing school work
D. Tourette's disorder
1. Description: appears between ages 2 and 15 and is characterized by recurrent involuntary and rapid movements affecting various parts of the body accompanied by vocal noises such as barks, grunts, or profanities
2. Implementation
   a. Assess **suicide** potential
   b. Remove dangerous objects from the environment
   c. Establish a trusting one-to-one relationship
   d. Maintain eye contact
   e. Protect the client from harm by providing a helmet or protective padding
   f. Allow the child to have a favorite toy or other object
   g. Provide positive reinforcement for appropriate behaviors
   h. Set limits on socially inappropriate or manipulative behaviors
   i. Encourage the client to confront tension and frustration before they emerge as inappropriate behaviors
   j. Provide noncompetitive group situations

XIV. Psychosexual Alterations

A. Sexuality
1. One's sense of being a sexual individual
2. Includes how one looks, behaves, and relates to others
B. Alterations in sexual expression
1. Heterosexuality—male/female sexual relationships
2. Homosexuality—sexual attraction to a member of the same sex
3. Bisexuality—sexual attraction to and activity with both sexes
4. Transvestism—obsession with clothing of the opposite sex
C. Alterations in sexual behavior
1. Transsexualism: feeling that one's sex is inappropriate and desiring to acquire sexual characteristics of the opposite sex
2. Exhibitionism: sexual urges and fantasies and exposing genitals to strangers
3. Fetishism: using nonliving objects for sexual gratification
4. Pedophilia: desiring sexual activity with a child under age 13
5. Sexual masochism: Sexual gratification that involves receiving pain
6. Sexual sadism: Sexual gratification that involves inflicting pain

7. Voyeurism: sexual gratification through observing others disrobing or engaging in sexual activity
8. Zoophilia: intense sexual arousal or desire with animals
9. Frotteurism: intense sexual arousal or desire when rubbing against a nonconsenting person

D. Implementation
   1. Assessment of sexual history and precipitating event for sexual disorder
   2. Encourage the client to explore personal beliefs
   3. Provide a nonjudgmental attitude
   4. Provide supportive psychotherapy
   5. Initiate psychoanalysis as prescribed

PRACTICE QUESTIONS

1. The nurse is caring for a client who has bipolar disorder with aggressive social behavior. Which of the following activities is most appropriate for this client?
   1 Ping-Pong
   2 Writing
   3 Chess
   4 Basketball

2. A client is admitted to the hospital with a diagnosis of major depression—severe, single episode. The nurse collects data on the client and identifies that a major concern is the client's altered nutrition related to poor nutritional intake. The most appropriate nursing intervention related to this concern is
   1 Explain to the client the importance of a good nutritional intake
   2 Weigh the client three times per week, before breakfast
   3 Report the nutritional concern to the psychiatrist and obtain a nutritional consult as soon as possible
   4 Consult with the nutritionist, offer the client several small frequent meals per day, and schedule brief nursing interactions with the client during these times

3. In planning activities for the depressed client, especially during the early stages of hospitalization, which of the following plans is best?
   1 Provide an activity that is quiet and solitary in nature to avoid increased fatigue, i.e., working on a puzzle or reading a book
   2 Plan nothing until the client asks to participate in milieu
   3 Offer the client a menu of daily activities and insist that the client participate in all of them
   4 Provide a structured daily program of activities and encourage the client to participate

4. The depressed client verbalizes feelings of low self-esteem and self-worth typified by statements such as "I'm such a failure . . . I can't do anything right." The best nursing response is

1 To tell the client that this is not true; that we all have a purpose in life
2 To remain with the client and sit in silence; this will encourage the client to verbalize feelings
3 To reassure the client that you know how the client is feeling and that things will get better
4 To identify recent behaviors or accomplishments that demonstrate skill ability

5. A depressed client is ready for discharge. The nurse feels comfortable that the client has a good understanding of the disease process when the client states
   1 "I'll never let this happen to me again. I won't let my boss or my job or my family get to me!"
   2 "It's important for me to eat well, exercise, and to take my medication. If I begin to lose my appetite or not sleep well, I've got to get in to see my doctor."
   3 "I've learned I am a good person and that I am worthy of giving and receiving love. I don't need anyone; I have myself to rely on!"
   4 "I don't know what happened to me. I've always been able to make decisions for myself and for my business. I don't ever want to feel so weak or vulnerable again!"

6. The nurse collects data on a client with the admitting diagnosis of bipolar affective disorder—mania. The symptom presentation that requires the nurse's immediate intervention is
   1 The client's outlandish behaviors and inappropriate dress
   2 The client's grandiose delusions of being a royal descendent of King Arthur
   3 The client's nonstop physical activity and poor nutritional intake
   4 The client's constant, incessant talking, which includes sexual innuendoes and teasing staff

7. The female client in a manic state emerges from her room. She is topless and is making sexual remarks and gestures toward staff and peers. The best initial nursing response is
   1 Quietly approach the client, escort her to her room, and assist her in getting dressed
   2 Approach the client in the hallway and insist that she go to her room
   3 Confront the client on the inappropriateness of her behaviors and offer her a time-out
   4 Ask the other clients to ignore her behavior; eventually she will return to her room

8. The nurse reviews the activity schedule for the day and believes the best activity that the manic client could participate in is
   1 Brown-bag luncheon and a book review
   2 Tetherball
   3 Paint by number activity
   4 Deep breathing and a progressive relaxation group

9. A client who is delusional says to the nurse, "The federal guards were sent to kill me." The nurse's best response is
   1 "The guards are not out to kill you."
   2 "I don't believe this is true."
   3 "I don't know anything about the guards. Do you feel afraid that people are trying to hurt you?"
   4 "What makes you think the guards were sent to hurt you?"

10. A woman comes into the emergency department in a severe state of anxiety following a car accident. The most important nursing intervention is
   1 Remain with the client
   2 Put the client in a quiet room
   3 Teach the client deep breathing
   4 Encourage the client to talk about her feelings and concerns

11. A male client with delirium becomes agitated and confused in his room at night. The best initial intervention by the nurse is
   1 Use a nightlight and turn off the television
   2 Keep the television on during the night and a soft light
   3 Move the client next to the nurses' station
   4 Play soft music during the night, and maintain a well-lit room

12. The nurse is collecting data on a client who is actively hallucinating. Which of the following nursing statements is most therapeutic at this time?
   1 "I talked to the voices you're hearing and they won't hurt you now."
   2 "I can hear your voice and she wants you to come to dinner."
   3 "Sometimes people hear things or voices others can't hear."
   4 "I know you feel 'they are out to get you' but it's not true."

13. The nurse is caring for a client with a diagnosis of depression. The nurse monitors for signs of constipation and urinary retention, knowing that these problems are most likely due to
   1 Inadequate dietary intake and dehydration
   2 Lack of exercise and poor diet
   3 Poor dietary choices
   4 Psychomotor retardation and side effects of medication

14. The client is admitted to the inpatient unit and is being considered for electroconvulsive therapy (ECT). The client appears calm but the family is hypervigilant and anxious. The client's mother begins to cry and states, "My son's brain will be destroyed. How can the doctor do this to him?" The nurse's best response is

   1 "It sounds as though you need to speak to the psychiatrist."
   2 "Your son has decided to have this treatment. You should be supportive of him."
   3 "Perhaps you'd like to see the ECT room and speak to the staff."
   4 "It sounds as though you have some concerns about the ECT procedure. Why don't we sit down together and discuss any concerns you may have."

15. The nurse is caring for a client who has been treated with long-term antipsychotic medication. As part of the nursing care plan, the nurse monitors for tardive dyskinesia (TD). In the event that TD occurs, the nurse most likely observes
   1 Abnormal movements and involuntary movements of the mouth, tongue, and face
   2 Abnormal breathing through the nostrils accompanied by a "trill"
   3 Severe headache, flushing, tremor, and ataxia
   4 Severe hypertension, migraine headache, and "marbles in the mouth" syndrome

16. The client who is diagnosed with pedophilia and was recently paroled as a sex offender, says, "I'm in treatment and I have served my time; now this group has posters of me all over the neighborhood telling about me with my picture on it." Which of the following is the most appropriate response by the nurse?
   1 "You understand that people fear for their children but you're feeling unfairly treated?"
   2 "When children are hurt as you hurt them, people want you isolated."
   3 "You seem angry but you have committed serious crimes against several children, so your neighbors are frightened."
   4 "You're lucky it doesn't escalate into something pretty scary after your crime."

17. The nurse is discharging a client with a history of command hallucinations to harm self or others. The nurse instructs the client about interventions for hallucinations and anxiety. The nurse knows the client understands this teaching when the client says
   1 "My medications won't make me anxious."
   2 "I can call my therapist when I'm hallucinating so that I can talk about my feelings and plans and not hurt anyone."
   3 "I'll go to a support group and talk so that I don't hurt anyone."
   4 "I won't get anxious or hear things if I get enough sleep and eat well."

18. The nurse observes that a client is psychotic, pacing, agitated, and presenting aggressive gestures. The client's speech pattern is rapid and affect is belligerent. Based on these observations, the nurse's immediate priority of care is to

1 Provide safety for the client and other clients on the unit

2 Offer the client a less stimulated area to calm down and gain control

3 Provide the clients on the unit with a sense of comfort and safety

4 Assist staff in caring for the client in a controlled environment

19. The nurse is caring for a male client diagnosed with catatonic stupor. The client is lying on the bed with the body pulled into a fetal position. The most appropriate nursing intervention is which of the following?

1 Leave the client alone and intermittently check on him

2 Take the client into the dayroom with other clients so they can help watch him

3 Sit beside him in silence with occasional open-ended questions

4 Ask direct questions to encourage talking

20. The mother of a teenage client with an anxiety disorder is concerned about her daughter's progress upon discharge. She states that her daughter "stashes food, eats all the wrong things that make her hyperactive," and "hangs out with the wrong crowd." In helping the mother prepare for her daughter's discharge, the nurse instructs her to

1 Restrict the daughter's socializing time with her friends

2 Consider taking time from work to help her daughter readjust to the home environment

3 Restrict the amount of chocolate and caffeine products in the home

4 Keep her daughter out of school until she can adjust to the school environment

21. A client is admitted with a diagnosis of depression. The nurse develops a plan of care for the client. Which of the following activities is most appropriate to include in the plan of care?

1 Provide an activity that is quiet and solitary in nature to avoid increased fatigue, such as working on a puzzle or reading a book

2 Plan nothing until the client asks to participate in milieu

3 Offer the client a menu of daily activities and insist the client participate in all of them

4 Provide a structured daily program of activities and encourage the client to participate

22. The client is unwilling to go out of the house for fear of "doing something crazy in public." Because of this fear, the client remains homebound except when accompanied outside by the spouse. The nurse analyzes this information and determines that the diagnosis is

1 Social phobia

2 Agoraphobia

3 Claustrophobia

4 Hypochondria

23. The client reports that crying spells have been a major problem over the past several weeks, and that the doctor said that depression is probably the reason. The nurse observes that the client is sitting slumped in the chair and the clothes that the client is wearing are not fitting well. The nurse interprets that further data collection should focus on

1 Sleep patterns

2 Onset of the crying spells

3 Weight loss

4 Medication compliance

24. The client with the diagnosis of major depression becomes more anxious on the unit, reports sleeping poorly, and seems to be more irritable with staff and family. The nurse interprets the client's behavior as

1 This client is at increased risk for suicide

2 This is a normal response to hospitalization

3 The client is dealing with pertinent issues

4 The client may need some time off the unit

25. Which of the following data does the nurse determine as indicating that the client is experiencing a major depressive episode?

1 The client is a male

2 The client states, "Since my wife died last week, I've been waking up hours before I should and I'm tired all day."

3 The client uses marijuana.

4 The client states, "The last 4 weeks I'm doing all the things I used to do but I'm not enjoying them."

26. A client was admitted to a medical unit with acute blindness. Many tests are performed and there seems to be no organic reason why this client cannot see. The nurse later learns that the client became blind after witnessing a hit-and-run car accident, when a family of three was killed. The nurse suspects that the client may be experiencing a

1 Psychosis

2 Conversion disorder

3 Dissociative disorder

4 Repression

27. The manic male client announces to everyone in the dayroom that a stripper is coming to perform this evening. When the psychiatric aide firmly states that this will not happen, the manic client becomes verbally abusive and threatens physical violence to the aide. Based on the analysis of this situation, the nurse determines that the most appropriate next action is to

1 With assistance, escort the manic client to his room and administer haloperidol (Haldol) PRN

2 Tell the client that smoking privileges are revoked for 24 hours

3 Orient the client to time, person, and place
4 tell the client that the behavior is not appropriate

28. The nurse is preparing a client for electroconvulsive therapy (ECT), which is scheduled for the following morning. Which of the following is not a component of the plan of care?
   1 Withhold food and fluids for 4 hours prior to the treatment
   2 Have the client void before the procedure
   3 Remove dentures and contact lenses prior to the procedure
   4 Administer tapwater enemas on the evening before the procedure

29. The nurse is caring for a client with a diagnosis of agoraphobia. Which of the following behaviors does the nurse expect the client to describe when communicating with the client about the disorder?
   1 A need to wash hands several times before eating a meal
   2 A fear of leaving the house
   3 A fear of speaking in public
   4 A fear of riding in elevators

30. An agoraphobic client has been diagnosed with major depression. The nurse notes that the client is not eating adequately and at times refuses to eat. To meet the client's nutritional needs, the nurse plans to
   1 Force foods and fluids
   2 Provide small, frequent meals
   3 Provide snacks and meals as requested
   4 Tell the client that social activities will be restricted unless food is consumed

ANSWERS

1. **2**

RATIONALE: Solitary activities that require a short attention span with mild physical exertion are the most appropriate activities initially with a client who is exhibiting aggressive behavior. Writing (journaling), walks with staff, and finger painting are activities that minimize stimuli and provide a constructive release for tension. Competitive games should be avoided because they can stimulate aggression and increase psychomotor activity.
TEST-TAKING STRATEGY: Knowledge of nursing interventions to meet the needs of the manic (aggressive) client is required to answer this question. Options 1, 3, and 4 are similar in that they are activities that the client cannot do alone. Option 2 is an activity that the client can do alone. It is the option that is different.
LEVEL OF COGNITIVE ABILITY: Application
PHASE OF NURSING PROCESS: Planning
CLIENT NEEDS: Psychosocial Integrity
CONTENT AREA: Mental Health
REFERENCE
Varcarolis, E. (1998). *Foundations of psychiatric-mental health nursing* (3rd ed.). Philadelphia: W. B. Saunders, p. 606.

2. **4**

RATIONALE: Change in appetite is one of the major symptoms of depression, coupled with depressed mood, increased fatigue, feelings of worthlessness, diminished ability to think or indecisiveness, and psychomotor agitation or retardation. Offering the client several small, frequent meals and the nurse's presence at that time to support, encourage, or perhaps even feed the client is an effective application of knowledge regarding the disease process and how it may affect the client.
TEST-TAKING STRATEGY: Option 4 is the only option that addresses the altered nutrition concretely and designs methods in which the client will feasibly increase the nutritional intake. Eliminate option 1 because the client is experiencing poor concentration; hence, even if the client does understand the rationale, the client still may not be able to complete tasks. Weighing the client does not address how to increase nutritional intake. Reporting to the psychiatrist and the nutritionist is to some degree correct, but lacks the method as to how one might increase food intake.
LEVEL OF COGNITIVE ABILITY: Application
PHASE OF NURSING PROCESS: Implementation
CLIENT NEEDS: Physiological Integrity
CONTENT AREA: Mental Health
REFERENCE
Varcarolis, E. (1998). *Foundations of psychiatric mental health nursing* (3rd ed.). Philadelphia: W. B. Saunders. p. 566.

3. **4**

RATIONALE: A depressed person often suffers with depressed mood and is often withdrawn. Also, the person experiences difficulty concentrating, loss of interest or pleasure, low energy, fatigue, and feelings of worthlessness and poor self-esteem. The plan of care needs to provide successful experiences in a stimulating yet structured environment.
TEST-TAKING STRATEGY: The depressed client requires a structured/stimulating program. Options 1 and 2 are too "restrictive" and offer little or no structure and stimulation. Option 3 is eliminated because the word "all" is in the selection. Option 4 is the only reasonable selection.
LEVEL OF COGNITIVE ABILITY: Application
PHASE OF NURSING PROCESS: Planning
CLIENT NEEDS: Psychosocial Integrity
CONTENT AREA: Mental Health
REFERENCE
Varcarolis, E. (1998). *Foundations of psychiatric mental health nursing* (3rd ed.). Philadelphia: W. B. Saunders. p. 566.

4. **4**

RATIONALE: Feelings of low self-esteem and worthlessness are common symptoms of the depressed client. An effective plan of care is to provide successful experiences for the client that are challenging but will not be met with failure to enhance the client's personal self-esteem. Reminders of the client's past accomplishments or personal successes are ways to interrupt clients' negative self-talk and distorted cognitive view of themselves.

TEST-TAKING STRATEGY: Communication blocks are evident in options 1 and 3 as the nurse gives advice or devalues the client's feelings. Option 2, silence, may be interpreted as agreement. Option 4 provides the client with information based upon fact and testing automatic negative thoughts.
LEVEL OF COGNITIVE ABILITY: Application
PHASE OF NURSING PROCESS: Implementation
CLIENT NEEDS: Psychosocial Integrity
CONTENT AREA: Mental Health
REFERENCE
Varcarolis, E. (1998). *Foundations of psychiatric mental health nursing* (3rd ed.). Philadelphia: W. B. Saunders. p. 566.

5. **2**

RATIONALE: The exact cause of depression is not known but it is believed to be related to a biochemical disruption of neurotransmitters in the brain. Diet, exercise, and medication are recognized treatment of the disease process.
TEST-TAKING STRATEGY: Option 2 is the only answer that incorporates a holistic treatment approach: good nutrition, exercise, and medication as well as the client's knowledge of the signs of possible relapse. Options 1, 3, and 4 offer no insight into the disease process. In addition, option 1 reflects possible blaming or personal failure; option 3, an unwillingness to reach out to others.
LEVEL OF COGNITIVE ABILITY: Comprehension
PHASE OF NURSING PROCESS: Evaluation
CLIENT NEEDS: Psychosocial Integrity
CONTENT AREA: Mental Health
REFERENCE
Varcarolis, E. (1998). *Foundations of psychiatric-mental health nursing* (3rd ed.). Philadelphia: W. B. Saunders. pp. 563–566.

6. **3**

RATIONALE: Mania is a mood characterized by excitement, euphoria, hyperactivity, excessive energy, decreased need for sleep, and impaired ability to concentrate or complete a single train of thought. It is a period when the mood is predominantly elevated, expansive, or irritable. All selections reflect a client's possible symptomatology. Option 3, however, clearly presents a nursing problem, which compromises one's physiological integrity and needs to be addressed immediately (Maslow's hierarchy of needs).
TEST-TAKING STRATEGY: All four options reflect symptomatology related to a manic state. The stem of the question asks for an immediate intervention. Option 3 indicates a potential disruption in the client's physiological status. Use Maslow's hierachy of needs theory to assist in answering the question.
LEVEL OF COGNITIVE ABILITY: Comprehension
PHASE OF NURSING PROCESS: Data Collection
CLIENT NEEDS: Psychosocial Integrity
CONTENT AREA: Mental Health
REFERENCE
Varcarolis, E. (1998). *Foundations of psychiatric mental health nursing* (3rd ed.). Philadelphia: W. B. Saunders. p. 602.

7. **1**

RATIONALE: A person who is experiencing mania lacks insight and judgment, has poor impulse control, and is highly excitable. The nurse must take control without creating increased stress or anxiety to the client. A quiet, firm approach while distracting the client (walking her to her room and assisting her to get dressed) achieves the goal of having her dressed appropriately and preserving her psychosocial integrity.
TEST-TAKING STRATEGY: The goal of the interaction is to have the client dress appropriately. Option 4 is immediately eliminated. Although options 1, 2, and 3 are all similar, "insisting" the client go to her room may meet with a great deal of resistance; confronting the client and offering her a consequence of time-out may be meaningless to her.
LEVEL OF COGNITIVE ABILITY: Application
PHASE OF NURSING PROCESS: Implementation
CLIENT NEEDS: Psychosocial Integrity
CONTENT AREA: Mental Health
REFERENCE
Varcarolis, E. (1998). *Foundations of psychiatric mental health nursing* (3rd ed.). Philadelphia: W. B. Saunders. p. 606.

8. **2**

RATIONALE: A person who is experiencing mania is overactive, full of energy, lacks concentration, and has poor impulse control. The client needs an activity that will allow him or her to use excess energy, yet not endanger others during the process.
TEST-TAKING STRATEGY: Options 1, 3, and 4 are relatively sedate activities that require concentration, a quality lacking in the manic state. Such activities may lead to increased frustration and anxiety for the client. Tetherball is an exercise that uses the large muscle groups of the body and is a great way to expend the increased energy this client is experiencing. Review the appropriate interventions for a manic client now if you had difficulty with this question.
LEVEL OF COGNITIVE ABILITY: Application
PHASE OF NURSING PROCESS: Planning
CLIENT NEEDS: Psychosocial Integrity
CONTENT AREA: Mental Health
REFERENCE
Varcarolis, E. (1998). *Foundations of psychiatric mental health nursing* (3rd ed.). Philadelphia: W. B. Saunders. p. 606.

9. **3**

RATIONALE: Disagreeing with delusions may make the client more defensive and the client may cling to the delusions even more. It is most therapeutic for the nurse to empathize with the client's experience.
TEST-TAKING STRATEGY: Use therapeutic communication techniques with the client experiencing delusions. Eliminate options 1 and 2 because they are similar and are statements that disagree with the client. Option 4 is encouraging discussion regarding the delusion. Review communication techniques with the client experiencing delusions now if you had difficulty with this question.
LEVEL OF COGNITIVE ABILITY: Application
PHASE OF NURSING PROCESS: Implementation
CLIENT NEEDS: Psychosocial Integrity
CONTENT AREA: Mental Health
REFERENCE
Varcarolis, E. (1998). *Foundations of psychiatric mental health nursing* (3rd ed.). Philadelphia: W. B. Saunders. pp. 191, 640.

10. **1**

RATIONALE: If a client is left alone with severe anxiety, he or she may feel abandoned and become overwhelmed. Placing the client in a quiet room is also indicated but the nurse must stay with the client. It is not possible to teach clients deep breathing or relaxation until anxiety decreases.

Encouraging the client to discuss concerns and feelings would not take place until the anxiety has decreased. **TEST-TAKING STRATEGY:** Note the key words "most important" and "severe." This question requires you to prioritize. Eliminate options 3 and 4 first, knowing that these actions are not possible when the client is in a severe state of anxiety. From the remaining options, the best action is to remain with the client.
LEVEL OF COGNITIVE ABILITY: Application
PHASE OF NURSING PROCESS: Implementation
CLIENT NEEDS: Psychosocial Integrity
CONTENT AREA: Mental Health
REFERENCE
Varcarolis, E. (1998). *Foundations of psychiatric mental health nursing* (3rd ed.). Philadelphia: W. B. Saunders. p. 349.

11. **1**

RATIONALE: It is important to provide a consistent daily routine and a low stimulating environment when the client is disorientated. Noise levels including radio and television may add to the confusion and disorientation. Moving the client next to the nurses' station is not the initial action.
TEST-TAKING STRATEGY: Note the key word "initial" in the stem of the question. Eliminate options 2 and 4 first because they are similar. Focusing on the key word will easily direct you to option 1. Review measures related to the client with delirium now if you had difficulty with this question.
LEVEL OF COGNITIVE ABILITY: Application
PHASE OF NURSING PROCESS: Implementation
CLIENT NEEDS: Psychosocial Integrity
CONTENT AREA: Mental Health
REFERENCE
Haber, J., Krainovich-Miller, B., McMahon, A., & Price-Hoskins, P. (1997). *Comprehensive psychiatric nursing* (5th ed.). St. Louis, MO: Mosby–Year Book. p. 676.

12. **3**

RATIONALE: It is important for the nurse to let the client know that what the client is saying is not understood by the nurse. It is not appropriate to reinforce the client's altered reality. Allow the client to express concerns but reinforce the reality, not the delusions. The nurse will want to avoid confronting the client but will want to say such supportive things as, "This must be very frightening to you" or "It's difficult to understand all that you are experiencing right now."
TEST-TAKING STRATEGY: Read each option carefully and note that options 1, 2, and 4 all indicate reinforcement to the client that the voices are real. Option 3 is the only statement that indicates reality. Review nursing interventions related to the client who is hallucinating now if you had difficulty with this question.
LEVEL OF COGNITIVE ABILITY: Application
PHASE OF NURSING PROCESS: Implementation
CLIENT NEEDS: Psychosocial Integrity
CONTENT AREA: Mental Health
REFERENCE
Glod, C. A. (1998). *Contemporary psychiatric-mental health nursing.* Philadelphia: F. A. Davis. pp. 324–328.

13. **4**

RATIONALE: Constipation can be related to inadequate food intake, lack of exercise, and poor diet; however, it would not account for urinary retention. Side effects of medications is the only choice that can satisfy both complaints of constipation and urinary retention.
TEST-TAKING STRATEGY: Options 1, 2, and 3 are all similar and address diet. Option 4 relates to both constipation and urinary retention. If you had difficulty with this question, take time now to review interventions for a client with depression and the effects of medications prescribed for this disorder.
LEVEL OF COGNITIVE ABILITY: Comprehension
PHASE OF NURSING PROCESS: Data Collection
CLIENT NEEDS: Physiological Integrity
CONTENT AREA: Mental Health
REFERENCE
Varcarolis, E. (1998). *Foundations of psychiatric mental health nursing* (3rd ed.). Philadelphia: W. B. Saunders. p. 567.

14. **4**

RATIONALE: Basic therapeutic communication techniques are addressed in this question. Therapeutic communication fosters an active collaborative process that facilitates problem solving, change, learning, and growth.
TEST-TAKING STRATEGY: Basic understanding of therapeutic communication is being tested. Options 1, 2, and 3 avoid dealing with the client/family concerns. Furthermore, option 2 sounds punitive toward the family. In option 4 the nurse encourages the family and client to verbalize fears and concerns. Once the nurse has heard these, the nurse can then help to allay these fears and impart information.
LEVEL OF COGNITIVE ABILITY: Application
PHASE OF NURSING PROCESS: Implementation
CLIENT NEEDS: Psychosocial Integrity
CONTENT AREA: Mental Health
REFERENCE
Varcarolis, E. (1998). *Foundations of psychiatric mental health nursing* (3rd ed.). Philadelphia: W. B. Saunders. p. 579.

15. **1**

RATIONALE: Tardive dyskinesia (TD) is a severe reaction associated with long-term use of antipsychotic medication. The clinical manifestations of TD are abnormal movements (dyskinesia) and involuntary movements of the mouth, tongue ("fly catcher" tongue), and face. In its more severe form, TD involves fingers, arms, trunk, and respiratory muscles. When this occurs, the medication is discontinued.
TEST-TAKING STRATEGY: Knowledge regarding the clinical manifestations of TD is required to answer this question. Options 2, 3, and 4 do not identify the characteristics of TD. If you had difficulty with this question, take time now to review the characteristics associated with TD.
LEVEL OF COGNITIVE ABILITY: Comprehension
PHASE OF NURSING PROCESS: Data Collection
CLIENT NEEDS: Physiological Integrity
CONTENT AREA: Mental Health
REFERENCE
Glod, C. A. (1998). *Contemporary psychiatric-mental health nursing.* Philadelphia: F. A. Davis. pp. 116–120.

16. **1**

RATIONALE: The use of the therapeutic communication techniques of focusing and verbalizing the implied is the most therapeutic communication because it assists the client to clarify thinking and to look at what the client is really saying. Option 1 is the only option that reflects the use of therapeutic communication techniques.
TEST-TAKING STRATEGY: Use therapeutic communication techniques to answer the question. Eliminate option 2

first. This option is straightforward but somewhat insensitive and anxiety provoking. Eliminate option 3 because it is not therapeutic. It does not help the client express feelings. Option 4 is incorrect because it is threatening and does not help the client express feelings.
LEVEL OF COGNITIVE ABILITY: Application
PHASE OF NURSING PROCESS: Implementation
CLIENT NEEDS: Psychosocial Integrity
CONTENT AREA: Mental Health
REFERENCE
Glod, C. A. (1998). *Contemporary psychiatric-mental health nursing.* Philadelphia: F. A. Davis. pp. 58–60; 445–459.

17. 2

RATIONALE: There may be an increased risk for impulsive and/or aggressive behavior if a client is receiving command hallucinations to harm (self) or others. Clients should be asked if they have intentions to hurt themselves or others. Talking about auditory hallucinations can interfere with subvocal muscular activity associated with a hallucination.
TEST-TAKING STRATEGY: Use the process of elimination. Options 1, 3, and 4 are all interventions that a client can do to aid wellness. Option 2 is a specific agreement to seek help and evidences self-responsible commitment and control over own behavior.
LEVEL OF COGNITIVE ABILITY: Comprehension
PHASE OF NURSING PROCESS: Evaluation
CLIENT NEEDS: Psychosocial Integrity
CONTENT AREA: Mental Health
REFERENCE
Haber, J., Krainovich-Miller, B., McMahon, A., & Price-Hoskins, P. (1997). *Comprehensive psychiatric nursing* (5th ed.). St. Louis: Mosby–Year Book. pp. 580, 592–593.

18. 1

RATIONALE: Safety to the client and other clients is the priority. Option 1 is the only response that addresses the client and other clients' safety needs. Option 2 addresses the client's needs. Option 3 addresses other clients' needs. Option 4 is not client centered.
TEST-TAKING STRATEGY: Use Maslow's hierarchy of needs theory to prioritize. Note the words "belligerent," "agitated," and "aggressive." Safety is the key issue. Option 1 is the global response and addresses the safety of all.
LEVEL OF COGNITIVE ABILITY: Application
PHASE OF NURSING PROCESS: Implementation
CLIENT NEEDS: Safe, Effective Care Environment
CONTENT AREA: Mental Health
REFERENCE
Carson, V., & Arnold, E. (1996). *Mental health nursing: The nurse-patient journey.* Philadelphia: W. B. Saunders. p. 348.

19. 3

RATIONALE: Clients who are withdrawn may be immobile and mute, and require consistent, repeated approaches. Intervention includes establishment of interpersonal contact. Communication with withdrawn clients requires much patience from the nurse. The nurse facilitates communication with the client by sitting in silence, asking open-ended questions, and pausing to provide opportunities for the client to respond.
TEST-TAKING STRATEGY: Eliminate option 1 because you would not leave the client alone. Option 2 relies on other clients to care for this client and this is an inappropriate expectation. Asking direct questions to this client is not

therapeutic. Option 3 is the best action because it provides for client supervision and communication as appropriate.
LEVEL OF COGNITIVE ABILITY: Application
PHASE OF NURSING PROCESS: Implementation
CLIENT NEEDS: Psychosocial Integrity
CONTENT AREA: Mental Health
REFERENCE
Haber, J., Krainovich-Miller, B., McMahon, A., & Price-Hoskins, P. (1997). *Comprehensive psychiatric nursing* (5th ed.). St. Louis: Mosby–Year Book. pp. 582, 593.

20. 3

RATIONALE: It is strongly recommended that clients with anxiety disorder abstain from or limit their intake of caffeine, chocolate, and alcohol. These products have the potential of increasing anxiety. Options 1 and 4 are unreasonable and are an unhealthy approach. It may not be realistic for a family member to take time from work.
TEST-TAKING STRATEGY: Eliminate similar distractors. Options 1, 2, and 4 are concerned with monitoring or curtailing the client's physical activities, whereas option 3 addresses preparation of the environment. Option 3 also focuses on the concern or issue expressed in the question.
LEVEL OF COGNITIVE ABILITY: Application
PHASE OF NURSING PROCESS: Implementation
CLIENT NEEDS: Health Promotion and Maintenance
CONTENT AREA: Mental Health
REFERENCE
Varcarolis, E. (1998). *Foundations of psychiatric mental health nursing* (3rd ed.). Philadelphia: W. B. Saunders. p. 471.

21. 4

RATIONALE: A depressed person often suffers with depressed mood and is withdrawn. Also, the person experiences difficulty concentrating, loss of interest or pleasure, low energy, fatigue, and feelings of worthlessness and poor self-esteem. The plan of care needs to provide successful experiences in a stimulating yet structured environment.
TEST-TAKING STRATEGY: The depressed client requires a structured and stimulating program. Options 1 and 2 are too "restrictive" and offer little or no structure and stimulation. Option 3 is eliminated because of the word "all" in the option. Option 4 is the only reasonable option that will provide a safe and effective environment.
LEVEL OF COGNITIVE ABILITY: Application
PHASE OF NURSING PROCESS: Implementation
CLIENT NEEDS: Psychosocial Integrity
CONTENT AREA: Mental Health
REFERENCE
Varcarolis, E. (1998). *Foundations of psychiatric mental health nursing* (3rd ed.). Philadelphia: W. B. Saunders. p. 566.

22. 2

RATIONALE: Agoraphobia is a fear of open spaces and the fear of being trapped in a situation from which there may not be an escape. Agoraphobia includes the possibility of experiencing a sense of helplessness or embarrassment if an attack occurs. Avoidance of such situations usually results in reduction of social and professional interactions. Social phobia focuses more on specific situations such as the fear of speaking, performing, or eating in public. Claustrophobia is a fear of closed-in places. Clients with hypochondriacal symptoms focus their anxiety on physical complaints and are preoccupied with their health.
TEST-TAKING STRATEGY: Knowledge regarding the specific types of phobias and associated client behaviors is

required to answer this question. If you had difficulty with this question, take time now to review phobia types and associated client behaviors.

LEVEL OF COGNITIVE ABILITY: Comprehension
PHASE OF NURSING PROCESS: Data Collection
CLIENT NEEDS: Psychosocial Integrity
CONTENT AREA: Mental Health
REFERENCE
O'Toole, M. (1997). *Miller-Keane encyclopedia & dictionary of medicine, nursing, & allied health* (6th ed.). Philadelphia: W. B. Saunders. p. 1242.

23. **3**

RATIONALE: All of the options are possible issues to address; however, the weight loss is the first item that needs assessment since an obvious ill fit of clothing could signify a substantial problem with physiological integrity. The client has told the nurse that the crying spells have been a problem, and medication has not been mentioned in the information given. Sleep is affected by depression and should be addressed; however, weight loss is the most important with the data given.

TEST-TAKING STRATEGY: Use the process of elimination and Maslow's hierarchy of needs to answer the question. Since all of the information is important to assess at some point, the nurse must decide which has priority with the given situation. Significant weight loss is the most serious physiological concern.

LEVEL OF COGNITIVE ABILITY: Comprehension
PHASE OF NURSING PROCESS: Data Collection
CLIENT NEEDS: Physiological Integrity
CONTENT AREA: Mental Health
REFERENCE
Johnson, B. S. (1997). *Psychiatric mental health nursing: Adaptation and Growth* (4th ed.). Philadelphia: Lippincott-Raven. pp. 545–546.

24. **1**

RATIONALE: The behaviors mentioned may be manifested by the client who is contemplating suicide. Many of these symptoms are symptoms of the depressed client; however, with this client these behaviors have increased. Hospitalization may actually lessen these symptoms in the depressed client since a feeling of hope or relief may occur once treatment begins. Facing issues may be traumatic, but this is not the best answer for the question. Time off the unit for this client could put the client at risk for injury. Only when anxiety and irritability can be controlled could the client safely leave the unit.

TEST-TAKING STRATEGY: Identify the client behaviors addressed in the question. Use the process of elimination as well as Maslow's hierarchy of needs to assist in answering the question. Of the options presented, option 1 is the priority. If you had difficulty with this question, take time now to review the characteristics and client behaviors related to suicide.

LEVEL OF COGNITIVE ABILITY: Comprehension
PHASE OF NURSING PROCESS: Data Collection
CLIENT NEEDS: Psychosocial Integrity
CONTENT AREA: Mental Health
REFERENCE
Carson, V., & Arnold, E. (1996). *Mental health nursing: The nurse-patient journey.* Philadelphia: W. B. Saunders. pp. 932–936.

25. **4**

RATIONALE: Major depression occurs twice as frequently in females as in males. Reacting to loss by experiencing altered sleep for 1 week is a normal grief response whereas early morning awakening that extends over 2 weeks along with other symptomatology constitutes major depression. Although depression is often associated with substance abuse, in and of itself it does not constitute a major depression. Option 4 is the correct answer because it describes anhedonia (loss of pleasure in activities previously or usually enjoyed) that has extended over 3 weeks, a cardinal criterion for major depression according to *DSM-IV.*

TEST-TAKING STRATEGY: Knowledge of the epidemiology of and criteria for major depression will assist you to analyze the options accurately. Use the process of elimination in selecting the correct option. If you were unfamiliar with the content, you might be able to determine the correct option by considering the time frame noted in the option, which is one of the factors to be considered in the criteria for major depression according to *DSM-IV.* Take time now to review the assessment data related to depression if you had difficulty with this question.

LEVEL OF COGNITIVE ABILITY: Comprehension
PHASE OF NURSING PROCESS: Data Collection
CLIENT NEEDS: Psychosocial Integrity
CONTENT AREA: Mental Health
REFERENCE
Varcarolis, E. (1998). *Foundations of psychiatric mental health nursing* (3rd ed.). Philadelphia: W. B. Saunders. p. 566.

26. **2**

RATIONALE: A conversion disorder is the alteration or loss of a physical function that cannot be explained by any known pathophysiological mechanism. It is thought to be an expression of a psychological need or conflict. In this scenario, the client witnessed an accident that was so psychologically painful, the client became blind. A dissociative disorder is a disturbance or alteration in the normally integrative functions of identity, memory, or consciousness. Psychosis is a state in which a person's mental capacity to recognize reality, communicate, and relate to others is impaired, thus interfering with the person's capacity to deal with life demands. Repression is a coping mechanism in which unacceptable feelings are kept out of awareness.

TEST-TAKING STRATEGY: Knowledge regarding defense mechanisms is required to answer the question. The key to the answer lies in the fact that the client evidences no organic reason to account for the blindness, hence a conversion disorder. If you had difficulty with this question, take time now to review this disorder.

LEVEL OF COGNITIVE ABILITY: Comprehension
PHASE OF NURSING PROCESS: Data Collection
CLIENT NEEDS: Psychosocial Integrity
CONTENT AREA: Mental Health
REFERENCE
Carson, V., & Arnold, E. (1996). *Mental health nursing: The nurse-patient journey.* Philadelphia: W. B. Saunders. pp. 697, 963–964.

27. **1**

RATIONALE: The client is at risk for injury to self and others and therefore should be escorted out of the dayroom. Hyperactive and agitated behavior usually responds to haloperidol. Antipsychotic medications are useful to manage the manic client; lithium takes 1 to 3 weeks to become effective. Option 2 may increase the agitation that already exists in this client. Orientation will not halt the behavior. Telling the client that the behavior is not appropriate has already been attempted by the aide.

TEST-TAKING STRATEGY: Use Maslow's hierarchy of needs and the process of elimination to answer the question. Look for the response that promotes safety of the client, other clients, and staff. Knowledge of psychopharmacology is helpful to answer this question correctly. If you had difficulty with this question, take time now to review the appropriate interventions in dealing with a manic client.
LEVEL OF COGNITIVE ABILITY: Application
PHASE OF NURSING PROCESS: Implementation
CLIENT NEEDS: Psychosocial Integrity
CONTENT AREA: Mental Health
REFERENCE
Wilson, H. S., & Kneisl, C. R. (1996). *Psychiatric nursing.* (5th ed.). Reading, MA: Addison-Wesley. pp. 347, 349.

28. **4**

RATIONALE: Enemas are not a component of the pretreatment care for a client scheduled for ECT. Options 1, 2, and 3 are a part of the pretreatment plan. Additionally, an informed consent is required and the nurse should teach the client and family what to expect with ECT and allow the client to discuss feelings regarding the procedure.
TEST-TAKING STRATEGY: Knowledge regarding the pretreatment care for the client scheduled for ECT is required to answer this question. If you had difficulty with this question, take time now to review this procedure.
LEVEL OF COGNITIVE ABILITY: Application
PHASE OF NURSING PROCESS: Planning
CLIENT NEEDS: Physiological Integrity
CONTENT AREA: Mental Health
REFERENCE
Varcarolis, E. (1998). *Foundations of psychiatric mental health nursing* (3rd ed.). Philadelphia: W. B. Saunders. p. 579.

29. **2**

RATIONALE: Agoraphobia is a fear of leaving the house and experiencing panic attacks when doing so. Option 1 describes an obsessive-compulsive behavior. Option 3 describes a social phobia. Option 4 describes claustrophobia.

TEST-TAKING STRATEGY: Knowledge regarding the various types of phobias is necessary to answer this question. Focus on the key word "agoraphobia." This focus will assist in directing you to option 2. If you had difficulty with this question, take time now to review the various types of phobias.
LEVEL OF COGNITIVE ABILITY: Comprehension
PHASE OF NURSING PROCESS: Data Collection
CLIENT NEEDS: Psychosocial Integrity
CONTENT AREA: Mental Health
REFERENCE
Carson, V., & Arnold, E. (1996). *Mental health nursing: The nurse-patient journey.* Philadelphia: W. B. Saunders. p. 706.

30. **2**

RATIONALE: A depressed client may eat small amounts of food rather than large amounts that may be overwhelming to them. If clients becomes overwhelmed, they may respond by withdrawing further. Providing snacks and meals when the client requests them will not ensure adequate nutritional intake. Forcing foods and fluids and telling the client that social activities will be restricted will cause further withdrawal in the client. Option 4 is also a demeaning action.
TEST-TAKING STRATEGY: Focus on the issue of the question, meeting the client's nutritional needs. Eliminate option 4 first as the most inappropriate action. Forcing foods and fluids will cause further client withdrawal. Eliminate option 3 next because this action will not ensure nutritional intake. Take time now to review nursing interventions that will meet the nutritional needs of a client with depression if you had difficulty with this question.
LEVEL OF COGNITIVE ABILITY: Application
PHASE OF NURSING PROCESS: Planning
CLIENT NEEDS: Psychosocial Integrity
CONTENT AREA: Mental Health
REFERENCE
Varcarolis, E. (1998). *Foundations of psychiatric mental health nursing* (3rd ed.). Philadelphia: W. B. Saunders. p. 563.

BIBLIOGRAPHY

Carson, V., & Arnold, E. (1996). *Mental health nursing: The nurse-patient journey.* Philadelphia: W. B. Saunders.

Fortinash, K., & Holoday-Worret, P. (1996). *Psychiatric-mental health nursing.* St. Louis: Mosby–Year Book.

Glod, Carol A. (1998). *Contemporary psychiatric-mental health nursing.* Philadelphia: F. A. Davis.

Haber, J., Krainovich-Miller, B. McMahon, A., & Price-Hoskins, P. (1997). *Comprehensive psychiatric nursing* (5th ed.). St. Louis: Mosby–Year Book.

Johnson, B. S. (1997). *Psychiatric mental health nursing: Adaptation and Growth* (4th ed.). Philadelphia: Lippincott-Raven.

Luckmann, J. (1997). *Saunders manual of nursing care.* Philadelphia: W. B. Saunders.

O'Toole, M. (1997). *Miller-Keane encyclopedia & dictionary of medicine, nursing, & allied health* (6th ed.). Philadelphia: W. B. Saunders.

Stuart, G. W. & Laraia, M. T. (1998). *Principles and practice of psychiatric nursing* (6th ed.). St. Louis: Mosby–Year Book.

Varcarolis, E. (1998). *Foundations of psychiatric mental health nursing* (3rd ed.). Philadelphia: W. B. Saunders.

Wilson, H. S., & Kneisl, C. R. (1996). *Psychiatric nursing* (5th ed.). Reading, MA: Addison-Wesley.

CHAPTER 62

Addictions

. . . .

I. Eating Disorders

A. Description: characterized by uncertain self-identification and grossly disturbed eating habits

B. Compulsive overeating
1. Binge-like overeating without purging
2. Food consumption is out of the individual's control and occurs in a stereotyped fashion
3. Client may be repulsed by eating, and the eating relieves tension but does not produce pleasure
4. Is aware that eating patterns are abnormal and feels depressed after eating
5. Eats secretly during a binge and consumes high-calorie, easily digestible food
6. Repeatedly tries to diet but without success
7. Lacks interest in exercise programs and feels helpless and hopeless about weight
8. When experiencing guilt, anger, depression, boredom, loneliness, inadequacy, or ambivalence, responds by eating

C. Anorexia nervosa
1. Description
   a. The onset is often associated with a stressful life event
   b. The client has an altered or inappropriate idea of obesity
   c. Body image is distorted, and the client has a disturbed self-concept
   d. Preoccupied with foods that prevent weight gain and has a phobia against foods that produce weight gain
   e. The eating disorder can be life-threatening
   f. Death can occur from starvation, **suicide,** or electrolyte imbalance
2. Data collection
   a. Refusal to eat and appetite denial
   b. Weight loss
   c. Feelings of lack of control
   d. Self-induced vomiting and self-administered enemas
   e. Exercises compulsively
   f. Overachiever and perfectionist
   g. Decreased temperature, pulse, and blood pressure
   h. Gastrointestinal (GI) disturbances such as constipation
   i. Scaly, dry skin
   j. Sleep disturbances
   k. Electrolyte imbalances
   l. Hormone deficiencies
   m. Amenorrhea for at least three consecutive menstrual periods
   n. Teeth and gum deterioration
   o. Cyanosis and numbness of extremities
   p. Esophageal varices from vomiting
   q. Bone degeneration

D. Bulimia nervosa
1. Description
   a. The client indulges in eating binges followed by purging behaviors
   b. Most clients remain within a normal weight range but feel that their lives are dominated by the eating-related conflict
2. Data collection
   a. Consumes high-calorie, easily digested food in secret
   b. Binge-purge syndrome
   c. Attempts to lose weight through diets, vomiting, enemas, cathartics, and amphetamines or diuretics
   d. Preoccupied with body shape and weight
   e. Guilt about secretive eating
   f. Mood swings
   g. Low self-esteem
   h. Needs to control yet experiences feelings of powerlessness or loss of control
   i. Poor interpersonal relationships
   j. Overuse of laxatives and diuretics
   k. Loss of tooth enamel and dental decay
   l. Stomach ulcers and electrolyte imbalances
   m. Esophageal varices from vomiting
   n. Rectal bleeding
   o. Cardiac disease and hypertension
   p. Self-mutilating behavior
   q. Thoughts and attempts at **suicide**

E. Implementation
1. Identify the client's nutritional status
2. Assist the client in identifying precipitators of the eating disorder

978

3. Encourage the client to state feelings about the eating behavior
4. Be accepting and nonjudgmental, expressing neither approval nor disapproval of the behavior
5. Encourage behavior modification techniques
6. Provide praise and positive reinforcement for accomplishments
7. Supervise the client during mealtimes and for a specified period after meals
8. Provide a pleasant, relaxed environment for eating
9. Monitor for signs of physical complications related to the eating disorder
10. Record intake and output (I&O)
11. Weigh the client daily at the same time, using the same scale, after the client voids; when weighing the client make certain that the client is wearing the same clothing when the previous weight was taken
12. Monitor elimination patterns
13. Monitor and limit the client's activity level
14. Encourage the client to participate in diversional activities
15. Monitor the client's **suicide** potential
16. Administer antidepressant medication as prescribed
17. Encourage psychotherapy as prescribed and refer the client to support groups

II. Substance Abuse Disorders

A. Description: behavioral changes associated with regular substance **abuse** that affects the central nervous system (CNS)
B. Substance dependence (Box 62–1)
1. Pattern of repeated use of a substance, which usually results in tolerance, withdrawal, and compulsive drug-taking behavior
2. The client takes substances in larger amounts and over longer periods of time than was intended
3. The client has the desire to cut down but has unsuccessful efforts to decrease or discontinue use
4. Daily activities revolve around the use of a substance

BOX 62–1. CAGE Screening Test for Substance Abuse

C—Have you ever felt the need to *cut* down on your drinking/drug use?
A—Have you ever been *annoyed* at criticism of your drinking/drug use?
G—Have you ever felt *guilty* about something you have done when you have been drinking or taking drugs?
E—Have you ever had an *eye-opener*, taking drugs first thing in the morning to get going or to avoid withdrawal symptoms?

C. Substance tolerance: The need for increased amounts of the substance to achieve the desired effect
D. Substance **abuse**
1. Client continues to use substance
2. Client experiences recurrent, significant harmful consequences related to the use of substances
3. Client has legal problems related to substance **abuse**
E. Substance withdrawal: occurs when blood levels decrease in an individual with prolonged heavy use of a substance
F. Precipitating factors of substance **abuse**
1. Rebellion and peer group pressure in adolescence
2. Pleasure-seeking experience as the substance decreases the physical and emotional pain
3. Depression
G. Dysfunctional behaviors of clients with substance **abuse**
1. Insensitive to self and others
2. Manipulative
3. Impulsiveness
4. Anger, including physical and verbal **abuse**
5. Avoidance of relationships
6. Sense of self-importance and requiring special treatment
7. Denial; blaming everything but the substance
8. Codependence, modifying self-behaviors and response to others
9. Low self-esteem
10. Depression

III. Alcohol Abuse

A. Description
1. Alcohol is a CNS depressant affecting all body tissues
2. Physical dependence is a biological need for alcohol to avoid physical withdrawal symptoms
3. Psychological dependence is a craving for the subjective effect of alcohol
B. Risk factors
1. Biological predisposition
2. Depressed and highly anxious characteristics
3. Low self-esteem
4. Poor self-control
5. History of rebelliousness, poor school performance, delinquency
6. Poor parental relationships
C. Data collection
1. Slurred speech
2. Uncoordinated movements
3. Unsteady gait
4. Restlessness
5. Belligerence
6. Confusion
7. Sneaking drinks, drinking in the morning, and experiencing blackouts
8. Binge drinking

    9. Arguments about drinking
   10. Missing work
   11. Increased tolerance to alcohol
   12. Intoxication, with blood alcohol levels greater than or equal to 0.1%

D. Physical symptoms
   1. Hepatitis, cirrhosis of the liver
   2. Esophagitis, gastritis, pancreatitis
   3. Anemias, immune system dysfunction
   4. Brain damage
   5. Peripheral neuropathy
   6. Cardiac disorders
   7. Telangiectasia
   8. Acne rosacea

E. Psychological symptoms
   1. Depression
   2. Irritability, hostility
   3. Suspiciousness
   4. Rationalization
   5. Isolation
   6. Decrease in inhibitions
   7. Decrease in self-esteem
   8. Denial that a problem exists

IV. Alcohol Withdrawal

A. Description
   1. Occurs when an addicted person stops ingesting alcohol
   2. Can occur 6 to 8 hours after drinking has ended or decreased, and symptoms can last 5 days or longer
   3. Alcohol withdrawal is highly individual, and some clients experience mild withdrawal symptoms requiring minimal medical supervision; others experience severe symptoms that can be life-threatening

B. Stages of withdrawal
   1. Stage 1
     a. May begin 6 to 8 hours after ingestion or significant decrease in usual consumption of alcohol
     b. Anxiety
     c. Anorexia
     d. Insomnia
     e. Tremors
     f. Hypervigilance
     g. Nausea and vomiting
     h. Headache
     i. Increased pulse and blood pressure
     j. Depression
   2. Stage 2
     a. May begin 8 to 12 hours after the last ingestion of a significant decrease in usual consumption of alcohol
     b. Profound confusion
     c. Gross tremors
     d. Nervousness
     e. Disorientation
     f. Nightmares
     g. Illusions
     h. Auditory and visual hallucinations

   3. Stage 3
     a. May begin 12 to 48 hours after the last ingestion or significant decrease in usual consumption of alcohol
     b. Severe hallucinations
     c. Grand mal seizures
   4. Stage 4
     a. May begin 3 to 5 days after the last ingestion or significant decrease in usual consumption of alcohol
     b. Confusion, disorientation, clouding of consciousness, and delirium
     c. Hypertension, diaphoresis, tachycardia
     d. Visual and tactile hallucinations
     e. Fluctuating levels of consciousness
     f. Fever (103° to 104°F)
     g. Tremors
     h. Tachycardia
     i. Severe psychomotor activity and agitation
     j. Sleeplessness
     k. Hallucinations
     l. A medical emergency

C. Implementation
   1. Initiate seizure precautions
   2. Chlordiazepoxide (Librium) may be prescribed for withdrawal and anticonvulsive effects
   3. Diazepam (Valium) or pentobarbital (Phenobarbital) may be prescribed to produce sedation and control withdrawal
   4. Phenytoin (Dilantin) may be prescribed to prevent seizures
   5. Thiamine (vitamin B_1) may be prescribed for malnutrition and to prevent Wernicke's encephalopathy
   6. Magnesium sulfate may be prescribed to increase the effectiveness of thiamine (vitamin B_1) and to help reduce postwithdrawal seizures
   7. Increase fluid intake; monitor intake and output
   8. Monitor vital signs frequently
   9. Orient the client frequently; maintain minimal stimuli
   10. Approach the client in an accepting, nonjudgmental manner
   11. Assist the client to use assertive techniques rather than manipulation to meet needs
   12. Set limits on manipulative behavior
   13. Direct the client to focus on the substance **abuse** problem
   14. Limits the client's blame-placing or rationalizing to explain the substance **abuse** problem
   15. Encourage the client to participate in group therapy and support groups
   16. Encourage the client to attend weekly Alcoholics Anonymous (AA) meetings

D. Complications associated with chronic alcohol use
   1. Vitamin deficiencies
   2. Vitamin B deficiency causing peripheral neuropathies

3. Thiamine deficiency causing Korsakoff's syndrome
4. Severe memory problems
5. Wernicke's encephalopathy, causing confusion, ataxia, and abnormal eye movements

E. Disulfiram (Antabuse) therapy
  1. Description
    a. An alcohol deterrent used for alcoholic dependence
    b. The medication sensitizes the client to alcohol and a reaction occurs if alcohol is ingested
    c. The client must abstain from alcohol for at least 12 hours before the initial dose is administered
    d. The client must avoid drinking for 14 days after antabuse therapy has been discontinued; otherwise the client is at risk for disulfiram-alcohol reaction
  2. Negative physiological responses
    a. Throbbing headache
    b. Flushing
    c. Nausea and excessive vomiting
    d. Diaphoresis
    e. Dizziness
    f. Blurred vision and confusion
    g. Hypotension
    h. Dyspnea
    i. Palpitations and tachycardia
    j. Chest pain
  3. Client education
    a. Educate regarding the effects of the medication
    b. Instruct the client that the effects of medication may occur for several days after discontinuance
    c. Ensure that the client agrees to abstain from alcohol and any alcohol-containing substances
    d. Instruct the client to avoid substances such as cough medicines, rubbing compounds, vinegar, mouthwashes, and aftershave lotions

V. Hallucinogens (Box 62–2)

A. Causes psychosis, with distorted perception, heightened sense of awareness, grandiosity, hallucinations, mystical experiences, and distortions of time and space
B. May harm self when under influence
C. No withdrawal syndrome when discontinued,

BOX 62–3. Opiates

Opium
Heroin
Meperidine hydrochloride (Demerol)
Morphine sulfate
Codeine sulfate
Methadone (Dolophine)
Hydromorphone (Dilaudid)
Fentanyl (Sublimaze)

---

but flashbacks may occur for several months after use stops
D. Bad trips may result in panic and unpredictable psychotic behaviors

VI. Marijuana

A. Causes altered state of awareness, relaxation, and mild euphoria
B. Decreases inhibitions
C. Decreases motivation from prolonged use
D. Can precipitate psychosis in susceptible individuals
E. Physiological effects include slowed reflexes
F. Causes drying of mucous membranes and reddening of eyes

VII. Opiates (Box 62–3)

A. Description
  1. Cause mental and physical deterioration
  2. High risk for infection with HIV virus or hepatitis virus if taken intravenously
  3. Cause decreased response to pain, respiratory depression, constriction of pupils, euphoria, apathy, impaired judgment
B. Opiate withdrawal
  1. Methadone blocks the action of opiates and may be used to assist with withdrawal
  2. Signs of withdrawal include anxiety; yawning; diaphoresis; cramping; rhinorrhea; achiness and muscle twitching; anorexia; insomnia; increased temperature, respiration, and blood pressure; nausea and vomiting; diarrhea; and restlessness
  3. Overdose of opiates can lead to coma, respiratory depression, and death

---

BOX 62–2. Hallucinogens

Lysergic acid diethylamide (LSD)
Phencyclidine piperidine (PCP)
Mescaline (peyote)
Psilocybin

BOX 62–4. Sedatives and Depressants

Amobarbital (Amytal)
Phenobarbital (Nembutal)
Secobarbital (Seconal)
Chloral hydrate (Noctec)
Glutethimide (Doriden)
Meprobamate (Equanil)
Benzodiazepines

VIII. Sedatives and Depressants (Box 62-4)

A. Description
   1. Act as a depressant, sedative, and hypnotic
   2. Cause physical and psychological dependence
   3. Cause euphoria
   4. Can cause depression and hostility
   5. Impaired judgment and lack of coordination can occur
   6. Slurring of speech
   7. Tolerance can develop
B. Withdrawal: causes increased temperature, tachycardia, postural hypotension, insomnia, tremors, agitation, apprehension, weakness, grand mal seizures, and psychosis

IX. Stimulants (Box 62-5)

A. Description
   1. Stimulants lead to alertness and extra energy and are used in obesity and narcolepsy; also used for hyperactive children
   2. Effects can include euphoria, hyperactivity, insomnia, anorexia and weight loss, tachycardia and hypertension, psychotic behavior
   3. Psychological dependence and tolerance can occur
   4. Sudden death has been associated with cocaine **abuse**
B. Withdrawal
   1. Crash
   2. Depression
   3. Lack of energy

X. Antianxiety Medications (Box 62-6)

A. Description
   1. Cause physical and psychological addictiveness
   2. Cause relaxation, drowsiness, ataxia, and hypotension
   3. Withdrawal can produce seizures
B. Withdrawal
   1. Initiate seizure precautions

   2. Increase fluids; monitor I&O
   3. Monitor vital signs
   4. Orient the client frequently; maintain minimal stimuli
   5. Approach the client in an accepting and nonjudgmental manner
   6. Direct the client's focus to the substance **abuse** problem
   7. Identify with the client situations that precipitate angry feelings
   8. Limit the client's blame-placing or rationalizing to explain the substance **abuse** problem
   9. Assist the client to use assertive techniques rather than manipulation to meet needs
   10. Set limits on manipulative behavior and verbal and physical **abuse**
   11. Hold the client firmly to reasonable limits, consistently reinforcing rules, with reasonable consequences for breaking rules; hold the client accountable for all behaviors
   12. Assist the client to explore strengths and weaknesses
   13. Encourage time out if the client is losing control
   14. Encourage the client to participate in unit activities
   15. Encourage the client to participate in group therapy and support groups
   16. See Box 62-7 for a list of therapies
   17. Box 62-8 delineates nursing care for clients during withdrawal

PRACTICE QUESTIONS

1. The nurse is caring for a female client who was recently admitted for anorexia nervosa. When the nurse enters the room the client is engaged in rigorous push-ups. Which of the following nursing actions is most appropriate?
   1 Allow the client to complete her exercise program
   2 Tell the client that she is not allowed to exercise rigorously
   3 Interrupt the client and offer to take her for a walk
   4 Interrupt the client and weigh her immediately

2. The nurse is assigned to care for a client with anorexia nervosa. The nurse is monitoring the behavior of the client and understands that the client with anorexia nervosa manages anxiety by
   1 Always reinforcing self-approval
   2 Having the need to always make the right decision
   3 Engaging in immoral acts
   4 Observing rigid rules and regulations

3. The nurse is assisting in developing a plan of care for the client hospitalized with bulimia nervosa. The nurse understands that which of the following is not a component of the plan of care?
   1 Monitoring I&O
   2 Monitoring electrolyte levels
   3 Observing for excessive exercise-type activity
   4 Checking for the presence of laxatives and diuretics in the client's belongings

4. The nurse is assigned to care for a client at risk for alcohol withdrawal. Which of the following symptoms alerts the nurse to the potential for delirium tremors (DTs)?
   1 Fever, hypertension, changes in level of consciousness, and hallucinations
   2 Hypotension, stupor, agitation, headache, and auditory hallucinations
   3 Vomiting, ataxia, muscular rigidity, and tactile hallucinations
   4 Coarse hand tremor, agitation, hallucinations, and hypotension

5. The spouse of a client admitted to the mental health unit for alcohol withdrawal says to the nurse, "I should get out of this bad situation." The best response by the nurse is
   1 "I agree with you. You should get out of this situation."
   2 "What do you find difficult about this situation?"
   3 "Why don't you tell your husband about this?"
   4 "This is not the best time to make that decision."

6. The nurse is caring for a client who has a history of opioid abuse and is monitoring the client for signs of withdrawal. Which of the following observations, if made by the nurse, is indicative of the clinical manifestations associated with withdrawal from opioids?
   1 Increased blood pressure (BP) and pulse with low-grade fever, yawning, restlessness, anxiety, craving, diarrhea, and mydriasis
   2 Tachycardia, mild hypertension, fever, sweating, nausea, vomiting, and marked tremors
   3 Increased appetite, irritability, anxiety, restlessness, increased appetite, and altered concentration
   4 Depressed feelings, high drug craving, fatigue with a desire to sleep or altered sleep (insomnia or hypersomnia), agitation, and paranoia

7. The nurse is caring for a client who is suspected to be dependent on drugs. Which of the following is most appropriate for the nurse to ask when collecting data from the client regarding drug abuse?
   1 "Why did you get started on these drugs?"
   2 "How long did you think you could take these drugs without someone finding out?"
   3 "How much do you use and what effect does it have on you?"
   4 The nurse does not ask any questions in fear that the client is in denial and will throw the nurse out of the room.

8. A client who has been drinking alcohol on a regular basis admits to having "a problem." The client is asking for assistance with the problem. The nurse encourages the client to attend which of the following community groups?
   1 Al-Anon
   2 Alcoholics Anonymous
   3 Families Anonymous
   4 Fresh Start

9. The client with a diagnosis of anorexia nervosa, who is in a state of starvation, is in a two-bed room. A newly admitted client will be assigned to this client's room. The nurse who is assisting in planning care for the client with anorexia nervosa knows that which of the following is not an appropriate choice for this client's roommate?
   1 A client with pneumonia
   2 A client with a fractured leg
   3 A client who is able to care for self
   4 A client who will need minimal assistance with care

10. The client has been hospitalized and has participated in substance abuse therapy group sessions. Upon discharge, the client has consented to participate in Alcoholics Anonymous (AA) community groups. Which of the following statements by the client best indicates to the nurse that the client has assimilated therapy session topics, cop-

ing response styles, and has processed information effectively for self-use?

1 "I know I'm ready to be discharged; I feel like I can say no and leave a group of friends if they are drinking—no problem."
2 "This group has really helped a lot. I know it will be different when I go home. But I'm sure that my family and friends will all help me like the people in this group have. They'll all help me. I know they will. They won't let me go back to old ways."
3 "I'm looking forward to leaving here; I know that I will miss all of you. So I'm happy and I'm sad, I'm excited and I'm scared. I know that I have to work hard to be strong and that everyone isn't going to be as helpful as you people."
4 "I'll keep all my appointments; go to all my AA groups. I'll do everything I'm supposed to. Nothing will go wrong that way."

11. The nurse is assigned to care for a client at risk for alcohol withdrawal. The nurse monitors the client knowing that the early signs of withdrawal will develop within how much time after cessation or reduction of alcohol intake?
1 Within 6 to 8 hours
2 After several hours
3 In 1 week
4 In 2 to 3 weeks

12. The nurse determines that the wife of an alcoholic client is benefiting from attending an Al-Anon group when the nurse hears the wife say
1 "My attendance at the meetings has helped me to see that I provoke my husband's violence."
2 "I no longer feel that I deserve the blame my husband inflicts on me."
3 "I can tolerate my husband's destructive behaviors now that I know they are common with alcoholics."
4 "I enjoy attending the meetings because they get me out of the house and away from my husband."

13. A female client with anorexia nervosa is a member of a support group. The client verbalizes that she would like to buy some new clothes but her finances are limited. Group members brought some used clothes to the client to replace the client's old clothes. The client believed that the new clothes were much too tight and reduced her calorie intake to 800 calories daily. The nurse identifies this behavior as
1 Normal
2 Indicative of the client's ambivalence
3 Evidence of the client's altered/distorted body image
4 Regression

14. A hospitalized client with a history of alcohol abuse tells the nurse, "I am leaving now. I have to go. I don't want any more treatment. I have things that I have to do right away." The client has not been discharged. In fact, the client is scheduled for an important diagnostic test to be performed in 1 hour. After discussing the client's concerns with the client, the client dresses and begins to walk out of the hospital room. The most appropriate nursing action is
1 Restrain the client until the physician can be reached
2 Call security to block all exit areas
3 Tell the client that they cannot return to this hospital again if they leave now
4 Call the nursing supervisor

15. The nurse is collecting data from a client with a diagnosis of bulimia nervosa. The nurse understands that which of the following is not a characteristic finding in this disorder?
1 Enlarged parotid glands
2 Dental erosion
3 Electrolyte imbalances
4 Body weight well below ideal range

ANSWERS

1. **3**

RATIONALE: Clients with anorexia nervosa are frequently preoccupied with rigorous exercise and push themselves beyond normal limits to work off caloric intake. The nurse must provide for appropriate exercise as well as place limits on rigorous activities. Options 1, 2, and 4 are inappropriate.
TEST-TAKING STRATEGY: Focus on the key words "most appropriate." Recalling that the nurse needs to set firm limits with clients who have this disorder will easily direct you to the correct option. If you had difficulty with this question, take time now to review interventions for the client with anorexia nervosa.

LEVEL OF COGNITIVE ABILITY: Application
PHASE OF NURSING PROCESS: Implementation
CLIENT NEEDS: Physiological Integrity
CONTENT AREA: Mental Health
REFERENCE
deWit, S. (1998). *Essentials of medical-surgical nursing* (4th ed.). Philadelphia: W. B. Saunders. p. 606.

2. **4**

RATIONALE: Clients with anorexia nervosa have the desire to please others. Their need to be correct or perfect interferes with rational decision-making processes. These clients are moralistic. Rules and rituals help the clients manage their anxiety.
TEST-TAKING STRATEGY: Eliminate options 1 and 2 because of the absolute word "always." Option 3 is not a

characteristic of anorexia nervosa. Review these characteristics now if you had difficulty with this question.
LEVEL OF COGNITIVE ABILITY: Comprehension
PHASE OF NURSING PROCESS: Data Collection
CLIENT NEEDS: Psychosocial Integrity
CONTENT AREA: Mental Health
REFERENCE
deWit, S. (1998). *Essentials of medical-surgical nursing* (4th ed.). Philadelphia: W. B. Saunders. p. 606.

3. 3

RATIONALE: Excessive exercise is a characteristic of anorexia nervosa, not a characteristic of clients with bulimia. Frequent vomiting, in addition to laxative and diuretic abuse, may lead to dehydration and electrolyte imbalances. Options 1, 2, and 4 are appropriate interventions in the plan of care.
TEST-TAKING STRATEGY: Note the key word "not." Note the similarities between options 1, 2, and 4 in that they directly or indirectly infer concern about fluid and electrolyte balance. Review the characteristics associated with bulimia nervosa now if you had difficulty with this question.
LEVEL OF COGNITIVE ABILITY: Comprehension
PHASE OF NURSING PROCESS: Planning
CLIENT NEEDS: Physiological Integrity
CONTENT AREA: Mental Health
REFERENCE
deWit, S. (1998). *Essentials of medical-surgical nursing* (4th ed.). Philadelphia: W. B. Saunders. p. 606

4. 1

RATIONALE: The symptoms associated with DTs typically include anxiety, insomnia, anorexia, hypertension, disorientation, visual or tactile hallucinations, changes in level of consciousness, agitation, fever, and delusions.
TEST-TAKING STRATEGY: Knowledge regarding the clinical manifestations associated with DTs is required to answer this question. Review each option carefully to ensure that all of the symptoms are contained in the correct option. Review these symptoms now if you had difficulty with this question.
LEVEL OF COGNITIVE ABILITY: Comprehension
PHASE OF NURSING PROCESS: Data Collection
CLIENT NEEDS: Physiological Integrity
CONTENT AREA: Mental Health
REFERENCE
Varcarolis, E. (1998). *Foundations of psychiatric mental health nursing* (3rd ed.). Philadelphia: W. B. Saunders. p. 766.

5. 2

RATIONALE: The best response is one that encourages the client to problem solve. Giving advice implies that the nurse knows what is best and can also foster dependency. The nurse should not agree with the client or request that the client provide explanations.
TEST-TAKING STRATEGY: Use therapeutic communication techniques. Note that the client of the question is the spouse. Eliminate option 3 because of the word "why." Eliminate option 1 because the nurse is agreeing with the client. Eliminate option 4 because this option places the client's feelings on hold. Option 2 is the only option that addresses the client's feelings.
LEVEL OF COGNITIVE ABILITY: Application
PHASE OF NURSING PROCESS: Implementation

CLIENT NEEDS: Psychosocial Integrity
CONTENT AREA: Mental Health
REFERENCE
Varcarolis, E. (1998). *Foundations of psychiatric mental health nursing* (3rd ed.). Philadelphia: W. B. Saunders. p. 191.

6. 1

RATIONALE: Opioids are CNS depressants. They generally cause drowsiness and the feeling of being out of touch with the world. Option 2 describes withdrawal from alcohol. Option 3 describes withdrawal from nicotine. Option 4 describes withdrawal from cocaine.
TEST-TAKING STRATEGY: Focus on the issue of the question, the clinical manifestations associated with withdrawal from opioids. If you had difficulty with this question, take time now to review the manifestations associated with opioid withdrawal.
LEVEL OF COGNITIVE ABILITY: Comprehension
PHASE OF NURSING PROCESS: Data Collection
CLIENT NEEDS: Physiological Integrity
CONTENT AREA: Mental Health
REFERENCE
Glod, C. (1998). *Contemporary psychiatric-mental health nursing.* Philadelphia: F. A. Davis. pp. 290–297.

7. 3

RATIONALE: It is best for the nurse to attempt to elicit information by being nonjudgmental and direct. Option 1 is incorrect because it is judgmental, off focus, and reflects the nurse's bias. Option 2 is incorrect because it is judgmental, insensitive, and aggressive. Option 4 is incorrect because it indicates passivity on the nurse's part and uses rationalization to avoid the therapeutic nursing intervention.
TEST-TAKING STRATEGY: Focus on the issue of the question and use therapeutic communication techniques. This will easily direct you to option 3. If you had difficulty with this question review the appropriate data collection techniques for the client with a drug abuse problem.
LEVEL OF COGNITIVE ABILITY: Comprehension
PHASE OF NURSING PROCESS: Data Collection
CLIENT NEEDS: Psychosocial Integrity
CONTENT AREA: Mental Health
REFERENCE
Glod, C. (1998). *Contemporary psychiatric-mental health nursing.* Philadelphia: F. A. Davis. pp. 289–293.

8. 2

RATIONALE: Alcoholics Anonymous is a major self-help organization for the treatment of alcoholism. Option 1 is a group for families of alcoholics. Option 3 is for parents of children who abuse substances. Option 4 is for nicotine addicts.
TEST-TAKING STRATEGY: If you are unfamiliar with these support groups, note the relationship between "drinking" in the question and "alcoholics" in the correct option. Familiarize yourself with the purpose of specific support groups now if you had difficulty with this question.
LEVEL OF COGNITIVE ABILITY: Application
PHASE OF NURSING PROCESS: Implementation
CLIENT NEEDS: Health Promotion and Maintenance
CONTENT AREA: Mental Health
REFERENCE
deWit, S. (1998). *Essentials of medical-surgical nursing* (4th ed.). Philadelphia: W. B. Saunders. p. 1014.

9. 1

RATIONALE: The client who has been starving has a compromised immune system. Having a roommate with pneumonia would put the client at risk for infection. Options 2, 3, and 4 are appropriate roommates for this client. **TEST-TAKING STRATEGY:** Note the key words "in a state of starvation" and "not." Eliminate options 3 and 4 first because they are similar. Recall that the priority needs of the client with anorexia nervosa are physiological. This should direct you to option 1. Review care to the client with anorexia nervosa if you had difficulty with this question. **LEVEL OF COGNITIVE ABILITY:** Application **PHASE OF NURSING PROCESS:** Planning **CLIENT NEEDS:** Safe, Effective Care Environment **CONTENT AREA:** Mental Health **REFERENCE** deWit, S. (1998). *Essentials of medical-surgical nursing* (4th ed.). Philadelphia: W. B. Saunders. p. 606.

10. 3

RATIONALE: In option 3, the client is expressing real concern and ambivalence about discharge from the hospital. The client also demonstrates reality in the statement. Option 1 indicates client denial. In option 2, the client is relying heavily on others. In option 4, the client is concrete and procedure-oriented; again, the client states that "nothing will go wrong that way" if the client follows all the directions. **TEST-TAKING STRATEGY:** Use the process of elimination and select the option that identifies the most realistic client verbalization. This will easily direct you to option 3. **LEVEL OF COGNITIVE ABILITY:** Comprehension **PHASE OF NURSING PROCESS:** Evaluation **CLIENT NEEDS:** Psychosocial Integrity **CONTENT AREA:** Mental Health **REFERENCE** deWit, S. (1998). *Essentials of medical-surgical nursing* (4th ed.). Philadelphia: W. B. Saunders. p. 1012.

11. 1

RATIONALE: Early signs of alcohol withdrawal develop within a few hours after cessation or reduction of alcohol and peak after 24 to 48 hours. **TEST-TAKING STRATEGY:** Note the key word "early." This will assist in directing you to option 1. If you are unfamiliar with the manifestations associated with alcohol withdrawal, take time now to review. **LEVEL OF COGNITIVE ABILITY:** Comprehension **PHASE OF NURSING PROCESS:** Data Collection **CLIENT NEEDS:** Physiological Integrity **CONTENT AREA:** Mental Health **REFERENCE** Varcarolis, E. (1998). *Foundations of psychiatric mental health nursing* (3rd ed.). W. B. Saunders. pp. 765–766.

12. 2

RATIONALE: Al-Anon support groups are a protected, supportive opportunity for spouses and significant others to learn what to expect and to obtain excellent pointers about successful behavioral changes. Option 2 is the most healthy response because it exemplifies an understanding that the alcoholic partner is responsible for his behavior and cannot be allowed to blame family members for loss of control. In option 1, the nonalcoholic partner should not feel responsible when the spouse loses control. Option 3 indicates that the wife remains codependent. Option 4 indicates that the group is being seen as an escape, not a place to work on issues. **TEST-TAKING STRATEGY:** Use the process of elimination. Identify the client of the question and identify the option that most directly addresses the issue of the question, that is, benefiting from attending an Al-Anon group. Review the purpose of this type of support group now if you had difficulty with this question. **LEVEL OF COGNITIVE ABILITY:** Comprehension **PHASE OF NURSING PROCESS:** Data Collection **CLIENT NEEDS:** Psychosocial Integrity **CONTENT AREA:** Mental Health **REFERENCE** Varcarolis, E. (1998). *Foundations of psychiatric mental health nursing* (3rd ed.). W. B. Saunders. p. 774.

13. 3

RATIONALE: Altered/distorted body image is a concern with clients with anorexia nervosa. Although the client may struggle with ambivalence and present with regressed behavior, the client's coping pattern relates to the basic issue of distorted body image. The nurse should address this need in the support group. **TEST-TAKING STRATEGY:** Focus on the information provided in the question to determine that the issue relates to a distorted body image. This will easily direct you to option 3. If you had difficulty with this question, take time now to review characteristics associated with the client with anorexia nervosa. **LEVEL OF COGNITIVE ABILITY:** Comprehension **PHASE OF NURSING PROCESS:** Data Collection **CLIENT NEEDS:** Psychosocial Integrity **CONTENT AREA:** Mental Health **REFERENCE** deWit, S. (1998). *Essentials of medical-surgical nursing* (4th ed.). Philadelphia: W. B. Saunders. p. 606.

14. 4

RATIONALE: A nurse can be charged with false imprisonment if a client is made to wrongfully believe that they cannot leave the hospital. Most health care facilities have documents that the client is asked to sign that relate to the clients' responsibilities when they leave against medical advice (AMA). The client should be asked to sign this document before leaving. The nurse should request that the client wait to speak to the physician before leaving but if the client refuses to do so, the nurse cannot hold the client against his or her will. Restraining the client and calling security to block exits constitutes false imprisonment. Any client has a right to health care and cannot be told otherwise. **TEST-TAKING STRATEGY:** Keeping the concept of false imprisonment in mind, eliminate options 1 and 2 because they are similar. Eliminate option 3 knowing that any client has a right to health. Review the points related to false imprisonment now if you had difficulty with this question. **LEVEL OF COGNITIVE ABILITY:** Application **PHASE OF NURSING PROCESS:** Implementation **CLIENT NEEDS:** Safe, Effective Care Environment **CONTENT AREA:** Mental Health **REFERENCE** Varcarolis, E. (1998). *Foundations of psychiatric mental health nursing* (3rd ed.). W. B. Saunders. p. 781.

15. **4**

RATIONALE: Clients with bulimia nervosa may not initially appear to be physically or emotionally ill. They are often at or slightly below ideal body weight. On further inspection, the client demonstrates enlargement of the parotid glands with dental erosion and caries if the client has been inducing vomiting. Electrolyte imbalances are present.
TEST-TAKING STRATEGY: Knowledge regarding the characteristics noted in bulimia nervosa will assist in answering this question. Option 4 is a characteristic sign of anorexia nervosa not bulimia nervosa. Review the characteristics of these disorders now if you had difficulty with this question.
LEVEL OF COGNITIVE ABILITY: Comprehension
PHASE OF NURSING PROCESS: Data Collection
CLIENT NEEDS: Physiological Integrity
CONTENT AREA: Mental Health
REFERENCE
Varcarolis, E. (1998). *Foundations of psychiatric mental health nursing* (3rd ed.). Philadelphia: W. B. Saunders. p. 816.

BIBLIOGRAPHY

deWit, S. (1998). *Essentials of medical-surgical nursing* (4th ed.). Philadelphia: W. B. Saunders.

Glod, C. (1998). *Contemporary psychiatric-mental health nursing.* Philadelphia: F. A. Davis.
Varcarolis, E. (1998). *Foundations of psychiatric mental health nursing* (3rd ed.). Philadelphia: W. B. Saunders.

CHAPTER 63

Crisis Theory and Intervention

. . . .

I. Crisis Intervention Therapy

A. Description
1. **Crisis** is a temporary state of disequilibrium
2. Decision making and problem solving are inadequate
3. Treatment is immediate, supportive, and directly responsive to immediate **crisis** to assist the client and/or the family through the stressful situation
B. Phases of a **crisis**
1. Phase 1: external precipitating event
2. Phase 2
   a. Perception of threat
   b. Increase in anxiety
   c. Client may cope or resolve **crisis**
3. Phase 3
   a. Failure of coping
   b. Increasing disorganization
   c. Physical symptoms emerge
   d. Relationship problems
4. Phase 4
   a. Mobilization of internal and external resources
   b. Resolutions related to precrisis functioning include functioning at a higher level, at the same level, or at a lower level
C. **Crisis** intervention
1. Treatment is immediate, supportive, and directly responsive to the immediate **crisis**
2. Feelings of the client are acknowledged
3. Goal-directed intervention
4. Provides opportunities for expression and validation of feelings
5. Connections are made between the meaning of the event and the **crisis**
6. Explores alternative **coping mechanisms** and tries out new behaviors

II. Grieving

A. Description

1. A normal human process that occurs in response to a loss
2. Progresses through various stages and the entire process may take up to 3 years
B. Data collection
1. Crying, depression
2. Guilt and anger
3. Fatigue and lethargy
4. Insomnia
5. Agitation
6. Anorexia
7. Ambivalence
8. Somatic complaints
9. Sense of detachment and unreality
10. Denial
C. Implementation
1. Explain the normal stages of the grieving process to the client
2. Monitor the client's progress through the grieving process
3. Encourage the client to express feelings about the loss and its significance on life
4. Encourage expression of angry feelings
5. Assist the client to make appropriate future plans related to changes caused by the loss
6. Encourage the client to work through the feelings associated with the loss

III. Affective (Mood) Disorders

A. Description
1. Illnesses that affect mood, ranging from elation or agitation to extreme sadness, emotional isolation
2. Types of mood disorders may include depressive disorders, suicidal behavior, and bipolar (manic depressive) disorders
3. Can be maladaptive and incapacitating in nature
B. Precipitating factors
1. Loss, which can be real or imagined and

related to the person, status, self-esteem, a body part or function
2. Major life events related to disruption of life patterns, conflict, or the entrance or exit of significant persons
3. Role changes, such as marriage or divorce, parenting, or employment status
4. Disruption in coping skills
5. Physical changes due to medical illness or debilitating condition or drug-induced

IV. Depression

A. Description
1. Affects feelings, thoughts, and behaviors
2. Can occur after a loss, including loss of self-esteem, the end of a significant relationship, the death of a loved one, or a traumatic event
3. The loss is followed by grief and mourning, and if this process does not resolve, depression results
4. Depression may be mild, moderate, or severe
5. Treatment includes antidepressant medication and electroconvulsive therapy (ECT)

B. Mild depression
1. Triggered by an external event; the experience follows the normal grief reaction
2. Lasts less than 2 weeks
3. Feeling sad, let down, or disappointed
4. Mild alterations in sleep patterns
5. Feeling less alert
6. Irritability
7. Disinterested in spending time with others
8. Increased use of alcohol or drugs

C. Moderate depression
1. Persists over time
2. The person experiences a sense of change and often seeks help
3. Despondent and gloomy
4. Low self-esteem and social withdrawal
5. Helplessness and powerlessness
6. May experience intense anxiety and anger
7. Diurnal variation—may feel better at a certain time of day, such as in the morning
8. Slow thought processes and difficulty concentrating
9. Rumination—persistent thinking about and discussion of a particular subject
10. Negative thinking and suicidal thoughts
11. Sleep disturbances
12. Anorexia, weight loss, and fatigue
13. Somatic complaints
14. Increased use of alcohol or drugs

D. Severe depression
1. Intense and pervasive
2. Guilt and worthlessness
3. Flat affect and decreased speech
4. May show agitation and pace about
5. Poor posture and unkempt appearance
6. Self-destructive thoughts; however, client may lack energy to act on thought
7. Social withdrawal

8. Poor concentration and overwhelmed by simple tasks
9. Severe psychomotor retardation
10. Anorexia and marked weight loss
11. Constipation and urinary retention
12. Lack of sexual interest
13. Diurnal variation—the person feels worse in the morning and better as the day goes on
14. Delusions and hallucinations

E. Implementation
1. Altered thought processes
   a. Encourage the client to discuss losses or changes in life situation
   b. Encourage the client to express sadness or anger and allow adequate time for verbal responses
   c. Assist in developing short-term goals
   d. Encourage the use of problem solving and positive thinking
   e. Limit decision making
   f. Spend short periods throughout the day with the client
   g. Be on time when a schedule is planned with the client
   h. Sit in silence with clients who are not verbalizing
   i. Use simple, concrete words when communicating
   j. Avoid a cheerful attitude
2. Risk for self-harm
   a. Assess for **suicide** clues and intervene to provide safety precautions as necessary
   b. Ask client directly, "Have you thought of hurting yourself?"
   c. Assess lethality of plans
   d. Do not leave alone for extended periods
   e. If client has a suicidal plan, place on one-to-one supervision
3. Activity intolerance
   a. Encourage daily exercise
   b. Assist with activities of daily living (ADLs) if client is unable to perform
   c. Begin with one-to-one activities
   d. Provide activities for easy mastery to increase self-esteem and assist in alleviating guilt feelings
   e. Provide activities that require little orientation (card games, drawing)
   f. Engage in gross motor activities (walking)
   g. Eventually bring client into small group activities, then large groups
4. Altered nutrition
   a. Ensure adequate nutrition
   b. Offer small, high-caloric, high-protein snacks and fluids throughout the day
   c. Stay with the client during meals
   d. Weigh the client weekly
   e. Monitor bowel patterns for constipation
5. Sleep pattern disturbance
   a. Ensure adequate sleep
   b. Provide rest periods after activities

c. Encourage the client to dress and stay out of bed during the day
d. Provide relaxation measures at bedtime
e. Decrease environmental stimuli at bedtime
f. Spend time with the client before bedtime

V. Suicidal Behavior

A. Description
   1. Suicidal clients characteristically have feelings of worthlessness, guilt, and hopelessness that are so overwhelming that they feel unable to go on with life and unfit to live
   2. The nurse caring for a depressed client always considers the possibility of suicide
B. High-risk groups
   1. Those with a history of previous **suicide attempts**
   2. Family history of **suicide attempts**
   3. Adolescents
   4. Disabled or terminally ill older adults
   5. Clients with personality disorders
   6. Clients with organic brain syndrome or dementia
   7. Depressed or psychotic clients
   8. Substance abusers
C. Clues
   1. Giving away personal, special, and prized possessions
   2. Canceling social engagements
   3. Making out or changing a will
   4. Taking out or changing insurance policies
   5. Positive or negative changes in behavior
   6. Poor appetite
   7. Sleeping difficulties
   8. Feelings of hopelessness
   9. Difficulty concentrating
   10. Loss of interest in activities
   11. Client statements that indicate an intent to attempt **suicide**
   12. Sudden calmness or improvement in a depressed client
   13. Client questions about poisons, guns, or other lethal objects
D. Data collection
   1. The plan
      a. Does the client have a plan?
      b. What is the plan, how lethal is the plan, and how likely is death to occur?
      c. Does the client have the means to carry out the plan?
   2. Client history of attempts
      a. **Suicide attempts** in the past and the outcomes
      b. Was the client accidentally rescued?
      c. Have the past attempts and methods been the same, or have methods increased in lethality?
   3. Psychosocial
      a. Is the client alone or alienated from others?
      b. Is hostility or depression present?

c. Do hallucinations exist?
d. Is substance **abuse** present?
e. Any recent losses or physical illness?
f. Any environmental or lifestyle changes?
E. Implementation
   1. Initiate **suicide** precautions
   2. Remove harmful objects
   3. Do not leave client alone
   4. Provide a one-to-one supervision at all times
   5. Provide a nonjudgmental, caring attitude
   6. Assist with the development of a contract, which is written, dated, and signed and indicates alternative behavior at times of suicidal thoughts
   7. Encourage the client to talk about feelings and to identify positive aspects about self
   8. Encourage active participation in own care
   9. Keep client active by assigning simple tasks
   10. Check that visitors do not leave harmful objects in the client's room
   11. Identify support systems
   12. Do not allow the client to leave the unit unless accompanied by staff member
   13. Continue to assess the client's **suicide** potential

VI. Abusive Behaviors

A. Anger
   1. A feeling of annoyance that may be displaced onto an object or person
   2. Is used to avoid anxiety and gives a feeling of power in situations in which the person feels out of control
B. Violence: the physical force that is threatening to the safety to self and others
C. Aggression: can be harmful and destructive when not controlled
D. Data collection
   1. History of violence or self-harm
   2. Poor impulse control and low tolerance of frustration
   3. Defiant and argumentative
   4. Verbal threats
   5. Increased pacing and agitation
   6. Muscle rigidity
   7. Flushed face
   8. Glaring
   9. Loud voice
E. Implementation
   1. Acknowledge anger
   2. Set limits on behavior
   3. Listen actively and assist the client to deal with consequences of anger
   4. Provide safety for expressing anger and safety to others
F. **Restraints** and **seclusion**
   1. Description
      a. Physical **restraints**: any manual method or mechanical device, material, or equipment that inhibits free movement
      b. **Seclusion**: the last step in a process to

maximize safety to a client and others in which a client is placed alone in a specially designed room for protection and close supervision

   c. Chemical **restraints:** medications given for a very specific purpose of inhibiting a specific behavior or movement; have an impact on the client's ability to relate to the environment

  2. Use of **restraints** and **seclusion**

   a. Should never be used as punishment or for the convenience of the staff

   b. The least restrictive means of **restraint** for the shortest duration should be used

   c. Used when behavior is physically harmful to the client or others

   d. Used when alternative or less restrictive measures are insufficient in protecting the client or others from harm

   e. Used when the client anticipates that a controlled environment would be helpful and requests **seclusion**

   f. Requires a written order of a physician, which must be reviewed and renewed every 24 hours and must specify the type of **restraint** to be used

   g. In an emergency, the client may be placed in **seclusion** or **restraint;** a written or verbal order is obtained as soon as possible thereafter

   h. Laws require the consent of the client unless an emergency situation exists and can be documented

   i. The client must be removed from **restraints** when safer and quieter behavior is observed

   j. While in **restraints,** the client must be protected from all sources of harm

   k. The nurse must document the behavior leading to **restraint** or **seclusion** and the time the client is placed in and released from **restraint** or seclusion

   l. The client in **restraint** or seclusion must be assessed every 15 to 30 minutes for physical needs, safety, and comfort, these observations are also documented

VII. Family Violence

A. Description

  1. The violence begins with threats or verbal or physical minor assaults, and the victim attempts to comply with the requests of the abuser

  2. The abuser loses control and becomes destructive and harmful while the victim attempts to protect him- or herself; the abuser then becomes loving and attempts to make peace

  3. The behavior may be an attempt for closeness and companionship

  4. The abuser believes that violence is normal

and that the victim is responsible for the **abuse**

  5. Outsiders are not aware of what is happening in the family, and when outsiders try to intervene, the family feels assaulted

  6. Family members are socially isolated and lack autonomy and trust among each other

  7. Caring and intimacy in the family are absent

  8. Family members expect other members in the family to meet their needs but none are able to do so

  9. The abuser threatens to abandon the family

B. Characteristics of abuser

  1. Impaired self-esteem

  2. Strong dependency needs

  3. Narcissistic and suspicious

  4. History of sexual **abuse** during childhood

  5. Perceive victims as their property and believe that they are entitled to **abuse** them

C. Characteristics of victims

  1. Feel trapped, dependent, helpless, and powerless

  2. Depressed

  3. Low self-esteem and blame themselves for the problems

D. Implementation

  1. Assess situations associated with family violence

  2. Assess for evidence of physical injuries

  3. Ensure privacy and confidentiality during data collection and provide a nonjudgmental and empathic approach to foster trust

  4. Family dysfunction is resolved with prescribed therapies, such as individual therapy, psychotherapy, counseling, group therapy, and support groups to assist family members to develop coping strategies

  5. Ensure that the victim is not left alone with abuser

  6. Assist victims to understand their participation in the **abuse**

  7. Assist the victim to develop self-protective abilities and other problem-solving abilities

  8. Provide support and assistance in coping with contacting the legal system

  9. Assist the family to identify an access to community and personal resources

VIII. Child Abuse (refer to Chapter 28 for information regarding child abuse)

IX. Elder Abuse (refer to Chapter 65 for information regarding elder abuse)

X. Rape

A. Description

  1. Engaging another person in sexual intercourse through the use of force and without the consent of the sexual partner

  2. The victim is not required by law to report the rape

  3. The victim is often blamed by others and

often receives no support from significant others

4. Acquaintance rapes involve someone known to the victim

5. Statutory rape is the act of sexual intercourse with someone under the age of legal consent even if there is consent from the minor

B. Data collection

1. Obtain the date of the last menstrual period

2. Determine form of birth control used and last act of intercourse before rape

3. Duration of intercourse, orifices violated, and penile penetration

4. Use of condom by the perpetrator

5. Feelings of shame, embarrassment, humiliation, anger, and revenge

6. Fear of telling others for fear of not being believed

C. Implementation

1. Encourage the client not to shower, bathe, douche, or change clothing until examined

2. Assist with pelvic examination and obtaining specimens to detect for semen

3. Preserve any evidence

4. Treat physical injuries

5. Provide for client safety

6. Assist the client to refrain from self-blame

7. Refer to **crisis** intervention and support groups

PRACTICE QUESTIONS

1. The nurse is reviewing the health care record of a client admitted to the psychiatric unit. The nurse notes that the admission nurse has documented that the client is experiencing anxiety as a result of a situational crisis. The nurse determines that this type of crisis could be caused by
   1 A fire that destroyed the client's home
   2 A recent rape episode experienced by the client
   3 The death of a loved one
   4 Witnessing a murder

2. The nurse is gathering data from a client in crisis. When determining the client's perception of the precipitating event that led to the crisis, the most appropriate question to ask is
   1 "What leads you to seek help now?"
   2 "Who is available to help you?"
   3 "What do you usually do to feel better?"
   4 "With whom do you live?"

3. The nurse assists in developing a plan of care for the client in a crisis state. When developing the plan, the nurse considers which of the following?
   1 Presenting symptoms in a crisis situation are similar for all individuals experiencing a crisis
   2 A crisis state indicates that the individual is suffering from an emotional illness
   3 A crisis state indicates that the individual is suffering from a mental illness

   4 A client's response to a crisis is individualized and what constitutes a crisis for one person may not constitute a crisis for another person

4. The nurse observes that a client with a potential for violence is agitated, pacing up and down the hallway, and is making aggressive and belligerent gestures at other clients. Which of the following statements is most appropriate to make to this client?
   1 "What is causing you to become agitated?"
   2 "You need to stop that behavior now!"
   3 "You will need to be restrained if you do not change your behavior."
   4 "You will need to be placed in seclusion!"

5. During a conversation with a depressed client on an inpatient unit, the client says to the nurse, "My family would be better off without me." The nurse's best response is
   1 "Everyone feels this way when they are depressed."
   2 "Have you talked to your family about this?"
   3 "You sound very upset. Are you thinking of hurting yourself?"
   4 "You will feel better once your medication begins to work."

6. The nurse is caring for an older adult client who has recently lost her husband. The client says, "No one cares about me anymore. All the people I loved are dead." Which of the following responses by the nurse is the most therapeutic?
   1 "That seems rather unlikely to me."
   2 "You must be feeling all alone at this point."
   3 "I don't believe that and neither do you."
   4 "Right! Why not just pack it in?"

7. The nurse is planning care for a client who is being hospitalized because the client has been displaying violent behavior and is at risk for harm to others. Which of the following is not a component of the plan of care?
   1 Keep the door to the client's room open when with the client
   2 Assign the client to a room at the end of the hall to avoid disturbing the other clients
   3 Face the client when providing care
   4 Ensure that a security officer is within the immediate area

8. Which behaviors observed by the nurse might lead to the suspicion that the depressed female adolescent client may be suicidal?
   1 The client becomes angry while speaking on the telephone and slams the receiver down on the hook
   2 The client runs out of the therapy group, swearing at the group leader and runs to her room
   3 The client gets angry with her roommate

when the roommate borrows the client's clothes without asking

4 The client gives away a prized CD and a cherished autographed picture of the performer

9. A client is admitted to the psychiatric unit following a serious suicidal attempt by hanging. The nurse's most important aspect of care is to maintain client safety. This is accomplished best by
   1 Assigning a staff member to the client who will remain with the client at all times
   2 Admitting the client to a seclusion room where all potentially dangerous articles are removed
   3 Removing the client's clothing and placing the client in a hospital gown
   4 Requesting that a peer remain with the client at all times

10. The police arrive at the emergency room with a client who has seriously lacerated both wrists. The initial nursing action is to
    1 Examine and treat the wound sites
    2 Secure and record a detailed history
    3 Encourage and assist client to ventilate feelings
    4 Administer an antianxiety agent

11. The nurse receives a telephone call from a male client who states that he wants to kill himself and has a bottle of sleeping pills in front of him. The best nursing action is to
    1 Insist that the client give you his name and address so that you can get the police there immediately
    2 Keep the client talking and allow the client to ventilate feelings
    3 Use therapeutic communications, especially the reflection of feelings
    4 Keep the client talking and signal to another staff member to trace the call so that appropriate help can be sent

12. The nurse is caring for a client with severe depression. Which of the following activities is most appropriate for this client?

1 Paint by number
2 A puzzle
3 Drawing
4 Checkers

13. The client in a severe major depressive episode is unable to address activities of daily living. The most appropriate nursing intervention is to
   1 Feed, bathe, and dress the client as needed until the client can perform these activities independently
   2 Structure the client's day so that adequate time can be devoted to the client's assuming responsibility for the activities of daily living
   3 Provide the client with choices and the consequences to the failure to comply with the expectation of maintaining activities of daily living
   4 Have the client's peers confront the client about how the noncompliance in addressing activities of daily living affects the milieu

14. An elderly male client who is a victim of elder abuse and the family have been attending weekly counseling sessions. Which of the following statements, if made by the abusive family member, indicates that they have learned positive coping skills?
   1 "I will be more careful to make sure that my father's needs are met."
   2 "I am so sorry and embarrassed that the abusive event occurred. It won't happen again."
   3 "I feel better able to care for my father now that I know where to obtain assistance."
   4 "Now that my father is moving into my home, I will need to change my ways."

15. The nurse is assisting in planning care for a client being admitted to the nursing unit who attempted suicide. Which of the following priority nursing interventions does the nurse include in the plan of care?
   1 Check whereabouts of the client every 15 minutes
   2 Suicide precautions with 30-minute checks
   3 One-to-one suicide precautions
   4 Ask that the client report suicidal thoughts immediately

ANSWERS

1. **3**

RATIONALE: A situational crisis arises from external rather than internal sources. External situations that could precipitate crisis include loss of or change of a job, the death of a loved one, abortion, a change in financial status, divorce, the addition of new family members, pregnancy, and severe illness. Options 1, 2, and 4 identify adventitious crisis. An adventitious crisis is not a part of everyday life, is unplanned, and is accidental.

TEST-TAKING STRATEGY: Knowledge regarding the types of crisis situations is required to answer this question. You should be able to eliminate options 1, 2, and 4 because of the nature of their similarity. If you had difficulty with this question, review the types of crisis now.
LEVEL OF COGNITIVE ABILITY: Comprehension
PHASE OF NURSING PROCESS: Data Collection
CLIENT NEEDS: Psychosocial Integrity
CONTENT AREA: Mental Health
REFERENCE
Varcarolis, E. (1998). *Foundations of psychiatric mental health nursing* (3rd ed.). Philadelphia: W. B. Saunders. pp. 368–369.

2. **1**

RATIONALE: A nurse's initial task when gathering data from a client in crisis is to assess the individual or family and the problem. The more clearly the problem can be defined, the better the chance a solution can be found. Option 1 will assist in determining data related to the precipitating event that led to the crisis. Options 2 and 4 identify situational supports. Option 3 identifies personal coping skills.

TEST-TAKING STRATEGY: Note the key words "precipitating event." Focus on these key words when selecting the correct option. Eliminate options 2 and 4 because these data will determine support systems. Eliminate option 3 because this question would be asked when determining coping skills.

LEVEL OF COGNITIVE ABILITY: Application
PHASE OF NURSING PROCESS: Data Collection
CLIENT NEEDS: Psychosocial Integrity
CONTENT AREA: Mental Health
REFERENCE
Varcarolis, E. (1998). *Foundations of psychiatric mental health nursing* (3rd ed.). Philadelphia: W. B. Saunders. pp. 370–371.

3. **4**

RATIONALE: Although each crisis response can be described in similar terms as far as presenting symptoms are concerned, what constitutes a crisis for one person may not constitute a crisis for another person because each is a unique individual. Being in the crisis state does not mean that the client is suffering from an emotional or mental illness

TEST-TAKING STRATEGY: Eliminate option 1 because of the word "all." Next eliminate options 2 and 3 because a crisis does not indicate "illness." Review the characteristics of a crisis state now if you had difficulty with this question.

LEVEL OF COGNITIVE ABILITY: Comprehension
PHASE OF NURSING PROCESS: Planning
CLIENT NEEDS: Psychosocial Integrity
CONTENT AREA: Mental Health
REFERENCE
Varcarolis, E. (1998). *Foundations of psychiatric mental health nursing* (3rd ed.). Philadelphia: W. B. Saunders. p. 367.

4. **1**

RATIONALE: The best statement is to ask the client what is causing the anger. This will assist the client to become aware of the behavior and may assist the nurse in planning appropriate interventions for the client. Option 2 is demanding behavior, which could cause increased agitation in the client. Options 3 and 4 are threats to the client and are inappropriate.

TEST-TAKING STRATEGY: Eliminate option 2 because of the demand that it places on the client. Eliminate options 3 and 4 because they indicate threats to the client. Review appropriate nursing actions for the violent client now if you had difficulty with this question.

LEVEL OF COGNITIVE ABILITY: Application
PHASE OF NURSING PROCESS: Implementation
CLIENT NEEDS: Psychosocial Integrity
CONTENT AREA: Mental Health
REFERENCE
Varcarolis, E. (1998). *Foundations of psychiatric mental health nursing* (3rd ed.). Philadelphia: W. B. Saunders. p. 301.

5. **3**

RATIONALE: Clients who are depressed may be at risk for suicide. It is critical for the nurse to assess suicidal ideation and plan. Ask the client directly if a plan for self-harm exists.

TEST-TAKING STRATEGY: Use therapeutic communication techniques. Option 3 is the only option that deals directly with the client's feelings. Additionally, clients at risk for suicide need to be directly assessed regarding the potential for self-harm.

LEVEL OF COGNITIVE ABILITY: Application
PHASE OF NURSING PROCESS: Implementation
CLIENT NEEDS: Psychosocial Integrity
CONTENT AREA: Mental Health
REFERENCE
Varcarolis, E. (1998). *Foundations of psychiatric mental health nursing* (3rd ed.). Philadelphia: W. B. Saunders. p. 192.

6. **2**

RATIONALE: The client is experiencing loss and is feeling hopeless. The most therapeutic response by the nurse is the one that attempts to translate words into feelings.

TEST-TAKING STRATEGY: This question tests your knowledge of the therapeutic communication that will assist the client to express the loneliness that the client is feeling. In option 1 the nurse is voicing doubt that is often used when a client verbalizes delusional ideas. In option 3 the nurse is disagreeing with the client, which implies that the nurse has passed judgment on the client's ideas or opinions. In option 4 the nurse uses sarcasm, which gives advice and is nontherapeutic as a nursing response.

LEVEL OF COGNITIVE ABILITY: Application
PHASE OF NURSING PROCESS: Implementation
CLIENT NEEDS: Psychosocial Integrity
CONTENT AREA: Mental Health
REFERENCE
Stuart, G. W., & Laraia, M. T. (1998). *Principles and practice of psychiatric nursing.* (6th ed.). St. Louis: Mosby–Year Book. p. 17.

7. **2**

RATIONALE: The client should be placed in a room near the nurses' station and not at the end of a long, relatively unprotected corridor. The nurse should not isolate self with a potentially violent client. The door to the client's room should be kept open and the nurse should never turn away from the client. A security officer or another staff member should be within immediate call should a suspicion of violence be imminent.

TEST-TAKING STRATEGY: Note the key word "not" in the stem of the question. Keeping in mind that safety is the issue, you should easily be able to select the correct option. If you had difficulty with this question, review guidelines in caring for the violent client.

LEVEL OF COGNITIVE ABILITY: Application
PHASE OF NURSING PROCESS: Implementation
CLIENT NEEDS: Safe, Effective Care Environment
CONTENT AREA: Mental Health
REFERENCE
Varcarolis, E. (1998). *Foundations of psychiatric mental health nursing* (3rd ed.). Philadelphia: W. B. Saunders. p. 305.

8. **4**

RATIONALE: A depressed, suicidal client often "gives" away that which is of value as a way of saying good-bye and wanting to be remembered. Options 1, 2, and 3 identify acting-out behaviors.

TEST-TAKING STRATEGY: Options 1, 2, and 3 are similar in that they deal with anger and "acting-out behaviors," which are often typical of any adolescent. Option 4 is differ-

ent in nature and an action that could indicate that the client may be saying good-bye.
LEVEL OF COGNITIVE ABILITY: Comprehension
PHASE OF NURSING PROCESS: Data Collection
CLIENT NEEDS: Psychosocial Integrity
CONTENT AREA: Mental Health
REFERENCE
Varcarolis, E. (1998). *Foundations of psychiatric mental health nursing* (3rd ed.). Philadelphia: W. B. Saunders. p. 730.

9. **1**

RATIONALE: Hanging is a serious suicide attempt. The plan of care must reflect action that will promote the client's safety. Constant observation status (one to one) with a staff member who is never less than an arm's length away is the best selection.
TEST-TAKING STRATEGY: Eliminate option 2 because seclusion is not the best intervention. Eliminate option 4 next because the responsibility to safeguard a client is not the peer's responsibility. Eliminate option 3 because removing one's clothing will not maximize all possible safety strategies. Review nursing interventions for the client at risk for suicide now if you had difficulty with this question.
LEVEL OF COGNITIVE ABILITY: Application
PHASE OF NURSING PROCESS: Planning
CLIENT NEEDS: Safe, Effective Care Environment
CONTENT AREA: Mental Health
REFERENCE
Varcarolis, E. (1998). *Foundations of psychiatric mental health nursing* (3rd ed.). Philadelphia: W. B. Saunders. p. 736.

10. **1**

RATIONALE: The initial nursing action is to examine and treat the self-inflicted injuries. Injuries from lacerated wrists can lead to a life-threatening situation. Other interventions may follow after the client has been treated medically.
TEST-TAKING STRATEGY: Use Maslow's hierarchy of needs theory to prioritize. Physiological needs come first. Option 1 addresses the physiological need.
LEVEL OF COGNITIVE ABILITY: Application
PHASE OF NURSING PROCESS: Implementation
CLIENT NEEDS: Physiological Integrity
CONTENT AREA: Mental Health
REFERENCE
deWit, S. (1998). *Essentials of medical-surgical nursing* (4th ed.). Philadelphia: W. B. Saunders. p. 28.

11. **4**

RATIONALE: In a crisis, the nurse must take an authoritative, active role to promote the client's safety. A bottle of sleeping pills in front of a client who verbalizes he wants to kill himself is a crisis. The client's safety is of prime concern. Keeping the client on the phone and getting help to the client is the best intervention.
TEST-TAKING STRATEGY: Although each of the options may seem appropriate, the best option is option 4. It is the most global response and encompasses every necessary action. The word "insist" may anger the client and he or she might hang up. Option 2 lacks the authoritative action stance of securing the client's safety. Using therapeutic communication is important, but overuse of "reflection" may sound uncaring or superficial and is lacking direction/solutions to the immediate problem of the client's safety.
LEVEL OF COGNITIVE ABILITY: Comprehension
PHASE OF NURSING PROCESS: Implementation
CLIENT NEEDS: Safe, Effective Care Environment

CONTENT AREA: Mental Health
REFERENCE
Varcarolis, E. (1998). *Foundations of psychiatric mental health nursing* (3rd ed.). Philadelphia: W. B. Saunders. p. 737.

12. **3**

RATIONALE: Concentration and memory are poor in severe depression. When a client has a diagnosis of severe depression, the nurse needs to provide activities that require little concentration. Activities that have no right or wrong choices or decisions minimize opportunities for clients to put themselves down.
TEST-TAKING STRATEGY: Knowledge of the nursing interventions that are indicated when working with clients who are depressed is required to assist you in answering this question. It is important to remember that clients with depression have difficulty concentrating and need activities that require little concentration. You must carefully select the option that meets this criterion.
LEVEL OF COGNITIVE ABILITY: Application
PHASE OF NURSING PROCESS: Implementation
CLIENT NEEDS: Psychosocial Integrity
CONTENT AREA: Mental Health
REFERENCE
Varcarolis, E. (1998). *Foundations of psychiatric mental health nursing* (3rd ed.). Philadelphia: W. B. Saunders. p. 566.

13. **1**

RATIONALE: The symptoms of major depression include depressed mood, loss of interest or pleasure, changes in appetite and sleep patterns, psychomotor agitation or retardation, fatigue, feelings of worthlessness/guilt, diminished ability to think or concentrate, and recurrent thoughts of death. Often the clients do not have the energy or interest to complete activities of daily living. Frequently, severely depressed clients are unable to perform even the simplest of activities of daily living. The nurse assumes this role and completes these tasks with the client. In doing so, the nurse establishes a therapeutic relationship as the nurse demonstrates respect and acceptance of the client and contributes to fostering the client's self-esteem.
TEST-TAKING STRATEGY: Note the key words "severe major depressive episode." Eliminate options 2 and 3 because the client lacks the energy and motivation to do these independently. In addition, option 3 may lead to increased feelings of worthlessness as the client fails to meet expectations. Option 4 will increase the client's feelings of poor self-esteem and unworthiness.
LEVEL OF COGNITIVE ABILITY: Application
PHASE OF NURSING PROCESS: Implementation
CLIENT NEEDS: Psychosocial Integrity
CONTENT AREA: Mental Health
REFERENCE
deWit, S. (1998). *Essentials of medical-surgical nursing* (4th ed.). Philadelphia: W. B. Saunders. p. 1002.

14. **3**

RATIONALE: Elder abuse is sometimes the result of family members who are being expected to care for their aging parents. This care can cause the family to become overextended, frustrated, or financially depleted. Knowing where to turn in the community for assistance in caring for aging family members can bring much needed relief. Using these alternatives is a positive alternative coping strategy that many families take advantage of.

TEST-TAKING STRATEGY: The stem of the question asks for a coping strategy. Only option 3 is a means of coping with the issues. The other responses are statements of good faith or promises which may or may not be kept in the future. Only option 3 outlines a definitive plan for how to handle the pressure associated with the father's care.
LEVEL OF COGNITIVE ABILITY: Comprehension
PHASE OF NURSING PROCESS: Evaluation
CLIENT NEEDS: Psychosocial Integrity
CONTENT AREA: Mental Health
REFERENCE
Varcarolis, E. (1998). *Foundations of psychiatric mental health nursing* (3rd ed.). Philadelphia: W. B. Saunders. p. 408.

15. **3**

RATIONALE: One-to-one suicide precaution is required for the client who has attempted suicide. Options 1 and 2 may be appropriate but not at the present time considering the situation. Option 4 may also be an appropriate nursing intervention, but the priority is stated in option 3. The best option is constant supervision so that the nurse may intervene as needed if the client attempts to cause harm to self.
TEST-TAKING STRATEGY: Note the key word "priority" in the stem of the question. Options 1 and 2 can be easily eliminated. Focusing on the key word will easily direct you to option 3. Review interventions for the suicidal client now if you had difficulty with this question.
LEVEL OF COGNITIVE ABILITY: Application
PHASE OF NURSING PROCESS: Implementation
CLIENT NEEDS: Safe, Effective Care Environment
CONTENT AREA: Mental Health
REFERENCE
deWit, S. (1998). *Essentials of medical-surgical nursing* (4th ed.). Philadelphia: W. B. Saunders. p. 1005.

BIBLIOGRAPHY

deWit, S. (1998). *Essentials of medical-surgical nursing* (4th ed.). Philadelphia: W. B. Saunders.

Glod, C. A. (1998). *Contemporary psychiatric-mental health nursing.* Philadelphia: F. A. Davis.

Hodgson, B., & Kizior, R. (2000). *Saunders nursing drug handbook 2000.* Philadelphia: W. B. Saunders.

Stuart, G. W., & Laraia, M. T. (1998). *Principles and practice of psychiatric nursing.* (6th ed.). St. Louis: Mosby–Year Book.

Varcarolis, E. (1998). *Foundations of psychiatric mental health nursing* (3rd ed.). Philadelphia: W. B. Saunders.

CHAPTER 64

Psychiatric Medications

I. Selective Serotonin Reuptake Inhibitors (SSRI) (Box 64–1)

A. Description
1. Produces the inhibition of serotonin uptake
2. Produces an antidepressant response

B. Side effects
1. Nausea
2. Diarrhea
3. Central nervous system (CNS) stimulation
4. Dry mouth
5. Photosensitivity
6. Insomnia
7. Headache
8. Nervousness
9. Dizziness
10. Weight loss

C. Implementation
1. Monitor vital signs
2. Monitor weight
3. Initiate safety precautions, particularly if dizziness occurs
4. Instruct the client to take a single morning dose to prevent insomnia
5. Administer with a snack or with meals, which reduces the risk of dizziness and light-headedness
6. Monitor the suicidal client especially during improved mood and increased energy levels
7. For clients on long-term therapy, monitor liver and renal function tests
8. Monitor WBC and neutrophil counts and discontinue the medication, as prescribed, if levels fall below normal

---

BOX 64–1. Selective Serotonin Reuptake Inhibitors (SSRIs)

Fluoxetine hydrochloride (Prozac)
Sertraline hydrochloride (Zoloft)
Paroxetine (Paxil)
Nefazodone (Serzone)
Trazodone (Desyrel)

---

9. If priapism (painful, prolonged penile erection) occurs, discontinue medication immediately and notify the physician
10. Instruct the client to change positions slowly to avoid hypotensive effect
11. Instruct the client to avoid alcohol
12. Instruct the client to report any visual changes to the physician

II. Tricyclic and Second-Generation Antidepressants (Box 64–2)

A. Description
1. Blocks the reuptake of norepinephrine and serotonin at the presynaptic neuron
2. Used to treat depression
3. May reduce seizure threshold
4. May reduce effectiveness of antihypertensive agents
5. Concurrent use with alcohol or antihistamines can cause CNS depression
6. Concurrent use with MAO inhibitors can cause hypertensive **crisis**

B. Side effects
1. Anticholinergic effects
2. Dry mouth
3. Decreased GI motility and constipation
4. Difficulty voiding
5. Dilated pupils and blurred vision
6. Photosensitivity
7. Cardiovascular disturbances
8. Tachycardia
9. Orthostatic hypotension
10. Dysrhythmias
11. Sedation
12. Weight gain
13. Anxiety, restlessness, and irritability
14. Decreased or increased libido with ejaculatory and erection disturbances

C. Implementation
1. Instruct the client that the drug may take several weeks to produce the desired effect
2. Client response may not occur until 2 to 4 weeks after the first dose

> **BOX 64–2. Tricyclic and Second-Generation Antidepressants**
>
> Clomipramine hydrochloride (Anafranil)
> Amitriptyline hydrochloride (Elavil)
> Imipramine hydrochloride (Tofranil)
> Norpramine (Desipramine)
> Nortriptyline hydrochloride (Pamelor, Aventyl)
> Perphenazine and amitriptyline (Triavil)
> Doxepin hydrochloride (Sinequan)
> Chlordiazepoxide and amitriptyline (Limbitrol)
> Bupropion (Wellbutrin)
> Fluoxetine (Prozac)
> Trazodone (Desyrel)
> Amoxapine (Afenidid)

3. Monitor for compliance of therapy
4. Monitor the suicidal client especially during improved mood and increased energy levels
5. Instruct the client to change positions slowly to avoid hypotensive effect
6. Monitor the pattern of daily bowel activity
7. Monitor for urinary retention by bladder palpation
8. For clients on long-term therapy, monitor liver and renal function tests
9. Administer with food or milk if GI distress occurs
10. Administer the entire daily oral dose at one time, preferably at bedtime
11. Instruct the client on fluoxetine (Prozac) to take the medication early in the day to avoid interfering with sleep
12. Instruct the client to avoid alcohol and nonprescription medications to prevent adverse drug interactions
13. Instruct the client to avoid driving and other activities requiring alertness
14. When the medication is discontinued, it should be tapered gradually

III. Monoamine Oxidase Inhibitors (MAOIs)
(Box 64–3)

A. Description
1. Inhibits monoamine oxidase enzyme, which is present in the brain, blood platelets, liver, spleen, and kidneys
2. Inhibition of the MAO enzyme metabolizes amines, norepinephrine, and serotonin; the concentration of these amines increases
3. Used for depression in clients who have not

> **BOX 64–3. Monoamine Oxidase Inhibitors (MAOIs)**
>
> Isocarboxazid (Marplan)
> Phenelzine sulfate (Nardil)
> Tranylcypromine sulfate (Parnate)

responded to other antidepressant therapy, including electroconvulsive shock therapy
4. Concurrent use with amphetamines, antidepressants, dopamine, epinephrine, guanethidine, levodopa, methyldopa, nasal decongestants, norepinephrine, reserpine, tyramine-containing foods, and vasoconstrictors may cause hypertensive **crisis**
5. Concurrent use with narcotic analgesics may cause hypertension or hypotension, coma, or seizures

B. Side effects
1. Postural hypotension
2. Restlessness
3. Insomnia
4. Dizziness
5. Lethargy
6. Weakness
7. GI upset
8. Dry mouth
9. Weight gain
10. Peripheral edema
11. Anticholinergic effects
12. CNS stimulation including anxiety, agitation, and mania
13. Delay in ejaculation

C. Hypertensive **crisis**
1. Hypertension
2. Occipital headache radiating frontally
3. Neck stiffness and soreness
4. Nausea and vomiting
5. Sweating
6. Fever and chills
7. Clammy skin
8. Dilated pupils
9. Palpitations
10. Tachycardia or bradycardia
11. Constricting chest pain

D. Implementation
1. Monitor blood pressure frequently for hypertension
2. Monitor for signs of hypertensive **crisis**
3. If palpitations or frequent headaches occur, discontinue the medication and notify the physician
4. Administer with food if GI distress occurs
5. Instruct the client that the medication effect may be noted during the first week of therapy but maximum benefit may take up to 3 weeks
6. Instruct the client to report headache, neck stiffness, or soreness immediately
7. Instruct the client to change positions slowly to prevent orthostatic hypotension
8. Instruct the client to avoid caffeine or over-the-counter preparations such as weight-reducing pills, or medications for hay fever and colds
9. Monitor for client compliance with medication administration
10. Instruct clients to carry a Medic-Alert card

BOX 64–4. Tyramine Foods to Avoid

Cheese, especially aged except cottage cheese
Sour cream
Pickled herring
Avocados
Bananas
Papaya
Broad beans
Figs
Overripe fruit
Brewer's yeast
Meat extracts and tenderizers
Yogurt
Sausage, bologna, pepperoni, salami
Soy sauce
Raisins
Red wine, beer, sherry
Beef or chicken liver
Caffeine such as coffee, tea, or chocolate

indicating that they are taking an MAOI medication
11. Avoid administering the medication in the evening because insomnia may result
12. MAO inhibitors should be tapered and discontinued 7 to 14 days before surgery
13. When the medication is discontinued, it should be discontinued gradually
14. Instruct the client to avoid foods that require bacteria/molds for their preparation/preservation or those that contain tyramine (Box 64–4)

IV. Antimanic Medications (Box 64–5)

A. Description
1. Affects cellular transport mechanism; alters both the presynaptic and postsynaptic events affecting serotonin, thus enhancing serotonin function
2. Concurrent use with diuretics, fluoxetine, methyldopa, or nonsteroidal anti-inflammatory medications increases lithium reabsorption by the kidney, or inhibits lithium excretion, either of which increases the risk of lithium toxicity
3. Acetazolamide, aminophylline, phenothiazines, sodium bicarbonate, and increased sodium intake may increase renal excretion of lithium, reducing its effectiveness
4. The therapeutic dose is only slightly less than the amount producing toxicity
5. The therapeutic drug serum level is 0.5 to 1.3 mEq/L

BOX 64–5. Antimanic Medications

Lithium carbonate (Eskalith, Lithane, Lithobid)
Lithium citrate (Cibalith-S)

6. The causes of an increase in lithium level include decreased sodium intake, fluid and electrolyte loss associated with severe sweating, dehydration, diarrhea, diuretic therapy or illness, and overdose
7. Serum lithium levels should be checked every 1 to 2 months or whenever any behavioral change suggests altered serum levels
8. Blood samples to check serum lithium levels should be drawn in the morning, 12 hours after the last dose
B. Side effects
1. Polyuria
2. Polydipsia
3. Anorexia
4. Nausea
5. Dry mouth
6. Mild thirst
7. Weight gain
8. Abdominal bloating
9. Soft stools or diarrhea
10. Fine hand tremors
11. Inability to concentrate
12. Muscle weakness
13. Lethargy
14. Fatigue
15. Headache
16. Hair loss
C. Implementation
1. Monitor the suicidal client especially during improved mood and increased energy levels
2. Administer medication with food to minimize GI irritation
3. Instruct the client to maintain a fluid intake of 6 to 8 glasses of water a day
4. Instruct the client to avoid excessive amounts of coffee, tea, or cola, which have a diuretic effect
5. Instruct the client to maintain an adequate salt intake
6. Do not administer diuretics while the client is taking lithium
7. Instruct the client to avoid alcohol
8. Instruct the client to avoid over-the-counter medications
9. Instruct clients that they may take a missed dose within 2 hours of the scheduled time; otherwise, they should skip the missed dose and take the next dose at the scheduled time
10. Instruct the client not to adjust dosage without consulting the physician because lithium should be tapered off and not discontinued abruptly
11. Instruct the client about the signs and symptoms of lithium toxicity
12. Instruct the client to notify the physician if polyuria, prolonged vomiting, diarrhea, or fever occurs
13. Instruct the client that the therapeutic response to the medication will be noted in 1 to 3 weeks

14. Monitor lithium levels, electrocardiogram (ECG), renal function tests, and thyroid tests

D. Lithium toxicity
   1. Description
      a. Occurs when ingested lithium cannot be detoxified and excreted by the kidneys
      b. Occurs when serum lithium level exceeds 1.5 mEq/L
   2. Mild toxicity
      a. Serum lithium level of 1.5 to 2.0 mEq/L
      b. Apathy
      c. Lethargy
      d. Diminished concentration
      e. Mild ataxia and muscle weakness
      f. Coarse hand tremors
      g. Slight muscle weakness
   3. Moderate toxicity
      a. Serum lithium level of 2.0 to 2.5 mEq/L
      b. Nausea
      c. Vomiting
      d. Severe diarrhea
      e. Mild to moderate ataxia and incoordination
      f. Slurred speech
      g. Tinnitus
      h. Blurred vision
      i. Muscle twitching
      j. Irregular tremor
   4. Severe toxicity
      a. Serum lithium level above 2.5 mEq/L
      b. Nystagmus
      c. Muscle fasciculations
      d. Deep tendon hyperreflexia
      e. Visual or tactile hallucinations
      f. Oliguria or anuria
      g. Impaired level of consciousness (LOC)
      h. Grand mal seizure or coma leading to death
   5. Implementation for lithium toxicity
      a. Hold lithium and notify the physician
      b. Monitor vital signs and LOC
      c. Monitor cardiac status
      d. Prepare to obtain lithium level; electrolyte, blood urea nitrogen (BUN), and creatinine counts; and CBC counts
      e. Monitor for suicidal tendencies and institute **suicide** precautions

V. Antianxiety or Anxiolytic Medications
(Box 64–6)

A. Description
   1. Depresses the central nervous system (CNS), thereby increasing the effects of gamma-aminobutyric acid (GABA), which produces relaxation and may depress the limbic system
   2. Benzodiazepines have anxiety-reducing (anxiolytic), sedative-hypnotic, muscle-relaxing, and anticonvulsant actions
B. Side effects
   1. Daytime sedation
   2. Ataxia

BOX 64–6. Benzodiazepines

Diazepam (Valium)
Alprazolam (Xanax)
Clorazepate (Tranxene)
Oxazepam (Serax)
Flurazepam (Dalmane)
Temazepam (Restoril)
Triazolam (Halcion)
Lorazepam (Ativan)
Estazolam (ProSom)
Chlordiazepoxide (Librium)
Clonazepam (Klonopin)
Halazepam (Paxipam)
Ketazolam (Loftran)
Prazepam (Centrax)
Quazepam (Doral)

---

   3. Dizziness
   4. Headaches
   5. Blurred or double vision
   6. Hypotension
   7. Tremor
   8. Amnesia
   9. Slurred speech
   10. Urinary incontinence
   11. Constipation
   12. Paradoxical CNS excitement
C. Acute toxicity
   1. Somnolence
   2. Confusion
   3. Diminished reflexes and coma
   4. Flumazenil (Mazicon), a benzodiazepine antagonist, administered IV, will reverse benzodiazepine intoxication in 5 minutes
   5. Clients being treated for an overdose of benzodiazepines may experience agitation, restlessness, discomfort, and anxiety
D. Implementation
   1. Monitor for motor responses such as agitation, trembling, and tension
   2. Monitor for autonomic responses such as cold, clammy hands and sweating
   3. Monitor for paradoxical CNS excitement during early therapy, particularly in the elderly and debilitated
   4. Monitor for visual disturbances because the medications can worsen glaucoma
   5. Monitor liver and renal function tests and blood counts
   6. Reduce the medication dose as prescribed for older adult clients and for clients with impaired liver function
   7. Initiate safety precautions because older adult clients are at risk for falling when taking these medications for sleep or anxiety
   8. Assist with ambulation if drowsiness or light-headedness occurs
   9. Instruct the client that drowsiness usually disappears during continued therapy
   10. Instruct clients to avoid tasks that require

alertness until the response to the medication is established

11. Instruct clients to avoid alcohol
12. Instruct clients not to take other medications without consulting the physician
13. Instruct clients not to abruptly withdraw the medication

E. Withdrawal
   1. To lessen withdrawal symptoms, the dosage of benzodiazepines should be tapered gradually over 2 to 6 weeks
   2. Abrupt or too rapid withdrawal results in
      a. Restlessness
      b. Irritability
      c. Insomnia
      d. Hand tremors
      e. Abdominal or muscle cramps
      f. Sweating
      g. Vomiting
      h. Seizures

VI. Disulfiram (Antabuse) Therapy (Refer to Chapter 62 for information regarding this therapy)

VII. Medications for Insomnia and Anxiety (Box 64–7)

A. Description
   1. Depresses the reticular activating system by promoting the inhibitory synaptic action of the neurotransmitter GABA
   2. Used for short-term treatment of insomnia or for sedation to relieve anxiety, tension, and apprehension
B. Side effects
   1. Confusion
   2. Irritability
   3. Allergic reactions
   4. Agranulocytosis
   5. Thrombocytopenic purpura
   6. Megaloblastic anemia
C. Overdose
   1. Tachycardia
   2. Hypotension
   3. Cold and clammy skin

BOX 64–7. Barbiturates

Amobarbital (Amytal)
Aprobarbital (Alurate)
Butabarbital (Butisol)
Pentobarbital (Nembutal)
Phenobarbital (Luminal)
Secobarbital (Seconal)
Busparone (BuSpar)
Chloral hydrate (Noctec)
Ethchlorvynol (Placidyl)
Hydroxyzine hydrochloride (Atarax)
Meprobamate (Equanil)
Zolpidem tartrate (Ambien)

---

4. Dilated pupils
5. Weak and rapid pulse
6. Signs of shock
7. Depressed respirations
8. Absent reflexes
9. Coma and death may result from respiratory and cardiovascular collapse

D. Withdrawal
   1. Severe withdrawal symptoms begin within 24 hours after the medication is discontinued in an individual with severe drug dependence
   2. Gradual withdrawal is used to detoxify a dependent person
   3. Anxiety
   4. Insomnia
   5. Nightmares
   6. Daytime agitation
   7. Tremors
   8. Delirium
   9. Convulsions
E. Implementation
   1. Administer lower doses as prescribed for elderly clients
   2. Medications should be used with caution in clients who are suicidal or have a history of drug **addiction**
   3. Maintain safety by supervising ambulation and using side rails at night
   4. Instruct the client to take medication as directed
   5. Instruct clients to avoid driving or operating hazardous equipment if drowsiness, dizziness, or unsteadiness occurs
   6. Instruct clients to avoid alcohol
   7. For insomnia, instruct the client to take medication 30 minutes before bedtime
   8. Instruct the client that a hangover effect may occur in the morning
   9. Instruct the client not to abruptly discontinue the medication
   10. Instruct the client taking chloral hydrate (Noctec), to take the medication with food or a full glass of water, fruit juice, or ginger ale to improve the taste and to prevent gastric irritation

VIII. Antipsychotic Medications (Box 64–8)

A. Description
   1. Improves the thought processes and behavior of clients with psychotic symptoms, especially those with schizophrenia
   2. Blocks dopamine receptors in the brain, thereby reducing the psychotic symptoms
   3. Blocks the chemoreceptor trigger zone and vomiting center in the brain, producing an antiemetic effect
   4. Phenothiazines lower the seizure threshold
   5. Antipsychotics should not be given with other antipsychotic or antidepressant medications
B. Side effects
   1. Anticholinergic effects

BOX 64–8. Antipsychotic Medications

PHENOTHIAZINES

Chlorpromazine hydrochloride (Thorazine)
Promazine hydrochloride (Sparine)
Triflupromazine (Vesprin)
Fluphenazine hydrochloride (Prolixin)
Perphenazine (Trilafon)
Prochlorperazine maleate (Compazine)
Acetophenazine maleate (Tindal)
Trifluoperazine hydrochloride (Stelazine)
Mesoridazine besylate (Serentil)
Thioridazine hydrochloride (Mellaril)

NONPHENOTHIAZINES

Droperidol (Inapsine)
Haloperidol (Haldol)
Loxapine (Loxitane)
Chlorprothixene hydrochloride (Taractan)
Thiothixene hydrochloride (Navane)

OTHER ANTIPSYCHOTICS

Clozapine (Clozaril)
Molindone hydrochloride (Moban)
Risperidone (Risperdal)

  2. Dry mouth
  3. Increased heart rate
  4. Urinary retention
  5. Constipation
  6. Hypotension
  7. Drowsiness
  8. Blood dyscrasias
  9. Pruritus
  10. Photosensitivity
C. Extrapyramidal syndrome
  1. Parkinsonism
    a. Tremors
    b. Masklike facies
    c. Rigidity
    d. Shuffling gait
  2. Dystonia
    a. Facial grimacing
    b. Abnormal or involuntary eye movements
  3. Akathisia
    a. Restlessness
    b. Constant moving about
  4. Tardive dyskinesia
    a. Protrusion of the tongue
    b. Chewing motion
    c. Involuntary movement of the body and extremities
D. Implementation
  1. Monitor vital signs
  2. Monitor for extrapyramidal syndrome
  3. Monitor for symptoms of neuroleptic malignant syndrome
  4. Monitor urine output
  5. Monitor serum glucose level
  6. Note that clients taking antipsychotic medications may require long-term medication for parkinsonian symptoms

  7. For oral use, the liquid form might be preferred because some clients hide tablets to avoid taking them
  8. Administer medication with food or milk to decrease gastric irritation
  9. Note that the absorption rate is faster with the liquid form
  10. Avoid skin contact with liquid concentrates to prevent contact dermatitis
  11. Protect liquid concentrates from light
  12. Dilute liquid concentrates with fruit juice
  13. Inform the client that a full therapeutic effect of the medication may not be evident for 3 to 6 weeks following initiation of therapy; however, an observable therapeutic response may be apparent after 7 to 10 days
  14. Inform client that phenothiazines may cause a harmless pinkish to red-brown urine
  15. Instruct the client to use sunscreen, hats, and protective clothing when outdoors
  16. Instruct clients to avoid alcohol or other CNS depressants
  17. Instruct clients to change positions slowly to avoid orthostatic hypotension
  18. Instruct clients to report signs of agranulocytosis including sore throat, fever, and malaise
  19. Instruct the client to report signs of liver dysfunction including jaundice, malaise, fever, and right upper abdominal pain
  20. When discontinuing antipsychotics, the medication dosage should be reduced gradually to avoid sudden recurrence of psychotic symptoms

IX. Neuroleptic Malignant Syndrome

A. Description
  1. A potentially fatal syndrome that may occur at any time during therapy with neuroleptic medications (antipsychotic or antischizophrenic medications)
  2. Although it is rare, it is more commonly seen at the initiation of therapy, after clients are changed from one medication to another, after a dosage increase, or when a combination of medications is used
B. Data collection
  1. Difficult or fast breathing
  2. Tachycardia or irregular pulse rate
  3. Fever
  4. High or low blood pressure
  5. Increased sweating
  6. Loss of bladder control
  7. Skeletal muscle rigidity
  8. Pale skin
  9. Excessive weakness or fatigue
  10. Altered level of consciousness
  11. Seizures
  12. Severe extrapyramidal side effects
  13. Difficulty swallowing
  14. Excessive salivation

15. Oculogyric **crisis**
16. Dyskinesia
17. Elevated WBC count
18. Elevated liver function tests
19. Elevated CPK level
C. Implementation
1. Notify the physician
2. Monitor vital signs
3. Initiate safety and seizure precautions
4. Discontinue neuroleptic medication
5. Monitor level of consciousness
6. Administer antipyretics as prescribed
7. Use a cooling blanket to lower the body temperature
8. Monitor electrolytes and monitor IV fluids as prescribed

PRACTICE QUESTIONS

1. The nurse has administered a dose of diazepam (Valium) to the client. The nurse takes which of the following most important actions before leaving the room?
   1 Drawing the shades closed
   2 Putting up the side rails on the bed
   3 Giving the client a bedpan
   4 Turning the volume on the television set down

2. The nurse is assisting in preparing a teaching plan for the client who is taking lithium carbonate (Eskalith). Which of the following is not a component of the teaching plan?
   1 Lithium blood levels must be monitored very closely
   2 Stop taking the medication if excessive diarrhea, vomiting, or diaphoresis occurs
   3 Take the lithium with meals
   4 Decrease fluid intake while taking the lithium

3. The client with a psychotic disorder is being treated with haloperidol (Haldol). Which of the following indicates the presence of a toxic effect of this medication?
   1 Hypotension
   2 Nausea
   3 Excessive salivation
   4 Blurred vision

4. Buspirone hydrochloride (BuSpar) is prescribed for a client with an anxiety disorder. The nurse instructs the client regarding the medication. The nurse informs the client that which of the following is characteristic of this medication?
   1 The medication can produce a sedating effect
   2 Tolerance can occur
   3 The medication is addicting
   4 Dizziness and nervousness may occur

5. Neuroleptic malignant syndrome is suspected in a client who is taking chlorpromazine (Thorazine). Which of the following medications does the nurse prepare in anticipation of being prescribed to treat this adverse reaction related to the use of chlorpromazine?
   1 Phytonadione (vitamin K)
   2 Bromocriptine (Parlodel)
   3 Enalapril maleate (Vasotec)
   4 Protamine sulfate

6. The nurse is caring for a hospitalized client who has been taking clozapine (Clozaril) for the treatment of a schizophrenic disorder. The nurse evaluates the laboratory studies that have been prescribed for the client. Which of the following laboratory studies does the nurse specifically review to monitor for an adverse reaction associated with the use of this medication?
   1 WBC count
   2 Platelet count
   3 Cholesterol level
   4 Blood urea nitrogen

7. Disulfiram (Antabuse) is prescribed for a client who is seen in the psychiatric health care clinic. The nurse is collecting data on the client and is providing instructions regarding the use of this medication. Which of the following data is most important for the nurse to obtain before administering this medication?
   1 When the last alcoholic drink was consumed
   2 A history of diabetes insipidus
   3 A history of hyperthyroidism
   4 When the last full meal was consumed

8. The nurse is collecting data on a client, and the client's spouse reports that the client is taking donepezil hydrochloride (Aricept). Which of the following disorders does the nurse suspect that this client may have based on the use of this medication?
   1 Dementia
   2 Obsessive-compulsive disorder
   3 Seizure disorder
   4 History of schizophrenia

9. Fluoxetine hydrochloride (Prozac) is prescribed for the client. The nurse provides instructions to the client regarding the administration of the medication. Which of the following statements if made by the client indicates an understanding regarding the administration of the medication?
   1 "I should take the medication right before bedtime."
   2 "I should take the medication with my evening meal."
   3 "I should take the medication at noon time with an antacid."
   4 "I should take the medication in the morning when I first arise."

10. The nursing student is assigned to care for a client with a diagnosis of schizophrenia. Haloperidol (Haldol) is prescribed for the client. The nursing

instructor asks the student to describe the action of the medication. Which of the following statements if made by the nursing student indicates an understanding of the action of this medication?

1. "It blocks the uptake of norepinephrine and serotonin."
2. "It blocks the binding of dopamine to the postsynaptic dopamine receptors in the brain."
3. "It is a serotonin reuptake blocker."
4. "It inhibits the breakdown of released acetylcholine."

11. A client receiving lithium carbonate (Eskalith) complains of loose, watery stools and difficulty walking. The nurse expects the serum lithium level to be which of the following?
    1. 0.7 mEq/L
    2. 1.0 mEq/L
    3. 1.3 mEq/L
    4. 1.7 mEq/L

12. When teaching a client who is being started on imipramine hydrochloride (Tofranil), the nurse informs the client that the desired effects
    1. May start during the first week of administration
    2. May start during the second week of administration
    3. May not occur for 2 to 3 weeks of administration
    4. May not occur until after a month of administration

13. A client receiving thioradazine (Mellaril) complains of feeling very "faint" when trying to get out of bed in the morning, The nurse recognizes this complaint as a symptom of
    1. Psychosomatic symptoms
    2. Cardiac dysrhythmias
    3. Respiratory insufficiency
    4. Postural hypotension

14. A client who is on lithium carbonate (Eskalith) therapy is scheduled for surgery. The nurse informs the client that
    1. The medication will be discontinued several days before surgery and resumed by injection in the immediate postoperative period
    2. The medication is to be taken until the day of surgery and resumed by injection immediately postoperatively
    3. The medication will be discontinued 1 to 2 days before the surgery and resumed as soon as full oral intake is allowed
    4. The medication will be discontinued a week before the surgery and resumed a week postoperatively

15. The client receiving tricyclic antidepressants arrives at the mental health clinic. Which observa-

tion indicates that the client is correctly following the medication plan?
    1. Reports sleeping 12 hours per night and 3 to 4 hours during the day
    2. Arrives at the clinic neat and appropriate in appearance
    3. Reports not going to work for the past week
    4. Complains of not being able to "do anything" anymore

16. The nurse is performing a follow-up teaching session with a client discharged 1 month ago. The client is taking fluoxetine (Prozac). What information is important for the nurse to gather regarding the adverse effects related to the medication?
    1. Problems with excessive sweating
    2. Gastrointestinal dysfunctions
    3. Cardiovascular symptoms
    4. Problems with mouth dryness

17. The client taking buspirone hydrochloride (BuSpar) for 1 month returns to the clinic for a follow-up visit. Which of the following manifestations indicates medication effectiveness?
    1. No report of alcohol withdrawal symptoms
    2. No paranoid thought processes
    3. No rapid heartbeat or anxiety
    4. No thought broadcasting or delusions

18. A client taking lithium carbonate (Eskalith) reports vomiting, abdominal pain, diarrhea, blurred vision, tinnitus, and tremors. The lithium level is checked as a part of the routine follow-up. The level is 3 mEq/L. The nurse knows this level is
    1. Normal
    2. Slightly above normal
    3. Excessively below normal
    4. Toxic

19. A client is placed on chloral hydrate (Noctec) for short-term treatment. What nursing action indicates a clear understanding of the major side effect of this medication?
    1. Monitor neurological signs every 2 hours
    2. Monitor blood pressure (BP) every 4 hours
    3. Instruct the client to call for ambulation assistance
    4. Lower the bed and clear a path to the bathroom at bedtime

20. The client admitted to the hospital gives the nurse a bottle of clomipramine (Anafranil). The nurse notes that the medication has not been taken by the client in 2 months. What behaviors observed in the client validate noncompliance with this medication?
    1. Frequent handwashing with hot soapy water
    2. Complaints of hunger and fatigue
    3. A pulse rate below 60 bpm
    4. Complaints of insomnia

21. An adult client is administered haloperidol (Haldol) IM BID. After 3 days of therapy, which of the following should be implemented first at the beginning of the nursing shift?
    1 Check vital signs, compare the data, and record
    2 Assess the physical safety of other unit clients
    3 Monitor the client's nutritional intake
    4 Assess the client's orientation and delusional status

22. Diphenhydramine hydrochloride (Benadryl) is used in the treatment of allergic rhinitis for a hospitalized client with a chronic psychotic disorder. This medication will not be continued at home because the nurse is aware that
    1 Allergic symptoms are short term
    2 Poor compliance causes this medication to fail to reach its therapeutic blood level
    3 Addictive properties are enhanced in the presence of psychotropic medications
    4 This medication promotes long-term extrapyramidal symptoms

23. The client arrives at the health care clinic and tells the nurse that he has been doubling the daily dosage of bupropion (Wellbutrin) to aid him in getting better faster. Which ongoing data collection is required based on this information?
    1 Monitor for orthostatic hypotension
    2 Monitor for seizure activity
    3 Monitor for weight gain
    4 Monitor for insomnia

24. Immediately after taking a routine evening dose of alprazolam (Xanax), a client says, "I'm not sure I should have taken that stuff.' The best response by the nurse is
    1 "You are afraid of the media claims about this medication."
    2 "Your depression will fade once the medication begins to work."
    3 "Anxiety is expected with any new experience."
    4 "Lets talk about how you feel about Xanax for a while."

25. The physician orders phenobarbital sodium (Luminal) 10 mL by mouth daily. The medication bottle is labeled 15 mg/5 mL. What will the nurse administer?
    1 15 mg
    2 30 mg
    3 18.2 mL
    4 36.4 mL

26. A client is discharged on phenobarbital sodium (Luminal) 200 mg PO daily. Which of the following statements, if made by the client, reflects an accurate understanding of safety precautions with this medication?
    1 "I can take my medication at any time daily."
    2 "Using a daily dosing system container is critical to the prevention of an overdose."
    3 "Drinking one beer may change the way my medication works."
    4 "I must take my medication with food if I need to."

27. Fluphenazine (Prolixin) is administered to a client daily. The nurse prepares a plan of care for the client. Which of the following does the nurse include in the plan of care?
    1 Monitor the blood pressure every 2 hours
    2 Review the WBC results daily
    3 Offer a frequent snack between meals
    4 Offer hard candy or gum periodically

28. A depressed client who is on tranylcypromine sulfate (Parnate) has been instructed on diet. The nurse feels confident that the client understands the diet when given a choice of foods at a restaurant. The client selects
    1 Pepperoni pizza, salad, and cola
    2 Roasted chicken, roasted potatoes, and beer
    3 Pickled herring, french fries, and milk
    4 Fried haddock, baked potato, and cola

29. A client is being treated for her depression with amitriptyline hydrochloride (Elavil). During the initial phases of treatment, the most important nursing intervention is
    1 Ordering the client an MAO–tyramine-free diet
    2 Recognizing that frequent blood levels are in order because there is a narrow range between therapeutic and toxic blood levels of this drug
    3 Obtaining baseline postural BP on the client before administering the drug, especially during the initial days of treatment
    4 Assessing the client for anticholinergic effects

30. A client who is on lithium carbonate (Eskalith) will be discharged at the end of the week. In formulating a discharge teaching plan, the nurse instructs the client that it is most important
    1 To avoid soy sauce, wine, and aged cheese
    2 To take the medication only as prescribed because it can become addicting
    3 To check with the psychiatrist before using any over-the-counter medications or prescription drugs
    4 To have lithium levels checked every 2 weeks

ANSWERS

1. **2**

RATIONALE: Diazepam is a sedative/hypnotic with anti-convulsant and skeletal muscle–relaxant properties. The nurse should institute safety measures before leaving the client's room to ensure that the client does not injure self. The most frequent side effects of this medication are dizziness, drowsiness, and lethargy. For this reason, the nurse puts the side rails up on the bed before leaving the room to prevent falls. Options 1, 3, and 4 may be helpful measures that provide a comfortable, restful environment. However, option 2 is the one that provides for the client's safety needs.

TEST-TAKING STRATEGY: Note that the stem of the question contains the key words "most important." This tells you that more than one or all of the options may be partly or totally correct. Use Maslow's hierarchy of needs to prioritize your response. Physiological and safety needs come first.

LEVEL OF COGNITIVE ABILITY: Application
PHASE OF NURSING PROCESS: Implementation
CLIENT NEEDS: Safe, Effective Care Environment
CONTENT AREA: Pharmacology
REFERENCE
Deglin, J., & Vallerand, A. (1999). *Davis's drug guide for nurses* (6th ed.). Philadelphia: F. A. Davis. p. 263.

2. **4**

RATIONALE: Because therapeutic and toxic dosage ranges are so close, lithium blood levels must be monitored very closely, more frequently at first, then once every several months. The client should be instructed to stop taking the medication and inform the physician if excessive diarrhea, vomiting, or diaphoresis occurs. Lithium is irritating to the gastric mucosa; therefore, it should be taken with meals. A normal diet and normal salt and fluid intake (1500 to 3000 mL per day or six 12-oz glasses) should be maintained because lithium decreases sodium reabsorption by the renal tubules, which could cause sodium depletion. A low sodium intake causes an increase in lithium retention and could lead to toxicity.

TEST-TAKING STRATEGY: Note the key word "not" in the stem of the question. Remember that generally it is important that clients be taught to maintain an adequate fluid intake. This principle will easily direct you to option 4. Review the client teaching points related to the administration of this medication now if you had difficulty with this question!

LEVEL OF COGNITIVE ABILITY: Application
PHASE OF NURSING PROCESS: Planning
CLIENT NEEDS: Health Promotion and Maintenance
CONTENT AREA: Pharmacology
REFERENCE
Hodgson, B., & Kizior, R (2000). *Saunders nursing drug handbook 2000*. Philadelphia: W. B. Saunders.

3. **3**

RATIONALE: Toxic effects include extrapyramidal symptoms such as marked drowsiness and lethargy, excessive salivation and a fixed stare, akathisia, acute dystonias, and tardive dyskinesia. Hypotension, nausea, and blurred vision are occasional side effects.

TEST-TAKING STRATEGY: Knowledge regarding the toxic effects and the side effects is required to answer this question. Using the process of elimination, the best selection is option 3, "excessive" salivation, because the question asks for a toxic effect. If you had difficulty with this question, review this medication now.

LEVEL OF COGNITIVE ABILITY: Comprehension
PHASE OF NURSING PROCESS: Data Collection
CLIENT NEEDS: Physiological Integrity
CONTENT AREA: Pharmacology
REFERENCE
Hodgson, B., & Kizior, R (2000). *Saunders nursing drug handbook 2000*. Philadelphia: W. B. Saunders.

4. **4**

RATIONALE: Buspirone is used in the management of anxiety disorders. The advantages of buspirone is that it is not sedating, tolerance does not develop, and it is not addicting. The medication has a more favorable side effect profile than do the benzodiazepines. Dizziness, nausea, headaches, nervousness, light-headedness, and excitement, which generally are not major problems, are side effects of the medication.

TEST-TAKING STRATEGY: Knowledge regarding the side effects and the advantages of buspirone is required to answer this question. If you are unfamiliar with this medication and its use, take time now to review.

LEVEL OF COGNITIVE ABILITY: Application
PHASE OF NURSING PROCESS: Implementation
CLIENT NEEDS: Physiological Integrity
CONTENT AREA: Pharmacology
REFERENCE
Varcarolis, E. (1998). *Foundations of psychiatric mental health nursing* (3rd ed.). Philadelphia: W. B. Saunders. p. 1005.

5. **2**

RATIONALE: Bromocriptine is an antiparkinsonian prolactin inhibitor used in the treatment of neuroleptic malignant syndrome. Vitamin K is the antidote for warfarin overdose. Protamine sulfate is the antidote for heparin overdose. Enalapril is an angiotensin-converting enzyme (ACE inhibitor), and an antihypertensive that is used in the treatment of hypertension.

TEST-TAKING STRATEGY: Knowledge regarding the treatment for neuroleptic malignant syndrome is required to answer this question. If you are unfamiliar with the various medications used as antidotes or treatments for various syndromes, take time now to review.

LEVEL OF COGNITIVE ABILITY: Comprehension
PHASE OF NURSING PROCESS: Planning
CLIENT NEEDS: Physiological Integrity
CONTENT AREA: Pharmacology
REFERENCE
Varcarolis, E. (1998). *Foundations of psychiatric mental health nursing* (3rd ed.). Philadelphia: W. B. Saunders. p. 1008.

6. **1**

RATIONALE: Hematological reactions can occur in the client taking clozapine, and include agranulocytosis and mild leukopenia. The WBC count should be assessed prior to initiating treatment and should be monitored closely during the use of this medication. The client should also be monitored for signs indicating agranulocytosis, which may include sore throat, malaise, and fever.

TEST-TAKING STRATEGY: Knowledge regarding the adverse effects that can occur in association with the use of

clozapine is required to answer this question. If you are unfamiliar with these adverse reactions and the laboratory studies that need to be closely monitored, take time now to review.
LEVEL OF COGNITIVE ABILITY: Comprehension
PHASE OF NURSING PROCESS: Data Collection
CLIENT NEEDS: Physiological Integrity
CONTENT AREA: Pharmacology
REFERENCE
Varcarolis, E. (1998). *Foundations of psychiatric mental health nursing* (3rd ed.). Philadelphia: W. B. Saunders. pp. 1009–1010.

7. 1

RATIONALE: Disulfiram is used as an adjunct treatment for selective clients with chronic alcoholism who want to remain in a state of enforced sobriety. Clients must abstain from alcohol intake for at least 12 hours before the initial dose of the medication is administered. The most important assessment is to determine when the last alcoholic intake occurred. The medication is used with caution in clients with diabetes mellitus, hypothyroidism, epilepsy, cerebral damage, nephritis, and hepatic disease. It is also contraindicated in severe heart disease, psychosis, or hypersensitivity related to the medication.
TEST-TAKING STRATEGY: Knowledge regarding the use of this medication is required to answer this question. Knowing that the medication is used as an adjunct treatment for selective clients with chronic alcoholism will assist in directing you to option 1 as the correct answer. If you are unfamiliar with this medication, take time now to review.
LEVEL OF COGNITIVE ABILITY: Comprehension
PHASE OF NURSING PROCESS: Data Collection
CLIENT NEEDS: Physiological Integrity
CONTENT AREA: Pharmacology
REFERENCE
Varcarolis, E. (1998). *Foundations of psychiatric mental health nursing* (3rd ed.). Philadelphia: W. B. Saunders. p. 1012.

8. 1

RATIONALE: Donepezil is a cholinergic agent that is used in the treatment of mild to moderate dementia of the Alzheimer's type. It enhances cholinergic functions by increasing concentration of acetylcholine. It slows the progression of Alzheimer's disease. Options 2, 3, and 4 are incorrect.
TEST-TAKING STRATEGY: Knowledge regarding the use of donepezil is required to answer this question. If you are unfamiliar with this medication, take time now to review.
LEVEL OF COGNITIVE ABILITY: Comprehension
PHASE OF NURSING PROCESS: Data Collection
CLIENT NEEDS: Physiological Integrity
CONTENT AREA: Pharmacology
REFERENCE
Varcarolis, E. (1998). *Foundations of psychiatric mental health nursing* (3rd ed.). Philadelphia: W. B. Saunders. p. 1012.

9. 4

RATIONALE: Fluoxetine is administered in the early morning without consideration to meals. Options 1, 2, and 3 are incorrect.
TEST-TAKING STRATEGY: Knowledge regarding client instructions related to the use of fluoxetine is required to answer this question. If you are unfamiliar with the use of this medication and the client teaching points, take time now to review.
LEVEL OF COGNITIVE ABILITY: Comprehension

PHASE OF NURSING PROCESS: Evaluation
CLIENT NEEDS: Health Promotion and Maintenance
CONTENT AREA: Pharmacology
REFERENCE
Varcarolis, E. (1998). *Foundations of psychiatric mental health nursing* (3rd ed.). Philadelphia: W. B. Saunders. pp. 1013–1014.

10. 2

RATIONALE: Haloperidol acts by blocking the binding of dopamine to the postsynaptic dopamine receptors in the brain. Imipramine hydrochloride blocks the reuptake of norepinephrine and serotonin. Donepezil hydrochloride inhibits the breakdown of released acetylcholine. Fluoxetine hydrochloride is a potent serotonin reuptake blocker.
TEST-TAKING STRATEGY: Knowledge regarding the action of haloperidol is required to answer this question. If you are unfamiliar with this medication, take time now to review.
LEVEL OF COGNITIVE ABILITY: Comprehension
PHASE OF NURSING PROCESS: Evaluation
CLIENT NEEDS: Physiological Integrity
CONTENT AREA: Pharmacology
REFERENCE
Varcarolis, E. (1998). *Foundations of psychiatric mental health nursing* (3rd ed.). Philadelphia: W. B. Saunders. pp. 1012–1015.

11. 4

RATIONALE: The therapeutic serum level of lithium is 1.0 to 1.5 mEq/L for clients with acute mania and 0.8 to 1.2 mEq/L for maintenance levels. Serum lithium concentrations of 1.5 to 2.0 mEq/L may produce vomiting, diarrhea, drowsiness, incoordination, coarse hand tremors, muscle twitching, ECG T-wave depression, and mental confusion.
TEST-TAKING STRATEGY: Knowledge regarding lithium carbonate and serum lithium levels is required to answer the question. Take time now to review this information.
LEVEL OF COGNITIVE ABILITY: Comprehension
PHASE OF NURSING PROCESS: Data Collection
CLIENT NEEDS: Physiological Integrity
CONTENT AREA: Pharmacology
REFERENCE
Varcarolis, E. (1998). *Foundations of psychiatric mental health nursing* (3rd ed.). Philadelphia: W. B. Saunders. p. 1017.

12. 3

RATIONALE: The therapeutic effects of administration of imipramine hydrochloride may not occur for 2 to 3 weeks after the antidepressant therapy has been initiated.
TEST-TAKING STRATEGY: Knowledge regarding the therapeutic effects of imipramine hydrochloride is required to answer this question. Take time now to review this information. Client information regarding the medication needs to be thorough and accurate.
LEVEL OF COGNITIVE ABILITY: Application
PHASE OF NURSING PROCESS: Implementation
CLIENT NEEDS: Physiological Integrity
CONTENT AREA: Pharmacology
REFERENCE
Hodgson, B., & Kizior, R. (2000). *Saunders nursing drug handbook 2000.* Philadelphia: W. B. Saunders. p. 522.

13. 4

RATIONALE: Neuroleptic medications can cause postural hypotension. The client needs to be taught to get out of

bed and to rise from a sitting position slowly because of this untoward effect related to the medication.
TEST-TAKING STRATEGY: The key phrase in the question is "feeling faint." This phrase will direct you to the correct option. Postural hypotension is a common complaint of clients taking neuroleptic medications.
LEVEL OF COGNITIVE ABILITY: Comprehension
PHASE OF NURSING PROCESS: Data Collection
CLIENT NEEDS: Psychosocial Integrity
CONTENT AREA: Pharmacology
REFERENCE
Hodgson, B., & Kizior, R. (2000). *Saunders nursing drug handbook 2000*. Philadelphia: W. B. Saunders. p. 985.

14. **3**

RATIONALE: The client who is on lithium carbonate must be off the medication from 1 to 2 days before the surgery and can resume the medication when full oral intake is ordered after the surgery.
TEST-TAKING STRATEGY: Use the process of elimination to answer the question. Lithium carbonate is an oral medication. It cannot be given as an injection. Therefore, eliminate options 1 and 2. Option 4 identifies an unreasonable period of time. Therefore, select option 3.
LEVEL OF COGNITIVE ABILITY: Application
PHASE OF NURSING PROCESS: Implementation
CLIENT NEEDS: Physiological Integrity
CONTENT AREA: Pharmacology
REFERENCE
Hodgson, B., & Kizior, R. (2000). *Saunders nursing drug handbook 2000*. Philadelphia: W. B. Saunders. p. 598.

15. **2**

RATIONALE: Depressed individuals will sleep for long periods, are not be able to go to work, and feel as if they cannot "do anything." Once they have had some therapeutic effect from their medication, they will report resolution of many of these complaints as well as demonstrate an improvement in their appearance.
TEST-TAKING STRATEGY: Use the process of elimination to answer the question. The symptoms stated in options 1, 3, and 4 are all symptoms of depression. The improvement in appearance indicates a therapeutic response to the medication, thus compliance with the medication regimen.
LEVEL OF COGNITIVE ABILITY: Comprehension
PHASE OF NURSING PROCESS: Evaluation
CLIENT NEEDS: Physiological Integrity
CONTENT AREA: Pharmacology
REFERENCE
Varcarolis, E. (1998). *Foundations of psychiatric mental health nursing* (3rd ed.). Philadelphia: W. B. Saunders. p. 572.

16. **2**

RATIONALE: The presence of excessive sweating and dry mouth are not associated side effects of this medication. The most common adverse reactions related to this medication include central nervous system and GI system dysfunction. Fluoxetine affects the GI system by causing nausea and vomiting, cramping, and diarrhea.
TEST-TAKING STRATEGY: Knowledge regarding the side effects and adverse reactions related to fluoxetine is required to answer this question. Take time now to review this information if you had difficulty with this question.
LEVEL OF COGNITIVE ABILITY: Comprehension

PHASE OF NURSING PROCESS: Data Collection
CLIENT NEEDS: Physiological Integrity
CONTENT AREA: Pharmacology
REFERENCE
Hodgson, B., & Kizior, R. (2000). *Saunders nursing drug handbook 2000*. Philadelphia: W. B. Saunders. p. 431.

17. **3**

RATIONALE: Buspirone hydrochloride is not recommended for the treatment of drug or alcohol withdrawal, thought disorders, or schizophrenia. Buspirone is most often indicated for the treatment of anxiety and aggression.
TEST-TAKING STRATEGY: Read all four options carefully. Use the process of elimination. Knowledge regarding the use of buspirone hydrochloride will direct you to the correct option. Take time now to review this medication if you had difficulty with this question.
LEVEL OF COGNITIVE ABILITY: Analysis
PHASE OF NURSING PROCESS: Evaluation
CLIENT NEEDS: Physiological Integrity
CONTENT AREA: Pharmacology
REFERENCE
Hodgson, B., & Kizior, R. (2000). *Saunders nursing drug handbook 2000*. Philadelphia: W. B. Saunders. p. 131.

18. **4**

RATIONALE: Routine maintenance serum levels are 0.8 to 1.2 mEq/L. Mild to moderate lithium intoxication occurs at 1.5 to 2.0 mEq/L. Levels of less than 0.4 mEq/L do not produce a therapeutic effect. Severe toxic levels are reached at levels greater than 2.5 mEq/L. Lithium toxicity requires immediate medical attention with lavage and possible peritoneal dialysis or hemodialysis.
TEST-TAKING STRATEGY: Knowledge regarding lithium carbonate and serum lithium levels is required to answer the question. Take time now to review this information.
LEVEL OF COGNITIVE ABILITY: Comprehension
PHASE OF NURSING PROCESS: Data Collection
CLIENT NEEDS: Physiological Integrity
CONTENT AREA: Pharmacology
REFERENCE
Hodgson, B., & Kizior, R. (2000). *Saunders nursing drug handbook 2000*. Philadelphia: W. B. Saunders. p. 598.

19. **3**

RATIONALE: Monitoring neurological signs every 2 hours is not indicated. This medication does not cause serious neurological impairment. Blood pressure decreases to critical levels are rare in the absence of other BP problems. There may be residual daytime sedation and impairment of motor coordination; therefore, instruct the client to call for ambulation assistance.
TEST-TAKING STRATEGY: Read the options carefully. The time frames identified in options 1 and 2 are not necessary in this situation. Risk for injury is the issue of the question. The bedtime precautions in option 4 allows the client to ambulate independently, placing the client at risk. This leaves option 3 as the correct answer.
LEVEL OF COGNITIVE ABILITY: Application
PHASE OF NURSING PROCESS: Planning
CLIENT NEEDS: Safe, Effective Care Environment
CONTENT AREA: Pharmacology
REFERENCE
Hodgson, B., & Kizior, R. (2000). *Saunders nursing drug handbook 2000*. Philadelphia: W. B. Saunders. p. 198.

20. **1**

RATIONALE: Handwashing is a common obsessive-compulsive behavior. Clomipramine is commonly used in the treatment of this disorder. Weight gain is a common side effect of taking this medication. Tachycardia is an often seen side effect. Sedation may be a side effect. Insomnia may be an infrequent side effect.

TEST-TAKING STRATEGY: Knowledge regarding the purpose of this medication is required to answer the question. From this point, use the process of elimination to select the correct option. Review the purpose of this medication now if you had difficulty with this question.

LEVEL OF COGNITIVE ABILITY: Analysis
PHASE OF NURSING PROCESS: Data Collection
CLIENT NEEDS: Physiological Integrity
CONTENT AREA: Pharmacology
REFERENCE

Hodgson, B., & Kizior, R. (2000). *Saunders nursing drug handbook 2000.* Philadelphia: W. B. Saunders. p. 237.

21. **4**

RATIONALE: Haloperidol is used to treat psychotic features in clients. Vital signs are routine and not specific to this situation. Physical safety of other clients is not a direct assessment of this client. Monitoring nutritional intake has no specific value as outlined in this situation. Hallucinations, delusions, and altered thought processes may cause clients to be a danger to themselves and others.

TEST-TAKING STRATEGY: Review the situation for data that gives clues to acuity and urgency. Note that the question asks for the "first" action. Identify the client of the question and eliminate option 2. Vital signs and nutritional status are routine observations in this situation and may be delayed until potential crisis assessments are performed.

LEVEL OF COGNITIVE ABILITY: Comprehension
PHASE OF NURSING PROCESS: Implementation
CLIENT NEEDS: Physiological Integrity
CONTENT AREA: Pharmacology
REFERENCE

Hodgson, B., & Kizior, R. (2000). *Saunders nursing drug handbook 2000.* Philadelphia: W. B. Saunders. p. 486.

22. **3**

RATIONALE: Allergic symptoms may be constant as long as allergens are present. Poor compliance may be a problem in psychotic clients. This variable is not a priority in this situation. Diphenhydramine may become addictive when used with psychiatric medications. Diphenhydramine may be used as a primary management tool for extrapyramidal symptoms and mild medication-induced movement disorders.

TEST-TAKING STRATEGY: Knowledge regarding the properties of diphenhydramine hydrochloride is required to answer this question. This knowledge will assist in directing you to the correct option. Take time now to review this medication if you had difficulty with this question.

LEVEL OF COGNITIVE ABILITY: Comprehension
PHASE OF NURSING PROCESS: Planning
CLIENT NEEDS: Physiological Integrity
CONTENT AREA: Pharmacology
REFERENCE

Hodgson, B., & Kizior, R. (2000). *Saunders nursing drug handbook 2000.* Philadelphia: W. B. Saunders. p. 331.

23. **2**

RATIONALE: Bupropion does not cause significant orthostatic blood pressure changes. Seizure activity is common in dosages greater than 300 mg daily. Bupropion frequently causes a drop in body weight. Insomnia is a side effect, but seizure activity causes a greater client risk.

TEST-TAKING STRATEGY: Knowledge regarding the medication bupropion is required to answer the question. Note that the question asks for the assessment that is required. This information will assist in directing you to the correct option. Take time now to review this medication if you had difficulty with this question.

LEVEL OF COGNITIVE ABILITY: Comprehension
PHASE OF NURSING PROCESS: Data Collection
CLIENT NEEDS: Physiological Integrity
CONTENT AREA: Pharmacology
REFERENCE

Hodgson, B., & Kizior, R. (2000). *Saunders nursing drug handbook 2000.* Philadelphia: W. B. Saunders. p. 130.

24. **4**

RATIONALE: The nurse adds anxiety to the client by mentioning media concerns. Alprazolam is used to treat anxiety, not depression. Clichéd responses do not express genuine concern. The nurse should focus on assessing the reason for the client's concern and provide teaching for this client.

TEST-TAKING STRATEGY: Identify the communication tools and communication blocks noted in the options. Use the process of elimination to assist you in selecting the correct option. Always address the client's feelings first, as noted in the correct option.

LEVEL OF COGNITIVE ABILITY: Application
PHASE OF NURSING PROCESS: Implementation
CLIENT NEEDS: Psychosocial Integrity
CONTENT AREA: Pharmacology
REFERENCE

Hodgson, B., & Kizior, R. (2000). *Saunders nursing drug handbook 2000.* Philadelphia: W. B. Saunders. p. 27.

25. **2**

RATIONALE: 15 mg are administered in each 5 mL of the medication. 10 mL of medication is administered with each dose. $15 \times 2 = 30$ mg.

TEST-TAKING STRATEGY: This is a simple math calculation. However, be careful in reading the dose prescribed and the label on the medication bottle when calculating the medication dosage.

LEVEL OF COGNITIVE ABILITY: Application
PHASE OF NURSING PROCESS: Implementation
CLIENT NEEDS: Physiological Integrity
CONTENT AREA: Pharmacology
REFERENCE

Hodgson, B., & Kizior, R. (2000). *Saunders nursing drug handbook 2000.* Philadelphia: W. B. Saunders. p. 1201.

26. **3**

RATIONALE: Taking the medication at the same time daily is a good medication administration policy. Dose containers are helpful, not critical to prevent dose omissions. Hypnotics should be used with caution to prevent additive effects with other central nervous system agents. The medication may be taken without regard to meals.

TEST-TAKING STRATEGY: Read the stem of the question carefully. Use the process of elimination in answering

the question. Remember, alcohol should not be consumed when taking hypnotics.
LEVEL OF COGNITIVE ABILITY: Comprehension
PHASE OF NURSING PROCESS: Evaluation
CLIENT NEEDS: Health Promotion and Maintenance
CONTENT AREA: Pharmacology
REFERENCE
Hodgson, B., & Kizior, R. (2000). *Saunders nursing drug handbook 2000.* Philadelphia: W. B. Saunders. pp. 815–816.

27. **4**

RATIONALE: Dry mouth is a common side effect. Frequent mouth rinsing with water, sucking on hard candy, and chewing gum will alleviate this common side effect. Hypotension and hypertension are rare side effects of fluphenazine. Leukopenia is common but not viewed as a serious health threat, and the WBC is not obtained on a daily basis. Weight gain is a common side effect and frequent snacks will enhance this problem.
TEST-TAKING STRATEGY: Knowledge regarding side effects related to this medication is required to answer the question. Eliminate options 1 and 2. It is unlikely that the client needs BP monitoring every 2 hours or that a WBC will be drawn daily. Offering a frequent snack is not specific. Review the common side effects related to fluphenazine now if you had difficulty with this question.
LEVEL OF COGNITIVE ABILITY: Application
PHASE OF NURSING PROCESS: Planning
CLIENT NEEDS: Physiological Integrity
CONTENT AREA: Pharmacology
REFERENCE
Hodgson, B., & Kizior, R. (2000). *Saunders nursing drug handbook 2000.* Philadelphia: W. B. Saunders. p. 434.

28. **4**

RATIONALE: Tranylcypromine sulfate is an MAO inhibitor used to treat depression. A tyramine-restricted diet is required while on this medication to avoid hypertensive crisis, a life-threatening side effect of the medication. Foods to be avoided are meats prepared with tenderizer, smoked or pickled fish, beef or chicken liver, and dry sausage (salami, pepperoni, bologna). In addition, figs, bananas, aged cheese, yogurt and sour cream, beer, red wine and other alcoholic beverages, soy sauce, yeast extract, chocolate, caffeine, and aged, pickled, fermented, or smoked foods need to be avoided. Many over-the-counter medications also include tyramine and must be avoided as well.
TEST-TAKING STRATEGY: A knowledge of the MAO inhibitor medications and the foods and medications that are to be avoided is necessary to answer this question. Take time now to review these medications if you had difficulty with this question!
LEVEL OF COGNITIVE ABILITY: Comprehension
PHASE OF NURSING PROCESS: Evaluation

CLIENT NEEDS: Health Promotion and Maintenance
CONTENT AREA: Pharmacology
REFERENCE
Hodgson, B., & Kizior, R. (2000). *Saunders nursing drug handbook 2000.* Philadelphia: W. B. Saunders. p. 1012.

29. **3**

RATIONALE: Amitriptyline hydrochloride is a tricyclic antidepressant often used to treat depression. The client may experience sedation, dry mouth, constipation, and blurred vision. These are annoying at best and can seem debilitating at worst. However, these are transient and will diminish with time. More commonly, orthostatic changes can produce hypotension and tachycardia. This can be frightening to the client and dangerous (as it may result in dizziness and the client falling). The client must be instructed to move slowly from a lying to a sitting to a standing position to avoid injury if these changes are experienced.
TEST-TAKING STRATEGY: Knowledge of the tricyclic medications is required to answer this question. If you had difficulty with this question, take time now to review this medication.
LEVEL OF COGNITIVE ABILITY: Application
PHASE OF NURSING PROCESS: Implementation
CLIENT NEEDS: Physiological Integrity
CONTENT AREA: Pharmacology
REFERENCE
Hodgson, B., & Kizior, R. (2000). *Saunders nursing drug handbook 2000.* Philadelphia: W. B. Saunders. p. 49.

30. **3**

RATIONALE: Lithium is recognized as the medication of choice to treat manic-depressive illness. Its exact mechanism of action remains speculative; however, an equilibrium of sodium (Na) and potassium (K) must be maintained to maintain therapeutic effects. Lithium competes with Na in the cell. Many over-the-counter medications contain Na, and often prescription medications (diuretics) change the Na:K ratios of the cell, thus affecting lithium concentrations and the therapeutic levels of the medication.
TEST-TAKING STRATEGY: A knowledge base relating to this medication is required. Food restriction (tyramine-restricted diet) is associated with MAO inhibitors. Antianxiety agents (not lithium) are generally addictive. Lithium blood levels are recommended but are generally every 3 to 4 months. Recall that the Na:K ratio must be maintained for lithium to remain effective. A disruption of these two electrolytes can lead to lithium toxicity.
LEVEL OF COGNITIVE ABILITY: Application
PHASE OF NURSING PROCESS: Planning
CLIENT NEEDS: Health Promotion and Maintenance
CONTENT AREA: Pharmacology
REFERENCE
Hodgson, B., & Kizior, R. (2000). *Saunders nursing drug handbook 2000.* Philadelphia: W. B. Saunders. p. 598.

BIBLIOGRAPHY

Clark, J., Queener, S., & Karb, V. (1997). *Pharmacologic basis of nursing practice* (5th ed.). St. Louis: Mosby–Year Book.
Deglin, J., & Vallerand, A. (1999). *Davis's drug guide for nurses* (6th ed.). Philadelphia: F. A. Davis.

Hodgson, B., & Kizior, R. (2000). *Saunders nursing drug handbook 2000.* Philadelphia: W. B. Saunders.
Kee, J., & Hayes, E. (1997). *Pharmacology: A nursing process approach* (2nd ed.). Philadelphia: W. B. Saunders.
Varcarolis, E. (1998). *Foundations of psychiatric mental health nursing.* (3rd ed.). Philadelphia: W. B. Saunders.

UNIT XX

....

The Gerontological Client

PYRAMID TERMS

Abuse—The willful infliction of pain, injury, or mental anguish. Unreasonable confinement or willful deprivation of services, including medical care. Abuse can include failure to prevent injury, verbal assaults, the demand to perform demeaning tasks, theft, or mismanagement of personal belongings.

Aging—The biopsychosocial process of change occurring between birth and death.

Alzheimer's Disease—An irreversible form of dementia. Individuals with Alzheimer's disease experience cognitive deterioration and progressive loss of ability to carry out the activities of daily living. The client experiences a steady decline in physical and mental functioning that frequently requires caregivers to seek outside resources for assistance.

Dementia—Organic syndrome identified by gradual and progressive deterioration in intellectual functioning. Long- and short-term memory loss occurs, with impairment in judgment, abstract thinking, problem-solving ability, and behavior.

Results in a self-care deficit. The most common type of dementia is Alzheimer's disease.

Depression—A functional disorder of mood that is not linked with aging. The depression may be precipitated by losses related to aging. Depression can be manifested by cognitive impairment or may be the cause of a decline in mental status. Depression can be identified by feelings of sadness, hopelessness, and worthlessness and a decreased interest in activities.

Exploitation—Illegal or improper use of the individual's resources.

Gerontology—The study of the process of aging.

Neglect—The lack of providing services necessary for physical or mental health.

Self-Neglect—The person chooses to avoid medical care or other services that could improve optimal function. Unless declared legally incompetent, an individual has the right to refuse care.

PYRAMID TO SUCCESS

The Pyramid to Success focuses on safety issues, the prevention of injury, restraints, abuse and neglect, depression, dementia, and Alzheimer's disease. Pyramid points also focus on methods of communication, particularly when deficits exist. When a question is presented on NCLEX-PN, if an age is identified in the case of the question, note the age. If the age represents an elderly client, use gerontological nursing concepts when answering the question.

NURSING PROCESS

DATA COLLECTION

Vision and hearing
Ability to communicate
Food and fluid intake
Arm and leg function
Basic activities of daily living
Skin integrity
Bowel and bladder function
Risk for infection
Risk for injury
Environmental hazards
Mental status
Social support systems

PLANNING	IMPLEMENTATION	EVALUATION
The client uses measures that will assist with orientation.	Assess visual abilities and for the presence of cataracts. Monitor for hearing loss. Use methods and devices that will assist with sensory deficits. Orient to environment.	The client remains oriented.
The client consumes adequate food and fluids.	Assess nutritional status including weight and hydration. Offer and provide frequent snacks, considering client's personal and cultural preferences.	The client maintains appropriate weight and hydration status. Nutrition and hydration are within normal, expected limits.
The client uses adaptive devices safely for mobility.	Assess upper and lower extremities and the ability to ambulate. Instruct client in the safe use of assistive devices for mobilization.	The client achieves an optimal level of physical mobility.
The client communicates needs. The client performs some measures of care to self.	Maintain and enhance self-care abilities. Assist with activities of daily living. Supervise self-care. Support self-functioning to maintain independence.	The client maintains optimal level of independence.
Client remains free of skin breakdown as a result of immobility.	Turn and reposition client. Monitor skin integrity. Instruct client in the importance of turning and repositioning.	The client's skin remains intact.
The client establishes a toileting routine. The client determines causes of urinary and bowel dysfunction. The client identifies practices that may contribute to bowel dysfunction.	Assess urinary and bowel function. Identify bowel habits. Identify factors that affect normal bowel function. Provide measures to promote normal urinary and bowel function. Instruct the client in measures to eliminate bowel dysfunction.	The client adheres to the prescribed bladder and bowel program. The client uses measures to eliminate bowel dysfunction. The client demonstrates normal urinary and bowel patterns.
Vital signs remain within baseline.	Assess for the risk of infection. Monitor vital signs and for signs of infection.	The client remains free from infection.
The client identifies behaviors that can cause injury. The client avoids injuries.	Determine the client's ability related to safety and functional self-care. Maintain safety precautions. Institute measures to prevent falls. Place the bed in the low position. Provide handrails in bathrooms and halls. Ensure that rooms are uncluttered. Provide adequate, nonglare lighting.	The client remains free of injury.

PLANNING	IMPLEMENTATION	EVALUATION
The client performs behaviors that are appropriate.	Monitor for disorientation. Assess mental status and for memory changes. Establish trust. Encourage psychosocial activity.	The client demonstrates optimal thought processes.
PLANNING	IMPLEMENTATION	EVALUATION
The client and family participate in developing the plan of care. The client and family identify methods of coping.	Involve the client and significant others in planning care. Determine the degree of impact that the disability may have on independence. Ensure that care options selected fit within the person's lifestyle. Display nonjudgmental attitudes. Assist in selecting activities for the client that maintain self-identity and lifelong interests. Encourage attending activities to maintain social interaction. Encourage verbalization about the past. Identify available support systems. Assist to provide resources to the family to obtain respite care.	The client and/or family identify resources and support services available.

CLIENT NEEDS

SAFE, EFFECTIVE CARE ENVIRONMENT

Advance directives
Client rights and advocacy
Confidentiality
Continuity of care
Informed consent
The use of restraints
Appropriate procedures for safety
Accident prevention

HEALTH PROMOTION AND MAINTENANCE

Aging process
Expected body image changes
Family systems
Lifestyle choices
The prevention and early detection of disorders associated with aging
The importance of safety, exercise, and nutrition
The safe use of medications
The importance of follow-up visits to the physician

PSYCHOSOCIAL INTEGRITY

Coping mechanisms
Grief and loss
Religious and spiritual resources
Sensory/perceptual alterations
Changes and adjustment in role function
Situational role changes
Adjustment to potential deterioration in physical and mental health and well-being
Loss of relationships
The threat to independent functioning
Abuse and neglect
The use of resources for the client and family

PHYSIOLOGICAL INTEGRITY

Assistive devices
Elimination
Mobility and immobility
Nutrition and oral hydration
Personal hygiene
Rest and sleep
Safe medication administration
Alterations in body systems and the related risks due to the aging process

BIBLIOGRAPHY

Cox, H., Hinz, M., & Lubno, M., et al. (1997). *Clinical applications of nursing diagnosis: Adult, child, women's, psychiatric, gerontic, and home health considerations* (3rd ed.). Philadelphia: F. A. Davis.

deWit, S. (1998). *Essentials of medical-surgical nursing* (4th ed.). Philadelphia: W. B. Saunders.

Hill, S., & Howlett, H. (1997). *Success in practical nursing: Personal and vocational issues* (3rd ed.). Philadelphia: W. B. Saunders.

Leahy, J., & Kizilay, P. (1998). *Foundations of nursing practice: A nursing process approach*. Philadelphia: W. B. Saunders.

Luckmann, J. (1997). *Saunders manual of nursing care*. Philadelphia: W. B. Saunders.

National Council of State Boards of Nursing (1998). *National Council detailed test plan for the NCLEX-PN examination*. Chicago: Author.

O'Toole, M. (Ed.). (1997). *Miller-Keane encyclopedia & dictionary of medicine, nursing, & allied health* (6th ed.). Philadelphia: W. B. Saunders.

Tyson, R. (1999). *Gerontological nursing care*. Philadelphia: W. B. Saunders.

CHAPTER 65

Care of the Gerontological Client

I. Physiological Changes of Aging (Box 65–1)

A. Integumentary system
1. Loss of pigment in hair and skin
2. Increased nail thickness and decreased nail growth
3. Thinning of the epidermis with easy bruising and tearing of the skin
4. Loss of elasticity and subcutaneous fat
5. Reduction in blood flow to the skin
6. Decreased skin turgor
7. Wrinkling of the skin
8. Dry, itchy, cracked skin
9. Inadequate sweating
10. Seborrheic and keratosis formation

B. Neurological system
1. Changes in mental status
2. Slowed reflexes and loss of balance
3. Dizziness and syncope
4. Slight tremors and difficulty with fine motor movement
5. Changes in sleep patterns, such as decreased total sleep with earlier risings
6. Increased susceptibility to hypothermia and hyperthermia

C. Musculoskeletal system
1. Posture and stature changes, causing a decrease in height
2. Kyphosis of the dorsal spine
3. Muscle mass decreases and muscles atrophy
4. Joint capsule components deteriorate
5. Bone brittleness increases
6. Deep tendon reflexes decrease

7. Mobility, range of motion, flexibility, and stability decrease
8. Stiffness increases
9. Physical strength and muscular coordination decrease
10. Gait changes, with shortened step and wider base

D. Cardiopulmonary system
1. Diminished energy and endurance
2. Lowered tolerance to exercise
3. Decreased stretch and compliance of the chest wall
4. Decreased rib mobility and lung tone
5. Decreased strength and function of respiratory muscles
6. Decreased size and number of alveoli
7. Decreased compliance of the heart; heart valves become thicker and more rigid
8. Decreased efficiency of blood return to the heart and decreased cardiac output
9. Increase in blood pressure
10. Susceptibility to postural hypotension

E. Hematologic and immune systems
1. Hemoglobin and hematocrit levels remain within normal range but average toward the low end of normal
2. Lymphocyte counts tend to be lower
3. Decreased resistance to infection and disease
4. Prone to clotting abnormalities

F. Gastrointestinal system
1. Decreased appetite, thirst, and intake
2. Decreased need for calories
3. Difficulty chewing (if dental problems exist) and swallowing food
4. Decreased stomach-emptying time
5. Digestive disturbances
6. Increased tendency toward constipation
7. Decreased absorption of carbohydrates, proteins, fats, and vitamins
8. Decreased lean body weight
9. Hiatal hernias common

BOX 65–1. Classification of Late Adulthood

Young old: 65–74 years
Middle old: 75–84 years
Old old: 85–99 years
The elite old: 100 years or more

G. Endocrine system
   1. Decreased secretion of hormones, with specific changes related to each hormone function
   2. Decreased metabolic rate
   3. Decreased glucose tolerance
   4. Resistance to insulin on peripheral tissues
H. Renal system
   1. Decreased kidney size, function, and ability to concentrate urine
   2. Decreased glomerular filtration rate
   3. Decreased capacity of the bladder
   4. Increased residual urine and increased incidence of infection and incontinence
   5. Impaired medication excretion
I. Reproductive system
   1. Decreased testosterone production and decreased size of testes
   2. Changes in the prostate leading to urinary problems
   3. Decreased secretion of hormones with the cessation of menses
   4. Vaginal changes including decreased muscle tone and lubrication
J. Special senses
   1. Decreased visual acuity
   2. Decreased accommodation
   3. Decreased peripheral vision and increased sensitivity to glare
   4. Increased adjustment time to changes in light
   5. Presbyopia and cataract formation
   6. Loss of hearing ability
   7. Inability to discern taste of food
   8. Decreased smell acuity
   9. Changes in touch

II. Psychosocial Aspects of Aging (Box 65–2)

A. Changes in role function
B. Adjustments to retirement and loss of income
C. Changes in social life
D. Adjustment to potential deterioration in physical and mental health and well-being
E. Loss of relationships
F. Threat to independent functioning
G. Coping with change and new life situations
H. Coping with stress of caring for dependent loved ones
I. Coping with loss

BOX 65–2. Concerns of the Older Population

Adequate income
Functional limitations from chronic illness and disability
Ability to maintain independence
Becoming a burden to loved ones
Isolation
Dependence on governmental and social systems
Access to social support systems

III. Elder Abuse and Neglect

A. Description
   1. Involves physical, psychological, financial, and social **abuse**
   2. Can involve a violation of client's rights
   3. Individuals at most risk include those that are dependent, usually because of confusion, immobility, or the need for personal hygiene
   4. Factors that contribute to **abuse** and **neglect** include long-standing family violence, caregiver stress, and the individual's increasing dependence
B. **Abuse**
   1. The willful infliction of pain, injury, or mental anguish
   2. Unreasonable confinement or willful deprivation of services, including medical care
   3. Can include failure to prevent injury, verbal assaults, the demand to perform demeaning tasks, theft, or mismanagement of personal belongings
C. **Neglect:** the lack of providing services necessary for physical or mental health
D. **Self-Neglect**
   1. The person chooses to avoid medical care or other services that would improve optimal functioning
   2. Unless declared legally incompetent, an individual has the right to refuse care
E. **Exploitation:** illegal or improper use of the individual's resources
F. Data collection
   1. Abrasions, lacerations, and bruises
   2. Burns
   3. Sprains, fractures, or dislocations
   4. Pressure sores
   5. Injuries inconsistent with history
   6. Frequent falls
   7. Untreated medical problems
   8. Inappropriate dress and poor hygiene
   9. Excessive drowsiness
   10. Over- or undermedication
   11. Malnutrition and dehydration
   12. Expression of fear in response to touch
G. Implementation
   1. Check client for signs of **abuse** and **neglect**
   2. All states mandate reporting cases of **abuse** and **neglect**
   3. Protective services need to be initiated
   4. Monitor for dysfunctional family systems and promote family functioning and self-care

IV. Use of Restraints

A. Physical restraints used to prevent injury are to be avoided, and alternative methods to provide safety must be implemented prior to the use of physical restraints
B. A physician's order must be obtained for the use of restraints
C. Discuss the use of restraints with the client and family

D. Obtain client/family consent for the use of restraints
E. Use the least restrictive device for restraint
F. Use only restraints that have been manufactured as a safety restraint
G. Observe the client frequently, and monitor for alterations in skin integrity and in circulation as a result of the restraints
H. Restraints need to be removed at frequent intervals to assess for complications and to allow for mobility and range of motion
I. Always follow the institutional policy regarding the use of restraints

V. Medications

A. Major problems with prescriptive medications include adverse affects, medication interactions, medication errors, noncompliance, and cost
B. Determine the use of over-the-counter medications
C. The use of medications should be kept to a minimum and doses should begin at one-third to one-half of normal adult doses (medications with the shortest half-life should be prescribed if possible)
D. Closely monitor for adverse effects (particularly in clients taking multiple medications) because of the increased risk for medication toxicity
E. Avoid the use of medications with anticholinergic effects
F. Note that a common sign of an adverse reaction in the elderly is an acute change in mental status
G. Advise the client to use one pharmacy and notify the consulting physicians of medications taken
H. Administration of medications
  1. Check for mouth dryness because medication may stick and dissolve in the mouth
  2. Place the client in a sitting position when administering medication
  3. Crush tablets if necessary and give with textured food (nectar, applesauce) if not contraindicated
  4. Do not crush enteric-coated tablets and do not open capsules
  5. Administer liquid preparations if the client has difficulty swallowing tablets
  6. If administering a suppository, do not insert suppository immediately after removing from the refrigerator; a suppository may take longer to dissolve because of decreased body core temperature
  7. When administering parenteral (SC, IM) medication, monitor the site because it may ooze medication or bleed because of decreased tissue elasticity
  8. Do not use an immobile limb for administering parenteral (SC, IM) medication
  9. Monitor client compliance with taking prescribed medications
  10. Monitor for safety in correctly taking medications
  11. Use a medication cassette to facilitate proper administration of medication

VI. Decubiti

A. Description
  1. An impairment of skin integrity
  2. Localized areas of necrosis of the skin and subcutaneous tissue due to pressure
  3. Prevention of skin breakdown is a major role of the nurse, particularly when caring for the bedridden or immobile client
B. Data collection (Table 65–1)
C. Implementation
  1. Institute measures to prevent decubiti
  2. Monitor for an alteration in skin integrity
  3. Relieve or remove pressure on the skin
  4. Turn and reposition the immobile client every 2 hours or more frequently if necessary
  5. Ambulate the client if possible
  6. Provide active and passive exercises every 8 hours
  7. Keep the skin clean and dry and the sheets wrinkle-free
  8. Apply moisture barrier as prescribed to protect the skin
  9. Use assistive devices to prevent pressure such as an alternating air pressure mattress or sheepskin padding
  10. Monitor the nutritional status of the client and provide adequate nutritional intake to promote tissue integrity

Table 65–1. Stages of Decubiti

Stage 1	Stage 2	Stage 3	Stage 4
A reddened area that returns to normal skin color after 15–20 minutes of pressure relief, such as turning the client to another position; the skin is intact, and the area is red and does not blanche with external pressure.	Area in which the top layer of skin is missing; the ulcer usually is shallow with a pinkish red base, and a white or yellow eschar may be present.	Deep ulcers that extend into the dermis and subcutaneous tissues; white, gray, or yellow eschar is usually present at the bottom of the ulcer, and the ulcer crater may have a lip or edge; purulent drainage is common.	Deep ulcers that extend into muscle and bone; foul-smelling; eschar is brown or black; purulent drainage is common.

VII. Dementia

A. Description
  1. Organic syndrome with progressive deterioration in intellectual functioning
  2. Long- and short-term memory loss occurs with impairment in judgment, abstract thinking, problem-solving ability, and behavior
  3. Results in a self-care deficit
  4. The most common type of **dementia** is **Alzheimer's disease**

B. **Alzheimer's disease**
  1. An irreversible form of **dementia**
  2. Individuals with **Alzheimer's disease** experience cognitive deterioration and progressive loss of ability to carry out the activities of daily living
  3. The client experiences a steady decline in physical and mental functioning that frequently requires caregivers to seek outside resources for assistance

C. Data collection
  1. Memory impairment
  2. Indifferent and occasionally irritable
  3. Restlessness and pacing
  4. Decrease in orientation
  5. Impaired cognitive function

D. Implementation
  1. Identify and reinforce retained skills
  2. Assist the client and family members to manage memory deficits and behavior changes
  3. Encourage family members to express feelings about caregiving
  4. Provide caregiver support and identify the resources and support groups available
  5. Provide continuity of care
  6. Orient the client to the environment
  7. Furnish the environment with familiar possessions
  8. Monitor activities of daily living
  9. Remind the client how to perform self-care activities
  10. Maintain independence
  11. Provide consistent routines
  12. Provide exercise such as walking with an escort
  13. Avoid activities that tax the memory
  14. Allow plenty of time to complete a task
  15. Use constant encouragement in a step-by-step approach
  16. Acknowledge the client's feelings
  17. Provide activities that distract and occupy time such as listening to music, coloring, and watching TV
  18. Provide mental stimulation with simple games or activities

E. Implementation for specific behaviors
  1. Wandering
    a. Provide a safe environment
    b. Prevent unsafe wandering
    c. Provide close supervision
    d. Close and secure doors
    e. Use identification bracelets and electronic surveillance devices
  2. Communication
    a. Adapt to the communication level of the client
    b. Use a firm volume and low pitch to communicate
    c. Use a calm and reassuring voice
    d. Use pantomime gestures if the client is unable to understand spoken words
    e. Use slow, clear, verbal communication techniques
    f. Use short words and simple sentences
    g. Call the client by name, identify self, and wait for a response
    h. Ask only one question at a time and give one direction at a time
    i. Repeat questions if necessary but do not rephrase
    j. Stand directly in front of the client and maintain eye contact
    k. Be alert to feelings and emotions expressed by the client
  3. Impaired judgment
    a. Eliminate from the environment throw rugs, toxic substances, dangerous electrical appliances, or any other objects that can present a risk of injury
    b. Reduce hot water heater temperature
  4. Altered thought processes
    a. Place a calendar and clock in a visible place
    b. Call the client by name
    c. Use familiar objects in the room
    d. Maintain familiar routines
    e. Make tasks simple
    f. Allow time for the client to complete a task
    g. Allow the client to reminisce
  5. Altered sleep patterns
    a. Allow the client to wander in a safe place until they become tired
    b. Prevent shadows in the room
    c. Avoid the use of hypnotics because they cause confusion and aggravate the sundown effect
  6. Agitation
    a. Identify the precipitant of the agitation
    b. Reassure the client
    c. Remove items that can be hazardous during the time of agitation
    d. Approach the client slowly and calmly from the front, then speak, gesture, and move slowly
    e. Remove the client to a less stressful environment
    f. Use touch gently
    g. Do not argue with the client or restrain the client
    h. Distract the client with questions about the problem and gradually turn the attention to something else

◆ **VIII. Depression**

A. Description
   1. A functional disorder of mood that is not linked with **aging**
   2. The **depression** may be manifested by cognitive impairment or may be the cause of a decline in mental status; often associated with physical problems
   3. **Depression** can be identified by feelings of sadness, hopelessness, worthlessness, and a decreased interest in activities
B. Data collection
   1. Difficulty concentrating
   2. Feelings of inadequacy and sadness
   3. Difficulty sleeping or excessive sleeping
   4. Weight gain or loss
   5. Constipation
   6. Loss of interest in activities
   7. Decreased endurance and energy
   8. Preoccupation with physical health
   9. Thoughts of death or suicide
C. Implementation
   1. Monitor for signs associated with **depression**
   2. Monitor for the risk of suicide and notify the physician
   3. Implement safety precautions for suicide risk
   4. Provide and reinforce positive experiences
   5. Provide a variation in daily schedule
   6. Allow the client to talk and reminisce
   7. Maintain reality

◆ **IX. Pain**

A. Description
   1. Pain can occur from numerous causes and most often occurs from degenerative changes in the musculoskeletal system
   2. The failure to alleviate pain in the older client can lead to functional limitations affecting their ability to function independently
B. Data collection
   1. Restlessness or agitation
   2. Moaning or crying
   3. Verbal reporting of pain
C. Implementation
   1. Monitor the client for signs of pain
   2. Identify the precipitating factor and pattern of pain
   3. Monitor the impact of pain on activities of daily living
   4. Provide pain relief through measures such as distraction, relaxation, massage, and biofeedback
   5. Administer pain medication as prescribed and instruct the client in their use
   6. Evaluate the effects of pain-reducing measures

X. Impaired Mobility

A. Description
   1. Usually occurs secondary to multiple types of problems and diseases
   2. Impaired mobility can occur due to decreased physical function related to cardiovascular, pulmonary, musculoskeletal, or neurological disease, or accidents
B. Data collection
   1. Existing disease processes
   2. Ambulation
   3. Ability to care for self
C. Implementation
   1. Identify risk of injury
   2. Determine cause of mobility restriction
   3. Monitor mobility restrictions related to disease processes
   4. Identify limitations related to all self-care activities
   5. Determine the best assistive aid or adaptive device for the client
   6. Demonstrate and monitor the safe use of the assistive device
   7. Provide range of motion to prevent deformities and contractures
   8. Provide rest periods between activities and in the afternoon
   9. Break up activities to last no longer than 20 minutes
   10. Perform activities that require a high level of energy in the morning
   11. Maintain activity through exercise and guided activities
   12. Monitor skin for integrity
   13. Monitor respiratory status and encourage deep breathing to promote lung expansion
D. Assistive devices (see Chapter 56)
   1. Canes
   2. Hemicanes or quadripod canes
   3. Walkers

XI. Fractured Hip

A. Description
   1. Bone is broken inside the joint (intracapsular), or the fracture can occur at the greater trochanter (extracapsular) outside the joint
   2. Fractured hips occurring in the elderly are most likely due to a fall
B. Data collection
   1. Cause of fall
   2. Safety
   3. Pain and swelling at the site
   4. Asymmetry of hip
   5. X-ray to confirm fracture
C. Implementation (see Chapter 56)

XII. Pneumonia

A. Description: the causes of pneumonia in the older client include the effects of the **aging** process on the respiratory system, weakness and the inability to cough, malnutrition, and the use of medications

B. Data collection
1. Acute change in mental status
2. Confusion
3. Cough
4. Elevated temperature
5. Dyspnea and tachypnea
6. Chest pain
7. Chest x-ray confirmation
C. Implementation
1. Monitor vital signs
2. Administer oxygen and respiratory therapy as prescribed
3. Administer antibiotics as prescribed
4. Provide adequate nutrition and hydration
5. Provide adequate rest with some progressive activity
6. Mobilize the bed rest client as soon as possible
7. Encourage the client to receive immunization against influenza and pneumococcal pneumonia to prevent infection

XIII. Nutritional Intake

A. Description
1. Physiological requirements decrease with age
2. The older client is at risk for inadequate nutritional and fluid intake due to inability to prepare food, loss of dentition, loss of appetite, lack of exercise, loss of taste and smell, loss of interest in eating, **depression**, or lack of financial resources
B. Data collection
1. Appetite and hydration status
2. Body weight
3. Ability to feed self
4. Ability to chew and swallow
5. Fluid and calorie intake
6. Ability to prepare food and the resources to shop
C. Implementation
1. Assess food likes and dislikes
2. Monitor intake of food and fluids
3. Monitor for signs of dehydration and malnutrition
4. Monitor body weight
5. Assess ability to chew or swallow
6. Provide small, frequent nutritious drinks and meals
7. Assess the ability to shop for and prepare food
8. Provide resources necessary to supply the client with adequate food

XIV. Constipation

A. Description
1. Constipation is the most frequent complaint of older people regarding bowel function
2. Normal elimination does not occur because of a structural problem or disease state
B. Data collection
1. Frequency of defecation
2. Usual time for defecation
3. Dietary habits
4. Use of laxatives or enemas
C. Implementation
1. Determine the cause of constipation
2. Reestablish typical bowel habits
3. Promote comfort and privacy during defecation
4. Increase fluid intake
5. Add fiber to the diet
6. Provide anal lubricant and stool softeners as prescribed
7. Use suppositories sparingly, limiting type to glycerin or Dulcolax as prescribed
8. Use enemas sparingly, limiting the use to small cleansing enemas such as Fleet, as prescribed
9. Avoid the use of mineral oil because of problems associated with the absorption of fat-soluble vitamins and the risk of aspiration

XV. Diarrhea

A. Description
1. Frequent defecation of loose or liquid stools
2. Infections may cause diarrhea
3. Fecal impaction may cause overflow diarrhea, with stool oozing around the impaction
4. Antibiotic-associated diarrhea, such as that caused by *Clostridium difficile*, is a problem for older individuals, particularly if they are hospitalized
B. Data collection
1. Frequency and usual time of defecation
2. Dietary habits
3. Use of laxatives or enemas
4. Stool oozing
5. Signs of dehydration
C. Implementation
1. Identify causative factor
2. Initiate interventions as prescribed based on causative factor
3. Monitor I&O and for signs of dehydration
4. Increase dietary bulk and fiber
5. Monitor skin around the anal area

XVI. Urinary Incontinence

A. Description
1. The involuntary release or leakage of urine
2. The physiological changes that occur in the kidney and bladder as a result of the **aging** process may lead to the urinary incontinence problems experienced by some older clients; however, incontinence is not a normal aging change
B. Data collection
1. Contributing factors
2. Fluid intake
3. Urinary incontinence or retention patterns
4. Signs of urinary infection such as burning, frequency, foul odor, or confusion
5. Urinalysis results

C. Implementation
   1. Monitor I&O
   2. Monitor urinary patterns
   3. Identify contributing factors such as a bladder infection, the distance to bathroom, difficulty ambulating or removing clothing, or coughing, sneezing, or laughing
   4. Establish toileting schedule such as every 2 hours, or before and after activities, meals, sleep, and rest periods
   5. Provide easy access to the bathroom
   6. Ensure adequate fluid intake
   7. Provide a protection plan for accidents to avoid embarrassment
   8. Instruct the client about the use of incontinence aids such as pads or briefs
   9. Provide skin care and monitor for skin breakdown
   10. Teach perineal (Kegel) exercises to control stress and urge incontinence

XVII. Impaired Vision and Hearing

A. Description
   1. Due to the physiological changes that occur with the **aging** process, clients develop decreased visual and hearing acuity
   2. Loss of sight and hearing, cataracts, glaucoma, and presbyopia can develop
B. Data collection
   1. Risk for injury
   2. Ability to see and hear adequately
   3. The need for assistive devices
   4. Frequently asking people to repeat statements
   5. Better understanding of speech when in small groups
   6. Avoiding large groups
   7. Withdrawing from social interactions
   8. Straining to hear; shouting in conversation
   9. Turning head to favor one ear or leaning forward
   10. Failing to respond when not looking in the direction of the sound
   11. Answering questions incorrectly
   12. Raising the volume of the television or radio
   13. Ringing in the ears
   14. Irritability
C. Implementation
   1. Impaired vision
      a. Alert the client when approaching
      b. When speaking to the client who has limited sight, use a normal tone of voice
      c. Orient the client to the environment
      d. Use a focal point and provide further orientation to the environment from that focal point
      e. Allow the client to touch objects in the room
      f. Use the clock placement of foods on the meal tray to orient the client
      g. When ambulating, allow the client to grasp your arm at the elbow and keep the arm close to your body so the client can detect the direction of movement; instruct the client to remain one step behind you when ambulating
      h. Provide radios, TVs, and clocks that give the time orally
      i. Promote independence as much as possible
   2. Impaired hearing
      a. Use written words if the client is able to see, read, and write
      b. Talk in a room without distracting noises
      c. Talk in lower tones, because shouting is not helpful
      d. Move close to the client and speak slowly and clearly
      e. Use telephone amplifiers
      f. Use flashing lights that are activated by a ringing telephone or doorbell
      g. Use specially trained dogs that help the client to be aware of sound and to alert the client to potential dangers
      h. Use lip reading and sign language, which combines speech with hand movements that signify letters, words, or phrases
      i. Encourage the client to wear glasses when talking to someone to improve vision for lip reading
      j. Face the client when speaking
      k. Provide plenty of light in the room
      l. Get the attention of the client before you begin to speak
      m. Keep hands and other objects away from the mouth when talking to the client
      n. Validate with the client the understanding of statements made by asking the client to repeat what was said
      o. Rephrase sentences and repeat information
      p. Move closer to the better hearing ear
   3. Hearing aids (Box 65–3)
      a. Encourage the client to start using the hearing aid slowly to develop the

---

BOX 65–3. Client Instructions in the Use of a Hearing Aid

Clean the ear mold with mild soap and water
Avoid excessive wetting, and keep the hearing aid dry
Clean the ear cannula of the hearing aid with a toothpick or pipe cleaner
Turn off the hearing aid and remove the battery when not in use
Keep extra batteries on hand
Keep in a safe place
Avoid dropping and avoid exposure of hearing aid to extremes of heat and cold
Adjust the volume to the minimal hearing level to prevent feedback squeaking
Prevent hair sprays, oils, or other hair and face products from coming in contact with the receiver

recognition of hearing via the hearing aid device

b. Teach the client to concentrate on the sounds that are to be heard and to filter out background noise

PRACTICE QUESTIONS

1. The nurse is assigned to care for an elderly client with hearing loss. The nurse plans care knowing that the elderly
   1 Are often distracted
   2 Respond to low-pitched tones
   3 Have middle-ear changes
   4 Develop moist cerumen production

2. An elderly client is admitted to the hospital with a diagnosis of malnutrition. The nurse is told that blood will be drawn to determine if the client has a protein deficiency. The nurse understands that which of the following blood tests will be done?
   1 Creatinine
   2 Transferrin
   3 Calcium
   4 Sodium

3. The nurse is assigned to care for an elderly client. To reduce the risk of aspiration during meals, the nurse positions the client
   1 Upright in a chair
   2 On the left side in bed
   3 In a low Fowler's position with legs elevated
   4 On the right side in bed

4. The nurse is assigned to care for an elderly client who is receiving nutrition via a nasogastric tube. Prior to administering the feeding, the priority nursing action is
   1 Check the placement of the tube
   2 Check the last time medications were given
   3 Check the time of the last feeding
   4 Warm the feeding to 103°F

5. An elderly hypertensive client is taking lisinopril (Prinivil, Zestril) 10 mg PO QID. The nurse reinforces instructions to the client regarding the medication. Which statement if made by the client indicates that further teaching is necessary?
   1 "I will take the pill after breakfast each day."
   2 "I need to change my position slowly."
   3 "If I get a bad headache, I should call my doctor."
   4 "I can skip a dose once a week."

6. Which of the following clients would most likely be a victim of elder abuse?
   1 A 90-year-old woman with advanced Parkinson's disease
   2 A 68-year-old man with newly diagnosed cataracts
   3 A 70-year-old woman with early diagnosed Lyme disease

4 A 75-year-old man with moderate hypertension

7. An elderly female client tells the nurse that she is afraid that she will fall while going to the bathroom at night. Which suggestion, if made by the nurse, indicates that the nurse understands the visual changes affecting the elderly?
   1 "Use a bell to call your daughter if you need to get up."
   2 "Keep a nightlight on in the bedroom and bathroom."
   3 "Use a commode in your bedroom at night."
   4 "Limit your fluid intake during the day."

8. The nurse is caring for a client with Alzheimer's disease who is agitated. The nurse plans which intervention to calm this agitated client?
   1 Playing a radio
   2 Turning the lights out
   3 Putting an arm around the client's waist
   4 Encouraging group participation

9. The nurse is assisting in planning group activities. Which of the following activities best promotes health and maintenance among older adults?
   1 Gardening every day for an hour
   2 Cycling three times a week for 20 minutes
   3 Sculpting once a week for 40 minutes
   4 Walking three to five times a week for 30 minutes

10. The nurse is caring for an elderly client with a diagnosis of myasthenia gravis. Which statement if made by the client indicates to the nurse that further teaching is necessary?
    1 "I can change the time of my medication on the mornings that I feel strong."
    2 "I rest each afternoon after my walk."
    3 "If I get abdominal cramps and diarrhea, I should call my doctor."
    4 "I cough and deep breathe many times during the day."

11. The nurse is assigned to care for an elderly client. Which of the following activities performed by the nurse fosters reminiscence in the client?
    1 Displaying calendars and clocks
    2 Encouraging client participation in pottery class
    3 Setting up a pet therapy session
    4 Having storytelling time

12. The nurse is caring for an immobile elderly client who is on bed rest. The nurse plans care knowing that which of the following problems would have the highest priority for the client?
    1 Oral mucous membrane irritation
    2 Respiratory congestion
    3 Impaired memory
    4 Loneliness

13. The nurse is caring for an elderly client at home. Which situation in the home noted by the nurse requires immediate attention?
    1 An operable smoke detector
    2 A prefilled medication tray
    3 Unsecured scatter rugs
    4 Cleared exit passageways

14. The nurse is encouraging an elderly female client's participation in recreational therapy. What nursing intervention does the nurse consider performing first?
    1 Change the client's soiled disposable brief
    2 Have the client's nails manicured
    3 Have the client's hair washed and cut
    4 Ask the client to wear supportive shoes

15. Which statement, if made by an elderly client, indicates to the nurse that further teaching about bowel elimination is necessary?
    1 "I drink 6 to 8 glasses of water per day."
    2 "I walk 1 to 2 miles per day."
    3 "I need to decrease fiber in my diet."
    4 "I have a bowel movement every other day."

16. Which of the following situations, if practiced by a nurse, portrays ageism?
    1 Accepting differences among older adults
    2 Allowing older adults to make decisions
    3 Informing the elderly of their rights
    4 Advising older adults to forgo aggressive treatment

17. The nurse plans to monitor an elderly client for medication toxicity knowing that which of the following age-related body changes may cause medication toxicity?
    1 Decreased cough efficiency and decreased vital capacity
    2 Decreased lean body mass and decreased glomerular filtration rate
    3 Decreased salivation and decreased gastrointestinal motility
    4 Decreased muscle strength and loss of bone density

18. The nurse is caring for an elderly male client who resides in a nursing home. The nurse plans which of the following to encourage autonomy in the client?
    1 Scheduling his barber appointments
    2 Allowing him to choose social activities
    3 Decorating his room
    4 Planning his meals

19. The nurse is caring for an elderly client who is terminally ill. Which of the following clinical signs indicates to the nurse that death may be imminent?
    1 Cold, clammy skin and irregular noisy breathing
    2 Eupnea and normal body temperature
    3 Presence of swallowing reflex and active bowel sounds
    4 Rubor and paresthesias

20. The nurse plans care for an elderly client knowing that the elderly client is less able to regulate hot and cold bodily changes because of alterations in the activity of the
    1 Parotid glands
    2 Thymus gland
    3 Pineal gland
    4 Sweat glands

21. The nurse is caring for an elderly client who is a widow. Which behavior, if engaged in by the client, indicates ineffective coping?
    1 Requesting to visit her husband's grave once a month
    2 Participating in a senior citizens program
    3 Looking at old snapshots of her family
    4 Neglecting her personal grooming

22. When communicating with an elderly client who is hearing impaired, the nurse initially
    1 Stands in front of the client
    2 Exaggerates lip movements
    3 Obtains a sign language interpreter
    4 Pantomimes and writes the client notes

23. The nurse is providing instructions to an elderly client regarding measures to improve sleep. Which statement, if made by the client, indicates that further teaching is necessary?
    1 "I will drink hot chocolate before bedtime."
    2 "I have stopped smoking cigars."
    3 "I swim three times a week."
    4 "I read for 40 minutes before bedtime."

24. The nurse is caring for an elderly male client at home. The nurse observes that the client is confined by his daughter-in-law to his room. When the nurse suggests he walk to the den and join the family, he says, "I'm in everyone's way. My son needs for me to stay here." The most appropriate action for the nurse to take is to
    1 Suggest to the client and family that they consider a nursing home for the client
    2 Suggest appropriate resources to the client and family such as respite care and senior citizens groups
    3 Say nothing as it is best for the nurse to remain neutral and wait to be asked for help
    4 Say to the daughter-in-law, "Confining your father to his room is inhuman."

25. The nurse is caring for an elderly male client at home. The nurse notes that the client has several bruises on his back, hips, and chest. The medication count and the client's mental status indicate that he is receiving too much sedation. The client says, "My son gets tired having to tend to me at night. I'm always wet and it's all my fault. My

son can't help being a little rough." Which of the following responses by the nurse is most appropriate?

1 "You're saying that when you're incontinent at night, you feel at fault and that you feel your son can't help being rough?"
2 "Oh, he can't, can he? I intend to report this abusive behavior to the police."
3 "Well, I know you feel that you're a bother but you pay your way and then some. I'll talk with your son and clear this right up."
4 "Let's not dwell on this. After all, you are doing quite well and maybe we can arrange for you to go to a nursing home on the weekends."

26. The nurse has reviewed the record of an assigned elderly client. Which of the following data indicates a potential complication associated with the skin of an aging client?
1 Wrinkling, baldness, and gray hair
2 Thinning and loss of elasticity in the skin
3 Deepening of expression lines, and wrinkling
4 Crusting of the skin

27. The nurse has reviewed the record of an assigned elderly client. Which of the following data indicates a potential complication associated with age-related changes in the musculoskeletal system?

1 Decrease in height
2 Decrease in lean body mass
3 Overall sclerotic lesions
4 Changes in structural bone tissue

28. The nurse has reviewed the record of an assigned older adult client. Which of the following data indicates a potential complication associated with the eyes of older adult clients?
1 Vision is 20/20
2 Irregular lens or cornea
3 Vision is 20/30
4 Lens opacity

29. The nurse is assigned to care for a client with a diagnosis of Alzheimer's disease. Which of the following does the nurse most likely expect to note when collecting data about the client?
1 Inability to talk
2 One-sided paralysis
3 Disorientation
4 Urinary and fecal incontinence

30. The nurse is caring for an elderly immobilized client. Which nursing intervention will prevent respiratory complications in the client?
1 Monitoring vital signs every shift
2 Decreasing oral fluid intake
3 Changing the client's position every 2 hours
4 Instructing the client to bear down every hour and hold the breath

ANSWERS

1. **2**

RATIONALE: Presbycusis refers to the age-related irreversible degenerative changes of the inner ear leading to decreased hearing acuity. These changes cause a decreased response to high-frequency sounds. Low-pitched tones of voice are more easily heard and interpreted by the elderly. Options 1, 3, and 4 are incorrect.
TEST-TAKING STRATEGY: Knowledge regarding the physiological changes that occur with hearing among the elderly is required to answer this question. If you had difficulty with this question, take time now to review the characteristics of presbycusis.
LEVEL OF COGNITIVE ABILITY: Comprehension
PHASE OF NURSING PROCESS: Planning
CLIENT NEEDS: Physiological Integrity
CONTENT AREA: Adult Health/Ear
REFERENCE
deWit, S. (1998). *Essentials of medical-surgical nursing* (4th ed.). Philadelphia: W. B. Saunders. p. 959.

2. **2**

RATIONALE: Serum transferrin is an iron-transport protein that can be measured directly or calculated as an indirect measurement of total iron-binding capacity. When serum transferrin is less than 100, the level of protein depletion is severe. The blood creatinine, calcium, or sodium levels do not measure protein.
TEST-TAKING STRATEGY: Use the process of elimination. The key word in the question is "protein." The only option that refers to the analysis of protein is option 2. Take time now to review these laboratory tests if you had difficulty with this question.
LEVEL OF COGNITIVE ABILITY: Comprehension
PHASE OF NURSING PROCESS: Data Collection
CLIENT NEEDS: Physiological Integrity
CONTENT AREA: Fundamental Skills
REFERENCE
Chernecky, C., & Berger, B. (1997). *Laboratory tests and diagnostic procedures* (2nd ed.). Philadelphia: W. B. Saunders. p. 647.

3. **1**

RATIONALE: It is preferable to get clients out of bed and sitting in a chair for meals. This position facilitates chewing and swallowing and prevents reflux of stomach contents. Options 2, 3, and 4 do not identify positions that will reduce the risk of aspiration.
TEST-TAKING STRATEGY: Focus on the issue of the question, "reduce the risk of aspiration." This should easily direct you to option 1. Also note the similarity between options 2, 3, and 4. Review measures that will prevent aspiration now if you had difficulty with this question.
LEVEL OF COGNITIVE ABILITY: Application
PHASE OF NURSING PROCESS: Implementation

CLIENT NEEDS: Physiological Integrity
CONTENT AREA: Fundamental Skills
REFERENCE
Tyson, R. (1999). *Gerontological nursing care*. Philadelphia: W. B. Saunders. p. 456.

4. 1

RATIONALE: Before administering a feeding, the nurse checks the placement of the tube by aspirating gastric contents and measuring the pH. Formulas are administered at room temperature. Options 2 and 3, although useful data, are not priority actions.
TEST-TAKING STRATEGY: Focus on the issue of the question and use the ABCs, airway, breathing, and circulation, to answer the question. In order to prevent the complication of aspiration, the priority is to verify accurate placement of the tube. Take time now to review the principles related to nasogastric tube feedings if you had difficulty with this question.
LEVEL OF COGNITIVE ABILITY: Application
PHASE OF NURSING PROCESS: Implementation
CLIENT NEEDS: Physiological Integrity
CONTENT AREA: Fundamental Skills
REFERENCE
Leahy, J., & Kizilay, P. (1998). *Foundations of nursing practice: A nursing process approach*. Philadelphia: W. B. Saunders. p. 781.

5. 4

RATIONALE: Lisinopril is an antihypertensive, angiotensin-converting enzyme (ACE) inhibitor. Adverse effects include headache, dizziness, fatigue, orthostatic hypotension, tachycardia, and angioedema. Specific client education points include taking one pill a day, not skipping or stopping the medication without consulting the physician, and monitoring for side effects and adverse reactions. The client should notify the physician if side effects occur.
TEST-TAKING STRATEGY: Note the key words "further teaching is necessary." Remembering that clients should never skip doses of medication will easily direct you to option 4. If you had difficulty with this question, take time now to review this medication.
LEVEL OF COGNITIVE ABILITY: Comprehension
PHASE OF NURSING PROCESS: Evaluation
CLIENT NEEDS: Health Promotion and Maintenance
CONTENT AREA: Pharmacology
REFERENCE
Hodgson, B., & Kizior, R. (1999). *Saunders nursing drug handbook 1999*. Philadelphia: W. B. Saunders. pp. 596–598.

6. 1

RATIONALE: The typical abuse victim is a woman of advanced age with few social contacts and at least one physical or mental impairment that limits the ability to perform activities of daily living. In addition, this client lives alone or with the abuser and depends on the abuser for care.
TEST-TAKING STRATEGY: Note the key words "most likely." Use the process of elimination and identify the client that is most defenseless as a result of the disease process. If you had difficulty with this question, take time now to review content related to elder abuse.
LEVEL OF COGNITIVE ABILITY: Comprehension
PHASE OF NURSING PROCESS: Data Collection
CLIENT NEEDS: Psychosocial Integrity

CONTENT AREA: Mental Health
REFERENCE
Tyson, R. (1999). *Gerontological nursing care*. Philadelphia: W. B. Saunders. p. 84.

7. 2

RATIONALE: Because it takes longer to adapt to changes from dark to light and vice versa, older people are at a greater risk of falls and injuries. Clients should be instructed to keep a nightlight on in the bedroom and bathroom to prevent an unsafe environment. Any place where there is a sudden change from dark to light or from light to dark can be dangerous. Options 1 and 3 do not promote independence. Limiting fluid intake can cause dehydration in the elderly.
TEST-TAKING STRATEGY: Focus on the issue of the question, the physiological eye changes that occur in the elderly. Using the process of elimination will easily direct you to option 2. Review the physiological changes that occur in the elderly now if you had difficulty with this question.
LEVEL OF COGNITIVE ABILITY: Comprehension
PHASE OF NURSING PROCESS: Evaluation
CLIENT NEEDS: Physiological Integrity
CONTENT AREA: Fundamental Skills
REFERENCE
deWit, S. (1998). *Essentials of medical-surgical nursing* (4th ed.). Philadelphia: W. B. Saunders. p. 291.

8. 3

RATIONALE: Nursing interventions for the Alzheimer's client who is angry, frustrated, or agitated include decreasing environmental stimuli, approaching the client calmly and with assurance, not demanding anything from the client, and distracting the client. It is important that the nurse reach out, touch, hold a hand, put an arm around the waist, or in some way maintain physical contact.
TEST-TAKING STRATEGY: Use the process of elimination. Playing a radio may increase stimuli and turning the lights out may produce more agitation. Clients with Alzheimer's disease would not be a candidate for group work if they are agitated. Calmly touching clients or putting an arm around their waist tends to distract them and decrease their agitation, frustration, or anger.
LEVEL OF COGNITIVE ABILITY: Application
PHASE OF NURSING PROCESS: Planning
CLIENT NEEDS: Psychosocial Integrity
CONTENT AREA: Fundamental Skills
REFERENCE
Tyson, R. (1999). *Gerontological nursing care*. Philadelphia: W. B. Saunders. pp. 451–452.

9. 4

RATIONALE: Exercise and activity are essential for health promotion and maintenance in the older adult and to achieve an optimal level of functioning. Approximately half of the physical deterioration of the elderly is caused by disuse rather than by the aging process or disease. One of the best exercises for an older adult is walking, progressing to 30-minute sessions three to five times each week. Swimming and dancing are also beneficial.
TEST-TAKING STRATEGY: Focus on the key words "best promote." Options 1, 2, and 3, although possible activities, are not the best activities. Option 4 is the best exercise for

an older adult. Review health promotion in the elderly now if you had difficulty with this question.
LEVEL OF COGNITIVE ABILITY: Comprehension
PHASE OF NURSING PROCESS: Planning
CLIENT NEEDS: Health Promotion and Maintenance
CONTENT AREA: Fundamental Skills
REFERENCE
Tyson, R. (1999). *Gerontological nursing care*. Philadelphia: W. B. Saunders. p. 181.

10. **1**

RATIONALE: The client with myasthenia gravis should be taught that timing of anticholinesterase medication is critical. It is important to instruct the client to administer the medication on time to maintain a chemical balance at the neuromuscular junction. If not given on time, the client may become too weak to swallow. Options 2, 3, and 4 include all the necessary information that the client requires to understand how to maintain health with this neurological degenerative disease.
TEST-TAKING STRATEGY: Use the process of elimination. Basic principles related to medication administration will easily direct you to option 1. Clients should not adjust dosage and medication times. If you had difficulty with this question, take time now to review the guidelines related to medication administration.
LEVEL OF COGNITIVE ABILITY: Comprehension
PHASE OF NURSING PROCESS: Evaluation
CLIENT NEEDS: Health Promotion and Maintenance
CONTENT AREA: Adult Health/Neurological
REFERENCE
deWit, S. (1998). *Essentials of medical-surgical nursing* (4th ed.). Philadelphia: W. B. Saunders. p. 383.

11. **4**

RATIONALE: Older adults who like to retell stories or past events need to be provided the opportunity to do so. This is called life review or reminiscence. Option 1 indicates reality orientation techniques. Options 2 and 3 indicate socialization and physical activity.
TEST-TAKING STRATEGY: Use the process of elimination. Note the relationship between "fosters reminiscence" in the question and "storytelling time" in the correct option. If you had difficulty with this question, take time now to review reminiscence therapy.
LEVEL OF COGNITIVE ABILITY: Application
PHASE OF NURSING PROCESS: Implementation
CLIENT NEEDS: Psychosocial Integrity
CONTENT AREA: Mental Health
REFERENCE
Taylor, C., Lillis, C., & Lemone, P. (1997). *Fundamentals of nursing: The art and science of nursing care* (3rd ed.). Philadelphia: Lippincott–Raven. p. 161.

12. **2**

RATIONALE: The client on bedrest is at risk for respiratory complications. Although options 1, 3, and 4 may be important problems to address, option 2 identifies airway, the highest priority.
TEST-TAKING STRATEGY: Use Maslow's hierarchy of needs theory and the ABCs—airway, breathing, and circulation. This will easily direct you to option 2. Airway is the priority.
LEVEL OF COGNITIVE ABILITY: Comprehension

PHASE OF NURSING PROCESS: Planning
CLIENT NEEDS: Physiological Integrity
CONTENT AREA: Fundamental Skills
REFERENCE
Taylor, C., Lillis, C., & Lemone, P. (1997). *Fundamentals of nursing: The art and science of nursing care* (3rd ed.). Philadelphia: Lippincott–Raven. p. 278.

13. **3**

RATIONALE: Some of the causes of trauma in an elderly client include an unsteady gait, the presence of unsecured scatter rugs, cluttered passageways, inoperable smoke detectors, and medication administration errors.
TEST-TAKING STRATEGY: Note the key words "requires immediate attention." Use the process of elimination. There is one unsafe situation among the options, the presence of unsecured scatter rugs. In order to prevent falls, these rugs need to be secured. The other options presented all ensure safety for the client.
LEVEL OF COGNITIVE ABILITY: Comprehension
PHASE OF NURSING PROCESS: Data Collection
CLIENT NEEDS: Safe, Effective Care Environment
CONTENT AREA: Fundamental Skills
REFERENCE
Taylor, C., Lillis, C., & Lemone, P. (1997). *Fundamentals of nursing: The art and science of nursing care* (3rd ed.). Philadelphia: Lippincott–Raven. p. 534.

14. **1**

RATIONALE: According to Maslow's hierarchy of needs theory, lower needs must be met before a person can focus on higher ones. Client needs may be prioritized according to the following needs: physiological, safety, love and belonging, self-esteem, and self-actualization. Option 1 addresses a physiological need.
TEST-TAKING STRATEGY: Use the process of elimination and do not read into the question. Basic physiological needs are a priority in administering nursing care. Although options 2, 3, and 4 address the client's needs, the priority is to keep the client clean and dry and to avoid embarrassment.
LEVEL OF COGNITIVE ABILITY: Application
PHASE OF NURSING PROCESS: Implementation
CLIENT NEEDS: Physiological Integrity
CONTENT AREA: Fundamental Skills
REFERENCE
Taylor, C., Lillis, C., & Lemone, P. (1997). *Fundamentals of nursing: The art and science of nursing care* (3rd ed.). Philadelphia: Lippincott–Raven. p. 278.

15. **3**

RATIONALE: Adequate dietary fiber is one of the most important factors in aiding bowel function. The retention of water by the fiber has the ability to soften stools and promote regularity. Fluids and exercise facilitate bowel elimination. Also remember that the client's elimination pattern is individual.
TEST-TAKING STRATEGY: Note the key words "further teaching is necessary." Use the process of elimination and general knowledge regarding measures to promote bowel elimination. Review these measures now if you had difficulty with this question.
LEVEL OF COGNITIVE ABILITY: Comprehension
PHASE OF NURSING PROCESS: Evaluation

CLIENT NEEDS: Health Promotion and Maintenance
CONTENT AREA: Fundamental Skills
REFERENCE
Leahy, J., & Kizilay, P. (1998). *Foundations of nursing practice: A nursing process approach*. Philadelphia: W. B. Saunders. p. 928.

16. 4

RATIONALE: Ageism is a form of prejudice, in which older adults are stereotyped by characteristics found in only a few members of their group. Options 1, 2, and 3 are supportive roles that the nurse engages in when dealing with the elderly. Option 4 suggests that the nurse does not think the elderly are worthy of aggressive treatment and demonstrates ageism.
TEST-TAKING STRATEGY: Use the process of elimination and focus on the issue of the question. Understanding the definition of ageism will easily direct you to option 4. If you are not familiar with this term, take time now to review.
LEVEL OF COGNITIVE ABILITY: Comprehension
PHASE OF NURSING PROCESS: Implementation
CLIENT NEEDS: Psychosocial Integrity
CONTENT AREA: Fundamental Skills
REFERENCE
Taylor, C., Lillis, C., & Lemone, P. (1997). *Fundamentals of nursing: The art and science of nursing care* (3rd ed.). Philadelphia: Lippincott–Raven. p. 165.

17. 2

RATIONALE: The elderly client is at risk to develop medication toxicity because of decreased lean body mass and age-associated decreased glomerular filtration rate. Options 1, 3, and 4 do not contribute to medication toxicity.
TEST-TAKING STRATEGY: Use the process of elimination and knowledge regarding the physiological changes associated with aging. Note that option 2 is the only option that addresses renal excretion. If you had difficulty with this question, take time now to review the physiological changes associated with aging.
LEVEL OF COGNITIVE ABILITY: Comprehension
PHASE OF NURSING PROCESS: Planning
CLIENT NEEDS: Physiological Integrity
CONTENT AREA: Fundamental Skills
REFERENCE
Black, J., & Matassarin-Jacobs, E. (1997). *Medical-surgical nursing: Clinical management for continuity of care* (5th ed.). Philadelphia: W. B. Saunders. p. 93.

18. 2

RATIONALE: Autonomy is the personal freedom to direct one's own life as long as it does not impinge on the rights of others. Loss of autonomy, and therefore independence, is a very real fear among the elderly. To promote independence in clients, it is essential to give them choices. Option 2 is the only option that allows the client to be a decision maker.
TEST-TAKING STRATEGY: Use the process of elimination. Note the similarity between options 1, 3, and 4. If you had difficulty with this question, take time now to review the definition of autonomy.
LEVEL OF COGNITIVE ABILITY: Application
PHASE OF NURSING PROCESS: Planning
CLIENT NEEDS: Safe, Effective Care Environment
CONTENT AREA: Fundamental Skills

REFERENCE
Tyson, R. (1999). *Gerontological nursing care*. Philadelphia: W. B. Saunders. p. 228.

19. 1

RATIONALE: The clinical signs of impending or approaching death include inability to swallow, pitting edema, decreased gastrointestinal and urinary tract activity, bowel and bladder incontinence, loss of motion, sensation, and reflexes, cold or clammy skin, cyanosis, lowered blood pressure, noisy or irregular respirations, and Cheyne-Stokes respirations.
TEST-TAKING STRATEGY: Use the process of elimination and eliminate options 2 and 3 as these identify normal findings. Option 4 does not imply approaching death. If you had difficulty with this question, take time now to review the signs associated with impending or approaching death.
LEVEL OF COGNITIVE ABILITY: Comprehension
PHASE OF NURSING PROCESS: Data Collection
CLIENT NEEDS: Physiological Integrity
CONTENT AREA: Fundamental Skills
REFERENCE
Taylor, C., Lillis, C., & Lemone, P. (1997). *Fundamentals of nursing: The art and science of nursing care* (3rd ed.). Philadelphia: Lippincott–Raven. p. 784.

20. 4

RATIONALE: Sweat glands control temperature regulation. As aging progresses, alterations in sweat gland activity make the glands less effective in temperature regulation, so the aging person is less able to regulate hot and cold bodily changes. The parotid glands are responsible for the drainage of saliva, which plays an important role in digestion. The pineal gland is a major site of melatonin biosynthesis. The thymus gland plays an immunologic role throughout life.
TEST-TAKING STRATEGY: Use the process of elimination. Note the relationship between "hot and cold bodily changes" in the question and "sweat glands" in the correct option. If you had difficulty with this question, take time now to review the functions of the glands identified in each option.
LEVEL OF COGNITIVE ABILITY: Comprehension
PHASE OF NURSING PROCESS: Planning
CLIENT NEEDS: Physiological Integrity
CONTENT AREA: Fundamental Skills
REFERENCE
deWit, S. (1998). *Essentials of medical-surgical nursing* (4th ed.). Philadelphia: W. B. Saunders. p. 895.

21. 4

RATIONALE: Coping mechanisms are behaviors used to decreased stress and anxiety. Typical coping behaviors include physical activity and exercise, smoking and drinking, lack of eye contact, and withdrawal. In response to a death, ineffective coping is manifested by an extreme behavior that in some instances may be harmful to the individual either physically or psychologically.
TEST-TAKING STRATEGY: Use the process of elimination and note the key words "ineffective coping." Options 1, 2, and 3 are positive activities that the individual is engaging in to get on with her life. Option 4 is indicative of a behavior that identifies an ineffective coping behavior in the grieving process.
LEVEL OF COGNITIVE ABILITY: Comprehension

PHASE OF NURSING PROCESS: Evaluation
CLIENT NEEDS: Psychosocial Integrity
CONTENT AREA: Fundamental Skills
REFERENCE
Taylor, C., Lillis, C., & Lemone, P. (1997). *Fundamentals of nursing: The art and science of nursing care* (3rd ed.). Philadelphia: Lippincott–Raven. pp. 760, 796.

22. 1

RATIONALE: The nurse should ensure that the hearing impaired client can see the nurse when speaking by providing adequate lighting and by standing in front of the client. The nurse should enunciate words clearly but not exaggerate lip movements. If the client is profoundly hearing impaired and uses signing, a sign language interpreter should be obtained. If a client cannot understand by reading lips, the nurse should try using gestures, pantomiming, or writing notes.
TEST-TAKING STRATEGY: Note the key word "initially." To communicate effectively with a hearing-impaired client, the nurse first makes sure that the client can see her or him. There are no data in the question to indicate that options 2, 3, or 4 are necessary interventions. If you had difficulty with this question, take time now to review nursing interventions for the hearing impaired.
LEVEL OF COGNITIVE ABILITY: Application
PHASE OF NURSING PROCESS: Implementation
CLIENT NEEDS: Physiological Integrity
CONTENT AREA: Fundamental Skills
REFERENCE
Tyson, R. (1999). *Gerontological nursing care*. Philadelphia: W. B. Saunders. p. 170.

23. 1

RATIONALE: The client should avoid caffeinated beverages and stimulants such as tea, cola, and chocolate before bedtime. The client should exercise regularly because exercise enhances sleep. Smoking is avoided. Reading before bedtime can assist in inducing sleep.
TEST-TAKING STRATEGY: Focus on the key words "further teaching is necessary." Options 2, 3, and 4 are positive responses, indicating that the client has learned about ways of improving sleep. Option 1 indicates that the client does not know that chocolate is a stimulant and will interfere with a good night's rest. Review items to avoid before bedtime now if you had difficulty with this question.
LEVEL OF COGNITIVE ABILITY: Comprehension
PHASE OF NURSING PROCESS: Evaluation
CLIENT NEEDS: Physiological Integrity
CONTENT AREA: Fundamental Skills
REFERENCE
deWit, S. (1998). *Essentials of medical-surgical nursing* (4th ed.). Philadelphia: W. B. Saunders. p. 1000.

24. 2

RATIONALE: Assisting clients and families to become knowledgeable of available community support systems is a role of the nurse. The suggestion to commit the client to a nursing home is premature. While the data provided tells you this elder requires nursing care, you don't know the extent of nursing care. Observing that the client has begun to be confined to his room makes it necessary for the nurse to intervene legally and ethically, so option 3 is not appropriate and is passive in terms of advocacy. Option 4 is incorrect and judgmental.

TEST-TAKING STRATEGY: Note the key words "most appropriate." Use the process of elimination and principles related to ethical and legal issues to answer the question. If you had difficulty with this question, take time now to review the role of the nurse in providing support to the family.
LEVEL OF COGNITIVE ABILITY: Application
PHASE OF NURSING PROCESS: Implementation
CLIENT NEEDS: Safe, Effective Care Environment
CONTENT AREA: Fundamental Skills
REFERENCE
Tyson, R. (1999). *Gerontological nursing care*. Philadelphia: W. B. Saunders. p. 216.

25. 1

RATIONALE: Option 1 summarizes and focuses upon the content of the client's message and restates so the client can hear himself making excuses about his son's physical abuse. The elder who is abused classically excuses the abuser. In option 2, the nurse is sarcastic and, without further investigation, moves to report the incident. In option 3, the nurse confirms the client's fear that he is a "bother," begins to insinuate that his son is using his money, and that this situation will be cleared up just by the nurse's talking with the client's son. Option 4 is incorrect because it advocates avoiding the issue.
TEST-TAKING STRATEGY: Use therapeutic communication techniques to answer the question. Option 1 is the only statement that reflects these techniques. If you had difficulty with this question, take time now to review therapeutic communication techniques and the blocks to communication.
LEVEL OF COGNITIVE ABILITY: Application
PHASE OF NURSING PROCESS: Implementation
CLIENT NEEDS: Psychosocial Integrity
CONTENT AREA: Mental Health
REFERENCE
Tyson, R. (1999). *Gerontological nursing care*. Philadelphia: W. B. Saunders. p. 216.

26. 4

RATIONALE: The normal physiological changes that occur in the skin of older adults includes thinning of the skin, loss of elasticity, deepening of expression lines, and wrinkling. Baldness and graying of the hair occur. Crusting of the skin indicates a potential complication.
TEST-TAKING STRATEGY: Note the key words "potential complication." Use the process of elimination and knowledge regarding normal expected findings to assist in directing you to the correct option. Review these normal findings and those that indicate a complication now if you had difficulty with this question.
LEVEL OF COGNITIVE ABILITY: Comprehension
PHASE OF NURSING PROCESS: Data Collection
CLIENT NEEDS: Physiological Integrity
CONTENT AREA: Adult Health/Integumentary
REFERENCE
Matteson, M. A., McConnell, E. S., & Linton, A. D. (1997). *Gerontological nursing: Concepts and practice* (2nd ed.). Philadelphia: W. B. Saunders. pp. 176–179.

27. 3

RATIONALE: Sclerotic lesions occur as bone resorption increases and results in replacement of original bone with fibrous material. This condition occurs in Paget's disease, an age-related disorder. Options 1, 2, and 4 identify normal age-related changes in the musculoskeletal system.

TEST-TAKING STRATEGY: Note the key words "potential complication." Use knowledge regarding normal expected findings to assist in directing you to the correct option. Review these normal findings and those that indicate a complication now if you had difficulty with this question.

LEVEL OF COGNITIVE ABILITY: Comprehension
PHASE OF NURSING PROCESS: Data Collection
CLIENT NEEDS: Physiological Integrity
CONTENT AREA: Adult Health/Musculoskeletal
REFERENCE
Matteson, M. A., McConnell, E. S., & Linton, A. D. (1997). *Gerontological nursing: Concepts and practice* (2nd ed.). Philadelphia: W. B. Saunders. pp. 197–200.

28. **4**

RATIONALE: One of the eye conditions that occurs in the older adult is cataracts. Cataracts result in a loss of opacity of the crystalline lens, causing visual disturbances. Options 1, 2, and 3 do not identify problems that can occur in the older adult. Option 1 describes normal vision. Option 2 describes an astigmatism. Option 3 describes near normal vision.

TEST-TAKING STRATEGY: Note the key words "older adult client" and "potential complication." Recalling that cataracts is a condition associated with the older adult client will easily direct you to option 4. Review problems that occur in the older adult client now if you had difficulty with this question.

LEVEL OF COGNITIVE ABILITY: Comprehension
PHASE OF NURSING PROCESS: Data Collection
CLIENT NEEDS: Physiological Integrity
CONTENT AREA: Adult Health/Eye
REFERENCE
Matteson, M. A., McConnell, E. S., & Linton, A. D. (1997). *Gerontological nursing: Concepts and practice* (2nd ed.). Philadelphia: W. B. Saunders. p. 360.

29. **3**

RATIONALE: In Alzheimer's disease, memory impairment and disorientation occur. Options 1, 2, and 4 are not findings associated with this disease.

TEST-TAKING STRATEGY: Recalling that Alzheimer's disease is a form of dementia will easily direct you to option 3. If you had difficulty with this question, take time now to review this important content and the assessment findings associated with the disease.

LEVEL OF COGNITIVE ABILITY: Comprehension
PHASE OF NURSING PROCESS: Data Collection
CLIENT NEEDS: Physiological Integrity
CONTENT AREA: Fundamental Skills
REFERENCE
Luckmann, J. (1997). *Saunders manual of nursing care.* Philadelphia: W. B. Saunders. pp. 578, 713–717.

30. **3**

RATIONALE: The nurse should check the client's vital signs every 4 hours to identify an elevated temperature that suggests infection. The nurse encourages fluid intake to loosen secretions and thus enable the client to expectorate more easily. Frequent position change helps to mobilize lung secretions and prevent pooling. It is important to encourage coughing and deep breathing to mobilize lung secretions. Clients should be instructed to avoid the Valsalva maneuver or any activity involving holding the breath.

TEST-TAKING STRATEGY: Note the key words "prevent respiratory complications." Use the process of elimination. Changing the position of the immobilized client every 2 hours will help prevent pooling of lung secretions. Options 1, 2, and 4 do not assist the client to improve ventilatory efforts. Review these measures now if you had difficulty with this question.

LEVEL OF COGNITIVE ABILITY: Application
PHASE OF NURSING PROCESS: Implementation
CLIENT NEEDS: Physiological Integrity
CONTENT AREA: Fundamental Skills
REFERENCE
Tyson, R. (1999). *Gerontological nursing care.* Philadelphia: W. B. Saunders. p. 306.

BIBLIOGRAPHY

Black, J., & Matassarin-Jacobs, E. (1997). *Medical surgical nursing: Clinical management for continuity of care* (5th ed.). Philadelphia: W. B. Saunders.

Chernecky, C., & Berger, B. (1997). *Laboratory tests and diagnostic procedures* (2nd ed.). Philadelphia: W. B. Saunders.

deWit, S. (1998). *Essentials of medical-surgical nursing* (4th ed.). Philadelphia: W. B. Saunders.

Hodgson, B., & Kizior, R. (1999). *Saunders nursing drug handbook 1999.* Philadelphia: W. B. Saunders.

Leahy, J., & Kizilay, P. (1998). *Foundations of nursing practice: A nursing process approach.* Philadelphia: W. B. Saunders.

Luckmann, J. (1997). *Saunders manual of nursing care.* Philadelphia: W. B. Saunders.

Matteson, M. A., McConnell, E. S., & Linton, A. D. (1997). *Gerontological nursing: Concepts and practice* (2nd ed.). Philadelphia: W. B. Saunders.

Taylor, C., Lillis, C., & Lemone, P. (1997). *Fundamentals of nursing: The art and science of nursing care* (3rd ed.). Philadelphia: Lippincott–Raven.

Tyson, R. (1999). *Gerontological nursing care.* Philadelphia: W. B. Saunders.

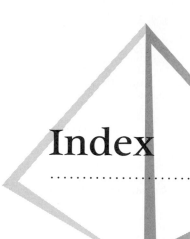

Index

Note: Page numbers in *italics* refer to figures; page numbers followed by t refer to tables; page numbers followed by b refer to text in boxes.